Drinking Water and Health

SAFE DRINKING WATER COMMITTEE

Advisory Center on Toxicology
Assembly of Life Sciences
National Research Council

NATIONAL ACADEMY OF SCIENCES
Washington, D.C. 1977

NOTICE: The project that is the subject of this report was approved by the Governing Board of the National Research Council, whose members are drawn from the Councils of the National Academy of Sciences, the National Academy of Engineering, and the Institute of Medicine. The members of the Committee responsible for the report were chosen for their special competences and with regard for appropriate balance.

This report has been reviewed by a group other than the authors according to procedures approved by a Report Review Committee consisting of members of the National Academy of Sciences, The National Academy of Engineering, and the Institute of Medicine.

At the request of and funded by the
U.S. Enviornmental Protection Agency
Contract no. 68-01-3139

Library of Congress Catalog Card Number: 77-089284
International Standard Book Number: 0-309-02619-9

Available from

Printing and Publishing Office
National Academy of Sciences
2101 Constitution Ave.
Washington, D.C. 20418

Printed in the United States of America

Contents

Preface

This volume presents the findings of a study of the potentially harmful effects that impurities in water may have on the health of those who drink it. The study was conducted by the Committee on Safe Drinking Water of the National Research Council, supported by a contract between the Environmental Protection Agency and the National Academy of Sciences.

Several factors combined to place an unusually heavy burden on all those who participated in this effort. At the outset, the purpose, scope, and duration of the study were defined in the Safe Drinking Water Act of 1974 in such a way as to require the Administrator of the Environmental Protection Agency not only to arrange for the study to be performed, but to make prompt use of the findings as the scientific basis for revision or ratification of the Interim Primary Drinking Water Regulations that were promulgated under the Act. These requirements, of necessity, imposed a severe restriction on the time available to the participants. It was also apparent that the application of modern methods of analysis had greatly expanded and diversified our knowledge of the occurrence of trace impurities in water and was continuing to do so much more rapidly than the rate of accumulation of information about their toxicity. This necessitated a careful and laborious scrutiny of a large and diverse segment of the scientific literature. Furthermore, the central effort of the study, namely, assessment of the long-term biological effects of ingesting the variety of different materials that are present in trace amounts in drinking water, made severe demands on our ability to apply the contemporary knowledge of toxicology and epidemiology to quantitative estimation of the risks to public health in terms that would be useful in framing regulations. In recognition of these limitations, it was concluded that the intent of Congress and the possibilities inherent in the body of scientific knowledge on which we could draw could best be reconciled in terms of the interpretation of the scope of the study given in Appendix A.

To carry out the work of the study, the principal subdivisions of the subject matter were assigned to subcommittees, each of which was chaired by a member of the Safe Drinking Water Committee, which, in turn, was responsible for the general direction of the study (see Appendix B). We are most grateful to all those members of the scientific community who served on these committees, meeting as frequently as the task required, and whose written contributions form the basis for this report.

It is a pleasure also to express, on behalf of the entire study group, a special note of thanks to the staff: Dr. Riley D. Housewright, Mr. J. P. T. Pearman, Dr. Robert Golden, Mrs. Susan Chen, and Mr. Ralph C. Wands, whose informed and tireless efforts ably supported the committees, not only in the planning and conduct of the study, but also by procuring the various bibliographic and consulting services that proved to be required. In this connection we are grateful to the International Agency for Research on Cancer for helping to assess the potential carcinogenicity of organic compounds found in drinking water; and to Ms. Libbey Smith, Ms. Judith L. Mullaney, Ms. Florence Carleton, Dr. Penelope Crisp, and Dr. Lana Skirboll, all of whom assisted in an extensive search of the scientific literature.

We acknowledge with gratitude the assistance of all those outside consultants who supplied information for our consideration, and the help of many members of the staff of the Environmental Protection Agency, especially Dr. Edgar A. Jeffrey and his successor, Dr. Joseph Cotruvo, and Dr. Robert Tardiff and Mr. Lee McCabe, who helped to place at our disposal the information available within that agency.

Organization of meetings and the labor of preparing manuscripts was made easier by the dedicated secretarial services of Mrs. Delores Banks, Ms. Helen Harvin, Mrs. Merle Morgan, and Ms. Carol Fisher.

Last, but not least, we thank the members of the public who took the trouble to submit suggestions for our consideration and expressed to us their views and concerns at our public meetings.

GERARD A. ROHLICH, *Chairman*
Safe Drinking Water Committee

Drinking Water and Health

Historical Note

As noted by Baker (1949), the quest for pure water began in prehistoric times. Recorded knowledge of water treatment is found in Sanskrit medical lore and in Egyptian inscriptions. Pictures of apparatus to clarify liquids (both water and wine) have been found on Egyptian walls dating back to the fifteenth century B.C. Boiling of water, the use of wick siphons, filtration through porous vessels, and even filtration with sand and gravel, as means to purify water, are methods that have been prescribed for thousands of years. In his writings on public hygiene, Hippocrates (460-354 B.C.) directed attention principally to the importance of water in the maintenance of health, but he also prescribed that rain water should be boiled and strained. The cloth bag that he recommended for straining became known in later times as "Hippocrates' sleeve."

Public water supplies, already developed in ancient times, assumed added importance with the progressive increase in urbanization. But though they were clearly beneficial in distributing water of uniform quality, large numbers of people ran the risk of suffering adverse effects when the water was unsafe to drink.

The first clear proof that public water supplies could be a source of infection for humans was based on careful epidemiological studies of cholera in the city of London by Dr. John Snow in 1854 (Snow, 1855). Although Snow's study of the contaminated Broad Street pump is the most famous, his definitive work concerned the spread of cholera through water supplied by the Southwark and Vauxhall Company and the

Lambeth Company. The former obtained its water from the Thames at Battersea, in the middle of London in an area almost certainly polluted with sewage, whereas the Lambeth Company obtained its water considerably upstream on the Thames, above the major sources of pollution. In one particular area served by these two companies, containing about 300,000 residents, the pipes of both companies were laid in the streets, and houses were connected to one or the other sources of supply. Snow's examination of the statistics of cholera deaths gave striking results. Those houses served by the Lambeth Company had a low incidence of cholera, lower than the average for the population of London as a whole, whereas those served by the Southwark and Vauxhall Company had a very high incidence. As the socioeconomic conditions, climate, soil, and all other factors were identical for the populations served by the two companies, Snow concluded that the water supply was transmitting the cholera agent. Snow's study, a classic in the field of epidemiology, is even more impressive when it is realized that at the time he was working, the germ theory of disease had not yet been established.

During the seventeenth to the early nineteenth centuries, a number of improvements in water supply were made, most of them related to improvements in filtration to remove the turbidity of waters. During this same period, the germ theory of disease became firmly established as a result of research by Louis Pasteur, Robert Koch, and others, and in 1884 Koch isolated the causal agent of cholera, *Vibrio cholera*.

Importance of Water Filtration

In 1892, a study of cholera by Koch in the German cities of Hamburg and Altona provided some of the best evidence of the importance of water filtration for protection against this disease (Koch, 1894). The cities of Hamburg and Altona both received their drinking water from the Elbe River, but Altona used filtration, since its water was taken from the Elbe below the city of Hamburg and hence was more grossly contaminated. Hamburg and Altona are contiguous cities, and in some places the border between the two follows a contorted course. Koch traced the incidence of cholera in the 1892 epidemic through these two cities, with special attention directed to the contiguous areas. In such areas it was assumed that climate, soil, and other factors would be identical, the principal variable being the source of water. The results of this study were clear-cut: Altona, even with an inferior water source, had a markedly lower incidence of cholera than Hamburg. Since by this time it was well established that cholera was caused by intestinal bacteria excreted in large numbers in the feces, it was concluded that the role of filtration was to remove the contaminating bacteria from the water.

In the United States, cholera was not a problem after the mid-nineteenth century; the waterborne disease of particular concern was typhoid fever. In England, William Budd had shown by the mid-nineteenth century that typhoid fever was a contagious disease, and the causal agent was isolated and identified by Eberth in 1880 and Gaffky in 1884 (Wilson and Miles, 1957). Although the causal agent, now called *Salmonella typhi*, is transmitted in a variety of ways, one of the most significant is by drinking water.

Experiments on water filtration were carried out in the United States during the late 1880's and early 1890's, notably by the Massachusetts State Board of Health experiment station established in 1887 at the city of Lawrence. At this station the treatment of water as well as sewage was considered by an interdisciplinary group that included engineers, chemists, and biologists. A leader in this work was W. T. Sedgwick, a professor at the Massachusetts Institute of Technology (MIT), and MIT's influence on water-supply research remained strong throughout the first quarter of the twentieth century. Much of the history of this work has been reviewed by Whipple (1921) and in the two editions of Hazen's book (1907, 1914); the technical aspects are discussed and clearly illustrated by Johnson (1913). One important technological advance that made water filtration adaptable even to rather turbid sources of water was the use of chemical-coagulation filtration processes, patented about 1884 by the brothers J. W. and I. S. Hyatt.

While the Lawerence experiments were going on, an epidemic of typhoid swept through the city, hitting especially hard at those parts that were using the Merrimac River as its water supply. As a result, the city of Lawrence built a sand filter, and its use led a marked reduction in the typhoid fever incidence. As reported by Hazen (1907), the death rate from typhoid fever in Lawrence dropped 79% when the 5-yr periods before and after the introduction of the filter were compared. Of additional interest was a reduction in the general death rate (all causes) of 10%, from 22.4 to 19.9 per 1,000 living.

Another major series of filtration experiments were made in 1895–1897 at Louisville, Ky., where the source of water was the muddy and polluted Ohio River. These experiments were successful, and from an engineering point of view were of importance because they showed that it was possible to treat source waters of a rather poor quality (the Merrimac River at Lawrence may have been polluted, but at least it was a clear water, making filtration rather easier.) The success of the Louisville experiments and the other studies led to rapid establishment of filters as a means of water purification; by 1907 Hazen could list 33 cities in the United States, some of comparatively large size, which were using mechanical filters, and 13 cities that were using slow sand filters. As discussed by Hazen, filtration led to an elimination of turbidity and color from the water, and to a removal of about 99% of the bacteria present. At that time these conditions were considered as a standard by which the quality of a treated water should be judged. As Hazen states: "There is no final reason for such standards. They have been adopted by consent because they represent a purification that is reasonably satisfactory and that can be reached at a cost which is not burdensome to those who have to pay for it . . . . There is no evidence that the germs (characteristic of sewage pollution) so left in the water are in any way injurious. Certainly if injurious influence is exercised it is too small to be determined or measured by any methods now at our disposal." This last statement is of considerable importance when considered in the light of the important advance in water purification practice yet to come, chlorination.

An excellent overview of the relationship between water quality and typhoid fever incidence was published at about this time by Fuertes (1897). He gathered typhoid fever statistics for a large number of cities in North America and Europe and grouped the data by type of source water and water treatment.

Chlorination, The Most Significant Advance in Water Treatment

Although a reading of Hazen's 1907 book might lead one to conclude that excellent water quality had been well established by filtration, the most important technological advance in water treatment was yet to come. The introduction of chlorination after 1908 provided a cheap, reproducible method of ensuring the bacteriological quality of water. Chlorination has come down to us today as one of the major factors ensuring safety of our drinking water.

Calcium hypochlorite was manufactured industrially for use as a bleaching powder and was used in paper mills and textile industries. It was a cheap chemical, and hence readily adaptable to use on the large scale necessary for drinking water. The first practical demonstration in the United States of its use in water supply was at the filter plant of the Chicago Stock Yards, where it was introduced by Johnson in the fall of 1908 (Johnson, 1913).

The use of chlorination in an urban water supply was introduced in Jersey City, N.J., in the latter part of 1908. The circumstances surrounding the Jersey City case are of some interest from a historical point of view and will be briefly reviewed. Jersey City received its water from a private company that used a large reservoir at Boonton, an impoundment of the Rockaway River. The water was supplied to the city unfiltered, although some settling took place in the reservoir. Several years before 1908 the city raised the contention that the water being supplied was not at all times pure and wholesome for drinking, as was required by the terms of its contract with the private company. At certain times of the year, the water in the reservoir became polluted as a result of sewage influx from communities on the river above the reservoir. Rather than undergo the expense of a filtration plant, or attempt to control the sewage influx from the various communities, the private company chose to introduce a chlorination system. The results were dramatic. A marked drop in total bacterial count was obtained, and at a cost far lower than any other procedure. After many months of operation, further testimony before the court was held, to determine whether the company was meeting its contract, and the court decided that the evidence was favorable to the company. As stated by the court examiner: "I do therefore find and report that this device [chlorination] is capable of rendering the water delivered to Jersey City pure and wholesome for the purposes for which it is intended and is effective in removing from the water those dangerous germs which were deemed by the decree to possibly exist therein at certain times."

The dramatic effect that chlorination had on water-supply problems is well illustrated by comparing the first and second editions of Hazen's book (1907 and 1914). In the first edition, barely any mention of disinfection is made (merely a remark about ozone being too expensive), but in the second edition Hazen waxes enthusiastic about the advantages of chlorination. As he says, chlorination could be used "at a cost so low that it could be used in any public waterworks plant where it was required or advantageous . . . . When the advantages to be obtained by this simple and inexpensive treatment became realized, as a result of the publicity given by the Jersey City experience, the use of the process extended with unprecedented rapidity, until at the present (1914) the greater part of the water supplied in cities in the United States is treated in this way or by some substitute and equivalent method."

Interestingly from the point of view of the present report, the introduction of chlorination also changed markedly the established ideas about water-quality standards: "The use of methods of disinfection has changed these standards radically. By their use it has been found possible to remove most of the remaining bacteria so that the water supplied can be as easily and certainly held within one-tenth of one percent of those in the raw water, as it formerly could be held within one percent . . . . Even today the limit has not been reached. It may be admitted that the time will come when a still higher degree of bacterial efficiency will be required. Present conditions do not seem to demand it, but we must expect that in some time in the future conditions will arise which will make it necessary. When additional purification is required it can be furnished." (Hazen, 1914).

The importance of Hazen's book is that Hazen was a major consulting engineer for a wide variety of water works, and was very influential in recommending treatment methods. Chlorination was introduced at about the time that adequate methods of bacteriological examination of water had developed, permitting an objective evaluation of the efficiency of treatment. This evaluation was not based on the incidence of typhoid fever directly, but was based on an indirect evaluation using bacterial or coliform counts.

Soon after chlorination was introduced, it was possible to obtain firm epidemiological evidence that cities chlorinating water had lowered incidences of typhoid fever (G. C. Whipple, 1921). Filtration was introduced in 1906 and chlorination in 1908, and both led to marked reductions in the incidence of typhoid fever. Another dramatic example derives from observations at Wheeling, W.Va., in 1917-1918 (Gainey and Lord, 1952). The incidence of typhoid fever in Wheeling was 155-200 per 100,000 during these years. Chlorination was introduced in the latter part of 1918, with the result that during the first 3 months of 1919 only seven cases were recorded. For 3 weeks during April 1919 chlorination was discontinued, with the result that the number of cases increased to 21, or a 300% increase. Chlorination was continued thereafter, and only 11 cases were recorded for the last 6 months of the year. Other examples of this sort could be cited (Gainey and Lord, 1952).

Summary

We thus see that by the beginning of World War I the essential features of water purification techniques were known, and their worth had been well established. Since that time there have been many refinements made at an engieering level, but no changes in the basic concepts. It is clear that the prime motivation for the development and introduction of purification methods has been to protect the public health, with special concern for controlling the spread of typhoid fever. An ancillary consideration has been esthetics, showing concern for the appearance, taste, and odor of the water.

One point worth emphasizing is that the availability of adequate treatment methods has influenced the standards for drinking water. This point was implied in the books by Hazen (1907 and 1914), but is most clearly seen in the preamble to the 1925 Federal Standards, which superseded the brief 1914 Standards (see Standard Methods, 7th edition, 1933, p. 136, for the complete 1925 Standards). The following quote is relevant:

> The first step toward the establishment of standards which will insure the safety of water supplies conforming to them is to agree upon some criterion of safety. This is necessary because "safety" in water supplies, as they are actually produced, is relative and quantitative, not absolute. Thus, to state that a water supply is 'safe' does not necessarily signify that absolutely no risk is ever incurred in drinking it. What is usually meant, and all that can be asserted from any evidence at hand, is that the danger, if any, is so small that it cannot be discovered by available means of observation. Nevertheless, while it is impossible to demonstrate the absolute safety of a water supply, it is well established that the water supplies of many of our large cities are safe in the sense stated above, since the large populations using them continuously have, in recent years, suffered only a minimal incidence of typhoid fever and other potentially waterborne infections. Whether or not these water supplies have had any part whatsoever in the conveyance of such infections during the period referred to is a question that cannot be answered with full certainty; but the total incidence of the diseases has been so low that even though the water supplies be charged with responsibility for the maximum share which may reasonably be suggested, the risk of infection through them is still very small compared to the ordinary hazards of everyday life.

At present other considerations make it necessary [for us] to be less confident than was the 1925 Committee on Standards. Typhoid fever and cholera are dramatic diseases whose causal agents are transmitted by the water route. Typhoid fever statistics have provided some of the best evidence of the efficacy of treatment systems, but it should be kept in mind that other diseases, not so easily diagnosed, might also be kept under control at the same time. The so-called Mills-Reincke theorem held that, for every death from waterborne typhoid, there were several deaths from other diseases for which the causal agents were transmitted by water (Shipple, 1921). At present, the incidence of typhoid fever in the United States is so low that no useful information on the effectiveness of recent changes in water-purification practices can be obtained from an examination of the statistics. During the years 1946-1970, there were 53 outbreaks of waterborne infectious disease due to typhoid, but there were 297 outbreaks due to other bacterial or viral agents, including 178 outbreaks of gastroenteritis of undetermined etiology (Craun and McCabe, 1973). Of the outbreaks, 71 percent resulted from contamination of private water systems, but most of the illness (83%) was associated with community water systems. During the period 1946-1960 there were 70 outbreaks of waterborne disease in communities served by public utilities (Weibel *et al.*, 1964), of which only 6 were typhoid fever. When data during this period for the number of outbreaks are examined, the incidence of typhoid is even lower—103 cases out of a total of 19,928 (for a percentage of 0.5%). Even considering that typhoid is more likely to be fatal than infectious hepatitis or gastroenteritis of unknown etiology, the Mills–Reincke theorem does seem to have considerable merit. Thus, the rationale that has been used in devising standards for microbiological contaminants (see quotation above from the 1925 Standards) does not necessarily hold up on careful examination. The coliform standards may have ensured freedom from typhoid fever, but we do not have the same assuredness that they have guaranteed freedom from other infections. Even granted that most of the outbreaks reported have occurred because of breakdowns in the proper functioning of water systems, the results show that intestinal infections other than typhoid are common and, because of their often ill-defined nature, may be improperly diagnosed. Finally, only "outbreaks" find their way into public health statistics, whereas sporadic, random cases of gastroenteritis generally go unreported. The epidemiological significance of the present microbiological standards warrants continuing investigation to bring about further refinements in meeting the goal of maximum protection of public health.

REFERENCES

Baker, M.N. 1949. The Quest for Pure Water. Am. Water Works Assoc., New York.

Craun, G.F., and L. J. McCabe. 1973. Review of the causes of waterborne-disease outbreaks. J. Am. Water Works Assoc. 65:74.

Fuertes, J.H. 1897. Water and public health. John Wiley, New York.

Gainey, P.L., and T.H. Lord. 1952. Microbiology of water and sewage. Prentice-Hall, Inc., New York.

Hazen, A. 1907. Clean water and how to get it, 1st ed. John Wiley, New York.

Hazen, A. 1914. Clean water and how to get it, 2d ed. John Wiley, New York.

Johnson, G.A. 1913. The purification of public water supplies. U.S. Geol. Surv. Water-Supply Paper 315.

Koch, R. 1894. Professor Koch on the Bacteriological Diagnosis of Cholera, Water-filtration and Cholera, and the Cholera in Germany during the Winter of 1892-93. Translated by G. Duncan David Douglas, publisher, Edinburough.

Snow, J. 1855. A reprint of two papers by John Snow, M.D., 1936. The Commonwealth Fund, New York.

Weibel, S.R., F.R. Dixon, R.B. Weidner, and L.J. McCabe. 1964. Waterborne-disease outbreaks, 1946-60. J. Am. Water Works Assoc. 56:947-958.

Whipple, G.C. 1921. Fifty years of water purification. *In* M.P. Ravenel, ed. A Half Century of Public Health, pp. 161-180. American Public Health Association, New York. (Reprinted 1970 by the Arno Press and the *New York Times*.)

I

Approach to the Study

INTRODUCTION

In this chapter the general approach, principles, and criteria adopted in the study are discussed in outline. Considerations that entered into evaluations of the effects on health of the various contaminants of drinking water are described, together with the reasons for selecting the subjects that were studied. The findings of the study are not summarized comprehensively in this section; each succeeding chapter includes a summary of the relevant conclusions and recommendations. A short summary of the principal conclusions of the study is given in Appendix C.

The study was undertaken by the NAS–NRC to meet the needs expressed in the Safe Drinking Water Act (PL 93-523), which requires the Environmental Protection Agency to promulgate national drinking water standards and, for the first time, regulations for enforcing them. The Act also directs the Administrator of the Environmental Protection Agency to arrange with the National Academy of Sciences, or other appropriate organization, to study the adverse effects on health attributable to contaminants in drinking water. Although the high quality of drinking water in the United States is recognized throughout the world, the law is an expression by the Congress of the concern of many citizens about maintaining the quality of public water supplies in this country.

The reader should not equate the size of this report or that of any of its chapters with the Committee's assessment of the magnitude of the challenge to public health that may be due to the presence of particular constituents in drinking water in the United States. Several factors have contributed to the length of this report: The Safe Drinking Water Act defined the scope of the study in encyclopedic terms and consequently the length of some of the chapters reflects the large number of topics and substances that it was necessary to consider. Other chapters deal with subjects that are complex and about which there are uncertainties, conflicting opinions, and inconclusive or incomplete data. The relevant studies, assumptions, methodologies, health effects, and research recommendations for each group of constituents required detailed consideration from several points of view before balanced judgments could be achieved. In some cases brevity had to be sacrificed to reach this objective within a reasonable time.

The primary purpose of the study was to assess the significance of the adverse effects that the constituents of drinking water may have on public health. The economic or technological feasibility of controlling the concentration of these constituents was outside the scope of the study.

The health effects associated with some methods of disinfection were noted, but the relative effectiveness and potential hazards associated with the various methods of water disinfection were not evaluated.

Application of analytical methods of great sensitivity has, in recent years, expanded our knowledge of the occurrence and diversity of impurities in drinking water. However, information about the biological results of chronic ingestion, at low dose rates, of most of these substances is acquired slowly because the bioassays that are usually required may take two or more years to complete. Although new approaches to the problem of estimating chronic adverse health effects may, in the future, ease this difficulty, the current knowledge on which this study is based is insufficient to assess all the contaminants of drinking water. The results reported here must therefore be considered as a contribution to an effort that should be continued.

Besides the known constituents of drinking water, some were also considered that it would be plausible to expect to be present, even though they have not yet been detected in water. (Certain pesticides used in large quantities fall into this category.)

In our review of water constituents, we have attempted to take into account not only their identities, concentrations, and toxicities, but also to consider other questions, such as:

1. What reason is there for concern about the material? What risks are associated with its presence in water?
2. How does the material get into water?
3. What sources are there other than water?

4. What contaminants need to be controlled?
5. Are there special places or persons at higher than average risk?
6. Are there essential nutritional requirements for this material?
7. In view of the data at hand, can one say that this is a material that causes temporary ill effects? Permanent ill-effects? Reversible effects?
8. In view of these effects—and their reversibility (or lack of it)—is it possible to set "no-observed-adverse-health-effects" levels?
9. For materials with special health benefits, what concentrations will maximize these benefits, while keeping the health risk associated with them at an acceptably low level?
10. What additional information is required to resolve the outstanding problems?

Many of the constituents of drinking water are natural materials, and enter water from the rocks and the soil and the air. Some are the natural waste products of men or animals. Others are artificial or synthetic materials, made and used for special purposes, that inadvertently find their way into water. Yet others occur naturally, but have become more widely distributed in populated areas as a result of industrial and agricultural activity.

WATER CONSUMPTION

In this study, a quantity of 2 liters per day has been taken to be the average amount of water consumed per person. This is also the amount used by EPA to calculate the current interim standards. Daily consumption of water is a function of temperature, humidity, physical activity, and other factors that vary widely. The average per capita water (liquid) consumption per day as calculated from a survey of nine different literature sources was 1.63 liters (NAS, 1974; McNall and Schlegal, 1968; Wolf, 1958; Guyton, 1968; Evans, 1941; Bourne and Kidder, 1953; Walker *et al.*, 1957; Randall, 1973; Pike and Brown, 1975). However, the larger volume of 2 liters/day was adopted as representing the intake of the majority of water consumers. We estimate that most of those who consume more than 2 liters per day still are afforded adequate protection, because the margin of safety estimated for the contaminants is sufficient to offset excess water consumption. Nevertheless, consideratioin should be given to establishing some standards on a regional or occupational basis, to take extremes of water consumption into account.

RISK AND SAFETY

The hazards of ingesting chemical pollutants in drinking water have been assessed in two general ways: with laboratory toxicity studies and epidemiological studies. The aim of studies of both types is to provide information about the risk to man. Risk constitutes only half of the equation; the other half is benefit to the exposed population. It is not possible to guarantee a risk-free society. The scientific methods and criteria we have used for evaluating long-term effects and risks in man are described in Chapter II, "Chemical Contaminants: Safety and Risk Assessment" and in the chapters concerning each group of contaminants.

Most of the experimental results on which the current knowledge of toxicity rests are based on observed effects on man and animals of doses and dose rates that are much larger than those that correspond to the usual concentrations of harmful materials in drinking water. There is, consequently, great uncertainty in estimating the magnitude of the risk to health that ingestion of contaminants in water may produce. An additional problem is to take into account the combined effects of two or more contaminants.

The theoretical and experimental bases for extrapolating estimations of risk to low levels of dose have been reviewed, and some principles are proposed to guide the conduct of this and similar studies.

MICROBIOLOGICAL CONTAMINANTS

Outbreaks of waterborne disease are reported to the National Center for Disease Control (CDC) by state health departments. In addition, EPA obtains information about additional outbreaks from state water-supply agencies. Both CDC and EPA are aware that data on waterborne outbreaks have limitations and must be interpreted with caution. The data collected represent only a small part of a larger public health problem. The number and kind of reported outbreaks and of some etiologies may depend upon the interest or capabilities of a particular state health department or individual. They do not reflect the actual number of outbreaks, cases, or etiologies of disease associated with drinking water.

Many small outbreaks are not reported to state health departments. There is no law or regulation requiring state authorities to report all gastroenteritis cases to CDC. In 1975, CDC reported 24 waterborne disease outbreaks involving 10,879 cases. No etiologic agent was found for the two largest outbreaks (Sewickley, Pa., 5,000 cases and Sellersburg,

Ind., 1,400 cases). In fact, no etiologic agent was identified in 17 of the 24 outbreaks. These 17 outbreaks accounted for 9,760 cases, or 89%, of the total reported in 1975.

Conclusions in the microbiology chapter, based on epidemiological data, are subject to the limitations of the reporting system and to our limited ability to identify etiologic agents in outbreaks known to be associated with drinking water.

The microbiological contaminants selected for consideration in this report are those for which there is epidemiological or clinical evidence of transmission by drinking water. They include a variety of bacteria, viruses, and protozoa. Methods of detecting these contaminants of drinking water were reviewed, and the quantitative relationships between dose levels and infectivity were examined. Because current drinking water standards place major emphasis on detection of microbiological contaminants, attention was devoted to the validity and health significance of microbiological standards.

PARTICULATE CONTAMINANTS

Finely divided solid particles of mineral and organic composition are commonly found suspended in some drinking water, particularly those supplies that do not practice coagulation and filtration. To discover whether or not the long-term ingestion of these materials in water is likely to produce adverse effects on human health, their occurrence, composition, and properties were reviewed.

This review indicated that many kinds of particulate matter may indirectly, through adsorption, facilitate the transport of toxic substances and pathogenic organisms and affect the efficiency of disinfection. Particles of organic composition also may indirectly give rise to chlorinated compounds by reaction with chlorine in water treatment.

Only in the case of particles derived from asbestos minerals, however, are there grounds for suspecting that direct effects on human health could be involved. Fibrous particles of asbestos minerals are known to be associated with increased incidence of cancer, including gastrointestinal cancer, among workers who inhale asbestos-laden air. Experiments on the inhalation of asbestos mineral fibers by animals have also demonstrated a carcinogenic effect. The particulate matter in drinking water often includes similar particles.

Although epidemiological studies have not indicated an increase with time in cancer death rates that can be ascribed to fibrous contamination of the drinking water, these negative findings do not exclude the possibility that such an increase may be detected in the future, because many cancers have long induction periods.

For these and other reasons, detailed elsewhere, it is believed to be important that research on the analysis of fibrous mineral particles in water, and on the toxicity of these materials when ingested, should be strongly pursued.

INORGANIC SOLUTES

The Interim Primary Drinking Water Regulations list maximum allowable concentrations for six metallic elements—barium, cadmium, chromium, lead, mercury, and silver. Ten additional metals were reviewed in this study—beryllium, cobalt, copper, magnesium, manganese, molybdenum, nickel, tin, vanadium, and zinc. Sodium, which is also a metal, was considered separately, because the problems it poses are quite distinct from those associated with the other metallic substances. In addition, the effects on health of several other inorganic constituents of drinking water were studied. These include arsenic, selenium, fluoride, nitrate, and sulfate. The relationship between water hardness and health also received attention.

The sources of inorganic ions in groundwater, surface water, water-treatment chemicals, and from the storage and distribution system are considered along with the health effects resulting from the total intake from food, air, and water.

ORGANIC SOLUTES

Of the 298 volatile organic compounds so far identified in drinking water, 74 were selected for detailed study along with 55 pesticides. A compound was selected for consideration if any of the following criteria applied:

1. Experimental evidence of toxicity in man or animals, including carcinogenicity, mutagenicity, and teratogenicity.
2. Identified in drinking water at relatively high concentration.
3. Molecular structure closely related to that of another compound of known toxicity.
4. Pesticide in heavy use; potential contaminant of drinking water supplies.
5. Listed in the Safe Drinking Water Act or National Interim Primary Drinking Water Regulations.

The evaluation of toxicity was based on a critical review of the scientific literature. The available data were of variable quality and quantity and, in some instances, inadequate for proper assessment of toxicity. In those cases where sufficient data were available, professional judgment was used to determine which compounds are carcinogenic, mutagenic, teratogenic, and noncarcinogenic.

The limitations that are inherent in the extrapolation of high-dose animal bioassay data to low-dose human exposure and the difficulty of making predictions for species that may have different metabolic rates and pathways for handling carcinogens, or different target-organ responses, are well known. Such risk assessment and extrapolation procedures are further compromised by the limited information that is available concerning the mechanisms by which these agents act (such as initiators, promoters, and modifiers) and the almost total lack of data regarding the potential synergistic and antagonistic interactions of these agents with each other and with other environmental agents. The risk of ingesting known or suspected carcinogens was estimated by the methods described in Chapter II. These methods are based on an assumption that there is no threshold in the dose-response relationship. The risk-estimate approach may provide unique advantages for other areas of toxicologic evaluation.

The more traditional approach of combining the maximum no-observed-adverse-effect level with an uncertainty (safety) factor to calculate an acceptable daily intake (ADI) was used for agents that were not considered to be known or suspected carcinogens and for which there was adequate toxicity data from prolonged ingestion studies in man or animals. Several alternative terms other than ADI were considered, but it was concluded that the introduction of new terms might lead to confusion and that the use of a widely recognized and generally acceptable term would be preferable for this report. Although the ADI has been used previously as an internationally established standard for the toxicological evaluation of food additives and contaminants, the concept is applicable to other cases of exposure by ingestion. The ADI is an empirically derived value that reflects a particular combination of knowledge and uncertainty concerning the relative safety of a chemical. The uncertainty factors used to calculate ADI values in this report represent the level of confidence that can be justified on the basis of the animal and human toxicity data. ADI values were not calculated for agents where the data were considered to be inadequate.

Since the calculation of the ADI values is based on the total amount of a chemical ingested, the ADI values calculated in this report do not represent the safe level for drinking water.

Little or no data are available on the toxicity of many organic compounds identified in drinking water. There is a need to determine which of these compounds should be subjected to extensive toxicity testing. Some of the criteria used for developing the order in which compounds should be tested are:

1. The relative concentrations of the compounds and the number of people likely to be exposed.
2. The number of supplies in which they occur.
3. Positive responses in *in vitro* mutagen screening systems.
4. Positive responses in *in vitro* prescreening systems for potential carcinogens (mammalian cell transformations).
5. Similarity of the chemical structure of the test compound with that of other compounds having defined toxic properties (i.e., structure-activity relationships).
6. Relationships of dose from water to total body burden.

RADIOACTIVE CONTAMINANTS

Because the presence of ionizing radiation is one of the standard features of the earth's surface, the adverse effects on health that may be ascribed to radioactive contaminants of drinking water were assessed in relation to the average background radiation dose, from all sources, of 100 mrem per year.

Previous estimations of the biological effects of the background radiation on human health were reviewed in the light of more recent scientific knowledge and used to calculate the magnitude of three kinds of adverse health effects that radiation can produce; namely, developmental and teratogenic effects on the fetus, genetic disease, and somatic (principally carcinogenic) effects.

When these estimates are related to the concentrations of radionuclides that are commonly found in drinking water, it is seen that consumption of 2 liters of water per day contributes such a small fraction to the total radiation background that the incidence of developmental, teratogenic, and genetic disorders is not increased enough for the change to be detectable.

Where somatic effects are concerned, it is estimated that the radionuclides in drinking water typically account for less than 1% of the incidence of cancers that may be attributed to the natural background of radiation. Only certain bone-seeking radionuclides (chiefly radium), in a few regions, reach concentrations in drinking water that are high enough to cause a significant increase in the incidence of bone cancer.

SUSCEPTIBLE SUBGROUPS AND OTHER CONSIDERATIONS

Groups that are more susceptible than the normal population are considered in the chapters on various classes of contaminants.

This report is concerned only with water used for drinking. Although all contaminants may cause problems when present in water used in health care facilities, the health hazards associated with such diverse uses of water as in humidifiers, kidney dialysis units, laundries, heating and cooling equipment, or many special uses that require further treatment of tap water, have not been considered. References and summaries of the scientific literature in this field have been published by DeRoos *et al.* (1974).

REFERENCES

Bourne, G.H., and G.W. Kidder, eds. 1953. Biochemistry and Physiology of Nutrition, vol. 1. Academic Press, New York.

DeRoos, R.L., V.R. Oviatt, A.G. DuChene, and N.J. Vick. 1974. Water use in biomedical research and health care failities—A presentation of article summaries. National Institutes of Health, Department of Health, Education, and Welfare, Contract no. NIH-ORS-72-2111.

Evans, C.L. ed. Starling's Principles of Human Physiology, 8th ed. Lea and Febiger, Philadelphia.

Federal Register, Wednesday, December 24, 1975, vol. 40, no. 248.

Guyton, A.C. 1968. Textbook of Medical Physiology, 3d ed. W.B. Saunders Co., Philadelphia.

McNall, P.E., and J.C. Schlegel. 1968. Practical thermal environmental limits for young adult males working in hot, humid environments. ASHRAE Transactions 74:225-235.

National Academy of Sciences-National Research Council. 1974. Recommended Dietary Allowances, 8th ed. Washington, D.C.

Pike, R.L., and M. Brown. 1975. Minerals and Water in Nutrition—An Integrated Approach, 2d Ed. John Wiley, New York.

Randall, H.T. 1973. Water, electrolytes and acid base balance. *In* R.S. Goodhart and M.E. Shils, eds. Modern Nutrition in Health and Disease. Lea and Febiger, Philadelphia.

Walker, B.S., W.C. Boyd, and I. Asimov. 1957. Biochemistry and Human Metabolism, 2d ed. Williams & Wilkins Co., Baltimore.

Wolf, A.V. 1958. Body water. Sci. Am. 99:125.

II

Chemical Contaminants: Safety And Risk Assessment

The hazards of ingesting pollutants in drinking water can be assessed in two general ways: with studies of toxicity in the laboratory and with epidemiological studies. Studies in the laboratory may employ a variety of experimental systems, ranging from chemical effects of pollutants on DNA, through exposure of bacterial or mammalian cells in culture, to lifetime feeding studies on experimental animals. They are prospective studies, in which relatively small numbers of cells or animals are exposed to characterized pollutants at known concentrations. Epidemiological studies deal with human populations. Their design is constrained by external circumstances, and they involve large numbers of people whose exposure to the pollutant in question is commonly uncertain and confounded by exposure to other pollutants.

The aim of studies of both types is to allow the risk to man to be estimated. The first can give precise information on relatively high risks related to individual pollutants in this or that animal species—to which human exposure and risk may be compared. The second can provide less precise information on the human risk related to one pollutant (isolated, it is hoped, from other pollutants).

Toxicity data obtained from laboratory animals will generally have to be relied on for estimating human risk, if we are to control human exposure to carcinogens. Epidemiological studies have discovered causes of disease and can buttress, supplement, or contradict laboratory data. Imaginative comparisons between laboratory and epidemiological data are of the utmost importance, particularly in the area of metabolic pathways and fate of chemicals found to be carcinogens in animals.

Efforts to develop rapid assays for mutagenesis and carcinogenesis have recently been greatly expanded. Methods that show promise include tests for mutagenicity that make use of bacterial, cell transformation, and organ culture systems. There appears to be high positive correlation between mutagenicity, as determined by some of these methods, and carcinogenicity in agents already studied (McCann *et al.*, 1975; McCann and Ames, 1976; Ames, 1976). The utility of these rapid methods will depend on experimental demonstration that their results are well correlated with those obtained from conventional long-term studies of carcinogenicity with well-designed animal systems. High priority should be given this research because it offers a reasonable probability of success in a relatively short time and at lower cost than long-term testing, and there is an urgent need for a primary screen for selecting compounds for long-term assay (DHEW, 1977).

The committee is fully conscious of these modern methods for determining genetic and physiological phenomena. Their use, when appropriate, and their further development is strongly encouraged.

Pollutants in water have many different effects. At one extreme, they can impart a disagreeable taste or odor. This is quickly perceived by the community, and the process of characterization and identification of the offending pollutant is generally prompt and fairly straightforward. At the other extreme, the effects on human health of a carcinogen present in drinking water will probably go undetected, particularly if it produces only a modest increase in the incidence of a common cancer.

The major toxicological and epidemiological efforts should therefore be directed to characterizing and identifying pollutants whose biological effects include chronic, irreversible, and progressive diseases, such as cancer. It is necessary to develop risk estimates for large human populations of varied susceptibilities that are exposed to small concentrations of such toxic pollutants, including carcinogens.

The development of safety factors for pollutants whose toxic effects are reversible and nonprogressive involves empirical calculations based on past history of use and concentrations that appeared safe for the public. These safety factors are usually applied to the highest dose or concentration at which no adverse effect was observed. The chosen dose or concentration is divided by a "safety factor" that varies over a wide range, depending on the adequacy of the data.

Whether or not the "safety factor" approach can be used with pollutants that cause chronic, irreversible, and progressive disease in laboratory animals is controversial. Those who argue for safety factors, and thereby thresholds, find it inconceivable that very small concentrations can cause a cancer to develop, claiming that body defenses can surely protect at doses smaller than the threshold value. Those who argue that safety factors are inadequate and that almost no thresholds can be determined, or theoretically developed, suggest that even one or a very few molecular events have a finite probability of initiating a successful malignant or neoplastic transformation in a cell, and that this can lead to a lethal cancer. Although one malignant cell can lead to death by cancer, many liver or kidney cells can be killed or damaged (but not malignantly transformed), without causing any detectable disease. Furthermore, man is never exposed to one carcinogen at a time, but is exposed to low concentrations of many at the same time.

Accordingly, we have adopted a "nonthreshold" approach for estimating risks from pollutants that have been shown to be carcinogenic in laboratory animals.

Demonstration that a pollutant is carcinogenic, and application of nonthreshold risk estimates to it, do not imply that its use must be prohibited. Such a proscription might itself give rise to even greater risks to health or other disadvantages. In some cases, a net risk must be estimated, and society must attempt to use the pollutant in such a way as to minimize risk and maximize benefit. Nowhere is this better illustrated than in the use of chlorination to disinfect water. Chlorination controls pathogenic organisms, but introduces chloroform, which is carcinogenic in animal-test systems. Methods must be devised to minimize concentrations of chloroform and chlorinated hydrocarbons, from whatever source, in drinking water. But before alternative methods for control of pathogenic organisms are instituted, toxicological studies must show that they are as effective as, and pose no greater risk than, chlorination. We perceive that society is willing to accept some risks to health if the attendant benefits are demonstrably greater.

Drinking water contains low concentrations of many chemicals, some of which, if ingested for a long time, could have delayed toxic effects. The insidious effect of chronic exposure to low doses of toxic agents is difficult to recognize, because often there are few early warning signs and, when signs are ultimately observed, the effects may have become irreversible. Subchronic toxicology studies may not offer reliable means for assessment of long-term toxic effects in animals, let alone extrapolation to chronic effects in man; hence, different considerations have to be applied in assessing risk. The methods and principles of acute toxicology do not offer any easy, straightforward methods for extrapolation of such experimental data to calculate risks for large human populations.

Two important questions must be answered: What assay procedures are required for a valid assessment of chronic toxicity of chemicals in experimental animals? How can the data from such procedures be extrapolated to estimate risks in humans? In dealing with these questions, we use the specific risk of cancer as our major example, although other toxicities are considered. This report seeks to summarize the state of the art in extrapolating to man the results of experiments on animals, chiefly in relation to carcinogenesis.

EFFECTS ON HEALTH

The purpose of drinking-water standards is to ensure protection from acute poisoning and from long-term, or "chronic," effects. In recent years, numerous short-duration, presumptive tests *in vitro* have been developed that may help to predict carcinogenesis. Nonetheless, studies of chronic toxicity continue to be required for safety evaluations. These are necessary because there is no general way to predict carcinogenic effects on the basis of the observed short-term effects of chemical-biological interactions. [The significance to health of the finding that a pollutant is mutagenic in the new test systems is unknown (See Drake, 1975; DHEW, 1977). But, because evidence of the correlation between mutagenicity and carcinogenicity continues to accumulate, we suggest that a conservative safety factor be provisionally applied to the mutagenicity data and that, if new information (such as the results of a reliable carcinogenicity study) is lacking 4 yr from the time a mutagenicity study is completed, nonthreshold methods be used to establish risk.]

Chronic exposures and chronic effects are different (Casarett, 1975). The former means frequent ingestion over a long period of time. The latter implies injury that persists, either because the injury is irreversible or progressive, or because the exposure is prolonged and the rate of new injury exceeds the rate of repair. Chronic exposure in animals is generally considered to be at least half the life span. In man, it can be much less.

Injury from chronic exposure may occur in at least three ways: by accumulation of the chemical to a critical concentration at sites of action sufficient to induce detectable injury; by accumulation of injury until physiological reserves can no longer compensate (i.e., repair is never complete); or after a long, latent period beginning with an exposure that has an unrecognized biological effect, and precipitates the eventual appearance of injury. In the first case, knowledge of the kinetics of chemical absorption, metabolism, and excretion obtained in short-term studies may allow computation of the amount of the toxic chemical that will accumulate in long-term use. Such investigations will improve the usefulness of long-term, low-dose, chronic-exposure studies. To predict chronic accumulation, or latent development, of injury from the results of short-term tests requires knowledge of the kinetics of injury and repair. There are few, if any, substances for which such understanding is at hand.

Reversibility of Chemical Injury

Reversible effects disappear after exposure ends. The time required for return to normal should be a small fraction of the remaining lifetime of an organism. During the period of return to normal, the organism must be at no greater risk (than one that was never exposed) of further or other damage from other sources. For some effects, reversibility may be qualified by the normal lifetime of a specific cell or macromolecule that serves as the end point of the effect. A nonreversible effect is one in which the damage does not regress completely, or may progress after exposure ceases.

Some effects of toxic chemicals are unmistakably irreversible. They include terata, malignant tumors, mutations in offspring of exposed animals, and some neurological changes. These are gross manifestations of specific chemical-cell interactions, and it is possible, or probable, that there are early reversible effects, either in the cellular process first affected or at intervening stages. Prediction of adverse effects from short-term studies is possible if the critical dose and the rate-limiting factors that determine reversibility are known. Without this knowledge, evaluation of toxicity will generally deal more with the possibility of irreversible effects than with speculatively reversible effects.

Net reversibility varies from one tissue, species, strain, or individual to another. It is generally impossible to measure the specific processes involved in injury and repair in the standard toxicity-evaluation study. However, measurements of reversibility in short-term studies should provide useful information that may allow extrapolation to the longer term.

The predictive value of such tests does not necessarily depend on the persistence of the chemical in the test organism. If the chemical produces a reversible effect and then is rapidly detoxified or excreted, it may be possible to compute the doses or schedules of exposure that would not produce cumulative and ultimately nonreversible or irreversible effects (see definitions below). But other factors might be overriding. For example, rapid reversibility after a single dose might not indicate the rate of reversal after repeated doses, if the first dose, in addition to the measured effect, altered the repair process or processes responsible for detoxification (Murphy, 1967). To evaluate repeated-dose effects, subchronic- and chronic-exposure studies should include groups of animals that are removed from exposure at selected intervals during the experiment. The rate of reversal of effects in these animals can be measured at intervals, or at some critical time after exposure ceases.

If the chemical persists in the organism, quantification of rates of reversal is more complicated. Data are needed on absorption and disposition to correspond with data on rates and reversal of effects.

Perspectives and Perceptions of Effects

Whether an effect is reversible, nonreversible, or irreversible might be shown by experiments (or epidemiological studies) that include observations during exposure-free "recovery"periods similar to those made at the end of the exposure period. Nonreversible and irreversible injuries are of greater concern than reversible injuries in evaluating human health effects. However, frequently recurring reversible injury may lead to greater morbidity than a nonreversible or irreversible injury that appears only late in life. Characterization of an effect as reversible implies that there is a dose below which health will not be compromised. This assumes, of course, that any subliminal cellular injury that is responsible for the manifest effect is also reversible. Full understanding of thresholds, margins of safety or safety factors, and extrapolations of estimated risk requires understanding the underlying cellular mechanisms of injury.

An alternative to the safety-factor approach for reversible toxicity may be considered. The nonthreshold approach is attractive partly because of the idea that one transformed cell could lead to fatal neoplastic disease. What number of damaged (but not transformed) or killed kidney, liver, or lung cells is compatible with a healthy life? If these numbers, or fractions of total organs, could be estimated for a number of species, including man, and if experimental dose-response curves for fractional damage to all vital organs could be obtained, the numbers of damaged cells that are compatible with health could be estimated. This might constitute an initial approach to the development of rational risk estimates for toxic effects other than cancer. Clearly, a major research effort is needed.

Where it was once common to refer to "no-effect doses" of chemicals and "safe" doses, it is now more appropriate to speak of "no-observed-adverse-effect" doses and "acceptable risk" when describing permissible use or exposure to chemicals. This change has been accompanied by an increasing concern for the health of the most susceptible individuals in the population, besides that of the average individual. Many scientists now distinguish between injuries produced by chemicals for which there is likely to be a threshold dose and effects (e.g., carcinogenesis and mutagenesis) for which there is likely to be either no threshold dose or no way presently known to estimate one for large, heterogeneous populations. [A report of another committee of the National Academy of Sciences expresses some doubt about the validity of the threshold concept for any type of biological effect (NAS, 1975); see also Drake *et al.*, 1975, and Hoel *et al.*, 1975.] From another point of view, Weil (1972), considering statistics and judgment in safety evaluation, wrote: "No matter what the biological effect, at some concentrations under some sets of conditions, a dose level must exist below which no biological damage will occur during the life-span of the great majority of men. No matter how small the dose, however, one, or a few, of millions of subjects may exhibit the critical response."

It is more prudent to treat some kinds of toxic effects that may be self-propagating or strictly cumulative, or both, as if there were no threshold and to estimate the upper limits of risk for any given exposure. Included among these are effects that result from an initial, chemically induced alteration in cellular genetics that is transmitted by cell propagation. Carcinogenesis and mutagenesis are examples in which a single cell transformation has the theoretical potential for irreversibility, which might involve self-propagation, even in the absence of further exposure.

Other injuries may become self-propagating—e.g., advanced stages of cirrhosis—but they are usually preceded by detectable injury that is reversible. The initial effects should have a dose-response threshold, inasmuch as the nature of cellular injury that precedes them can be detected while the injury is still reversible.

Some forms of injury may be strictly cumulative, because the cells in which they occur are not repaired or replaced. (For example, destruction of enough neurons leads to a decrease in central nervous system function.)

Congenital malformations appear to be irreversible. In this case, injury occurs from exposure during only a brief period. In addition, it is probable that a threshold dose could be estimated from adequate experimental or epidemiological data.

Current knowledge of the proper principles for extrapolating toxicological data from high dose to low dose, and from one species to another, is inadequate. Nonetheless, standards for drinking water must be developed. Whenever possible, a maximal no-observed-adverse-effect dosage should be identified. Three major categories of effects should be considered, and different ways of arriving at standards can be proposed for each.

Irreversible (Self-Propagating) Effects

(These are likely to become life-threatening even after exposure has ceased)

1. Genetically self-propagating effects, e.g., somatic or germ-cell mutation that culminates in a malignant neoplasm or is transmitted to later generations: Assume no threshold, assume a linear dose-response at low doses, and estimate risk. Set standard at something other than zero only if exposure cannot be eliminated by reasonable means, or if material has no safer substitute, and if it has great utility or social value. An acceptable degree of risk arrived at by a case-by-case consideration involving numerous scientific, technological, economic, and societal issues and values should determine the permitted dose.

Nonreversible Effects

1. Effects that are sequels to probably detectable, reversible injury, but that may become self-propagating (such as cirrhosis): If a threshold can be demonstrated, use it as an upper limit, with application of an appropriate safety factor. If not, proceed as in "Irreversible Effects."

2. Death of irreplacable cells, cumulative with continued exposure, e.g., central nervous system disease, as in exposure to methyl mercury. If a threshold can be demonstrated, use it as an upper limit, with application of an appropriate safety factor. If not, proceed as in "Irreversible Effects."

Reversible Effects

1. Life-threatening or major morbidity, e.g., inhibition of a vital enzyme system. If a threshold can be demonstrated, use it as an upper limit. If not, proceed as in "Irreversible Effects."

2. Minor morbidity, e.g., sensory irritation without histological change. Determine the range of sensitivities and choose an upper limit low enough to minimize occurrence in the population.

3. No detectable functional or sensory decrement, but possibly predictive precursor of more serious effect, e.g., plasma cholinesterase inhibition, or small increase in liver enzymes in plasma. Proceed as in 2.

IRREVERSIBLE TOXICITY

Many factors make the assessment of long-term health risks to human populations difficult—for example:

1. The sensitivity of the test systems used to detect carcinogenic effects depends on the number of animals used in each test and on the duration of their survival.
2. Any series of experiments will yield false-positive and false-negative results.
3. Detection of neoplastic changes in treated animals requires extensive gross and microscopic examination of many tissues by trained people.
4. Time, resources, and money required to conduct an adequate test are all substantial.

Controversies have arisen because of the above problems and because of inadequate testing for long-term effects. False-positive results can cause unnecessary public concern and the removal of useful materials from the market, and false-negative results can endanger the health of large groups of people. Long-term effects are particularly difficult to detect and treat because they are discovered only after many years, by which time they are often irreversible.

The main question to be answered is: "Within the limitations of present-day capabilities, what are the minimal requirements for an adequate test (on experimental animals) of the long-term effects of potentially toxic agents, and how can these results be used to estimate possible risk to the human population?"

Summary of Principles for Extrapolating Animal Toxicity To Humans

Despite wide gaps in our knowledge of the metabolism and ultimate fate of chemicals in man, properly conducted experiments will yield results that can improve our estimates of the risk to human populations from long-term exposures.

Many mechanisms for chemical carcinogenesis have been postulated. If the mechanism involves somatic mutation or alteration, there is no threshold dose for long-term exposure; if the mechanism is unknown, it is prudent to assume that DNA damage is involved. The idea that there is a "safe" dose of such chemicals may be conceptually valid, but *"safety" cannot be established by any experimental method now available.* Every dose should be regarded as carrying some risk. A "most probable risk" can be estimated by appropriate statistical treatment of the results of experiments on animals, and once the benefits of use of a chemical have been defined and estimated, it is possible to weigh the health risks against the health benefits. The balance between them should then be the overriding consideration in regulating the amounts of such substances in the environment.

The method used in classical toxicology for determining safe doses for short-term exposure of humans to drugs is to estimate a maximum exposure that is tolerated without adverse effects in a group of animals, and to apply a safety factor. This procedure is valid only for estimating the risk of reversible toxic effects. "No-observed-adverse-effect dose" is a better term, because it makes clear that the exposure can often be a function of the size of the experiment—the larger the experiment, the lower this dose can be.

Studies in laboratory animals must be used to predict the safety of environmental chemicals. Human epidemiological studies cannot be used to predict nor assure safety, for several reasons:

1. Epidemiology cannot tell what effects a material will have until after humans have been exposed. One must not conduct what might be hazardous experiments on man.
2. If exposure has been ubiquitous, it may be impossible to assess the effects of a material, because there is no unexposed control group. Statistics of morbidity obtained before use of a new material can sometimes be useful, but when latent periods are variable and times of introduction and removal of materials overlap, historical data on chronic effects are usually unsatisfactory.
3. It is usually difficult to determine doses in human exposures.
4. Usually, it is hard to identify small changes in common effects, which may nonetheless be important if the population is large.
5. Interactions in a "nature-designed" experiment usually cannot be controlled.

With the possible exception of arsenic and benzene, the known human carcinogens are carcinogenic in some laboratory species. Therefore, animal studies of carcinogenesis in laboratory animals are useful for predicting effects in man.

Thus, for ethical and practical reasons, data derived by using animals for toxicity testing are essential for protecting the public from harmful effects of new chemicals in the environment and probably also necessary for evaluating the potential harm of "old" chemicals. By the same token, epidemiological surveillance studies are necessary for detecting the errors that will surely arise from use of the animal studies alone. Thus, epidemiological studies are both a last line of defense and a means for verifying and adjusting the conclusions from animal studies.

The General Problem Of Extrapolation

The knowledge and insight that provide a basis for more successful extrapolation are rapidly increasing. The value of tests on laboratory animals is most easily estimated when the chemical agents tested are ultimately administered to, or confront man in a manner similar to the animal exposure, as in the drug-development process. The sequence of animal tests of a new chemical agent, after toxicological studies, continues with studies conducted in order to determine: the mechanism through which the laboratory animals respond to the agent, the nature of its metabolism in tissues and organs, and the rates and routes of elimination of the agent and its derivatives. Thus, damage observed in an organ of an animal provides clues that lead to an understanding of the metabolism and organ involvement of the substance in humans. Similarities and differences between humans and animals can be noted, and the validity of the laboratory-animal test systems can be better estimated. This approach is most useful for observing early effects that occur soon after the substance is administered. The use of such data for assessing long-term effects in humans has many difficulties.

When a mouse or man is exposed to a chemical, a number of events can occur that can greatly influence the final reaction, which may appear as the observed toxic effect. These events include: absorption; distribution and storage; metabolism, excretion, and reabsorption; arrival at the site of action; reaction with the biological receptor; and interaction with other constituents of the environment. They can be compared among various animal species and among strains and individuals. Anatomical, biochemical, physiological, pharmacological, and pathological differences and similarities can and have been identified, and there have been efforts to characterize systematically the differences and similarities between species for some compounds and classes of compounds. These are appropriate subjects for research.

Chemicals to which man is exposed can be divided into two classes: those deliberately administered for therapeutic, diagnostic, or nutritive purposes, which contribute to health, and those with uses that do not directly benefit health, but reach man through a variety of routes.

To some extent, the acute toxicity of the first class can be observed directly in man. If the chemicals are already in use, the laboratory-animal toxicity tests provide a type of pre-screening or early warning system. However, chemicals of the second class are generally not tested in man, and their potential hazard can be estimated only through laboratory animal testing, epidemiological studies, or observation.

Extrapolation of data from laboratory animals to man is difficult to treat in a systematic and comprehensive fashion. Although vast amounts of data have been accumulated on the toxicity of compounds in animals and the effects of drugs and other chemicals on human health, experiments that generate the data tend to be so diverse that comparison is usually impossible. Good quantitative data on the toxicity of compounds in man are rare. Most commonly, there is neither knowledge of the amount of a chemical to which man was exposed nor of the incidence and severity of toxic effects.

Toxicologists rely heavily on "experience" for successful extrapolation of toxicity data to man. Unfortunately, experience is interpreted differently by different people and thus is a variable guide. For some of the most serious toxic effects, it can also be very misleading. For example, some cancers may take decades to develop in man after exposure to a carcinogen, so it is difficult for investigators to develop experience that will permit them to link exposure to ultimate effect. Tests for mutagenic effects in the human population are inadequate today, and it is possible that such effects from chemicals are already appearing. However, who has had enough "experience" to infer that man has changed because of some specific chemical in, say, the last 50 yr? Statistical observation of small changes is usually difficult. For example, if 20% of all pregnant women used a chemical that caused stillbirths in 5% of the women who used it, the resulting increase in stillbirths would be 1% ($0.20 \times 0.05 = 0.01$), and it is likely that it would not even be noticed. If 5% of all pregnant women used a chemical that caused a delayed effect in 20% of their offspring, this also would probably escape notice. Even if the chemical caused a 10% increase in a most common form of cancer in the offspring of the 5% of women (e.g., cancer of the colon, which would mean an increase of 200 deaths per year), the effect would very likely go undetected.

Specific Problems In Extrapolation

Experiments on laboratory animals are generally performed under highly standardized conditions, with controlled diet, temperature, humidity, and light-dark cycles, and usually with genetically homogeneous animals, such as inbred mice, rats, or beagles. Thus, one obtains reasonably precise and reproducible information on the toxicity of a substance under specified conditions, in animals from specific genetic pools. However, large and diverse segments of the human population may be exposed to the compound. Humans are not genetically homogeneous: They live under various environmental conditions, they eat a great variety of foods, and they are exposed to large and increasing numbers of substances. We would like to protect the whole population—its most sensitive members as well as the average. Therefore, environmental and genetic variability must be considered in the process of extrapolation.

Man is generally exposed to toxic pollutants in the water supply through his gastrointestinal tract, and laboratory animals should be exposed in the same way. However, some problems inherent in the use of animals must be kept in mind when one is using animal studies to predict the carcinogenic potential of a substance for man.

SIZE OF ANIMALS

Size tends to determine the rate of distribution of substances in the body; in large animals, they are distributed more slowly and tend to persist longer. In general, large animals metabolize compounds more slowly than do small animals. Large mammals have many more susceptible cells; thus, if the carcinogenic event is rare, it would be more likely to occur in a large mammal than in a small one (a mouse experiment using 1,600–2,000 animals represents about the same number of susceptible cells as are contained in one man). Obviously, however, a mouse is not the equivalent of a very small man; nor is a man the equivalent of a very large mouse. In the mouse, the ratio of cardiac output per minute to blood volume is 1:1. In man, the ratio is 1:20. Thus, blood circulates approximately 20 times as rapidly in a mouse as in a man. (This difference is not a peculiar species difference, but typifies the differences between very small and relatively large animals.) The implication is that the time a substance spends in the plasma (excluding metabolism) is longer in a larger mammal than in a smaller one. Thus, for the same milligram-per-kilogram dose, human tissues are exposed to a substance for a much longer time than mouse tissues. This is consistent with data obtained in studies of anticancer drugs, which showed that—on a milligram-per-kilogram basis—a mouse required 12 times as much drug to respond as did man, a rat 6 times as much, and a dog and a monkey 2–3 times as much. When the data were expressed on a milligram-per-square-meter basis, the differences between species were sharply reduced. In addition, the cell-division rate is greater in small animals: e.g., the cycle time of mouse gut or marrow cells is about half that of man. The life span of a man is 35 times that of a mouse. Thus, there are many more cell divisions in man, and therefore a greater opportunity for neoplastic change.

These observations suggest that small mammals that are routinely used for toxicity testing are often more resistant than man to toxic compounds. This implies that small animal systems are likely to produce many false-negative results, and has important implications for establishing safety factors or using "conservative" techniques for extrapolation.

NUMBER OF ANIMALS

The number of exposed animals is important. Typically, about 10^2–10^3 experimental animals are tested, whereas the population of humans to be protected may be 10^8–10^9.

The human population is genetically heterogeneous, whereas test populations of animals, as a rule, are relatively inbred. Genetic traits can affect many aspects of susceptibility to pollutants.

Selectivity influences the test-animal population in that only healthy, vigorous animals are started on test, whereas the exposed human population may contain subpopulations that are ill and weak.

ENVIRONMENTAL DIFFERENCES

Nutritional differences and the physical environment (heat, light, ionizing radiation, etc.) can affect response to pollutants. The chemical environment—from drugs to air pollutants—with its overwhelming number and types of substances, provides the possibility for synergistic toxicity. Synergistic effects have occurred with therapeutic drugs, are well known in experimental carcinogenesis, and are an ever-present danger.

ABSORPTION

Rates of absorption of chemicals through the gastrointestinal tract are generally comparable in laboratory animals and man. The barriers within the gastrointestinal tract and the cell membranes, which prevent the free passage of organic compounds, are quite similar among mammalian species. These barriers are either the cells themselves or the intercellular junctions, which are "closed" or "tight" and which, in general, force substances to move through cells, rather than between them. It should be recognized, however, that there are differences between one animal and another and between man and animal. The ratio of surface area to volume in the gastrointestinal tract, and the transit time through it, often differ among and within species. These factors affect absorption. The pH differs in various parts of the gastrointestinal tract in different species; this can affect the absorption of some partially ionized compounds. The possibility that intact proteins can be absorbed in neonates of some species suggests that absorption in the neonate can be nonspecific.

The presence of *bacteria* in the gastrointestinal tract can affect absorption indirectly. Bacteria may convert the original substance into one that is more or less absorbable, and thus alter the apparent toxicity of a chemical, or they may convert a nontoxic substance into a toxic one. For example, reduction of nitrate to nitrite permits the formation of highly carcinogenic nitrosamines by reaction with secondary amines from the diet. The bacterial populations in the gastrointestinal tract vary between species and within species, and in the same individual from time to time, often changing with changes in diet.

DISTRIBUTION AND STORAGE

Once a compound is absorbed, it is distributed throughout the body, largely by the *circulatory system.* This gives the opportunity for binding to plasma protein or tissue, and storage in such depots as fat and bone. There can also be *differences between species* with respect to plasma protein and tissue binding. These differences do not seem to be of major importance, but small mammals, such as mice, tend to bind substances less extensively than man. Research on such subjects as storage depots is needed.

METABOLIC DIFFERENCES

The primary organs that *metabolize substances* are the liver, the lungs, and the kidneys. With respect to hepatic metabolism—often considered to be the most important—small mammals generally metabolize substances more rapidly than large mammals, and herbivores more rapidly than carnivores. There are other interspecific differences; this is a field in which research is active.

EXCRETION AND REABSORPTION

There are few comparable data contrasting renal or hepatic *excretory rates of substances* in mice, rats, dogs, monkeys, and man. What data there are suggest that small mammals excrete compounds via the kidneys considerably more rapidly than large mammals. There are too few data to show systematic differences in hepatic excretion and the extent of reabsorption after hepatic excretion. Some substances are excreted through the hepatic system more rapidly by rodents than by dogs and other large animals. After excretion via the bile, reabsorption from the gastrointestinal tract may occur.

DIFFERENCES IN RECEPTOR SITES

The action of *cellular and intracellular membranes* is also of concern. An unaltered substance or its metabolites, after distribution through the body, must pass through a variety of cellular and intracellular membranes to arrive at the site of action. Many of these membranes are of major importance in determining the ultimate toxicity of the substance. The blood-brain and blood-testicular barriers, for instance, effectively modulate the chemical composition of the fluid surrounding the central nervous system cells and the developing sperm cells. These barriers can also avert or delay the arrival of potentially toxic compounds at the sites of action. Similarly, the placenta acts as a barrier between the maternal circulation and the developing fetus. In addition to the passive barriers, active-transport systems influence the movement of foreign organic compounds. This is a subject in which research is moving rapidly, and there is a great need for unified systematic theories on interspecific relationships. In general, if a substance reaches a site of action, the ultimate toxic reaction seems to be consistent among species. Development of a lesion will then follow this reaction. With some of the more serious manifestations, such as malignant change and mutagenic change, development of a lesion may depend on the extent of damage (e.g., severely damaged cells will die; generation time of the cells and rates of repair processes may be affected). For instance, the generation time of the rapidly proliferating cell population in the mouse is about half of that in man; therefore, cancer is likely to appear earlier in the mouse.

Design Of Laboratory Experiments On Animals

In designing assay procedures, the route and type of human exposure should be duplicated as closely as possible. Because it is often impossible, *a priori,* to determine specific susceptibility—and because man may often be the most susceptible species—more than one species of laboratory animal should be used. Short-lived species, such as rats and mice, should be chosen so that tests can be completed in a short time. Doses should be selected for long-term studies, so that exposure to the test substance causes little or no weight loss or shortening of life of animals under test. Sufficiently great exposures in animals need to be used to compensate for the possibly higher sensitivity of the human population and the uncertainties involved in extrapolation. However, the dose should not be so high as to produce acute toxic effects.

Some *logical and statistical considerations* in the design and conduct of the animal experiments affect the extrapolation. Two major considerations are the *structure* of the experiments—how many doses, how spaced, inbred vs. outbred animals—and the *size* of the experiment—how many animals at each dose. If several doses are used, it may be possible to derive a dose-response relationship.

The faith that can be placed in an experimental result is also related to the size of the experiment. An experiment using 1,000 animals that shows no untoward effects at a high dose elicits much more confidence that there truly is no effect than does an experiment using 10 animals—even if it is conducted at a similarly high dose. A low response rate, 1–2%, is almost impossible to establish with an experiment that uses fewer than 500 animals. If the animals were spread out among several doses (some of which might give a 0.1% or 0.01% response), the number of animals needed to yield reliable figures would be in the hundreds of thousands.

Man is genetically heterogeneous and lives in a heterogeneous environment, so some experimenters feel more confident in their extrapolations if there are non-inbred animals in their experiments. Using such animals generally requires larger experiments to give reproducible results. One approach to this problem is to conduct many experiments, in several species, using inbred animals of each species.

Current Capability to Extrapolate

More and more patterns that are useful for extrapolation to man are being recognized and can be identified in the course of studying pharmacological disposition of a substance. Most of the differences that have been observed suggest that man is more sensitive than the usual experimental animal, and this must be kept in mind in establishing permissible exposures for humans.

There are great difficulties in comparing the median animal to the not-so-average man. Man is not genetically homogeneous and is usually exposed to a much wider range of environmental conditions than the usual experimental animal. Differences in environmental factors are known to affect the toxicity of a substance. Differences in the genetic makeup of the individual can affect toxicity. These must be considered in the extrapolation of laboratory-animal toxicity data to man. We must predict for, and protect, the highly sensitive individual as well as the average or median person. Because of the multitude of man-made chemicals, the different habits and life-styles of populations, and the different eating habits of populations, there is considerable variation in the intake of, or exposure to, environmental pollutants. These must also be considered in establishing permissible exposures to environmental agents.

In the last decade, large genetic differences in metabolism of toxic agents have been found in man, and study of these effects has led to a new branch of pharmacology—pharmacokinetics. The range of variability is illustrated by the observation that, in a group of about 20 patients, the steady-state plasma concentrations of two tricyclic antidepressants varied by about 30-fold, and the half-time of disappearance from the plasma varied about 10-fold (Hammer and Sjoqvist, 1967). Also, the plasma concentration of isonicotinic acid hydrazide has been found to vary by a factor of almost 100 in different people, and this appears to be genetically controlled (Weber, 1976).

Many examples of unexpected toxic reactions to therapeutic agents have been caused by interactions of compounds that were normally safe when given alone (Conney and Burns, 1972). The likelihood that such synergistic interactions will occur with environmental pollutants is high. An early and striking example of unexpected synergistic interactions (hypertensive crisis) occurred in patients who, while taking monoamine oxidase inhibitors, ate cheese that contained bioactive amines. Although theoretically predictable, this effect had not been suggested in the literature before it was observed in patients.

Many sources of variation within the population of any species, such as age, sex, pregnancy, disease, can affect the response to foreign substances. An example is the difference between sexes in metabolism and toxicity of acetylsalicylic acid (Menguy *et al.,* 1972).

In addition, such environmental variables as temperature, lighting, barometric pressure, humidity, and diet are known to affect the toxicity of environmental pollutants. For example, the oral absorption of pentobarbital is greatly altered by the prior ingestion of a small cheese sandwich. In this case, peak pentobarbital concentration in plasma is diminished by about 50%, and the duration of the effective plasma concentration is doubled (Bush *et al.,* 1966).

Another difficulty in extrapolating from laboratory animals to man is the dose-duration problem. The lifetime of a mouse is about 2 yr. A man's life expectancy is close to 70 yr, and a woman's 5 yr longer. Because man usually excretes compounds more slowly than mice, this means that man, with a very small daily intake, can develop a greater accumulation of a compound over many years.

It is currently impossible to estimate the effects of all the genetic and environmental variability in the human population.

Although gains are being made in predicting effects of pollutants in man, safety testing must, for the present, continue to rely on the results of administration of high doses of substances in test animals to provide a basis for protecting the human population.

THRESHOLDS

Biological Considerations

Whether or not a particular effect follows a dose-response relationship that has a threshold depends entirely on the mechanism of the effect. Many effects have thresholds. For example, the gastrointestinal-radiation syndrome, acute drug toxicity, and radiation or drug control of some tumors all have dose-response curves that show thresholds. The curves are sigmoid, and below a particular dose there is zero probability of producing the effect, because it requires many independent occurrences and will not occur until the number of such events exceeds some critical value. The gastrointestinal-radiation (or drug) syndrome is a case in point. An animal will not die until the number of intestinal crypt cells that have been killed exceeds some value that is critical to the integrity of the organ. Any radiation or drug dose that kills fewer cells than this critical number can be considered to be "safe" (at least for this one syndrome).

We are used to thinking in terms of thresholds and sigmoid dose-response curves. For example, if it costs $4,000 to buy an automobile, we do not imagine that we will have a 50% chance of buying the same vehicle for $2,000. If 100 aspirin tablets constitute a lethal dose, we do not calculate that we will have a 1% chance of dying if we swallow a single tablet. Because we know the mechanisms underlying these events, we expect thresholds to the dose-response curves, and indeed they are evident.

However, other effects may well *not* have threshold dose-effect relationships. If an effect can be caused by a single hit, a single molecule, or a single unit of exposure, then the effect in question cannot have a threshold in the dose-response relationship, no matter how unlikely it is that the single hit or event will produce the effect. Mutations in prokaryotic and eukaryotic cells can be caused by a single cluster of ion pairs produced by a beam of ionizing radiation. We would expect that mutations can be caused by a single molecule or perhaps group of molecules in proximity to the DNA. The necessary conclusion from this result is that the dose-response relationship for radiation and chemical mutagenesis cannot have a threshold and must be linear, at least at low doses.

It is one step further to correlate mutagenesis with carcinogenesis. Nevertheless, the evidence is strong that there is a close relationship between the two (McCann *et al.*, 1975; McCann and Ames, 1976; Ames, 1976; DHEW, 1977).

We therefore conclude that, if there is evidence that a particular carcinogen acts by directly causing a mutation in the DNA, it is likely that the dose-response curve for carcinogenesis will not show a threshold and will be linear with dose at low doses.

CONSIDERATION OF THE DOSE-RESPONSE RELATIONSHIP

In considering the possibility of thresholds for carcinogenesis, it is important to understand that there is no agent, chemical or physical, that induces a form of cancer in man that does not occur in the absence of that agent. In other words, when there is exposure to a material, we are not starting at an origin of zero cancers. Nor are we starting at an origin of zero carcinogenic agents in our environment. Thus, it is likely that any carcinogenic agent added to the environment will act by a particular mechanism on a particular cell population that is *already being acted on by the same mechanism to induce cancers.* This reasoning implies that only if it acted by a mechanism entirely different from that already operating on the tissue could a newly added carcinogen show a threshold in its dose-response curve.

EXAMINATION OF EXPERIMENTAL DOSE-RESPONSE CURVES

The most extensive information on carcinogenesis both in experimental animals and in humans is with ionizing radiation (BEIR,1972). Although there is evidence implicating thresholds in some animal tissues (Walburg, 1974), thresholds have in general not been established for most tissues. If such thresholds exist, they occur at sufficiently low doses that it would require massive, expensive, and impracticable experiments to establish them. In view of the common finding—for example of a linear dose-response relationship (unaffected by dose-rate)—for cancer induction in animals by high LET radiation, it is unlikely that such thresholds exist. Linearity is not essential to the no-threshold argument since nonlinear, dose-response relationships do not necessarily imply the existence of thresholds.

Recent reviews by Barendsen (1975) and Brown (1976) suggest that the dose-response curve for mutation induction, the production of chromosome aberrations, and the induction of tumors in mammals is linear with low-LET radiation up to about 50–100 rads. Brown (1976) concluded from the available human data that this also applies to man. Such findings argue against a threshold for ionizing radiation. Because many carcinogenic agents act like radiation in producing mutations, chromosome aberrations, and cell killing, we see this as an additional argument against the likelihood of thresholds in the dose-response curves of these agents.

HETEROGENEITY OF THE POPULATION

The human population in the United States—the population we are trying to protect—is a large, diverse, and genetically heterogeneous group exposed to a variety of toxic agents. Genetic variability to carcinogenesis is well documented (Strong, 1976), and it is also known that individuals who are deficient in immunological competence (for genetic or environmental reasons) are particularly susceptible to some forms of cancer (Cottier *et al.,* 1974). It seems, therefore, that even if we were to postulate an average threshold for a particular cancer induced by a particular agent, we would in practice need a series of thresholds for different individuals. It would be extremely difficult to establish a single threshold.

We conclude from these arguments that, despite all the complexities of chemical carcinogenesis, thresholds in the dose-response relationships do not appear to exist for direct-acting carcinogens. If they do exist, they are unlikely to be detected and, hence, impossible to use. This means that there can be no totally "safe" exposure to a particular carcinogen, nor can the term "margin of safety" have any meaning. Any dose of a carcinogen must be considered to be associated with a risk, and even if that risk is vanishingly small, it must be estimated.

Statistical Considerations

Many quantitative theories of carcinogenesis that have been proposed relate the frequency of detectable tumors to the intensity of exposure to the carcinogen. The purposes of these theories are twofold: to elucidate the mode of action of the carcinogen and the nature of the neoplastic change, and to estimate—from animal experimentation—the risk to human populations exposed to environmental concentrations of the carcinogen.

One of the earliest quantitative theories was that of Iversen and Arley (Iversen and Arley, 1950; Arley and Iversen, 1952). Their model was basically a one-step transition process, in which a single "normal" cell is regarded as having some probability of being transformed to a cancer cell. Iversen and Arley assumed that this transition probability was a linear function of the amount of the carcinogen, the intercept of this linear function representing the background or spontaneous transition probability, as would be obtained if none of the carcinogen were present. After transition to a cancer cell, Iversen and Arley assumed, growth of the clone could be represented by a pure birth process with a birth rate independent of the initial amount of the carcinogen. It was assumed that the clone would become a detectable tumor when it reached a given size. This model is commonly referred to as the one-hit model and implies that the expected number of tumors within a lifetime will depend only on the total dose and not on the pattern of exposure. The mathematical forms of several hit-theory models have been reviewed by Turner (1975), including generalizations that take account of variations in susceptibility and the number of critical targets.

Both Nordling (1953) and Stocks (1953) carried the Iversen-Arley model a step further when they proposed theories in which a single cell can generate a tumor only after it has undergone more than one change or mutation; these could be termed multievent theories of carcinogenesis. They assumed that, within some time-frame, the probabilities of transition from one state to the next were the same and proportional to both time and the concentration of the carcinogen. Like Iversen and Arley, Nordling and Stocks assumed that the growth time of the tumor (after the last event had occurred) was either independent of the carcinogen or negligible. When the number of necessary changes is about 6 or 7, this model yields age-specific, cancer-incidence rates that are proportional to the fifth or sixth power of age and in this respect is consistent with human incidence data. However, the model also predicts that cancer incidence is proportional to the same high powers of the concentration of the carcinogen; this is not in agreement with the results of human and animal data. To avoid this discrepancy, Armitage and Doll (1954, 1961) modified the theory of Nordling and Stocks by assuming that the probabilities of transition between events were not all equal. They also assumed that only some of the transitional events depended on the carcinogen and that the remainder had a probability of spontaneous transition independent of the concentration of the carcinogen in question. With this modification, the model became consistent with both human and animal data that showed tumor incidence as related to either dose or the square of dose, but not higher powers. It should be noted that the theories of Nordling, Stocks, and Armitage and Doll are based on the concept that carcinogenesis has a single-cell origin, whereas a theory proposed by Fisher and Holloman (1951) is multicellular in concept.

They proposed that a tissue of N cells must contain at least K cells that have undergone some transformation if a tumor is to occur in the tissue. This theoretical approach leads to a model very similar in form to the multievent model. Other multievent theories have been proposed that incorporate the concepts of cell death or loss of ability to divide (Burch, 1960), and modifications that permit cells in intermediate stages to grow more rapidly than normal (Armitage and Doll, 1957).

Crump *et al.* (1976) discussed many of these models of carcinogenesis from the viewpoint of low-dose kinetics. They made two basic assumptions: that the cancer process is single-cell in origin, possibly with multiple steps between initiation and complete alteration, and that the growth period of the completely altered cell is basically independent of the degree of exposure. For direct carcinogenic processes, in which the agent or its metabolite acts at the cellular level to produce an irreversible change, they concluded that most models of carcinogenesis will be linear for low doses. In addition, they showed that, if it can be assumed that the environment contains carcinogens that act in conjunction with the test agent, then all the models thus far proposed will be linear for low doses.

In all these theories, the emphasis is mainly on the stochastic nature of the changes involved in the carcinogenesis process. The role played by the carcinogen is considered to a much lesser degree. It is commonly assumed that transitional events in the process that are attributable to the carcinogen occur with probabilities proportional to the degree of exposure. This is undoubtedly a gross oversimplification of the actual process. The actual exposure is no doubt modified by absorption, distribution, metabolism, and excretion of the chemical substance, and the effective exposure should probably be the actual concentration of the carcinogen at and within the target cells. Other factors that may affect delivery of the carcinogen to intracellular compartments are membrane permeability and enzyme binding. Therefore, the "effective dose" may well be some complex function of the actual exposure and the biochemical and physiological characteristics of the host. Most of these mathematical models incorporate the dose as it is actually administered in animal experiments or human exposure. The function relating administered dose to "effective dose," if it is not a simple case of proportionality, can have a profound effect on the dose-response relationship. As a simple example, consider a linear model relating dose (effective dose) to response. If the effective dose is proportional to the administered dose, then a linear model obtains for administered dose versus response. If the dose relationship is concave, which would obtain if the incremental increase in effective dose decreases with higher doses, then the relationship between administered dose and response would also be concave. Thus, the various dose-response curves that have been observed may not be indicative of different carcinogenic processes once the agent has reached the target cell, but rather may indicate different functions relating administered dose to effective dose. This problem will probably relate more to chemical carcinogenesis, as opposed to radiation-induced cancer.

Even if a normal cell has been transformed to some intermediate stage in the carcinogenic process, this would not necessarily mean that cancer must occur. Cell repair or recovery or some other response from the immune mechanisms may be sufficient to stop or reverse the process before the final stage is reached. In addition, the death of these transformed cells may occur before the process has a chance to continue toward the eventual cancer. This is one of the major arguments in favor of the existence of a threshold. However, if there is some probability that these recovery mechanisms will not complete their role before the occurrence of another event or transformation, this type of threshold will not exist.

Thresholds may be considered from two viewpoints—an "actual" threshold, which is an exposure below which any carcinogenic response attributable to the specific agent is impossible, and a "practical" threshold, which is an exposure below which an attributable carcinogenic response is highly unlikely. In discussing carcinogenic thresholds, Mantel (1963) has argued that it is immaterial whether or not "actual" thresholds exist, and that one should consider the "practical" thresholds when estimating human risk. Mantel and Bryan (1961) stated that a risk of cancer of 1 in 10^8 could be thought of as a "practical" threshold and that efforts should be made to estimate exposures that would produce no more than this risk. Using mathematical models that relate the latency period (time between initiation of exposure and appearance of cancer) to the exposure, Jones (1976) suggested that a "practical" threshold could be defined as an exposure for which the latency period is beyond the normal life span.

Experimental or observational evidence of the existence of an "actual" threshold is usually presented in the form of a dose-response graph, in which the percentage of animals with tumors or the average number of tumors per animal is plotted against the dose of the carcinogen. Either the existence of doses that do not lead to an increase in tumor incidence over controls, or the extrapolation of such curves to low doses that apparently would result in no tumor increase, is cited as an indication of the existence of a threshold below which no response is possible. This type of reasoning is an exercise in self-deception.

In the first case, failure to observe positive responses does not guarantee that the probability of response is actually zero. From a statistical viewpoint, zero responders out of a population of size N is consistent at the 5% significance level with an actual response probability between zero and approximately $3/N$ (e.g., when $N = 100$ and zero responders are observed, the true probability of response may be as high as 3%).

In the second case, when an observed plot of dose against tumors is extrapolated downward to find a no-effect dose, it is assumed that the observed dose-response relationship, usually linear, will obtain throughout the entire spectrum of doses and that one threshold exists for the entire population at risk. The assumption of linearity throughout the entire dose spectrum can easily lead to erroneous conclusions. For example, consider the true dose-response relationship shown by the dashed curve in Figure II-1.

This curve is convex, which would be consistent with a multievent theory of carcinogenesis in which more than one event is affected by the carcinogenic agent. This type of convex dose-response relationship, when sampled in an animal experiment over only a part of the dose range, could be thought to imply the existence of a threshold if simple linear extrapolation is used. If the animal experiment is performed at doses between A and B, one could conclude that a threshold exists at dose d_1; if the experiment is performed at doses between B and C, the conclusion could be that a higher threshold exists at dose d_2. In fact, with convex dose-response curves, simple linear extrapolation will always imply the existence of a threshold, if the experiment is performed over any range of doses that appears to produce linearity between dose and response.

In addition, the assumption of one threshold is unrealistic. It is much more likely that, if thresholds do exist, not all members of the population have the same one. The human population is a very diverse, genetically heterogeneous group that is exposed in different degrees to a large variety of toxic agents. Many different disorders may affect the frequency of mutational events in specific tissues. Disorders characterized by chromosomal instability have been found to be predisposed to malignancy. Patients with xeroderma pigmentosum are highly susceptible to ultraviolet-induced skin cancer, and it has been found that they have deficient DNA repair mechanisms (Robbins *et al.*, 1974). In Bloom's syndrome, there is an immune deficiency and increased risk of leukemia and cancer of the colon (German, 1972). These systems may provide a model in which the risk of mutation and subsequent malignancy after exposure to an environmental carcinogen may be genetically determined. If malignancy is the result of a series of mutational events, there must be subpopulations at various degrees of risks or with various thresholds for the carcinogenic agent. Therefore, the search for thresholds should not be

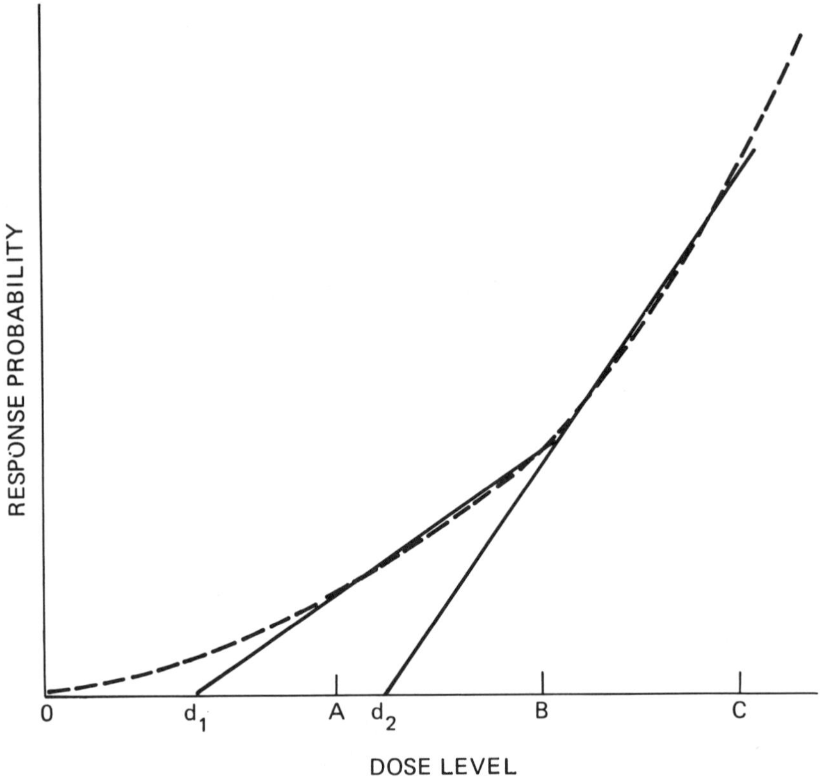

FIGURE II-1 Linear extrapolation from a convex dose–response curve.

a search for one specific no-effect dose applicable to all members of the population at risk; rather, the problem is to find many thresholds for each of the subgroups within the population.

This variability in thresholds or susceptibility to carcinogenic agents has been shown by Mantel *et al.* (1961) to induce an increased convexity in dose-response curves at low doses. They demonstrated that a linear dose-response curve with a fixed threshold will become convex at low exposures, if the individual thresholds are allowed to vary. Therefore, the extrapolation of observed dose-response curves, when the individual thresholds actually vary in the population, will, at best, simply lead to the average threshold of the population at risk. This estimate of the average threshold will have little practical utility, because many members of the population will have individual thresholds below this value. In addition, if we are willing to assume that threshold variability is the likely state in nature, then from a statistical viewpoint it is practically impossible to distinguish between mathematical models that hypothesize different thresholds and multievent models that hypothesize no thresholds, because the shapes of the two models can be very similar, and in some cases identical. For example, a one-hit, dose-response model with a threshoid may be written as,

$$P(d|\lambda) = \begin{cases} 0 & d < \lambda \\ 1 - e^{-\alpha(d-\lambda)} & d \geqslant \lambda \end{cases}$$

where $P(d|\lambda)$ represents the dose-induced response rate at a dose level d and λ is the threshold below which no response can occur. If we assume that the population consists of individuals with different thresholds, and that these thresholds vary according to some probability distribution $F(\lambda)$, then the variable-threshold model is simply the convolution of $P(d|\lambda)$ with $F(\lambda)$,

$$P(d) = \int_{\Lambda} P(d|\lambda) dF(\lambda)$$

If, for computational simplicity, we choose $F(\lambda)$ to be an exponential probability distribution, then this variable-threshold model takes the mathematical form,

$$P(d) = 1 - \frac{e^{-\alpha d} - \alpha/\beta\, e^{-\beta d}}{1 - \alpha/\beta}$$

The interesting aspect of this particular mathematical model is that, as the ratio α/β approaches unity, the model becomes

$$P(d) = 1 - (1 - \alpha d) e^{-\alpha d}$$

which is the mathematical form of a two-hit model for dose response.

Discrimination among these models on the basis of animal experiments is often impossible. These three models were fitted to data from an experiment by Terracini *et al.* (1967), in which dietary concentrations of dimethylnitrosamine (DMN) of 0–20 ppm were fed to female rats. The experiment was continued for 120 weeks, and the appearance of liver tumors was the response variable. The data are shown in the following table.

DMN in Diet (ppm)	0	2	5	10	20
Number responders/at risk	0/29	0/18	4/62	2/5	15/23
Response rate	0.0%	0.0%	6.5%	40%	65%

The fixed-threshold and variable-threshold models, in addition to the two-hit model, all fit these data equally well. There is no statistical basis on which to prefer one over the others. Experimental results like these, although appearing to give evidence of a threshold, will provide no statistical evidence either in favor of, or opposed to, the existence of such thresholds. Therefore, statistical analysis of standard animal carcinogenicity experiments is not—and probably will never be—in a position to resolve the threshold question. There are too many "biologically reasonable" mathematical models, both implying and denying the existence of thresholds, that will fit the observed results.

The quantitative theories of carcinogenesis that have been proposed are all stochastic. They consider the probabilistic aspects of the occurrence of some series of events. If one is willing to assume that these events have transition probabilities that can be affected by the carcinogen (no matter how small the concentration); that the systems of distribution and metabolism have some chance of allowing some amount of the carcinogenic agent to reach the target cells (no matter how small the chance or the amount); and that the repair and recovery systems may not do a perfect job (no matter how small the chance that this will happen), then there will be no exposure that will have a zero probability of leading to a cancer.

In addition, when considering the possibility of carcinogenic thresholds, one should keep in mind that no agent has been found to induce a type of cancer that has not been previously described. It is possible, perhaps even likely, that many carcinogenic agents act by the same mechanism on the same target cells. This would imply that, inasmuch as there are many carcinogenic agents in our everyday environment, some additional carcinogen could act in a simple additive manner and thus that any exposure would simply be added to the background. This means that for a population already exposed to carcinogenic agents, any additional carcinogen would simply increase the expected tumor incidence in a continuous manner, no matter how low the exposure to the additional agent. Therefore, despite all the complexities of the mechanisms of chemical carcinogenesis, because of genetic variation among members of the population at risk and because statistical analysis cannot resolve the question one way or the other, the search for an "actual" carcinogenic threshold is probably fruitless, and any human exposure to a carcinogen should be considered to be associated with some risk, no matter how small that risk may be. The current mathematical models that relate exposure to attributable risk are, at best, extremely crude. Much work needs to be done to refine these theories.

HIGH-DOSE TO LOW-DOSE EXTRAPOLATION

Dose-Response Models

Animal experiments must be performed at doses high enough to produce tumors, and environmental concentrations must be low enough to produce few, if any, tumors. Therefore, to estimate the probability of response at dose levels outside the experimental range, it is necessary to make an assumption concerning the form of the dose-response relationship at low doses. As noted above, many quantitative theories of carcinogenesis have been proposed that relate the occurrence of detectable tumors to both the quantity and the duration of exposure to the carcinogenic agent. Most of these theories start with the premise that the carcinogenic process consists of one or more stages that occur at the cellular level, but that not all of these stages are related to the carcinogen. These stages may be cell mutations or other biological or chemical events and may be monocellular or multicellular in origin. The probability of transition to an event related to the carcinogen is assumed to be proportional to the exposure. The exact nature and causes of these events are largely unknown. However, the most important aspect of these quantitative theories of carcinogenesis is that most of them lead to mathematical models for which the probability of tumor occurrence is generally related to a polynomial function of dose. For low exposure, the region of most importance, they are all well approximated by a simple linear function of dose (Iversen and Arley, 1950; Fisher and Holloman, 1951; Muller, 1951; Nordling, 1953). This class of dose-response models may be considered as models that are "linear at low dose." Other mathematical dose-response models have been proposed for this problem of extrapolating from high doses to low doses, the most notable being the log-probit method of Mantel and Bryan (1961). These types of models have little biological justification in what is known about the carcinogenic process. In addition, some require use of preselected parameters chosen without regard to the particular experimental situation or results. A dose-response model selected for extrapolation purposes should, at the very least, be consistent with current knowledge of the carcinogenic process.

The mathematical models that relate dose to response rate fall into two categories: dichotomous-response models, for which the important experimental fact is whether a particular condition, such as a malignant tumor, is present by a particular time (in chronic exposure experiments, this time is usually the animal's normal lifetime); and time-to-response models, for which the actual time to occurrence of the particular condition is known for each animal in the experiment. (For the latter type of model, the relationship of time since initiation of exposure, to response can be ascertained together with the relationship between exposure and response). Each type of model is completely specified, except for some unknown parameters that are to be estimated from the experimental results. These estimates and the functional form of the assumed dose-response model will provide an estimate of the risk attributable to the carcinogen at any desired dose.

In the dichotomous-response situation, the multievent theory of carcinogenesis proposed by Armitage and Doll (1961) leads to a mathematical model that relates the probability of response $P(d)$ to the dose d by

$$P(d) = 1 - e^{-(\lambda_0 + \lambda_1 d + \lambda_2 d^2 + \ldots + \lambda_k d^k)}$$

where k represents the number of transitional events in the carcinogenic process that are related to the carcinogen under test and $\lambda_0, \lambda_1, \lambda_2, \ldots, \lambda_k$ are unknown nonnegative parameters. As with the other "linear-at-low-dose" models, for small enough values of the exposure d, this dose-induced response rate will be approximately equal to $\lambda_1 d$ (assuming that λ_0 is the "background" rate). Therefore, in extrapolating from high dose levels to low doses, the risk attributable to the carcinogen, after correcting for background, will depend on the magnitude of the coefficient, λ_1.

When estimating risk with this model, the function is to be fitted to the experimental data by some such procedure as maximal likelihood (Guess and Crump, 1976). A point estimate of the attributable risk may be obtained from the model with the estimated parameters, but to incorporate the vagaries of random sampling, it would be prudent to include the upper-statistical confidence limit on this risk estimate.

Appropriateness of Data for Low-Dose Extrapolation

Before extrapolation is attempted, considerable attention must be given to the appropriateness of the experimental data. Bioassay procedures must be of high quality in order to avoid misleading risk estimates. Also, oral administration of the carcinogen is necessary, because we are concerned with estimating the risks associated with drinking-water consumption. The experimental animals should receive a lifetime administration of the carcinogen, because this corresponds to the human situation that we are attempting to estimate. It is not correct to assume that the tumor yield in a partial lifetime study will be equivalent to a lifetime study with the same total dose. This follows from the multistage models for carcinogenesis which assume that the cancer-incidence rate is proportional to a power (often 3 to 5) of duration of exposure. It may be possible to extrapolate from partial to full-lifetime exposure, but it must be done on a sound biological basis.

Serious problems also develop from the actual data generated by the assay. These problems have to do with the need for some observed dose-response information. Often, the experimental doses are very high, and this produces cancers in almost all the experimentally treated animals. This may be because the assay protocols are designed for the determination of carcinogenicity, and not for low-dose extrapolation and dose-response estimation. If all of the treated animals produce high incidences of tumors, one has no useful idea of where the dose-response curve actually is (particularly the lower convex portion of the curve). The true dose-response curve could be badly underestimated—even with the use of a straight-line extrapolation. Therefore, one must have some information concerning doses at which the tumor incidence is in the lower convex portion of the dose-response curve.

Although low-dose extrapolations are out of the question for high-incidence data, one can calculate some relative dose information that can be used in expressing concerns over possible adverse health effects. Essentially, the exposure that is of interest in man is converted to the equivalent dose in animal study. The ratio of the lowest experimental dose to the equivalent human dose is then calculated. Clearly, the closer this ratio is to unity, the greater the concern.

One final point should be made. The extrapolations should generally be conducted on total tumor yields, as opposed to specific tumor types, because we wish to estimate total cancer risk in man.

INTERACTIONS

A major concern in carcinogenesis, and in assessing the safety of a single material, lies in the answer to the question "How does this material behave in the presence (or absence) of other materials?" Is the response to two materials the sum of the individual responses? Do the effects come about as if doses were added? Is there more (or less) than additivity? Do some things cancel each other out?

Some experience in man begins to give answers to these questions. The few known interactive effects in man are related to exposures to cigarette smoking combined with some other exposure—industrial or social. These are the combined effects of: cigarette smoking (inhaled); asbestos exposure (Selikoff, 1968); inhalation of radon, as in the case of the uranium miners (Lundin, 1971); and the use of alcohol (Rothman, 1972). All of these show risks that are more than additive. For example, the heavy smoker has about two times the risk of the nonsmoker of dying of cancer of the oral cavity. The heavy drinker-heavy smoker has about 15 times the risk of the nonsmoker, nondrinker. Reports from Great Britain support the idea that the recent reduction in male lung cancer mortality, particularly in Greater London, with small changes in cigarette smoking and large changes in air pollution have come about through an interaction between urban air pollution and cigarette smoking (Lawther, 1976).

Animal experimentation (Berenblum, 1947) showed an initiator-promoter effect, in which each material applied separately (to the skin of test animals) had little or no carcinogenic effect. The two materials, applied in the appropriate sequences, however, were highly carcinogenic. At one time it appeared that there were materials that were purely initiators (they started the process) and there were others that were purely promoters (they moved the process along to frank cancer). More recent views suggest that some materials are both initiators and promoters, sometimes acting as one, sometimes as the other, and sometimes as both, giving a "complete" carcinogen (Berenblum, 1974).

The exact nature of initiation and promotion is not clear, and there is evidence that there is initiation-inhibition as well (Falk, 1971). Thus, it may be possible that the carcinogenic effect of one material may be inhibited by another material. Genetic susceptibility can be included in the initiator-promoter model. Increased genetic susceptibility may be providing an initiator step, while increased genetic resistance will look like initiation-inhibition. Some instances of this are evident in man. For example, ultraviolet radiation leads to skin cancer, mostly in people with fair skin, light hair and light eyes (Urbach, 1969). We know that these latter characteristics are genetically determined and so we speak of genetic susceptibility. Dark-skinned, dark-eyed, dark-haired people have genetic resistance. It is not nearly so obvious, nor do we know the genetics involved, in the case of the higher susceptibility to breast cancer among women from "breast cancer families." Women who come from families where a mother, sisters, or the fathers' sister(s) have breast cancer are at higher (twofold to threefold) risk than women from non-breast-cancer families (Lilienfeld, 1963). There is nothing so obvious nor so directly involved as skin pigmentation to give any leads here.

A possibly unifying concept concerning interactions is the "fertile ground" idea. If the carcinogen falls on fertile ground, it will lead to cancer growth. If not, no cancer. This implies a whole set of questions about the nature of the "fertile ground." Some animal experimentation seems to imply that, with the induction of mammary tumors in the rat by hormonal stimulation, the ground is made fertile by earlier viral infection (Shellabarger, 1976). Similar results seem to be shown in the induction of (mouse) cancers through the combination of malaria infection and exposure to the Moloney mouse-tumor virus (Wedderburn, 1970). A similar mechanism has been suggested for the development of Burkitt's lymphoma in children in East Africa, in malaria infection associated with appropriate viral infection (Morrow, 1976).

Another way that fertile ground can arise is through a deficiency interaction. Here, the absence of some element, material, or vitamin may reduce the ability of repair mechanisms, so that a level of a carcinogen that produces little or no cancer in a population capable of repair produces much cancer in a population of repair-deficient individuals. An example is the high cancer rate in Xeroderma pigmentosum patients—people with a low ability for DNA repair (Robbins, 1974; Cleaver, 1968). A similar mechanism (on a grosser level) may be involved in the high incidence of cancer of the esophagus in central Asians, whose bread and tea diet may not contain the elements necessary to permit repair of tissue affected by low levels of a nonidentified carcinogen (Mahboubi, 1973).

Much of the classical toxicology of dose-response assumes a distribution of sensitivities in a population. Individuals with thresholds lower than the dose given will respond by developing the condition. Individuals with higher thresholds will not. The existence of dose-response curves that are not simple step-functions (zero response at dose d, 100% response at dose $d + e$, where e is some very small increment of dose) suggests these host-environment interactions. Individuals with high gluathione and sulfhydryl levels in their livers may be able to "handle" (to metabolize to some nonactive form) toxicants much better than individuals with low levels (Gillette, 1974).

According to Brown (1975), no carcinogen has been found to induce a cancer of an entirely new, never-before-seen histological type. A possible explanation of this is that many carcinogencic agents or processes act through the same ultimate mechanism in the same target cells. He writes " . . . since there are many carcinogenic agents in our . . . environment, [a new] carcinogen could act in a simple, additive manner and thus any level of exposure would . . . be added to the . . . existing background." This kind of interaction phenomenon has important implications for the models used in extrapolation. It implies that these models may not assume any threshold for a new material in a world already populated by many carcinogens. It also leads to the conclusion by Crump *et al.* (1976) that "all models of carcinogenesis thus far proposed will be linear at low doses."

The discovery of interactions will require more sophisticated experimental techniques than are now being used. Testing combinations of materials multiplies the number of tests that must be done (100 materials, tested two at a time, will require $100 \times 99/2!$ tests;—tested three at a time will require $100 \times 99 \times 98/3!$ tests). New techniques for multiple testing will have to be developed. Uncovering deficiency interactions will require entirely new and different approaches.

SUMMARY—Chemical Contaminants: Safety and Risk Assessment

Large populations are repeatedly exposed to potentially toxic contaminants in the drinking water—in minute amounts over many months or years, or over whole lifetimes. Delayed, essentially irreversible, effects can occur. Methods and criteria of classical, conventional toxicology do not offer reliable means for assessing long-term toxic effects such as carcinogenesis in man by extrapolation from animal data; hence, novel considerations have to be applied in assessing risk.

The insidious effects of chronic exposure to low doses of toxic agents is difficult to recognize, because there are few, if any, early warning signs and, when signs are ultimately observed, they often imply irreversible effects. For example, cancer induction in experimental animals, even with the most potent carcinogenic chemicals, requires at least several months and in many instances a whole lifetime. There are as yet no easy, straightforward methods for extrapolating even chronic-exposure experimental data to calculate risks to large human populations. Teratogenic effects are easier to establish by animal experimentation, but there are similar uncertainties in extrapolating to human populations. Mutagenic effects are difficult to assess experimentally in mammals, and such effects are particularly insidious, in that they appear only in later generations.

Various measures used in assessing acute toxicity—such as LD_{10}, LD_{50}, and maximal tolerated dose—are generally found to be quantitatively similar among most animals. On the basis of dose-per-unit of body surface, toxic effects in man are in the same range as those in experimental animals, such as mouse, rat, hamster, dog, and monkey. On a body-weight basis, man is generally more vulnerable than the experimental animal, probably by a factor of 6–12. Comparative studies have shown generally that absorption, metabolism, and excretion of various drugs are slower, dose-for-dose, in man; that there is greater retention of such drugs; and that higher concentrations occur in body fluids and tissues in man than in small mammals. With an awareness of these quantitative differences, appropriate safety factors can be applied to calculate relatively safe therapeutic dosages for man. These methods and principles of classical toxicology are useful for assessing toxic effects that are reversible and nonprogressive. They are much less useful in dealing with the problems of chronic irreversible toxicity or the effects of long-term exposure. This subject has not been considered widely in the past.

From the review of available information, two major questions emerge: "What types of experimental-assay procedures are required for a valid assessment of chronic toxicity of chemicals in experimental animals?" "How can such data be extrapolated to estimate risks in humans?" In dealing with these questions, our recommendations are restricted to a specific risk—namely, cancer—with the understanding that the same considerations will apply at least partially to the problems of mutagenesis and teratogenesis. Furthermore, we consider only carcinogens whose mechanisms involve somatic mutations.

Some principles that underlie efforts to assess the irreversible effects of long-continued exposure to carcinogenic substances at low dose rates are outlined below.

Principle 1

EFFECTS IN ANIMALS, PROPERLY QUALIFIED, ARE APPLICABLE TO MAN

This premise underlies all of experimental biology and medicine, but because it is continually questioned with regard to human cancer, it is desirable to point out that cancer in men and animals is strikingly similar. Virtually every form of human cancer has an experimental counterpart, and every form of multicellular organism is subject to cancer, including insects, fish, and plants. Although there are differences in susceptibility between different animal species, between different strains of the same species, and between individuals of the same strain, carcinogenic chemicals will affect most test species; and there are large bodies of experimental data that indicate that exposures that are carcinogenic to animals are likely to be carcinogenic to man, and vice versa.

Evidence that circumstances leading to cancer induction in humans are also applicable to experimental animals stems from the very first observation of chemical carcinogenesis—the appearance of cancer of the scrotum in chimney sweeps, observed by the British surgeon, Percival Pott, in 1775. It was not until modern times that a substance implicated in human cancer was found to be carcinogenic in animals, when the Japanese scientists, K. Yamagiwa and K. Ichikawa, found in 1915 that extracts from coal tar cause cancer when applied to the skin of experimental animals. Many pure carcinogenic chemicals have since been isolated from a wide variety of "tars" derived from incomplete combustion of organic matter, such as coal, wood, and tobacco. There is little doubt that these and other chemicals, alone or in combination, are responsible for the greatly increased incidence of lung cancer among smokers. With the possible exception of arsenic and benzene, all known carcinogens in man are also carcinogenic in some species, although not in all that have been tested.

Principle 2

METHODS DO NOT NOW EXIST TO ESTABLISH A THRESHOLD FOR LONG-TERM EFFECTS OF TOXIC AGENTS

With respect to carcinogenesis, it seems plausible at first thought, and it has often been argued, that a threshold must exist below which even the most toxic substance would be harmless. Unfortunately, a threshold cannot be established experimentally that is applicable to a total population. A time-honored practice of classical toxicology is the establishment of maximal tolerated (no-effect) doses in humans based on finding a no-observed-adverse-effect dose in chronic experiments in animals, and to divide this dose by a "safety factor" of, say, 100, to designate a "safe" dose in humans. There is no scientific basis for such estimations of safe doses in connection with carcinogenesis. For example, even if *no* tumors are obtained in an assay of 100 animals, this means only that at a 95% confidence level, the true incidence of cancer in this group of animals is less than 3%. Even if we were to carry out the formidable task of using 1,000 animals for assay and no tumors appeared, we could only be 95% sure that the true incidence were less than 0.3%. Obviously, 0.3% is a very high risk for a large human population.

In fact, there are no valid reasons to assume that false-negative results of carcinogenicity tests are much less frequent than false-positive ones. To dismiss all compounds that did not induce tumors in one or two mouse and rat experiments as noncarcinogenic is wrong. Labeling as "carcinogens" all substances that gave rise to increased incidence of tumors is justified only if there is conclusive evidence of a causal relationship. The "relative risk" of compounds that are not found to induce tumors in animal experiments must also be considered. But this requires evaluation of data other than those collected in chronic toxicity studies on rodents.

Experimental procedures of bioassay in which even relatively large numbers of animals are used are likely to detect only strong carcinogens. Even when negative results are obtained in such bioassays, it is not certain that the agent tested is unequivocally safe for man. Therefore, we must accept and use possibly fallible measures of estimating hazard to man. This reasoning leads us to the statement of Principles 3 and 4.

Principle 3

THE EXPOSURE OF EXPERIMENTAL ANIMALS TO TOXIC AGENTS IN HIGH DOSES IS A NECESSARY AND VALID METHOD OF DISCOVERING POSSIBLE CARCINOGENIC HAZARDS IN MAN

The most commonly expressed objection to regulatory decisions based on carcinogenesis observed in animal experiments is that the high dosages to which animals are exposed have no relevance in assessment of human risks. It is therefore important to clarify this crucial issue. Practical considerations in the design of experimental model systems require that the number of animals used in experiments on long-term exposure to toxic materials will always be small, compared with the size of the human populations similarly at risk. To obtain statistically valid results from such small groups of animals requires the use of relatively large doses so that effects will occur frequently enough to be detected. For example, an incidence as low as 0.01% would represent 20,000 people in a total population of 200 million and would be considered unacceptably high, even if benefits were sizable. To detect such a low incidence in experimental animals directly would require hundreds of thousands of animals. For this reason, we have no choice but to give large doses to relatively small experimental groups and then to use biologically reasonable models in extrapolating the results to estimate risk at low doses. Several methods of making such calculations have been considered and used, but we think that the best method available to us today is to assume that there is no threshold, and that the incidence of tumors is directly proportional to dose. However, it is important to recognize that such calculations may give either too small or too large an estimate risk. The actual risk to humans might be even greater over a human lifetime, because it is about 35 times that of a mouse; and there is evidence that the risk of cancer increases rapidly with the length of exposure. Moreover, experimental assays are conducted under controlled dietary and environmental conditions with genetically homogeneous animals, whereas humans live under diverse conditions, are genetically heterogeneous, and are likely to include subpopulations of unusual susceptibility.

It should be emphasized that these general considerations give only a *minimal* estimate of human risk; moreover, they do not take into consideration differences in susceptibility between species. For example, beta-naphthylamine is well established as a human carcinogen on the basis of epidemiologic studies of occupationally exposed workers, whereas experiments have not shown it to be carcinogenic in the hamster, which is relatively resistant.

Not all substances that cause a given incidence of cancer in the rat are equally carcinogenic for man. This means that chronic-toxicity studies, which are imperfect assay systems for carcinogenicity testing, should not be used as the sole criterion in the assessment of risk.

Principle 4

MATERIAL SHOULD BE ASSESSED IN TERMS OF HUMAN RISK, RATHER THAN AS "SAFE" OR "UNSAFE"

The limitations of the current experimental techniques do not allow us to establish safe doses, but with the help of statistical methods we may be able to estimate an upper limit of the risk to human populations. To calculate such a risk, we need data to estimate population exposure; a valid, accurate, precise, and reproducible assay procedure in animals; and appropriate statistical methods. Several general guidelines may be presented. First, no rigid, generally applicable procedure can be recommended for testing all toxic agents. Substances differ too much in their overall effects, and the design of appropriate assays will ultimately have to be left to the well-informed judgment of expert investigators. If substances that affect large populations are found to be carcinogenic, experiments of much wider scope may have to be conducted to obtain more detailed information on their possible effects in humans. As a pragmatic guideline, it would be desirable to test a compound for carcinogenicity in at least two species, such as the mouse and the rat, and the strains of animals used should have a rather low incidence of spontaneous tumors under the conditions of the test. It is important to include "positive" controls, with known carcinogens, under the same conditions used for the test animals. This has been a point of considerable controversy.

Experiments should be conducted over as much of the lifetime of the experimental animal as possible. The highest dose should be the maximum that is tolerated without shortening the lifespan through causes other than cancer. Every animal, whether it dies during the exposure period or is sacrificed at the end of the experiment, should be examined grossly and microscopically, and all toxic effects (not only cancer) should be noted.

Risk constitutes but half the essential comparison that should be made in the assessments of human hazard; the other half is benefit to the exposed population of the agent for which hazard has been identified. Decisions cannot involve merely the risk. Statements of benefits should include the nature, extent, and recipient of the benefit. Technology has always been associated with some risk. But the acceptability of risk should depend on the specific benefits derived, the nature of the population exposed, and the availability of practical alternatives.

It is not possible to guarantee a risk-free society; nor is a risk-free society necessarily the best society. It is often necessary to accept the risks of chemicals—such as drugs and pesticides—when the benefits warrant their use. Risks imposed on persons who gain no benefits are generally not acceptable. Personal choice and personal values enter into the risk-benefit comparison. For major benefits—for example, in the treatment of otherwise incurable or incapacitating diseases—much higher risks are allowable than otherwise. An important principle in risk-benefit assessment is that each person must be allowed the widest possible choice—supported by full information on risks, as well as benefits—so that intelligent choices may be made.

The benefit portion of the equation should be well defined by knowledgeable experts, and based on data at least as good as the risk data. It is important, therefore, that the benefit-risk comparisons be established with the active cooperation of people who are qualified to assess the usefulness of a substance and the consequences to those in need of it, as well as to the population at large.

Finally, mankind is already exposed to many carcinogens whose presence in the environment cannot be easily controlled. In view of the nature of cancer, the long latent period of its development, and the irreversibility of chemical carcinogenesis, it would be highly improper to expose the general population to an increased risk if the benefits were small, questionable, or restricted to limited segments of the population.

Principles To Be Used for Noncarcinogens and Nonmutagens

The nature and reversibility of the toxic effect must be considered.

For carcinogens that are not shown to be mutagens, some sort of extrapolation must be postulated.

For noncarcinogens for which it seems likely that there are thresholds for toxic effects, the acceptable dose should be below the threshold. If a threshold cannot be shown, the acceptable dose must be related to the data from animal experimentation and consideration of the seriousness of the toxic effects, as well as the likelihood and ease of reversibility, the variability of the sensitivity of the exposed population, and the economic and health-related importance of the material.

RESEARCH RECOMMENDATIONS

Research must be supported to develop an understanding of the mechanisms by which water pollutants produce toxic effects. This includes pharmacokinetics, toxication-detoxication mechanisms, and biochemical and pathological mechanisms of action.

Estimates of margin of safety can be made more precisely and rationally as more is known about what happens to a chemical in the body and what the chemical or its metabolites do to the body. The results of such research also are necessary to develop rapid, inexpensive, accurate screening tests for various critical forms of toxicity.

It is recognized that much of this research is going on, but the Committee is convinced that more must be done. In protecting the population of the United States from environmental pollution there is no more important or potentially productive effort than the support of this kind of research. Since these studies are long-term in nature and must be closely coupled to basic biomedical research, they should be supported primarily by research rather than regulatory agencies.

There are many research needs in the field of chronic disease epidemiology. Manpower is in critically short supply. There are critical problems of data resources.

Research on statistical methods and mathematical models for estimating low dose effects should be encouraged. Statistical work is pratically nonexistent for effects other than carcinogenesis. Although a considerable effort has been expended on dose-response estimation for carcinogenesis, very little has been done on species variability and susceptible subgroups. This area could at least be studied from an empirical standpoint so that there would be a better understanding of the precision of low-dose risk estimates.

These recommendations are summarized below:

1. Studies of the physiological and biochemical mechanisms by which the toxic substances in water produce their effects.

2. Development of rapid, inexpensive, and precise tests to identify substances that may produce important toxic effects at low doses and dose rates.

3. Epidemiological studies of chronic disease.

4. Research on statistical methods and analytical models for describing and estimating the effects of long exposure to low doses of toxic substances. Studies should not be limited to carcinogenesis and should consider, also, differences between species, and particularly sensitive subgroups in the population.

REFERENCES

Ames, B.N. 1976. Carcinogenicity tests. (Letters) Science 191:241–245.

Arley, N., and S. Iversen. 1952. On the mechanism of experimental carcinogenesis. VI. Hit theory interpretation of some experiments of Berenblum and Shubiko Acta Path. Microbiol. Scand. 31:164–171.

Armitage, P., and R. Doll. 1954. The age distribution of cancer and a multi-stage theory of carcinogenesis. Br. J. Cancer 8:1–12.

Armitage, P., and R. Doll. 1957. A two-stage theory of carcinogenesis in relation to the age distribution of human cancer. Br. J. Cancer 11:161–169.

Armitage, P., and R. Doll. 1961. Stochastic models for carcinogenesis. *In* Proceedings of the Fourth Berkeley Symposium on Mathematical Statistics and Probability, vol. 4, pp. 19–38. University of California Press, Berkeley and Los Angeles.

Barendsen, G.W. 1975. The effectiveness of small doses of ionizing radiations for the induction of cell reproductive death, chromosomal changes and malignant transformation. Presented at 5th Symposium on Microdosimetry, Verbania Pallanza, Italy, Sept. 22.

Berenblum, I., and P. Shubik. 1947. A new quantitative approach to the study of the stages of chemical carcinogenesis in the mouse's skin. Br. J. Cancer 1:383–391.

Berenblum, I. 1974. Carcinogenesis as a Biological Problem. North Holland Publ. Co., Amsterdam/Oxford. 376 pp.

Brown, C.C. 1975. Personal Communications.

Brown, J.M. 1976. Linearity versus nonlinearity of dose-response for radiation carcinogenesis. Health Physics 31:231–245.

Burch, P.R.J. 1960. Radiation carcinogenesis: A new hypothesis. Nature 185:135–142.

Bush, M.T., G. Berry, and A. Hume. 1966. Ultra-short-acting barbiturates as oral hypnotic agents in man. Clin. Pharmacol. Ther. 7:373–378.

Casarett, L.J., and J. Doull, eds. 1975. Toxicology:The Basic Science of Poisons, pp. 11–25. Macmillan Publ. Co., New York.

Cleaver, J.E. 1968. Defective repair replication of DNA in xeroderma pigmentosum. Nature 218:652–656.

Conney, A.H., and J.J. Burns. 1972. Metabolic interactions among environmental chemicals and drugs. Science 178:576–586.

Cottier, H., M.W. Hess, H.U. Keller, P. Luscieti, and B. Sordat. 1974. Immunological deficiency states and malignancy. *In* Interaction of Radiation and Host Immune Defense Mechanisms in Malignancy. Proceedings of a Conference at Greenbrier, West Virginia, March, pp. 30–44.

Crump, K.S., D.G. Hoel, C.H. Langley, and R. Peto. 1976. Fundamental carcinogenic processes and their implications for low dose risk assessment. Cancer Res. 36: 2973–2979.

DHEW. 1977. Approaches to determining the mutagenic properties of chemicals: Risk to future generations. Report of Committee to Coordinate Toxicology and Related Programs, Department of Health, Education and Welfare. Obtainable from: Box 12233, Research Triangle Park, N.C.

Drake, J., Chairman. 1975. Environmental mutagenic hazards, Committee 17 Report. Science 187:503–514.

Falk, H.L. 1971. Anti-carcinogenesis—An alternative. *In* B.L. van Duuren and B.A. Rubin, eds. Inhibition of Carcinogenesis. Progress in Experimental Tumor Research 14:105–137. S. Karger, New York.

Fisher, J.C., and J.H. Holloman. 1951. A new hypothesis for the origin of cancer foci. Cancer 4:916–918.

German, J. 1972. Genes which increase chromosomal instability in somatic cells and predispose to cancer. Prog. Med. Genet. 8:61–101.

Gillette, J.R., J.F. Mitchell, and B.B. Brodie. 1974. Biochemical mechanism of drug toxicity. Ann. Rev. Pharmacol. 14:271–288.

Guess, H.A., and K.S. Crump. 1976. Low dose rate extrapolation of data from animal carcinogenicity experiments—Analysis of a new statistical technique. Math. Biosci. 32:15–36.

Hammer, W., and F. Sjoqvist. 1967. Plasma levels of monomethylated tricyclic antidepressants during treatment with ipramine-like compounds. Life Sci. 6:1895–1903.

Hoel, D.G., D.W. Gaylor, R.L. Kirschstein, U. Saffiotti, and M.A. Schneiderman. 1975. Estimation of risks of irreversible, delayed toxicity. J. Toxicol. Environ. Health 1:133–151.

Iversen, S., and N. Arley. 1950. On the mechanism of experimental carcinogenesis. Acta Pathol. Microbiol. Scand. 27:773–803.

Jones, H. 1976. Dose-effect relationships in carcinogenesis and the matter of threshold of carcinogenesis. Presented at the NIEHS Conference on the Problems of Extrapolating the Results of Laboratory Animal Data to Man and of Extrapolating the Results from High Dose Level Experiments to Low Dose Level Exposures, Pinehurst, N. C., March 10–12.

Lawther, P.J., and R.E. Waller. 1976. Air pollutants and lung cancer—Recent trends in England and Wales. Presented at the Cold Spring Harbor Symposium.

Lilienfeld, A.M. 1963. The epidemiology of breast cancer. Cancer Res. 23:1503–1513.

Lundin, F.E., J.K. Wagoner, and V.E. Archer. 1971. Radon Daughter Exposure and Respiratory Cancer. Quantitative and Temporal Aspects. NIOSH/NIEHS Joint Monograph 1. U.S. Department of Health, Education, and Welfare.

Mahboubi, E., J. Kmet, P.J. Cook, N.E. Day, P. Ghadirian, and S. Salmasizadeh. 1973. Oesophageal cancer studies in the Caspian Littoral of Iran: The Caspian cancer registry. Br. J. Cancer 28:197–214.

Mantel, N., and W.R. Bryan. 1961. Safety testing of carcinogenic agents. J. Nat. Cancer Inst. 27:455–470.

Mantel, N., W.E. Heston, and J.M. Gurian. 1961. Thresholds in linear dose-response models for carcinogenesis. J. Nat. Cancer Inst. 27:203–215.

Mantel, N. 1963. Symposium on chemical carcinogenesis. Part IV. The concept of threshold in carcinogenesis. Clin. Pharmacol. Therap. 4:104–109.

McCann, J., E. Choi, E. Yamasaki, and B. N. Ames. 1975. Detection of carcinogens as mutagens in the *Salmonella*/microsome test: Assay of 300 chemicals. Proc. Nat. Acad. Sci. 72:5135–5139.

McCann, J., and B. N. Ames. 1976. Detection of carcinogens as mutagens in the *Salmonella*/microsome test: Assay of 300 chemicals: Discussion. Proc. Nat. Acad. Sci. 73:950–954.

Menguy, R., L. Desbaillets, W.F. Masters, and S. Okabe. 1972. Evidence for a sex-linked difference in aspirin metabolism. Nature 239:102–103.

Morrow, R.H., A. Kisuule, M.C. Pike, and P.G. Smith. 1976. Burkitt's lymphoma in Mengo Districts of Uganda: Epidemiologic features and their relationship to malaria. J. Nat. Cancer Inst. 56:479–483.

Muller, H.J. 1951. Radiation damage to the genetic material. Sci. Prog. 7:93–94.

Murphy, S.D. 1967. Malathion inhibition of esterases as a determinant of malathion toxicity. J. Pharmacol. Exp. Ther. 156:352–365.

National Academy of Sciences-National Research Council. Division of Medical Sciences. 1972. The Effects on Populations of Exposure to Low Levels of Ionizing Radiation. Washington, D.C. 217 pp.

National Academy of Sciences. 1975. Principles for Evaluating Chemicals in the Environment. Washington, D.C. 454 pp.

Nordling, C.O. 1953. A new theory on the cancer inducting mechanism. Br. J. Cancer 7:68–72.

Robbins, J.H., K.H. Kraemer, M.A. Lutzner, B.W. Festoff, and H.G. Coon. 1974. Xeroderma pigmentosum. An inherited disease with sun sensitivity, multiple cutaneous neoplasms, and abnormal DNA repair. Ann. Int. Med. 80:221–248.

Rothman, K.J., and A.Z. Keller. 1972. The effect of joint exposure to alcohol and tobacco on risk of cancer of the mouth and pharynx. J. Chron. Dis. 25:711–716.

Selikoff, I.J., E.C. Hammond, and J. Churg. 1968. Asbestos exposure, smoking and neoplasia. J. Am. Med. Assoc. 204:106–112.

Shellabarger, C.J. 1976. Modifying factors in rat mammary gland carcinogenesis. *In* J.M. Yuhas, R.W. Tennant, and J.D. Regan, eds. Biology of Radiation Carcinogenesis, pp. 31–43. Raven Press, New York.

Stocks, P. 1953. A study of the age curve for cancer of the stomach in connection with a theory of the cancer producing mechanism. Br. J. Cancer 7:407–417.

Strong, L.C. 1976. Susceptible subgroups. Presented at the NIEHS Conference on the Problems of Extrapolating the Results of Laboratory Animal Data to Man and of Extrapolating the Results from High Dose Level Experiments to Low Dose Level Exposures. Pinehurst, N.C., March 10–12.

Terracini, B., P.N. Magee, and J. Barnes. 1967. Hepatic pathology in rats on low dietary levels of dimethylnitrosamine. Br. J. Cancer 21:559–565.

Turner, M.D. 1975. Some classes of hit-theory models. Math. Biosci. 23:219–235.

Urbach, F. 1969. Biological Effects of Ultraviolet Radiation. Pergamon Press, Oxford, England.

Walburg, H.E., Jr. 1974. Experimental radiation carcinogenesis. *In* J. T. Lett, H. Adler, and M. Zelle, eds. Advances in Radiation Biology, vol. 4, p. 209–254. Academic Press, New York.

Weber, W.W. 1976. Genetic variability and extrapolation from animals to man: Some perspectives on susceptibility to chemical carcinogenesis fom aromatic amines. Presented at the NIEHS Conference on the Problems of Extrapolating the Results of Laboratory Animal Data to Man and of Extrapolating the Results from High Dose Level Experiments to Low Dose Level Exposures, Pinehurst, N.C., March 10–12.

Wedderburn, N. 1970. Effect of concurrent malarial infection on development of virus-induced lymphoma in Balb/c mice. Lancet 2:1114–1116.

Weil, C.S. 1972. Statistics vs. safety factors and scientific judgment in the evaluation of safety for man. Toxicol. Appl. Pharmacol. 21:454–463.

Wittemore, A., and J.B. Keller. Quantitative Theories of Carcinogenesis. In press.

Yamagiwa, K., and K. Ichikawa. 1915. Experimentelle Studie über die Pathogenese der Epithelialgeschwulste. Mitt. Med. Fak. Tokio 15:295–344.

III

Microbiology of Drinking Water

The principal microbiological contaminants found in drinking water of the United States are bacteria, viruses, and pathogenic protozoa. Each is considered in a separate section of this chapter. Helminths are included along with the protozoa. Little information is available on mycoplasma, pathogenic yeast, and pathogenic fungi in drinking water. Microbiological contaminants, such as fungi and algae, do not seem to be important causes of waterborne disease, although they are sometimes associated with undesirable tastes and odors.

EPIDEMIOLOGY

The average annual number of waterborne-disease outbreaks in the United States reported since 1938 is shown in Figure III-1 (Center for Disease Control, 1976b). There was a decrease in the number of outbreaks during the late 1930's and 1940's, but this trend was reversed in the early 1950's. There has been a pronounced increase in the outbreaks reported by the Center for Disease Control (CDC) in Atlanta, Georgia, since 1971. The reason for this apparent increase is not entirely clear, but it could be either the result of improved reporting or an overloading of our treatment plants with source water of increasingly lower quality. Since 1971, the CDC, the Environmental Protection Agency (EPA), state epidemiologists, and engineers in state water-supply surveillance agencies have cooperated in the annual reporting of outbreaks. The purposes of such

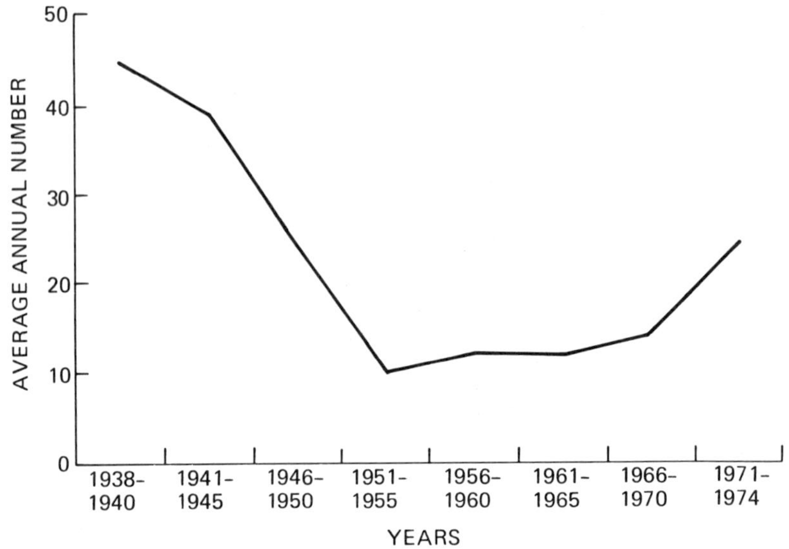

FIGURE III-1 Average annual number of waterborne disease outbreaks, 1938–1975.

reports are to control disease by identifying contaminated water sources and purifying them, and to increase knowledge of disease causation. The roles of many microbial agents, including, for example, *Yersinia enterocolitica* and mycoplasma, remain to be clarified.

The most important waterborne infectious diseases that occurred in 1971-1974 are listed in Table III-1. The etiologic agent was determined in only 53% of 99 disease outbreaks that involved 16,950 cases (Craun *et al.* 1976). The remainder were characterized as "acute gastrointestinal illness of unknown etiology."

Shigellosis was the most commonly identified bacterial disease (2,747 cases) in 1971-1974. Most of the cases were associated with non-municipal water systems. Four typhoid fever outbreaks affected 222 people and involved semipublic and individual water systems.

In 1974, 28 waterborne-disease outbreaks, comprising 8,413 cases, were reported to the Center for Disease Control (1976a). The largest was an outbreak of giardiasis that occurred in Rome, N.Y., with an estimated 4,800 cases. The second largest involved about 1,200 cases caused by *Shigella sonnei*. In the third largest, which involved 615 cases of acute gastrointestinal illness, the etiologic agent was not definitely determined, but *Yersinia enterocolitica* was suspected. The fourth largest was caused by *Shigella sonnei* and involved 600 persons. Nineteen states reported at least one outbreak. Craun *et al.* (1976) stated that "this probably reflects the level of interest in investigating and reporting in different states rather than the true magnitude of the problem within the state."

Semipublic water systems were associated with 55% of the outbreaks and accounted for 32% of the total cases in 1971-1974. Municipal systems accounted for 31% of the outbreaks, but 67% of the cases. Individual systems accounted for 14% of the outbreaks and only 1% of the cases, but outbreaks associated with individual systems probably are under-reported, as opposed to those associated with municipal and semipublic systems.

Deficiencies in treatment and contamination of groundwater were responsible for a majority of the outbreaks (65%) and cases (63%) in 1971-1974. Inadequate or interrupted chlorination was involved in 31% of the outbreaks and 44% of the cases.

Craun *et al.* (1976) have drawn attention to the large number of waterborne disease outbreaks involving travelers. In 1971-1974, 49 (72%) of the 68 outbreaks that occurred in connection with semipublic and individual systems affected travelers, campers, visitors to recreational areas, or restaurant patrons; and 86% of the 49 outbreaks occurred during April–September.

Outbreaks on cruise ships are excluded from the above tabulations, but they are of interest and should be mentioned because they involve the traveling public. For example, in June 1973, about 90% of 655 passengers and 35% of 299 crew were affected by an outbreak of acute gastroenteritis. An epidemiological investigation identified *Shigella flexneri* type 6 among early cases, and contaminated water and ice aboard the ship were implicated as vehicles of transmission (Center for Disease Control, 1973). In 1975, outbreaks of diarrhea on 8 ships affected between 9% and 61% of the passengers. In most of these outbreaks the causal agents and vehicles

TABLE III-1 Etiology Of Waterborne Outbreaks and Cases, 1971–1974

Disease	Outbreaks	Cases
Gastroenteritis	46	7,992
Giardiasis	12	5,127
Shigellosis	13	2,747
Chemical poisoning	9	474
Hepatitis-A	13	351
Typhoid fever	4	222
Salmonellosis	2	37
TOTAL	99	16,950

of transmission were unknown; water was identified as the vehicle in one of them (Center for Disease Control, 1976b).

In 1975, 24 waterborne disease outbreaks involving 10,879 cases were reported to the Center for Disease Control (1976b). No etiologic agent was found for the two largest outbreaks (Sewickley, Pa.—5,000 cases and Sellersburg, Ind.—1,400 cases). The third largest outbreak, involving over 1,000 persons, occurred at Crater Lake National Park, Oreg. Enterotoxigenic *E. coli* was isolated from residents of the park who became ill, and from the park's water supply.

Seventeen of the 24 outbreaks and about 90% of the cases reported to CDC were designated as "acute gastrointestinal illness." This category includes cases characterized by gastrointestinal symptoms for which no specific etiologic agent was identified. Cases resulting from water treatment deficiencies (2,695) or deficiencies in the water distribution system (6,961) accounted for almost 89% of the total cases in 1975. As in the past, most of the cases occurred in the spring and summer.

The reported numbers of outbreaks and illnesses represent only a portion of the true totals. Craun *et al.* (1976) called attention to the outbreak at Richmond Heights, Fla., in 1974 as an example of why good disease surveillance is necessary and of the way in which many illnesses may go unnoticed. Initially, only 10 cases of shigellosis in this outbreak were recognized by authorities. An epidemiologic investigation revealed that approximately 1,200 illnesses actually occurred. This large outbreak might not have been detected if local health authorities had not been conducting shigellosis surveillance. In another outbreak, some 1,400 residents of Sellersburg, Ind. (31% of the town's population) experienced gastroenteritis. The high attack rate, rapid onset of the outbreak, review of water sampling data, and the town-wide survey suggested that the illness was waterborne, but no bacterial or viral pathogens or chemical toxins were found in the town water supply. Until improved detection and reporting systems are in use, the available epidemiological data will represent only a small fraction of the waterborne-disease problems in this country.

BACTERIA

The principal bacterial agents* that have been shown to cause human intestinal disease associated with drinking water are: *Salmonella typhi*,

*Nomenclature in this report follows the 8th edition of Bergey's *Manual of Determinative Bacteriology* (Buchanan and Gibbons, 1974).

typhoid fever; *Salmonella paratyphi-A*, paratyphoid fever; *Salmonella* (other species and a great number of serotypes), salmonellosis, enteric fever; *Shigella dysenteriae*, *S. flexneri*, and *S. sonnei*, bacillary dysentery; *Vibrio cholerae*, cholera; *Leptospira* sp., leptospirosis; *Yersinia enterocolitica*, gastroenteritis; *Francisella tularensis*, tularemia; *Escherichia coli* (specific enteropathogenic strains), gastroenteritis; and *Pseudomonas aeruginosa*, various infections. Several other organisms have been associated with gastroenteritis, such as those in other genera of the Enterobacteriaceae: *Edwardsiella*, *Proteus*, *Serratia*, and *Bacillus*.

Number of Cells Required to Infect

In attempting to assess the hazards in drinking water, it is important to know how many viable pathogenic cells are necessary to initiate an infection. McCullough and Eisele (1951a,b,c,d) found that a dose of 10^6-10^8 salmonellae per person was necessary for most strains, although 10^5 cells of some strains could infect. More recent studies by Dupont, Hornick, and associates on selected enteric bacterial pathogens are summarized in Table III-2. Some enteric pathogens are highly virulent, causing infection when relatively few cells are administered (e.g., *Shigella flexneri* and *S. dysenteriae*), whereas others require large numbers to infect (e.g., *Salmonella typhosa* and *Vibrio cholerae*).

Virulence is a genetic trait and can vary markedly from strain to strain (Meynell, 1961). Phenotypic variation in virulence can occur within a given clone. A small percentage of the cells in a population may be unusually virulent (Meynell, 1961; Meynell and Meynell, 1965). Thus, it does not always follow that because large numbers of cells are required for infection in feeding trials, that large numbers in drinking water are necessary to cause infection. Some few individuals may become infected by small numbers of unusually virulent cells. Recent evidence also indicates the possibility of genetic transfer of virulence from invading microbes into the resident intestinal population, providing another means by which small numbers of organisms might initiate a disease state.

The consequences of an increasing prevalance in livestock and their excreta of coliform organisms containing infectious plasmids and giving rise to clinical conditions were not examined in detail because of time constraints and their lack of immediate relevance to standard setting. Similarly, the consequences of adding antibiotics to animal and poultry feed and the enhanced hazards of spreading drug-resistant organisms were not examined.

The infecting dose also varies with the age and general health of the

TABLE III-2 Infective Doses For Man of Bacterial Enteric Pathogens

	Subjects Infected/Total Tested								
Enteric Pathogen Dose: Viable Cells	10^1	10^2	10^3	10^4	10^5	10^6	10^7	10^8	10^9
Shigella dysenteriae									
Strain M131	1/10	2/4	7/10	5/6					
Strain A-1		1/4		2/6					
Shigella flexneri									
Srain 2A#		6/33[a]	33/49[b]	66/87	15/24				
Strain 2A##				1/4	3/4	7/8	13/19	7/8	
Salmonella typhi									
Strain Quailes			0/14		32/116		16/32	8/9	40/42
Vibrio cholerae									
Strain Inaba									
With $NaHCO_3$				11/13		45/52		2/2	
No $NaHCO_3$				0/2		0/4	0/4	2/4	1/2
Enteropathogenic *E. coli*									
Strain 4608				0/5		0/5		4/8	

SOURCES: *Shigella dysenteriae*: Levine *et al.*, 1973; *Shigella flexneri*: Dupont *et al.*, 1972b; Dupont *et al.*, 1969; *Salmonella typhi*: Hornick *et al.*, 1970; *Vibrio cholerae*: Cash *et al.*, 1974; Enteropathogenic *E. coli*: Dupont *et al.*, 1971.

[a]Dose: 1.8×10^2.

[b]Dose: 5×10^3.

host population (MacKenzie and Livingstone, 1968). Infants and the aged may be particularly susceptible. Previous exposure to a given pathogen is important, in that coproantibodies may prevent infection with a strain that is generally present in the population, whereas a new serotype introduced into the water supply may present an increased hazard.

Not all strains of *Shigella* are highly virulent. Shaughnessy *et al.* (1946) determined infecting doses of four strains of *Shigella* while studying immunization in volunteers. They found that infectivity in mice could not be directly correlated with infectivity in humans and that doses of 10^9 organisms or higher were needed to produce human infection. In their extensive studies to develop a *Shigella* vaccine, Hornick, DuPont, and associates observed the infective dose for several strains. With *S. flexneri* 2A, 30 of 39 volunteers became ill from a dose of 10^5-10^8 organisms

(DuPont *et al.*, 1969). They showed that *Shigella* must penetrate the intestinal mucosa to produce symptoms of classic dysentery and that addition of bicarbonate facilitated this process. Two vaccine strains of *S. flexneri* 2A, a hybrid of a *Shigella* mutant, *E. coli*, and a streptomycin-dependent strain, could be safely administered orally in doses of 10^{10} organisms or higher (DuPont *et al.*, 1972a). A virulent strain could cause symptoms in doses of as few as 180 organisms (DuPont *et al.*, 1972b). With *Shigella dysenteriae* 1 (Shiga strain)—an organism that has two pathogenic modes, invasiveness and enterotoxin elaboration—the infecting dose in man was shown to be as low as 10 organisms (Levine *et al.*, 1973).

With such high infectivity of *Shigella*, why are waterborne outbreaks not more common? One possibility is that *Shigella* survives poorly in water. Wang *et al.* (1956) pointed out that, in a number of bacillary dysentery outbreaks involving water, the organism was not, or could not be, isolated. Over several years of studying irrigation water in Colorado, Wang *et al.* (1956) and Dunlop *et al.* (1952) were not successful in isolating shigellae, although salmonellae were frequently isolated. The survival of shigellae in water appears to be shorter than that of many other bacteria; Dolivo-Dobrovolskiy and Rossovskaya (1956) found *Shigella* survival times of only 0.5-4.0 h during the warmest time of the year. However, enteric pathogens may survive much longer times in lake or river sediment than in free waters, and resuspension of such pathogen-loaded sediments at a later time may introduce a "slug" of bacteria into the waters that is not completely removed by treatment systems.

Estimation of Disease Potential by Direct Quantitation of Bacterial Pathogens

The detection of bacterial pathogens in water polluted with human or animal fecal matter is relatively easy when large numbers of organisms are present (American Public Health Association, 1975). Pathogenic bacteria have been isolated from relatively clean reservoirs, rivers, streams, and groundwater; large samples, concentration techniques, and often elaborate laboratory procedures are used. However, detecting the presence of these pathogenic organisms in processed and disinfected water is far more difficult.

Scientific literature presents a vast array of media and methods for direct pathogen detection in finished water (Geldreich, 1975). The greatest emphasis has been on the *Salmonella-Shigella* group of enteric organisms. Numerous modifications of well-known media are used for pre-enrichment, enrichment, selective inhibition, and isolation, and there are many recommended modifications of incubation temperature and time. Some methods use the classic most-probable-number (MPN) procedure for quantification; others use membrane filtration. Reviews of proposed procedures may be found in the *Journal of the Water Pollution Control Federation* (Geldreich, 1968, 1969, 1970b; Van Donsel, 1971; Reasoner, 1972, 1973, 1974, 1975). A recent review appeared in the fourteenth edition of *Standard Methods* (American Public Health Association, 1975).

There are serious limitations to the use of direct isolation of specific pathogenic bacteria for evaluating water quality. First, there is no single procedure that can be used to isolate and identify all these microorganisms. Second, only for salmonellae are the available procedures sufficiently accurate; the methods for other major pathogens—such as *Shigella*, *Vibrio*, and *Leptospira*—are inadequate. Third, none of the available procedures is applicable to quantitative isolation of small numbers of pathogens in drinking water. Fourth, even if procedures could be recommended, it is doubtful whether laboratories doing *routine* bacteriologic studies of water would have the expertise to carry out the procedures reliably.

In outbreaks caused by gross contamination, the standard procedures would be of value. Recently, Reasoner and Geldreich (1974) reviewed several of the rapid-detection methods proposed for water and concluded that the cost per test, although perhaps higher than for conventional procedures, must be tolerated for potable-water quality assessment in emergency situations created by natural disasters, treatment breakdown, or rupture in the distribution network. None of these procedures would provide protection to the public as great as that provided by the currently used indicator organism, the coliform.

Indicator Organisms

The term "indicator organism," as used in water microbiology, means: a microorganism whose presence is evidence that pollution (associated with fecal contamination from man or other warm-blooded animals) has occurred. Indicator organisms may be accompanied by pathogens, but do not necessarily cause disease themselves.

As noted above, pathogens are usually more difficult to grow, isolate, and identify than indicator organisms, and often require special media and procedures. Indicator organisms, rather than the actual pathogens, are used to assess water quality because their detection is more reliable and less time-consuming. Pathogens appear in smaller numbers than indicator organisms and are therefore less likely to be isolated. An indicator organism should have the following characteristics:

- Applicable to all types of water.
- Present in sewage and polluted waters when pathogens are present.
- Number is correlated with the amount of pollution.
- Present in greater numbers than pathogens.
- No aftergrowth in water.
- Greater survival time than pathogens.
- Absent from unpolluted waters.
- Easily detected by simple laboratory tests in the shortest time consistent with accurate results.
- Has constant characteristics.
- Harmless to man and animal.

No organism or group of organisms meets all these criteria, but the "coliform group" of organisms fulfills most of them.

ESCHERICHIA COLI AND THE COLIFORM GROUP

Escherichia coli is commonly found in the human intestine. It is not normally a pathogen, although pathogenic strains are known. Physiologically, *E. coli* and members of the genera *Salmonella* and *Shigella* are quite similar. All are classified as enteric bacteria of the family Enterobacteriaceae (Cowan, 1974). They are facultatively anaerobic, and are able to ferment sugars with the production of organic acid and gas. These three genera carry out a type of fermentation called "mixed-acid fermentation," but differ in a number of physiological characteristics. Many physiological differences between various enteric bacteria are known (Ewing and Martin, 1974), but at the beginning of the twentieth century this was not so. In the early days of water bacteriology, some simple operational distinctions were necessary. The lactose-fermentation test became the prime diagnostic tool: *E. coli* ferments lactose with the formation of acid and gas; *Salmonella* and *Shigella* do not ferment lactose.

One source of confusion is the necessity to distinguish between *E. coli* and the "coliform group" of bacteria. Although the taxonomy of bacteria is constantly undergoing revision (see Buchanan and Gibbons, 1974, for the latest version), the genus *Escherichia* is well defined. It is distinguished from other mixed-acid fermenters of the Enterobacteriaceae primarily on the basis of sugar-fermentation reactions, motility, production of indole from tryptophan, lack of urease, inability to utilize citrate as sole carbon source, and inhibition of growth by potassium cyanide. However, the "coliform group" is not so precisely defined. The "coliform group," as defined in *Standard Methods* (American Public Health Association, 1975), comprises all "aerobic and facultative anaerobic, gram-negative, non-spore-forming, rod-shaped bacteria which ferment lactose with gas formation within 48 hr at 35 C." This is not a taxonomic grouping, but an operational one that is useful in water-supply and sewage-treatment practice. It includes organisms in addition to *E. coli*, most importantly *Klebsiella pneumoniae* and *Enterobacter aerogenes*, which are not mixed-acid fermenters. The entry of the term "coliform" into sanitary bacteriology was associated with a policy established by H. E. Jordan when he became editor of the *Journal of the American Water Works Association*; he stated that he would substitute "coliform" for "*E. coli*" in papers submitted to him (Jordan, 1937).

Although most isolates classifiable as *Escherichia* by modern methods ferment lactose, about 5-9% of them do not (Ewing and Martin, 1974). No isolates of the genus *Salmonella*, either in the species *S. typhi* or in other species, produce gas from lactose (Ewing and Martin, 1974); therefore, a water sample containing *Salmonella* and a lactose-negative *E. coli* would be negative on the coliform test and would probably be discarded without further examination, because of the definition of "coliform." Even if glucose were substituted for lactose in a coliform analysis, a significant fraction of organisms would be missed, inasmuch as about 9% of isolates of *Escherichia* do not form gas from glucose (Ewing and Martin, 1974).

Because there are two procedures—the multiple-tube-dilution or most-probable-number (MPN) technique, and the membrane-filter (MF) technique—the coliform group of organisms requires two definitions (American Public Health Association, 1975). On the basis of the MPN technique, the group consists of all aerobic and facultatively anaerobic, gram-negative, non-spore-forming, rod-shaped bacteria that ferment lactose with formation of gas within 48 h at 35°C. On the basis of the MF technique, the group consists of all organisms that produce a dark colony (generally purplish-green) with a metallic sheen within 24 h of incubation on the appropriate culture medium; the sheen may cover the entire colony or appear only in a central area or on the periphery. These two groups are not necessarily the same, but they have the same sanitary significance.

If the coliform group is to be used as an indicator of fecal pollution of water, it is important to know that the coliforms do not lose viability in the water environment faster than pathogenic bacteria, such as salmonel-

TABLE III-3 Comparative Die-Off Rates (Half-Time)[a] of Fecal Indicator Bacteria and Enteric Pathogens

Bacteria	Half-time (h)	Number of strains
Indicator Bacteria		
Coliform (avg.)	17.0-17.5	29
Enterococci (avg.)	22.0	20
Streptococci (from sewage)	19.5	
S. equinus	10.0	1
S. bovis	4.3	1
Pathogenic bacteria		
Shigella dysenteriae	22.4	1
S. sonnei	24.5	1
S. flexneri	26.8	1
S. enteritidis, paratyphi A&D	16.0–19.2	2
S. enteritidis, typhimurium	16.0	1
S. typhi	6.0	2
V. cholerae	7.2	3
S. enteritidis, paratyphi B	2.4	1

[a]Time required for 50% reduction in the population. From McFeters *et al.* (1974).

lae and shigellae. Little information exists on the survival of bacteria in finished water, and the data on other types of water are scattered and fragmentary. McFeters *et al.* (1974) recently reviewed previous work and presented their own data on die-off of intestinal pathogens in well water. As seen in Table III-3, die-off rates for pathogens and coliforms are approximately the same. Earlier work on the survival of salmonellae in water was reviewed by McKee and Wolf (1963).

Another factor to be considered is the relative sensitivity of coliforms and bacterial pathogens to disinfection. Although this subject has been studied little recently, the older work (Butterfield et al., 1943; Butterfield and Wattie, 1946; Wattie and Chambers, 1943) indicated that there was essentially no difference between these different organisms in sensitivity to disinfection. This is not true when the coliform group is compared with viral pathogens. Viruses survive longer than bacterial pathogens (Colwell and Hetrick, 1976).

SOME DEFICIENCES OF COLIFORMS AS INDICATOR ORGANISMS

Coliforms meet many of the criteria for an ideal indicator organism previously listed; however, there are some deficiencies. There is aftergrowth in water—some strains do not disappear, but adapt to the new environment, and may become part of the natural flora. They are often found in waters, having entered through storm runoff. And they do not have constant characteristics; it is this property more than any other that has recently caused some water bacteriologists to question the continued use of coliforms as indicator organisms. False-negative and false-positive test results are not uncommon. The following summarizes the objections which have been raised by workers to the continued use of coliforms:

- Atypical lactose reactions, the concern of bacteriologists as early as 1899 (Parr, 1939), have occurred.
- Coliforms may be suppressed by high populations of other organisms, especially in untreated groundwater (Allen and Geldreich, 1975) or where there is no free residual chlorine (Geldreich *et al.*, 1972).
- Coliforms do not represent a homogeneous group; it has been suggested (Dutka, 1973) that the definition of "coliform" include any organism defined by Edwards and Ewing (1972) as Enterobacteriaceae (this might require the addition of the oxidase test to the definition of the group, because all Enterobacteriaceae are oxidase-negative).
- The genus *Aeromonas* is a common cause of false-positive results in warm weather (Bell and Vanderpost, 1973; Ewing *et al.*, 1961; Ptak *et al.*, 1973). These can be eliminated by the use of the oxidase test, since *Aeromonas* is oxidase-positive and coliforms are oxidase-negative.
- False-negative results by strains that are unable to ferment lactose can give an unwarranted sense of security.

In the final analysis, testing for coliform, while not perfect bacteriologically, is still the most reliable indicator of the possible presence of fecal contamination and therefore of the pathogens that may be present in water.

OTHER INDICATOR ORGANISMS

Because of certain limitations of the coliform group as general indicators of water quality, workers have continually searched for better indicator organisms. No other organism has been found that is better than the coliform group, but it is pertinent to mention briefly some of these other indicators (Geldreich, 1975). Fecal coliforms (defined as those organisms which develop on media incubated at 44.5°C) have frequently been used in stream and lake pollution work, but are not suitable as indicators of drinking water quality because the number of fecal coliforms is considerably lower in source waters than total coliforms, making the test less sensitive. Fecal streptococci (defined as those organisms able to grow on medium containing sodium azide) have been used in water pollution work, but have not proven suitable for drinking water analysis because of low recovery rates, poor agreements between various methods, and uncertainty as to their significance in water. Several other organisms have been suggested as indicators but have found even less acceptance: *Clostridium perfringens, Bifidobacterium, Pseudomonas, Staphylococcus*. It would be undesirable and extremely risky to substitute any organism for the coliform group now, although research studies that compare other indicator organisms with coliforms are warranted.

RAPID METHODS FOR COLIFORM COUNTS

There is great need for a rapid method of coliform counts which could give results in a shorter time than the 18-24 h required by the membrane-filter method. A rapid method would permit early detection of system problems, and would considerably increase public health protection. Correlation of any rapid method used with accepted standards methods is essential, at least to the degree that the MF and MPN methods correlate. Unfortunately, no suitable rapid method for drinking water exists at present, but we will mention several methods briefly, in order to encourage research in this area.

One theoretically-feasible method would be a direct microscopic method, in which coliform cells would be concentrated on a membrane filter and stained by a specific staining procedure. The most commonly suggested staining procedure has been the use of fluorescent antibodies specific for the coliform organisms (Danielsson, 1965; Ginsburg *et al.*, 1972). Unfortunately, this method is unlikely to succeed because there are at least 145 serotypes of *E. coli*, plus several more for the *Klebsiella* and *Enterobacter* group, so that a polyvalent antibody containing all of these antibodies would be necessary. Also, the number of cells in drinking water is likely to be so low that inconveniently long observation times would be necessary for quantifying the organisms present. Another disadvantage is that fluorescent antibodies might not distinguish living cells from dead, so that nonviable cells (perhaps resulting from a disinfection treatment) would also be counted.

Another rapid method that was suggested involves the use of radioactively labeled lactose and measurement of the radioactive CO_2, liberated as a result of metabolism of the coliforms. This procedure was first suggested by Levin *et al.* (1961) and has been studied further by Scott *et al.* (1964). The EPA in Cincinnati (Reasoner and Geldreich, 1974) is currently attempting to improve this method. One of the desirable features of such a method is that it could be automated and run on-line. A disadvantage of the system is that, at present, it is not sensitive enough to detect 10 or fewer organisms after 6 h of incubation. It seems unlikely that such a method could ever be made sensitive enough to detect single coliform cells in 100-ml water samples, so that it probably will never replace standard methods, but it might prove useful in process control in large water systems.

The EPA at Cincinnati has also developed a 7-h fecal coliform test, employing a membrane filter technique (Reasoner and Geldreich, 1974). Several other rapid methods which have been under study can be found in: Cady and Dufour (1974); DeBlanc *et al.* (1971); and Newman and O'Brien (1975).

SAMPLING FOR THE COLIFORM TEST

Water bacteriologists and sanitary engineers agree that the weakest link in the chain of water-monitoring and -testing is the collection of the sample. Too often this is left to the semiskilled or untrained worker.

The USEPA Interim Regulations (*Federal Register*, Dec. 24, 1975) follow the USPHS 1962 Drinking Water Standards: the number of required samples per month is based on the population served. Prior to 1925, when water quality standards were under the jurisdiction of the Treasury Department, bacterial sampling was left to the discretion of the local health and water utility officials and varied widely according to local practices and the capacity of the laboratory. This, of course, was unsatisfactory, and was so recognized by responsible water utility people.

In 1941, a conference was called by the USPHS to revise the drinking water quality standards, and among the subjects under consideration were the frequency of sampling, the location of the sampling points, and the increased number of samples from the distribution system rather than from the plant final effluent. The deliberations of this 1941 conference, which resulted in the adoption of new Standards in 1942, can be found in the *Journal of the American Water Works Association*: 1941, 33:1804; 1942, 35:135; 1942, 35:93; and 1941, 35:2215-2226.

The principal changes adopted by the U.S. Public Health Service in 1941 were as follows:

1. The number of samples to be examined monthly from the distribution system would depend on the population served. During this discussion, the quality of the source water, the treatment procedure, the sanitary condition of the distribution lines, and the daily volume delivered to the consumers were also considered. Apparently, these latter

factors made the final decision so complicated that in the final standard, only the size of the population served was used to decide on sampling frequency.

2. The detection of potential hazards in the distribution system due to faulty plumbing, cross-connection, post-contamination, and faulty plant and distribution system operation was included in the standards.

Samples were to be taken from representative points throughout the distribution system, with the frequency to be such as to determine the bacteriological quality of the water. The minimum number of samples per month was to be determined from the graph appearing in the *Journal of the American Water Works Association* (35:93-104, 1942). Apparently, this graph became the basis of the 1962 standards and the present interim regulations. According to F. Donald Maddox, Chief, Water Supply Systems Section, Region V, USEPA (personal communication to Walter Ginsburg), the subject of sample frequency was again discussed by the Committee that revised the 1962 Drinking Water Standards, and no changes were made. It is Maddox's opinion that the original 1942 curve was based on a number of water supply systems of different sizes which were known to have good treatment facilities and to be sampling at what was considered to be adequate frequency. The curve was plotted using these selected cities as a base line.

Richard L. Woodward, who served on the 1946 and 1962 Standards revision committees (personal communication to Walter Ginsburg) bears out the contention that the decision as to the number of samples to be examined was based on these elements of expert judgement.

One inherent weakness of this frequency graph has been discussed in the *Federal Register* (Dec. 24, 1975, p. 59568). It concerns the question of preparing monthly coliform averages from monthly percentages of positive samples. When four or fewer samples are examined each month, and one sample exceeds 4/100 ml, there is no way that the monthly average can conform to the recommended standards, even though the other three samples are negative. The regulations give the states the authority to average over a 3-month period when four or fewer samples are the required rate, but this hardly affords a community the protection it needs when the water system is doing a poor job of treatment.

The Community Water Supply Survey by the USEPA in 1969 (McCabe *et al.*, 1970) showed that 85% of the systems surveyed did not collect the required minimum number of samples. Such improper sampling frequency is one of the most abused requirements. This can cause problems in the distribution system to go undetected (Geldreich, 1971; Miller, 1975).

In light of this discussion, it is clear that considerable research is necessary, with modern statistical methods, to develop better sampling protocols for water systems that serve different populations.

COLIFORM STANDARDS

United States Standards

The first U.S. national standards for bacteriological water quality were established in 1914 (Public Health Reports, 1914). These standards were specifically applicable to water used on interstate carriers, but were adopted quite early (formally or informally) by many states. Morse and Wolman (1918) concluded that the standards are not precise and accurate indices of quality, but simply a convenient mode of analysis for comparative purposes that must be used with considerable caution.

It is obvious that with drinking water that meets the standards there is no absolute assurance of the absence of pathogens, only confidence that their presence is unlikely; hence, the probability of waterborne-disease transmission is decreased. The decline in morbidity and mortality from some diseases, such as cholera, typhoid fever, salmonellosis, and shigellosis, provides some evidence of the validity of this confidence, although some of the decline may be due to the generally better health of the population, making people less susceptible to infection.

The latest standards adopted by the PHS were those of 1962 (U.S. Public Health Service, 1962). Although none of the bacteriological numerical values was changed, a major procedural revision was made; the membrane-filter technique was accepted as an equivalent alternative to the multiple-tube-dilution (MPN) technique that had been in use since 1914. The MF standard was set at one coliform/100 ml.

The interim regulations of the EPA (*Federal Register*, Dec. 25, 1975) have broadened the applicability of the standards to all public water systems, specified a sample size of 100 ml when the MF technique is used, and modified the required frequency of sampling. A monthly mean of less than one coliform/100 ml is still the standard.

International Standards

Although many countries have their own drinking-water standards, two standards have international status—the World Health Organization European Standards (World Health Organization, 1970) and the International Standards (World Health Organization, 1971). In their preparation, individual national standards were considered.

The International Standards are proposed as "minimal standards which are considered to be within the reach of all countries throughout the world at the present time" (World Health Organization, 1970). They distinguish between piped supplies (roughly equivalent to the EPA definition of community public systems) and individual or small community supplies (comparable with the EPA definition of noncommunity systems) and between water leaving the treatment plant and that in the distribution system. For treated, disinfected supplies, water entering the distribution system should be of such quality that no coliform bacteria can be demonstrated (by the specified procedures) in 100 ml of water. For undisinfected water, the samples should yield no *E. coli* and three or fewer coliforms/100 ml. Within the distribution system, the standards are specified that "(1) Throughout any year, 95% of samples should not contain *E. coli* in 100 ml; (2) No sample should contain more than 10 coliform organisms per 100 ml; and, (3) Coliform organisms should not be detectable in 100 ml of any two consecutive samples." In nonpiped systems, the coliform count should not exceed 10/100 ml.

The European Standards are comparable to the International standards, but do not distinguish—in terms of quality—between disinfected and undisinfected water. The standard of 95% of 100-ml samples—showing no coliform bacteria throughout a year—"corresponds to an average density of about one coliform organism in 2 liters of water." Despite the numerical differences between the U.S. and the international standards, it is the intent of both sets of standards that coliform bacteria be absent from drinking water, to provide protection against disease.

STATISTICAL LIMITS

In discussing numerical standards of bacteriological quality of drinking water, the accuracy and the statistical limits of the tests must be considered. In using the classical, multiple-tube-fermentation test for coliform bacteria, it has been recognized that the procedure itself has a large inherent error (Morse and Wolman, 1918). A more recent discussion of these limits (Prescott *et al.*, 1946) concluded that "because of the marked inaccuracy of the dilution MPN method . . . any tendency toward fictitious accuracy in expressing the result should be discouraged." Table III-4, reproduced from *Standard Methods for the Examination of Water and Wastewater* (American Public Health Association, 1975), clearly shows this.

The membrane filter technique, because it is equivalent statistically to a plate count, has a much smaller error. Thomas and Woodward (1955)

TABLE III-4 MPN Index and 95% Confidence Limits for Various Combinations of Positive and Negative Results, Using Five 10–ml Samples

No. of Tubes Giving Positive Reaction out of 5 of 10 ml Each	MPN Index per 100 ml	95% Confidence Limits	
		Lower	Upper
0	< 2.2	0	6.0
1	2.2	0.1	12.6
2	5.1	0.5	19.2
3	9.2	1.6	29.4
4	16.	3.3	52.9
5	>16.	8.0	Infinite

From American Public Health Association (1975).

compared the two methods and concluded "that, on the average, the former MPN gave higher indications of density by a factor of 1.0-1.9 with an average of 1.3 for the specific technics used. . . . However, the difference is not regarded as important from a practical viewpoint because of the inherent lack of precision of the individual MPN value." —and that, "With nearly all of the samples listed, the precision attained with a single filter was found to be two to five times greater than that of a 5-5-5-tube MPN" (note that the drinking water standards require only 5 tubes at one dilution with a corresponding greater lack of precision).

THE HEALTH SIGNIFICANCE OF THE COLIFORM TEST

Several pathogens, notably those in the genus *Shigella*, are able to initiate infection in humans even when introduced in very low numbers. Because it is not feasible to assay for bacterial pathogens directly in water, it is important to consider the utility of the coliform test in ensuring the bacteriologic safety of drinking water.

A direct approach to assessing the significance of the coliform count would be to obtain evidence of a correlation between numbers of coliforms and numbers of pathogenic bacteria (e.g., salmonellae or shigellae). One attempt to seek such a correlation was the study of Kehr and Butterfield (1943). Although imperfect, this is the only study found that attempts to relate the coliform count directly to disease incidence. In the discussion below, this study is analyzed in some detail in order to present a picture of the approach necessary to place the coliform standard on a firmer scientific basis. (It is perhaps of historical interest that the motivation for their study was an adverse decision by the Illinois Supreme Court as to the value of the coliform count in indicating that water is unsafe.)

The approach used by Kehr and Butterfield involved two aspects. First, data on the relative proportions of *Salmonella typhosa* and coliforms in various types of water (such as river, sewage, and sludge) were obtained from the literature, and the numbers of *S. typhosa* per 10^6 coliforms were calculated. These data, obtained from cities throughout the world, were then plotted on the ordinate on log-log paper, with typhoid fever morbidity on the abscissa (Figure III-2). An approximately straight line was obtained. The point here was that the excretion rate of coliforms would be the same in a healthy as in a sick population, but that the latter would also excrete typhoid bacteria. Kehr and Butterfield then considered the stability of the *E. coli-S. typhosa* ratio and showed that *S. typhosa* and coliforms died off at approximately the same rate during sewage treatment, during self-purification in streams and lakes, and during drinking-water purification. The stability of this ratio is not surprising, when it is considered that *S. typhosa* and coliforms are members of the same group of bacteria and are likely to show similar tolerance and sensitivities to environmental influences.

From the data in Figure III-2 and from recorded waterborne outbreaks of typhoid fever, Kehr and Butterfield estimated a minimal infecting dose of *S. typhosa* for the general population and the percentage of persons infected by that dose. In doing this, these workers considered only epidemics of typhoid fever of a diffuse nature, i.e., characterized by a low attack rate but spread over a fairly large population. Kehr and Butterfield wrote that such epidemics were common at the time. Outbreaks with high attack rates, in which infection could arise more or less directly from carrier or patient discharge, were not considered, in order to avoid situations not likely to involve drinking water. In the diffuse typhoid epidemics, a common observation is the additional widespread occurrence of nontyphoid gastrointestinal disturbances. Considering the frequency of occurrence of the diffuse pattern of epidemics, and the data on concentrations of *S. typhosa* found in sewage and polluted waters (as given in Figure III-2), Kehr and Butterfield concluded that it would be unlikely in such an outbreak for a person to drink more than a single typhoid bacterium, or at most only a few, and that a single typhoid organism could produce infection in a small percentage of the general population. This conclusion is consistent with studies in experimental animals, which have shown that infection can be initiated by single bacterial cells (Meynell, 1961; Meynell and Meynell, 1965).

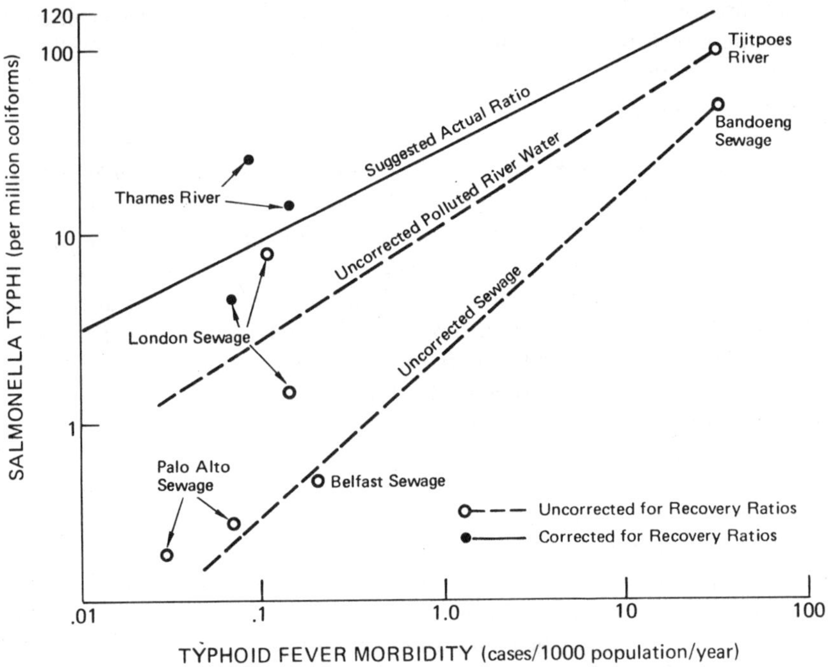

FIGURE III-2 Ratio of *Salmonella typhi* per million coliforms for varying typhoid fever morbidity rates. From Kehr and Butterfield (1943).

But this conclusion is not unequivocal. Populations of bacteria, even if derived from the same clone, can have a range of infectivities, and populations of humans have a range of susceptibilities. Thus, although a single cell may initiate an infection, not every cell-host contact will lead to infection. When the pathogenic bacterial population is diluted by a large volume of drinking water and spread over a large population, there is a probability that an appropriately virulent cell will reach a susceptible person. This is the situation that Kehr and Butterfield considered in their analysis of diffuse waterborne typhoid epidemics.

If the hypothesis that a single typhoid bacterium is infective can be accepted, then it is possible to consider the significance of the typhi:coliform ratio in drinking water. Assume that a water plant is treating source water with a typhi:coliform ratio of $10{:}10^6$, corresponding roughly to the ratio found in many polluted surface waters. Assuming equal destruction of typhoid bacteria and coliforms during treatment, if the finished water contained one coliform/100 ml (a reasonable possibility, even in many well-run plants), then the probability of consuming one typhoid bacterium when drinking a liter of water would be 10^{-5}; or, put another way, 10 people in a population of 1,000,000 could be infected. In an attempt to verify this, Kehr and Butterfield analyzed a number of epidemics of waterborne disease of the diffuse type, and concluded that the observed incidence of infection was consistent with this hypothesis. Thus, it was concluded that water which does not meet the coliform standard (one coliform/100 ml) can be responsible for waterborne disease, both gastroenteritis and typhoid fever.

Even more important, this analysis raises the question of whether water that *meets* the standard might bear disease-causing organisms. It is a simple exercise in arithmetic to convince oneself that this could be the case, inasmuch as drinking water with less than one coliform/100 ml, thus meeting the standards, could well have pathogenic organisms. Suppose that, instead of analyzing 100 ml of water, 1 liter were analyzed, and one coliform was found. This would be a coliform count of 0.1/100 ml, equivalent to one typhoid infection per 1,000,000 people (assuming the same typhi:coliform ratio as in the previous paragraph). Since the incidence of nonspecific gastroenteritis can be expected to be higher than that of typhoid, water that meets the present coliform standard *may* be the bearer of disease. However, existing epidemiologic data and reporting systems would not permit detection of such waterborne incidents, because the number of organisms would be below the detection limits of current surveillance methods.

The epidemiologic work of Stevenson (1953) added much weight to the rationale of establishing a coliform standard for drinking-water sources. His analyses showed that if raw water has fewer than 1,000 coliforms/100 ml, then it would be very likely that the salmonellae in finished water would be below infective levels.

Gallagher and Spino (1968) challenged the validity of the standards and stated that "summarized data from several stream surveys over the past few years showed little apparent correlation between quantities of total or fecal coliforms and the probable isolation of salmonellae." Geldreich (1970a) challenged their conclusion, on the basis of fecal coliform detections that showed a correlation between coliform numbers and salmonellae isolations. He showed from numerous previous studies that, when fecal coliforms were 200/100 ml or more, there was a finite probability of isolating salmonellae. Smith and Twedt (1971) corroborated these data in a study of two Michigan rivers.

There are well-known epidemiologic histories of the presence of bacterial pathogens when the coliform index was low. Boring *et al.* (1971) reported that *Salmonella typhimurium* outnumbered coliforms by a factor of 10 in the Riverside, California outbreak. Similarly, a report by Seligmann and Reitter (1965) showed that index organisms can be low in the presence of pathogens. These sporadic reports of the failure of the index-organism concept emphasize the need for more research on pathogen detection.

CONCLUSION ON COLIFORM STANDARD

Thus, we conclude that the current coliform standard is of value in protecting against frank outbreaks of bacterial diseases, but it may not protect against low levels of virulent pathogens. It is clear that further protection could be achieved by analyzing larger samples for coliforms. More important than analysis of larger water samples for the protection of the public health—more frequent sampling, especially at more points throughout the distribution system—should be considered.

It has been reported repeatedly in the literature that the presence of any type of coliform organism in drinking water is undesirable. The regulations essentially demand that coliform-free water be distributed to consumers. Wolf (1972) has ably summarized: "The drinking water standard presently in use (approximately one coliform per 100 ml) is, in a sense, a standard of expedience. It does not entirely exclude the possibility of acquiring an intestinal infection. It is attainable by the economic development of available water supplies, their disinfection, and, if need be, treatment in purification works by economically feasible methods. It is not a standard of perfection."

It is not clear that the coliform standard provides comparable protection against virus disease. In fact, available information indicates that viruses may survive considerably longer than coliform bacteria outside the human host, and that the infectious dose may be very small (see section on viruses).

Good engineering and public health practices emphasize the need for using raw water of the highest possible quality, and for providing adequate sanitary-survey information. Bacteriological testing—or the imposed use of bacteriological standards—are adjuncts, not replacements for good-quality raw water, proper water treatment, and integrity of the distribution system. The present coliform standards appear adequate to protect public health when: raw water is obtained from a protected source, is appropriately treated, and is distributed in a contamination-free system. Current coliform standards are not applicable for water reclaimed directly from wastewater.

The Standard Plate Count

The standard plate count (SPC) for drinking water, as described in *Standard Methods* (American Public Health Association, 1975), is the plating of small quantities (usually 1.0 or 0.1 ml) of a properly collected water sample in a nutrient agar medium (plate count tryptone glucose extract agar) and incubating aerobically for a fixed period at a prescribed temperature (35°C for 24 h or 20°C for 48 h).* The SPC is often referred to by other names, such as "total count," "viable count," "plate count," "bacterial count," "water plate count," and "total bacterial count." The organisms that develop into colonies on the agar plates represent a portion of the total population of bacteria in the water. This portion contains the bacteria that grow in the prescribed time in the specific environment provided. Although the method described is standard, there is no universal agreement on the acceptable concentration of organisms in drinking water. The most common allowable bacterial numbers used by health departments, water-supply agencies, and local jurisdictions vary from 100/ml to 500/ml of colony-forming units.

Geldreich (1973) has summarized several ways in which a standard based upon fecal-organism detection alone may not provide adequate health protection. Information gained from continued surveillance of water supplies by a standard plate count would provide an added degree of health protection. Even though water treatment is adequate and chlorine disinfection is provided, quality could deteriorate in the distribution system as a result of growth of organisms other than detectable coliforms. Finished water containing floc, or unfiltered turbid waters, may carry organisms past the disinfection treatment, or the organisms may be protected by association with larger forms of life, such as nematodes (Chang *et al.*, 1960). Changes in water pressure in the distribution lines may cause release of organisms from protected areas, dead ends, or protecting materials in the system.

Geldreich *et al.* (1972) and Geldreich (1973) also reviewed the phenomenon of suppression of fecal organisms by the presence of large populations of organisms in common genera whose members normally show up in standard plate counts. These genera include *Pseudomonas*, *Bacillus*, *Streptomyces*, *Micrococcus*, *Flavobacterium*, *Proteus*, and various yeasts. It was concluded that the presence of 1,000 noncoliform organisms

*In most tap waters, the number of organisms capable of growing at 20°C is considerably higher than the number growing at 35°C. It is unlikely that most organisms growing at 20°C will also grow at 35-37°C, and hence could not be pathogenic to man. A 20°C count could still be of value in water works practice, in providing information about filtration efficiency and about possible contamination of groundwater supplies.

per ml could suppress the growth of coliforms. Geldreich (1973) speculated that this type of suppression of coliforms below detectable concentrations may have occurred in the Riverside, Calif., *Salmonella typhimurium* outbreaks, where coliform analyses did not reveal the contamination (Boring *et al.*, 1971). Plate counts over 500/ml also seemed to make detection of salmonellae and shigellae very difficult in a bacteriologic study of potable water in Karachi, Pakistan (Ahmed *et al.*, 1967). Although the genera of organisms detected by the SPC may not be harmful or dangerous to normal humans when present in drinking water in low numbers, under special circumstances (such as during therapy), these organisms are known to produce severe acute or chronic human infections (Geldreich *et al.*, 1972). Geldreich (1973) proposed that a 500/ml limit be placed on the standard plate count and that immediate investigation of water treatment and distribution systems be undertaken whenever the limits were exceeded. He recommended that water supplies be monitored routinely—at least every 3 months—to maintain the baseline data on the general bacterial population. A summary from Geldreich's (1973) paper follows.

It should be clearly understood that the standard plate count is not a substitute for total coliform measurements of the sanitary quality of potable water. Rather, the use of a standard plate count limitation will:

1. Provide a method of monitoring for changes in the bacteriological quality of finished water in storage reservoirs and distribution systems.
2. Indirectly limit the occurrence and magnitude of *Pseudomonas*, *Flavobacterium* and other secondary pathogenic invaders that could pose a health risk in the hospital environment.
3. Reduce problems in the detection of low densities of total coliforms due to interference by noncoliform bacteria.
4. Monitor the effectiveness of chlorine throughout the distribution network and provide a warning of filter effluent-quality deterioration and the occurrence of coliform breakthrough.
5. Indicate the existence of sediment accumulation in the distribution network that provides a protective habitat for the general bacterial population.

Finally, the noncoliform bacterial population can be controlled by removing sediment and slime deposits from the distribution network followed by continuous application of chlorine in sufficient dosage to insure the maintenance of a free residual throughout the system.

It should be emphasized that a standard plate count of 500/ml is attainable by water systems. Control of the general bacterial population in a variety of public water-supply distribution systems was demonstrated by Geldreich (1973), with a chlorine residue of approximately 0.3 mg/liter. In 60% of 923 water systems, standard plate count densities of 10/ml or less were obtained.

Although it is difficult to document, it is probably true that among the reasons for the decline in use of the standard plate count for drinking water are—the cost of the test, the lack of trained people to perform the number of tests needed, the difficulty of implementing and monitoring the laboratories needed, the resistance that would occur among the small and isolated water-plant operators, and similar issues. Although these are valid criticisms, they do not speak to the basic question of whether a regular system of plate-count surveillance would provide a tool for assessing the health hazards of water.

CONCLUSIONS ON STANDARD PLATE COUNT

The standard plate count is a valuable procedure for evaluating the bacterial quality of drinking water. Ideally, standard plate counts should be performed on samples taken throughout systems. The SPC has major health significance for surface-water systems that do not use flocculation, sedimentation, filtration, and chlorination, and for those groundwater systems that do no chlorination. When it is used, the sampling frequency should be at least 10% of the frequency of the coliform analysis, except that at least one sample should be collected and analyzed each month.

The scientific information available makes it reasonable to establish the upper limit of the SPC initially at 500/ml, as developed in 35°C, 48-h plate count procedure (using the procedures prescribed by *Standard Methods* (American Public Health Association, 1975.)

RECOMMENDATIONS FOR RESEARCH ON BACTERIAL CONTAMINANTS

A research program is needed to increase the value of the relatively simple bacteriological tests in controlling the sanitary quality of drinking water. The program should include:

1. Epidemiological studies of water quality and health, with application of more sensitive methods for detecting pathogens in drinking water and better reporting of outbreaks of waterborne disease.
2. Development of membrane-filtration methods to allow testing of larger samples and to reduce interference by overgrowth and disinfectants.
3. Improvement of procedures for making total plate counts and study

of the utility of such tests for assessing the health hazards of drinking water.

4. Research on more rapid and sensitive methods for detecting pathogens and the use of such methods for monitoring the quality of water.

VIRUSES

Viruses differ fundamentally from other microrganisms that may occur in water. They are transmitted as submicroscopic, inert particles that are unable to replicate or adapt to environmental conditions outside a living host. These particles, or virions, have the potential to produce infections, and sometimes disease, in people who ingest them with drinking water. A viral particle eventually loses its infectivity with the passage of time, and with exposure to the rigors of its environment.

The viruses important to human health that are most likely to be transmitted by drinking water are the enteric viruses. These are primarily parasites of a portion of the intestinal tract. The stomach and duodenum are seldom affected by viruses, partly because of unfavorable conditions. Acid and proteolytic secretions predominate in the stomach; these and bile empty into the duodenum. Only viruses that can withstand such conditions will remain infectious and thus able to implant further down the digestive tract.

The most important human enteric viruses are the enteroviruses (i.e., acid-stable picornaviruses), reoviruses, parvoviruses, and adenoviruses (Fenner *et al.*, 1974). The virions of all these groups are roughly spherical, acid-stable, and lack envelopes. All are relatively stable in the environment outside the host organism. Enterovirus particles are small (20-30 nm) and contain single-stranded ribonucleic acid (RNA). Reovirus particles are medium-sized (70-80 nm) and contain double-stranded RNA. Parvovirus particles are small and contain single-stranded deoxyribonucleic acid (DNA). Adenovirus particles are medium-sized and contain double-stranded DNA. Hepatitis A (infectious hepatitis) is transmitted by particles that closely resemble those of the enteroviruses (Provost *et al.*, 1975).

Unlike bacteria, the viruses are obligate intracellular parasites and cannot replicate in a cell-free medium. Many viruses can be grown in cultured cells *in vitro*. Some transmitted to man by water, most notably the virus of hepatitis A, have not yet been cultivated *in vitro*.

Ordinarily, viruses are detected and enumerated on the basis of their infectivity in cell culture or experimental animals. Testing of viruses for infectivity was greatly advanced by the finding that animal cells grown *in vitro* would support the replication of human viruses (Enders *et al.*, 1949). Infectivity resides in the nucleic acid portion of the virus particle. When a suspension of infectious particles is inoculated into a culture of susceptible cells, the particles are engulfed by, or penetrate, host cells, and the cells produce progeny virus. Death of the cells often results.

If diffusion of the progeny virus particles is restricted by gelling the medium in which the cells are maintained, cell death occurs in a localized area called a "plaque." Such a plaque can be initiated by one viral particle, so that plaque enumeration has become an important method to measure animal viruses (Dulbecco, 1952; Dulbecco and Vogt, 1954). However, a plaque is not always initiated by a single viral particle, and many viral suspensions contain more aggregates than single particles (Sharp *et al.*, 1975); so the plaque-forming unit (PFU) is not an absolute basis for determining the numbers of viral particles.

Knowledge of viruses was acquired much more rapidly after the advent of cell-culture techniques. Nevertheless, transmission of enteric viruses by water had already been surmised by the time cell cultures became available.

History of the Enteric Viruses

The first reported epidemic of poliomyelitis in the United States occurred in New England (Putnam and Taylor, 1893). Caverly's (1896) observation that many cases had occurred in the Otter Creek Valley in Vermont suggested that the disease might be waterborne.

The poliomyelitis virus had been thought to infect people by the nasopharyngeal route. Kling (1929) found more virus in patients' stools than in their throats, but his findings were not generally accepted. Later, Harmon (1937) reported isolating virus by inoculating monkeys with colonic washings of four patients whose nasopharynxes yielded no virus. It was evident that infantile paralysis was not a strictly neurotropic disease and that the causative agent was strongly associated with the human intestines.

The picture was complicated by the presence of yet-unidentified agents other than the polioviruses in stools. The criterion of neuronophagia, seen in the spinal cords of inoculated monkeys, did not reliably distinguish the polioviruses from these other agents. In 1948, Dalldorf and Sickles reported isolating viruses from the stools of children by inoculation into suckling mice. The original stool specimens came from Coxsackie, N.Y., but "coxsackieviruses" were soon being discovered in many other locations.

When cell cultures became available, tests of stool suspensions began to yield viruses that were neither polioviruses nor coxsackieviruses (Robbins *et al.*, 1951). The isolations of many such viruses were not clearly associated with any disease; these agents were eventually designated "enteric cytopathic human orphan" (ECHO) viruses. The National Foundation for Infantile Paralysis convened a committee to identify and classify these new viruses (Committee on the ECHO Viruses, 1955. The echoviruses were later classified with the polioviruses and coxsackieviruses to form the enterovirus group, members of which are numbered serially (Committee on the Enteroviruses, 1957, 1962).

The reoviruses were originally designated as members of the ECHO group. In 1959, Sabin suggested the term "reovirus" to apply to three serologic types of viruses that had common properties that differed from those of the echoviruses. The reoviruses are common in wastewater; 80% of the viruses that were isolated from wastewater by England *et al.* (1967) were reoviruses. The reoviruses have been recovered from persons with a wide variety of illnesses, but in no case has their etiologic role been established unequivocally (Horsfall and Tamm, 1965).

The adenoviruses (Rowe *et al.*, 1953) have produced large outbreaks of acute respiratory disease in military populations, and were a serious problem during World War II (Klein, 1966). They produce sporadic infections in the general population but are not often associated with overt disease. They occur frequently in sewage and wastewater and might thus contaminate drinking water. Their significance to the health of the general public is uncertain.

Probably the most important viral disease sometimes transmitted by water is hepatitis A. The disease was first described by Lurman in 1885. Its most common route of transmission is fecal-oral, primarily by person-to-person contact. In addition to water and personal contact, the disease is sometimes transmitted by food. The largest epidemic of hepatitis known to have been transmitted by water occurred in 1956 in Delhi, India; it was estimated that more than 30,000 cases occurred after sewage contamination of drinking water (Anonymous, 1957; Melnick, 1957). The virus has never been cultivated in cell culture, so that all available evidence about the transmission of infectious hepatitis by polluted drinking water is epidemiologic. Mosley (1967) suggested that the incidence of waterborne infectious hepatitis is grossly underreported, but estimated that less than 1% of the cases of this disease result from transmission by water.

Viruses that are still unidentified may also be responsible for waterborne disease, since there are many episodes of waterborne gastroenteritis and diarrhea of unknown etiology. Taylor *et al.* (1972)

listed gastroenteritis as the most common waterborne disease, on the basis of number of outbreaks during 1961-1970. It is not clear which of the enteric viruses, if any, produce this common illness.

Epidemiology

Knowledge that a virus is shed in feces and may persist for a short time in wastewater is not proof that it is transmitted by water. Clearly, not every virus that is present in feces is waterborne. Viruses transmitted by a fecal–oral cycle can always be transferred directly from person to person, but this requires close contact. Several of the enteric viruses are known to be transmitted by water, but only some of the time.

Eight outbreaks of poliomyelitis in Europe and North America were eventually attributed to transmission by water, but Mosley (1967) believed that only one of them was adequately documented. This occurred in "Huskerville," Nebr., in 1952; at least 45 people were made ill after contamination of a municipal water system.

The viral disease most frequently reported to be transmitted by water is hepatitis A (infectious hepatitis). Viral hepatitis became a reportable disease in the United States in January 1952, but the two types of hepatitis (i.e., infectious and serum hepatitis) were not separately notifiable until 1966.

The viral etiology of infectious hepatitis and transmission of the virus through water were adduced by Neefe and Stokes in 1945. Published reports of 50 hepatitis A outbreaks, attributed to contaminated drinking water, were summarized by Mosley (1967), who found the evidence of transmission by water to be convincing in only 30 of the 50 outbreaks cited.

Craun *et al.* (1976) reported 13 outbreaks of waterborne hepatitis that affected 351 people during 1971-1974. Although hepatitis A has been implicated epidemiologically in some 66 waterborne outbreaks since 1946 (Table III-5), there is no evidence of its transmission through correctly operated conventional water-treatment systems, except where defects in the distribution system have been found to be the source of contamination (Craun, 1976). About 40,358 cases of hepatitis were reported in 1974 (Center for Disease Control, 1974), but only a small fraction of these cases was transmitted by water.

Epidemiologists have techniques that permit a decision as to whether an outbreak is waterborne or foodborne. These techniques require adequate and thorough reporting of the outbreak and a follow-up of infected individuals, to determine opportunities for contact with the

TABLE III-5 Waterborne Outbreaks of Hepatitis A by Source of Contamination, 1946–1974

Cause	Municipal Systems	Semipublic and Individual Systems
Untreated surface water	1	10
Untreated groundwater	4	26
Inadequate or interruption of disinfection	3	5
Contamination through distribution system	11	1
Insufficient data to classify	3	2
TOTAL	22	44

disease agent. Since most waterborne outbreaks involve breakdowns or deficiencies in water-treatment systems, they are usually signalled as waterborne by their localization in one city or district and by evidence from coliform counts of unsafe water.

Hepatitis A infections also result from the consumption of contaminated shellfish (Denis, 1974; Dismukes *et al.*, 1969; Dougherty and Altman, 1962; Gard, 1957; Mason and McLean, 1962; Roos, 1956; and Ruddy *et al.*, 1969). Much information involving shellfish has been derived from studies with enteric viruses other than the hepatitis agent. Clams (Hoff and Becker, 1969; Koff *et al.*, 1967; Liu *et al.*, 1966b), oysters (DiGirolamo *et al.*, 1970; Hedstrom and Lycke, 1964; and Metcalf and Stiles, 1965), and mussels (Bellelli and Leogrande, 1967; Bendinelli and Ruschi, 1969; and Duff, 1967) have been implicated. In water polluted with human feces, the shellfish accumulate enteric viruses (Liu *et al.*, 1967; Metcalf and Stiles, 1965; and Mitchell *et al.*, 1966), including the hepatitis virus. Humans have become infected by eating improperly cooked shellfish (DiGirolamo *et al.*, 1970; Koff and Sear, 1967; Koff *et al.*, 1967; and Mason and McLean, 1962). The shellfish themselves do not become infected (Chang *et al.*, 1971); rather, the virus is confined largely to their digestive tracts (Liu *et al.*, 1966b; Metcalf and Stiles, 1968). If the shellfish are removed to water that is not polluted, they will eventually free themselves of the virus (Liu *et al.*, 1966a; Metcalf and Stiles, 1968; and Seraichekas *et al.*, 1968).

Neither the common cold nor gastroenteritis is a reportable disease; these are probably the two most common (in the order named) human illnesses. Gastroenteritis has been called "sewage poisoning," "summer flu," and 'unspecified diarrhea." Symptoms include nausea, vomiting, and diarrhea. No single etiologic agent has been identified; comparable illnesses may be caused by *Shigella sonnei, Salmonella typhosa*, enteropathogenic *Escherichia coli*, and *Giardia lamblia*, as well as nonbacterial agents (Craun and McCabe, 1973). The "Norwalk agent" (Kapikian *et al.*, 1972) and other viruses may eventually take their places among the known etiologic agents of gastroenteritis, but some questions as to how viruses may cause gastroenteritis have not yet been answered (Blacklow *et al.*, 1972). Infants whose intestines are infected with oral poliomyelitis vaccine virus do not show the symptoms of gastroenteritis.

There have been two outbreaks of gastroenteritis in the United States (one of which led to hepatitis) in which enteric viruses were recovered from the drinking water. In Michigan, restaurant patrons who drank unchlorinated well water became ill within 30 h (Mack *et al.*, 1972). Records showed that the well water had been contaminated with coliform organisms several times during the previous 6 months. No coliforms were detected initially in a 50-ml sample of the water. After 9.46 liters (2.5 gal) were concentrated by ultracentrifugation, both *Escherichia coli* and poliovirus 2 were recovered from the sample. No salmonellae or shigellae were recovered. A second 9.46-liter sample was tested after chlorination, but neither *E. coli* nor poliovirus could be recovered. In Dade County, Fla., the same migrant labor camp that had a water-associated typhoid outbreak in February 1973 (Pfeiffer, 1973) was the site of an outbreak of hepatitis A in March 1975 (Wellings *et al.*, 1976). Samples of the chlorinated water taken at the camp nursery, rectal swabs from children in the nursery, and water from the evaporation pond all yielded echovirus. Poliovirus also was isolated from the evaporation-pond water.

The present status of hepatitis A has been summarized as follows by Craun *et al.* (1976):

> There were thirteen outbreaks of waterborne viral hepatitis, affecting 351 people during 1971-1974. Over the past several years, there has been considerable controversy regarding the existence of viruses in treated water supplies and the possible health consequences. Hepatitis A has been epidemiologically-implicated in 66 waterborne outbreaks since 1946, and the data can be examined to determine how these outbreaks occurred (Table III-5). Of the 22 outbreaks occurring in municipal systems, three resulted from either inadequate or interrupted disinfection, and five were related to the use of contaminated, untreated surface or groundwater. Half (eleven) of the outbreaks in municipal systems, however, occurred as the result of contamination of the distribution system, primarily through cross-connections and backsiphonage. There is no evidence, however, that the hepatitis A virus has been transmitted through correctly-operated, conventional water-treatment systems, except where distribution defects have been found as the source of the contamination. For the semipublic and individual systems, the use of contaminated, untreated groundwater was the important factor responsible for outbreaks of hepatitis-A.

The cited epidemiological and laboratory evidence presents some paradoxes. The virus of hepatitis A has been shown, epidemiologically, to be transmissible in water, but has not been isolated in the laboratory from water samples. Gastroenteritis is transmissible in water; however, at least some of the time the disease is not caused by virus. Clearly, more research is needed to resolve these problems.

Recovery and Identification of Viruses

FACTORS INFLUENCING RECOVERY

More than 100 different serological types of human enteric viruses may appear in wastewater (Berg, 1973). The chance that one or more of these viruses will appear in a community source of potable water is steadily increasing, as demands on available water make reuse increasingly necessary (Berg *et al.*, 1976). According to an EPA study of 155 cities that use surface-water supplies, 1 of every 30 gal that enter water-treatment plants has already passed through the wastewater system of a community that is upstream (Culp *et al.*, 1973). With the increasing use of renovated water, there is a need for methods that can detect the enteric viruses that might occur in raw or finished water.

Detection methods based on virus infectivity are more sensitive than immunochemical procedures, because more virus is needed to produce a perceptible immunochemical reaction than would ordinarily be needed to infect a cell culture. The amount of virus present in polluted surface-waters may vary over a wide range. A calculated value of 38 plaque-forming units (PFU) per gal, based on virus-shedding by children under 15 yr old, was derived from data analyzed by Clarke *et al.* (1964). A total of 330 PFU/gal was recovered from a stream receiving wastewater effluent (Grinstein *et al.*, 1970). The available data suggest that raw potable water sources, subject to pollution from wastewater discharges, may contain significant numbers of enteric viruses.

Conventional treatment of a water supply (coagulation, sedimentation, filtration, and disinfection) to produce finished water is expected to result in removal or inactivation of a minimum of 6 $\log_{10}$ of virus (Clarke, 1976). Barring gross contamination of finished water, only low numbers of viruses are likely to occur in properly treated supplies. Such small amounts of virus are likely to be detected only by highly efficient methods.

The general quality of the water is important in virus recovery. Turbidity, organic matter, pH, salts, and heavy metals all influence virus recovery. Both organic and inorganic solids suspended in water can adsorb viruses (Schaub and Sagik, 1975). In the testing of large volumes of water containing suspended solids, virus adsorption to these solids complicates the recovery process. Sample clarification that results in removal of the solids may also result in removal of virus. Deliberate use of solids for recovery of virus may not always succeed, because of failure to desorb the virus (Berg, 1973).

Organic material in water may influence the virus-recovery process by interfering with the ability of the virus to adsorb to a collecting surface (Wallis and Melnick, 1967a). The interference results in loss of the virus through penetration of the collecting surface. Organic matter can also protect the virus. Entrapment of enteric virus in fecal clumps would call for special procedures to disrupt the clumps, and thus release the virus.

Acid pH and metal cations are known to enhance adsorption of the virus to clay particles (Carlson *et al.*, 1968) and to membrane–filter surfaces (Wallis and Melnick, 1967b). Desorption of virus is favored by a pH of 9-11 and by the presence of organic substances (Cliver, 1967).

Knowledge of the influence of these factors can be used to avoid loss of the virus during sample collection, or can be applied to procedures to promote the recovery of the virus from water.

In summary, detectability of waterborne viruses is limited by: the low concentrations in which the virus occurs, the presence of interfering substances in the water, adsorption or entrapment of the naturally occurring virus, and inadequacies in the laboratory host systems (cell lines, experimental animals) in which isolation must ultimately take place.

CELL-CULTURE SYSTEMS FOR DETECTION

The types and quantities of viruses that can be detected depend on which cell cultures are used and how virus activity is manifested (plaquing versus cytopathology). Primary-monkey-kidney, or human embryonic-kidney cell cultures were originally recommended for maximal efficiency in detecting enteric viruses (Lee *et al.*, 1965). One established primate cell line (BGM) was more sensitive than primary primate cultures in detecting viruses in water (Dahling *et al.*, 1974). In another study, 31 echoviruses were recovered in human, diploid-embryonic lung cells, but not in monkey-kidney cells (Zdrazilek, 1974). A cell line that may eventually reduce the need for suckling mice in detecting cosackievirus A has been evaluated by Schmidt *et al.*(1975). Plaquing (agar overlay) and cytopathic (liquid overlay) methods in combination were recommended for isolation of as many enteric viruses as possible (Hatch and Marchetti, 1975). The

TABLE III-6 Enteric Viruses and Host Systems Required for Isolation of Virus

		Host System				
		Primate		Human		Mice[e]
Virus Group	Number	Primary[a]	Continuous[b]	Primary[c]	Continuous[d]	
Enteroviruses						
Polioviruses	3	+	+	+	±	
Coxsackievirus A[1]	23					+
Coxsackievirus B	6	+	+	+	±	
Echoviruses[2]	31	+	+	+	±	
Reoviruses	3	+	+	+	±	
Adenoviruses	31			+	±	
Hepatitis A[3]	3?					
Gastroenteritis viruses[3,4]	?					

[1]Coxsackieviruses A-7, 9, 16, and perhaps others may be isolated in cell culture systems.
[2]Human diploid-embryonic lung cultures were reported useful for isolation.
[3]No acceptable host-cell system for routine laboratory use has been developed.
[4]Identified as acute infectious nonbacterial gastroenteritis agents (AING).

[a]Primary monkey-kidney, African Green monolayers (PMK-AG).
[b]Buffalo-Green monkey-kidney monolayers (BGM).
[c]Primary human embryonic-kidney monolayers (HEK).
[d]Diploid human embryonic-lung monolayers (HEL).
[e]Swiss mice, 4 days of age or less.

Ideal host system use for maximum virus recoveries includes: (1) PMK-AG, agar and liquid enterovirus, and reovirus, overlay media; (2) HEK, agar and liquid enterovirus overlay media; (3) HEL liquid overlay medium; and (4) suckling mice.

enteric viruses and the host systems that are required to isolate them are shown in Table III-6.

The best available combination of laboratory host systems will not detect the virus of hepatitis A and will miss other viruses. Cultures that are susceptible to a given virus may differ in sensitivity, and wild strains of a virus may fail to form plaques (or to produce cytopathology in the same way) as laboratory strains.

RECOVERY PROCEDURES FOR VIRUS IN FINISHED WATER

There are extensive reviews of methods for recovering waterborne viruses (Hill *et al.*, 1971; Sobsey, 1976). Present methods seem generally adequate for recovery of enteroviruses, but perhaps not of reoviruses and adenoviruses (Fields and Metcalf, 1975).

Representative recoveries of virus from seeded water-samples are shown in Table III-7. Although there is no universal method for concentrating all enteric viruses from water, some methods are quite effective for some of the enteric viruses in some types of water. Flowthrough-filter adsorption-elution systems and ultrafiltration methods with anisotropic, polymeric membranes in tangential-flow systems are the best for recovery of small quantities of enterovirus in large volumes of treated or finished water. Virus concentration from water by adsorption to precipitable salts or polyelectrolytes, aqueous polymer two-phase separation, reverse osmosis, hydroextraction, continuous-flow ultracentrifugation, and forced-flow electrophoresis methods can generally be applied only to samples of a few liters. Therefore, they are not suited to recovery of a low number of infectious units of virus from large samples of water.

IDENTIFICATION OF VIRUSES RECOVERED FROM WATER

Serologic methods for virus identification are often based on virus infectivity. In the serum-neutralization test, infectivity is blocked by the action of a homologous antibody. Neutralization tests, using combination pools of enterovirus equine antisera, are one of the reliable ways of identifying an enterovirus isolate (Melnick *et al.*, 1973). These tests are usually completed within 48-72 h in cell cultures, after recovery of the isolate and passage in cell culture. The total time required for completion of all these procedures depends on virus growth-rates and may vary from a few days to weeks.

Immunochemical methods have been evaluated as a more rapid means of virus identification. Immunofluorescence (Katzenelson, 1976) and immunoenzymatic (Kurstak and Morisset, 1974) procedures have been tested. These procedures are based on antigen–antibody interactions whose results can be seen sooner than the visible cytopathic effects required for interpretation of serum-neutralization tests.

The concept of an indicator bacterium was discussed in some detail earlier in this report. Indicator bacteria are organisms that, although not pathogenic in themselves, are constantly present in intestinal discharges, so that their detection in the environment constitutes a signal for possible fecal pollution. Is it possible to consider certain viruses as indicator viruses? Such indicator viruses might provide a clue to the inadequacy of source-waters, or water-treatment systems, in terms of virus contamina-

TABLE III-7 Representative Virus Recoveries Cited for Methods Used to Recover Enteric Viruses from Water[1]

Recovery System	Tested	Initial Volume (liters)	Final Volume (ml)	Test Virus	Initial Virus Concentration (PFUL/l)	Virus Recovery (Percent)	References
Alginate ultrafilter	tap	10.0	1.5	P	1×10^5	66	Gartner, 1967
	tap	5.0	3.0	P2	1×10^5	40	Nupen, 1970
	various	0.1	2.0	P1	?	95–100	Foliguet *et al.*, 1973
Aluminum hydroxide	saline	1.0	1.0	P1,E7	100–200	82	Wallis and Melnick, 1967[b]
	sewage	10.0	30.0	C33	1×10^5	50	Lal and Lund, 1974
Ferric hydroxide	river	4.0	2–3[a]	P3	1–9	25–30	Schafer, 1971
PE60	tap	95–378	10.0	P1	0.26–11	74	Wallis *et al.*, 1970
	saline	1.0	5.0	T2	$17–6.5 \times 10^6$	25	Sorber *et al.*, 1972
Bentonite	sewage	1.0	10.0	P1	?	48	Moore *et al.*, 1974
Iron Oxide	tap	0.5	100.0	CA9	1×10^5	86	Rao *et al.*, 1968
Polymer two-phase	sewage	0.2	4–5	P3	2.5×10^8	99	Lund and Hedstrom, 1966
	saline	2–3	1.2–8.4	P1	0.65–200	87	Shuval *et al.*, 1969
	tap	1.0	14.0	P2	2×10^6	22	Nupen, 1970
	deionized	0.12	?	E6	170	35	Grindrod and Cliver, 1970
Ultrafiltration	distilled	38–113	50	P1	87	66	Sweet *et al.*, 1974

Reverse Osmosis	filtered tap	10–20	100–200	P1	42–1057	0–32	Sweet *et al.*, 1974
Hydroextraction	distilled	1.0	10	P1	570–5.7 × 10^4	21–51	Shuval *et al.*, 1967
Filter adsorption–elution	tap	1.0	1.0	CA9	12	24	Cliver, 1967
	sewage	3.7	4.0	P1	1 × 10^6	80	Wallis and Melnick, 1967[a]
	river	0.5	10.0	P1	62	92	Rao and Labzoftsky, 1969
	filtered tap	5.0	10.0	P1	1.6–160	64	Fattal *et al.*, 1973
	tap & estuary	378	2–3	P1	0.063–0.51	43	Hill *et al.*, 1972
	tap	567–1,134	3.0[b]	P1	0.09–180	61	Wallis *et al.*, 1972
	tap	378	10.0	P1	1–6.6	77	Sobsey *et al.*, 1973
	coastal	95	10.0	P1	9–1,200	63	Metcalf *et al.*, 1974[a]

P 1, 2, or 3 = Poliovirus 1, 2, or 3
E7 = Echovirus 7
C33 = Coxsackievirus B3
T2 = Bacteriophage (Coliform) T2
CA9 = Coxsackievirus A9
E6 = Echovirus 6

[a]Two-step procedure; second step by polymer two-phase method.
[b]Two-step procedure; second step concentration by PE60.

[1]Data shown were selected from tables appearing in *Methods for Detecting Enteric Viruses in Water and Wastewater*, pp. 138–188. Proc. International Conference on Viruses in Water, Mexico City, 1974. American Public Health Association, Washington, D.C. 1976.

tion or removal, and hence could be useful in the control of waterborne virus disease.

If a rapid serologic-identification test were available, it might be adaptable to detection of some indicator virus whose presence has correlated with that of other enteric viruses. The polioviruses (which are common in wastewater and easy to detect) have been proposed as indicators of other enteric viruses that are more difficult or impossible to detect by laboratory methods. A rapid immunochemical method for detecting polioviruses might be attainable, but this does not validate the use of polioviruses as indicators. Although polioviruses are the most common group of enteric viruses recovered from polluted waters, they are not always predominant or even present among the enteric viruses in field samples (Grinstein *et al.*, 1970; Metcalf *et al.*, 1974b). Because recovery methods are essentially the same, whether for polioviruses or for all the enteric viruses, there is little to be gained by adopting such an indicator virus now.

SENSITIVITY OF THE FLOWTHROUGH METHOD

Laboratory-based trials of flowthrough equipment and methods, using at least 100 gal of tapwater experimentally contaminated with poliovirus, regularly yielded positive results from 500-gal samples that contained 3-5 PFU/100 gal, and sometimes only 1-2 PFU/100 gal (Hill *et al.*, 1976). Members of the reovirus, echovirus, and coxsackievirus groups A and B, at inputs of 1 PFU/gal or less, were also recovered when 100 or 500 gal of water were sampled. Emphasis was placed on ability to recover small quantities of virus in large volumes of finished water. Performance at extremely low concentrations of virus was considered a better index of the merits of a method than high-percentage recoveries based on very large test doses. The success of the laboratory trials has led to inclusion of flowthrough procedures in the fourteenth edition of *Standard Methods for the Examination of Water and Wastewater* (1975) as a tentative method for finished water.

PERSPECTIVES IN TESTING LARGE-VOLUME SAMPLES

Some of the assets of the flowthrough method may also be viewed as liabilities. The portable concentrator permits the testing of large-volume samples without transporting great quantities of water to the laboratory; however, a probable consequence is that the laboratory virologist is not answerable for the validity of the field-sampling procedures. The method enables detection of as little as 1 PFU of virus in a 100-gal water sample, but the authenticity and significance of a positive test result is questionable when very few PFU are found. The method can detect only viruses for which susceptible tissue cultures or laboratory animals are available, so that the agents of hepatitis A and most viral gastroenteritides will be missed. The vaccine polioviruses have the highest overall probability of occurrence and detection, but they do not themselves constitute a threat to human health. The vaccine polioviruses, when compared to coliform organisms, may constitute a more sensitive or valid indicator of the threat of waterborne virus pathogens; however, this kind of comparison should be made only after more coliform tests have been performed on much larger samples than 100 ml. Both the flowthrough method of virus collection and larger-volume coliform tests may have a future as standard methods for discretionary, intensive testing of finished water; neither should be regarded as a routine monitoring method for on-line quality control.

Health Effects of Viruses in Drinking Water

Large numbers of enteric viruses are present in some human feces and, therefore, in wastewater. These viruses may not be completely removed or inactivated by wastewater treatment, so they may be discharged to surface water that serves as another community's raw-water source (Clarke *et al.*, 1964). If the viruses are not completely removed or inactivated by water treatment, they may be ingested. People infected by these ingested viruses do not always become ill, but disease is a possibility in persons infected with the agent of hepatitis A or any of the other enteric viruses. Several diseases involving the central nervous system, and more rarely the skin and heart, are caused by the better-characterized enteroviruses: polioviruses, coxsackieviruses, and echoviruses. Some reoviruses and parvoviruses have been implicated in nonbacterial gastroenteritides. More than 100 serotypes of enteric viruses are known and are recovered from wastewater from time to time (Davis *et al.*, 1967). Sporadic occurrences of echoviruses and coxsackieviruses in a susceptible population may result from transmission of the viruses through water, but this has yet to be proven.

Poliovirus infection by the oral route has been studied to some extent, especially in connection with the development of attenuated poliomyelitis vaccines for orally administration. The remainder of the enteric viruses have been used only to a small extent in research of this kind. In the few studies of other orally administered viruses, there was usually no attempt to determine how much virus was needed to produce infection, or even how much virus was being administered.

Some of the particles in any collection of virus are perceptibly defective. The rest apparently possess all the constituents necessary to initiate infection of a cell and, by successive replication, of a host organism; such a particle might be described as "nondefective."

A nondefective virus particle, inoculated into a culture of susceptible cells, may or may not cause an infection. Incipient infections may be aborted in one way or another, so the number of apparently nondefective particles greatly exceeds the number of tissue-culture infections they can produce. Schwerdt's (1957) ratios of particles to tissue-culture doses (the quantities of virus required to produce perceptible infections in a tissue-culture, whether the infections are perceived by cytopathic effects, plaque formation, or some other manifestation) were about 36:1 to over 100:1, whereas Joklik and Darnell (1961) reported a ratio of approximately 250:1. The latter study showed that the particles that had not succeeded in initiating infections were not defective; but the ways in which incipient infections were seen to abort would not account for an infectivity ratio as high as 250:1.

However, only one poliovirus particle ordinarily infects a cell. Thousands of nondefective, genetically identical progeny particles are produced in replication. Once a cell is infected, its neighbors in a culture are virtually certain to become involved. Nevertheless, if small numbers of nondefective particles have been inoculated at the outset, infection of a first cell is unlikely to occur.

Poliovirus infection by the oral route had to be studied during development of the "live-virus" poliomyelitis vaccines. Sabin found that nonhuman primates could not be substituted for man in such investigations, because of species differences in the relative susceptibility of the intestines to poliovirus infection. He reported that, if fewer than 10^5 tissue-culture doses of vaccine poliovirus were ingested by a human, the virus would bypass the pharynx, but would infect the intestines (1957).

Ratios of physical particles to oral, infectious doses for man, comparable with those for tissue-culture doses, have not been reported. Orally administered poliovirus doses have therefore been expressed in terms of tissue-culture doses, even though infections of these two host systems have never been shown to be analogous. Indeed, the disagreement (Bodian, 1957; Sabin, 1957) over which intestinal cells are responsible for replication of poliovirus still seems to be unresolved. Horstmann (1961) described 10^5 tissue-culture doses as "an average minimal reliable dose for most strains," and thought it remarkable that some strains would infect by the oral route when fewer than 10^4 tissue-culture doses had been ingested.

The subjects in several of the early poliomyelitis-vaccine trials were

TABLE III-8 Results of Feeding Various Quantities of Poliomyelitis Vaccine to Infants

Dose	No. Infected/ No. Fed	Percent Infected	References
PFU[a]			
0.2	0/2	0	Koprowski, 1956
2	2/3	66	Koprowski, 1956
20	4/4	100	Koprowski, 1956
5.5×10^6	16/18	89	Holguin *et al.*, 1962
TCD_{50}[b]			
$10^{3.5}$	28/97	29	Lepow *et al.*, 1962
$10^{4.5}$	42/96	46	Lepow *et al.*, 1962
$10^{5.5}$	48/84	57	Lepow *et al.*, 1962
$10^{6.6}$	12/20	60	Krugman *et al.*, 1961
$10^{7.6}$	15/20	75	Krugman *et al.*, 1961
$10^{3.5}$	208/308	68	Warren *et al.*, 1964
$10^{5.5}$	133/169	79	Warren *et al.*, 1964
1	3/10	30	Katz and Plotkin, 1967
2.5	3/9	33	Katz and Plotkin, 1967
10	2/3	67	Katz and Plotkin, 1967
$10^{5.5}$	4/8	50	Gelfand *et al.*, 1960
$10^{7.5}$	9/9	100	Gelfand *et al.*, 1960

[a]Plaque-forming units.
[b]TCD_{50} = Tissue culture dose 50%.

infants in their first few days or months of life. They included babies born to mothers who had various serum concentrations of antibody against polioviruses. The criterion of infection was the shedding of the virus in the infant's feces after 1 week. Though large amounts of virus were often administered, not all vaccinated infants became infected. The findings of several investigators are summarized in Table III-8. A study by Koprowski (1956) showed that two of three children, each fed 2 PFU of vaccine poliovirus in enteric-coated capsules, became infected. Plotkin and Katz (1967) presented data that they believe demonstrated a parity between the quantity of vaccine poliovirus needed to infect a tissue-culture and that which will infect a human subject by the oral route. Studies by others indicated a need for more than 10^4 tissue-culture doses of vaccine in infants (Gelfand *et al.*, 1961).

The available data on polioviruses have important limitations; unfortunately, far less information seems to be available concerning infectivity, by the oral route, of other intestinal viruses. The dose of coxsackievirus B5 that would infect 50% of newborn mice to which it was administered by the oral route was between 10^2 and 10^3 tissue-culture doses in studies by Loria *et al.* (1974). Their criterion of infection was disease, so they were measuring the pathogenic dose, rather than the infecting dose. No other reports of attempts to determine the minimal infecting dose of ingested human intestinal viruses seem to be available—whether for humans or other species—in terms of tissue-culture doses.

In sum, poliovirus infection at the cellular level appears to be initiated by a single nondefective particle. If the ratio of nondefective particles to infections is the same for ingested virus, this is fortuitous: the yet-to-be-identified cells in the intestines to which the particles must attach may be either more or less susceptible than tissue-culture cells, just as the susceptibility of different tissue-culture cells may vary. Counts of virus particles are not likely to be useful in this application, and some important intestinal viruses cannot be enumerated in tissue-cultures at all. There is no valid basis for establishing a no-effect concentration for viral contamination of finished drinking water.

Virus Removal in Water Treatment

When viral disease occurs in association with a drinking-water supply, one first has to consider the possibility that cross-contamination or back-siphonage may have admitted waste water into the distribution system. However, this source will not be discussed here; the integrity of water-distribution systems is a technological, rather than a virological, problem. If the integrity of a system is not maintained, the most immediate consequences are more likely to involve enteric bacteria than viruses.

Alternatively, viruses may occur in a community's raw water supply as a result of intended or inadvertent "recycling" of wastewater. If viruses are not removed or inactivated (a virus is said to be inactivated when it loses its ability to produce infection) in the treatment of the water, disease may occur among those who drink the finished product. The required degree of virus removal or inactivation cannot be stated explicitly, because of lack of good information as to how much virus must be ingested to cause disease. When goals in virus removal are considered, it is also important to remember that less than 1% of water consumed by a community is used internally by humans; more than 40 gal of water per person per day are used for household purposes (Witt *et al.*, 1975).

One would like to know what amounts of virus might occur in raw water at the point of intake. Most reports of virus in raw water are not quantitative: for example, Foliguet *et al.* (1966a) reported detecting enteroviruses in 13 of 162 raw-water samples tested in France during 1961-1963, but one cannot determine the volume of water that each sample represented. The highest virus concentrations measured at or near water intakes by Berg (1973) were somewhat less than 0.2 PFU/liter of water. Available data (Chang 1968) indicate that 30 PFU/liter constitutes a "reasonable virus load in moderately polluted water." One would hope to remove or inactivate all viruses before the treated drinking water were considered "finished."

Berg (1973) has offered to resolve this difficulty by requiring that reclaimed and other potable water be disinfected so as to destroy at least 12 logarithmic units of a reference virus at 5°C and that the finished water be tested frequently to ensure that there is not more than 1 PFU in a 100-gal (379-liter) sample of the final product. An apparatus that will accommodate such samples has been developed. Recently, 4 of 12 samples (100-105 gal, or 379-397 liters each) of finished water from a modern, well-operated plant serving 600,000 people in Fairfax County, Va. were shown to contain 1-4 PFU of poliovirus each (T.G. Metcalf, unpublished data). The public-health significance of such findings is uncertain. The infectious dose of poliovirus by the oral route is not yet known, and the detected virus was apparently of vaccine origin and therefore nonpathogenic. Any virus detected in finished drinking water may indicate that other viruses, not detectable by laboratory techniques, are also present; however, no outbreak of human illness has been associated with the water supply that was examined.

The detection of very few tissue-culture doses of virus in extremely large samples does not yet support the adoption of a numerical specification for the volume of finished water from which detectable virus must be absent, or for the projected viricidal effectiveness of a disinfection process. Safety of drinking water, from the virus standpoint, cannot at present be defined in numerical terms.

None of the unit operations and processes used today in the treatment of water supplies were devised originally to remove or destroy viruses. Still, almost all these treatments have some antiviral effect. The potential antiviral effectiveness of disinfection (chlorination) probably exceeds that of all other available treatments combined. Any treatment for which there are substantial data to indicate ability to remove at least 50% of incident-viruses will be considered here. Many of the data have been obtained from bench-scale studies with experimentally inoculated model viruses. Accurate measurement of virus removal (by a treatment being evaluated) is possible only if the initial concentrations of viruses are very high. The required concentrations of viruses would not occur naturally in water destined for human consumption (except in reclaimed wastewater), and would be difficult to attain by adding laboratory viruses to pilot-scale batches of water. Such experiments are conducted under more closely controlled conditions than may be attainable in practice, and the aggregation that is always present in virus suspensions may differ in degree between inoculated virus and naturally occurring virus. Results will not be reported here to a greater degree of precision than seems reasonable to expect in practice.

COAGULATION AND SETTLING

An early step in the treatment of raw water often includes coagulating suspended solids and allowing them to settle to the bottom of a tank. The supernatant water is then collected for further treatment. Substances added to induce coagulation may include primary flocculants (such as aluminum sulfate and ferric chloride,), coagulant aids (polyelectrolytes), acids, alkalis, and even clay used for supplemental turbidity. Four recent, extensive studies indicated that virus removal from 90% to well above 99% can be achieved by coagulation and settling under carefully controlled conditions (Foliguet and Doncoeur, 1975; Manwaring *et al.*, 1971; Schaub and Sagik, 1975; and Thorup *et al.*, 1970). Either aluminum sulfate or ferric chloride proved a good primary flocculant for virus removal. Polycationic coagulation aids were useful in removing virus, but anionic or nonionic polyelectrolytes probably would not be effective. Clays are sometimes added, to ensure formation of a visible floc to which virus may adsorb. Organic matter in the water interfered with virus removal by coagulation and settling; this effect may be prevented by prechlorination or preozonation. Finally, it should be noted that the virus removed had not been inactivated. Virus adsorbed to floc was quite capable of causing infection.

FILTRATION AND SORPTION

Virus particles are too small to be retained mechanically on sand, or on most alternate media used in water filtration. Virus retention by such media depends on association of the virus with suspended matter that is large enough to be trapped mechanically, or by direct sorption of free virus particles to the surface of the filter medium.

When sand filtration follows coagulation and settling in the treatment scheme, viruses that sorbed onto fine floc particles can be retained efficiently by sand (Foliguet and Doncoeur, 1975). Virus removal by the filter ranges from 90% to more than 99%, with the very highest figures resulting when the virus was poorly removed by previous settling of the floc. Sand, by itself, is reputed to be a poor medium for removing viruses from water (Chang, 1968). However, Lefler and Kott (1974) removed more than 99% of their model viruses by slow sand filtration when the suspending water contained calcium chloride and magnesium chloride at 0.01 N.

Diatomaceous earth has been evaluated by Brown *et al.* (1974) as a filter medium for removing viruses from water. The medium was coated with ferric hydroxide or a synthetic polymer developed for water treatment. The model virus was removed from dechlorinated tapwater (pH 9.5) to the extent of approximately 98%, but the process was less effective at a lower pH (6.7-6.8), or in the absence of coating. It is not clear whether this filtration process was intended principally to follow or to supplant the coagulation and settling-steps in water treatment.

Activated carbon is another possible sorbant medium for removing viruses. Cliver (1971) found that retention of virus on the medium could be 90% initially, but was apparently lower after a column had been operated for some time. Relatively little desorption seemed to occur when water, rather than wastewater, was treated.

The possibility of virus desorption from a filter-medium, or of resuspension of floc to which virus has adsorbed, must always be considered in evaluating treatments such as those described above. None of these treatments appears to inactivate the virus that has been retained. Indeed, if any of these treatments proves less effective in practice than was indicated in bench-scale studies, it may well be because of desorption or resuspension, rather than inadequate initial retention of virus.

WATER-SOFTENING

Softening of water at the treatment plant may inactivate virus, rather than simply remove it. Sproul (1971) summarized research in his laboratory that showed modest virus removal with straight-lime softening, and more than 99% removal with sodium hydroxide precipitation of magnesium ions, with excess lime-soda ash softening. He used the term "inactivation" to describe this removal, but he compared data from his and other laboratories which indicated that viral infectivity is lost only in some cases at a pH near 11, which occurs in excess lime-soda ash softening.

DISINFECTION

If all of the treatments described above were applied sequentially to raw water, one could expect a total of 6 logarithmic units of virus removal or destruction, without recourse to chemical disinfection. However, chemical disinfection seems to be more reliable than the other treatments. Most chemical disinfectants that are effective against viruses are strong oxidizing agents. The general principles of action of these substances on viruses have been discussed by various authors, not all of whom reached the same conclusions. Liu *et al.* (1971) emphasized differences in resistance among the groups of enteric viruses (as well as the importance of clumping of virus particles) as a source of confusion in interpreting inactivation data. Given the contact times likely to be used, these differences are probably not critical to the success of an efficient disinfectant. However, Krusé *et al.* (1971) emphasized that not all slowly effective forms of disinfectants can be made to accomplish their task by extending contact time. Treatment prior to terminal disinfection accomplishes two purposes—reducing the virus load and preparing water for more effective terminal disinfection, by removal of interfering substances.

CHLORINATION

Chlorine, applied in its elemental form or as hypochlorite, is the standard of disinfection against which others are compared. Depending on the pH of the water and on the presence of ammonia, the chlorine may take the form of HOCl, OCl^-, Cl_2, or chloramines. The viricidal effectiveness of these forms apparently decreases in the order listed.

Neefe *et al.* (1947) studied chlorine inactivation of the virus of infectious hepatitis (in drinking water that was given to human volunteers). The results were not quantitative, but they showed that, if viruses were added (as a suspension of infectious feces) to water that was then coagulated and filtered, a chlorine dose sufficient to yield a free residue of 0.4 mg/l after 30 min of contact would render the virus noninfectious for the volunteers. Nothing has been done to refute or augment these findings in the intervening period of almost 30 yr.

Clarke and Kabler (1954) showed that coxsackievirus A2 was inactivated more slowly by chlorine at a pH of 9 than at a pH of 7, and more slowly at 3-6°C than at 27-29°C. Not surprisingly, the inactivation rate also depended on the concentration of free chlorine (hypochlorous acid and hypochlorite ion). Kelly and Sanderson (1958, 1960) extended these results to other human enteroviruses and showed that the antiviral action of chloramines is a great deal slower than that of free chlorine.

Clarke *et al.* (1956) found adenovirus 3 to be more susceptible to chlorine than the enteroviruses; destruction rate of the former was said to be comparable to that of *Escherichia coli*. Liu *et al.* (1971) showed that the reoviruses were even more chlorine-sensitive than the adenoviruses, and that some of the differences in chlorine sensitivity among enteroviruses might be related to the degree of aggregation of the viruses in suspension.

The aggregation always seen in virus suspensions imposes significant limits on the predictability of virus inactivation (Sharp *et al.*, 1975).

Hypochlorous acid, which predominates below a pH of 7.5, is more active against viruses than is hypochlorite ion (Chang, 1968). When the water contains nitrogenous substances, chlorine should be added to the "breakpoint," beyond which any further added chlorine will be free to inactivate viruses (Krusé *et al.*, 1971). Chlorine dioxide (ClO_2) may offer some advantages over other forms of chlorine because it is less reactive with ammonia, and less affected by temperature and pH (Chang, 1968).

BROMINATION

Bromine has been studied (to a limited extent) as an alternative to chlorine in inactivating waterborne virus (Taylor and Johnson, 1974). It is clearly effective, and it may be somewhat less subject than chlorine to "demand" losses in use. Bromamine, for instance, is capable of significant virus inactivation. More study will be required before bromine can be considered likely to supplant chlorine as a general disinfectant. It does have advantages for some specialized uses.

IODINATION

Iodine is also capable of inactivating enteroviruses in water under controlled conditions (Berg *et al.*, 1964). Although relatively high doses may be required, Chang (1968) suggested that iodine may be useful in special situations. Studies by Olivieri *et al.* (1975) on the comparative modes of action of the halogens on a small bacterial virus (f2) indicated that iodine reacts with the coat protein, whereas chlorine probably inactivates the viral nucleic acid.

OZONATION

Ozone is finding increasing use as a water disinfectant and is proving effective against viruses. Although Majumdar *et al.* (1973) found that ozone was relatively ineffective against poliovirus when the disinfectant was present at less than 1 mg/liter, Katzenelson *et al.* (1974) found ozone to be faster and more effective than chlorine against poliovirus, even at concentrations as low as 0.3 mg/liter. Ozone does seem to offer significant advantages as an antiviral disinfectant for water. Its most conspicuous liability is that its activity cannot be sustained in the water all the way to the consumer, so that it does not provide any protection against post-treatment contamination.

Effectiveness of Water Treatments

Virus may occur in some raw water; standard treatments, such as coagulation and settling followed by rapid sand filtration (if carefully performed under practical conditions) could remove a combined total of 6 logarithmic units of virus present. Viruses removed in these ways are not inactivated.

A virus that is still present can be inactivated by chemical disinfection. Ozone and chlorine seem most clearly suited to community use for water disinfection. With raw water that sometimes contained virus, both ozone and chlorine were found to produce finished water in which viruses could not be detected by the methods used (Foliguet *et al.*, 1966b). In general, it appears that current treatment technology, diligently applied, can consistently produce finished water in which viruses are not likely to pose a threat to public health (Clarke *et al.*, 1974).

The theoretical model for virus removal or inactivation by each treatment assumes that a zero concentration of virus will never be attained. This implies that testing ever-larger samples of finished water will, in some instances, result in detection of a virus. If the presence of virus in finished water results from undertreatment of virus-contaminated raw water, treatment should be intensified (to include coagulation, settling, filtration, and chemical disinfection, such as breakpoint chlorination, if these are not already being done), and efforts should be made to alleviate the contamination of raw water.

Bacterial Indicators and Viruses in Drinking Water

It should be clear from the preceding discussion that virologic tests are not "routine" in the sense that many bacteriological methods are routine. Can bacteriological methods be of any value in ensuring the virological safety of drinking water?

Viruses differ fundamentally from bacteria in size and in biological properties. Decreases in concentrations of bacterial indicators during water treatment ought not to be expected to correlate directly with virus removal or inactivation. Competent execution of water-treatment methods ultimately determines the safety of the finished product.

In the event of a treatment break or a loss of integrity of the distribution system, the presence of excessive turbidity, coliforms, or standard plate counts will indicate the existence of an unsafe situation and a possible viral hazard. Even though these indicators are only incidentally correlated with the presence of virus in drinking water, they are important, because they will evoke remedial action. Detection of viruses themselves in drinking water will take at least 2 days, in the case of gross contamination, and 1-2 weeks under most circumstances. The results of virological tests on contaminated water are unlikely to be known before human illness occurs. Microbiological indicators may have a limited correlation with viral contamination, but they and chlorination afford more protection to public health than does any available alternative approach to routine monitoring of finished water.

Conclusions

1. The presence of infective virus in drinking water is a potential hazard to the public health, and there is no valid basis on which a no-effect concentration of viral contamination in finished drinking water might be established.

2. Continued testing for viral contamination of potable water should be carried out with the facilities and skills of a wide variety of research establishments, both inside and outside the government, and methodology for virus testing should be improved.

3. The bacteriological monitoring methods currently prescribed or recommended in this report (coliform count and standard plate count) are the best indicators available today for routine use in evaluating the presence in water of intestinal pathogens including viruses.

Research Recommendations

1. Improved methods should be developed for recovery, isolation, and enumeration of viruses from water supplies.

2. A laboratory method should be devised for detecting the virus of hepatitis A in potable water.

3. More should be learned about the etiology of viral gastroenteritis; special attention should be given to detection methods for gastroenteritis viruses that are transmissible through water.

4. The amount of virus that must be ingested in drinking water to produce infections and disease should be determined for several different enteric viruses.

5. Additional research should be conducted on the ability of various water-treatment methods to remove or inactivate viruses. Low-cost modifications to increase the reliability and effectiveness of existing methods should be sought.

PATHOGENIC PROTOZOA AND HELMINTHS

Eggs and cysts of parasitic protozoa and helminths are deposited in the environment with excreta, and may enter water supplies. Water-purification processes have not been developed on the basis of considerations related to these organisms; but, fortuitously, the introduction of flocculation, filtration, and chlorination of water have been successful in diminishing the extent to which water serves as a source of parasitic infection. Perhaps more than water treatment, sanitary sewerage systems have diminished the spread of various intestinal helminths. Eggs of these helminths are not easily killed in sewage-treatment processes (Newton *et al.*, 1948; Greenberg and Dean, 1958; World Health Organization, 1964). Since there is a tendency for helminth eggs to be concentrated in sewage sludges, there is some concern when sludges are used in agriculture (Greenberg and Dean, 1958; World Health Organization, 1964). There are specific drinking-water problems with protozoan parasites, such as *Entamoeba histolytica*, the cause of amebic dysentery and amebic hepatitis, and *Giardia lamblia*, a flagellate about whose pathogenicity there is no longer any serious doubt (Moore *et al.*, 1969; Wolfe, 1975; Wanner *et al.*, 1963; Zamcheck *et al.*, 1963; and, Brandborg *et al.*, 1967). The waterborne-disease outbreak with the largest number of cases reported to have occurred in the United States in 1974 was due to *Giardia lamblia* (Center for Disease Control, 1976a).

Attention will be focussed here on the protozoan organisms that represent a threat to human health. The intestinal helminths will be considered, especially in terms of the characteristics that make then susceptible to elimination from sewage effluents and that also make them unlikely to be found in raw or finished water.

Protozoa

Parasitic protozoa replicate in the human host, and may be responsible for severe disease. *Entamoeba histolytica* (Craig, 1934; World Health Organization, 1969) has been found to be responsible for severe outbreaks of dysentery. It is also capable of setting up chronic infections in the human host, with the eventual development of abscesses of the liver and occasionally other organs. *Giardia lamblia* is not so severe a pathogen, but is responsible for gastrointestinal disturbances, flatulence, diarrhea, and discomfort. Both these organisms are able—on occasion—to penetrate our sanitary barriers.

AMEBIASIS

During the period 1946-1970, there were five reported outbreaks of amebiasis due to *Entamoeba histolytica* transmitted by water. Four of these outbreaks were related to private distribution systems, and involved a total of 50 clinical cases. The well-studied South Bend outbreak in 1953, in which there were at least 750 infections and 30 clinical cases, with 4 fatalities, was due to sewage contamination of a private water supply to a factory (LeMaistre *et al.*, 1956). One outbreak involved a public system and accounted for 25 cases (Craun and McCabe, 1973). Before 1946, there were two major amebiasis outbreaks due to contaminated water. The well-known Chicago epidemic of 1933 was traced to cross-connections between sewage and water lines in a hotel (Bundesen *et al.*, 1936). The Mantetsu-apartment-building outbreak in 1947 (Ritchie and Davis, 1948) in Tokyo was similarly traced to sewage contamination of water due to faulty distribution systems.

FACULTATIVELY PARASITIC AMEBAE

In recent years, a relatively large number of cases of meningoencephalitis have been reported as caused by free-living, facultatively parasitic amebae of the genera *Naegleria*, *Hartmanella*, and *Acanthamoeba*. Most of these cases have been related to swimming in fresh water ponds or swimming pools. However, more recently (Baylis *et al.*, 1936; Robert and Rorke, 1973) *Naegleria fowleri* and *Acanthamoeba* sp. have been isolated from tapwater in association with cases of primary amebic meningoencephalitis. It is possible that the occurrence of these fresh water amebae will increase in surface water because of the leaching of fertilizers from agricultural lands, and the other factors that are contributing to accelerated eutrophication of ponds and lakes. Viable cysts, identified as *Naegleria* and *Hartmanella* species, have been found in 8 of 15 finished-water supplies in a survey of large-city supplies across the United States (Robert and Rorke, 1973). The cyst densities were low, about 10-15/gal. Little is known about the characteristics of the cysts and trophozoites of these organisms. It seems likely that the cysts will be at least as resistant to chlorine as those of the parasitic amebae and flagellates. Therefore, considerable emphasis must be placed on flocculation and filtration processes, in order to to remove these organisms from the waters in which they may be proliferating.

GIARDIASIS

Giardiasis is emerging as a major waterborne disease. The largest outbreak of giardiasis in the United States occurred in Rome, N.Y. (Center for Disease Control, 1975). There were 395 cases of symptomatic giardiasis identified by stool examinations in the 7-month period from November 1, 1974, to June 7, 1975. A random household survey, conducted during one week in early May 1975, identified 150 stool-positive cases of giardiasis among 1,421 persons. On the basis of the survey data, the attack rate was 10.6%, and more than 4,800 persons may have been ill; a larger number probably harbored asymptomatic infections. Ten samples of the raw water were collected with a large-volume water sampler and were fed to 10 pathogen-free beagle puppies, of which 2, fed from different samples, became infected. The Center for Disease Control's diagnostic parasitology laboratory identified one *G. lamblia* cyst in one of the water samples. The Rome water-supply system did not maintain a free chlorine residual, but used only combined residual disinfection of surface water. Information on this and other *Giardia* outbreaks is reported in Foodborne and Waterborne Disease Outbreaks, Annual Summary 1974, Center for Disease Control (1976a).

Veazie (1969) noted the occurrence of some 50,000 cases of gastroenteritis in Portland from October 1954 to March 1955. Some of these cases were attributed to infection with giardiae. A report of this outbreak appeared in the form of a letter to the editor in the *New England Journal of Medicine*, after publication of the study on the Aspen outbreak (Moore *et al.*, 1969). Waterborne outbreaks of giardiasis in the United States numbered 14 between 1969 and 1975 and involved at least 700 diagnosed cases. Of these, 12 outbreaks occurred during the period 1971-1974 (Craun 1975) and involved over 300 people. This apparent increase in incidence may be due to greater awareness on the part of physicians; much publicity was accorded to outbreaks of *Giardia* infections among tourists in Leningrad, starting in 1970. According to Schulz (1975), a questionnaire survey of 1,419 travelers to the USSR showed that 324 (23%) had acquired giardiasis. The mean time between entry into the USSR and the appearance of symptoms was 14 days, and the illness lasted 6 weeks. Leningrad was identified as the site of infection, and attack rates were highest among travelers who drank tapwater.

All the U.S. outbreaks involving municipal systems, except for a large outbreak at Aspen, Colorado, in 1965-1966, have been associated with surface-water sources where disinfection was the only treatment. At Aspen, it is apparent that wells that served as a source of water for part of the community were contaminated from old, broken sewer lines that passed close to them (Moore *et al.*, 1969).

Helminths

In the United States the most important intestinal worms that are transmitted in drinking water include *Ascaris lumbricoides*, the stomach worm; *Trichuris trichiura*, the whipworm; *Ancylostoma duodenale* and *Necator americanus*, the hookworms; and *Strongyloides stercoralis*, the threadworm. All of these are nematodes, or roundworms. The stomach worm and whipworm are transmitted directly from one host to another by their eggs, after the eggs have had an opportunity to develop outside the body; the development involves the formation of an infective larva from the embryo contained in the egg. The hookworms live in the soil, grow, and undergo two molts, until they reach a stage which is infectious to man. They usually gain entry into their new host by penetrating the skin and then wandering through the body until they mature in the intestinal tract. The threadworm, like the hookworm, produces an infective larva that invades through the skin. It has the option of passing through one or several free-living generations before producing infective larvae; therefore, it can expand the number of infective larvae derived from each egg.

In addition to the nematodes described above, there is one cestode, or flatworm, that takes up residence in the human intestinal tract when it can. This worm is *Hymenolepis nana*, the dwarf tapeworm. It is the only one of the cestodes infecting humans that has a direct life cycle; i.e., the egg serves as the infecting agent by the oral route. The larva and adult develop from the egg. The adult produces a string of proglottides, up to 200; eggs are produced in each. The gravid proglottides often rupture in the intestinal tract of the host, setting the eggs free. The eggs are immediately infective when passed in the feces.

All other important helminthic parasites of man require intermediate hosts for the development of larval stages infective to man. Except for the guinea worm, *Dracunculus medinensis*, which develops as an infective larva in the water flea, *Cyclops*, the ingestion of water is a minor factor in the spread of these parasites from host to host. *D. medinensis* is not endemic in the United States.

The eggs of the stomach worm and the whipworm measure $60 \times 45\ \mu m$ and $52 \times 23\ \mu m$, respectively. Hookworm and threadworm eggs are similar in size. The egg of the dwarf tapeworm is about $44 \times 37\ \mu m$. All of these eggs are denser than water. They are also of such a size that they can be entrapped in sewage-treatment plants and in the sand filters of water-purification plants. However, motile larvae of the hookworms and of the threadworm are capable of moving through sand filters in water-purification plants, as has been shown to be the case with a number of free-living nematodes. Like the free-living nematodes, and possibly to a greater extent because infective larvae are resistant to the environment and do not ingest food, the larvae of these parasitic worms can be expected to survive usual chlorination procedures.

All the parasites considered above are soil-transmitted parasites. It is possible that surface runoff during heavy rains can bring eggs or larvae into raw-water sources. In treatment, however, their large size practically ensures that they will be entrapped in flocculation and filtration processes. Viable hookworm and threadworm larvae, because of their mobility, might be able to traverse sand filters. Because of an enormous dilution effect, and because even the larvae tend to settle out in water, one would be hard-put to attribute a human infection with one of these parasites to a water source, other than wells polluted from the surface. One other factor should be mentioned: the worm burden acquired by a host is directly related to the number of infective eggs or larvae to which the host is exposed; there is no replication of the worms in the definitive host. Therefore, the odds against the establishment of a serious worm infection in a human via a water-distribution system are extremely high. It is unlikely that the transmission of helminthic infections via water systems is significant.

Free-living nematodes that ordinarily are found in soil are occasionally washed into river water by heavy rains, and can pass rapid sand-filtration barriers and survive chlorination. These nematodes belong to the genera *Cheilobus*, *Diplogaster*, *Trilobus*, *Aphelenchus*, *Rhabditis*, and others. They are not parasitic and pose no direct threat to man. However, they are reported to produce a gummy substance, small quantities of which confer an unpleasant taste to finished water. Besides having this characteristic, the nematodes may pose a problem in that they are resistant to chlorine; free residual chlorine at 2.5-3.0 ppm failed to immobilize them in 120 m (Chang *et al.*, 1961). Because these nematodes ingest bacteria, it is conceivable that they could serve to protect pathogenic organisms from chlorine and therefore take them to the consumer. However, the chances of this appear small, because the nematodes pass the bacteria when they are active, and shed bacteria if they molt to a sheathed (resistant) stage. As examples of actively motile nematode larvae, such as infective hookworm and *Strongyloides* larvae, these nematodes indicate the ease with which such organisms can penetrate sand filters. Statistically, however, the chances are small that water-distribution systems contribute significantly to the spread of parasitic nematode infections, or that viable free-living nematodes will carry any significant numbers of bacterial pathogens past the disinfection systems.

Water-Treatment Practices and Parasite Removal

Cysts of *Entamoeba histolytica* are resistant to high concentrations of chlorine (Brady *et al.*, 1943; Stringer *et al.*, 1975). Concentrations of chlorine required to kill cysts in raw water in 20-30 m can exceed 9 ppm, depending on pH and other conditions; certainly, residual-chlorine concentrations in water-distribution systems are not adequate. *Giardia* cysts are also not reportedly destroyed by chlorination at conventional doses and contact times. It has been stated that they will survive 0.5 ppm for 30 m. Ozone, applied at 0.5 ppm, can kill 97% to more than 99% of cysts of *E. histolytica* suspended in tapwater (Newton and Jones, 1949). Bromine is a more effective cysticide than chlorine or iodine. At a pH of 4, a bromine residue at 1.5 ppm was needed to produce 99.9% cyst mortality in 10 m. The same degree of cyst destruction was achieved by iodine residue at 5 ppm and chlorine residue at 2 ppm, respectively. High pH's decrease the cysticide activity of all three halogens (Stringer *et al.*, 1975); however, the cysts of both these protozoans are of such size that flocculation and filtration can be expected to remove them from finished water (Anderson *et al.*, 1973). The cyst of *E. histolytica* measures 10-15 μm in diameter, and that of *G. lamblia* measures 9-12 $\times$ 6-9 μm. When outbreaks of *G. lamblia* have been traced to municipal water, the system has relied on disinfection, rather than including flocculation and filtration. This suggests that mechanical means of clarifying water are important as antiparasitic measures. Because the protozoan cysts are resistant to usual residual-chlorine concentrations maintained in the distribution system, the need for filtration is emphasized. It is also important to emphasize the danger of faulty distribution systems, even when relatively high residual-chlorine concentrations are maintained; cross-connection control is essential.

Conclusions

The principal pathogenic parasites that may escape our sanitary barriers in public water supplies are the protozoa *Entamoeba histolytica* and *Giardia lamblia*. The cysts of these organisms are not completely destroyed by the usual chlorination. Most cysts, however, will be removed by sedimentation and filtration through sand. Filters should be of adequate depth, and the rates of filtration and back-flushing should be adjusted, to ensure entrapment of cysts and to prevent turnover of the filter or channeling. Proper maintenance is essential. The greatest risks will occur in water systems that use only disinfection, and in contamination of water in the distribution system by sewage from broken lines or from cross-connections. Normal residual chlorine in such circumstances cannot kill cysts.

More study is needed to define the conditions required for destruction of *Giardia lamblia* cysts; little is known of their survival.

Occasionally, facultatively parasitic amebae can pass through the treatment processes and appear in finished water. Although these amebae can produce fatal encephalitides in man, the usual route of entry is the nasal passages, while a person swims in a pool or a pond of untreated or inadequately treated fresh water. The numbers of free-living ameba cysts found in finished water are small.

Entrapment of pathogenic bacteria by parasites and other metazoa, such as free-living nematodes, may lead to protection of the bacteria from disinfection. However, it appears unlikely—on the basis of the statistics of the occurrence of such organisms in finished water, the condition of the organisms seen, and the fact that viable nematodes are continually passing bacteria through their gut—that a significant number of pathogenic organisms would survive in finished water with an adequate residual disinfectant.

SUMMARY—MICROBIOLOGY OF DRINKING WATER

The incidence of enteric disease in the United States has been reduced by effective water treatment systems, but in 1974 the Center for Disease Control reported 28 waterborne disease outbreaks and 8,413 cases. In 1975 there were 24 outbreaks and 10,879 cases.

Very few of these outbreaks were caused by chemical poisoning. Most cases (6,832 or 81%) in 1974 were caused by microorganisms. The category designated "acute gastrointestinal illness" accounted for the largest number of cases (9,760) in 1975. These cases were characterized by symtoms for which no etiologic agent was identified. They account for approximately 90% of the total cases reported by the Center for Disease Control in 1975. Microorganisms account for most of the remaining cases.

Improved detection and reporting systems are needed to determine more accurately the incidence of waterborne diseases nationwide. Outbreaks occur that are not reported. The etiologic agent was not identified in 15% of the cases reported in 1974, and 90% of those reported in 1975. Improved alarm systems are needed.

In 1971-1974, deficiencies in treatment, such as inadequate or interrupted chlorination and contamination of groundwater, were responsible for a majority (65%) of the waterborne-disease outbreaks. In 1975, treatment deficiencies were responsible for most outbreaks; however, deficiencies in the distribution systems were responsible for the highest number of cases.

Bacteria

The control of waterborne epidemics still depends largely upon the control of infectious enteric diseases. Much of the success in this regard can be attributed directly to the use of chlorine as a disinfectant. Although the excessive use of chlorine in water treatment may result in the formation of several compounds that are known carcinogens for animals, and suspected carcinogens for humans, the advantages far outweigh this limitation.

Several substitutes for chlorine (e.g. ozone, chlorine dioxide, bromine, and iodine) that are also powerful oxidants and disinfectants have been suggested, but much more research is required before any of them can be recommended as a sole substitute for chlorine in water treatment. Questions concerning disinfection effectiveness, toxicity of by-products, and residual in the distribution system must be answered for proposed substitutes as well as for chlorine. It may be possible to reduce the concentrations of undesirable organic by-products of chlorination—without compromising disinfection—by changing the sequence or rate of chlorine addition in relation to other steps in water treatment. Partial use of other oxidizing agents, before chlorination, may also help to modify organic matter before significant amounts of chlorinated derivatives can be formed.

Good engineering and public health practices emphasize the need for using raw water of the highest possible quality. Bacteriological testing, or the imposition of bacteriological standards, are adjuncts to, not substitutes for, good–quality raw water, proper water treatment, and integrity of the distribution system. Application of the present coliform standards appears adequate to protect public health when raw water is obtained from a protected source, is appropriately treated, and is distributed in a contamination-free system.

Current coliform standards are not satisfactory for water reclaimed directly from wastewater. The meeting of current coliform standards is insufficient to protect public health for water reclaimed directly from waste water, or for water containing several percent of fresh sewage effluent. For such raw-water supplies, standards for viable virus content,

Clostridium content, or total bacterial count should be developed and applied as a supplement to coliform standards.

The standard plate count is not a substitute for total coliform measurements of the sanitary quality of potable water; it is, however, a valuable procedure for assessing the bacterial quality of drinking water. Ideally, standard plate counts (SPC) should be performed on samples taken throughout the systems. The SPC has major health significance for surface-water systems that do not use flocculation, sedimentation, filtration, and chlorination, and for those groundwater systems that do not include chlorination.

Viruses

The bacteriological monitoring methods currently prescribed (coliform count, standard plate count) are the best indicators available today for routine use in determining the probable levels of viruses in drinking water. The best available water treatment technology, if diligently applied, should provide a high degree of assurance that viruses injurious to human health are absent from finished drinking water. However, because knowledge of the scale of potential viral contamination is scanty, and because there is no rigorous basis for establishing a harmless level of viral concentration in water, research on the problems of viral contamination should be strongly supported. In particular, the following subjects deserve special attention:

1. Methods for testing of potable water for viral contamination.
2. Methods for recovery, isolation, and evaluation of viruses (especially hepatitis A).
3. Specific etiology of viral gastroenteritis.
4. Methods for evaluating and improving effectiveness of present water treatments to remove or inactivate viruses.
5. The amount of virus that must be ingested to produce infections and disease should be determined for several different enteric viruses.

Parasites

The most important waterborne parasitic diseases in the United States are amoebiasis and giardiasis. Outbreaks of amoebiasis appear to have resulted from sewage contamination in the distribution systems. Giardiasis, which in recent years has become a major problem in some areas, appears to be associated with inadequately treated surface waters.

The cysts of both of these parasites are more resistant to chlorine than are bacteria, but flocculation and filtration can remove them. Nevertheless, knowledge of the vulnerability of all of these organisms to disinfection is incomplete, and, in particular, the conditions necessary for destruction of Giardia cysts require further study. The same considerations apply to a few other parasitic protozoa that, although rare, have been identified in public water systems.

Metazoan parasites (helminths, nematodes) that can be present in raw water will be controlled in public water supplies by well-regulated flocculation, filtration, and disinfection.

Testing

One of the greatest deficiencies of customary methods for evaluating the bacteriological quality of water is that results from tests are unknown until after the sampled water has already entered the distribution system and been used. Successful regulation of the microbiological quality of drinking water therefore depends on the use of raw water supplies of relatively invariant high quality. Sudden invasions of contamination are unlikely to be detected promptly enough to prevent exposure and, in addition, may overwhelm the corrective treatments.

Nevertheless, it is essential that present methods of microbiological testing be continued, in order to validate the effectiveness of disinfection, and for detecting defects within the system.

REFERENCES

Ahmed, Z., I.A. Poshini, and M.A. Siddiqui. 1967. Bacteriological examination of drinking water of Karachi and isolation of enteric pathogens. Pakistan J. Sci. Ind. Res. 7:103-110.

Allen, M.J., and E.E. Geldreich. 1975. Bacteriological criteria for groundwater quality. Ground Water 13:45-52.

Anderson, K., A. Jamieson, J.B. Jadin, and E. Willaert. 1973. Primary amoebic meningeoencephalitis. Lancet 1:672.

Anonymous. 1957. Infectious hepatitis in Delhi (1955-56): A critical study. Ind. J. Med. Res. 45(Suppl.). 155 pp.

Baylis, J.R., O. Gullans, and B.K. Spector. 1936. The efficiency of rapid sand filters in removing cysts of amoebic dysentery organisms from water. Public Health Rep. 51:1567-1575.

Bell, J.B., and J.M. Vanderpost. 1973. Comparion of membrane filtration methods in the isolation of "coliforms." Proc. 16th Conf. Great Lakes Res., pp. 15-20. International Association for Great Lakes Research. Braun-Bromfield, Ann Arbor.

Bellelli, E., and G. Leogrande. 1967. Ricerche batteriologiche e virologiche sui mitili. Ann. Sclavo 9:820-828.

Bendinelli, M., and A. Ruschi. 1969. Isolation of human enterovirus from mussels. Appl. Microbiol. 18:531-532.

Berg, G. 1973. Reassessment of the virus problem in sewage and in surface and renovated waters. *In* S.H. Jenkins, ed. Progress in Water Technology, Vol. 3, pp 87-94. Pergamon, Oxford.

Berg, G., H.L. Bodily, E.H. Lennette, J.L. Melnick, and T.G. Metcalf. 1976. Viruses in Water. Proceedings of the International Conference on Viruses in Water, Mexico City, 1974. American Public Health Association, Washington, D.C.

Berg, G., S.L. Chang, and E.K. Harris. 1964. Devitalization of microorganisms by iodine. 1. Dynamics of the devitalization of enteroviruses by elemental iodine. Virology 22:469-481.

Blacklow, N.R., R. Dolin, D.S. Fedson, H. Dupont, R.S. Northrup, R.B. Hornick, and R.M. Chanock. 1972. Acute infectious nonbacterial gastroenteritis: etiology and pathogenesis. Ann. Intern. Med. 76:993-1008.

Bodian, D. 1957. Mechanisms of infection with polioviruses. *In* Cellular biology, nucleic acids and viruses, Vol. 5, pp. 57-72. Special Publications of the New York Academy of Sciences.

Boring, J.R., III, W.T. Martin, and L.M. Elliott. 1971. Isolation of Salmonella typhimurium from municipal water, Riverside, Calif., 1965. Am. J. Epidemiol. 93:49-54.

Brady, F.J., M.F. Jones, and W.L. Newton. 1943. The effect of chlorination of water on viability of cysts of Entamoeba histolytica. War Med. 3:409-419.

Brandborg, L.L., C.B. Tankersley, S. Gottlieb, M. Barancik, and V.E. Sartor. 1967. Histological demonstration of mucosal invasion by Giardia lamblia in man. Gastroenterology 52:143-150.

Brown, T.S., J.F. Malina, Jr., B.D. Moore, and B.P. Sagik. 1974. Virus removal by diatomaceous earth filtration. *In* J.F. Malina, Jr., and B.P. Sagik, eds. Virus Survival in Water and Wastewater Systems, pp. 129-144. Center for Research in Water Resources, University of Texas at Austin.

Buchanan, R.E., and N.E. Gibbons, eds. 1974. Bergey's Manual of Determinative Bacteriology, 8th ed. Williams & Wilkins, Inc., Baltimore.

Bundesen, H.N., J.I. Connolly, I.D. Rawlings, A.E. Gorman, G.W. McCoy, and A.V. Hardy. 1936. Epidemic amebic dysentery. Nat. Inst. Health Bull. no. 166. 187 pp.

Butterfield, C.T., E. Wattie, S. Megregian, and C.W. Chambers. 1943. Influence of pH and temperature on the survival of coliforms and enteric pathogens when exposed to free chlorine. Public Health Rep. 58:1837-1866.

Butterfield, C.T., and E. Wattie. 1946. Influence of pH and temperature on the survival of coliforms and enteric pathogens when exposed to chloramine. Public Health Rep. 61:157-192.

Cady, P., and S.W. Dufour. 1974. Automated detection of microorganism metabolism and growth by impedance measurements. Abstracts, 74th Meeting of the American Society for Microbiology, Chicago, Ill. No. E. 43.

Carlson, G.F., Jr., F.E. Woodard, D.F. Wentworth, and O.J. Sproul. 1968. Virus inactivation on clay particles in natural waters. J. Water Pollut. Control Fed. 40:R89-106.

Cash, R.A., S.I. Music, J.P. Libonati, M.J. Snyder, R.P. Wenzel, and R.B. Hornick. 1974. Response of man to infection with Vibrio cholerae. I. Clinical, serologic and bacteriologic responses to a known inoculum. J. Infect. Dis. 129:45-52.

Caverly, C.S. 1896. Notes of an epidemic of acute anterior poliomyelitis. J. Am. Med. Assoc. 26:1-5.

Center for Disease Control. 1973. Morbidity and Mortality Weekly Report 22:217. U.S. Department of Health, Education and Welfare, Atlanta, Ga.

Center for Disease Control. 1974. Morbidity, and Mortality in the United States. Vol. 23 No. 53. Year ending Dec. 28. U.S. Department of Health, Education and Welfare, Atlanta, Ga.

Center for Disease Control. 1975. Giardiasis—In residents of Rome, New York and in U.S. travelers to the Soviet Union. Morbidity and Mortality Weekly Report 24(43):366, 371. U.S. Department of Health, Education and Welfare, Atlanta, Ga.

Center for Disease Control. 1976a. Foodborne and Waterborne Disease Outbreaks, Annual Summary 1974. Publication no. (CDC) 76-8185. U.S. Department of Health, Education and Welfare. Atlanta, Ga.

Center for Disease Control. 1976b. Foodborne and Waterborne Disease Outbreaks, Annual Summary 1975. Publication no. (CDC) 76-8185. U.S. Department of Health, Education and Welfare. Atlanta, Ga.

Chang, P.W., O.C. Liu, L.T. Miller, and S.M. Li. 1971. Multiplication of human enteroviruses in northern quahogs. Proc. Soc. Exp. Biol. Med. 136:1380-1384.

Chang, S.L. 1961. Viruses, amebas and nematodes and public water supplies. J. Am. Water Works Assoc. 53:288-296.

Chang, S.L. 1968. Water borne viral infections and their prevention. Bull. WHO 38:401-414.

Chang, S.L., G. Berg, N.A. Clarke, and P.W. Kabler. 1960. Survival and protection against chlorination of human enteric pathogens in free-living nematodes isolated from water supplies. Am. J. Trop. Med. Hyg. 9:136-142.

Chang, S.L., R.L. Woodward, and P.W. Kabler. 1960. Survey of free-living nematodes and amebas in municipal supplies. J. Am. Water Works Assn. 52:613-168.

Clarke, N.A. 1976. Personal Communication with T.G. Metcalf.

Clarke, N.A. and P.W. Kabler. 1954. Inactivation of purified Coxsackie virus in water by chlorine. Am. J. Hyg. 59:119-127.

Clarke, N.A., R.E. Stevenson, and P.W. Kabler. 1956. The inactivation of purified type 3 adenovirus in water by chlorine. Am. J. Hyg. 64:314-319.

Clarke, N.A., E.W. Akin, O.C. Liu, J.C. Hoff, W.F. Hill, Jr., D.A. Brashear, and W. Jakubowski. 1975. Virus study for drinking-water supplies. J. Am. Water Works Assoc. 67:192-197.

Clarke, N.A., G. Berg, P.K. Kabler, and S.L. Chang. 1964. Human enteric viruses in water: Source, survival and removability. Proceedings of the International Conference, London, 1962. Adv. Water Pollut. Res. 2:523-536.

Clarke, N.A., W.F. Hill, Jr., and W. Jakubowski. 1974. Detection of viruses in water: Tentative standard method. Proceedings, Second Annual Water Technology Conference, American Water Works Association, December 1-4, 1974, Dallas, Texas.

Cliver, D.O. 1967. Enterovirus detection by membrane chromatography. *In* G. Berg, ed. Transmission of Viruses by the Water Route, pp. 139-141. Interscience, New York.

Cliver, D.O. 1971. Viruses in water and wastewater: Effects of some treatment methods. *In* V. Snoeyink and V. Griffin, eds. Virus and Water Quality: Occurrence and Control, Proceedings of the Thirteenth Water Quality Conference, vol. 69, no. 1, pp. 149-157. University of Illinois Bulletin, Urbana.

Colwell, R. R., and F. M. Hetrick. 1976. Annual Report, Office of Naval Research. *In* A.L.H. Gameson, ed. Discharge of Sewage from Sea Outfalls. Proc. Symp. August 27 - Sept. 2, 1974. Pergamon Press. 455 pp.

Committee on the ECHO Viruses. 1955. Enteric cytopathogenic human orphan (ECHO) viruses. Science 122:1187-1188.

Committee on the Enteroviruses. 1957. The enteroviruses. Am. J. Public Health 47:1556-1566.

Committee on the Enteroviruses. 1962. Classification of human enteroviruses. Virology 16:501-504.

Cowan, S.T. 1974. Enterobacteriaceae. *In* R.E. Buchanan and N.E. Gibbons, eds. Bergey's Manual of Determinative Bacteriology, 8th ed., pp. 290-293. Williams & Wilkins, Baltimore.

Craig, C.F. 1934. Amebiasis and Amebic Dysentery. Charles C Thomas, Springfield, Ill. 315 pp.

Craun, G.F. 1975. Microbiology—Waterborne outbreaks. J. Water Poll. Control Fed. 47:1566-1581.

Craun, G.F., and L.J. McCabe. 1973. Review of the causes of waterborne-disease outbreaks. J. Am. Water Works Assoc. 65:74-84.

Craun, G.F., L.J. McCabe and J.M. Hughes. 1976. Waterborne Disease Outbreaks in the U.S. 1971-1974. J. Am. Water Works Assoc. 68:420-424.

Culp, G.L., R.L. Culp, and C.L. Hamann. 1973. Water resource preservation by planned recycling of treated wastewater. J. Am. Water Works Assoc. 65:641-647.

Dahling, D.R., G. Berg, and D. Berman. 1974. BGM, a continuous cell line more sensitive than primary rhesus and African green kidney cells for the recovery of viruses from water. Health Lab. Sci. 11:275-282.

Dalldorf, G., and G.M. Sickles. 1948. Unidentified, filterable agent isolated from the feces of children with paralysis. Science 108:61-62.

Danielsson, D. 1965. A membrane filter method for the demonstration of bacteria by fluorescent antibody technique. 1. A methodological study. Acta Pathol. Microbiol. Scand. 63:597-603.

Davis, B.D., R. Dulbecco, H.N. Eisen, H.S. Ginsberg, and W.B. Wood. 1967. Microbiology. Harper and Row, New York. 1464 pp.

Denis, F. 1974. Les virus pathogenes pour l'homme dans les eaux de mer et dans les mollusques: Survie-Recherche-Bilan. Med. Mal. Infect. 4-6 bis:325-334.

DeBlanc, H.J., Jr., F. DeLand, and H.N. Wagner, Jr. 1971. Automated radiometric detection of bacteria in 2967 blood cultures. Appl. Microbiol. 22:846-849.

Di Girolamo, R., J. Liston, and J.R. Matches. 1970. Survival of virus in chilled, frozen and processed oysters. Appl. Microbiol. 20:58-63.

Dismukes, W.E., A.L. Bisno, S. Katz, and R.F. Johnson. 1969. An outbreak of gastroenteritis and infectious hepatitis attributed to raw clams. Am. J. Epidemiol. 89:555-561.

Dolivo-Dobrovolskiy, L.B., and V.S. Rossovskaya. 1956. The problem of the survival of dysentery bacteria in reservoir water. Gig. Sanit. 1956(6): 52-55. Cited in Biol. Abstr. 34: 13898 (1958).

Dougherty, W.J., and R. Altman. 1962. Viral hepatitis in New Jersey 1960-1961. Am. J. Med. 32:704-716.

Duff, M.F. 1967. The uptake of enteroviruses by the New Zealand marine blue mussel Mytilus edulis aoteanus. Am. J. Epidemiol. 85:486-493.

Dulbecco, R. 1952. Production of plaques in monolayer tissue cultures by single particles of an animal virus. Proc. Nat. Acad. Sci. USA 38:747-752.

Dulbecco, R., and M. Vogt. 1954. Plaque formation, and isolation of pure lines with poliomyelitis viruses. J. Exp. Med. 99:167-182.

Dunlop, S.G., R.M. Twedt, and W.L.L. Wang. 1952. Quantitative estimation of Salmonella in irrigation water. Sewage Ind. Wastes 24:1015-1020.

Dutka, B.J. 1973. Coliforms are an inadequate index of water quality. J. Environ. Health 36:39-46.

DuPont, H.L., S.B. Formal, R.B. Hornick, M.J. Snyder., J.P. Libonati, D.G. Sheahad, E.H. LaBrec, and J.P. Kalas. 1971. Pathogenesis of Escherichia coli diarrhea. New Engl. J. Med. 285:1-9.

DuPont, H.L., R.B. Hornick, A.T. Dawkins, M.J. Snyder, and S.B. Formal. 1969. The response of man to virulent Shigella flexneri 2a. J. Infect. Dis. 119:296-299.

DuPont, H.L., R.B. Hornick, M.J. Snyder, J.P. Libonati, S.B. Formal, and E.J. Gangarosa. 1972a. Immunity to shigellosis. I. Response of man to attenuated strains of Shigella. J. Infect. Dis. 125:5-11.

DuPont, H.L., R.B. Hornick, M.J. Snyder, J.P. Libonati, S.B. Formal, and E.J. Gangarosa. 1972b. Immunity in shigellosis. II. Protection induced by oral live vaccine or primary infection. J. Infect. Dis. 125:12-16.

Edwards, P.R., and W.H. Ewing. 1972. Identification of Enterobacteriaceae, 3rd ed. Burgess Publishing Co., Minneapolis.

Enders, J.F., T.H. Weller, and F.C. Robbins. 1949. Cultivation of Lansing strain of poliomyelitis virus in cultures of various human embryonic tissue. Science 109:85-87.

England, B., R.E. Leach, B. Adame, and R. Shiosaki. 1967. Virologic assessment of sewage treatment at Santee, California. *In* G. Berg, ed. Transmission of Viruses by the Water Route, pp. 401-417. Interscience, New York.

Ewing, W.H., and W.J. Martin. 1974. Enterobacteriaceae. *In* E.H. Lennette, E.H. Spaulding, and J.P. Truant, eds. Manual of clinical microbiology, pp. 189-221. American Society for Microbiology, Washington, D.C.

Ewing, W.H., R. Hugh, and J.G. Johnson. 1961. Studies on the Aeromonas group. U.S Department of Health, Education, and Welfare Public Health Service. Communicable Disease Center, Atlanta, Ga.

Fattal, B., E. Katzenelson, M. Nevo, and H.I. Shuval. 1973. Evaluation of different methods for the detection and concentration of small quantities of viruses in water. Proc. Fourth Scientific Conference, Israel Ecological Soc., Tel-Aviv, April 8-9, pp. A49-A69.

Favero, M.S. and C.H. Drake. 1964. Comparative study of microbial flora of iodinated and chlorinated pools. Public Health Rep. 79:251-257.

Fenner, F., B.R. McAuslan, C.A. Mims, J. Sambrook, and D.O. White. 1974. The Biology of Animal Viruses, 2nd ed. Academic Press, New York.

Fields, H.A., and T.G. Metcalf. 1975. Concentration of adenovirus from seawater. Water Res. 9:357-364.

Foliguet, J.M., and F. Doncoeur. 1975. Elimination des enterovirus au cours du traitement des eaux d'alimentation par coagulation-flocculation-filtration. Water Res. 9:953-961.

Foliguet, J.M., J. Lavillaureix, and L. Schwartzbrod. 1973. Viruses and water. II. General review of the methods available to detect viruses in water. Rev. Epidemiol. Med. Soc. Sante Publ. 21:185-259.

Foliguet, J.M., L. Schwartzbrod, and O.G. Gaudin. 1966a. La recherche des virus dans les eaux d'egout, de surface et d'alimentation en Meurthe-et-Moselle. II. Resultats quantitatifs et qualificatifs definitifs. Rev. Hyg. Med. Soc. 14:411-432.

Foliguet, J.M., L. Schwartzbrod, and O.G. Gaudin. 1966b. La pollution virale des eaux usees, de surface et d'alimentation; etude effectuee dans le departement francais de Meurthe-et-Moselle. Bull. WHO 35:737-749.

Gallagher, T.P., and D.F. Spino. 1968. The significance of numbers of coliform bacteria as an indicator of enteric pathogens. Water Res. 2:169-175.

Gard, S. 1957. General discussion. *In* F.W. Hartman, G.A. LoGrippo, J.G. Mateer, and J. Barron, eds. Hepatitis Frontiers, pp. 241-243. Little, Brown & Co. Boston.

Gartner, H. 1967. Retention and recovery of polioviruses on a soluble ultrafilter. *In* G. Berg, ed. Transmission of Viruses by the Water Route, pp. 121-127. Interscience Publishers, New York.

Geldreich, E.E. 1968. Literature review. Microbiology. J. Water Pollut. Control Fed. 40:1052-1068.

Geldreich, E.E. 1969. Literature review. Bacterial pathogen detection in water. J. Water Pollut. Control Fed. 41:1054.

Geldreich, E.E. 1970a. Applying bacteriological parameters to recreational water quality. J. Am. Water Works Assoc. 62:113-120.

Geldreich, E.E. 1970b. Literature review. Bacterial pathogen detection in water. J. Water Pollut. Control Fed. 42:1060-1062.

Geldreich, E.E. 1973. Is the total count necessary? Proc. Am. Water Works Assoc. Water Quality Technology Conference, pp. VII-1–VII-11, Cincinnati (Dec. 3-4, 1973).

Geldreich, E.E. 1975. Handbook for evaluating water bacteriology laboratories. Water Supply Research Laboratory, Cincinnati, Ohio. U.S. Environmental Protection Agency EPA-670/9-75-006:135-158.

Geldreich, E.E., H.D. Nash, D.J. Reasoner, and R.H. Taylor. 1972. The necessity of controlling bacterial populations in potable waters: Community water supply. J. Am. Water Works Assoc. 64:596-602.

Gelfand, H.M., D.R. LeBlanc, A.H. Holguin, and J.P. Fox. 1960. Preliminary report on susceptibility of newborn infants to infection with poliovirus strains of attenuated virus vaccine. *In* Second International Conference on Live Poliovirus Vaccines, pp. 308-314. Scientific Publication no. 50. Pan American Health Organization, Washington, D.C.

Gelfand, H.M., D.R. LeBlanc, J.P. Fox, and A. H. Holguin. 1961. The susceptibility of infants to infection with natural ("wild") and attenuated (vaccine) strains of polioviruses. *In* Poliomyelitis: Papers and Discussions Presented at the Fifth International Poliomyelitis Conference, Copenhagen, Denmark, July 26-28, 1960, pp. 285-289. Lippincott, Philadelphia.

Ginsburg, W. 1973. Improved total count techniques. *In* Proc. Am. Water Works Assoc. Water Quality Technology Conference, pp. VIII-I–VIII-8, Cincinnati (Dec. 3-4, 1973).

Ginsburg, W., B. Crawford, and J.J. Knipper. 1972. Filter-fluorescent antibody technique for rapid screening of indicator organisms. J. Am. Water Works Assoc. 64:499-505.

Greenberg, A.E. and B. H. Dean. 1958. The beef tapeworm, measly beef and sewage—A review. Sewage Ind. Wastes 30(3):262-269.

Grindrod, J. and D.O. Cliver. 1970. A polymer two-phase system adapted to virus detection. Archiv Ges. Virusforsch. 31:365-372.

Grinstein, S., J.L. Melnick, and C. Wallis. 1970. Virus isolations from sewage and from a stream receiving effluents of sewage treatment plants. Bull. WHO 42:291-296.

Harmon, P.H. 1937. The use of chemicals as nasal sprays in the prophylaxis of poliomyelitis in man. J. Am. Med. Assoc. 109:1061.

Hatch, M.H., and G.E. Marchetti. 1975. A comparative study of agar overlay and standard tissue culture methods for isolation of enteroviruses. Public Health Rep. 90:29-33.

Hedstrom, C.E., and E. Lycke. 1964. An experimental study on oysters as virus carriers. Am. J. Hyg. 79:134-142.

Hill, W.F., Jr., E.W. Akin, and W.H. Benton. 1971. Detection of Viruses in Water: A review of Methods and Application. *In* V. Snoeyink and V Griffin, ed. Virus and Water Quality: Occurrence and Control. Proceedings of the Thirteenth Water Quality Conference, vol. 69, no. 1, pp. 17-46. University of Illinois Bulletin, Urbana.

Hill, W.F., Jr., E.W. Akin, W.H. Benton, and T. G. Metcalf. 1972. Virus in water. II. Evaluation of membrane cartridge filters for recovering low multiplicities of poliovirus from water. Appl. Microbiol. 23:880-888.

Hill, W.F., Jr., W. Jakubowski, W.E. Akin, and N.A. Clarke. 1976. Detection of virus in water: Sensitivity of the tentative standard method for drinking water. Appl. Environ. Microbiol. 31:254-261.

Hoff, J.C., and R.C. Becker. 1969. The accumulation and elimination of crude and clarified poliovirus suspensions by shellfish. Am. J. Epidemiol. 90:53-61.

Holguin, A.H., J.S. Reeves, and H.M. Gelfand. 1962. Immunization of infants with the Sabin oral poliovirus vaccine. Am. J. Public Health 52:600-610.

Hornick, R.B., S.E. Greisman, T.E. Woodward, H.L. DuPont, A.T. Dawkins, and M.J. Snyder. 1970. Typhoid fever: pathogenesis and immunologic control. New Engl. J. Med. 283:686-691.

Horsfall, F.L., and I. Tamm. 1965. Viral and Rickettsial Infections of Man. Lippincott, Philadelphia. pp. 574.

Horstmann, D.M. 1961. Factors affecting optimum dosage levels of live poliovirus vaccines. *In* Poliomyelitis: Papers and Discussions Presented at the Fifth International Poliomyelitis Conference, Copenhagen, Denmark, July 26-28, 1960, pp. 304-310. Lippincott, Philadelphia.

Joklik, W.K., and J.E. Darnell, Jr. 1961. The adsorption and early fate of purified poliovirus in HeLa cells. Virology 13:439-447.

Jordan, H.E. 1937. Editorial statement—The coliform group of bacteria. J. Am. Water Works Assoc. 29:1999-2000.

Kapikian, A.Z., R.G. Wyatt, R. Dolin, T.S. Thornhill, A.R. Kalica, and R.M. Chanock. 1972. Visualization by immune electron microscopy of a 27-nm particle associated with acute infectious nonbacterial gastroenteritis. J. Virol. 10:1075-1081.

Katz, M., and S.A. Plotkin. 1967. Minimal infective dose of attenuated poliovirus for man. Am. J. Public Health 57:1837-1840.

Katzenelson, E. 1976. Virologic and engineering problems in monitoring viruses in water. *In* Viruses in Water. Proceedings of the International conference on Viruses in Water, pp. 152-164. Mexico City, 1974, American Public Health Association, Washington, D.C.

Katzenelson, E., B. Kletter, H. Schechter, and H.I. Shuval. 1974. Inactivation of viruses and bacteria by ozone. *In* A.J. Rubin, ed. Chemistry of Water Supply, Treatment and Distribution, pp. 409-421. Ann Arbor Science Publishers, Ann Arbor, Mich.

Kehr, R.W., and C.T. Butterfield. 1943. Notes on the relation between coliforms and enteric pathogens. Public Health Rep. 58:589-607.

Kelly, S., and W.W. Sanderson. 1958. The effect of chlorine in water on enteric viruses. Am. J. Public Health 48:1323-1334.

Kelly, S.M., and W.W. Sanderson. 1960. The effect of chlorine in water on enteric viruses. II. The effect of combined chlorine on poliomyelitis and Coxsackie viruses. Am. J. Public Health 50:14-20.

Klein, D.A., and S. Wu. 1974. Stress: A factor to be considered in heterotrophic microorganism enumeration from aquatic environments. Appl. Microbiol. 27:429-431.

Klein, M. 1966. Adenovirus. *In* J.E. Prier, ed. Basic Medical Virology, pp. 385-402. Williams & Wilkins Co., Baltimore.

Kling, C. 1929. Recherches sur l'epidemiologie de la poliomyelitis. Svenska Laksallsk. Handl. 55:23-48.

Koff, R.S. and H.S. Sear. 1967. Internal temperature of steamed clams. New Engl. J. Med. 276:737-739.

Koff, R.S., G.F. Grady, T.C. Chalmers, J.W. Mosley, B.L. Swartz, and the Boston Interhospital Liver Group. 1967. Viral hepatitis in a group of Boston hospitals. III. Importance of exposure to shellfish in a non-epidemic period. New Engl. J. Med. 276:703-710.

Koprowski, H. 1956. Immunization against poliomyelitis with living attenuated virus. Am. J. Trop. Med. Hyg. 5:440-452.

Krugman, S., J. Warren, M.S. Eiger, P.H. Berman, R.M. Michaels, and A.B. Sabin. 1961. Immunization with live attenuated poliovirus vaccine. Am. J. Dis. Child. 101:23-29.

Krusé, C.W., V.P. Olivieri, and K. Kawata. 1971. The enhancement of viral inactivation of halogens. *In* V. Snoeyink and V. Griffin, eds. Virus and Water Quality: Occurrence and Control. Proceedings of the Thirteenth Water Quality Conference, vol. 69, no. 1, pp 197-209. University of Illinois Bulletin, Urbana.

Kurstak, E., and R. Morisset. eds. 1974. Viral Immunodiagnosis. Academic Press, New York.

Lal, S.M., and E. Lund. 1976. Recovery of virus by chemical precipitation followed by elution. *In* Proceedings of the Seventh International Conference on Water Pollution Research, Paris, 1974, vol. 1, pp. 687-693. (Technical Papers, S.H. Jenkins, ed.) Pergamon, New York.

Lee, L.H., C.A. Phillips, M.A. South, J.L. Melnick, and M.D. Yow. 1965. Enteric virus isolation in different cell cultures. Bull. WHO 32:657-663.

Lefler, E., and Y. Kott. 1974. Virus retention and survival in sand. *In* J.F. Malina, Jr. and B.P. Sagik, eds. Virus Survival in Water and Wastewater Systems, pp. 84-91. Center for Research in Water Resources, University of Texas at Austin.

LeMaistre, C.A., R.W. Sappenfield, C. Culbertson, F.R.N. Carter, A.C. Offutt, H. Black, and M.M. Brooke. 1956. Studies of a waterborne outbreak of amebiasis, South Bend, Indiana. I. Epidemiological aspects. Am. J. Hyg. 64:30-45.

Lepow, M.L., R.J. Warren, V.G. Ingram, S.C. Dougherty, and F.C. Robbins. 1962. Sabin type I oral poliomyelitis vaccine. Effect of dose upon response of newborn infants. Am. J. Dis. Child. 104:67-71.

Levin, G.V., V.L. Stauss, and W.C. Hess. 1961. Rapid coliform organism determination with C^{14}. J. Water Pollut. Control Fed. 33:1021-1037.

Levin, G.V., E. Usdin, and A.R. Slonim. 1968. Rapid detection of microorganisms in aerospace water systems. Aerospace Med. 39:14-16.

Levine, Max. 1953. Should bacteriological standards for drinking water be reevaluated? J. Am. Water Works Assoc. 45:927-932.

Levine, M.M., H.L. DuPont, S.B. Formal, R.B. Hornick, A. Takeuchi, E.J. Gangarosa, M.J. Snyder, and J.P. Libonati. 1973. Pathogenesis of Shigella dysenteriae 1 (Shiga) dysentery. J. Infect. Dis. 127. 261-270.

Liu, O.C., H.R. Seraichekas, and B.L. Murphy. 1966a. Fate of poliovirus in northern quahaugs. Proc. Soc. Exp. Biol. Med. 121:601-607.

Liu, O.C., H.R. Seraichekas, and B.L. Murphy. 1966b. Viral pollution of shellfish. 1. Some basic facts of uptake. Proc. Soc. Exp. Biol. Med. 123:481-487.

Liu, O.C., H.R. Seraichekas, and B.L. Murphy. 1967. Viral depuration of the northern quahaug. Appl. Microbiol. 15:307-315.

Liu, O.C., H.R. Seraichekas, E.W. Akin, D.A. Brashear, E.L. Katz, and W.J. Hill, Jr. 1971. Relative resistance of twenty human enteric viruses to free chlorine in Potomac water. *In* V. Snoeyink and V. Griffin, eds. Virus and Water Quality: Occurrence and Control, Proceedings of the Thirteenth Water Quality Conference, vol. 69, no.1, pp. 171-195. University of Illinois Bulletin, Urbana.

Loria, R.M., S. Kibrick, and W.A. Broitman. 1974. Peroral infection with group B coxsackievirus in the newborn mouse: a model for human neonatal infection. J. Infect. Dis. 130:225-230.

Lund, E., and C.E. Hedstrom. 1966. The use of an aqueous polymer phase system for enterovirus isolations from sewage. Am. J. Epidemiol. 84:287-291.

Lurman, A. 1885. Eine Icterusepidemie. Berlin Klin. Wochschr. 22:20-23.

Mack, W.N., L. Yue-Shoung, and D.B. Coohon. 1972. Isolation of poliomyelitis virus from a contaminated well. Health Serv. Rep. 87:271-274.

MacKenzie, C.R., and D.J. Livingstone. 1968. Salmonellae in fish and food. S. Afr. Med. J. 42:999-1003.

Majumdar, S.B., W.H. Ceckler and O.J. Sproul. 1973. Inactivation of poliovirus in water by ozonation. J. Water Pollut. Control Fed. 45:2433-2443.

Manwaring, J.F., M. Chaudhuri, and R.S. Engelbrecht. 1971. Removal of viruses by coagulation and flocculation. J. Am. Water Works Assoc. 63:298-300.

Mason, J.O., and W.R. McLean. 1962. Infectious hepatitis traced to the consumption of raw oysters. An epidemiologic study. Am. J. Hyg. 75:90-111.

McCabe, L.J., and G.T. Craun. 1975. Status of waterborne diseases in the U.S. and Canada: Committee report. J. Am. Water Works Assoc. 67:95-98.

McCabe, L.J., J.M. Symons, R.D. Lee, and G.G. Robeck. 1970. Survey of community water supply systems. J. Am. Water Works Assoc. 62:670-687.

McCullough, N.B., and C.W. Eisele. 1951a. Experimental human salmonellosis. I. Pathogenicity of strains of Salmonella meleagridis and Salmonella anatum obtained from spray-dried whole egg. J. Infect. Dis. 88:278-289.

McCullough, N.B., and C.W. Eisele. 1951b. Experimental human salmonellosis. II. Immunity studies following experimental illness with Salmonella meleagridis and Salmonella anatum. J. Immunol. 66:595-608.

McCullough, N.B., and C.W. Eisele. 1951c. Experimental human salmonellosis. III. Pathogenicity of strains of Salmonella newport, Salmonella derby and Salmonella bareilly obtained from spray-dried whole egg. J. Infect. Dis. 89:209-213.

McCullough, N.B., and C.W. Eisele. 1951d. Experimental human salmonellosis. IV. Pathogenicity of strains of Salmonella pullorum obtained from spray-dried whole egg. J. Infect. Dis. 89:259-265.

McFeters, G.A., G.K. Bissonnette, J.J. Jezeski, C.A. Thomson, and D.G. Stuart. 1974. Comparative survival of indicator bacteria and enteric pathogens in well water. Appl. Microbiol. 27:823-829.

McKee, J.E. and H.W. Wolf, eds. 1963. Water Quality Criteria, 2nd ed. The Resources Agency of California State Water Resources Control Board, Publication no. 3-A (Reprint December, 1971). Sacramento.

Melnick, J.L. 1957. A waterborne urban epidemic of hepatitis. *In* F.W. Hartman, ed. Hepatitis Frontiers, pp. 211-225. Little Brown & Co., Boston.

Melnick, J.L., V. Rennick, B. Hampil, N. Schmidt, and H.H. Ho. 1973. Lyophilized combination pools of enterovirus equine antisera: Preparation and test procedures for the identification of field strains of 42 enteroviruses. Bull. WHO 48:263-268.

Merson, M.H., W.H. Barker, Jr., G.F. Craun, and L.J. McCabe. 1974. Outbreaks of waterborne disease in the United States 1971-1972. J. Infect. Dis. 129:614-615.

Metcalf, T.G., and W.C. Stiles. 1965. The accumulation of enteric viruses by the oyster, Crassostrea virginica. J. Infect. Dis. 115:68-76.

Metcalf, T.G., and W.C. Stiles. 1968. Viral pollution of shellfish in estuary waters. Am. Soc. Civil Eng. Sanit. Eng. Div. J. SA4:595-609.

Metcalf, T.G., C. Wallis, and J.L. Melnick. 1974a. Environmental factors influencing isolation of enteroviruses from polluted surface waters. Appl. Microbiol. 27:921-926.

Metcalf, T.G., C. Wallis, and J.L. Melnick. 1974b. Virus enumeration and public health assessments in polluted surface water contributing to transmission of virus in nature. *In* J.F. Malina, Jr. and B.P. Sagik, eds. Virus Survival in Water and Wastewater Systems, pp. 57-70. Center for Research in Water Resources, University of Texas at Austin.

Meynell, G.G. 1961. Phenotypic variation and bacterial infection. Symp. Soc. Gen. Microbiol. 11:174-195.

Meynell, G.G., and E. Meynell. 1965. Theory and Practice in Experimental Bacteriology, pp. 199-203. Cambridge University Press.

Miller, R.S. 1975. Check sampling for monitoring bacteriological quality. J. Am. Water Works Assoc. 67:28-32.

Mitchell, J.R., M.W. Presnell, E.W. Akin, J.M. Cummins, and O.C. Liu. 1966. Accumulation and elimination of poliovirus by the eastern oyster. Am. J. Epidemiol. 84:40-50.

Moore, B.E.D., L. Funderburg, and B. P. Sagik. 1974. Application of viral concentration techniques to field sampling. *In* J.F. Malina and B.P. Sagik, eds. Virus Survival in Water and Wastewater Systems, pp. 3-15. Center for Research in Water Resources, University of Texas at Austin.

Moore, G.T., W.M. Cross, D. McGuire, C.S. Mollohan, N.N. Gleason, G.R. Healy, and L.H. Newton. 1969. Epidemic giardiasis at a ski resort. New Engl. J. Med. 281:402-407.

Morse, R.B., and A. Wolman. 1918. The practicability of adopting standards of quality for water supplies. J. Am. Water Works Assoc. 5:198-228.

Mosley, J.W. 1967. Transmission of viral diseases by drinking water. *In* G. Berg, ed. Transmission of Viruses by the Water Route, pp. 5-23. Interscience Publishers, New York.

Neefe, J.R., and J.S. Stokes. 1945. An epidemic of infectious hepatitis apparently due to a waterborne agent. J. Am. Med. Assoc. 128:1063-1075.

Neefe, J.R., J.B. Baty, J.B. Reinhold, and J. Stokes, Jr. 1947. Inactivation of virus of infectious hepatitis in drinking water. Am. J. Public Health 37:365-372.

Newman, J.S., and R.T. O'Brien. 1975. Gas chromatographic presumptive test for coliform bacteria in water. Appl. Microbiol. 30:584-588.

Newton, W.L., and M.F. Jones. 1949. Effect of ozone in water on cysts of Endamoeba histolytica. Am. J. Trop. Med. 29:669-681.

Newton, W.L., W.B. Figgat, and S.R. Weibel. 1948. The effects of sewage-treatment processes upon ova and miracidia of Schistosoma japonicum. Sewage Works J. 20:657-664.

Nupen, E.M. 1970. Virus studies on the Windhoek waste water reclamation plant (southwest Africa). Water Res. 4:661-672.

Olivieri, V.P., C.W. Kruse, Y.C. Hsu, A.C. Griffiths, and K. Kawata. 1975. The comparative mode of action of chlorine, bromine, and iodine on f2 bacterial virus. *In* J.D. Johnson, ed. Disinfection—Water and Wastewater, pp. 145-162. Ann Arbor Science Publishers, Inc., Ann Arbor, Mich.

Parr, L.W. 1939. Coliform bactria. Bacteriol. Rev. 3:1-48.

Pfeiffer, K.R. 1973. The Homestead typhoid outbreak. J. Am. Water Works Assoc. 65:803-805.

Plotkin, S.A., and M. Katz. 1967. Minimal infective doses of viruses for man by the oral route. *In* G. Berg, ed. Transmission of Viruses by the Water Route, pp. 151-166. Interscience, New York.

Prescott, S.C., C.E.A. Winslow, and M.H. McCrady. 1946. Water Bacteriology with Special Reference to Sanitary Water Analysis. 6th ed. John Wiley & Sons, New York.

Provost, P.J., B.S. Wolanski, W.J. Miller, O.L. Ittensohn, W.J. McAleer, and M.R. Hilleman. 1975. Biophysical and biochemical properties of CR326 human hepatitis A virus. Am. J. Med. Sci. 270:87-92.

Ptak, D.J., W. Ginsburg, and B.F. Willey. 1973. Identification and incidence of Klebsiella in chlorinated water supplies. J. Am. Water Works Assoc. 65:604-608.

Putnam, J.J., and E.W. Taylor. 1893. Is acute poliomyelitis unusually prevalent this season? Boston Med. Surg. J. 129:509-510.

Rao, N.U., and N.A. Labzoffsky. 1969. A simple method for the detection of low concentrations of viruses in large volumes of water by the membrane filter technique. Can. J. Microbiol. 15:399-403.

Rao, V.C., R. Sullivan, R.B. Read, and N.A. Clarke. 1968. A simple method for concentrating and detecting viruses in water. J. Am. Water Works Assoc. 60:1288-1294.

Reasoner, D.J. 1972. Literature review. Microbiological pathogens in animals and their detection. J. Water Pollut. Control Fed. 44:1182-1193.

Reasoner, D.J. 1973. Literature review. Microbiology—Detection of bacterial pathogens and their occurrence. J. Water Pollut. Control Fed. 45:1278-1289.

Reasoner, D.J. 1974. Microbiology—Detection of bacterial pathogens and their occurrence. J. Water Pollut. Control Fed. 46:1395-1408.

Reasoner, D.J. 1975. Microbiology—Detection of bacterial pathogens and their occurrence. J. Water Pollut. Control Fed. 47:1581-1587.

Reasoner, D.J., and E.E. Geldreich. 1974. Rapid bacteriological methods. Proc. AWWA Water Quality Technology Conference, Dallas, Texas, pp. IX-1-IX-15.

Ritchie, L.S. and C. Davis. 1948. Parasitological findings and epidemiological aspects of epidemic amebiasis occurring in occupants of the Mantetsu apartment building, Tokyo, Japan. Am. J. Trop. Med. 28:803-816.

Robbins, F.C., J.F. Enders, T.H. Weller, and G.L. Florentino. 1951. Studies on the cultivation of poliomyelitis viruses in tissue culture. V. The direct isolation and serologic identification of virus strains in tissue culture from patients with nonparalytic and paralytic poliomyelitis. Am. J. Hyg. 54:286-293.

Robert, V.B., and L.B. Rorke. 1973. Primary amebic encephalitis, probably from Acanthamoeba. Ann. Int. Med. 79:174-179.

Roos, B. 1956. Hepatitepidemi spridd genom ostron. Svenska Lakartidn. 53:989-1003.

Rosen, L. 1965. Reovirus group. *In* F.L. Horsfall and I. Tamm, eds. Viral and Rickettsial Infections of Man, 4th ed. pp. 569-579. Lippincott, Philadelphia.

Rowe, W.P., R.J. Huebner, L.K. Gilmore, R.H. Parrott, and T.G. Ward. 1953. Isolation of a cytopathogenic agent from human adenoids undergoing spontaneous degeneration in tissue culture. Proc. Soc. Exp. Biol. Med. 84:570-573.

Ruddy, S.J., R.F. Johnson, J.W. Mosley, J.B. Atwater, M.A. Rossetti, and J.C. Hart. 1969. An epidemic of clam-associated hepatitis. J. Am. Med. Assoc. 208:649-655.

Sabin, A.B. 1957. Properties of attenuated polioviruses and their behavior in human beings. *In* Cellular Biology Nucleic Acids and Viruses, vol. 5, pp. 113-127. Special Publications of the New York Academy of Sciences.

Sabin, A.B. 1959. Reoviruses, a new group of respiratory and enteric viruses formerly classified as ECHO type 10 is described. Science 130:1387-1389.

Scarpino, P.V. 1971. Bacterial and viral analysis of water and waste water. *In* L.L. Ciacco, ed. Water and Water Pollution Handbook, vol. 2, pp. 639-761. Marcel Dekker, New York.

Scarpino, P.V., M. Lucas, D.R. Dahling, G. Berg, and S.L. Chang. 1974. Effectiveness of hypochlorous acid and hypochlorite ion in destruction of viruses and bacteria. *In* A.J.

Rubin, ed. Chemistry of Water Supply, Treatment and Distribution, pp. 359-368. Ann Arbor Science Publishers, Ann Arbor, Mich.

Schafer, E. 1971. Experimentelle Untersuchungen zur quantitativen Erfassung von Polio-Impfvirus Type II in Oberflachenwasser. GWF-Wasser/Abwasser 112:109-113.

Schaub, S.A., and B.P. Sagik. 1975. Association of enteroviruses with natural and artifically introduced colloidal solids in water and infectivity of solids-associated virions. Appl. Microbiol. 30:212-222.

Schmidt, N.J., H.H. Ho, and E.H. Lennette. 1975. Propagation and isolation of group A coxsackieviruses in RD cells. J. Clin. Microbiol. 2:183-185.

Schulz, M.G. 1975. Giardiasis. J. Am. Med. Assoc. 233:1383-1384.

Schwerdt, C.E. 1957. Physical and chemical characteristics of purified poliomyelitis virus. *In* Cellular Biology, Nucleic Acids and Viruses, vol. 5, pp. 157-166. Special Publications of the New York Academy of Sciences.

Scott, R.M., D. Seiz, and H.J. Shaughnessy. 1964. I. Rapid C^{14} test for coliform bacteria in water. II. Rapid C^{14} test for sewage bacteria. Am. J. Public Health 54:827-844.

Seligmann, R. and R. Reitler. 1965. Enteropathogens in water with low Esch. coli titer. J. Am. Water Works Assoc. 57:1572-1574.

Seraichekas, H.R., D.A. Brashear, J.A. Barnick, P.F. Carey, and O.C. Liu. 1968. Viral depuration by assaying individual shellfish. Appl. Microbiol. 16:1865-1871.

Sharp, D.G., R. Floyd, and J.D. Johnson. 1975. Nature of the surviving plaque-forming units of reovirus in water containing bromine. Appl. Microbiol. 29:94-101.

Shaughnessy, H.J., R.C. Olsson, K. Bass, F. Friewer, and S.D. Levinson. 1946. Experimental human bacillary dysentery. J. Am. Med. Assoc. 132:362-368.

Shuval, H.I., B. Fattal, S. Cymbalista, and N. Goldblum. 1969. The phase-separation method for the concentration and detection of viruses in water. Water Res. 3:225-240.

Shuval, H.I., S. Cymbalista, B. Fattal, and N. Goldblum. 1967. Concentration of enteric viruses in water by hydro-extraction and two-phase separation. *In* G. Berg, ed. Transmission of Viruses by the Water Route, pp. 45-55. Interscience, New York.

Smith, R.J., and R.M. Twedt. 1971. Natural relationships of indicator and pathogenic bacteria in stream waters. J. Water Pollut. Control Fed. 43:2200-2209.

Sobsey, M.D. 1976. Methods for detecting enteric viruses in water and wastewater, *In* G. Berg, H.L. Bodily, E.H. Lennette, J.L. Melnick, and T.G. Metcalf, eds. Viruses in Water, Proceedings of the International Conference on Viruses in Water, Mexico City, 1974. American Public Health Association, Washington, D.C.

Sobsey, M.D., C. Wallis, M. Henderson, and J.L. Melnick. 1973. Concentration of enteroviruses from large volumes of water. Appl. Microbiol. 26:529-534.

Sorber, C.A., B.P. Sagik, and J.F. Malina, Jr. 1972. Monitoring of low-level virus in natural waters. Appl. Microbiol. 22:334-338.

Sproul, O.J. 1971. Recent research results on virus inactivation by water treatment processes. *In* V. Snoeyink and V. Griffin, eds. Virus and Water Quality: Occurrence and Control, vol. 69, no. 1, pp. 159-169. Proceedings of the Thirteenth Water Quality Conference, University of Illinois Bulletin, Urbana.

Standard Methods for the Examination of Water and Wastewater. 1975. 14th Ed. American Public Health Association. Washington, D.C.

Sternberg, G.M. 1892. Manual of Bacteriology. William Wood and Co., New York.

Stevenson, A.H. 1953. Studies of bathing water quality and health. Am. J. Public Health 43:529-538.

Stringer R.P., W.N. Cramer, and C.W. Kruse. 1975. Comparison of bromine, chlorine and iodine as disinfectants for ameobic cysts. *In* J.D. Johnson, ed. Disinfection—Water and

Wastewater, Chapter 10, pp. 193-209. Ann Arbor Science Publishers, Inc., Ann Arbor, Mich.

Sweet, B.H., R.D. Ellender, and J.K.L. Leong. 1974. Recovery and removal of viruses from water utilizing membrane techniques. *In* Developments in Industrial Microbiology, vol. 15: Symposium: Detection of Viruses in Waste and Other Waters, August 1973, pp. 143-159. Proc. 30th General Meeting of the Society for Industrial Microbiology.

Taylor, A., Jr., G.F. Craun, G.A. Faich, L.J. McCabe, and E.J. Gangarosa. 1972. Outbreaks of waterborne diseases in the United States, 1961-1970. J. Infect. Dis. 125:329-331.

Taylor, D.G. and J.D. Johnson. 1974. Kinetics of viral inactivation by bromine. *In* A.J. Rubin, ed. Symposium on the Chemistry of Water Supply, Treatment and Distribution, Dallas, 1973, pp. 369-408. Ann Arbor Science Publishers, Ann Arbor, Mich.

Thomas, H.A., Jr., and R.L. Woodward. 1955. Estimation of coliform density by the membrane filter and the fermentation tube methods. Am. J. Public Health 45:1431-1437.

Thorup, R.T., F.P. Nixon, D.F. Wentworth, and O.J. Sproul. 1970. Virus removal by coagulation with polyelectrolytes. J. Am. Water Works Assoc. 62:97-101.

U.S. Environmental Protection Agency. 1975. NERC annual report. National Environmental Research Center, United States Environmental Protection Agency, Cincinnati, Ohio. EPA 670/9-75-002.

U.S. Treasury Department. 1914. Bacteriological standard for drinking water. Public Health Rep. 29:2959-2966.

U.S. Public Health Service. 1962. Drinking water standards. Public Health Service Publ. no. 956. U.S. Department of Health, Education and Welfare, Washington, D.C.

Van Donsel, D.J. 1971. Literature review. Microbiology-waterborne outbreaks. J. Water Pollut. Control Fed. 43:1221-1236.

Veazie, L. 1969. Epidemic giardiasis. N. Engl. J. Med. 281:853.

Wallis, C., and J.L. Melnick. 1967a. Concentration of viruses from sewage on Millipore membranes. Bull. WHO 36:219-225.

Wallis, C., and J.L. Melnick. 1967b. Concentration of viruses on aluminum and calcium salts. Am. J. Epidemiol. 85:459-468.

Wallis, C., A. Homma, and J.L. Melnick. 1972. Apparatus for concentrating viruses from large volumes. J. Am. Water Works Assoc. 64:189-196.

Wallis, C., J.L. Melnick, and J.E. Fields. 1970. Detection of viruses in large volumes of natural waters by concentration on insoluble polyelectrolytes. Water Res. 4:787-796.

Wang, W.L.L., S.G. Dunlop, and R.G. DeBoer. 1956. The survival of Shigella in sewage. I. An effect of sewage and fecal suspensions on Shigella flexneri. Appl. Microbiol. 4:34-38.

Wanner, R.G., F.O. Atchley, and M.A. Wasley. 1963. Association of diarrhea with Giardia lamblia in families observed weekly for occurrence of enteric infections. Am. J. Trop. Med. Hyg. 12:851-853.

Warren, R.J., M.L. Lepow, G.E. Bartsch, and F. C. Robbins. 1964. The relationship of maternal antibody, breast feeding and age to the susceptibility of newborn infants to infection with attenuated poliovirus. Pediatrics 34:4-13.

Wattie, E., and C.W. Chambers. 1943. Relative resistance of coliform organisms and certain enteric pathogens to excess lime treatment. J. Am. Water Works Assoc. 35:709-720.

Wellings, F.M., C.W. Mountain, A.L. Lewis, J.L. Nitzkin, M.S. Saslaw, and R.A. Graves. 1976. Isolation of an enterovirus from chlorinated tap water. J. Infect. Dis. (In press.)

White, G.C. 1975. Disinfection: The last line of defense for potable water. J. Am. Water Works Assoc. 67:410-413.

Witt, M., R. Siegrist and W.C. Boyle. 1975. Rural household wastewater characterization. *In* Proceedings of the National Home Sewage Disposal Symposium, Dec. 9-10, 1974, pp. 79-88. American Society of Agricultural Engineers, St. Joseph, Mich.

Wolf, H.W. 1972. The coliform count as a measure of water quality *In* R. Mitchell, ed. Water Pollution Microbiology. Wiley Interscience, New York.

Wolfe, M.S. 1975. Giardiasis. J. Am. Med. Assoc. 233:1362-1365.

World Health Organization. 1970. European Standards for Drinking-Water, 2nd ed. Geneva.

World Health Organization. 1971. International Standards for Drinking-Water, 3rd ed. Geneva.

World Health Organization. 1964. Soil-transmitted helminths: Report of a WHO Expert Committee on helminthiasis. WHO Tech. Report Series no. 277. Geneva.

World Health Organization. 1969. Amoebiasis: Report of a WHO Expert Committee. WHO Tech. Report Series no. 421. Geneva.

Zamcheck, N., L.C. Hoskins, S.J. Winawer, S.A. Broitman, and L.S. Gottlieb. 1963. Histology and ultrastructure of parasite and intestinal mucosa in Human giardiasis: Effect of Atabrine therapy. Gastroenterology 44:860.

Zdrazilek, J. 1974. Sensitivity of human diploid embryonic lung cells for isolation of Echoviruses from sewage. J. Hyg. Epidemiol. Microbiol. Immunol. 18:2-8.

IV

Solid Particles in Suspension

INTRODUCTION

In addition to dissolved substances, drinking water typically contains small amounts of very finely divided solid particles of several kinds. These particles, ranging in size from colloidal dimensions to about 100 μm, are composed of inorganic and organic materials that are derived from soils and rocks and from the debris of human activity with which the raw water has come in contact. They include clays, acicular or fibrous particles of asbestos minerals, and organic particles resulting from the decomposition of plant and animal debris in the soil.

Little is known about the effects that these suspended solids may have on the health of those who drink water that contains them. However, there is widespread concern over the biological effects of the asbestos mineral fibers that occur in water, since similar fibers are known to be carcinogenic when air heavily laden with them is inhaled for many years. In view of this concern that such fibers as occur in water may be injurious to health, their occurrence, characterization, analysis, and biological effects are reviewed in some detail.

No evidence has yet been discovered that either of the other classes of common particulate contaminants of drinking water—clays and organic colloids—has any direct effect on health. Nevertheless, it is possible that both may indirectly affect the quality of drinking water because they can adsorb a variety of toxic substances, bacteria, and viruses from solution or suspension and bind them more or less strongly. By such means these materials may serve to concentrate and transport some water pollutants and protect them from removal by water treatment.

For this reason, the properties of clays and organic particulates are also discussed, together with the tendency of chemicals, bacteria, and viruses to become concentrated at the surfaces of such particles.

Removal of suspended particles from water is briefly reviewed, together with the significance of measurements of turbidity as an index of water quality.

CLAY PARTICLES AND THEIR INTERACTIONS

Clay is usually defined on a particle-size basis, the upper limit being 2 μm diameter. Soils and sediments in nature will therefore have varying proportions of clay material containing clay-mineral components (usually the phyllosilicates), as well as nonclay-mineral material that may include a variety of substances such as iron and aluminum oxides and hydroxides, quartz, amorphous silica, carbonates, and feldspar. The clay minerals themselves are classified in Table IV-1 (Grim, 1968).

Clays are ubiquitous in soils and sediments derived from soils. They may be formed in soils during soil development through the weathering of various minerals, or they can be inherited essentially without change from the parent material upon which the soils are formed. Parent material, climate, topography, and vegetation determine the kinds of clays that are found. Hydrothermal activity may also lead to clay formation. As erosion acts on the landscape, clays may be suspended in water and carried until they are deposited by sedimentation. Most sedimentary rocks contain more or less clay as, for example, shales (almost exclusively clay), limestones, and sandstones.

A number of scientific techniques are useful for studying clays, but the most useful for identification and indication of relative abundance is X-ray diffraction. The diffraction properties of the various clay minerals, as well as the methods of treatment and sample preparation, can be found in publications of Grim (1968), Brown (1961), and Whittig (1965). Infrared spectroscopy is a valuable adjunct to X-ray diffraction in characterizing clays, and this subject has recently been reviewed by Farmer (1975). Infrared spectroscopy is the most powerful method for study of organic-clay interactions (Mortland, 1970; Theng, 1975). Other techniques useful in characterizing clays are electron microscopy (Gard, 1971), thermal methods (Mackenzie, 1957), and chemical analysis (Weaver and Pollard, 1973).

The layer-lattice clay minerals, in themselves, do not appear to have

TABLE IV-1 Classification of the Clay Minerals (Grim, 1968)

I. Amorphous
    Allophane group
II. Crystalline
    A. Two-layer type (sheet structures composed of units of one layer of silica tetrahedrons and one layer of alumina octahedrons)
        1. Equidimensional
            Kaolinite group
            Kaolinite, nacrite
        2. Elongate
            Halloysite group
    B. Three-layer types (sheet structures composed of two layers of silica tetrahedrons and one central dioctahedral or trioctahedral layer)
        1. Expanding lattice
            a. Equidimensional
                Montmorillonite group (smectite)
                Vermiculite
                Montmorillonite, sauconite
            b. Elongate
                Montmorillonite group
                Nontronite, saponite, hectorite
        2. Nonexpanding lattice
            Illite group
    C. Regular mixed-layer types (ordered stacking of alternate layers of different types)
            Chlorite group
    D. Chain-structure types (hornblende-like chains of silica tetrahedrons linked together by octahedral groups of oxygens and hydroxyls containing Al and Mg atoms)
            Attapulgite
            Sepiolite
            Palygorskite

deleterious effects when ingested by humans. Some of them are, in fact, constituents of pharmaceuticals such as kaopectate (kaolinite). Other indications (some from folklore) suggest beneficial results from ingestion of clays. The effect of ingestion of fibrous clay minerals of the chain-structure types (e.g., attapulgite, palygorskite, sepiolite, sometimes called "asbestos"), is still open to question and is the subject of extensive study at the present time. If layer-lattice clay minerals have deleterious effects on human health, they are probably indirect, through adsorption, transport, and release of inorganic and organic toxicants, bacteria, and viruses.

Several reports have shown that concentrations of many pollutants are much higher in sediments of streams and lakes than in the waters with which they are associated. Clays and organic particulates are the materials chiefly responsible for such concentrations. Since clays are ubiquitous in many waters used as sources for human consumption, it is to be expected they will appear as particulate matter in some drinking waters and thus it is of interest to consider the kinds of interactions they have with dissolved materials. Considerable knowledge exists regarding the surface chemistry and adsorptive properties of clays, and thus, with information on the nature of a solute, it is possible to have some idea of their interaction. Clays are very adsorptive substances. The possibility exists that clays could act as vehicles for transport of toxic compounds through adsorption in one environment, followed by release of the toxic material when the clay entered a different environment.

It has been well established that some pesticides applied to watersheds can be adsorbed by soil components and subsequently removed into water by erosional processes (Bailey *et al.*, 1974; Nicholson, 1969; Nicholson and Hill, 1970).

Inorganic Pollutants

This classification of pollutants would include metal cations and some anions. Among the metal cations that have been found to be polluting some water and soils are Pb, Cr, Cu, Zn, Co, Mn, Ni, Hg, and Cd, while radioactive isotopes of Pu, Cs, and Sr, among others, offer potential threats as pollutants. On the other hand, anionic species such as phosphates, arsenate, borate, and nitrates are considered pollutants in some situations.

The interactions of metal cations with clays include adsorption by ion exchange, precipitation as hydroxides or hydrous oxides on clay surfaces, and adsorption as complex species. Obviously, pH and Eh are critical factors in determining the nature of the interactions between clays and some transition and heavy metal ions. Hodgson's review (1963) includes some reference to earlier work on clay interactions with some of the transition ions and heavy metals. Jenne (1968) has effectively described the various factors controlling the concentrations of transition cations in waters and soils, while Jenne and Wahlberg (1968) and Tamura (1962), among others, have considered the interaction of radionuclides with clays. Holdridge (1966) has reported adsorption studies of heavy metal cations on ball clay. With regard to phosphate, it is likely that its interactions with calcium ion and amorphous hydroxides of Fe^{3+} and Al^{3+} and with allophane are more important than adsorption by clay minerals in affecting its concentration in natural waters.

In addition to adsorption by simple ion exchange, much work indicates the retention of transition and heavy metals at clay mineral surfaces via precipitation of insoluble compounds, notably hydroxy and oxidehydroxy polymers. The incorporation of Al^{3+}, Mg^{2+}, and Fe^{3+} hydroxy polymers within the interlamellar space of swelling clays to form chlorite-like species is a well-known pedogenic process. It has also been shown that these brucite-gibbsite-like materials may often be withdrawn if the mineral is subjected to a different environment, usually one involving a change in pH. Gupta and Malik (1969) have reported the incorporation of Ni^{2+} in smectite to form a nickel-chlorite, while Blatter (1973) found similar reactions of smectite with Hg^{2+}. Thus it seems that many of these kinds of metal cations have the ability to form interlayer complexes in swelling clays. It would seem likely that in natural systems where the polluting species might be present in very low concentrations compared with other interlayer-forming species such as Al^{3+}, they might be incorporated within the gibbsite-like layer as it forms, in essentially isomorphous substitution for Al^{3+}, although reports of this phenomenon were not found. It would also appear that incorporation of a polluting metal cation within the intergrade clay is no guarantee that it might not again be released to the natural system when the clay, through erosion and deposition, is placed in a different environment where the interlayer material may be removed. This phenomenon has been shown for vermiculite-chlorite intergrades that, upon erosion from an acidic soil, are deposited in a calcareous freshwater lake or floodplain to form discrete vermiculite, within relatively short periods of time (Frink, 1969; Lietzke and Mortland, 1973).

The clay mineral vermiculite has a special affinity for K^+ ion, in which the ion is initially adsorbed in the interlamellar regions of the mineral and then trapped by collapse of the layer structure. The ion is thus removed from direct interaction with the surrounding solution. This process is called potassium fixation, but will occur with other ions of similar diameter to more or less extent. Cations that might be considered pollutants that undergo this reaction with vermiculite are Ba^{2+} and radioactive Cs^+.

The hydroxides and hydrous oxides of iron, manganese, and aluminum are often components of the clay fraction of sediments and have important effects on pollutant concentrations in natural waters. They often exist as coatings on the surfaces of other minerals and thus may exert chemical activity far out of proportion to their total concentrations. Jenne (1968) suggests that they furnish the principal control on the concentrations of heavy metals such as Co, Ni, Cu, and Zn through adsorption processes. The principal factors affecting adsorption and desorption of heavy metals from these kinds of particulates are pH, Eh, concentration of the metal in question, concentration of competing metals, and the effects of other adsorbents such as organic matter and clay minerals.

Organic Pollutants

These materials encompass a wide range of compounds, including pesticides, polychlorinated biphenyls, aromatic species of various kinds arising from industrial activity, and fluorine compounds in aerosols. Whether or not organic species adsorb or interact with clays depends upon the structure and properties of the compound and the nature of the clay and its exchangeable cations. Several mechanisms of interaction are possible and have been described in a number of recent reviews (Mortland, 1970; Bailey and White, 1970; Theng, 1974; and Rausell-Colom and Serratosa, 1975). Organic cations adsorb on clays by ordinary ion exchange and are usually preferred over the inorganic ions by the exchange complex because of their large size and high molecular weights.

Examples of organic compounds that are cationic and could be considered pollutants if transported outside their areas of application are the herbicides Paraquat and Diquat. These compounds are strong bases and are completely ionized in water. Other organic compounds, while neutral at the ambient pH of the solution phase, may become protonated after adsorption at the clay surface. The surface acidity of clays has been shown to be a considerably stronger proton donor system than pH measurements of the water-clay system would indicate. Thus, organic compounds containing basic nitrogen or carbonyl groups may become protonated, and therefore cationic, after adsorption at clay surfaces.

Another kind of organic-clay interaction is the coordination or ion-dipole type. Compounds with nitrogen, oxygen, sulfur, or olefinic groups have electron pairs that may be donated to electrophilic exchange cations to form complexes on the clay surface. In natural systems, an important consideration is the competitive effect of water for these adsorption sites. That is, the energy of ligand formation of an organic molecule with an exchange cation must be greater than the solvation energy of the cation in order to displace water molecules and obtain direct organic-cation coordination. In the laboratory these interactions are easily obtained by dehydration; however, in natural systems the competition of water is a major factor in determining whether or not these complexations occur. Nevertheless, it is likely that this kind of interaction does occur with some highly polar, electron-donating organic compounds. Another important factor is the nature of the exchange cation. Thus, for example, transition metal cations on the exchange complex, that have unfilled *d* orbitals, will interact strongly with electron-supplying groups of organic molecules.

Still another kind of organic-clay interaction is hydrogen bonding. These interactions can be classified into three types:

1. Hydrogen bonding between water molecules directly solvating exchangeable cations and polar functional groups, such as carbonyl, on organic molecules. The water molecules thus act as a "bridge" between the cation and organic species.
2. Hydrogen bonding between functional groups such as alcoholic and amino groups and oxygens of the silicate surfaces. Infrared spectroscopy has indicated that these are relatively weak bonds, being within the lower range of energies where hydrogen bonding is found.
3. Intermolecular hydrogen bonding between two organic species on the clay curface. Other factors involved in clay-organic interactions include physical forces and entropy effects.

With this general description of the interactions of organic species with clays, it is now appropriate to mention some special clay-organic properties that have relevance to organic pollutants. Many organic compounds, including aromatics and particularly the halogenated types such as DDT, chlorinated and brominated phenyls and biphenyls, are adsorbed to little if any extent on clay surfaces from aqueous solution. In the natural environment they are more likely to be adsorbed in organic components of soils and sediments. These materials usually have limited solubility in water, since they are hydrophobic. It is thus not surprising that they are not attracted to the hydrophilic surfaces of clays. The above discussion, however, suggests that, in natural systems, clay-organic complexes may act as adsorbing media for some organic pollutants that are not adsorbed at all by pure inorganic clays.

Another phenomenon that may take place when organic species are adsorbed at clay surfaces is that of catalytic alteration. This has particular relevance for organic pollutants since there is much interest in their fate in the environment. Much work has been reported on catalytic reactions on clays at high temperatures, but it is only recently that much attention has been paid to catalysis by clays in conditions resembling the natural environment. One mechanism by which clays can act as catalysts is via their Brönsted acidity. Examples of this are the hydrolysis of esters demonstrated by McAuliffe and Coleman (1955), the conversion of atrazine to hydroxyatrazine by Russell *et al.* (1968), the decomposition of alkylammonium ions by Chaussidon and Calvet (1965), and the hydrolysis of nitriles to amides by Sanchez *et al.* (1972). In many decomposition reactions involving Brönsted acidity, carbonium ion formation is undoubtedly involved. On the other hand, Lewis acid sites may exist in clays that also will catalyze many organic reactions. These sites (electron acceptors) may be part of the basic structure of the mineral itself as, for example, ferric iron within the octahedral layer or exposed aluminum on the edges of the minerals. In addition, some cations on exchange sites function in this capacity, particularly those of the transition metal group. Solomon *et al.* (1968) have demonstrated catalytic properties of Lewis sites located on edges of clay minerals. The activity of some transition metal cations on exchange sites has also been amply demonstrated as, for example, the decomposition of urea to ammonium ion when complexed with Cu^{2+}, Mn^{2+}, or Ni^{2+} smectite. No such reaction was noted for urea complexed with alkali metal or alkaline earth-saturated clay (Mortland, 1966). Aromatic molecules such as benzene will complex via pi electrons with clay minerals saturated with Cu^{2+}, under mildly desiccating conditions. Under more vigorous dehydrating conditions, a radical cation of benzene is formed that will react with molecular benzene to give polymers containing phenyl groups as well as fragmented benzene rings (Doner and Mortland, 1969). Anisole (methoxybenzene) will also form radical cations that react with molecular anisole to give 4,4′-dimethoxybiphenyl (Fenn *et al.*, 1973). Other cationic species with oxidizing abilities as great as Cu^{2+}, such as Vo^{2+} and Fe^{3+}, were also found to produce radical cations from some aromatic species with subsequent polymer formation (Pinnavaia *et al.*, 1974). These reactions suggest the possibility that some pollutant species adsorbed on clay surfaces may undergo similar reactions to form radical cations and subsequently interact with themselves, or other organic compounds with formation of different chemical derivatives. Thus, pollutant degradation or alteration on clays by oxidation-reduction reactions involving exchangeable transition-metal cations may be a real possibility in nature.

In addition to the degradation of atrazine to hydroxyatrazine, mentioned above, a number of other clay-catalyzed pesticide reactions have been reported. For example, Fleck and Haller (1945) report the conversion of DDT to DDE by kaolinite and smectite samples, preheated to 400°K. Also, degradation of heptachlor by palygorskite has been suggested by Malina *et al.* (1956). The degradation of the organic phosphate insecticide, ronnel, by clays heated to various temperatures has been reported by Rosenfield and van Valkenburg (1965). Organic phosphate pesticides have been observed by Mortland and Raman (1967) to be hydrolyzed in the presence of Cu^{2+}-montmorillonite by a coordination mechanism. The much weaker catalytic effects of Cu^{2+}-vermiculite, beidellite, and nontronite were attributed to reduced activity of the copper on these minerals, as compared with montmorillonite, due to charge location. While most of the degradation of pesticides in nature has been attributed to biological agencies, the above discussion would suggest that catalysis at mineral surfaces may also play a role.

Natural organic material in soils forms complexes with clays that exert important influences on the physical, chemical, and biological properties of the soil (Greenland, 1965, 1971). Since the exact chemical and physical nature of these organic materials is not known, the kinds of interaction they have with clays are less well known than those of well-defined organic compounds. However, some of the kinds of reactions described above are probably involved. It is obvious that clays eroded from soil surfaces into streams and lakes will probably be, to some degree, complexed with organic matter.

Humic acids, a constituent of soil organic matter, may be strongly adsorbed by clays, presumably by interaction with positive sites on the edges of clay particles or with polyvalent cations on the cation exchange complex acting as "bridges." Schnitzer and Kodama (1967) have shown that fulvic acid (another constituent of soil organic matter) adsorption depends on pH, and is greater under acid than alkaline conditions. This is to be expected, since the fulvic acid would be relatively undissociated at low pH but considerably more anionic at alkaline pH. Schnitzer and Kodama (1972) showed that fulvic acid is very strongly bound to Cu^{2+} on the exchange sites of montmorillonite through a coordination type of reaction. In addition, they have shown such adsorption is typical for any electrophilic cation on the exchange complex, particularly for ions of the transition metal group.

Summary

Pollutant concentrations are higher in sediments than in the waters with which they are associated. It should be recognized that the consequences of pollutant adsorption by clays may be very important in natural systems and may affect drinking water quality. Clay-pollutant complexes may be mobilized by erosion from the landscape, or form when eroded clay enters a stream containing a polluting species. If the complex survives water treatment and enters the drinking water system, it would then be available for ingestion by humans. In the adsorbed state on the clay surface the pollutant is probably not toxic, but the possibility exists that the pollutant might be released from the clay in the environment of the alimentary tract and thus exert toxic effects. Whether or not such a process might take place would depend on the complex in question, so that no generalities are possible. Information is completely lacking in this area, and thus research should be encouraged and supported.

ASBESTOS: NOMENCLATURE, OCCURRENCE AND REDISTRIBUTION IN WATER

Structure and Nomenclature

Asbestos is the name for a group of naturally occurring hydrated silicate minerals possessing fibrous morphology and commercial utility. This definition generally limits application of the term to the minerals chrysotile, some members of the cummingtonite-grunerite series, crocidolite, anthophyllite, and some members of the tremolite-actinolite series. Amosite is commonly used to refer to a cummingtonite-grunerite asbestos mineral, but it is a discredited mineral name (Rabbit 1948; Committee on Mineral Names, 1949).

Mode of occurrence and fiber length are important determinants of commercial value. Of the commercially mined and processed asbestos minerals, chrysotile accounts for about 95%, the remainder being amosite and crocidolite (May and Lewis, 1970). Crocidolite is the fibrous equivalent of riebeckite, and chrysotile belongs to the serpentine group of minerals, which contains other nonfibrous members (Deer *et al.*, 1970). Noncommercial deposits of asbestos minerals are also relatively common.

The standard definitions of the Glossary of Geology (American Geological Institute, 1972; second printing, 1973) are given below.

ASBESTOS: (a) a commercial term applied to a group of highly fibrous silicate minerals that readily separate into long, thin, strong fibers of sufficient flexibility to be woven, are heat resistant and chemically inert, and possess a high electric insulation, and therefore are suitable for uses (as in yarn, cloth, paper, paint, brake linings, tiles, insulation cement, fillers, and filters), where incombustible, nonconducting, or chemically resistant material is required. (b) a mineral of the asbestos group, principally chrysotile (best adapted for spinning) and certain fibrous varieties of amphibole (ex. tremolite, actinolite, and crocidolite). (c) a term strictly applied to the fibrous variety of actinolite. Syn: asbestos; amianthus; earth flax; mountain leather.

ASBESTIFORM: Said of a mineral that is fibrous, i.e. that is like asbestos.

ACICULAR (Cryst): Said of a crystal that is needlelike in form. cf: fascicular, sagenitic

FIBROUS: Said of the habit of a mineral, and of the mineral itself (e.g. asbestos), that crystallizes in elongated thin, needle-like grains, or fibers.

The nomenclature used in this report conforms generally to these definitions, subject only to the further qualifications that the term asbestos will not be used in its most restrictive sense (c, above);

asbestiform will not be used; and the terms acicular and fibrous are to be understood as discussed below.

The term asbestos has often been used in recent scientific literature to describe individual fibrous or acicular particles of microscopic and submicroscopic size. However, mineralogists and geologists have hastened to point out that the term should be used only as defined above, in reference to the minerals in bulk. Ampian (1976) considers the terms asbestos and asbestiform to be synonymous and that they then may only be used to apply to the bulk fibrous forms occurring in nature.

Asbestiform is often used to define the morphology of a mineral that is similar to asbestos, but does not necessarily occur in nature in a commercial deposit; to avoid ambiguity, the term will not be used here.

The terms acicular and fibrous are used here to characterize any mineral particle that has apparent crystal continuity, a length-to-width aspect ratio of 3 or more and widths in the micrometer or submicrometer range. Although the two terms are not strictly synonymous, the use here of either one to describe a mineral particle should be taken to imply the other, unless otherwise qualified.

Table IV-2 lists some of the naturally occurring minerals that can have, but do not always have, an acicular morphology. To this list could be added a number of synthetic fibers, although they are not naturally occurring minerals. Many of the minerals in Table IV-2 are common rock-forming minerals.

Properties of Asbestos Minerals

MINERALOGY

The asbestos minerals belong to the serpentine and amphibole groups, and the amphiboles are further divided into those of the orthorhombic crystal system (orthoamphiboles) and amphiboles of the monoclinic crystal system (clinoamphiboles). Table IV-3 summarizes the basic properties of the asbestos minerals.

Chrysotile is the asbestos mineral of the serpentine group. Its crystal structure is a double sheet, comprising a layer of silica tetrahedra and a layer of magnesia octahedra, arranged in a manner that is somewhat analogous to the alumina octahedra—silica tetrahedra layering of kaolinite. The way in which the sheet structure is modified to develop a fibrous morphology is, in detail, very complex; but in essence the modification can be imagined as a buckling of the double sheet, due to misfits, to form a hollow tube (Deer *et al.*, 1966). This central tube may or may not be filled with electron-opaque material, and the appearance of its

TABLE IV-2 List of Some Minerals That May Occur in Acicular-Fibrous Form. Major Element Stoichiometry Has Been Simplified in Many Cases.

Mineral	Formula
Silicates	
Epidote	$Ca_2FeAl_2O(Si_2O_7)OH\cdot(Si_2O_4)$
Lawsonite	$CaAl_2(OH)_2Si_2O_7\cdot H_2O$
Sillimanite (fibrolite)	Al_2SiO_5
Pectolite	$Ca_2NaH(SiO_3)_3$
Kyanite	Al_2SiO_5
Mullite	$3Al_2O_3\cdot 2SiO_2$
Diopside-hedenbergite	$Ca(Mg,Fe)(Si_2O_6)$
Enstatite	$MgSiO_3$
Wollastonite	$CaSiO_3$
Jadeite (Nephrite)	$NaAl(Si_2O_6)$
Anthophyllite	$(Mg,Fe)_7Si_8O_{22}(OH,F)_2$
Tremolite-actinolite	$Ca_2(Mg,Fe^2)_5(Si_8O_{22})(OH,F)_2$
Hornblende	$(Ca,Na,K_2)_{2-3}(Mg,Fe^2,Fe^3,Al)_5[Si_6(Si,Al)_2]O_{22}(OH,F)_2$
Crocidolite (glaucophane-riebeckite)	$Na_5Fe^3_2Fe^2_3(Si_8O_{22})(OH,F)_2$
Cummingtonite-grunerite	$(Fe,Mg)_7(Si_8O_{22})(OH)_2$
Eckermannite-arfvedsonite	$Na_3(Mg,Fe)_4Al(Si_8O_{22})(OH,F)_2$
Halloysite	$Al_2Si_2O_5(OH)_4$
Nontronite	$(Ca,Na)_{1.3}(Mg,Fe)_4(S;_{0.3}Al_{0.7})_8O_{20}(OH)_4\cdot nH_2O$
Palygorskite-attapulgite-sepiolite	$(Mg,Al)_5Si_8O_{22}(OH)_6\cdot 4H_2O$
Chrysotile (Serpentine)	$Mg_3Si_2O_5(OH)_4$
Talc	$Mg_6Si_8O_{20}(OH)_4$
Prehnite	$Ca_2Al(Al,Si_3O_{10})(OH)_2$
Natrolite	$Na_2(Al_2Si_3O_{10})\cdot 2H_2O$
Scolecite	$Ca(Al_2Si_3O_{10})\cdot 3H_2O$
Thomsonite	$NaCa_2((Al,Si)_5O_{10})_2\cdot 6H_2O$
Stilbite	$(Ca,Na_2,K_2)(Al_2Si_7O_{18})\cdot 7H_2O$
Mordenite	$(Na_2,K_2,Ca)(Al_2Si_{10}O_{24})\cdot 7H_2O$
Ferrierite	$(Na,K)_4Mg_2(Al_6Si_{30}O_{72})(OH)_2\cdot nH_2O$
Nonsilicates	
Cassiterite	SnO_2
Goethite-limonite	$FeO\,OH\cdot nH_2O$
Rutile	TiO_2
Nemalite (brucite)	$Mg(OH)_2$
Stibnite	Sb_2S_3
Bismuthinite	Bi_2S_3
Marcasite	FeS_2
Jamesonite	$2PbS\cdot Sb_2S_3$
Gypsum	$CaSO_4\cdot 2H_2O$
Celestite	$SrSO_4$
Alum	$KAl(SO_4)_2\cdot 12H_2O$
Aragonite	$CaCO_3$
Lublinite	$CaCO_3$
Siderite	$FeCO_3$
Apatite	$Ca_5(PO_4,CO_3)(OH,F)$
Vivianite	$Fe_3(PO_4)_2\cdot 8H_2O$

image under the electron microscope will be affected accordingly (Yada, 1967). The chemical composition of chrysotile shows comparatively little of the great variability that is found in the amphiboles.

Double chains of silica tetrahedra and metals, octahedrally linked, form the basic structural elements of the amphiboles. The net result is a prominent cleavage parallel to the double chain, and this generally produces an acicular or prismatic habit. Amphiboles show a wide range of chemical composition, reflecting the temperature, pressure, chemistry, and metamorphic history of formation. This wide variation in composition is due to substitution in the basic silica tetrahedra, and the ability of the crystal structure to accommodate a wide variety of different coordinating cations; the result is that all amphiboles, including the asbestos-forming amphiboles, show overlapping composition. Anthophyllite and cummingtonite also have overlapping chemical compositions, as do crocidolite, tremolite-actinolite, and hornblende. Analytical results in the literature often refer to "amphibole fibers," implying that these are understood to be derived from asbestos. However, many nonasbestos amphibole minerals form fibrous or acicular particles when finely divided.

SURFACE PROPERTIES

The surface areas of fibrous particles have an important bearing on coagulation and adsorption processes and hence on the ultimate fate of the particulates in the environment. The surface areas of UICC (Unio Internationale Contra Cancrum) reference samples have been measured, using both the nitrogen adsorption and the permeability methods (Rendall, 1970).

The specific surface of chrysotile is about twice that of the amphibole asbestos minerals. This difference may be due to the greater length-to-width ratio of chrysotile and its porous tubular morphology.

The isoelectric point, the pH at which the net surface charge of a mineral in an aqueous solution is zero, has been measured for chrysotile and cummingtonite. Chrysotile has an isoelectric point of 11.8, and the isoelectric point of cummingtonite is 5.2–6.0. Anthophyllite may have a value similar to that of chrysotile, and the other amphibole asbestos minerals may have values similar to those of cummingtonite (Parks, 1967). As the pH of the medium falls below the isoelectric point, the surface charge of suspended particles tends to become more positive. Therefore, in a typical drinking water, chrysotile particles should be more positively charged than those of the amphiboles. However, other suspended or

TABLE IV-3 Mineralogy of Common Asbestos Minerals

Name	Chrysotile	Anthophyllite	Cummingtonite-Grunerite	Crocidolite (Glaucophane-Riebeckite)	Ferroactinolite-Tremolite
Group	Serpentine	Amphibole	Amphibole	Amphibole	Amphibole
Structure	Sheet silicate	Double chain	Double chain	Double chain	Double chain
Composition	Mg_3 (Si_2O_5) $(OH)_4$ constant comp. (Trace Ni, Cr, Al, Fe^{+2},	$(Mg, Fe)_{5-6}$ Al_{1-2} $(Si_6$ $(Si, Al)_2O_{22})$ $(OH,F)_2$	(Mg_4Fe_3) (Si_8O_{22}) $(OH)_2$ to Fe_7 Si_8O_{22} $(OH)_2$ Mn common substituent	$Na_2Fe_3{}^{+2}Fe_2{}^{+3}$ (Si_8O_{22}) $(OH, F)_2$ Mg substitutes for Fe^{+2};	Ca_2 $(Mg, Fe^{+2})_5$ Si_8O_{22} $(OH, F)_2$ Al substitutes often; see hornblende

	basal cleavage	(210) : ($2\bar{1}0$) = 54.5°	(110) good (110) : ($1\bar{1}0$) = 55°	(110) good (110) : (110) = 56°	(110) good (110) : (110) = 56°
Crystal System	Monoclinic Cm	Orthorhombic Pn ma	Monoclinic C2/m	Monoclinic C2/m	Monoclinic C2/m
Cell Lattice Dimensions	a = 5.3 b = 9.2 c = 7.3 β = 90°	a = 18.5 b = 17.7 c = 5.3	a = 9.6 b = 18.3 c = 5.3 β = 102°	a = 9.8 b = 18.0 c = 5.3 β = 103°	a = 9.9 b = 18.1 c = 5.3 β = 105°
Occurrence	Low grade metamorphism of ultrabasic rocks	Metamorphic rocks	Metamorphosed Fe formations (retrograde and amphibolites)	In iron formation as metamorphic mineral	Actinolite in Fe formations Tremolite in metamorphosed calcareous rocks

dissolved materials can interact with the asbestos minerals and modify their charge.

MORPHOLOGY

Fibrils are the individual tubes of single crystals that bundle together to produce a fiber. Chrysotile fibers are usually curved and occur in open bundles, splitting into smaller individual fibrils. Therefore, it is often difficult to carry out repeatable size measurements. The fibrils have various diameters, but the average outer diameter is about 200 Å. Typical electron micrographs of chrysotile show cylinders, tube-in-tube, and cone-in-cone forms (Whittaker and Zussman, 1971). Quite frequently there is a median stripe of greater or less electron density, suggesting that there is a difference in the core compared to the sides of the fiber. A tubular structure, either void or filled with an electron-dense substance, is the simplest explanation of this observation (Yada 1967; Whittaker, 1966; Kehieker *et al.*, 1967; Whittaker and Zussman, 1971; House, 1967).

On the other hand, amphiboles are usually straight and show good cleavage edges parallel to the fiber length and often a second cleavage transverse to the length. The fiber width of UICC samples of anthophyllite often exceeds the fiber width of amosite, which, in turn, exceeds the average width of crocidolite. Approximate minimum fiber widths are: anthophyllite—2500 Å, amosite—1500 Å, and crocidolite—600 Å (Timbrell *et al.*, 1970).

Fiber-length distributions have been determined for the UICC reference samples (Rendall, 1970); laboratory experiments have shown that observed distributions depend to some extent on the method used to disperse the fibers for measurement (Timbrell and Rendall, 1972). Table IV-4 shows the distribution of fiber lengths by number in UICC reference samples, as determined from the analysis of Rendall (1970). When this distribution is compared to milled dusts, the UICC reference is seen to approach the lower limit of industrial dust in the case of amosite, and to approach the upper limit of industrial dust in the case of chrysotile (Rendall, 1970). Both in water and in air, the longer fibers (>2 μm) are much rarer in the general environment than in occupational settings.

SOLUBILITY

Acid dissolution of asbestos minerals has often been studied in order to test resistance to corrosion (Cotterell and Holt, 1972; Speil and Leineweber, 1969; Choi and Smith, 1971). In general, the resistance to

TABLE IV-4 Length Distribution of UICC Reference Samples (after Rendall, 1970)

Mineral Type	% by Number of Length Greater Than (μm): 0.2	0.5	1.0	2.0	5.0	10	25	50	100
Amosite	99.9	76.9	45.9	20.3	5.69	1.29	0.21	0.05	0.02
Anthophyllite	99.9	78.2	45.5	22.9	4.79	1.29	0.14		
Crocidolite	100	71.6	35.8	13.3	3.01	0.68	0.08	0.01	0.01
Chrysotile A (Rhodesian)	99.9	79.3	44.4	21.3	6.09	3.26	0.77	0.15	
Chrysotile B (Canadian)	100	69.4	36.0	16.2	3.00	1.24	0.31	0.07	

acid solution is chrysotile < < amosite < actinolite < crocidolite < anthophyllite < tremolite.

Occurrence of Asbestos and Fibrous Minerals

Fibrous minerals must be considered to be common wherever unconsolidated sediment occurs, because many of the common rock-forming minerals can have an acicular morphology (Cralley, *et al.*, 1969)

The wide variation in composition, and the crystallographic similarities, as well as the ubiquitous occurrence of fibrous or acicular minerals, make analysis of environmental samples most difficult. Most analytical studies consider only minerals of the asbestos group.

Asbestos minerals generally occur in metamorphic retrograde deposits. Chrysotile occurs in low-grade metamorphic deposits, and the amphiboles occur in slightly higher-grade metamorphic deposits. Metasomatism may be a key process in the formation of the asbestos minerals.

Deposits of commercial grade asbestos are mined in Canada and the United States. Chrysotile accounts for 95% of the world production with amosite and crocidolite accounting for most of the remainder. The largest-known deposits of chrysotile in the world are found in a belt 125 km by 10 km between Danville and Chaudiere, Quebec. Other Canadian deposits are found in northern Ontario (Matachawan), in northern British Columbia (Cassiar), and Newfoundland (Baie Verte). In the United States, extensive deposits are found in California, Vermont, Arizona, and North Carolina. The North Carolina deposits are amphiboles, whereas all the other deposits consist of chrysotile. Additional deposits, presently unexploited, are found in other states, notably Montana and Wyoming.

Uses and Redistribution

There are over 2000 recorded uses of asbestos minerals in the United States (May and Lewis). From this one can conclude that there will be a correlation between population and industrial activity and the concentration of asbestos in the environment. Higher concentrations of asbestos fibers are commonly found in the air and waters around metropolitan areas (Cunningham and Pontefract, 1971; Kay, 1973).

The following tabulation of uses of asbestos fibers, consisting almost entirely of chrysotile, is of the United States in 1968 (May and Lewis, 1970).

Construction		88%
Cement products	69%	
Floor tile	10%	
Paper products	7%	
Paint and caulking	2%	
Transportation		3%
Textiles		2%
Plastics		1%
Other		6%

Redistribtion of asbestos minerals to the environment depends on the extent to which the material is conserved or sequestered in the processes of mining, manufacturing and consumption. Emission factors, expressing the fractional loss of asbestos to the environment (on a mass to mass basis) from the various processes and uses, have been estimated in two different studies (Davis, 1970; Environment Canada, 1973), and are shown in Table IV-5.

When considering redistribution of asbestos in the environment, it is important to distinguish between the mass of material involved and a more pertinent consideration—the number of fibers of specified dimensions. Note that the production and use estimates, modified by the emission factors, give estimates of emission on a mass basis that can not be directly related to numbers of fibers of particular size ranges. (Size and number are discussed in the following sections on health effects.) Asbestos fibers occur in bundles, individual fibers, and fibrils and in varying size ranges in the environment. It is not possible, in a general sense, to relate mass to number.

The natural background concentrations of asbestos fibers in water and in air are not well known. Some minimum concentrations from remote areas suggest that concentrations of 10^4 to 10^6 fibers per liter represent approximate background figures for water, and an ambient air concentra-

TABLE IV-5 Emission Factors for Asbestos (Chrysotile) for the United States (Davis, 1970) and Canada (Environment Canada, 1973)

	Emission Factor (g/kg)	
	Canada	United States
Production		
Asbestos mining	4.0	4.5
Asbestos milling	6.0	42
Manufacturing		
Cement products	0.075	0.5
Floor tile	0.075	0.5
Paving	0.075	—
Coatings/caulking	0.075	0.5
Insulation	0.15	—
Friction materials	0.45	3.0
Plastics	0.075	—
Textiles	0.15	1.0
Paper	0.075	0.5
Miscellaneous	0.075	0.5
Consumption		
Construction industry	0.075	—
Sprayed insulation	5.0	5.0
Brake linings		
Installation	5.0	5.0
Wear	20	5.0

NOTE: Emission factor = mass of asbestos (g) emitted to environment per unit mass (kg) of asbestos in use.

tion of about 0.01 fiber/cc is an approximate background estimate for air. It may well be that these figures represent a lower limit of detection in a modern analytical laboratory surrounded by materials containing asbestos. In regions that are remote from industrial and populated areas, the median lengths of fibers found in water are generally less than those found in air. Median fiber lengths of $< 1\ \mu m$ are typical, and fibers greater than $2\ \mu m$ are uncommon in such cases (Durham and Pang, 1976; Kay, 1973). There are reports that asbestos fibers reach the environment by natural weathering (NAS-NRC, 1971), but this hypothesis has not been substantiated for areas where asbestos minerals occur naturally and that have not been disturbed by man.

Asbestos cement pipe is used in some localities to transport drinking water and there has been some concern over the release of fibers from these pipes (Wright, 1974). Studies have been carried out on the solubility of concrete and cement (Flentje and Schweitzer, 1955; Kristiansen, 1974). In general, almost all soft waters (alkalinity and hardness about 10^{-4} equivalents/liter) should dissolve calcium carbonate in the pipe, whereas hard waters typically would not do so. In addition to solubility studies, fiber analyses are being carried out in a pipe-loop laboratory as well as in asbestos cement pipe in soft water areas (EPA, 1975). Results are tentative at present, but they suggest that some fibers are emitted in corrosive waters.

Exposure of asbestos and other fibrous particle-forming minerals to redistribution may result from the presence of the material in a gangue. The best documented case of this kind of emission is that of the release of fibrous cummingtonite from taconite ore tailings into the Western arm of Lake Superior (Cook *et al.*, 1974). This amphibole occurs together with quartz, tremolite-actinolite, and other minor minerals in both fibrous and nonfibrous forms. A tabulation of the approximate emission rates of fibrous cummingtonite and associated materials gives:

Total emissions	70,000 metric tons/day
cummingtonite-grunerite concentration	40 wt. %
Fiber concentration, emissions	9×10^9 fibers/g dry wt.
	0.006 g of fiber/g dry wt.
Annual emissions	
total cummingtonite-grunerite	10 million metric tons
no. of fibers	2.3×10^{23}
weight of fibers	150,000 metric tons

It is interesting to note that the consumption of asbestos in the United States in 1968 was about 840,000 metric tons (May and Lewis, 1970) or about 5.5 times the fiber emissions into Lake Superior. If we assume that the average emission factor for asbestos is between 0.08 and 0.15 g/kg (Table IV-5), the total emissions of asbestos (chrysotile) in the United States can be estimated to be about equal to the fibrous emission into western Lake Superior cited above, on a mass basis.

The ultimate fate of the fibrous cummingtonite-grunerite is not well documented. The concentrations of cummingtonite-grunerite fibers in the western arm of Lake Superior are generally >10 million/liter. The central and eastern portions of Lake Superior have concentrations of 2-3 million fibers/liter, those in nearshore areas being somewhat higher (Kramer, 1976). In comparison, a number of inflowing streams have concentrations of 1 to 2 million fibers/liter. If the lake were homogeneously mixed, and no fibers were transported out of the lake, one would expect between 3 million and 5 million fibers/liter from measurements of the emission. From these calculations, one may estimate that 50% or more of the fibers are removed from suspension in the water of Lake Superior, presumably by sedimentation.

Topics for Research in Mineralogy

One of the more important questions is what differences, if any, exist between fibers derived from asbestos and those that arise from single crystals or cleavages of single crystals. Furthermore, it is important to be able to develop analytical methods to define these differences and to relate these differences to health effects. In a recent summary of the mineralogical aspects of this research, Zoltai (1976) concluded that 1) "the mechanism responsible for the development of asbestiform habit may be related to unique surface structures and properties of individual fibers that make up a bundle, 2) electron microscope studies of 'amosite' asbestos fibers reveal the presence of narrow bands of polysynthetic twinning and of triple chains interlayered with the usual double chain structure of the amphiboles, 3) most of the natural asbestos ('amosite') fibers have apparently orthorhombic optical properties at a scale of several microns, and 4) some natural asbestos contains adsorbed metals and compounds." Reasons for the development of fibrous habit are not known. Several workers have shown details of variations in structure in asbestos minerals, and these variations must be compared with small-scale cleavage fibers from nonasbestos deposits (Chisholm, 1973; Hartman, 1963; Hutchinson *et al.*, 1975; Ruud *et al.*, 1976).

ASBESTOS FIBER SAMPLING AND ANAYLSIS

Introduction

Several methods have been used to identify fibrous or acicular particulates of asbestos minerals and determine their concentrations in air, water, mineral samples and biological tissue. These include optical and electron microscopy, X-ray diffraction, and differential thermal analysis. Identification of fibers of asbestos origin and their estimation in water and tissue samples is difficult for a variety of reasons:

1. Asbestos mineral fibers in water are generally present in low mass concentrations even though the number density of fibers may be high.
2. Many analytical methods can not distinguish between fibers of asbestos origin and particles of other nonasbestos and nonfibrous minerals.
3. Mineral fibers present in water samples are generally smaller than can be resolved with the optical microscope, hence the electron microscope must be used.

Methods of estimating mineral fibers in water, and their limitations, are discussed below.

Optical Microscopy

Occupational exposure to asbestos fibers in air is monitored, in the United States, by collecting the fibers on contrast optical microscopy. For optical microscopy, asbestos fibers are defined as those particles of length greater than 5 μm and a length-to-diameter ratio of 3 to 1 or greater. This method may not be specific for asbestos mineral fibers (by fiber definition), nor can it detect fibers less than about 0.5 μm in diameter.

Petrographic microscopy may be used to identify asbestos mineral fibers greater than approximately 0.5 μm in diameter. With the polarizing microscope, various optical crystallographic measurements such as refractive index, extinction angles and sign of elongation may be made and compared with data reported for standard asbestos mineral reference samples.

Dispersion staining with polarized light has been reported as a method for identifying asbestos mineral fibers (Julian and McCrone, 1970). Dispersion staining colors may vary depending on the geographic area in which the asbestos was mined. Fibers less than 0.5 μm in diameter can not be identified by this method.

Asbestos fibers present in water and tissue samples are generally too small in diameter for analysis by any of the above optical microscopic methods.

Electron Microscopy

Both transmission and scanning electron microscopy have been used for mineral fiber identification and estimation. In addition to morphological observation, selected area electron diffraction and microchemical analysis may be used to identify fibers.

In addition to their superior resolving power, most modern transmission electron microscopes can be used to observe electron diffraction patterns. Crystalline materials diffract electrons in regular patterns that are indicative of their crystal structures. Visual observation of single fiber (single crystal) electron diffraction patterns may be used to differentiate chrysotile fibers from amphibole fibers (Langer *et al.*, 1974; Timbrell, 1970; Clark and Ruud, 1975). The hollow "central core" of chrysotile fibers may also aid in fiber identification but beam damage may cause this feature to disappear (Langer *et al.*, 1974). Other fibrous minerals may also have hollow cores.

The amphibole mineral fibers are generally straighter in appearance than those from chrysotile. Selected area diffraction patterns for the amphibole asbestos minerals may be similar in appearance; therefore, casual visual observation of these patterns is sufficient only for classification of the fiber as being "an amphibole asbestos" (Langer *et al.*, 1974; Cook *et al.*, 1974; Clark and Ruud, 1975). Electron diffraction patterns of asbestos amphibole minerals are sometimes streaked perpendicular to the fiber length. It is then necessary to study the intensity distribution of the spots within the layer lines to distinguish them from chrysotile.

In addition to visual observation of electron diffraction patterns for fiber identification, photographs can be made of the diffraction patterns and crystal "d" spacings measured from the photographic plates and calculated using the instrument camera constant (Timbrell, 1970). Both "spot" and polycrystalline patterns may be measured, but the precision of measurement is not nearly that obtainable with X-ray diffraction. It must be born in mind also that intensities are not the same as observed for X-ray powder patterns, and additional reflections may be present.

Although some laboratories are confident of their ability to perform positive fiber identification by electron microscopy with electron diffraction, the method is empirical and has not been rigorously tested. The possibility still remains that other nonasbestos mineral particles may sometimes give diffraction patterns characteristic of chrysotile, or of the fibrous amphiboles, in certain orientations in the electron beam.

Electron beam microchemical analysis may sometimes be used to distinguish microscopic minerals from other fibrous particles (Rubin and Magiore, 1974; Ferrell *et al.*, 1975; Maggiore and Rubin, 1973; Langer *et al.*, 1975). The most common system presently in use is the energy dispersive X-ray detector, in combination with a scanning or transmission electron microscope. X-ray wavelength dispersive analyzers and the conventional electron microprobe have been used; however, their routine application is limited due to data acquisition times, small particle size, and to other considerations discussed below.

Electron beam X-ray microanalysis coupled only with morphology has often been cited as a method for identifying microfibers (Rubin and Maggiore, 1974; Ferrell *et al.*, 1975). However, many scientists have criticized this technique as having several major faults (Ruud *et al.*, 1976). First, the elemental composition of amphibole minerals is variable, and seldom ideally stoichiometric. Furthermore many nonamphibole minerals are similar in composition to the asbestos amphiboles and sometimes produce microscopic fibers. Second, the chemistry of the environment, e.g., high ion water, can change the actual or apparent composition of the fiber by ion exchange or surface coating. Third, the variables affecting quantitative microanalysis are such that a plus or minus 10% elemental variance is not uncommon from a single prepared standard sample (Ferrell *et al.*, 1975). Electron microscopy with microchemical analysis for fiber identification is reliable only when combined with considerable knowledge of the mineralogy of the fiber source. Such knowledge is generally lacking in the case of water samples.

As has already been discussed, possession of proper elemental intensities by energy dispersive X-ray analysis is generally not sufficient for positive identification of fibers. For example, chrysotile, anthophyllite, and fibrous talc, which have similar elemental compositions, may be difficult to differentiate (Rubin and Maggiore, 1974; Ruud *et al.*, 1976). However, these materials may easily be distinguished using selected area electron diffraction (Ruud *et al.*, 1976; Langer *et al.*, 1975). Transmission electron microscopes equipped with energy dispersive X-ray detectors allow simultaneous observation of morphology, crystal structure, and elemental composition. These microscope systems have been used to study fibers of known asbestos origin as well as environmental and material samples (Cook *et al.*, 1974; Dement *et al.*, 1975). The probability of positive fiber identification (including amphibole minerals) is greatly enhanced with these techniques.

Identification and counting of fibrous or acicular particles in environmental and tissue samples has been accomplished by electron microscopy.

Langer *et al.* (1975) have reported a qualitative method for preparing tissue samples for electron microscopy. This method involves first dissolving the tissue in a 40% solution of potassium hydroxide followed by centrifuging. After centrifuging, the residue is dispersed in distilled water and a drop pipetted onto Formvar-coated 200-mesh electron microscope grids. Similar techniques have been used by Pontefract and Cunningham (1973).

Concentrations of fibrous or acicular particulates in environmental samples and biological tissue are usually expressed as fibers per unit volume or weight of sample (fibers/m^3,fibers/l, fibers/gm dry lung, etc.). These concentrations are determined by counting fibrous or acicular particles within calibrated areas on the electron microscope viewing screen or counting fibers in photographs. Fiber concentrations in water samples determined by laboratories using the same mounting techniques have been reported to vary by a factor of 2 to 3 (Cook *et al.*, 1974). Much larger variations have been reported between laboratories using different techniques (Brown et al., 1976).

The mass of chrysotile concentrations in environmental samples has also been determined using electron microscopy. This is accomplished by measuring the length and diameter (volume) of each fiber and calculating mass using the appropriate density (Selikoff *et al.*, 1972). The accuracy of this method has not been studied in detail.

X-Ray Diffraction

X-ray powder diffractometry is one of the standard mineralogical techniques used in the analysis of solid crystalline phases. X-ray diffraction has been widely used for identification and quantitation of fibers in bulk materials such as talc (Stanley and Norward, 1973; Rohl and Langer, 1974) and other industrial materials (Crable and Knott, 1966a, 1966b; Keenan and Lynch, 1970). X-ray diffraction has also been used to study amphibole asbestos contamination of water samples (Cook *et al.*, 1974). However application of X-ray diffraction to routine analysis of environmental samples has been limited. Birks *et al.* (1975) have reported a feasibility study concerning quantitative analysis of airborne asbestos. This technique, however, is still in the research phase and has not been developed to the reliability of a general analytical method.

It must be recognized that, with the exception of the technique described above, X-ray diffraction methods are not capable of differentiating between asbestos mineral fibers and their nonfibrous mineral counterparts. This fact, combined with the relatively low sensitivity, suggests that analysis of environmental samples by X-ray diffraction should be confirmed by electron microscopy.

Differential Thermal Analysis

Differential thermal analysis has been used to determine asbestos mineral fiber levels in talc samples (Schlez, 1974).

It has not been used for environmental samples because it has low sensitivity. Moreover, it is not capable of differentiating between asbestos fibers and their nonfibrous mineralogical polymorphs.

BIOLOGICAL EFFECTS OF ASBESTOS MINERALS

Epidemiological Findings

Numerous epidemiological studies have shown that occupational exposure to asbestos dust can lead to asbestosis (characterized primarily by pulmonary fibrosis); the formation of pleural plaques; a greatly increased risk of bronchogenic carcinoma; pleural mesothelioma; and peritoneal mesothelioma (Selikoff *et al.*, 1973; Newhouse, *et al.*, 1972; Elmes and Simpson, 1971; Selikoff and Churg, 1965; Bogovski *et al.*, 1973; and Lee, 1974). There is also evidence that the elevated risk of bronchogenic carcinoma as a result of occupational exposure to asbestos dust is largely (though perhaps not entirely) confined to cigarette smokers (Hammond *et al.*, 1975). Different types of asbestos may vary in their potency in relation to the effects mentioned above; but this has been difficult to evaluate owing to lack of precise information on degree of exposure, and various other problems.

Although there is little evidence concerning the possible effects of nonoccupational exposure, some cases of mesothelioma have been found among persons working in or living near shipyards and the wives of asbestos workers who handled the dusty clothes of their husbands (Newhouse and Thompson, 1965; Wagner *et al.*, 1960; Anderson *et al.*, 1976).

There has been much discussion of the possibility that the effects of inhaling asbestos mineral dust vary greatly with the length of the particles. However, no epidemiological evidence is available on this matter. The dust to which industrial workers are exposed typically consists of fibers varying in length from very long to extremely short. Fibers sufficiently large to be seen under a light microscope are invariably accompanied by large numbers of far smaller fibers.

It should be noted that all of the epidemiological evidence noted above has come from studies of people who have been exposed to dust from types of asbestos minerals that have been used commercially. There is no direct epidemiological evidence on the effects of various other types of fibrous minerals, some of which may perhaps find their way into drinking water.

The fact that exposure to air heavily polluted with asbestos mineral fibers often leads to the diseases mentioned above does not necessarily indicate that drinking water contaminated with an equally large number of such fibers may lead to the same diseases or perhaps some other diseases. (Site of cancer can vary depending upon the way in which individuals are subjected to a carcinogenic agent, for example: skin

TABLE IV-6 Observed vs. Expected Number of Deaths from Cancer of Several Sites among Two Groups of Workers Occupationally Exposed to Asbestos Dust. Data Provided by Selikoff, Hammond, Seidman, and Churg.

	Group #1. Asbestos Insulation Workers (United States and Canada)			Group #2. "Amosite" Asbestos Factory Workers (New Jersey)		
Site of Cancer	Obs. Deaths	Exp. Deaths	Ratio	Obs. Deaths	Exp. Deaths	Ratio
Buccal and pharnyx	15	7.87	1.91	6	2.04	2.94
Esophagus	14	5.38	2.60	0	1.36	—
TOTAL	29	13.25	2.19	6	3.40	1.76
Stomach	18	11.23	1.60	10	4.89	2.04
Colon-Rectum	47	28.64	1.64	16	7.65	2.09
TOTAL	94	53.12	1.77	32	15.94	2.01

exposure, inhalation, or ingestion.) However, the hypothesis is tenable to the degree that it cannot be ruled out of consideration without evidence to the contrary.

It is important to note that workers exposed to air containing large numbers of asbestos minerals fibers inevitably ingest such fibers. Many of the fibers that are inhaled are later propelled upward from the lungs and trachea, enter the mouth, and are then swallowed. Thus, fibers are brought into direct surface contact with the epithelial lining of the buccal cavity, esophagus, stomach, and intestines. For this reason, it is pertinent to inquire whether death rates from cancer arising in these tissues are higher among asbestos workers than in the general population, age, sex, and calendar-years of exposure being taken into consideration. This has been investigated by Selikoff, Hammond, Seidman, Churg, and their associates. The data shown in Table IV-6 were provided by these investigators. It shows, for each of two groups of workers, the observed and expected number of deaths from cancer of sites directly exposed to asbestos fibers by way of ingestion: buccal cavity and pharynx, esophagus, stomach, colon, and rectum. The two groups are described below.

Group #1. The entire membership of the insulation workers union in the United States and Canada was registered as of January 1, 1967 (17,800 men). Many characteristics of the men were recorded, including date of birth and onset of work with asbestos. These subjects have been traced through December 31, 1974.

Group #2. This group consisted of the entire workforce (1941–45) of a factory in an eastern U.S. city that manufactured "amosite" asbestos insulation materials (including insulating block and pipe covering and asbestos mattresses), for use by insulation workers in the construction industry, especially in ship construction and repair. The plant opened its doors in June 1941 and remained in business until November 1954. Very few of these production workers studied had had prior occupational exposure to asbestos. Between 1941 and the end of 1945, a total of 933 men were hired; of these, some worked for as little as one day, while others worked until 1954, when the plant closed. Of the 933 men, 881 (94.4%) were traced through December 31, 1973, and the remaining 52 were traced for a part of the period but later lost to follow-up.

For both groups, "observed," as shown in Table IV-6, means the number of men who were found to have died of the indicated cause during the period of observation. "Expected" numbers of deaths are based upon age-specific death rates for white males in the United States during each year of observation.

Group #1 was by far the larger of the two groups, and in consequence the figures are more stable statistically. In this group, the observed number of deaths was substantially higher than the expected number for cancer of each of the four sites. The findings were similar for Group #2, except in respect to cancer of the esophagus (zero observed versus 1.36 expected deaths).

In each of the two groups, the excess of observed over expected number of deaths (for all four sites of cancer combined) was highly significant statistically. It may be argued whether U.S. white males are an appropriate control group in relation to Group #2 (New Jersey "amosite" workers). Therefore, the expected numbers for Group #2 were recomputed based upon New Jersey mortality data. These expected numbers were a little higher than those shown in Table IV-6.

Similar findings in respect to gastrointestinal cancer have been reported by Mancuso (1965) and by Elmes and Simpson (1971). This, taken together with the data presented in Table IV-6, strongly suggests that ingestion of asbestos mineral fibers can result in an increased risk of cancer of several sites. If so, the degree of risk is probably highly dependent upon the number of fibers ingested and the duration of exposure. It may also depend upon the type and size of the fibers, as well as upon other agents to which the individuals have been exposed. For example, both smoking and alcohol increase the risk of cancer of the buccal cavity; and it is possible that exposure of the buccal mucosa to asbestos mineral fibers simply increases the risk of cancer occurring among persons also exposed to one or both of these other two factors.

As described elsewhere in this report, mineral fibers—varying in concentration from trace amounts to hundreds of thousands per liter, or more—are present in drinking water in various locations in the United States. The situation in Duluth, Minn. (as described elsewhere), is of special interest from an epidemiological point of view.

Studies of time trends in cancer death rates and incidence rates in Duluth (as compared with other cities) do not show any increases that could reasonably be attributed to the mineral fiber pollution of the drinking water of that city (Mason *et al.*, 1974; Levy, *et al.*, 1976).

Among persons occupationally exposed to asbestos dust, the increases in death rates from cancer of the stomach, colon, and rectum do not reach measurable proportions until many years after onset of exposure. The lapse of time since Duluth water was first heavily polluted with mineral fibers is not yet sufficient to have produced a significant increase in death rates from these cancers, even if it be assumed that the risk for residents of Duluth is as great as the risk for workers occupationally exposed to asbestos dust. If the risk is not so great—but still of important proportions—it will probably become apparent within another 5, 10, or 15 yr from now. An even lower risk might not become apparent for a much longer period of time—and then it would be difficult if not impossible to pinpoint the cause.

Experimental Studies

As discussed above, epidemiological studies of the population exposed have failed to detect any increase in gastrointestinal cancer that might be ascribed to the asbestos mineral fibers contained in some drinking water. But, since these results do not indicate conclusively that ingestion of water containing such fibers is without risk, and because these substances are widely distributed, it is important also to consider experimental evidence.

An Advisory Committee on Asbestos Cancers to the Director of the International Agency for Research on Cancer, meeting in 1972, considered whether there was evidence of an increased risk of cancer resulting from asbestos minerals present in water, beverages, food, or in the fluids used for the administration of drugs. They concluded that "such evidence as there is does not indicate any risk" (IARC, 1973). The group recommended that the effect of long-term ingestion of fibers of various sizes, shapes, and chemical compositions should be studied. The advisory committee's conclusion can hardly be taken as a categorical denial of risk, but rather reflected the inconclusive character of the evidence then available.

Published results attest to the difficulties experienced by many investigators in studying, by means of experiments with animals, the biological effects and behavior of inorganic fibrous materials in general, and asbestos mineral fibers in particular. Several different approaches have been taken to the design of such experiments, including administration of different types and preparations of asbestos minerals and glass fibers to several species of experimental animals, by ingestion (feeding), inhalation, surgical implantation and injection. Experiments have also been conducted to test the response to fibers of cell cultures *in vitro*. The results of some representative experiments of these kinds are reviewed below.

Westlake *et al.* (1965, 1974) fed chrysotile to rats and noted the presence of fibers of the material in many sites in the colonic epithelium and lamina propria; and Webster (1974), after feeding crocidolite to baboons, showed that small numbers of fibers appeared in the ashed tissue of the gut wall. Gross *et al.* (1974) reported no such penetration. Bolton and Davis (1976), reporting on the short-term effects of chronic ingestion of asbestos minerals by rats, found no sign of cell penetration by fibers or damage to the gut mucosa. They concluded that penetration of the gastrointestinal wall, if it occurred, must have been on a very small scale.

Pontefract and Cunningham (1973) reported that chrysotile, administered to rats intragastrically by direct injection, was later found to be distributed to other organs, and suggested that the material penetrated the digestive tract. Gross (1974) questioned this interpretation of the study on the grounds that the method of administration was likely to have produced contamination of other organs by leakage. Cunningham and Pontefract (1974) reported the appearance of asbestos mineral fibers in fetal organs after injection of asbestos into the femoral veins of pregnant Wistar rats. While none of these papers demonstrated transport of fibers across tissue boundaries, some included the suggestion that the reported deposition of the material in other organs implied that transport had occurred. Reports such as these have, without resolving the matter, lent interest to the question whether or not human ingestion of asbestos may be accompanied by similar effects.

Experimental investigations with animals of the toxic effects of asbestos mineral fibers have not yet led to the development of an experimental model system that reproduces the putative effects of ingestion of such fibers by man. Nevertheless, various animal studies on the toxicity of asbestos have been reported, and some large-scale feeding experiments are now in progress.

In the experimental studies by Wagner *et al.* (1974), using the UICC reference samples, no association was found between exposure to asbestos by inhalation and excess gastrointestinal cancers. Thus, this animal study did not duplicate the positive epidemiological findings previously discussed. The possible effects of ingested asbestos also were studied experimentally. Several animal feeding studies with asbestos are reported to have shown no increase in cancer with this route of exposure (Bonser and Clayson, 1967; Smith, 1973; and Gross *et al.*, 1974). The asbestos minerals tested included crocidolite, chrysotile, and "amosite." However, none of these studies would be considered adequate under modern constructs of chronic toxicity testing (National Academy of Sciences, 1975; Sontag *et al.*, 1976), and so the possibility of false negatives remains.

More recently, Gibel *et al.* (1976) fed filter material containing asbestos (20 mg/day) to 50 Wistar rats. This material was composed of asbestos (chrysotile, 53%), sulfated cellulose and a condensation resin. The authors reported 12 malignant tumors in the group that was fed the filter material, 2 malignant tumors in a control group, and 3 in a similar group of rats that were fed the same amount of a standard grade of talc. The 12 malignant tumors appearing in the group receiving the filter material comprised 1 lung carcinoma, 3 reticular cell sarcomas, 4 kidney carcinomas, and 4 liver carcinomas. In the control animals and the talc-fed animals the malignant tumors were all liver carcinomas. The average survival times were 441 days in the filter-fed group, 702 days in the controls and 649 days in the talc-fed group. The presence of other substances besides asbestos in the filter material and the manner of reporting the malignant tumor counts suggests that further studies are needed, with asbestos alone, before firm conclusions can be drawn from the results of this study.

A fundamental difficulty associated with these studies is that they seek to duplicate an effect in man by means of animal models that have neither been validated for the route of administration nor for the materials of interest. Negative results may be interpreted as indicating either the absence of the effect under investigation or, simply, as further proof that the model was not valid to start with. At present, the existing animal data base leaves the matter unresolved.

Results obtained from some experiments with animals by direct application of fibrous materials, and with *in vitro* systems, have been adduced to support the view that ingestion of drinking water containing mineral fibers should not be expected to lead to any observed increase in gastrointestinal cancer in the general population. These experiments are interpreted to show the dependence of biological effect on the size of fibers. In this approach, large quantities of mineral fibers, of various size distributions, are injected into the pleural or peritoneal cavity. Stanton *et al.* (1969) wrapped a plaque of fibrous material around the lung in their animal model studies. This discussion will be limited to the results reported with respect to a carcinogenic response.

The results obtained from these experiments, in which the material under investigation is deposited or applied directly, are limited by the statistics of their individual designs, methods of fiber preparation, and determination of fiber size distribution. They may be summarized as follows:

1. Tumor induction is related to fiber size, shape and durability, and not to the source of the fiber or its chemical composition (Stanton and Wrench, 1972; Stanton, 1973; Stanton *et al.*, 1977; Pott and Fredricks, 1972; Pott *et al.*, 1976).
2. In cell cultures, particles less than 20 μm in length do not induce growth of fibroblasts (Maroudas *et al.*, 1973).
3. Chrysotile containing particles less than 5 μm in length did not elicit a carcinogenic response (Smith, 1974; Smith *et al.*, 1972).
4. Defining a "significant" asbestos fiber as one less than 0.5 μm in diameter and greater than 10 μm in length, there was good agreement between the number of these "significant" fibers in an asbestos sample and its degree of carcinogenicity (Wagner *et al.*, 1973).
5. Man-made mineral fibers less than 1.5 μm in diameter and greater than 8 μm in length have the highest probability of inducing a biological response. The response appears to increase with increasing fiber length at fiber diameters less than 1.5 μm (Stanton *et al.*, 1977).

In contrast to the results summarized above, two other investigations appear to show a different dependence of biological effect on fiber length. In one of these, Pott *et al.* (1972) injected 100 mg of two different preparations of chrysotile intraperitoneally, one sample contained 95% of particles less than 5 μm in length and the other (a milled sample) contained 99% less than 3 μm in length. Both groups gave approximately the same tumor incidence, although the latency period was greater in the latter group. The data subsequently were reported in greater detail by Pott *et al.* (1974). In this, for the unmilled chrysotile, 78.7% of the fibers were less than 2 μm in length and 93.9% were less than 5μm in length; while for the milled sample, 97.4% were less than 2 μm in length and

99.8% were less than 5 μm in length. After administration of the unmilled chrysotile sample, the elapsed time to appearance of first tumor was 270 days with a tumor incidence of 37.5%, while for the milled chrysotile sample the time to appearance of first tumor was 400 days, with a tumor incidence of 30%. This study would indicate that both short and long fibers were carcinogenic, though the milled sample seems to have been somewhat less active than the unmilled one. But in the absence of information about the distribution of fiber diameters and the number per unit weight it is impossible to assign activity to a particular size class with certainty.

Another possible exception is contained in a paper by Wagner *et al.* (1976) describing experiments with glass fibers. In these experiments two different preparations of glass fibers were injected intrapleurally into experimental animals. The characteristics of the fiber preparations and the results are summarized below.

Characteristics of Glass Fibers

	Finer	Coarser
Diameter <0.5μm	99%	—
Diameter <1μm	—	17%
Median diameter (μm)	0.12	1.8
Length >20μm	2%	—
Length >50μm	—	10%
Median length (μm)	1.7	22
Results		
No. with mesothelioma	4/32	0/32
Absence of hyperplasia in mesothelial cells	1/32	12/32

The same weight (20 mg) of each material was used per animal, and there were about 1,000 times more fibers in the finer glass than in the coarser glass (Wagner *et al.*, 1976). The results indicate, therefore, that the finer sample contained more "active" fibers than did the coarser.

On the basis of the animal experiments noted above, it is possible to infer that, in these experimental systems, short fibers may be biologically unreactive, or less reactive, than longer ones. Since the majority of the fibers that are found in water are short (<5 μm), these may be similarly unreactive, and this may account for failure to detect any increased incidence of various gastrointestinal cancers related to ingestion of mineral fibers in water.

Another hypothesis can be offered for the inability to detect, in the general population, any increase in gastrointestinal cancers attributable to ingestion of asbestos mineral fibers in water. Assuming that the heavily exposed asbestos workers (who showed an excess gastrointestinal cancer rate) swallowed a large fraction of the fibers, of all sizes, that they inhaled, the dose so acquired would have been several orders of magnitude greater than that ingested in drinking water by members of the general population. It would therefore be expected that any excess gastrointestinal cancer due to fibers in water would be much smaller in the general population than that found in asbestos workers, and if sufficiently low might be very difficult to detect against the usual background incidence of cancers of the colon, sigmoid, and rectum, and less so for cancers of the esophagus and stomach.

The results of experiments on the chronic toxicity of asbestos mineral fibers fall very far short of rigorously clarifying the risk to health that may be associated with potable water—either qualitatively or quantitatively. Although no harmful effects of fibrous contamination of drinking water on the present state of public health have been demonstrated, it is possible, as noted in the discussion of the epidemiology, that they may be observed in the future.

The development of gastrointestinal cancers among the heavily exposed asbestos workers has been slow (20 to 30 yr or more), and the possibility of long-delayed effects of mineral fiber ingestion through water cannot be ignored. Research on the unresolved problems of the chronic effects of ingesting asbestos mineral fibers therefore merits strong support.

ORGANIC PARTICULATES IN WATER

The organic particulate matter found in natural water systems may be classified as follows:

1. Organic matter associated with soil particles.
2. Organic particles from effluent of sewage treatment facilities and industrial waste disposal facilities.
3. Plant and animal debris.
4. Microorganisms.
5. Organic colloids.

Microorganisms are discussed in Chapter III; the other categories are discussed below.

Organic Matter Associated with Soil Particles

The major part of the suspended material in most natural bodies of water is made up of soil particles derived from the land surface by erosion. The coarser sand and silt fractions consist mainly of inorganic rock and mineral fragments, many of which are, at least partially, coated with organic material. The clay-size fraction of most soils consists of clay minerals, metal oxides, hydrous metal oxides, and soil organic material (humus) in intimate contact with one another. As Gorbunov, Yerokhina, and Schchurina (1971) and Greenland (1971) have shown, the clay minerals in the A horizons of most soils are coated with organic matter, forming a so-called "clay-organic complex."

Greenland also found that hydrous oxides provide even more sites for adsorption of organic matter in soils than do micaceous clay minerals. Hydrous oxides also coat surfaces of clay mineral grains. It is therefore to a certain extent artificial to attempt to separate the effects of the organic and inorganic components of the soil particulate matter suspended in water. However, it is likely that in many instances the effect of the organic components is predominant.

In those instances in which the soil organic material (humus) forms coatings on the clay and oxide surfaces of soil particles, reactions between the coated particles and the environment external to the particles will to a large extent be governed by the physical and chemical properties of the humus. For example, the ion-exchange capacity and the adsorption properties of the particles will be strongly influenced by the ion-exchange capacity and the adsorption capacity of the humus coatings.

Both soluble and insoluble organic compounds are sorbed by humus. Ladd and Butler (1971) have shown that the humic and fulvic acid components of soil humus inhibit proteolytic enzymes by binding them. In addition to enzymes, humus strongly binds some pesticides and other organic compounds that are found in soils and natural waters. This sorption reduces the phytotoxicity of herbicides and often inhibits the degradation of many pesticides (Wershaw and Goldberg, 1972).

In order to understand the interactions of soil particles in natural water systems, it is necessary to consider briefly what is known about the chemical structure and physical-chemical properties of soil humus. Humus has been traditionally fractionated into three compounds: humic acid, fulvic acid, and humin. Humic acid is the component that is soluble in strong base but insoluble in strong acid, fulvic acid is soluble in both acid and base; and humin is insoluble in both acid and base.

Humic acids contain phenolic, quinoid, polycarboxylic aromatic acidic, and aliphatic groups, the aromatic groups predominating (Kononova, 1966; Felbeck, 1965, 1971; Scheffer and Ulrich, 1960; Steelink, 1963; Flaig, 1970). In addition to benzene carboxylic acid and phenolic groups, some authors have included fatty acid, protein, and polysaccharide groups. It has been assumed that these groups are joined together covalently by linkages such as ether, ester and carbon-carbon to form three-dimensional polymers of high molecular weight (Flaig, 1970).

Several recent studies indicate that this structural interpretation is not correct. Wershaw and Pinckney (1971, 1973a, 1973b) have shown that the most abundant humic acid fractions form aggregates in solution that are made up of relatively small molecules (molecular weights of several thousand or less). The degree of association of these molecules is a function of pH. Monahan, DeLuca, and Wershaw (1972) have found that the degree of aggregation of some of the fractions is also a function of concentration and that at low concentrations the molecules are dissociated. The presence of these aggregates will have a marked effect on the way humic acids interact with pollutants in natural water systems, and this will be discussed later.

Fulvic acids are generally believed to be similar in structure to humic acids but of lower molecular weight. It is apparent, however, that other groups of compounds, such as polysaccharides, proteins, and aminosugars are also included in many fulvic acid preparations (J. A. Leenheer, oral communications, 1974).

Alternating treatment of the humin fraction with strong mineral acids and strong bases generally renders most of the humin soluble in basic solutions (Kononova, 1966). From this Kononova has concluded that humins are humic acids that are bound by the mineral constituents of soils.

Humic substances have a large capacity for base exchange. Kononova (1966) has reviewed the exchange capacity of several different soils and has reported values from about 200 to over 500 milli-equivalents per 100 g for humic acids. The ion exchange capacities of humic acids depend on pH and are smaller at low pH values than at high pH values.

There has been a great deal of study lately on trace metals in natural water systems because of the effect that variations in the concentration of those metals can have on plant and animal health. Harding and Brown (1975) have studied the distribution of some selected trace metals in sediments of the Pamlico River estuary in North Carolina. They found the highest concentrations of trace elements in the mixed clay organic matter sediments in the center of the estuary. These high trace metals concentrations are apparently due to human activity. Concentrations 4 to 1,750 times normal background were detected. Their evidence suggests that the trace metals are scavenged from water entering the estuary by the clay and organic matter in the sediments. The suspended clay and organic matter in the water would also be expected to have high trace metal concentrations. Shimp *et al.* (1971) have found that the concentrations of bromine, chromium, copper, lead, and zinc increase with increasing organic carbon concentrations in recent sediments from southern Lake Michigan. They pointed out that: "High concentrations of these elements correlate more closely with the amounts of organic carbon present than with clay-size material, water depth, iron oxide or manganese oxide."

A significant portion of the cation exchange capacity of most soils and marine sediments is due to organic polyelectrolytes; in soils and sediment of high organic content, most of the exchange capacity can be attributed to organic polyelectrolytes (Schnitzer, 1965; Rashid, 1969). Schnitzer and Skinner (1965) found that both carboxyl and phenolic hydroxyl ligands react with polyvalent cations. Infrared studies by Rashid (1971) on marine humic acids confirmed the participation of carboxyl groups in exchange reactions with cations, but no evidence for the participation of phenolic hydroxyl groups was found.

Koshy and Ganguly (1969), Malcolm (1969), and Ong *et al.* (1970) have studied the formation of soluble humic acid-metal complexes. They found that the amount of metal ions that is complexed by humic acid increases with increasing pH. Although these authors did not offer an explanation for this behavior, it is reasonable to suppose that, with increasing pH, more disaggregation of the humic acid takes place, and more ligand sites are exposed for complexing with the metal ions. The metal ions may be bound both by ligands on a single molecule or ligands on more than one molecule. The metal ions may therefore act as bridges between molecules, causing aggregation (Sipos *et al.*, 1972).

In addition to interactions with metals, humic acids and other natural organic polyelectrolytes can interact strongly with other organic components in natural water systems. These interactions can be of two types: incorporation of organic molecules into humic acids during their formation, and reaction of organic compounds with humic acids after their formation.

Humic acids are generally considered to arise from the microbial degradation of organic debris. Martin and his co-workers (1972) have shown that some soil fungi can convert a wide variety of different organic substrates into phenolic and quinoid compounds and aromatic acids, which are then converted into humic acids.

Some studies have also revealed that some humic acid fractions have high free radical content. Steelink and Tollin (1967) and others have found free radicals both in soils and in humic acids isolated from soils. The evidence suggests that the radicals detected are quinoid radicals. Martin has not postulated a mechanism for the conversion of the phenols, quinones, and aromatic acids into humic acids, but it is likely that free radical polymerization reactions play a major role in this conversion.

The free radicals that polymerize into humic acid molecules probably arise either from enzymatic reactions or photolysis. Compounds that are either oxidized or reduced to free radicals may be derived either from plant and animal remains, or from sewage, pesticides, or other pollutants. The conditions for these oxidation-reduction reactions are undoubtedly present in many soil–water systems. Su and Zabik (1972) have studied the photolysis of the miticide *m*-(*n*,*N*-dimethylformamidine) phenyl *N*-methylcarbamate in water. They have shown that decomposition proceeds through the formation of free radicals. Similarly, Mazzocchi and Rao (1972) have found that radical intermediates are formed in the photolysis of the herbicides monuron and fenuron.

Bordeleau *et al.* (1972) have studied the degradation of phenylamide herbicides in soils. They found that azobenzenes and polyaromatic compounds are formed by a combination of enzymatic and chemical reactions, from the phenylamide herbicides. Chloroaniline groups are formed by acyl-amidase degradation of phenylamide herbicides. These chloroaniline groups are then transformed to stable chloroazobenzene residues by peroxidases. During the enzymatic degradation by peroxidase, free radical intermediates were detected by electron paramagnetic resonance. The free radicals produced in the above reactions could be incorporated into humic acids. The work of Khan and Schnitzer (1972) strongly suggests that different organic molecules are indeed incorporated in humic acid. They have succeeded in releasing a variety of hydrophobic organic compounds from a humic acid after exhaustive methylation with diazomethane. They were able to identify alkanes, fatty acids, dialkyl phthalates, and butyl adipate in the mixture of released compounds. These compounds comprised about 1% of the total humic acid weight. Previous extraction with organic solvents had released only a very small amount of the hydrophobic compounds. Khan and Schnitzer have proposed that humic acid has a molecular sieve type of structure that traps insoluble organic compounds. This mechanism implies that humic acid molecules form a three-dimensional network with suitable voids in which the hydrophobic molecules are adsorbed. Khan and Schnitzer apparently assume that methylation disrupts this structure and releases the entrapped compounds. The humic acids that were used by Khan and Schnitzer were extracted from soil with sodium hydroxide solution. During this type of extraction, disaggregation of the humic acid molecules will take place and most of the molecules trapped in the voids should be released. The compounds that they identified were apparently not released and therefore another mechanism must have been responsible for binding these molecules. The fact that methylation was required for release of the molecules strongly suggests that they were chemically bonded to functional groups in the humic acid polymers and could well have been incorporated into the humic acid polymer when it was formed.

The humic acid polymer, after formation, may participate in reactions which may be conveniently divided into the categories tabulated below. When considering these types of interactions it must be kept in mind that humic acids form molecular aggregates; changes in the degree of aggregation will probably modify these interactions.

Mechanisms of Interaction

Physical Interactions
- Adsorption
  - a. Hydrogen bonding
  - b. Van der Waals bonding

Chemical Interactions
- Chemisorption
- Coordination reactions
- Radical and other chemical reactions

Most organic pesticides are adsorbed by soil organic matter (Wershaw and Goldberg, 1972). A few studies of the mechanism of adsorption of particular pesticides by soil polyelectrolytes have been conducted. Sullivan and Felbeck (1968) and Li and Felbeck (1972) have proposed that the sorption of triazine herbicides is due either to hydrogen bonding or to ionic bonding or to both of these taking place simultaneously. Hsu and Bartha (1976) found that up to 90% of the 3,4-dichloraniline (DCA) derived from the biodegradation of phenylamide herbicides is adsorbed so strongly by soil organic matter that it is not extractable by solvents. The bound DCA is susceptible to acid and alkaline hydrolysis. The authors have concluded that this suggests that the nitrogen atom of the DCA is covalently bound to the carbon of a carbonyl group or to a quinoid ring of a humic acid molecule. Much more work is necessary, however, to elucidate the general principles of adsorption of pesticides by soil organic polyelectrolytes.

The evidence cited above for the strong adsorption of many pesticides by soil organics suggests that one would expect these pesticides to be associated with the sediments in rivers and lakes, and indeed this has been found to be the case.

Manigold and Loral (personal communication, 1976) have found in a study of the distribution of pesticides in rivers that the chlorinated hydrocarbon insecticides such as DDT are concentrated in the suspended sediments and that very little of these materials is found in solution in the water. A similar situation would be expected with the polychlorinated biphenyls and other hydrophobic pollutants in natural waters.

An example of chemisorption by humic acids appears to be found in the work of Perry and Adam (1971). They studied the incorporation of peptides into humic acid by allowing glycylglycine to react with humic acid at pH 8.5. They found that part of the amino nitrogen introduced into humic acid by this reaction could not be removed by hydrolysis with 6N HCL at 110°C for 24 hr. At least part of this unreleased amino nitrogen is probably bound to the humic acid by *N*-phenyl linkages. Although the mechanism of formation of these bonds has not been elucidated, this example illustrates the reactivity of humic acids and the strengths of the bonds formed. It also suggests that chemisorption accounts for much of the binding of amino acids, peptides, and proteins that has been observed in soils. Anderson (1958) has shown that the hydrolysis products of deoxyribonucleic acid (DNA) are released from humic acid by perchloric acid hydrolysis; he concluded from this that DNA is present in humic acid. The binding of enzymes to humic acids (Ladd and Butler, 1971; Mato *et al.*, 1971) is probably also due in part to the formation of bonds between amino nitrogen groups and reactive sites on the humic acid molecules. Undoubtedly, other types of reactions can also take place, some perhaps involving shared metal cations. A careful study of the interactions of humic acids with enzymes should give a new insight into the biochemical reactions that take place in soil-water systems.

Municipal and Industrial Wastes

Municipal and industrial waste disposal is a major source of organic particulate matter in natural waters that serve as sources for drinking water. The amount of particulate matter added by any particular waste disposal site is highly dependent on the amount of treatment that is given to the wastes (Litchfield, 1975; Soderquist, 1975; Gove and Gillman, 1975; Jewell *et al.*, 1975; Talbot, 1975; Pico, 1975; Macauley, 1975). Large quantities of organic and inorganic particulate wastes are also added to natural water from urban runoff and from combined sewer overflows (Field and Knowles, 1975). These sources supply large quantities of pollutants to natural waters during periods of heavy rainfall, so that the amount of pollution is highly variable. This makes it particularly difficult to predict the quality of the feed water into a drinking water plant that is being supplied with water from a source that is subject to intermittent pollution caused by storm runoff. In combined sanitary storm sewage systems untreated sanitary sewage may be discharged into a receiving stream during periods of high storm sewage flow.

Organic matter supplied to natural waters by sanitary sewage-treatment plants and treatment facilities for food-processing plants undergoes degradation relatively rapidly. However, some industrial products are much more persistent. Giger *et al.* (1974), in their study of the sediments in Lake Zug, Switzerland, found high concentrations of petroleum-derived hydrocarbons in the sediments near densely populated areas. They concluded that biodegradation of these hydrocarbons is retarded in the sediments.

Shelton and Hunter (1974) have studied the occurrence of oil pollutants in sediments. They found that the heavier petroleum fractions are concentrated in sediments. In the event of an oil spill, petroleum is adsorbed by the sediment in the area of the spill and slowly released. As time passes, the petroleum components remaining in the sediment will become heavier and heavier.

The fine-grained particulate matter found in rivers and lakes that drain heavily populated areas are generally high in organic carbon and in trace elements. Much of this material is derived from domestic and industrial waste disposal. For example, high concentrations of metals are often found in sewage sludge and in the organic particulates released by sewage treatment plants (Bruland *et al.*, 1974; Leland, Copenhaver, and Wilkes, 1975).

An example of high trace metal concentrations in suspended sediments of a heavily industralized drainage basin is found in southern Lake Michigan. Leland *et al.* (1973) have studied the distribution of trace metals in the bottom and suspended sediments in southern Lake Michigan. Their data show markedly higher concentrations of arsenic, bromine, chromium, copper, mercury, lead and zinc " . . . near the sediment water interface of fine-grained sediments than in underlying sediments of Southern Lake Michigan." They found that with the exception of bromine the trace element concentrations in the suspended sediments were equal to or higher than the concentrations in fine-grained surficial sediments. They concluded from this evidence that the high trace metal concentrations in the sediments are due to high concentrations in the suspended sediments that settle out in the lake. The highest concentrations of trace elements are in the central basin of the lake, where the finest sediments are found. Thus the smallest suspended particles, which do not settle out until they have reached the center of the lake, have the highest concentrations of trace metals. These sediments also have the highest organo-chlorine insecticide concentrations. Leland, Shukla, and Shimp (1973) found a positive correlation between the organic carbon concentration, iron oxide concentration, and trace metal concentrations in the sediments.

Since many of the communities around Lake Michigan take their drinking water from the lake, the high trace metal and pesticide concentrations in the suspended sediments could pose a problem if the coagulation and filtration processes used in water treatment are not adequate to remove them from the water.

When organic particulate matter containing high trace metal concentration is introduced into a natural body of water a new set of equilibrium equations will in general be required to represent the system. If the chemical composition of the water is different from that of the solutions in which the particulate matter acquired the trace metals, redistribution of metal ions between the water and the sediment phases will take place. This sediment will serve as a source of trace metals in water even after the source of pollution is removed.

Release of metals fixed to the suspended and bottom sediments may also take place by decomposition of the organic matter binding the metals in the sediment. DeGroot, DeGoeij, and Zegers (1971) have reported this phenomenon in the Rhine and Ems rivers. They found that most of the mercury and other heavy metals transported to the sea by the rivers are fixed to suspended particles of less than 16 μm in diameter. The metal ions remain fixed to the suspended particles in both of the rivers until the chemical composition of the river water is changed by mixing with seawater. Downsteam from the freshwater tidal zone of each of the rivers mercury, zinc, lead, chromium, arsenic, cobalt, and iron are lost from the sediments. The authors have attributed this to decomposition of the organic matter of the suspended sediment. Experiments performed in their laboratories suggest that the metals are released as organometallic complexes.

Muller and Forstner (1974) have questioned the conclusions of DeGroot, DeGoeij, and Zegers and claim that most of the reduction in heavy metal concentration in the sediments of the Rhine estuary is due to dilution of the sediments derived from the Rhine with cleaner North Sea sediments. However they do not totally discount the solubilization mechanism. At this time, however, it is not at all clear which conclusion is correct.

Organic Debris

Very little work has been done on debris from living organisms in streams. Lammers (1967) has used ultracentrifugation to isolate the suspended organic components of streams. In his later work (Lammers, 1975) he isolated the organic debris from the gut of living filter-feeding organisms. Lammers chose several different bivalves for this work. The use of the bivalves allows one to obtain integrated samples of the debris in the stream. The material isolated from the bivalves was then fractionated by ultracentrifugation. In both of the above papers Lammers deals mainly with the viruses, algae, and bacteria that he isolated; however, he does indicate that other organic particles, such as ribosomes, were also isolated.

A number of studies have shown that organisms in natural bodies of water concentrate hydrophobic pollutants, such as chlorinated hydrocarbon insecticides, in their tissue (Sodergran *et al.*, 1972). It would therefore be expected that some of the organic debris in natural waters would contain elevated levels of hydrophobic pollutants; however, there do not appear to be any studies in the literature that deal with this matter.

Organic Colloids

Organic polyelectrolytes that are very similar to the soil humic and fulvic acids have been isolated from surface and groundwaters. As Black and Christman (1963) point out, these materials will impart a brownish color to water if present in high enough concentration, and indeed many potable water supplies are colored. Day and Felbeck (1974) have shown that the fungus *Aureobasidium pullulans,* which is common in sewage, soils, and surfaces, exudes a substance similar to fulvic acid. Martin and his co-workers in a series of papers (see Haider *et al.*, 1972, and Martin *et al.*, 1972, for reviews of this work) have shown that soil microorganisms can form humic substances in two ways: by extracellular transformation of plant and animal constituents into humic compounds and by synthesis of humic precursors from aliphatic compounds. The most common precursors that Martin and his co-workers have detected are phenols that are polymerized by autoxidation or enzymatic reactions, or more likely by both pathways, into humic materials. Similar transformations in sewage and in surface waters would be expected. Thus we may expect that the degradation of many organic wastes will result in the formation of humic materials. During the polymerization process, it is possible that resistant pollutant molecules that have not been degraded by the microorganisms will be incorporated into the humic and fulvic acid polymers.

The first part of this discussion has been principally concerned with the relatively insoluble humic acid associated with soils. However, the humic acid salts of the more common monovalent cations are soluble in water. Wershaw and Pinckney (1973b) have demonstrated that these humic acid molecules form molecular aggregates in solution, the degree of aggregation depending on both pH and concentration. This aggregation phenomenon was detected both in humic acid fractions and in unfractionated salts. Fractionation apparently increased the chemical homogeneity of the fractions by comparison with the unfractionated salts. The aggregates that have been detected in the fractions therefore probably comprise molecules that are chemically more or less similar. However, in an unfractionated sample, the aggregates will contain a diversity of different types of molecules. Even molecules that are quite different from humic acids can be incorporated into the aggregates; Wershaw *et al.* (1969) have shown that the sodium salt of humic acid can solubilize DDT by incorporating DDT molecules into the sodium humate aggregates (micelles).

Undoubtedly, this mechanism is responsible for the transport of other relatively insoluble pollutants, besides DDT, in natural water systems. Ballard (1971) reported an apparent example of this mechanism at work in a natural system. He found that the urea salt or the ammonium salt of humic acid solubilized DDT and carried it down through a soil profile.

In addition to solubilization reactions, soluble humic acid salts and fulvic acids interact with metals to form colloidal organometallic complexes. Much of the early work on colloidal humic material-metal complexes was on iron complexes. Several workers have found that the oxidation of ferrous iron is greatly retarded in many natural waters that contain humic substances (Theis and Singer, 1974).

Whatever the reaction mechanism, it has been well established that humic material stabilizes both ferrous and ferric iron in natural water systems. This has important implications for water treatment, since the standard method of removing excess iron from water is to oxidize it with oxygen and allow it to precipitate as $Fe(OH)_3$. The presence of humic material inhibits these reactions.

A number of more general studies (Rashid and Leonard, 1973; Orlov and Yeroshicheva, 1967; Ong *et al.*, 1970) have shown that humic materials form complexes with copper, cobalt, manganese, nickel, zinc, iron, and aluminum, and solubilize these metals in natural water systems.

Cheam has reviewed the literature on the complexation of copper (II) by fulvic acid. The available evidence indicates that copper is chelated at a bidentate site consisting of a phenolic hydroxl group and an ionized carboxyl group.

Potable water supplies containing humic materials are often decolonized by chlorination. Rook (1974) has shown that chlorination of humic acid solutions in water results in the formation of haloforms, some of which are known or suspected to be carcinogenic (Nicholson, 1977). A survey for haloforms in the water of 80 cities, conducted by the EPA, showed that occurrence of trihalomethanes is widespread in finished drinking waters and is a direct result of chlorination (Stevens *et al.*, 1975; Symons, 1976). The risks that ingestion of these compounds may pose to human health are discussed in Chapter VI.

Summary

Natural organic polyelectrolytes (humic materials) play a major role in the binding and transport of pollutants in natural water systems. These reactions include: (1) adsorption of pesticides, enzymes, and other organic compounds; (2) free radical reactions including charge-transfer reactions between free radicals; (3) ion-exchange and complexation reactions between metal ions and ligands or trace organic polyelectrolytes; (4) solubilization reactions in which relatively insoluble compounds are rendered more soluble.

These reactions will lead to the binding of toxic metals and organic compounds to suspended colloidal particles in raw water supplies.

MICROORGANISMS AND SUSPENDED PARTICLES IN WATER

The tendency of microorganisms to form aggregates and to become concentrated at the surfaces of solid particles, rather than to be uniformly and individually dispersed, may have important consequences for their survival and for their reactions to the various processes of water treatment. It is doubtful that many of these microbial agglomerates will pass through an efficiently operating water-treatment process, but a large segment of the population ingests surface water that has had only partial treatment (i.e., disinfection). Under such circumstances these microbial agglomerates constitute potential health hazards.

Unfortunately, there is a lack of scientific information on either the survival of the bacterial component of these microbial-agglomerates after disinfection of surface waters or on their ability to disaggregate and produce infection in the human host after ingestion. Viral aggregates, on the other hand, have a higher resistance to disinfection than free virions and produce infection in susceptible hosts. (See Chapter III, "Microbiology," section on viruses.)

Although there is a large body of scientific information from laboratory and field studies on raw water sources with regard to bacterial and viral agglomerates, the same level of scientific attention has not been given to studies of the viability of these agglomerates in finished drinking water or, more importantly, on infection of the human host after ingestion of these agglomerates.

Particulate-Bacterial Interactions

A knowledge of aquatic and terrestrial habitats of microorganisms is essential to the understanding and resolution of problems that arise when man must use the same environment. Potable water, which may be regarded as an environment, has been developed by man out of natural aquatic microbial habitats that are continuously fed, in a microbial sense, from the terrestrial habitat. Pollution of these habitats by higher organisms adds to the natural microbial population already present. This pollution component of the microbial population supplies the more hazardous aspects to the potable water environment because these are the microbial members that have passed through man and other organisms and have, in some instances, been responsible for debilitation or death.

Studies of microbial aggregates in terrestrial environments that ultimately seed the raw water sources have been carried out by Brock (1966, 1974), Cameron (1965–1969), Rice *et al.* (1975), Henrici (1948), Schmidt (1968), Mallette (1963), and Kononova (1966). These studies demonstrated that the most extensive microbial growth takes place in nature on the surfaces of particles and inside loose flocs of solid particles. This occurs because the nutrients required for microbial growth are also adsorbed at the surfaces of these particles. Only a few microorganisms are found *free* in the soil solution or in raw water because of the lack of dissolved nutrients. Thus, chemical and microbiological analyses of water *per se* will not reveal the higher concentrations of organic nutrients and microorganisms present on the surfaces and inside sand, silt, or clay particles that have settled to lower water strata or to the bottom of the raw water sources. Some of the aggregates will be sequestered by sedimentation, but microbial particulates in lake and reservoir sediments remain viable and grow rapidly at the time of the spring inversion, when mixing with upper layers will cause some redistribution (Henrici, 1948; Boylen and Brock, 1973; Hendricks, 1973).

Mutual microbial interactions also occur, not only in association with inorganic and organic particulates, but also in their absence to form mixed microbial aggregates. Such mutualistic relationships may benefit both organisms in such ecological associations or show a graded series of symbioses of variable stability and specificity. Studies of these particulate interrelationships have been reviewed by Lederberg (1952) and investigated by Sharp and Church (1963) and Rice *et al.* (1975).

These mutualistic relationships allow microbial growth to take place in environments unsuitable for rapid growth of either member alone; this concept has implications for the survival and rapid growth of microorgnisms in nutrient-starved aquatic systems, e.g., potable water supplies.

Investigations of the physical–chemical attachment of microorganisms to sand, silt, and clays, the difficulties encountered in disaggregating these particulate complexes, and the conditions promoting migration of the aggregates into potable water supplies (deep wells in particular) have been reported by Stotzky (1965, 1966), Lammers (1967), Boyd *et al.* (1969), and Gray and Wilkinson (1965). Of the physical–chemical characteristics studied, Stotzky, in a series of publications, showed that cation exchange capacity (CEC) had an important effect on the binding of organisms to particles. Lammers isolated and fractionated various organic and inorganic particle species occurring in natural waters. Studies of this kind could help to elucidate the composition and concentration of microbial particulates in water.

Particulate-Viral Interactions in Water

River silt adsorbs viruses with moderate efficiency and does not relinquish them very easily. Berg (1973) showed experimentally that silt adsorbed up to 94% of poliovirus 1 from distilled water, but only 0.3 to 0.6% of the adsorbed virus could be eluted from the silt. He also showed that viruses were recovered more frequently from the silt filtered from river water than from the river water itself. Since viruses were not recovered so efficiently from silt as from water, there would appear to be much more virus adsorbed to the silt than suspended in the water. These studies on viral adsorption to sand, silt, clays, and organics (feces) to form particulates are consistent with what is known for bacterial aggregates.

To infect by ingestion of water, viruses must pass from their source (human and animal excreta) through two formidable barriers: sewage treatment and water treatment. In both processes, formation of large particulate–viral flocs are required for settling and filtration. Sewage or water treatment may inactivate the virus, but viruses may also survive in the settled sludge or on filters.

Aggregation and Survival

Several studies have demonstrated that the presence of particulate matter in water interferes with disinfection. Neefe *et al.* (1967), Walton (1961), Hudson (1962), Sanderson and Kelly (1962), Tracy *et al.* (1966), and Symons and Hoff (1975) have all shown this effect. The association between microorganism and particle appears to produce a resistant complex that is not easily dissociated.

Some aspects of the resistance to disinfection of viruses that have become associated with organic particulate material are illustrated by experiments reported by Symons and Hoff (1975) on the inactivation of aqueous suspensions of poliovirus 1. Purified suspensions of the free virus, washed suspensions of virus on the debris of cells in which it had been grown, and mixtures of suspensions of virus and uninfected cells were treated with HOCl at 3 mg/liter. The results indicated that preparations of free virus, either alone or mixed immediately with cell suspensions, were inactivated rapidly. By contrast, virus associated with cell debris, and virus mixed with a cell suspension and held overnight, were inactivated much more slowly. The authors note that the nature of the association between virus particles and cell debris, and the extent to which these preparations represent the conditions in which viruses occur in nature and in treated water, are unknown.

Melnick (1975) discusses the viral inactivation problems associated with the use of heat, formalin, chlorine, and other agents, in cases where tissue-culture techniques demonstrate viral inactivation (no PFU). If however, the virus is inoculated into an animal host, it may produce infection although no PFU's were demonstrated in tissue culture. (See also Chapter III, "Microbiology," section on viruses.) Viral particulates and aggregates form protective barriers to some of the internal virions of the aggregate. Thus the nucleic acid component of the virus is doubly protected against disinfecting (inactivating) agents by the viral protein coat and by the outer mass of virus particles in the aggregate.

Petrilli *et al.* (1974) used an experimental treatment plant to show that enteroviruses survived even though coliforms, *E. coli*, and fecal streptococci were eliminated after treatment of raw water by coagulation with ferric chloride, sedimentation, filtration through activated carbon or sand, and terminal chlorination. He also demonstrated survival of enterovirus in spring water that had been chlorinated sufficiently to destroy the coliforms and fecal streptococci that were also initially present. A review of viral problems facing water treatment plant operators is presented by Taylor (1974).

Conclusions

Investigations are required of the physical–chemical attachment of microorganisms to sand, silt, clays, and organic particles, and disaggregation of these particulate complexes. Viral aggregates are more resistant to disinfection than are separate viral particles. Fundamental information is needed on the interactions between the viable and nonviable components of particulates in drinking water and particularly on their resistance to disinfecion and to other water-treatment processes.

PARTICULATE REMOVAL AND TURBIDITY

Definitions and Occurrence

Some terms commonly used in water treatment practice are described here. *Turbidity* in water is caused by the presence of suspended matter such as clay, silt, nonliving organic particulates, plankton, and other microscopic organisms. Operationally, turbidity measurements are expressions of certain light scattering and absorbing properties of a water sample. *Color* in water is due primarily to the presence of natural organic matter; it may also be caused by certain industrial wastes and by some metallic complexes. Color is measured by determining light adsorption. Hence, colloidal particles can produce some color as it is operationally determined.

Filtration has been defined as the passage of a fluid through a porous medium to remove matter held in suspension. Particles ranging in size from a small fraction of a micrometer to several hundred micrometers can be removed by conventional packed-bed filters used in water treatment if appropriate chemical pretreatment is provided. *Coagulation* is a process in which colloidal particles are destabilized by the addition of suitable chemicals and then assembled into larger aggregates primarily by gentle fluid motion. *Sedimentation* is a process by which solids are separated from water by gravity. In conventional treatment for the removal of particulates, the solids in water are first coagulated into compact, fast-settling flocs. Most of these are then removed by sedimentation, after which the water is filtered to remove additional particulates.

Softening involves the removal of calcium and magnesium ions from water. Usually these are removed as solids, *viz*., calcium carbonate and magnesium hydroxide. Hence, water-softening plants have sedimentation and filtration facilities for the removal of these precipitates. Other solids in the raw water (e.g., clay) and other precipitates that may be formed in the softening process can then be removed by these solid-liquid separation processes.

A survey by the USPHS of municipal water facilities in communities with populations of 25,000 or more was summarized by Jenkins (1963). The population covered by this survey totaled 100,940,020 people. A minimum of 62% of this population received filtered water and hence was delivered water treated for the removal of particulates. This information has been revised and expanded to include more communities in a facilities survey by the EPA in the early 1970's. The results are presently being analyzed and summarized by EPA.

Removal of Particulates

MINERAL FIBERS

Pilot-scale filtration experiments for the removal of amphibole and chrysotile fibers from the Duluth water supply have been conducted (Black and Veatch, Consulting Engineers, 1975; Logsdon and Symons, 1975). Amphibole fibers were easily removed by coagulation and filtration. Considerable difficulties were encountered in removing the chrysotile fibers. These were small and may have been positively charged. Since conventional filters are able to remove submicroscopic particles (Yao *et al.*, 1971), and since conventional pretreatment chemistry (coagulation) is designed to destabilize negative particles, it is plausible that the surface characteristics of the chrysotile particles may hinder their removal by conventional filtration practice. Finally, it is important to note that the design, operation, and evaluation of water-treatment facilities for the removal of fibrous particles is seriously impaired by the time, effort, and expense required to detect these particles in water supplies.

CLAY

Direct evidence of the removal of clays from water supplies by coagulation and filtration is lacking, since clay particles are not detected directly in routine water analysis. It can be implied that clays are effectively removed since they comprise a significant portion of natural "turbidity," and conventional treatment plants are very effective in turbidity removal. This conclusion is substantiated by laboratory studies of the coagulation and filtration of clay suspensions. Studies of this type are numerous. For example, Packham (1965) and Black and Hannah

(1961) have demonstrated effective coagulation and sedimentation of kaolinite, montmorillonite, and other clay suspensions using aluminum sulfate for destabilization under conditions similar to those encountered in potable water treatment. Among many others, Ling (1955) and Adin and Rebhun (1974) demonstrated effective removal of clays from suspension by filtration after appropriate chemical pretreatment.

ORGANICS

Conventional processes for the removal of particulates are effective in removing color and many other organic macromolecules and particulates from water. Here again, laboratory studies provide the bulk of the available evidence. Hall and Packham (1965) have demonstrated that humic and fulvic acids can be coagulated by iron(III) and aluminum(III) salts. Humic acids were readily removed, but a significant fraction of the fulvic acid component was not removed by either coagulant. Similar results have been reported by others, including Black and Willems (1961) and Rook (1975).

MICROBIOLOGICAL PARTICULATES

Large microorganisms including algae and amoebic cysts are readily removed by filtration from properly pretreated water. Bacterial removals in excess of 99% are also achievable (ASCE *et al.*, 1969). More than 98% of poliovirus type 1 was removed by conventional coagulation and filtration (Robeck *et al.*, 1962). Complete (i.e., 100%) removal of microorganisms is not feasible, so that filtration is followed by disinfection with chlorine in conventional water treatment practice.

Possible Concerns

HALOMETHANES AND OTHER CHLORINATED ORGANICS

The natural humic substances are known to be precursors for the formation of chloroform and other halomethanes in water treatment. These may be colloidal, or adsorbed on other colloids such as clays. A recent study (Stevens *et al.*, 1975) has indicated that the rate and extent of chloroform production is reduced when chlorine is added to water containing humic substances after filtration, rather than before coagulation. Presumably, some organic materials (particulates, or solutes adsorbed on particulates) are removed by coagulation and filtration prior to chlorination. Hence, water treatment for particulate removal can lead indirectly to reduced chloroform production.

ENCASING OF MICROBIAL PARTICULATES

It has been proposed that pathogenic bacteria and viruses can be encased in gelatinous metal hydroxides during conventional coagulation processes. If these particles then pass through subsequent settling and filtration facilities, it has been further proposed that the hydroxide gel coatings can protect the pathogens from being inactivated by chlorination. It has also been proposed that natural organic substances can coat and protect pathogens from disinfection. These problems are addressed by Symons and Hoff (1975). Their preliminary evidence suggests that adsorption of virus particles on clays or coagulation of viruses by aluminum dulfate do not impair disinfection of poliovirus type 1 by chlorine. The presence of cell debris, however, significantly slowed the rate of disinfection. This problem requires additional research.

COAGULANT PRECIPITATES

The amorphous hydroxide flocs (e.g., aluminum hydroxide, ferric hydroxide) formed in many coagulation processes are reactive solids. They can, for example, adsorb trace metals and organic compounds. Hence, if they pass through filters and into the treated water, they may carry other substances with them. This is plausible, but conjectural.

POWDERED CARBON

Powdered activated carbon is frequently used for controlling taste and odor. If some of these carbon particles pass through the filters, they exert a chlorine demand and may also carry adsorbed substances with them. Some of these adsorbed substances might have been on the carbon before it was added to the water. EPA does not at this time have standards for carbon used during water treatment. The problem is at present hypothetical, i.e., no data are available.

ORGANIC COAGULANTS

Many synthetic organic materials have been approved for use in water treatment for removal of particulates. These have been examined and certified as nontoxic. The problem of the safety of polyelectrolytes is currently under review by EPA and FDA (Symons, 1976).

Turbidity

This consideration of turbidity as an indicator of potable water quality begins with an evaluation of the test itself. Two recent reviews are excellent (McCluney, 1975; Pickering, 1976). Turbidity determinations involve measurements of the light scattering and absorbing properties of a suspension. A variety of definitions, methods of measurement, instruments, standards, and units of measure have been used. Typically, the light scattered at an angle of 90° to an incandescent source beam is determined. The amount of light scattered depends on the number, size, shape, and refractive index of the particles, the wavelength spectrum of the incident light, and the geometry and detection characteristics of the turbidimeter.

A variety of standards (American Public Health Association, 1976) and instruments are in current use. However, each type of instrument will respond differently to the diversity of sizes, shapes, and types of particles found suspended in both raw and treated waters. Furthermore, depending on the method of standardization used, the same instrument can indicate different turbidities on a single water sample. Hence, it is important that the turbidity test be standardized to provide a sound base for the possible use of turbidity as an indicator of water quality and for other uses.

Since many pollutants in water are either particles themselves or are adsorbed on particles, and since particles absorb and scatter light, it is advantageous to consider turbidity as an indicator of water quality. In addition, there are indications that normally innocuous particles can, at least under some circumstances, protect pathogens from a disinfecting agent (Symons and Hoff, 1975). Finally, it is important to note that turbidity determinations are rapid, relatively inexpensive, and can be performed continuously by detectors *in situ*.

Measurements of turbidity do not give complete information about the size, number, mass, or type of the particles that scatter or absorb light. Small particles (those less than about 0.1 μm in maximum dimension, single viruses and many asbestos mineral particles) do not scatter much visible light and so are not detected by conventional measurements. Furthermore, larger particles can scatter light effectively but may be harmless; the presence of ice crystals in Arctic waters illustrates this point.

Conclusions

Many harmful substances in raw water supplies and in treated potable waters are either particulates themselves or adsorbed on solid particles.

These particles can be removed efficiently by conventional water treatment using coagulation, settling, and filtration processes.

Particles that pass through conventional coagulation and filtration plants in significant amounts do so because of inadequate design, operation, or control of these facilities. Some of these particles may be harmful in themselves. Most are innocuous, but have the potential of containing harmful substances.

The absence of a detectable turbidity does not guarantee that a water is free from harmful particulates. A determination that a water has a high turbidity does indicate the presence of particulate materials and is a cause for concern.

Turbidity is a collective parameter. It cannot replace specific tests for individual pollutants (e.g., Pb, asbestos); it can provide an indication that such tests should be performed. The nature of the particulates in a raw water supply should be determined, and removal accomplished when necessary, by treatment of the supply and appropriate source control.

The rapidity, low cost, and "*in situ*" features of turbidity measurement make it valuable for monitoring and operation of water-treatment plants. When high turbidities are observed in potable water supplies, particular attention should be given to the chlorine demand of the water and to the disinfection process.

Finally, the test itself must be standardized. This will involve the selection of a single light-scattering standard material or a single optical unit, and a standardized light source, instrument geometry, and detection system.

SUMMARY—SOLID PARTICLES IN SUSPENSION

Materials suspended in drinking water include inorganic and organic solids as finely divided particles of sizes ranging from colloidal dimensions to over 100 μm. Such particles may also have other substances and microorganisms attached to them.

Small particles of some materials, such as the asbestos minerals, may have the potential to affect human health directly when they are ingested, and there is widespread concern over the biological effects of such substances.

Many kinds of particles, though apparently harmless in themselves, may indirectly affect the quality of water by acting as vehicles for concentration, transport, and release of other pollutants.

Water treatment can often be effective in removing most of the particles suspended in it, but conventional methods of detecting the presence of particulate material by measurement of turbidity have serious deficiencies.

Direct Effects on Health

Particles of asbestos and other fibrous minerals occur in raw water; usually in a range of sizes from fractions of a micrometer to a few micrometers. Generally, there are fewer than 10 million fibers per liter, but waters are found with from less than 10,000 to more than 100 million fibers per liter. Some of the highest counts have been found near some cities. Fibers in drinking water are typically less than 1 μm long and fibers longer than 2 μm are uncommon. Identification and counting of fibers is difficult and time consuming, usually requiring the transmission electron microscope. The reported counts are highly variable, often differing from one count to the next by a factor of 10 or more.

Epidemiological studies of workers exposed to asbestos by inhalation have shown an increase in death rates from gastrointestinal cancer. With respiratory exposure it is likely that more fibers are swallowed than remain in the lungs. The workers studied were exposed to asbestos with a large range of fiber lengths. It is not clear whether fiber length is pertinent to the development of cancer in the digestive tract in humans.

Epidemiological studies of cancer death rates in Duluth, Minn., where the water supply has been contaminated with mineral fiber, have so far not revealed any increase with time, in comparison with death rates in other areas. Contamination of the Duluth drinking water began less than 20 yr ago, however, and since many cancers have long latency periods, these negative epidemiological findings do not exclude the possibility that an increase might appear within the next 5 to 15 yr.

Animal deposition model studies have shown that fiber length and diameter affect the carcinogenic response seen, the long thin fibers appearing to be the active ones. However, the relevance of these animal deposition models to the human experience is not clear. While some animal studies have shown penetration of the gastrointestinal epithelium, others have not.

It is not known whether other inorganic particulates that occur in water produce any direct effects on human health.

Indirect Effects on Health

The concentration of inorganic, organic and biological pollutants is usually much higher in the suspended solids and sediments of streams and lakes than in water. Clay, organic, and biological particulates, alone or in combination, are the materials chiefly responsible for such concentrations. Clay and organic particulates have large surface areas and strongly adsorb ions, polar and nonpolar molecules, and biological agents. Occurrence of these materials in water is a consequence of natural events, as well as human activity, and is common in many waters that people drink. Although many of the clay or natural organic particulates, in themselves, may not have deleterious effects when ingested by humans, they may exert important health effects through adsorption, transport, and release of inorganic and organic toxicants, bacteria, and viruses. The clay or organic complex with a pollutant may be mobilized by erosion from the land, or complexes may form when eroded particulate matter enters a stream containing pollutants. The atmosphere is also an important pathway. In the adsorbed state, organic and inorganic toxicants may be less active; however, the possibility exists that the toxicants may be released from the particulate matter in the alimentary tract and then exert toxic effects. It is not clear how complexes of particulate matter with viruses and bacteria behave in the gut. It is known, however, that some enzymes retain their activity when adsorbed on clay, and that viral-clay particulates are infectious in tissue culture and in animal hosts.

Turbidity as an Indicator

A high turbidity measurement is an indication that a water may produce an adverse health effect; however, a low turbidity measurement does not guarantee that a water is potable. Turbidity measurements do not indicate the type, number, or mass of particles in a water supply. Where particulates in water are suspected of being harmful, the particulate content should be identified and counted by more specific techniques. Such techniques may include biological, organic, inorganic, and fibrous particulate surveys.

Turbidity measurements are valuable for process control in water-treatment plants. However, the results obtained with present instruments, procedures, and units of measurement are not well correlated with particle concentrations and size distribution. The test itself must be standardized and refined to facilitate its use for this and other purposes.

Conclusions and Recommendations

Certain mineral fibers found in water are suspected of being harmful upon ingestion. The available data with respect to asbestos orally ingested through drinking water do not suggest an immediate hazard to public health. They do suggest that additional research, both experimental (using animals) and epidemiological, is required to determine the degree of hazard. Until new results become available, contamination of drinking water by mineral fibers should be kept to a minimum through the use of effective coagulation and filtration processes and other appropriate measures.

Because particulates are vehicles for concentration, transport, and release of pollutants, they may have indirect effects on health. Coagulation and filtration are effective methods of reducing particulate concentrations. Measurement of particulate content by turbidimetry is imprecise and cannot be relied upon as a sole indicator of the safety of an uncharacterized drinking water source.

Recommendations for Future Research

1. A survey of suspended particulate matter in raw and treated drinking water supplies in several "typical" communities is urgently needed as background information. This must be coupled with analysis of accompanying organic and inorganic material and microorganisms, as well as characterization of the particulates with respect to size, shape, composition, and adsorbed constituents.
2. Ingestion studies should be carried out with fibers of various types and size distributions in validated animal model systems.
3. Epidemiological studies of time trends in death rates should be conducted in areas that have high concentrations of mineral fibers in drinking water.
4. Electron microscopy procedures for detecting and counting asbestos fibers should be scrutinized with respect to their specificity, precision, and accuracy.
5. Information is required on the effects of inorganic, organic, and biological toxicants adsorbed on clay and organic particulates.
6. Development of improved and standardized methods for determining particle concentrations and size distributions by optical techniques, such as light scattering and absorption, should be supported.

REFERENCES

Clay Particles and their Interactions

Bailey, G.W., A.P. Barnett, W.R. Payne, Jr., and C.N. Smith. 1974. Herbicide runoff from four coastal plain soil types. EPA 660/2-74-017.

Bailey, G.W., and J.L. White. 1970. Factors influencing the adsorption, desorption and movement of pesticides in soil. Residue Rev. 32:29-92.

Blatter, C.L. 1973. Hg-complex intergrades in smectite. Clays Clay Min. 21:261-263.

Brown, G. 1961. The X-ray Identification and Crystal Structures of Clay Minerals. Mineralogical Society, London.

Chaussidon, J., and R. Calvet. 1965. Evolution of amine cations adsorbed on montmorillonite with dehydration of the mineral. J. Phys. Chem. 69:2265-2268.

Doner, H.E., and M.M. Mortland. 1969. Benzene complexes with Cu(II) montmorillonite. Science 166:1406-1407.

Farmer, V.C. 1975. The Infrared Spectra of Minerals. Mineralogical Society, London.

Farmer, V.C., and J.D. Russel. 1967. Infrared adsorption spectrometry in clay studies. Clays Clay Min. 15:121-142.

Fenn, D.B., M.M. Mortland, and T.J. Pinnavaia. 1973. The chemisorption of anisole on Cu-montmorillonite. Clays Clay Min. 21:315-322.

Fleck, E.E., and H.L. Haller. 1945. Compatibility of DDT with insecticides, fungicides and fertilizers. Ind. Eng. Chem. 37:403-405.

Frink, C.R. 1969. Chemical and mineralogical characteristics of eutrophic lake sediments. Soil Sci. Soc. Am. Proc. 33:369-372.

Gard, J.A. 1971. The Electron-Optical Investigation of Clays. Mineralogical Society, London.

Greenland, D.J. 1965. Interactions between clays and organic compounds in soils II. Soils Fertil. 28:521-532.

Greenland, D.J. 1971. Interactions between humic and fulvic acids and clays. Soil Sci. 111:34.

Grim, R.E. 1969. Clay Mineralogy. McGraw Hill Book Company, New York.

Gupta, G.C., and W.V. Malik. 1969. Transformation of montmorillonite to nickel chlorite. Clays Clay Min. 17:233-240.

Hodgson, J.D. 1963. Chemistry of the micronutrient in soils. Adv. Agron. 15:119-159.

Holdridge, D.A. 1969. The sorption of heavy-metal cations by ball clay. Proc. Int. Clay Conf. Israel 1:341-349.

Jenne, E.A. 1968. Controls on Mn, Fe, Co, Ni, Cu, and Zn concentrations in soils and water: the significant role of hydrous Mn and Fe oxides. Adv. Chem. 73:337-387.

Jenne, E.A., and J.S. Wahlberg. 1968. Role of certain stream-sediment components in radioion sorption. Geol. Prof. Pap. 433-F.

Lietzke, D.A., and M.M. Mortland. 1973. The dynamic character of a chloritized vermiculitic soil clay. Soil Sci. Soc. Am. Proc. 37:651-656.

Mackenzie, R.C. 1957. The Differential Thermal Investigation of Clays. Mineralogical Society, London.

Malina, M.A., A. Goldman, L. Trademan, and P.B. Polen. 1956. Deactivation of mineral carriers for stable heptachlor-dust formulations. J. Agr. Food Chem. 4:1038-1042.

McAuliffe, C., and N.T. Coleman. 1955. H-ion catalysis by acid clays and exchange resins. Soil Sci. Soc. Am. Proc. 19:156-160.

Mortland, M.M. 1966. Urea complexes with montmorillonite: An infrared absorption study. Clay Min. 6:143-156.

Mortland, M.M., and K.V. Raman. 1967. Catalytic hydrolysis of some organic phosphate pesticides by Copper (II). J. Agr. Food Chem. 15:163-167.

Mortland, M.M. 1970. Clay organic complexes and interactions. Adv. Agron. 22:75-117.

Nicholson, H. P. 1969. Occurrence and significance of pesticide residues in water. J. Wash. Acad. Sci. 59:4-5.

Nicholson, H.P., and D.W. Hill. 1970. Pesticide contaminants in water and mud and their environmental impact. *In* Relationship of Agriculture to Soil and Water Pollution. Cornell Univ. Conf. Agr. Waste Mangement. pp. 171-179.

Pinnavaia, T.J., P. Hall, S. Cady, and M.M. Mortland. 1974. Aromatic radical cation formation on the intracrystal surfaces of transition metal layer lattice silicates. J. Phys. Chem. 78:994-999.

Rausell-Colom, J.A., and J.M. Serratosa. 1975. Reaction of clays with organic substances. *In* Chemistry of Clays and Clay Minerals. Minerological Society, London. (in press)

Rosenfield, C., and W. Van Valkenburg. 1965. Decomposition of *O,o*-dimethyl 0-2, 4,5-trichlorophenyl phosphorothioate (ronnel) adsorbed on bentonite and other clays. J. Agr. Food Chem. 13:68-72.

Russell, J.D., G.W. Bailey, W.R. Payne, J.D. Pope, and J.I. Teasley. 1968. Mode of chemical degradation of *s*-triazines by montmorillonite. Science. 160:1340-1342.

Sanchez, A., A. Hidalgo, and J.M. Serratosa. 1972. Adsorption des nitriles dans la montmorillonite. Proc. Int. Clay Conf. Madrid 617:626.

Schnitzer, M., and H. Kodama. 1972. Reactions between fulvic acid and Cu^{2+}-montmorillonite. Clays Clay Min. 20:359-367.

Schnitzer, M., and H. Kodama. 1967. Reaction between a podzol fulvic acid and Na-montmorillonite. Soil Sci. Soc. Am. Proc. 31:632-636.

Solomon, D.H., and B.C. Loft. 1968. Reactions catalyzed by clay minerals. III. The mechanisms of spontaneous interlamellae polymerizations in aluminosilicates. J. Appl. Polymer. Sci. 12:1253-1262.

Tamura, T. 1962. Strontium reactions with minerals. Ground Disposal of Radioactive Wastes Conf. 2d, Chalk River Canada, Sept. 26-29, 1961. U.S. Atomic Energy Comm. TID-7628, Book 1, 187-197.

Theng, B.K.G. 1974. The Chemistry of Clay-Organic Reactions. Halstead Press, New York.

Weaver, C.E., and L.D. Pollard. 1973. The Chemistry of Clay Minerals. Elsevier Scientific Publishing Co., Amsterdam.

Whittig, L.D. 1965. Methods of Soil Analysis, vol. 1, pp. 671-696. Am. Soc. Agron. Inc., Madison, Wis.

Asbestos: Nomenclature, Occurrence, and Redistribution in Water

Ampian, S.G. 1976. Asbestos minerals and their nonasbestos analogs. *In* Review of Mineral-Fibers Session, Electron Microscopy of Microfibers. Pennsylvania State University, University Park, Pa.

Chisholm, J.E. 1973. Planar defects in fibrous amphiboles. J. Material Sci. 8:475-483.

Choi, I., and R.W. Smith. 1971. Kinetic study of dissolution of asbestos fibers in water. J. Colloid Interface. Sci. V. 40: 253-262.

Cook, P.M., G.E. Glass, and J.H. Tucker. 1974. Asbestiform amphibole minerals: detection and measurement of high concentrations in municipal water supplies. Science 185:853-855.

Committee on Mineral Names. 1949. Am. Min. 34:339.

Cotterell, K., and P.F. Holt. 1972. An examination of crocidolites from North West Cape and Transvaal Mines. Inst. Min. Metall. Trans. Sect. B. 81:169-171.

Cralley, L.J., R.G. Keenan, J.R. Lynch, and W.S. Lainhart. 1968. Source and identification of respirable fibers. J. Am. Ind. Hyg. Assoc. 29:129-135.

Cunningham, H.M. and R. Pontefract. 1971. Asbestos fibers in beverages and drinking water. Nature 232:332-333.

Davis, W.E. 1970. National inventory of sources and emissions of asbestos. NTIS PB 192252.

Deer, W.A., R.A. Howie, and J. Zussman. 1966. An Introduction to the Rock-forming Minerals. Longmans, London.

Durham, R.W., and T. Pang. 1976. Asbestiform fiber levels in Lakes Superior and Huron. Scientific Series no. 67. Inland Waters Directorate, Canada Centre for Inland Waters, Burlington, Ontario.

Environment Canada. 1973. National inventory of sources and emissions of asbestos. Report APCD 73-4, Air Pollution Control Directorate, Environment Canada, Ottawa.

EPA. 1975. Preliminary assessment of suspected carcinogens in drinking water. Interim Report to Congress. Environmental Protection Agency.

Flentje, M.E., and R.J. Schweitzer. 1955. Further study of solution effects on concrete and cement in pipe. J. Am. Water Works Assoc. 49:1441.

Hartman, P. 1963. Structure, growth and morphology of crystals. Z. Kristallog. 119:65-78.

House, R.F. 1967. Dispersion of asbestos. U.S. Pat. Office no. 3,586, 639.

Hutchinson, J.L., M.C. Irusteta, and E.J.W. Whittaker. 1975. High-resolution electron diffraction studies of fibrous amphiboles. Acta Crystallog. 31:794-801.

Kay, G. 1973. Ontario intensifies search for asbestos in drinking water. J. Water Pollut. Control Fed:33-35.

Kehieker, D.M. *et al.* 1967. Determination of elementary fiber size of chrysotile asbestos. Sov. Phys. Crystallog. 12:430-435.

Kramer, J.R. 1976. Fibrous cummingtonite in Lake Superior. Can. Min. 14:91-98.

Kristiansen, H. 1974. The extraction of calcium by soft water from prestressed concrete pipes. Vatten, 1:70.

May, T.C., and R.W. Lewis. 1970. Asbestos. *In* Mineral Facts and Problems. U.S. Bureau Mines Bulletin 650:851-865.

NAS-NRC. 1971. Airborne asbestos. Committee on Biologic Effects of Atmospheric Pollutants. National Research Council. (See also Environment Canada, 1973.)

Parks, G.A. 1967. Aqueous surface chemistry of oxides and complex oxide minerals. *In* W. Stuum, ed. Equilibrium Concepts in Natural Water Systems, Adv. Chem. no. 67, Am. Chem. Soc.

Rabbit, J.C. 1948. Am. Min. 33:263-323.

Rendall, R.E.G. 1970. The data sheets on the chemical and physical properties of the UICC standard reference samples. *In* H.A. Shapiro, ed. Pneumoconiosis. Oxford University Press.

Ruud, C.O., C.S. Barrett, P.A. Russell and R.L. Clark. 1976. Selected area electron diffraction and energy dispersive X-ray analysis for the identification of asbestos fibers, a comparison. Micron 7:115-132.

Timbrell, . 1970. Characteristics of the International Union Against Cancer Standard Reference Samples of Asbestos. *In* H.A. Shapiro, ed. Pneumoconiosis. Oxford University Press.

Timbrell, V., F. Pooley, and J.C. Wagner. 1970. Characteristics of respirable asbestos fibers. In H.A. Shapiro, ed. Pneumoconiosis. Oxford University Press.

Timbrell, V., and R.E.G. Rendall. 1972. Preparation of the UICC reference samples of asbestos. Powder Tec. 5:279-287.

Whittaker, E.J.W. 1966. Diffraction contrast in electron microscopy of chrysotile. Acta. Crystallog. 21:461-466.

Whittaker, E.J.W. and J. Zussman. 1971. The Serpentine Minerals. *In* J.A. Gard, ed. Electron Optical Investigations of Clays. The Mineralogical Society, London.

Yada, K. 1964. Study of chrysotile asbestos by a high resolution electron microscope. Acta Crystallog. 23:704-707.

Zoltai, Tibor, and J.H. Stout. 1976. Comments on asbestiform and fibrous mineral fragments, relative to Reserve Mining Company taconite deposits. Report to Minn. Pollution Control Agency, Minneapolis.

Wright, G.W. 1974. Does the use of asbestos-cement pipe for potable water systems cause a health hazard? J. Am. Water Works Assoc. 66:4-22.

Asbestos Fiber Sampling and Analysis

Beaman, D.R., and D.M. File. 1975. The quantitative determination of asbestos fiber concentrations. The Dow Chemical Company, unpublished report.

Berkley, D., J. Churg, I.J. Selikoff, and W.E. Smith. 1965. The detection and localization of asbestos fibers in tissue. Ann. N.Y. Acad. Sci. 132:48-63.

Berkley, C., A.M. Langer, and V. Baden. 1968. Instrumental analysis of inspired fibrous pulmonary particles. Trans. N.Y. Acad. Sci. 30:331-350.

Birks, L.S., M. Fatemi, J.V. Gilfrich, and E.T. Johnson. 1975. Quantitative analysis of airborne asbestos by x-ray diffraction. Feasibility Study AD-A007530, Naval Res. Lab., Washington, D.C.

Brown, A.L., Jr., W.F. Taylor, and R.E. Carter. 1976. The reliability of measures of amphibole fiber concentration in water. Environ. Res. 12:150-160.

Clark, R.L., and C.O. Ruud. 1975. Transmission electron microscopy standards for asbestos. Micron 5:270.

Cook, P.M., J.B. Rubin, C.J. Maggiore, and W.J. Nicholson. 1974. X-ray diffraction and electron beam analysis of asbestiform minerals in Lake Superior waters. *In* Trans. Inst. Electrical Electronic Eng. (in press).

Crable, J.V., and M.J. Knott. 1966a. Application of x-ray diffraction to the determination of chrysotile in bulk and settled dust samples. Am. Ind. Hyg. J. 27:383-387.

Crable, J.V., and M.J. Knott. 1966b. Quantitative x-ray diffraction analysis of crocidolite and amosite in bulk or settled dust samples. Am. Ind. Hyg. J. 27:449-453.

Dement, J.M., R.D. Zumwalde, and K.M. Wallingford. 1975. Asbestos fiber exposures in a hard rock gold mine. *In* Proc. N.Y. Acad. Sci. Conf. Occup. Carcinogenesis. Ann. N.Y. Acad. Sci. 271:345-352 (1976).

Ferrell, R.E., G.G. Paulson, and C.W. Walker. 1975. Evaluation of an SEMEDS method for identification of chrysotile. Scanning Electron Microscopy:537-546.

Julian, Y., and W.C. McCrone. 1970. Identification of asbestos fibers by microscopical dispersion staining. Microscope 18:1-10.

Keenan, R.G., and J.R. Lynch. 1970. Techniques for the detection, identification and analysis of fibers. Am. Ind. Hyg. J. 31:587-597.

Langer, A.M., A.D. Mackler, and F.D. Pooley. 1974. Electron microscopical investigation of asbestos fibers. Environ. Health Perspect. 9:63-80.

Langer, A.M., I. Rubin, and I.J. Selikoff. 1975. Electron microprobe analysis of asbestos bodies. Histochem. Cytochem. J. 20:735-740.

McCrone, W.C., and I.M. Stewart. 1974. Asbestos. American Laboratory, April.
McMillan, L.M., R.G. Stout, and B.F. Willey. 1977. Asbestos in raw and treated water: an electron microscopy study. Environ. Sci. Tech. 11:390-394.
Nicholson, W.J. 1974. Analysis of amphibole asbestiform fibers in municipal water supplies. Environ. Health Perspect. 9:165-172.
Pooley, F.D. 1972. Electron microsope characteristics of inhaled chrysotile asbestos fibre. Br. J. Ind. Med. 29:146-153.
Otiz, L.W., and B.L. Isom. 1974. Transfer technique for electron microscopy of membrane filter samples. Am. Ind. Hyg. Assoc. J.35:423-425.
OSHA. 1975. Occupational Safety and Health Standards. U.S. Department of Labor, Occupational Safety and Health Administraion. Fed. Reg. 29 CFR 1910.1001.
Rohl, A.N., and A.M. Langer. 1974. Identification and quantitation of asbestos in talc. Environ. Health Perspect. 9:95-109.
Rubin, I.B., and C.J. Maggiore. 1974. Elemental analysis of asbestos fibers by means of electron probe techniques. Environ. Health Perspect. 9:81-94.
Ruud, C.O., C.S. Barrett, P.A. Russell, and R.L. Clark. 1976. Selected area electron diffraction and energy dispersed x-ray analysis for the identification of asbestos fibers, a comparison. Micron 7:115-132.
Schlez, J.P. 1974. The detection of chrysotile asbestos at low levels in talc by differential thermal analysis. Thermochemica Acta 8:197-203.
Selikoff, I.J., W.J. Nicholson and A.M. Langer. 1972. Asbestos air pollution. Arch. Environ. Health 25:1-13.
Stanley, H.D., and R.E. Norward. 1973. The detection and identification of asbestos and asbestiform minerals in talc. *In* Proceedings Symp. on Talc, Washington, D.C., May 8, 1973. Bureau of Mines Information Circular 8639.
Timbrell, V. 1970. Characteristics of the UICC standard reference samples of asbestos. *In* H. Shapiro, ed. Pneumoconiosis. Oxford Univ. Press, London.

Biological Effects of Asbestos Minerals, Epidemiological Findings

Anderson, H.A., R. Lilis, S.M. Daum, A.S. Fischbein, and I.J. Selikoff. 1976. Household-contact asbestos neoplastic risk. Ann. N.Y. Acad. Sci. 271:311-323.
Bogovski, P., V. Timbrell, J.C. Gilson and J.C. Wagner, eds. 1973. Biological Effects of Asbestos. IARC Scientific Publication no. 8.
Elmes, P.C., and M. J. C. Simpson. 1971. Insulation workers in Belfast. 3. Mortality 1940-1966. Br. J. Ind. Med. 28:226-236.
Hammond, E.C., I.J. Selikoff, H. Seidman. 1975. Multiple interaction effects of cigarette smoking. Extrapulmonary cancer. *In* Proc. XI Int. Cancer Congress, Florence 1974, vol. 3, Cancer Epidemiology. Environ. Factors:147-150. Excerpta Medica, Amsterdam.
Lee, D.H.K., ed. 1974. Proceedings of the Joint NIEHS-EPA Conference on "Biological Effects of Ingested Asbestos," Durham, North Carolina, November 1973. Environ. Health Perspect. 9:113-338.
Levy, B.S., E. Sigurdson, J. Mandel, E. Laudon, and J. Pearson. 1976. Investigating possible effects of asbestos in city water: Surveillance of gastrointestinal cancer incidence in Duluth, Minnesota. Am. J. Epidemiol. 103:362-368.
Mancuso, T.F. 1965. Asbestos and neoplasia: Epidemiology: Discussion. Ann. N.Y. Acad. Sci. 132:589-594.
Masson, T.J., F.W. McKay, R.W. Miller. 1974. Asbestos-like fibers in Duluth water supply: Relation to cancer mortality. J. Am. Med. Assoc. 228:1019-1020.

Newhouse, M.L., G. Berry, J.C. Wagner, and M. E. Turok. 1972. A study of the mortality of female asbestos workers. Br. J. Ind. Med. 29:134-141.

Newhouse, M.L., and H. Thompson. 1965. Mesothelioma of the pleura and peritoneum following exposure to asbestos in the London area. Br. J. Ind. Med. 22:261-269.

Selikoff, I.J., and J. Churg, Co-chairmen. 1965. Biological effects of asbestos. Ann. N.Y. Acad. Sci. 132:1-766.

Selikoff, I.J., E.C. Hammond, and H. Seidman. 1973. Cancer risk of insulation workers in the United States. *In* Biological Effects of Asbestos. IARC Scientific Publication no. 8:209-216.

Wagner, J.C., C.A. Sleggs, and P. Marchand. 1960. Diffuse pleural mesothelioma and asbestos exposure in the North Western Cape Province. Br. J. Ind. Med. 17:260-271.

Biological Effects of Asbestos Minerals, Experimental Studies

Ampian, S.G. 1976. Asbestos minerals and their nonasbestos analogs. *In* Review of Mineral-Fibers Session, Electron Microscopy of Microfibers. Pennsylvania State University, University Park, Pa.

Bolton, R.E., and J.M.G. Davis. 1976. The short-term effects of chronic asbestos ingestion in rats. Ann. Occup. Hyg. 19:121-128.

Bouser, G.M., and D.B. Clayson. 1967. Feeding of blue asbestos to rats. 45th Annual Report, British Empire Cancer Campaign:242.

Cook, P.M., G.E. Glass, and J.H. Tucker. 1974. Asbestiform amphibole minerals: detection and measurement of high concentrations in municipal water supplies. Science 185:853-855.

Cunningham, H.M., and R. Pontefract. July 30, 1971. Asbestos fibers in beverages and drinking water. Nature 232:332-333.

Cunningham, H.M., and R.D. Pontefract. 1974. Placental transfer of asbestos. Nature 249:177-178.

Cunningham, H.M., R.D. Pontefract, and R.C. O'Brien. 1976. Quantitative relationship of fecal asbestos to asbestos exposure. J. Toxicol. Environ. Health 1:377-379.

Fears, T.R. 1976. Cancer mortality and asbestos deposits. Am. J. Epidemiol. 104:523-526.

Gibel, W., Kh. Lohs, K.H. Horn, G.P. Wildner, and F. Hoffmann. 1976. Tier experimentelle Untersuchungen über eine kanzerogene Wirkung von Asbestfiltermaterial nach oraler Aufnahme. Arch. Geschwulstforsch. 46:437-442.

Gross, P. 1974. Letter to ed.: Asbestos fibers in drinking water. J. Am. Med. Assoc. 229:767.

Gross, P., R.A. Harley, L.M. Swinburne, J.M.G. Davis, and W. B. Greene. 1974. Ingested mineral fibers. Do they penetrate tissue or cause cancer? Arch. Environ. Health. 29:341-347.

Hammond, E.C., and I.J. Selikoff. 1973. Relation of cigarette smoking to risk of death of asbestos associated disease among insulation workers in the United States. *In* Biological Effects of Asbestos. IARC Scientific Publication no. 8:312-377.

Harwood, C.F., and G. Yamate. 1975. The detection and quantification of asbestos present in the environment. *Presented at* Third International Conference on the Physics and Chemistry of Asbestos Minerals, Quebec.

IARC 1973. Report of the Advisory Committee on Asbestos Cancers to the Director of the International Agency for Research on Cancer. Br. J. Ind. Med. 30:180-186.

Kay, G. September, 1973. Ontario intensifies search for asbestos in drinking water. Water Pollut. Control 72:33-35.

Levy, B.S., E. Sigurdson, J. Mandel, E. Laudon and J. Pearson. 1976. Investigating possible effects of asbestos in city water: Surveillance of gastrointestinal cancer incidence in Duluth, Minnesota. Am. J. Epidemiol. 103:362-368.

Maroudas, N.G., C.H. O'Neill, and M.F. Stanton. April 14, 1973. Fibroblast anchorage in carcinogensis by fibres. Lancet 1:807-809.

Masson, T.J., F.W. McKay, and R.W. Miller. 1974. Asbestos-like fibers in Duluth water supply. Relation to cancer mortality. J. Am. Med. Assoc. 228:1019-1020.

NAS 1975. Priniciples for Evaluating Chemicals in the Environment. National Academy of Sciences, Washington, D.C.

Nicholson, W.J., and F.L. Pundsack. 1973. Asbestos in the environment. *In* Biological Effects of Asbestos. IARC Scientific Publication no. 8:126-130.

Pontefract, R.D., and H.M. Cunningham. 1973. Penetration of asbestos through the digestive tract of rats. Nature 243:352-353.

Pott, F., and K.H. Friedrichs. 1972. Tumors in rats by intraperitoneal injection of fibrous dusts. Naturwissenschaften 59:318.

Pott, F., F. Huth, and K.H. Friedrichs. 1972. Tumors of rats after L.P. injection of powdered chrysotile and benzo[a]pyrene. Zentrabl. Bakteriol. Parasitenkd. Infektionskr. Hyg., Abt. 1: Orig. Reihe B 155:463-469.

Pott, F., F. Huth, and K.H. Friedrichs. 1974. Tumorigenic effect of fibrous dusts in experimental animals. Environ. Health Perspect. 9:313-315.

Pott, F., F. Huth, and K.H. Friedrichs. April, 1976. Result of animal carcinogenesis studies after application of fibrous glass and their implications regarding human exposure. *In* Occupational Exposure to Fibrous Glass. A Symposium, Univ. of Maryland, College Park, Maryland, June 26-27, 1974:183-191. U.S. Department of Health, Education, and Welfare. N10SH 76-151.

Shabad, L.M., L.N. Pyleo, L.V. Krioosheeva, T.F. Kulagina, and B.A. Neminko. 1974. Experimental studies on asbestos carcinogenicity. J. Cancer Inst. 52:1175-1187.

Smith, W.E. 1973. Asbestos, talc and nitrites in relation to gastric cancer. Am. Ind. Hyg. Assoc. J. 34:227-228.

Smith, W.E. 1974. Experimental studies on biological effects of tremolite talc on hamsters. *In* Proc. Symp. on Talc, Washington, D.C., May 8, 1973. Bureau of Mines Information Circular 8639:43-48.

Smith, W.E., D.D. Hubert, and M.S. Badollet. 1972. Biologic differences in response to long and short asbestos fibers. Am. Ind. Hyg. Assoc. J. 33:A162.

Sontag, J.M., N.P. Page, and U. Saffiotti. 1976. Guidelines for Carcinogen Bioassay in Small Rodents. NCI Carcinogenesis Technical Report Series No. 1. Department of Health, Education, and Welfare Publication No. (NIH) 76-801.

Stanton, M.F. 1973. Some etiological considerations of fibre carcinogenesis. *In* Biological Effects of Asbestos. IARC Scientific Publication no. 8:289-294.

Stanton, M.F. 1974. Fiber carcinogenesis: Is asbestos the only hazard? J. Nat. Cancer Inst. 52:633-634.

Stanton, M.F., R. Blackwell, and E. Miller. 1969. Experimental pulmonary carcinogenesis with asbestos. Am. Ind. Hyg. Assoc. J. 30:236-244.

Stanton, M.F., M. Layard, A. Tegeris, E. Miller, M. May, and E. Kent. 1977. Carcinogenicity of fibrous glass: Pleural response in the rat in relation to fiber dimension. J. Nat. Cancer Inst. 58:587-603.

Stanton, M.F., and C. Wrench. 1972. Mechanisms of mesothelioma induction with asbestos and fibrous glass. J. Nat. Cancer. Inst. 48:797-821.

Wagner, J.C., G. Berry, J.W. Skidmore, and V. Timbrell. 1974. The effects of the inhalation of asbestos in rats. Br. J. Cancer 29:252-269.

Wagner, J.C., G. Berry, and J.W. Skidmore. April 1976. Studies of the carcinogenic effects of fiber glass of different diameters following intrapleural innoculation in experimental animals. *In* Occupational Exposure to Fibrous Glass. A Symposium, Univ. of Maryland, College Park, Maryland, June 26-27, 1974:193-197, U.S. Department of Health, Education, and Welfare. N10SH 76-151.

Wagner, J.C., G. Berry, and V. Timbrell. 1973. Mesotheliomata in rats after inoculation with asbestos and other materials. Br. J. Cancer 28:173-185.

Webster, I. 1974. The ingestion of asbestos fibers. Environ. Health Perspect. 9:199-202.

Westlake, G.E., H.J. Spjut, and M.N. Smith. 1965. Penetration of colonic mucosa by asbestos particles. An electron microscopic study in rats fed asbestos diets. Lab. Invest. 9:2029-2033.

Organic Particulates in Water

Anderson, G. 1958. Identification of derivatives of deoxyribonucleic acid in humic acid. Soil Sci. 86:196-174.

Ballard, T.M. 1971. Role of humic carrier substances in DDT movement through forest soil. Soil Sci. Soc. Am. Proc. 35:146-147.

Black, A.P., and R.F. Christman. 1963. Characteristics of colored surface waters. J. Am. Water Works Assoc. 55:753-770.

Bordeleau, L.M., J.D. Rosen, and R. Bartha. 1972. Herbicide-derived chloroazobenzene residues: Pathway of formation. J. Agr. Food Chem. 20:573-578.

Bruland, K.W., K. Bertine, M. Koide, and E.D. Goldberg. 1974. History of metal pollution in Southern California coastal zone. Environ. Sci. Tech. 8:425-432.

Cheam, V. 1973. Chelation study of copper (II): Fulvic acid system. Can. J. Soil Sci. 53:377-382.

Day, H., and G.T. Felback, Jr. 1974. Production and analysis of a humicacid-like exudate from the aquatic fungus Aureobasidium pullulans. J. Am. Water Works Assoc. 66:484-488.

De Groot, A.J., J.J.M. De Goeij, and C. Zegers. 1971. Contents and behavior of mercury as compared with other heavy metals in sediments from the River Rhine and Ems. Geologie en Mijnbouw. 50:393-398.

Felbeck, G.T., Jr. 1975. Structural chemistry of soil humic substances. Adv. Agron. 17:327-368.

Felbeck, G.T., Jr. 1971. Structural hypotheses of soil humic acids. Soil Sci. 111:43-48.

Field, R., and D. Knowled. 1975. Urban runoff and combined sewer overflow, J. Water Pollut. Control Fed. 47:1352-1369.

Flaig, W. 1970. Contribution a la connaissance de la constitution et de la synthese des acides humiques. Sci. Sol 1:39-72.

Giger, W., M. Reinhard, C. Schaffner, and W. Stumm. 1974. Petroleum-derived and idigenous hydrocarbons in recent sediments of Lake Zug, Switzerland. Environ. Sci. Tech. 8:454-455.

Gove, G.W. and I. Gellman. 1975. Paper and allied products. J. Water Pollut. Control Fed. 47:1402-1446.

Gorbunov, N.I., G.L. Yerokhina, and G.N. Shchurina. 1971. Relationship between soil minerals and humic substances, Pochvovedeniye 7:117-128.

Greenland, D.J. 1971. Interactions between humic and fulvic acids and clays. Soil Sci. 111:34-31.

Haider, K., J.P. Martin, Z. Filip, and E. Fustec-Mathon. 1972. Contribution of soil microbes to the formation of humic compounds. Proc. Int. Meet. Humic Substances:71-85.

Harding, C., and H.S. Brown. 1975. Distribution of selected trace elements in sediments of Pamlico River estuary, North Carolina. Environ. Geol.:181-191.

Hsu, T-S., and R. Bartha. 1976. Hydrolyzable and nonhydrolyzable 3,4-dichloroaniline-humus complexes and their respective rates of biodegradation. J. Agric. Food Chem. 24:118-122.

Jewell, W.J., J.B. Petersen, E.G. Srinath, W.T. Tseng, E.J. Kroeker, and E.C. McGriff, Jr. 1975. Agricultural wastes. Water Pollut. Control Fed. 47:1446-1465.

Khan, S.U., and M. Schnitzer. 1972. The retention of hydrophobic organic compounds by humic acid. Geochem. Cosmochim. Acta 36:745-754.

Kononova, M.M. 1966. Soil Organic Matter. Pergamon Press, New York.

Koshy, E., and A.K. Ganguly. 1969. Organic materials in the marine environments and their interactions with some metal ions. Bhabha Atomic Research Centre, Bombay, India.

Ladd, J.N., and J.H.A. Butler. 1971. Inhibition by soil humic acids of naive and acetylated proteolytic enzymes. Soil Biol. Biochem. 3:157-160.

Lammers, W.T. 1967. Biophysical limnology, separation of suspended and colloidal particles from natural water. Environ. Sci. Tech. 1:52-57.

Lammers, W.T. 1975. An investigation of colloidal organic particles isolated from different populations of bivalves. Verh. Int. Verein. Limnol. 19:1540-1545.

Leland, H.V., S. Shukla, and N.F. Shimp. 1973. Factors affecting distribution of lead and other trace elements in sediments of southern Lake Michigan. *In* C. Singer, ed. Trace Metals and Metal-Organic Interactions in Natural Waters, pp. 89-129.

Leland, H.V., E.D. Copenhaver, and D.J. Wilkes. 1975. Tidal pollution. Heavy metals and other trace elements. J. Water Pollut. Control Fed. 47:1635-1656.

Li, Gwo-Chen, and G.T. Felbeck, Jr. 1972. A study of the mechanism of atrazine adsorption by humic acid from muck soil. Soil Sci. 113:140-148.

Litchfield, J.H. 1975. Meat, fish, and poultry processing wastes. J. Water Pollut. Control Fed. 47:1381-1389.

Macauley, D.C. 1975. Chemicals and allied products. J. Water Pollut. Control Fed. 47:1515-1520.

Malcolm, R.L. 1969. A comparison of conditional stability constants of North Carolina humic and fulvic acids with Co(II) and Fe(III): Southeast. Geol. Soc. Am. Meet. Proc., April, Columbia, S.C.

Martin, J.P., K. Haider, and E. Bondietti. 1972. Properties of model humic acids synthesized by phenoloxidase and autoxidation of phenols and other compounds formed by soil fungi. Proc. Int. Meet. Humic Substances:171-186.

Mato, M.C., R. Fabregas, and J. Mendez. 1971. Inhibitory effect of soil humic acids on indoleacetic acidoxidase. Soil Biol. Biochem. 34:285-288.

Mazzocchi, P.H., and M.P. Rao. 1972. Photolysis of 3-(*p*-chlorophenyl)-1,1-dimethylurea (Monuron) and 3-phenyl-1,1-dimethylurea (Fenuron). J. Agr. Food Chem. 20:957-959.

Monahan, A.R., A.F. DeLuca, and R.L. Wershaw. 1972. Spectroscopic characterization of humic acid fractions in aqueous media. Am. Chem. Soc. Meet., Aug. 27-Sept. 1, New York.

Muller, G., and U. Forstner. 1974. Heavy metals in sediments of the Rhine and Elbe estuaries: Mobilization or mixing effect? Environ. Geol. 1:33-39.

Nicholson, A.A., O. Meresz, and B. Lemyk. 1977. Determination of free and total potential haloforms in drinking water. Anal. Chem. 49:814-819.

Ong, H.L., V.E. Swanson, and R.E. Bisque. 1970. Natural organic acids as agents of chemical weathering. U.S. Geol. Sur. Prof. Pap. 700-C:C130-C137.

Orlov, D.S., and N.L. Yeroshicheva. 1967. Interaction of humic acids with the cations of some metals. Soviet Soil Sci. S(570) Sa34E:1799-1806.

Perry, D.R., and W.A. Adams. 1971. The incorporation of glycylglycine into humic acid. Biochem. J. 125:29-30.

Pico, R.F. 1975. Dairy wastes. J. Water Pollut. Control Fed. 47:1513-1516.

Rashid, M.A. 1969. Contribution of humic substances to the cation exchange capacity of different marine sediments. Maritime Sediments 5:44-50.

Rashid, M.A. 1971. Role of humic acids of marine origin and their different molecular weight fractions in complexing di- and trivalent metals. Soil Sci. 111:298-306.

Rashid, M.A. and J.D. Leonard. 1973. Modifications in the solubility and precipitation behavior of various metals as a result of their interaction with sedimentary humic acid. Chem. Geol. 11:89-97.

Rook, J.J. 1974. Formation of haloforms during chlorination of natural waters. Water Treatment and Examination 23:234-243.

Scheffer, F., and B. Ulrich. 1960. Humus und humusdungung. *In* Lehrbuch der Agrikulturchemie und Bodenkunde. F. Enke, Stuttgart.

Schnitzer, M. 1965. Contribution of organic matter to the cation exchange capacity of soils. Nature 207:665-668.

Schnitzer, M., and S.I.M. Skinner. 1965. Organo-metallic interactions in soils: 4. Carboxyl and hydroxyl groups in organic matter and metal retention. Soil Sci. 99:278-284.

Shelton, T.B., and J.V. Hunter. 1974. Acrobic decomposition of oil pollutants in sediments. J. Water Pollut. Control Fed. 46:2172-2182.

Shimp, N.F., J.A. Schleicher, R.R. Ruch, D.B. Heck, and H.V. Leland. 1971. Trace element and organic carbon accumulation in the most recent sediments of southern Lake Michigan. Environmental Geology Notes no. 41.

Sipos, S., I. Dekany, and F. Szanto. 1972. Investigation of humic acids and metal humates with analytical ultracentrifuge. Acta Phys. Fasc. 3-4:253-257.

Södergren, A., Bj. Svensson, and S. Ulfstrand. 1972. DDT and PCB in south Swedish streams. Environ. Pollut. 3:25-36.

Soderquist. 1975. Fruit, vegetable, and grain processing wastes. J. Water Pollut. Control Fed. 47:1389-1398.

Steelink, C. 1963. What is humic acid? J. Chem. Ed. 40:379.

Steelink, C., and G. Tollin. 1967. Free radicals in soil. Soil Biochem. I:147-169.

Stevens, A.A., C.J. Slocum, D.R. Seeger, and G.G. Robeck. 1975. Chlorination of organics in drinking water. *In* Proceedings of Conference on Environmental Impact of Water Chlorination. Oak Ridge National Laboraory, Oak Ridge, Tenn.

Su, G.C.C., and M.J. Zabik. 1972. Photochemistry of bioactive compounds. Photolysis of (*N,N*-dimethylformamidine) phenyl *N*-methylcarbamate hydrochloride in water. J. Agr. Food Chem. 20:642-644.

Sullivan, J.D., Jr., and G.T. Felbeck, Jr. 1968. A study of the interaction of *S*-triazine herbicides with humic acids from three different soils. Soil Sci. 106:42-52.

Symons, J.M. 1976. Interim Treatment Guide for the Control of Chloroform and other Trihalomethanes. U.S. Environmental Protection Agency.

Talbot, R. 1965. Textile wastes. J. Water Pollut. Control Fed. 47:1465-1473.

Theis, T.L., and P.C. Singer. 1974. Complexation of iron(II) by organic matter and its effect on iron(II) oxygenation. Environ. Sci. Tech. 8:569-573.

Wershaw, R.L., P.J. Burcar, and M.C. Goldberg. 1969. Interaction of pesticides with natural organic material. Environ. Sci. Tech. 3:271-273.

Wershaw, R.L., and D.J. Pinckney. 1971. Association and dissociation of a humic acid fraction as a function of pH. U.S. Geol. Sur. Prof. Pap. 750-D: D216-D218.

Wershaw, R.L., and M.C. 1972. Interaction of organic pesticides with natural organic polyelectrolytes. Advances in Chemistry Series no. 111, Fate of Orgnic Pesticides in the Aquatic Environment, pp. 149-158. American Chemical Society.

Wershaw, R.L., and D.J. Pinckney. 1973a. The fractionation of humic acids from natural water systems. J. Res. U.S. Geol. Sur.

Wershaw, R.L. and D.J. Pinckney. 1973b. Determination of the association and dissociation of humic acid fractions by small angle X-ray scattering. J. Res. U.S. Geol. Sur.

Microorganisms and Suspended Particles in Water

Berg, G. 1973. Removal of viruses from sewage, effluents, and water. Bull. WHO 49:451-460.

Boyd, J.W., T. Yoshid, L.E. Vereen, R.L. Cada and S.M. Morrison. 1969. Bacterial response to the soil environment. Sanitary Engineering Papers, Colorado State Univ., Ft. Collins, No. 5:1-22.

Boylen, C.W., and T. D. Brock. 1973. Bacterial decomposition processes in Lake Wingra sediments during winter. Limnol. Oceanogr. 18:628.

Brock, T.D. 1966. Principles of Mcrobial Ecology. Prentice-Hall, N.J.

Brock, T.D. 1974. Biology of Microorganisms, 2d ed. Prentice-Hall, N.J.

Cameron, R.E. 1965-1969. Soil Studies-Micobial Habitats. NASA Publ. Space Programs Summaries, vol. IV. Jet Propulsion Laboratory, Pasadena, California.

Gray, G.W., and S.G. Wilkinson. 1965. The action of EDTA on *Pseudomonas aeruginosa*. J. Appl. Bacteriol. 28:153-164.

Hendricks, C.W. 1973. Measurement of baseline levels of enteric bacterial activity in river water. Louisiana State Univ. Rep. LSU-SG-73-01:245.

Henrici, A.T., and E.J. Ordal. 1948. The Biology of Bacteria. D.C. Heath, New York.

Hudson, H.E. 1962. High quality water production and viral disease. J. Am. Water Works Assoc. 54:1265-1272.

Kononova, M.M. 1966. Soil Organic Matter, 2d Engl. ed., pp. 51-52. Pergamon Press, New York.

Lammers, W.T. 1967. Separation of suspended and colloidal particles from natural water. Environ. Sci. Tech. 1:52-57.

Lederberg, J. 1952. Cell genetics and hereditary symbiosis. Physiol. Rev. 32:403-430.

Mallette, M.F. 1963. Validity of the concept of energy of maintenance. N.Y. Acad. Sci. 102:521-535.

Melnick, J.L. 1975. Proceedings 13th Water Quality Conference, Virus and Water Quality: Occurrence and Control. Univ. of Illinois and Illinois EPA.

Neefe, J.R., J.B. Baty, J.G. Reinhold, and J. Stokes. 1947. Inactivation of the virus of infectious hepatitis in drinking water. Am. J. Public Health 37:365-372.

Petrilli, F.L., P. Crovari, S. DeFlora, and A. Vannucci. 1974. The virological monitoring of water. I. Drinking water. Boll. 1st. Sieroter, Milan. 53:434-442.

Rice, C.W., I.L. Uydess, W.P. Hempfling, and W.V. Vishniac. 1975. Isolation of microorganisms from soil of the Antarctic "Dry Valleys". Abstr. Annual Meet. Am. Soc. Microbiol., New York City.

Sanderson, W.W., and S. Kelly. 1962. Discussion of Human Enteric Viruses in Water: Source, Survival and Removability, by N.A. Clarke, G. Berg, P.K. Kabler, and S.L. Chang, Int. Conf. Water Pollut. Res. London 1962. Pergamon Press, New York, 1964.

Schmidt, E.L. R.O. Bankole, and B.B. Bohlool. 1968. Fluorescent antibody approach to study of rhizobia in soil. J. Bacteriol. 95:1987-1992.

Sharp, J.J., and B.D. Church. 1963. Molecular mutualism among the marine protista. Bact. Proc. 996:47.

Stotzky, G. 1966a. Influence of clay minerals on microorganisms. II. Effect of various clay species, homoionic clays, and other particles on bacteria. Can. J. Microbiol. 12:831-848.

Stotzky, G. 1966b. Influence of clay minerals on microorganisms. III. Effect of particle size, cation exchange capacity, and surface area on bacteria. Can. J. Microbiol. 12:1235-1246.

Symons, J.M., and J.C. Hoff. 1975. Rationale for turbidity maximum contaminant level. 3d Water Quality Tech. Conf., Am. Water Works Assoc., Atlanta, Ga., December 8-10.

Taylor, F.B. 1974. Viruses: What is their significance in water supplies? J. Am. Water Works Assoc. 66(5):306-311.

Tracy, H.W., V.M. Camarena, and F. Wing. 1966. Coliform persistence in highly chlorinated waters. J. Am. Water Works Assoc. 58:1151.

Walton, G. 1961. Effectiveness of water treatment processes as measured by coliform reduction. U.S. Department of Health, Education, and Welfare, PHS Publ. no. 898.

Particulate Removal and Turbidity

Adin, A., and M. Rebhun. 1974. High-rate contact flocculation-filtration with cationic polyelectrolytes. J. Am. Water Works Assoc. 66:109-117.

American Public Health Association. 1976. Standard Methods for the Examination of Water and Wastewater, 14th ed., pp. 131-139.

American Society of Civil Engineers, American Water Works Association, Conference of State Sanitary Engineers, 1969, Water Treatment Plant Design, p. 122. American Water Works Association, Inc., New York.

Black and Veatch, Consulting Engineers. 1975. Direct Filtration of Lake Superior Water For Asbestiform Fiber Removal. Report No. EPA-670/2-75-0500, EPA, National Environmental Research Center, Cincinnati, Ohio.

Black, A.P., and S.A. Hannah. 1961. Electrophoretic studies of turbidity removal by coagulation with aluminum sulfate. J. Am. Water Works Assoc. 53:438-452.

Black, A.P., and D.G. Willems. 1961. Electrophoretic studies of coagulation for removal of organic color. J. Am. Water Works Assoc. 53:589-604.

Hall, E.S., and R.F. Packham. 1965. Coagulation of organic color with hydrolyzing coagulants. J. Am. Water Works Assoc. 57:1149-1166.

Jenkins, K.H. 1963. 1962 USPHS summary of municipal water facilities in communities of 25,000 or more. J. Am. Water Works Assoc. 55:1485-1492.

Ling, J.T. 1955. A study of filtration through uniform sand filters. Proc. Am. Soc. Civil Eng., Sanitary Engineering Division, 81:Paper no. 751.

Logsdon, G.S., and J.M. Symons. 1975. Removal of asbestiform fibers by water filtration. Water Supply Research Laboratory, EPA, Cincinnati, Ohio.

McCluney, W.R. 1975. Radiometry of water turbidity measurements. J. Water Pollut. Control Fed. 47:252-266.

Packham, R.F. 1965. Some studies of the coagulation of dispersed clays with hydrolyzing salts. J. Colloid Sci. 20:81-92.

Pickering, R.J. 1976. Measurements of 'turbidity' and related characteristics of natural waters. U.S. Geol. Sur. Open-File Rep. 76-153.

Robeck, G.G., N.A. Clarke, and K.A. Dostal. 1962. Effectiveness of water treatment processes in virus removal. J. Am. Water Works Assoc. 54:1275-1292.

Rook, J.J. 1975. Formation of and occurrence of haloforms in drinking water. Presented at 95th Annual Conference of the American Water Works Asociation, June 8-13, Minneapolis, Minn.

Stevens, A.A., C.J. Slocum, D.R. Seeger, and G.G. Robeck. 1975. Chlorination of organics in drinking water. Presented at Conference on the Environmental Impact of Water Chlorination, Oak Ridge Naional Laboratory, Oak Ridge, Tenn.

Symons, J.M. 1975. Personal communication.

Symons, J.M., and J.C. Hoff. 1975. Rationale for Turbidity Maximum Contaminant Level. Water Supply Research Division, U.S. Environmental Protection Agency, Cincinnati, Ohio.

Yao, K.M., M.T. Habibian, and C.R. O'Melia. 1971. Water and wastewater filtration: Concepts and applications. Environ. Sci. Tech. 5:1105-1112.

V

INORGANIC SOLUTES

TRACE METALS

Trace metals may be present in natural groundwater or surface water. The sources of these trace metals are associated with either natural processes or man's activities. Two important natural processes contributing trace metals to natural water are chemical weathering and soil leaching. The factors affecting the release of trace metals from primary materials and soil and their solution and stability in water are solubility, pH, adsorption characteristics, hydration, coprecipitation, colloidal dispersion, and the formation of complexes. Decaying vegetation can also affect the concentration of trace metals in water. Many plants are known to concentrate various elements selectively. As a result, trace metals may become available during the decay of the plants. Thus, the penetration and movement of rainwater through soil may pick up these available trace metals and affect the groundwater resource. Likewise, runoff resulting from rainfall may transport trace metals to surface-water.

Mining and manufacturing are other important sources of trace metals in natural waters. Several operations associated with the mining of coal and mineral ores can lead to the discharge of wastewater contaminated with trace metals or to the accumulation of spoiled material, which may be leached of trace metals by rainfall and reach either surface or groundwater. The discharge of industrial wastewater, such as that generated by plating and metal-finishing operations, may also be the source of trace metals in natural water.

The treatment of raw surface or groundwater to make it acceptable for public consumption may include the removal of trace metals. However, trace metals may be added to water as a result of the treatment and the subsequent distribution throughout a community. Depending on the quality of the raw water and the quality desired in the finished (treated) water, treatment may involve the use of chemicals, such as alum (aluminum sulfate), lime, and iron salts. The chemicals used are usually of commercial or technical grade with no exact composition, although the American Water Works Association has established standards for most chemicals used in the treatment of water supplies. Because of the possibility of impurities in the chemicals, it is conceivable that trace metals may be added to the water during treatment. A chemical itself, such as alum, may also contribute to the trace metal content of the finished water, depending on its solubility and the characteristics of the water.

The occurrence of corrosion in the distribution system may also add trace metals to finished water before it reaches the consumer. Common piping materials used in distribution systems are iron, steel, cement (reinforced concrete), asbestos cement, and plastic. Lead, copper, zinc, aluminum, and such alloys as brass, bronze, and stainless steel may also be used in addition to ferrous metals in pumps, small pipes, valves, and other appurtenances. Trace metals may be contributed to the water through corrosion products or simply by solution of small amounts of metals with which the water comes in contact.

Trace Metals in Water Samples Collected in the Distribution System or at Household Taps

The concentration of trace metals in water collected in the distribution system or at household taps is more relevant with respect to the quality of water being consumed by the public than is the raw water. The data in Table V-1, taken from the community water supply survey involving 969 public water supplies, indicate the levels of several selected elements in water samples collected in distribution systems. Chromium and silver were present in microgram quantities, while cadmium, lead, and barium were found to be in the milligram range (McCabe *et al.*, 1970).

The results of analyzing a number of tap-water samples, collected at homes in Dallas, Texas, for trace metals are given in Table V-2. In the unpublished report from which these data were taken, it was speculated that the high iron concentration was due to the use of steel water mains in the distribution system, whereas the high manganese concentration was the result of accumulation of sandy sediment in the distribution system. The high copper and zinc concentrations in the water samples were

TABLE V-1 Concentrations of Selected Trace Metals in 2,595 Distribution Water Samples

Element	Limit,[a] mg/liter	Maximum Concentration, mg/liter	Fraction of Samples Exceeding Limit, %
Barium	1.0	1.55	<0.1
Cadmium	0.01	3.94	0.1
Chromium (VI)	0.05	0.08	0.2
Lead	0.05	0.64	1.4
Silver	0.05	0.03	0

[a]USPHS Drinking Water Standards of 1962
(From McCabe *et al.*, 1970)

believed due to the household plumbing. "Local influences" was the reason cited for the high lead and nickel concentrations in the tap water.

Several studies have shown the combined effect of treatment and the distribution system on the trace-metal content of the water reaching consumers. A treatment plant handling 90 million gallons/day (90 mgd) and obtaining its raw water from the Allegheny River was studied with respect to barium, copper, and nickel (Shapiro *et al.*, 1960). This particular plant used sedimentation, slow sand filtration, and chlorination. Water samples were collected for analysis before and after chlorination and at a consumer's tap at a remote point in the distribution system. Nickel and copper occurred in significantly higher concentrations in the tap water compared with the treatment plant after chlorination—

TABLE V-2 Concentrations of Selected Trace Metals in Houschold Tap-Water Samples, Dallas, Texas

Element	No. Samples	Concentration, mg/liter			
		Average	Median	Maximum	Minimum
Cadmium	43	0.011	0.003	0.056	0.001
Chromium	36	0.004	0.003	0.020	0.001
Copper	43	0.037	0.029	0.164	0.004
Iron	35	0.093	0.088	0.274	0.031
Mercury	43	0.000115	0.000100	0.000885	0
Manganese	43	0.0037	0.004	0.008	0.001
Nickel	36	0.0109	0.010	0.023	0.005
Lead	43	0.0095	0.010	0.027	0
Zinc	43	0.0124	0.011	0.049	0.005

TABLE V-3 Comparison of Concentrations of Several Trace Elements in Raw and Tap Water of Three Cities in Sweden

Element	Raw-Water Concentration, μg/liter	Concentration Ratio, Tap; Raw		
		Malmo	Stockholm	Goteberg
Barium	1–3	6.7	4.0	0.5
Cadmium	0.02–0.3	2.5	0.5	1.0
Cobalt	0.1	0.7	1.0	3.0
Copper	2–13	0.5	0.2	0.4
Mercury	0.09–0.4	1.1	1.0	1.0
Zinc	8–28	4.5	2.8	1.4

(From Bostrom and Wester, 1967)

100 μg/liter vs. 30 μg/liter for nickel and 4,000 μg/liter vs. 90 μg/liter for copper. In the case of barium, the concentration was lower at the tap—40 μg/liter vs. 90 μg/liter. The concentration of copper in water was higher following chlorination (30 μg/liter before and 90 μg/liter after).

The effect of treatment and the distribution system on the concentration of trace metals was also studied in three cities in Sweden—Malmo, Stockholm, and Goteberg (Bostrom and Wester, 1967). A comparison of the raw and tap water concentration of six trace metals is shown in Table V-3.

The change in concentration of several trace metals in raw, finished, and tap water was studied in the Denver municipal system, which draws its raw water from a variety of sources and uses five treatment plants that are interconnected, which makes it impossible to determine the plant from which a tap-water sample is derived (Barnett *et al.*, 1969). The maximum:minimum ratio for most of the trace metals in the raw water varied from 1.5:1-6.5:1; higher ratios were observed for aluminum, iron, molybdenum, and zinc. A comparison of the concentrations of the trace metals in the tap and finished water, based on ratios, shows that there were both reductions and increases in the distribution system. As with the raw waters, the concentrations of trace metals in the tap-water samples showed considerable variation.

A distribution system in Seattle, Washington, was studied in an attempt to determine the severity and location of the corrosion that was known to be occurring (Dangel, 1975). The concentrations of several trace metals were determined in the raw water and in two samples collected at household taps. Standing samples were collected as soon as the tap was turned on; this represented water in contact with the household plumbing at least overnight. Running samples collected after bleeding the line for 30 s represented water from the distribution main. The corrosiveness of the system was recognized by the low pH and hardness of the water. A comparison of the concentrations of iron, copper, zinc, lead, and cadmium in the raw water with those in the standing water confirmed the corrosiveness of the water. However, after a comparison of the concentrations of the same trace metals in the standing and running samples, it was concluded that most of the metal pickup was occurring in the service lines connecting the distribution main to the buildings and in the inside plumbing. It was also noted that the corrosion products tested—the trace metals—correlated well with the materials in contact with the water.

Trace Metals in Finished Water Supplies

A survey of the mineral content of the water served to customers (finished water) in the 100 largest U.S. cities was made in 1962 (Durfor and Becker, 1964). The highest, median, and lowest concentrations are listed in Table V-4. The raw water used by these cities was either groundwater (wells and infiltration galleries) or surface water (streams, reservoirs, and lakes). The chemical quality of most groundwater supplies is stable, compared with

TABLE V-4 Maximum, Minimum, and Median Concentrations of Constituents of Finished Water in Public Water Supplies of 100 Largest Cities in United States

	Concentration, mg/liter		
Constituent	High	Median	Low
Iron	1.3	0.02	0.00
Manganese	2.5	0.00	0.00
Magnesium	120	6.25	0.00
Silica	72	7.1	0.00
	μg/liter		
Silver	7.0	0.23	ND
Aluminum	1,500	54	3.3
Barium	380	43	1.7
Chromium	35	0.43	0 2
Copper	250	8.3	<0.61
Molybdenum	68	1.4	ND
Nickel	34	<2.7	ND
Lead	62	3.7	ND
Vanadium	70	<4.3	ND

ND, not detected.
(From Durfor and Becker, 1964)

TABLE V-5 Frequency of Detection and Concentrations of Dissolved Trace Metals in 1,577 Raw Surface Waters in the United States (October 1, 1962–September 30, 1967)

Element	Frequency of Detection, %	Concentration, μg/liter Minimum	Maximum	Mean
Zinc	76.5	2	1,183	64
Cadmium	2.5	1	120	9.5
Iron	75.6	1	4,600	52
Molybdenum	37.7	2	1,500	68
Manganese	51.4	0.3	3,230	58
Aluminum	31.2	1	2,760	74
Beryllium	5.4	0.01	1.22	0.19
Copper	74.4	1	280	15
Silver	6.6	0. 1	38	2.6
Nickel	16.2	1	130	19
Cobalt	2.8	1	48	17
Lead	19.3	2	140	23
Chromium	24.5	1	112	9.7
Vanadium	3.4	2	300	40
Barium	99.4	2	340	43

(From Kopp, 1970)

that of streams, whose quality often varies seasonally and during flood periods. The mineral content of impounded water is generally less than that of water in streams.

In addition to the quality of the raw water, it is important to recognize that water-treatment practices can affect the concentration of trace metals in finished water. This can be seen from the data in Tables V-5 and V-6. The concentrations of several trace metals in surface water of the United States are summarized in Table V-5. Table V-6 gives values for finished municipal water after treatment. This summary of analyses performed on raw surface water and finished water indicates higher mean concentrations of iron, zinc, lead, copper, and aluminum in finished water. This broad comparison points to the possibility that trace metals are added to water during treatment. Barnett *et al.* (1969) cited such an instance in which the use of aluminum sulfate at a treatment plant increased the aluminum concentration in the finished water by a factor of 5. Shapiro *et al.* (1962) observed, in a study of Pittsburgh tap water, a considerable increase in the copper content between samples at the water-treatment plant and those taken in the distribution system. Nickel also showed a tendency to be higher in the distribution water samples than at the treatment plant; however, the opposite was true for barium.

In comparing the concentrations of several trace metals in raw water taken from the Thames River and finished water at two treatment plants using prechlorination, flocculation with alum, rapid sand filtration, and postchlorination, it was found that treatment had no effect on the cobalt concentration (Andelman and Shapiro, 1973). However, as a result of treatment, the concentrations of manganese and nickel in the finished water decreased, whereas those of copper and cadmium increased.

In addition, 83 water-supply systems in EPA Region V were examined for various organic and inorganic constituents (USEPA, 1975). Region V consists of Illinois, Indiana, Michigan, Minnesota, Ohio, and Wisconsin. The water supplies examined were selected jointly by the EPA and the states and consisted of 14 groundwater and 69 surface-water supplies. The concentrations of metals in the raw- and finished-water supplies included in the survey are summarized in Table V-7.

Occurrence of Trace Metals in Raw Water Supplies

In reporting the results of various water surveys, no attempt has been made to distinguish between different analytical methods used that may well have different sensitivities and precision.

TABLE V-6 Frequency of Detection and Concentrations of Trace Metals in 380 Finished Waters in the United States (October 1, 1962–September 30, 1967)

Element	Frequency of Detection, %	Concentration, μg/liter Minimum	Maximum	Mean
Zinc	77.0	3	2,010	79.2
Cadmium	0.2	12	12	12
Iron	83.4	2	1,920	68.9
Manganese	58.7	0.5	450	25.5
Copper	65.2	1	1,060	43
Silver	6.1	0.3	5	2.2
Lead	18.1	3	139	33.9
Chromium	15.2	1	29	7.5
Barium	99.7	1	172	28.6
Molybdenum	29.9	3	1,024	85.9
Aluminum	47.8	3	1,600	179.1
Beryllium	1.1	0.02	0.17	0.1
Nickel	4.6	1	490	34.2
Cobalt	0.5	22	29	26
Vanadium	3.4	14	222	46.1

(From Kopp, 1970)

TABLE V-7 Metal Concentration Ranges in Raw- and Finished-Water Supplies of 83 Cities in EPA Region V

Element	Concentration, μg/liter	
	Raw Water	Finished Water
Silver	<0.2–0.3	<0.2–0.3
Arsenic	<1.0–10.0	<1.0–50.0
Cadmium	<0.2–12	<0.2–0.4
Chromium	<5.0–17.0	<5.0–6.0
Copper	<5.0–200.0	<5.0–200.0
Iron	<20–330	<20–1,100
Magnesium	1,800–62,000	800–49,000
Manganese	<5.0–760	<5.0–350
Sodium	1,100–77,000	1,000–91,000
Lead	<2.0–30.0	<2.0–20.0
Selenium	<5.0	<5.0
Zinc	<5.0–210	<5.0–460

BARIUM

Barium was found in 99.4% of the surfacewater samples examined by Kopp and Kroner (1967). The range was 2-340 μg/liter, and the average was 43 μg/liter.

BERYLLIUM

The maximum beryllium concentration observed in 1961 by Durum and Haffty was less than 0.22 μg/liter in the Atchfalaya River at Krotz Springs, Louisiana. Kopp and Kroner (1967) noted the presence of beryllium in 5.4% of their samples, with concentrations ranging from 0.01 to 1.22 μg/liter and an average of 0.19 μg/liter.

CADMIUM

Groundwater contamination from electroplating operations has been reported by Lieber (1954) to cause cadmium concentrations of up to 3.2 mg/liter. In Illinois surface waters, 10 of 27 sampling stations on different watersheds had cadmium concentrations below 10 μg/liter; the maximum observed by Ackermann (1971) was 20 μg/liter. Of 112 samples of surface and groundwater in Canada examined, only four had detectable concentrations of cadmium, i.e., 10 μg/liter (Procter and Gamble, 1974). Kopp and Kroner (1967) reported that 2.5% of the surface-water samples examined in their study contained cadmium at 1-120 μg/liter, with a mean of 9.5 μg/liter. In a comprehensive study of U.S. rivers in 1974 (USGS, 1974), a maximum dissolved concentration of cadmium of 42 μg/liter was reported for the Tanana River in Alaska. Durum *et al.* (1971) reported cadmium concentrations of 1-10 μg/liter in 42% of the surface-water samples examined, with only 4% above 10 μg/liter; the maximum concentration was 130 μg/liter. High concentrations were reported to occur in densely populated areas. Durum (1974) reported a distinct regional pattern: areas with many pollution sources and higher rainfall were higher in cadmium.

CHROMIUM

Durum and Haffty (1961) reported a range of concentrations for chromium in U.S. rivers of 0.7 to 84 μg/liter. Kopp and Kroner (1967) detected chromium in 24.5% of the samples examined, with concentrations ranging from 1 to 112 μg/liter and averaging 9.7 μg/liter. In a study of surface and groundwater in Canada, all but two of 240 samples examined were below 50 μg/liter (Procter & Gamble, 1974). In 1974, a maximum dissolved chromium concentration of 30 μg/liter was recorded in water from the Pecos River, New Mexico; the Los Angeles River; and the Columbia River, Oregon (USGS, 1974). In a 1970 survey, 11 of 700 samples had chromium concentrations of 6 to 50 μg/liter, with none exceeding 50 μg/liter (Durum *et al.*, 1971). Ackermann (1971) reported chromium concentrations below 5 μg/liter for 18 of 27 river stations in Illinois; the maximum was 50 μg/liter.

COBALT

The limit of solubility of cobalt in normal river water is approximately 5 μg/liter, according to Durum *et al.* (1971), who reported that 37% of the river-water samples examined contained cobalt at 1-5 μg/liter, with less than 1% exceeding 5 μg/liter. A 1961 study showed a maximum of 5.8 μg/liter in the Mississippi River at Baton Rouge (Durum, 1961). A recent survey detected a maximum of 17 μg/liter in the Kentucky River at Lockport (USGS, 1974). Kopp and Kroner (1967) found cobalt in 2.8% of surface-water samples examined; the concentration ranged from 1 to 48 μg/liter, with a mean of 17 μg/liter.

COPPER

Copper has been observed to adsorb to colloidal material at alkaline pH (McKee and Wolf, 1963). Durum and Haffty (1961) found the maximum copper concentration in the Susquehanna River to be 105 μg/liter. Kopp and Kroner (1967) detected copper in 74.4% of the surface-water samples examined; the concentration ranged from 1 to 280 μg/liter, with a mean of 15 μg/liter. A recent survey detected a maximum of 40 μg/liter in the North Platte River (USGS, 1974). Analysis of 13 Canadian surface and groundwaters—including wells, rivers, and lakes—showed copper at 20-860 μg/liter, the maximum being recorded in Lake Ontario (Proctor & Gamble, 1974). Copper in excess of 100 μg/liter was reported in 8 of 27 Illinois streams, with a maximum of 260 μg/liter (Ackermann, 1971).

LEAD

Pickering and Henderson (1966) reported a maximum solubility of lead of 500 μg/liter in soft water and 3 μg/liter in hard water. Durum and Haffty (1961) reported a maximum lead concentration of 55 μg/liter in the St. Lawrence River at Levis, Quebec. In a more recent sampling of 727 U.S. sites, lead was found, at 1-50 μg/liter, in 63% of the surface-water samples examined (Durum *et al.*, 1971). However, lead was detected less frequently at U.S. Geological Survey benchmark stations than at locations in more developed areas.

In 1974, the Mississippi River at Vicksburg showed a maximum lead concentration of 29 μg/liter (USGS, 1974). Of 52 surface and groundwaters examined in Canada, 50 were found to have less than 10 μg/liter; the concentrations in the other two samples were 22 and 25 μg/liter (Procter & Gamble, 1974). In Illinois surface water, 25 of 27 river stations were found to have lead below 50 μg/liter; the other two had concentrations greater than 50 μg/liter (Ackermann, 1971). Kopp and Kroner (1967) found lead at 2-140 μg/liter, with a mean of 23 μg/liter in 19.3% of their surface water samples. Durum (1974) reported that the concentration of lead in water, like that of cadmium, can be correlated with urbanization and runoff.

MANGANESE

Durum and Haffty (1961) observed a maximum manganese concentration of 181-185 μg/liter in two different surface waters. The median for all samples was 20 μg/liter. Kopp and Kroner (1967) detected manganese in 51.4% of surface-water samples; the concentration ranged from 0.3 to

3,230 μg/liter, with a mean of 59 μg/liter. A maximum of 1,200 μg/liter was detected in two different surface waters in 1974 (USGS, 1974).

MERCURY

Durum *et al.* (1971) found dissolved mercury ranging from 0.1 to 4.3 μg/liter in 7% of the surface-water samples examined; in some cases, total mercury exceeded 5 μg/liter. According to a survey performed by Jenne (1972), only 4% of the surface waters examined showed mercury in excess of 10 μg/liter; most of these were small lakes and reservoirs. The same study reported that groundwater samples were below the limit of detection for mercury. In 1974, the Rio De La Plata, Puerto Rico, was observed to have a maximum dissolved mercury concentration of 2 μg/liter, and the James River in Virginia showed 1.6 μg/liter (USGS, 1974).

MOLYBDENUM

Durum and Haffty (1961) detected a maximum molybdenum concentration of 6.9 μg/liter in the Colorado River, Yuma, Arizona. In a more extensive survey, Kopp and Kroner (1967) found molybdenum in 32.7% of their surface-water samples; the concentration ranged from 2 to 1,500 μg/liter, with a mean of 68 μg/liter.

NICKEL

A maximum nickel concentration of 71 μg/liter was observed in the Hudson River at Green Island, New York (Durum and Haffty, 1961). Kopp and Kroner (1967) found nickel in 16.2% of surface-water samples: the concentration ranged from 1 to 130 μg/liter, with a mean of 19 μg/liter. In a study of 13 Canadian surface and groundwater resources, only one sample was found to have nickel above the detection limit of 100 μg/liter (Procter & Gamble, 1974). In a study of Illinois surface-waters, 24 river stations had nickel concentrations below 50 μg/liter, and 3 had concentrations of 50-530 μg/liter (Ackermann, 1971).

SILVER

Samples containing silver at approximately 1 μg/liter were noted by Durum and Haffty (1961) in the St. Lawrence River, Levis, Quebec, and in the Colorado River, Yuma, Arizona. Of the surface-water samples examined by Kopp and Kroner (1967), only 6.6% contained detectable amounts of silver; the concentration ranged from 0.1 to 38 μg/liter, with an average of 2.6 μg/liter.

VANADIUM

A high vanadium concentration of 6.7 μg/liter has been reported in the Sacramento River, Sacramento, California (Durum and Haffty, 1961). Kopp and Kroner (1967) observed detectable concentrations in 3.4% of the samples analyzed; the concentration ranged from 2 to 300 μg/liter, with an average of 40 μg/liter.

ZINC

The early studies of Durum and Haffty (1961) showed a maximum zinc concentration of approximately 144 μg/liter in the St. Lawrence River, Levis, Quebec. Kopp and Kroner (1967) found zinc in 76.5% of their surface-water samples: the concentration ranged from 2-1,183 μg/liter, with an average of 64 μg/liter. Durum *et al.* (1971) reported that zinc concentrations as high as 50 mg/liter could be found in surface water in mining areas, but that most samples had a concentration ranging from 10 to 50 μg/liter. Lazarus *et al.* (1970) reported the average concentration of zinc in rainfall of about 107 μg/liter. In 1974, a zinc concentration of 730 μg/liter was found in the North Platte River, Lisco, Nebraska (USGS, 1974). In a variety of surface and groundwater sources in Canada, the zinc concentration was found to be 20-110 μg/liter (Procter & Gamble, 1974). In a study of 27 Illinois surface-water sources, a maximum concentration of 2,000 μg/liter was observed (Ackermann, 1971). Durum (1974) reported that the concentration of zinc in surface water, like those of lead and cadmium, could be correlated with urbanization and runoff.

Geographical and Local Factors

Durum and Haffty (1961) studied 15 stations on various rivers. Considering 13 of the trace metals pertinent to this review, 3 of the 15 stations had the maximum concentrations of more than 1 element. The St. Lawrence River at Levis, Quebec, had the maximum concentrations of silver, lead, and zinc; the Colorado River at Yuma, Arizona, had the maximum concentrations of silver and molybdenum; and the Mississippi River at Baton Rouge, Louisiana, had the maximum concentrations of cobalt, iron, and manganese.

Kopp and Kroner (1967) presented data for 5 years for 16 major river basins in the United States. Table V-8 summarizes the basins in which the highest and lowest 5-yr means were reported. The variability between the high and low means is shown as a ratio; for example, the ratio for manganese shows more variability than that for any of the other trace metals for which there was a detectable minimal concentration. Table V-9 shows the highest and lowest observed concentrations of various trace metals in different surface and groundwaters, as reported in the references cited here. The possible frequency of detection is also given. For example, zinc will, in all probability, be found in 75% of all water samples examined for zinc from various locations, and its concentration will range from 2 to 50,000 μg/liter.

Removal Of Metals By Water-Treatment Processes

Beyond health considerations, the necessity of removing metals from drinking water is primarily a function of adequate surveillance and the development of analytical procedures capable of detecting trace concentrations. The need to remove metals raises the question of how effective the current water processes are in removing metals from a water supply. Most treatment processes in use today were not developed to remove trace concentrations of metal. Chemical coagulation-flocculation, for example, is used primarily to remove turbidity and color from raw water; and any significant removal of lead through coagulation with alum is secondary to the original objective. Every treatment plant that uses alum coagulation will vary with respect to its potential for removing lead, owing to differences in water characteristics and operating procedures.

Table V-10 indicates the potential of several different treatment processes for removing barium, cadmium, chromium, cobalt, copper, lead, magnesium, manganese, mercury, methylmercury, molybdenum, nickel, silver, tin, vanadium, and zinc. The treatment processes considered include chemical coagulation (alum and ferric chloride), lime softening (low lime and excess lime), the application of activated carbon, reverse osmosis, and ion exchange. Removal efficiencies have been rated semiquantitatively as "poor" ($<$30% removal), "fair" (30-60% removal), "good" (60-90% removal), and "very good" ($>$90% removal). Unfortunately, some studies have been performed whose published reports did not give percentage values for removal efficiencies. In these cases, efficiency was assigned on the basis of the written description.

CHEMICAL COAGULATION

Salts of trivalent aluminum and iron have long been used to remove color and turbidity from water. Two mechanisms for the removal of trace

TABLE V-8 Minimum and Maximum 5-Year Mean Concentrations and Their Occurrence

Metal	Low Mean, μg/liter	High Mean, μg/liter	High:Low Ratio	River Basins	
				Low Mean	High Mean
Zinc	16	205	12.8	California	Lake Erie
Cadmium	0	50	—	Tennessee Missouri Low Mississippi California Alaska	Lake Erie
Iron	19	173	9.1	North Atlantic	Western Gulf
Molybdenum	15	145	9.7	South East	Great Basin
Manganese	2.3	232	101	Western Great Lakes	Ohio River
Aluminum	11	333	30.3	Alaska	Western Gulf
Beryllium	0	0.28	—	Upper Miss. Southwestern Low Miss. Colorado Western Gulf California Great Basin Alaska	Ohio River

Copper	7	25	3.3	Western Great Lakes	Ohio River
Silver	0.3	5.8	19.3	Great Basin	Colorado
Nickel	3	56	18.7	Western Gulf	Lake Erie
Cobalt	0	36	—	Tennessee Western Gulf California Great Basin Alaska	Southwestern Low Miss.
Lead	4	39	9.8	Western Gulf California	Lake Erie Missouri
Chromium	4	25	6.3	South East Great Basin	Western Gulf
Vanadium	0	171	—	Tennessee Western Great Lakes Great Basin	Missouri
Barium	15	90	6.0	Western Great Lakes	Southwestern Low Mississippi

(From Kopp and Kroner, 1967)

TABLE V-9 Overall Minimum and Maximum Metal Concentrations in Groundwater and Surface Water and Probable Frequency of Detection

	Highest Observed Concentration, μg/liter	Lowest Observed Concentration, μg/liter	Probable Frequency of Detection,[a] %
Barium	340	2	99+
Beryllium	1.22	0.01	80
Cadmium	130	1	5–40
Chromium	112	0.7	25–66
Cobalt	48	1	5–40
Copper	860	1	75
Lead	140	1	25–66
Manganese	3,230	0.3	50
Mercury	10	0.1	10
Molybdenum	1,500	2	30
Nickel	530	1	25–66
Silver	38	0.1	10
Vanadium	300	2	5
Zinc	50,000	2	75

[a]Estimated upward from the best values reported in the literature, on basis of current analytical methods.

metals by aluminum and ferric salts have been proposed: chemisorption to insoluble $Al(OH)_3$ and $Fe(OH)_3$, and by association with organic matter and clays, which are normally removed in the coagulation-flocculation process (Singer, 1974).

Symons *et al.* (1975) used jar tests with Cincinnati tap water to which trace amounts of various metals were added and reported very good removal of cadmium with ferric sulfate when the pH of the solution was above 7.5. Removal of cadmium with alum was reported as only poor to fair. Removal of barium was expected because of the formation of insoluble barium sulfate. However, only poor results were achieved with ferric sulfate and alum, presumably because of the supersaturation of barium sulfate. Ferric sulfate and alum concentrations between 20 and 100 mg/liter removed only small amounts of inorganic mercury (II) and methylmercury. Slightly better results were obtained in removing inorganic mercury with ferric sulfate than with alum. Increased removal of inorganic mercury was observed when the suspended solids in the test water were increased. It was speculated that this increase was due to the adsorption of mercury to the particulate matter (Logsdon and Symons, 1973).

Using samples of tap water and wastewater with added doses of various metals, Nilsson (1975) found that lead and copper were removed very effectively by alum doses of 100 mg/liter when the pH was 6.5-7.0. Zinc, nickel, and cobalt were only slightly removed under those conditions. These results were explained by the insolubility of the metals at neutral pH. Lead and copper were suspected to be present as insoluble hydroxides, oxides, and carbonates, which are readily flocculated by alum.

Nordell (1961) noted that coagulation of colloidal oxides of iron and manganese with ferric salts may give favorable results. However, the preferred method of removal consists of aeration followed by settling and filtration if reduced species of iron and manganese are present, which is usually the case. Removing dissolved silica by treating surface waters with ferric sulfate may be effective. Aluminum removal to approximately 1 mg/liter may be achieved by coagulation with alum when the pH of the water is 5.5-6.5.

Poor removal of radiosotopes of chromium, molybdenum, and cobalt by chemical coagulation with Al(III) and Fe(III) salts has been reported by Straub (1964). Coagulant doses of approximately 20-100 mg/liter at neutral pH values were used in jar tests. Increased removal was demonstrated when artificial turbidity was added to the test water, indicating adsorption to the particulate matter.

LIME SOFTENING

The major objective of lime softening is the removal of hardness from water. Two types of softening processes are used: when the alkalinity of water is sufficiently high, the low-lime process is used, and the pH of the water is raised to approximately 9.5-10.5; when the alkalinity of water is low, excess lime may be used to remove hardness not associated with alkalinity, and the pH of the water may be raised to around 10.5-11.5. Removal of trace metals during either process may be due to precipitation as hydroxides at the increased pH or to chemisorption of the metals to calcium carbonate and magnesium hydroxide precipitates.

Symons *et al.* (1975) showed that, although removal of barium by coagulation was poor, good to very good results could be obtained with lime precipition. Cadmium removal with both the low- and excess-lime processes was in excess of 90%. The removal of methylmercury was described as poor and the removal of inorganic mercury was fair to good in studies of both lime processes with the jar test procedure. Additional results presented by the authors indicated that significantly better results were obtained for the removal of both methylmercury and inorganic mercury in a pilot-plant operation.

TABLE V-10 Removal of Metals by Water Treatment Processes

Metal	Chemical Coagulation: Alum	Chemical Coagulation: Ferric Salts	Lime Softening: Low pH 9.5–10′	Lime Softening: Excess pH 10.6–11.6	Activated Carbon	Reverse Osmosis	Ion Exchange
Ba	Poor[1]	Poor[1]	Good[1]	Good–V Good[1]	Poor[1]		V Good[5,6] Cation
Cd	Poor–Fair[1]	Good–V Good[1] pH >7.5	V Good[1]	V Good[1,2]	V Good[2]	V Good[4]	V Good[2] Cation
Cr	Poor[9]	Poor[9]		Poor[9]	V Good[2]	V Good[4]	V Good[2] Anion
Co	Poor[3,9] pH 6.5–7	Poor[9]	Good[3]		Good[12]		
Cu	Good[3] pH 6.5–7					V Good[4]	
Pb	Good[3] pH 6.5–7		V Good[7]	Poor–Fair[11]	Good[12]		V Good[6] Cation
Mg			Poor–Fair[8]	V Good[8]	V Good[4]		V Good[7] Cation
Mn		Fair–Good[10] high pH		Good[10]			Fouls Resins

Methyl Hg	Poor[1]	Poor[1]	Poor[1]	Poor[1]	V Good[13]		V Good[5] Cation
Inorganic Hg	Poor[1]	Fair[1]	Fair[1]	Good[1]	Good[1]		V Good[5]
Mo	Poor[9]	Poor[9]					
Ni	Poor[3] pH 6.5–7		Good[3]		Fair[12]	V Good[4]	
Ag				V Good[2]	V Good[2]	V Good[4]	Good[2] Cation
Sn					V Good[12]		
V					Fair–Good[12]		
Zn	Poor[3] pH 6.5–7		Good[3]		Poor–Fair[12]		

Removal Efficiencies

Poor = < 30 percent
Fair = 30–60 percent
Good = 60–90 percent
V Good = >90 percent

References

1. Symons *et al.*, 1975
2. Linstedt *et al.*, 1971
3. Nilsson, R., 1971
4. Furukawa, D. H., 1974
5. Logsdon and Symons, 1974
6. Semmers, M. J., 1975
7. Bowers, E., 1971.
8. Tuepker and Dye, 1971
9. Straub, C. P., 1964
10. Nordell, E., 1961
11. Naylor and Dague, 1975
12. Sigworth and Smith, 1972
13. Logsdon and Symons, 1973

Lime precipitation of municipal secondary effluent with added trace metals at a pH of 11 was shown to remove silver (50 μg/liter) and cadmium (10 μg/liter) in excess of 95% (Lindstedt *et al.*, 1971). Removal of chromium (50 μg/liter) was very poor. At a pH of 11, silver and cadmium were found to be present as insoluble hydroxides, and chromium as the soluble chromate, CrO_4^{-2}.

Nilsson (1971) demonstrated that—although cobalt, nickel, and zinc were poorly removed by chemical coagulation—lime precipitation at a pH of 9.5 was very effective in removing these metals from samples of tap water and wastewater to which they were added.

In a review of the chemistry of lime precipitation, Dye and Tuepker (1971) emphasized that the removal of magnesium was most effective with the excess-lime process. The removal of magnesium by the low-lime process is usually poor, because of the dissociation of magnesium hydroxide [$Mg(OH)_2$] at pH values below 10. Removal of iron by the low- and excess-lime processes and removal of manganese by the excess-lime process were reported to be incidental, because of the high pH associated with each process (Nordell, 1961). Naylor and Dague (1975) found that the excess-lime process with pH greater than 10.5 was unable to remove lead, either becuase of the physical character of the lead oxides or because of the presence of soluble lead hydroxide $Pb(OH)_3$. Very good removal of lead by the low-lime process was noted. The presence of suspended matter increased the removal of lead with both the low- and excess-lime processes.

ACTIVATED CARBON

Activated carbon is normally used to remove substances that cause taste, odor, and color in water. The use of activated carbon for removal of organic matter in general has been recognized. The removal of metals by activated carbon may be due to several mechanisms. Impurities in activated carbon, especially oxygen and sulfur, may play a significant role. Also surface oxides may act as weak-acid cation-exchange sites or sulfide groups may interact strongly with some metals resulting in chemisorption. Activated carbon may also act as a nucleation site for the precipitation of metals. On the other hand, trace metals associated with organic matter may be removed by interactions between the activated carbon and the organic matter. Activated carbon can also act as a reducing agent. Reduction of metal oxyanions—e.g., $Cr_2O_7^{-2}$ and MnO_4^{-2} to Cr(III) and Mn(II)—may result in the precipitation of the reduced species as oxides or hydroxides—$Cr(OH)_3$ and MnO_2 (Singer, 1974).

Logsdon and Symons (1973) and Symons *et al.* (1975) have reported that trace amounts of inorganic mercury and methylmercury can be removed effectively by activated carbon. The superior removal of methylmercury, compared with inorganic mercury, was attributed to interactions between the activated carbon and the methyl functional group. Poor removal of barium with activated carbon was reported.

Lindstedt *et al.* (1971) reported removal of silver, cadmium, and chromium (in excess of 95%) from municipal secondary effluents with activated carbon. The high degree of removal was attributed to a combination of mechanisms.

Sigworth and Smith (1972) extrapolated several years of data on removal of several metals from paper mill waste solutions by activated carbon to obtain what they felt to be reasonable removal efficiencies that may be expected in the treatment of drinking water. The data were collected for solutions having very high concentrations of metals and low pH values. The authors concluded that the removal of zinc would be poor under the extrapolated conditions, the removal of vanadium and nickel would probably be fair, and the removal of cobalt, iron, lead, and tin would probably be good.

REVERSE OSMOSIS

Reverse osmosis is used as a desalination or demineralization process. The ionic strength of water is reduced by forcing it to diffuse through a cellulose acetate membrane against the high osmotic pressure caused by ionic imbalance. Furukawa (1973) has reported the rejection (separation) of cadmium, chromium, copper, aluminum, iron, magnesium, nickel, and silver by reverse osmosis to be in excess of 98%.

ION EXCHANGE

Ion exchange involves the reversible exchange of ions between a solution and an exchange resin. Exchange resins are available to exchange either anions or cations. The for specific ions over other ions, according to the ionic charge, the hydrated ionic radius of the ions, and their concentration in solution.

Lindstedt *et al.* (1971) demonstrated the removal of silver and cadmium from municipal secondary effluents by a cation-exchange bed. Chromium VI was removed effectively by an anion-exchange bed when present as the metal oxyanion $HCrO_4^-$.

Semmens (1975) has observed very good removal of barium and lead by clinoptilolite, a cation-exchange resin. Very good removal of barium, methylmercury, and inorganic mercury have been reported by Logsdon and Symons (1973). Bowers (1971) noted the efficient removal of magnesium by ion exchange.

Although ion-exchange treatment can be designed for the removal of iron, manganese, and aluminum, the presence of these metals in water may impair the exchange capacity of a resin designed for the removal of other metals. Nordell (1961) stated that some removal of dissolved silica with a strongly basic anion resin is possible.

Analysis of Drinking Water for Trace Metals

The literature on chemical analyses of trace metals in natural fresh water is voluminous. Only the most pertinent publications will be discussed here.

Brown *et al.* (1970) have prepared a comprehensive manual that contains methods used by the U.S. Geological Survey to collect, preserve, and analyze water samples for dissolved mineral and gas content. Among the topics discussed are the selection of sampling sites, frequency of sampling, sampling equipment, sample preservation, laboratory equipment and techniques, accuracy and precision of the analysis, and reporting of results. The methods of analysis are applicable to a wide range of water, from that with trace concentrations of dissolved metals to that with high concentrations.

The National Environmental Research Center of the EPA at Cincinnati, Ohio, has published methods of chemical analysis of water and wastes (USEPA, 1971). The atomic-absorption method is suggested for the determination of aluminum, cadmium, chromium, copper, lead, magnesium, manganese, silver, and zinc; and the flameless atomic-absorption method is suggested for mercury. Method selection was based on the following criteria:

1. The method should measure the desired constituent with precision and accuracy sufficient to meet data needs in the presence of the interferences normally encountered in polluted water.
2. The method should utilize the equipment and skills normally available in the typical water-pollution control laboratory.
3. The method should be in use in many laboratories or have been sufficiently tested to establish its validity.
4. The method should be sufficiently rapid to permit routine use for the examination of a large number of samples.

Guidelines establishing test procedures for analysis of various pollutants in water were published in the *Federal Register* on October 16, 1973. They included references to 71 test procedures for measurement of pollutants for which limitations were specified under the Federal Water Pollution Control Act Amendments of 1972.

Several professional associations have recommended procedures for analysis of water samples for various trace metals. Such publications are *Standard Methods for the Examination of Water and Wastewater* (American Public Health Association, 1976), and *Annual Book of ASTM Standards* (American Society for Testing Materials, 1970).

In addition, many symposium volumes and handbooks have summarized the state of the art for the analysis of trace metals in aqueous solution. Those reviews can be found in Hume (1967), Boettner and Grunder (1968), Hemphill (1973), Cosgrove and Bracco (1973), and others.

Recent developments dealing with analytic methods for trace metals in waters are reviewed biannually in *Analytical Chemistry* and annually in *Journal of Water Pollution Control Federation* (Minear, 1975).

SAMPLE TREATMENT

For the determination of trace metals in fresh water, large volumes of sample are required. Caution must be exercised in the proper collection and treatment of water samples, if the analytic results are to reflect the actual conditions of the water sampled. Water samplers sometimes introduce serious contamination. In selecting sample containers, care must be taken to avoid containers whose interior surfaces contain active metal-binding sites or that may release contaminating metals into the water sample. Inert plastic containers are usually preferred to glass. Polyethylene bottles are generally satisfactory. Ediger (1973) recommended a cleaning procedure of soaking containers in a 2% nitric acid solution for 24 h and then rinsing several times with metal-free water.

Rapid changes may occur in the chemical composition of water samples during storage, owing either to the introduction of contaminants from the containers or to selective adsorption of metals onto the walls of containers. Trace metals in water are also subject to change because of biologic activity. Water samples are usually stabilized by the addition of dilute acid. The EPA recommends the addition of 3 ml of 50% nitric acid to each liter of filtered sample. For unfiltered samples, 5 ml of concentrated nitric acid is recommended. Other preservatives have been recommended for metals known to be unstable in aqueous solution, such as silver (West *et al.*, 1967) and mercury (Omang, 1971).

ANALYSIS

A general requirement in analytic chemistry is standardization of methods. Some methods that serve today as the legal standards in drinking-water quality control for trace metals are not sufficiently sensitive and accurate. The establishment of a method, moreover, does not guarantee that it will produce the same results when used by different analysts in different laboratories. A strong effort is required in evaluating and improving the analytic methods used in drinking water quality control.

The analysis of trace metals is intimately related to the setting and enforcement of drinking-water standards. The reliability and detectability of analytic methods may be the limiting factors in defining standards and maintaining surveillance. Methods must be reliable and provide a measurement of the species under consideration. Furthermore, in the case of effective monitoring programs, methods must be rapid and must have a reasonable cost.

In any trace analytic method, the first consideration is sensitivity. Because of the very low concentrations of some trace metals in natural water, methods should have sensitivities of a nanogram or less. Such methods may involve concentrating the sample; this should be avoided if possible. The stated sensitivity value for a particular method is generally not an exact figure. "Sensitivity" is sometimes defined as the concentration that yields a reading of 1% of full scale of the instrument; it is used in this manner in atomic absorption. The detection limits are usually defined as twice the background.

The specificity of an analytic method indicates the degree to which the method detects one element with no interferences from other elements that are present. Ideally, one would like methods that are specific for each element to be analyzed with few or no interferences.

Accuracy and precision of the procedures are important, but results will be less accurate and less precise as concentrations move into the micrograms-per-liter region. Each procedure should be checked for precision on real samples, and the data reported with respect to the standard deviation.

In selecting a method of water analysis for trace metals, sensitivity, speed, ease of operation, and relative lack of chemical interferences make the conventional and flameless atomic-absorption spectrophotometers instruments of choice. All analytic procedures recommended by the EPA and the U.S. Geological Survey for determining trace metals in water samples are based on atomic-absorption spectrophotometry. These instruments are generally available in analytic laboratories.

For general information on atomic-absorption analysis, books by Elwell and Gidley (1966), Slavin (1968), Ramirez-Munoz (1968), L'vov (1970), Price (1972), Reynolds and Aldous (1970), Kirkbridge and Sargent (1974), and Robinson (1975) are recommended.

Barium

OCCURRENCE

Barium, one of the alkaline earth metals, occurs naturally in almost all (99.4%) surface waters examined, in concentrations of 2-340 μg/liter, with an average of 43 μg/liter (Kopp and Kroner, 1967). The drainage basins with low mean concentration of barium (15 μg/liter) occur in the western Great Lakes, and the highest mean concentration of 90 μg/liter is in the southwestern drainage basins of the lower Mississippi Valley. Finished water of public systems frequently (99.7% of supplies examined) contains barium, at 1-172 μg/liter, with a mean of 28.6 μg/liter. The 100 largest cities (Durfor, 1964) of the United States had a median concentration of 43 μg/liter, with a maximum of 380 μg/liter, but 94% of all determinations were less than 100 μg/liter. Drinking water at the tap, as determined in 2,595 samples, had a maximum of 1,550 μg/liter; the maximum was found in one of only two samples that exceeded the interim standard of 1,000 μg/liter (McCabe, 1970).

CHEMICAL CHARACTERISTICS

Barium is slightly rarer than strontium in the earth's crust. It may replace potassium in some of the igneous rock minerals, especially feldspar. Barium sulfate (barite) is a common barium mineral of secondary origin. In stream water and most groundwater, only traces of the element are present.

The reason for the small amount of barium in solution is the low solubility of barium sulfate. Because natural water usually contains sulfate, only trace amounts of barium will dissolve. Barium sulfate is soluble in pure water at 20°C—barium at 1.6 mg/liter and sulfate at 1.1 mg/liter. The solubility of barium sulfate increases considerably in the presence of chloride and other anions. However, water containing sulfate at more than a few parts per million will not carry barium at more than a few parts per million (USGS, 1959).

METABOLISM

The metabolism of barium has been traced by radioisotope techniques and shown to be similar to that of calcium (Seaber, 1933; Bauer *et al.*, 1956). The digestive system is extremely permeable to barium, allowing for rapid transfer to and from the bloodstream (Bauer, 1957). The metal is transported in the plasma and disappears from the blood completely within 24 h.

Excretion of barium is different from that of calcium, in that the rate is greater in feces than in urine. In feces, 20% of barium is excreted in 24 h compared with 6% of calcium; in urine 7% of barium is excreted in 24 h compared with 0.9% of calcium.

HEALTH EFFECTS

No vital metabolic function has yet been found for barium, although it is believed to be beneficial for rats and guinea pigs under specific dietary conditions (Underwood, 1971).

Barium is highly toxic when soluble salts are ingested. Fatalities have occurred from mistaken use of barium salt rodenticide. The fatal dose of barium chloride for man has been reported to be about 0.8-0.9 g, or 550-600 mg of barium (Sollman, 1957).

Industrial exposure to barium oxide and sulfate dusts produces a benign pneumonoconiosis called "baritosis." Although barium poisoning is rare in industry, the potential from the more soluble forms is real. The American Conference of Governmental Industrial Hygienists set an airborn threshold limit value (TLV) for barium of 0.5 mg/m^3. The limit was based on several years of observation of workers at Los Alamos exposed to barium nitrate.

Acute barium poisoning exerts a strong, prolonged stimulant action on all muscles, including cardiac and smooth muscle of the gastrointestinal tract and bladder. Barium is capable of causing nerve block (deNo, 1946) and in small or moderate doses produces a transient increase in blood pressure by vasoconstriction (Gostev, 1944).

There has been no determination of the chronic effects of barium administered repeatedly over a long period, either in food or drinking water.

ANALYSIS

Conventional flame atomization does not have sufficient sensitivity to determine barium in most water samples; however, a barium detection limit of 10 μg/liter can be achieved, if a nitrous oxide flame is used. Renshaw *et al.* (1973) described a concentration procedure for barium that uses thenoyltrifluoroacetone–methylisobutylketone extraction at a pH of 6-8.

With a tantalum liner insert, the barium detection limit of the flameless atomic absorption procedure can be improved to 0.1 μg/liter (Renshaw, 1973).

CONCLUSIONS AND RECOMMENDATIONS

A drinking-water guideline was derived from the 8-h weighted maximum allowable concentration (TLV) in industrial air of 0.5 mg/m^3 set by the American Conference of Governmental Industrial Hygienists. It was assumed that, with an 8-h inhalation of 10 m^3 of air, the daily intake would be 5 mg of barium, of which 75% was absorbed in the bloodstream and 90% transferred across the gastrointestinal tract. Based on the above assumptions, it was reasoned that a concentration of about 2 mg/liter of water would be safe for adults. To provide added safety for more susceptible members of the population, such as children, a level of 1 mg/liter was recommended (Stockinger, 1958). There have been no long-range feeding studies to confirm the safety of this barium intake. The limit set in the USSR is 4 mg/liter of water. International and European standards do not list barium upper limits, because available information is insufficient.

It is rare to find sources of water that exceed a barium concentration of 1 mg/liter, although a concentration of 1.55 mg/liter has been recorded in drinking water. The 1975 *Analysis of Interstate Carrier Water Supply Systems* showed none exceeding the 1 mg/liter standard. Small numbers of people are known to be consuming well waters in Illinois, Kentucky, Pennsylvania, and New Mexico that are at, or exceed by 10 times, the standard for barium. It would be desirable to study any risk that might be associated with this chronic ingestion of barium.

Animal studies should be undertaken at least, to determine the toxic effects of long-term ingestion of barium at low concentrations.

Beryllium

OCCURRENCE

A relatively rare element, found chiefly in the mineral beryl (beryllium aluminum silicate), beryllium is not likely to occur in natural water in appreciable concentrations. Although the chloride and nitrate are very soluble and the sulfate moderately so, the carbonate and hydroxide are almost insoluble in cold water (McKee and Wolf, 1963).

Beryllium is used primarily in metallurgy to produce special alloys, in the manufacture of X-ray diffraction tubes and electrodes for neon signs, and in nuclear reactors (Browning, 1961). It is also used in rockets and in missile fuels. Cralley (1972) presented an extensive discussion of the many modern uses of beryllium metal, beryllium–copper alloys, beryllium oxide, and minor beryllium compounds. The consumption of beryl increased from 1,200 short tons in 1941 to 8,483 tons in 1969.

Using emission spectroscopy, Durum and Haffty (1961) measured beryllium in 59 samples of surface water from 15 rivers in the United States and Canada. The highest concentration observed was less than 0.22 μg/liter. Kopp and Kroner (1967) noted the presence of beryllium in 85% of their samples from the 15 major river basins of the conterminous United States; the concentration ranged from 0.01-1.22 μg/liter, with an average of 0.19 μg/liter. According to *Standard Methods* (APHA, 1976), beryllium has been reported to occur in U.S. drinking water at 0.01-0.7 μg/liter, with a mean of 0.013 μg/liter.

In a study of many groundwater samples from the western United States, beryllium was detected in only three highly acid mine waters. Beryllium discharged to ground water will not travel far in neutral solution, because it is rapidly adsorbed by the clay in the soil. In the eastern United States and in Siberia, surface water was reported to contain beryllium at 0.1-0.9 μg/liter. Pacific Ocean water contains 2-9 μg/liter (Griffitts *et al.*, 1976). According to the NAS-NAE report on water-quality criteria (NAS, 1973), the concentration of beryllium in seawater is only 6×10^{-4} μg/liter.

Food does not appear to be a significant source of human exposure to beryllium. According to Griffitts *et al.* (1976), "there is no evidence at present that beryllium is moving from soils into food or feed plants in the United States in amounts that are detrimental to plants, animals, or people." Furthermore, "the forms of beryllium in plants and their digestibility by animals have not yet been determined."

CHEMICAL CHARACTERISTICS

Although beryllium is in the same group of elements as the alkaline earth metals, it shares few properties with them. Beryllium replaces silica in the structure of some igneous rock minerals and is present as independent beryllium minerals in pegmatites, the most important of which is beryl. In the weathering process, beryllium (like aluminum) is concentrated in hydrolysates and does not go into solution to any appreciable degree. Beryllium is not likely to be found in natural water in greater than trace amounts, because of the relative insolubility of beryllium oxides and hydroxides at the normal pH range of such water. The solubility of the oxide is reported as about 20–70 μg/l in pure water at about 28°C. The sulfate and chloride of beryllium are very soluble, but would hydrolyze and lower the pH. In the presence of sodium hydroxide (high pH), beryllium hydroxide is soluble, probably because of the formation of anion complexes. The effects of other ions or cations on the solubility of beryllium are not known (USGS, 1959).

Some data on adsorption of trace quantities of beryllium in water by glass and plastic containers have been reported. At a pH of 3.5, there was no adsorption of beryllium by the container. However, at a pH of 7 and 8, there was considerable adsorption. Adsorption of beryllium by naturally occurring minerals is probably an important cause of the low concentrations in water, inasmuch as such adsorption seems to proceed effectively at pH values common in natural water.

METABOLISM

Absorption of beryllium from the digestive tract is slight (about 0.006% of that ingested), and excretion is fairly rapid (Browning, 1961).

HEALTH EFFECTS

In a comprehensive review, Pomelee (1953) reported that there was no indication that beryllium in any form is harmful when taken orally.

Inhalation of particles is by far the major hazard to humans from this metal. Beryllium has been incriminated in pulmonary ailments of workers exposed to beryllium dusts (Browning, 1961). Since the development, in about 1947, of spectrochemical techniques for detecting beryllium in air, there has been a substantial increase in the number of reported cases of beryllium poisoning.

No information was uncovered to indicate that beryllium is a beneficial or necessary component of human nutrition.

Rats were healthy after 2 yr on a diet that included beryllium sulfate at about 6.0 mg/day, equivalent to beryllium at 1.0 mg/kg of body weight per day. Four dogs showed no ill effects after 19 months of daily ingestion of beryllium sulfate at 10 mg/kg of body weight; 1 dog lost weight after 9-months and was killed for examination. No evidence of tissue damage was found (Pomelee, 1953). When mice were fed beryllium at 5.0 mg/liter in drinking water for life, slight effects on the body weight of females (but not males) were disclosed, and there were no effects on the life span and survival of either sex. These studies with mice indicated that beryllium is poorly absorbed through the gut and that ingestion is not a hazard (Schroeder and Mitchener, 1975). According to Stokinger (1972), the dietary LD_{50} of beryllium sulfate in rats after 172 days was 2,750 mg/kg of body weight per day. The beryllium metal in beryllium oxide eaten in the diet at 5.0% is so poorly absorbed that no effect on growth occurred over long periods of feeding. Beryllium sulfate did not interfere with growth until a concentration of 1.4% (14,000 mg/kg of diet) was reached.

With the data for 10 of the 15 river basins studied by Kopp and Kroner (1967), Berg and Burbank (1972) attempted to establish correlations between carcinogenic trace metals in water supplies and cancer mortality—8 metals compared with 34 types of cancer, for a total of 272 comparisons. At the 0.05 level of significance, they expected about 14 comparisons to show positive correlations. In fact, 28 positive correlations were found, 5 of which were associated with beryllium. When they studied these findings in further detail, however, especially with respect to bone cancer, the 5 correlations were not meaningful. Berg and Burbank concluded that the correlations were not consistent with a waterborne pattern and could be explained by other known factors.

The inclusion of beryllium in the work of Berg and Burbank (1972) was prompted by the fact that beryllium was the first metal to produce cancers in animals with any substantial frequency away from the site of administration. Stokinger (1972) noted that soluble beryllium sulfate is about equally toxic (in milligrams per kilogram of body weight) to rats, mice, dogs, monkeys, and rabbits, whether administered by inhalation, intratracheally, intravenously, or subcutaneously. When beryllium is transported via the bloodstream from its initial site of deposition, a significant part of the administered dose ends up in the skeleton, irrespective of the mode of administration. In the bones of animals, it has been shown to produce osteosarcoma; but this has been demonstrated only in animals and not yet in humans who have beryllium lung disease from inhaling beryllium dust (IARC, 1973).

According to Sterner and Eisenbud (1951), acute pneumonitis among human beings has been caused by exposures to beryllium in the atmosphere at concentrations of less than 1.0 to over 100 $\mu g/m^3$ of air. The symptoms of beryllosis include skin and lung diseases of variable severity. The reactions of people to a given exposure are said to vary widely, but apparently any person will show a reaction if time and degree of exposure are great enough.

It became apparent by 1947 that many cases of what was then thought to be pulmonary sarcoidosis were appearing among beryllium production workers as a result of inhalation of beryllium compounds and metallic dust. On the recommendations of an *ad hoc* advisory committee, the Atomic Energy Commission (AEC) established strict in-plant limits for beryllium in the atmosphere and much stricter limits for neighborhoods near AEC plants (Stokinger, 1972). Apparently, beryllosis is confined to the lungs, and beryllium is not translocated to other parts of the body. Any sputum that might be swallowed would get into the digestive tract, where beryllium has been shown to be relatively harmless. No unusual incidence of lung cancer has yet been found among workers exposed to beryllium, although sizable numbers had exposures more than 20 years ago. This experience indicates that, if beryllium proves to be carcinogenic in humans, it is of low potency (Stokinger, 1972).

ANALYSIS

According to *Standard Methods* (USEPA, 1976), atomic-absorption spectrophotometry and colorimetry are equally suitable for the determination of beryllium. Direct flame atomization offers a detection limit of 2 μg/liter. Sachdev and West (1969) have described a concentration procedure that uses solvent extraction with an oxine–acetylacetone–dithizone combination at a pH of 6.0. The detection limit can be lowered to 0.03 μg/liter when the graphite furnace is used for atomization. Chapman *et al.* (1974) have used flameless atomic absorption for beryllium analysis.

CONCLUSIONS AND RECOMMENDATIONS

Beryllium is relatively harmless when ingested in food and water, except at very large continuing dosages. It is present in natural surface water at concentrations generally less than 1.0 μg/liter, with averages of less than 0.2 μg/liter; hence, it presents no hazard in drinking water. The USSR has set a limit of 0.2 μg/liter, but the World Health Organization has not established any limit (Stoefen, 1973). The EPA has not promulgated any limit for beryllium in its *National Interim Primary Drinking Water Regulations* (1975). Beryllium is known to cause cancer in various species of laboratory animals, but to date has not been associated with human cancer. Because of the strong association of beryllium with cancer in animals a continuing effort should be made to study both through epidemiology and chronic low-level feeding studies the toxicology of beryllium.

Cadmium

The sources, distribution, metabolism, and toxicology of cadmium have been reviewed by Friberg *et al.* (1971, 1974, 1975), Underwood (1971), Nordberg, (1976), and Copenhaver *et al.* (1973).

OCCURRENCE

The principal industrial uses of cadmium are in electroplating, in pigment manufacture, and as a plasticizer, chiefly in polyvinylchloride. Cadmium occurs in zinc ores and is an important by-product in the metallurgy of zinc. Because cadmium is an impurity in zinc, cadmium should possibly receive some consideration when poor grades of zinc are used for galvanizing. The use of cadmium-plated containers in food- and beverage-handling materials is now prohibited by the Food and Drug Administration because acute cadmium poisoning has been recognized in man after consumption of food and particularly acidic beverages stored in cadmium-plated containers. Except where stated, estimates of intake and critical renal concentration are taken from *Cadmium in the Environment, II and III (1974, 1975).*

In streams and rivers, the concentration of cadmium tends to be higher in sediment than in filtered running water. From studies in Japan (Friberg, 1974) and upstate New York (Kubota *et al.*, 1974; Durum, 1974), it appears that most fresh water contains cadmium at less than 1 μg/liter. The U.S. Geological Survey reported that about 46% of samples contained detectable amounts—1 μg/liter or more. Regional differences are noted within the United States, with the higher concentrations found in runoff water in the Northeast, in some urbainzed areas in the South, and in the central states. This distribution pattern suggested to Durum that pollution sources and rainfall may be the major contributors of cadmium in river water.

Carbonate content and pH influence the stability and solubility of cadmium in water. It is least soluble at a pH of approximately 8-9 and becomes increasingly soluble as the pH decreases. But, the median concentration in surface water in most areas is less than the detection limit (<1 μg/liter of water). Durum used filtered samples and found that 4% of surface waters in the United States exceeded the 1962 USPHS drinking-water standard of 10 μg/liter. However, the USPHS National Community Water Supply study indicated that the drinking-water standard for cadmium was exceeded by only 0.1% of 969 water-supply systems tested, which served an estimated 18 million people. Craun and McCabe (1975) reported data on the interaction between soft water and accumulation of cadmium in the distribution systems for Boston and Seattle. This survey indicated that 13% of samples obtained in Boston showed a higher concentration at the tap than at the treatment plant. In Seattle, which has more acidic water, 51% of the sample showed an increase. Both running and standing samples were obtained. In Seattle, 7% of the samples exceeded the 10 μg/liter drinking-water standard; in the Boston area, none exceeded this standard.

There is a wide consensus that the cadmium content of food is the major source of cadmium for the general population. Friberg *et al.* (1974) estimated that the average daily intake for adults is approximately 50 μg. If this estimate is adjusted on a caloric basis for children consuming a similar diet, the intake at 2-3 years of age would be about one-third to one-half of the adult intake. There is a rather wide range in the estimates of cadmium intake in food. This may be due largely to difficulties in the measurement of trace amounts of cadmium. Because cadmium is a contaminant of superphosphate fertilizers and because of current plans to use sewage sludge for agricultural purposes, it is the consensus of most experts that the food supply should be carefully monitored for cadmium and other trace metals.

Although air cadmium concentrations may be high near lead, zinc, and cadmium smelters and refineries, it is generally about 1 ng/m^3 elsewhere.

Cigarette tobacco contains cadmium at about 1 ppm. Friberg (1974) has estimated that the smoking of one pack of cigarettes a day can contribute 2-4 μg of cadmium a day.

The best-described accident related to discharge of cadmium into water is the occurrence of Itai–Itai disease among residents along the Jintsu River in Japan (Friberg *et al.*, 1971). These residents were apparently exposed not only through the drinking of water, but also through the ingestion of rice grown in the contaminated water.

CHEMICAL CHARACTERISTICS

Elemental cadmium is present in rocks in much lower quantities than those reported for zinc. Only traces are likely to be found in natural water, but cadmium may be introduced in amounts significant from a health standpoint by solution from containers or tubing or by waste disposal.

Cadmium probably could be present only in small amounts in water with the normal alkaline pH, because of the low solubility of the carbonate and hydroxide. Cadmium hydroxide is soluble at about 1 mg/liter at 25°C. Exact data regarding solubility of the carbonate are not available. At a pH below about 4.5, the solubility of cadmium would be controlled by other factors and would probably be greater (USGS, 1959).

METABOLISM

The total daily intake of cadmium from air, water, food, and cigarettes is estimated to range between 40 μg/day (for nonsmoking rural residents who have negligible air exposure and consume a low-cadmium diet) and 190 μg/day (for smokers living in industrialized cities and consuming a high-cadmium diet).

Absorption from the digestive tract is thought to average about 10%. However, a number of factors, including dietary calcium, protein, and age, may have an important bearing on this. For the digestive-tract route of assimilation, the major organs of cadmium storage are the liver and renal cortex. The renal cortex may contain one-third of the total cadmium body burden. The biologic half-life of cadmium in these organs is variously estimated at 13 to 38 yr. Urinary excretion is low, from 1 to 9 μg/day. Because cadmium tends to accumulate, a more useful way of looking at the question is to consider the rate of accumulation. The human placenta is apparently highly impermeable to cadmium. The total body burden is estimated at 1 ng at birth and at 15–50 mg at the age of 50 years. This is consistent with an average accumulation of 0.9–1.8 μg/day. There is a major need for a more reliable estimate of the rate of cadmium accumulation.

The renal cortex is considered to be the critical organ for accumulation of cadmium from low-level dietary exposures, and the critical concentration for renal cortex is approximately 200 μg/g of tissue (wet weight) (Friberg *et al.*, 1974; Nordberg, 1976). At greater concentrations, irreversible renal injury may occur. In the outbreak of Itai–Itai disease on the Jintsu River, renal cortical cadmium concentration was estimated at 600-1,000 μg/g of tissue (wet weight) in those most severely (and irreversibly) affected. With an assumed water consumption of 1.5 liters/day, the average cadmium intake from water was estimated at 5 μg/day, or less than 10% of the total intake.

HEALTH EFFECTS

In industry, after overexposure to cadmium at high concentrations (50 $\mu g/m^3$) well in excess of that for the general population, bronchitis, emphysema, anemia, and renal stones have been found. Among the general population, gastrointestinal upsets similar to "food poisoning" have been reported in association with consumption of food or beverages conveyed in cadmium-plated vessels. Sporadic outbreaks of this sort occur when cadmium-plated vessels not intended for food are used to prepare lemonade and other acidic beverages for picnics and similar outings.

For the general population, the major route of absorption is through the gastrointestinal tract. The major effects are likely to be on the kidney. There is an extensive literature—reviewed by Friberg (1971, 1974, 1975), Nordberg (1976), and Sandstead (1974)—on this problem. Experimental data indicate that the zinc:cadmium ratio in the organs is an important determinant of cadmium toxicity (in most foodstuffs, the dietary ratio of cadmium to zinc is 1:100; it is highest in meat products and lowest in dairy products), and there is some evidence that the intake of sodium may also influence cadmium toxicity. There are no dose–response data. Limited autopsy data suggest that average renal cortical concentrations of cadmium in American and European populations are generally less than 50 $\mu g/g$ of tissue (wet weight)—less than the projected critical concentration by a factor of 4 or more.

In addition to the suspected interactions between cadmium, zinc, and calcium, recent experimental studies indicate that cadmium at very high doses can interfere with the activation of vitamin D in both liver and kidneys to the final active 1,25-dihydroxycholecalciferol (Nordberg, 1976; Sandstead, 1974). There is also evidence from animal studies that cadmium is implicated in the etiology of hypertension (Schroeder, 1965); the thresholds and dose–response relationships are unknown. There is some evidence that cadmium is carcinogenic in the rat, but no substantial evidence to implicate it with human cancer (IARC, 1973). Cadmium is known to be teratogenic in the rat following rather high (2–13 mg/kg) doses on specific days of gestation (Chernoff, 1973).

Another effect observed—at high doses in rats—is ease of producing testicular and ovarian necrosis when cadmium is given by injection. This same effect can be seen in rats (who can not vomit) with high oral doses.

There are no identified hypersusceptible segments of the human population. Although victims of Itai–Itai disease were predominantly multigravid, postmenopausal women, this does not mean that these alone are predisposing conditions. It should, however, be noted that, on a body weight basis, infants may have a higher intake of cadmium. If, in fact, calcium intake is an important protective factor, it is well to note that a significant proportion of the population from school age up is lactose-intolerant and may voluntarily reduce milk intake and hence calcium intake on this account. If, as appears likely from experimental studies, zinc is an important protective factor against cadmium toxicity, it is worth noting that preliminary evidence indicates that those with hemoglobin SS or SC have shown signs of zinc deficiency. Further studies in these groups appear warranted.

ANALYSIS

Direct flame atomization has a cadmium detection limit of 2 μg/liter. Most reported analyses, however, involve some form of concentration. The U.S. Geological Survey procedure (Brown *et al.*, 1970) recommends extracting the cadmium as an ammonium pyrrolidine dithiocarbamate at a pH of 2.8 with methylisobutylketone. Other concentration procedures have been described for fresh water (USEPA, 1971; Traversy, 1971; Kaminski, 1974; Kinrade and Van Loon, 1974; Kubota *et al.*, 1974; Korkisch and Sorio, 1975; Aldous *et al.*, 1975).

The sampling boat and Delves cup techniques have cadmium detection limits of 0.1 and 0.05 μg/liter, respectively. Using the graphite furnace to atomize the sample can improve detection to 0.005 μg/liter. Paus (1971) has used the graphite furnace to determine cadmium in lake water at concentrations of 0.5–2.5 μg/liter. Other methods have been reported by Dolinsek and Stupar (1973), Surles *et al.* (1975), and Rattonetti (1974). Barnard and Fishman (1973) have critically evaluated the use of the graphite furnace for cadmium determinations in fresh water.

For all types of biologic samples, the available data indicate that either background correction or extraction is essential when determinations are made by atomic-absorption spectrophotometry, owing to the enhancing effect of sodium on the cadmium signal. Although it has not been fully explored, it appears that electrochemical techniques may be more suitable, although somewhat less sensitive, because such measurements may be influenced, to a lesser degree, by matrix effects. Except on a large-group basis, it appears that the measurement of cadmium in blood and spontaneously voided urine is of relatively little value, because these measurements are not reliable indicators of the concentrations of cadmium in the organs, particularly in the renal cortex.

For the reasons stated above, one should scrutinize data carefully. It is likely that data obtained during the early years of atomic-absorption spectrophotometry are not reliable, because the background effect, particularly of sodium, was not appreciated at the time.

CONCLUSIONS AND RECOMMENDATIONS

There should be a comparison of the intakes of cadmium in various industrial and geographic regions and an attempt to correlate them with specific diseases. These kinds of correlations should also be done on autopsy samples. There is a need to analyze, particularly in soft-water areas, the accumulation of cadmium in drinking water at the tap. There is also a need for certified reference samples, such as the NBS bovine liver and orchard leaves. Interlaboratory comparisons, exchange of standards, and establishment of a reference method are also warranted. The possible effect of cadmium on vitamin D metabolism needs investigation. The available data do not suggest any need to change the present drinking-water standard of 10 μg/liter, although there is a clear need for data on soft, aggressive water areas.

Chromium

The NAS-NRC has recently (1974) completed an extensive review of the medical and biologic effects of chromium, which has been reviewed and excerpted for this report. Additional material has also been included when necessary.

OCCURRENCE

Durum and Haffty (1961) reported a range of concentrations for chromium in U.S. rivers of 0.7–84 μg/liter. Kopp and Kroner (1967) detected chromium in 24.5% of the samples examined, with concentrations ranging from 1–112 μg/liter and averaging 9.7 μg/liter. In a study of surface and groundwaters in Canada, all but two of 240 samples examined were below 50 μg/liter (Procter & Gamble, 1974). In 1974, a maximum dissolved chromium concentration of 30 μg/liter was recorded in water from the Pecos River, New Mexico; the Los Angeles River; and the Columbia River, Oregon (USGS, 1974). In a 1970 survey, 11 of 700 samples had chromium concentrations of 6–50 μg/liter, with none exceeding 50 μg/liter (Durum *et al.*, 1971). Ackermann (1971) reported chromium concentrations below 5 μg/liter for 18 of 27 river stations in Illinois; the maximum was 50 μg/liter.

CHEMICAL CHARACTERISTICS

The element chromium is amphoteric and can exist in water in several different states. It is present in minor amounts in igneous rocks and is much more abundant in basic and ultrabasic types than in the more silicic types of rocks. In attack by weathering, chromium in cationic form Cr(III) behaves somewhat like iron and is largely retained in resistates and hydrolysates. Very little chromium goes into solution. Natural water, therefore, would be expected to contain only traces of chromium as a cation, unless the pH were very low.

Chromium, under strongly oxidizing conditions, may be converted to the hexavalent state and occur as chromate anions. Natural chromates are rare and, when CrO_4^- is present in water, it is usually the result of pollution by industrial wastes. Fairly high concentrations of chromate anions are possible in water with normal pH (USGS, 1959).

A study by Schroeder and Lee (1975) indicated that the oxidation state of chromium may be altered in natural water. Because of the possibilities for oxidation of Cr(III) and reduction of Cr(VI), they concluded that water-quality standards should be based on *total* chromium, rather than on hexavalent chromium.

METABOLISM

Because of analytic problems related to the determination of chromium, data on the absorption and metabolism of chromium must be interpreted with caution. Trivalent chromium affects glucose metabolism, binds strongly with plasma albumin, and interacts with manganese in glucose metabolism (Hambridge, 1971).

In a study in which rats were administered trivalent chromium for a short time, there was no glucose metabolism effect, whereas administration for 15–120 days markedly affected glucose metabolism. Oversupply is reported to be no problem, and there appears to be a homeostatic mechanism for trivalent chromium involving a hepatic or intestinal transport system that rejects excessive accumulation.

Oral ascorbic acid converts hexavalent chromium to trivalent chromium, and, when given within an hour or two, reduces gastrointestinal tract injury from hexavalent chromium (Hambidge, 1971).

Glucose tolerance in man declines with age; as many as two-thirds of an elderly population sampled in the United States had an abnormal glucose tolerance test. Tissue chromium in the United States also declines with age (Streeten *et al.*, 1965).

The average daily intake of chromium in the United States varies widely due to diet and geography. Estimates range from 5 to 115 μg/day with an average of 60–65 μg/day (NAS, 1974) to 5–500 μg/day, with an average of 280 μg/day (Schroeder, 1970).

It has been reported that, regardless of dietary history or amount administered, only 0.5–3% of a given dose of trivalent chromium is available to the organism. The degree of absorption depends on the chemical form of the chromium and ranges from 0.1 to 1.2% of trivalent chromium salts to about 25% of the glucose tolerance factor.

Chromium is excreted in urine and feces with the urinary pathway accounting for 80%. Nearly all chromium in urine is present in the form of low-molecular-weight complexes: very little protein bound chromium is excreted. Estimates of excretion also vary between wide extremes. Mean 24-h urinary chromium excretion of 20 young adults was 8.4 μg with a range of 1.6 - 21 μg (NAS, 1974). Other estimates have shown an average urinary excretion from 3 to 160, μg/day with an average of 138 μg/day (Schroeder, 1970).

It is possible that pH plays a role in the physiologic distribution of hexavalent and trivalent chromium; the trivalent precipitates at physiologic pH and forms chromic hydroxide. Trivalent chromium may also precipitate with proteins (IARC, 1973).

According to Schroeder (1974), the background body burden of chromium in Americans is low and declines between the ages of 34 and 44. Body burdens of Africans, New Easterners, and Orientals are much higher. Thais had higher tissue chromium concentrations than any other group.

Organ distribution studies have been inconclusive. Results in rats given doses of chromium chloride showed the ovaries and spleen to have the highest uptake and, the kidneys and liver the next highest, with the lungs, heart, pancreas, and brain lower. But when chromium was given in the form of glucose tolerance factor, the results were different; the liver accumulated most, followed by the uterus, kidneys, and bone. In autopsies of humans, the highest accumulation has been in lungs; this suggests that humans are accumulating most chromium from the air, rather than from water or food (NAS, 1974).

HEALTH EFFECTS

Acute systemic poisoning from chromium may result from accidental exposures, from therapeutic uses of chromium, and from suicide attempts. Principal damage to the body is tubular necrosis of the kidney. Cats fed 50–1,000 mg/day of chromic phosphate for 80 days were not affected. Rats fed trivalent chromium at 25 ppm for 1 yr or 5 ppm for a lifetime were also not affected (NAS, 1974).

Hexavalent chromium chemicals can be tolerated by animals in low concentrations, especially when they are administered in feed or drinking water, in which the degree of absorption is a factor. For example, rats tolerated hexavalent chromium in drinking water at 25 ppm for a year, and dogs showed no effect of chromium as potassium chromate at 0.45–11.2 ppm over a 4-year period. Even higher concentrations have been reported by some investigators. However, larger doses of hexavalent chromium are highly toxic and may cause death, especially when injected intravenously, subcutaneously, or intragastrically (NAS, 1974, p. 82).

Chronic toxicity can be observed in several mammalian species with hexavalent chromium in the drinking water in concentrations of more than 5 mg/liter. At this concentration, the element was found to accumulate in rats, but it caused no changes in growth rate, food intake, or results of blood analysis. Even 25 mg/liter in the drinking water failed to produce changes in these characteristics or in the histologic appearance of the tissues after 6 months. Dogs tolerated hexavalent chromium in the water at up to 11.2 mg/liter for 4 years without ill effects. The minimal lethal dose in dogs is approximately 75 mg of chromium as sodium chromate, when injected intravenously. The salt causes acute hypertension, hypocholesterolemia, and hypoglycemia. Growing chickens showed no detrimental symptoms when they were fed 100 μg/g in diet (NAS, 1974, p. 29).

Although hexavalent chromium has long been recognized as a toxic substance, trivalent chromium is considered by most investigators to be relatively innocuous and even (in microgram amounts) essential to human health. Hexavalent chromium produces hemorrhage of the gastrointestinal tract after ingestion. Inhaled chromate may cause cancer of the respiratory tract in occupationally exposed individuals (IARC, 1973). It also produces ulceration on dermal exposure.

The chronic adverse effects most often considered in chromium toxicity are respiratory and dermatologic. It now appears that investigators agree on several points:

1. People who work with hexavalent chromium can develop cutaneous and nasal mucous-membrane ulcers, whereas exposure to trivalent chromium does not produce these effects.
2. People who work with hexavalent chromium compounds can develop contact dermatitis from these agents, and they react to patch and intracutaneous tests with nonirritant concentrations of potassium dichromate.
3. Hexavalent chromium in tissue is reduced to the trivalent form.
4. Hexavalent chromium has greater diffusibility and solubility in tissue than trivalent chromium.
5. Hexavalent chromium can readily penetrate membranes.
6. Trivalent chromium can readily bind with some proteins to form complexes (NAS, 1974, p. 72).

Atherosclerosis in relation to chromium has been of interest. Studies have indicated that atherosclerosis can be induced in animals by chromium-deficient diets (Hambridge, 1971).

With regard to carcinogenicity, intraosseous, intramuscular, subcutaneous, intrapleural, and intraperitoneal injections of chromium compounds have been reported to cause the development of sarcomas in rabbits, mice, and rats. There is some evidence that calcium chromate in the form of a pellet attached to the bronchial mucosa in rat lung may be carcinogenic, but there is no support for the view that it constitutes a carcinogenic hazard in human food (Sunderman, 1971). An IARC working group (1973) concluded "there is no evidence that non-occupational exposure to chromium constitutes a cancer hazard."

ANALYSIS

Both hexavalent and total chromium concentrations are commonly determined in water. Direct aspiration of samples into a flame is used to determine the total chromium content with a detection limit of 3 μg/liter. The U.S. Geological Survey (Brown *et al.*, 1970) has suggested a procedure for the determination of hexavalent chromium by extraction with ammonium pyrrolidine dithiocarbamate at a pH of 2.8. The same procedure is also used for the determination of total chromium after oxidation of any trivalent chromium present to the hexavalent state with potassium permanganate. Nix and Goodwin (1970) have used diethyldithiocarbamate for extraction of chromium.

Fernandez and Manning (1971), Barnard and Fishman (1973), and Surles *et al.* (1975) have used the graphite furnace to increase sample vaporization for the determination of total chromium; the detection limit is 0.1 μg/liter.

CONCLUSIONS AND RECOMMENDATIONS

The NAS chromium report offered recommendations for research. These were among the most pressing:

1. At present, only two analytic techniques can be successfully used for accurate quantitative determination of chromium at the low concentrations that exist in many environmental media, especially in plant and animal tissue-neutron activation and shielded-arc emission spectrography. Both methods are expensive and time-consuming and require considerable experience and thus are not applicable to large-scale environmental studies. Laboratory research, using the latest analytic instrumentation, is needed for the development of sensitive, accurate, and precise methods for the analysis of chromium that could be used by most laboratory investigators. . . .
2. Accurate background information on normal concentrations of chromium in various media is necessary for predicting trends.
3. The potential toxicity of chromium depends on its valence state. There are no techniques for estimating the concentration of chromium in relation to its valence state, especially in animal and plant tissue. Data of this type also would be extremely useful for understanding the biologic function and availability of chromium. . . .
4. Research is needed to ascertain the relation between exposure to airborne chromium and chromium concentrations in urine, blood, and other biologic

media, such as hair. If any relation is demonstrated, biologic standards for exposure may become possible. (NAS, 1974, pp. 112–113).

There is a strong link between airborne chromium and lung cancer, but there is no firm evidence to establish a relationship between non-occupational exposure by any other route. There is also evidence that chromium has an important role in maintaining glucose metabolism and may also be a factor in atherosclerosis. It is therefore possible that with the exception of occupational exposure a deficiency of chromium may be more of a problem.

The present interim drinking-water standard of 0.05 mg/liter is less than the no-observed-adverse-health-effect level. Consideration should be given to setting the chromium limit in terms of the hexavalent form. Extensive work is urgently needed to establish the role of dietary chromium with regard to atherosclerosis and glucose metabolism as well as its possible carcinogenic effects at low levels in lifetime feeding studies.

Cobalt

OCCURRENCE

Cobalt and its salts are used for making alloys, in nuclear technology, as pigments in the china and glass industry, and as binders in the tungsten–carbide tool industry. Cobalt may be divalent or trivalent. Solutions containing cobaltous ions (Co^{+2}) are relatively stable, but cobaltic ions (Cr^{+3}) are powerful oxidizing agents and are thus unstable in natural water. Cobaltous chloride, $CoCl_2$, is a highly soluble salt that is used in the manufacture of sympathetic ink, barometers, and hydrometers, as well as in galvanoplating, ceramics, and (as a feed supplement) salt licks for ruminant animals. Cobaltous nitrate, $Co(NO_3)_2$, is used in the manufacture of cobalt pigments and sympathetic ink and in decorating porcelain. Cobaltous sulfate, $CoSO_4$, a red crystalline substance that is readily soluble in water, is used in decorating and plating and for remedying cobalt deficiencies in cattle and sheep (McKee and Wolf, 1963).

Durum *et al.* (1971) examined more than 720 river-water samples during low flows in October 1970 in the 50 states and Puerto Rico; 37% contained traces of cobalt, in the range of 1.0–5.0 μg/liter; 54% contained cobalt below the detection limit, i.e., less than 1.0 μg/liter; 21 samples (2.9%) contained 6–9 μg/liter; 20 samples (2.8%) contained 10–19 μg/liter; 17 samples (2.4%) contained 20–39 μg/liter; and 6 samples (0.8%) contained 40–99 μg/liter.

In an earlier report, using emission spectroscopy on 59 samples of water from 15 rivers in the United States and Canada, Durum and Haffty (1961) found a maximum cobalt concentration of 5.8 μg/liter in the Mississippi River at Baton Rouge, Louisiana. Kopp and Kroner (1967) noted the presence of cobalt in only 2.8% of their samples from the 15 major river basins of the conterminous United States, with concentrations ranging from 1.0 to 48 μg/liter and a mean of 17 μg/liter.

In Russia, Barabannik *et al.* (1961) measured cobalt in two artesian supplies used for drinking water at Kiev. These wells vary from 89.6–261.5 m in depth. In the shallower wells, cobalt concentrations varied from 0.61 to 2.41 μg/liter, with an average of 1.32 μg/liter; in the deeper, the range was 0.43–1.4 μg/liter, with an average of 0.94 μg/liter.

Green leafy vegetables are the richest and most variable sources of cobalt in human diets; dairy products and refined cereals are among the poorest. Typical concentrations in food are 0.4–0.6 mg/kg (dry weight) in spinach, 0.2 in cabbage and lettuce, 0.01 in cornseed, and 0.003 in white flour. These figures indicate that the diet contributes far greater amounts of cobalt than are ever likely to be obtained from water.

CHEMICAL CHARACTERISTICS

Cobalt and nickel are very similar in chemical behavior. Both are present in igneous rocks in small amounts and are more prevalent in the basic and ultrabasic types than in silicic rocks. In the process of weathering, cobalt may be taken into soluton more readily than nickel, but it is adsorbed to a great extent by the hydrolysate or oxidate sediments. Cobalt may be taken into solution in small amounts through bacteriological activity similar to that causing solution of manganese.

METABOLISM

Cobalt is part of the vitamin B_{12} molecule and as such is an essential nutrient. Ruminants can synthesize their own vitamin B_{12} if they are given cobalt orally. A wide margin of safety (well over 100) exists between the required and toxic doses for sheep and cattle (NAS, 1973). Nonruminants, such as humans, require preformed vitamin B_{12}, in which the one cobalt atom per molecule accounts for only 4.34% of the total molecular weight of the vitamin. The requirement of humans for cobalt in the form of vitamin B_{12} is about 0.13 μg/day (USFDA, 1975).

HEALTH EFFECTS

According to Underwood (1973), cobalt has a low order of toxicity in all species studied. Daily doses of 3 mg/kg of body weight (about 1,000 times normal) can be tolerated by sheep for many weeks without harmful effects.

Using the data on 10 of the 15 river basins studied by Kopp and Kroner (1967), Berg and Burbank (1972) examined correlations between potentially carcinogenic trace metals in water supplies and cancer mortality among humans. Cobalt showed no correlation with any of the 34 different types of cancer studied.

Cobalt has been severely indicted as a toxicant when added to beer to promote the formation of foam (USFDA, 1975). Clusters of congestive heart failure deaths were observed in Quebec, Canada; Omaha, Nebraska; and Leuven, Belgium among heavy beer drinkers about 1965. Cobalt salts had been added to the beer at cobalt concentrations of 1.2–1.5 mg/liter (Underwood, 1973). At such concentrations, the consumption of 24 pints a day would supply only about 15 mg of cobalt sulfate—well below the amount that can be taken with impunity by normal people. In fact, cobalt salts have been used therapeutically at up to 300 mg/day without cardiotoxic effects. The episodes were clearly attributed to the cobalt: the toxicity was no longer observed when the cobalt was removed. Research has since shown that the addition of cobalt to ethanol results in toxicity which is greater than the additive effects of feeding the materials separately (USFDA, 1975b).

In an attempt to provide additional evidence to validate the USSR requirement for cobalt in water, Krasovskii and Fridlyand (1971) performed experiments on 380 white mice, albino rats, and guinea pigs, with various oral doses of cobaltous chloride, nitrate, sulfate, and acetate. The LD_{50} of cobaltous chloride was 80 mg/kg of body weight for albino rats and 55 mg/kg for guinea pigs. Aqueous solutions of cobalt at 2.5, 0.5, and 0.05 mg/kg of body weight were administered orally for 6 days/week for 7 months. Cobalt poisoning at 2.5 mg/kg was manifested in disturbed conditioned reflexes and alterations in hematopoiesis. The effects on other metabolic processes and overall resistance were less pronounced. The animals treated with 0.5 mg/kg exhibited only mild and transient polycythemia and a decrease in phagocytic activity of leukocytes. At 0.05 mg/kg, there were no effects on the characteristics investigated.

According to the FDA report (USFDA, 1975), acute cobalt toxicity in some animals has been demonstrated only at very high doses—e.g., in chickens at 50 mg/kg of diet per day and in sheep at 6 mg/kg of body weight per day. At doses under 5 mg/kg of diet (or under 2 mg/kg of body weight) no adverse effects were noted. At higher dosages, a loss of appetite, loss of weight, and debilitation were observed. However, intravenous injection of cobalt (at less than 1.0 mg/kg of body weight) causes death. The mechanisms of cobalt's toxic action are not well understood.

Long-term toxicity in humans was observed primarily in children when cobalt was given to correct anemia (USFDA, 1975). Between 1955 and 1961, more than four incidents involving more than 10 children were reported. Children between the ages of 3 months and 12 years became ill as a result of cobalt administration with iron in a commercial preparation. The most common observations were the development of goiter and decreased thyroid function. Increased cardiac rate, increased respiration rate, skin changes, and blood lipid changes were also noted. All symptoms were reversed when cobalt therapy was discontinued. The dosages at which these conditions were observed were between 1 and 6 mg/kg of body weight per day.

ANALYSIS

With detection limits at 10 μg/liter, cobalt in fresh water is not normally detectable by direct flame atomization; a concentration step is usually required for cobalt determination in water. The U.S. Geological Survey (Brown *et al.*, 1970) uses the APDC solvent extraction procedure, in which the cobalt–APDC complex is extracted at a pH of 2.8 with methylisobutylketone. Similar procedures with APDC have been reported (Brooks *et al.*, 1967; Traversy, 1971; Kinrade and Van Loon, 1974; Aldous *et al.*, 1975). Extractions with diethyldithiocarbamate (Nix and Goodwin, 1970) and dithizone (Sachdev and West, 1969) have also been described. Paus (1971) has used the graphite furnace to enhance atomization of the cobalt in fresh water; the detection limit is 0.4 μg/liter.

CONCLUSIONS AND RECOMMENDATIONS

Cobalt in natural and treated water has been observed only in trace concentrations—one-hundredth or less of the amounts occurring naturally in foods. It is an essential element for ruminants, in that it allows them to take vitamin B_{12} internally. Apart from its content in vitamin B_{12}, it provides no known nutritional benefit to humans. In doses in excess of 1 mg/kg of body weight it may pose a health hazard to humans, especially children and older people suffering from other ailments. Cobalt acts with alcohol to produce severe cardiac effects at concentrations as low as about 1.2–1.5 mg/liter of beer. The USSR has set a limit of 1.0 mg/liter of water (Stoefen, 1973).

The Interim Primary Drinking Water Regulations do not limit cobalt, nor has the WHO recommended a limit on its International or European Standards.

Because the maximum no-adverse-health-effect concentration is more than an order of magnitude greater than that found in any natural-water or drinking-water supply, there appears to be no reason at present to regulate the concentration of cobalt in drinking water.

Copper

OCCURRENCE

Copper is frequently found in suface water and some groundwater. Copper was detected in 74.4% of over 1,500 river- and lake-water samples in the United States at concentrations up to 280 μg/liter (Kopp and Kroner, 1970). A recent survey detected a maximum of 40 μg/liter in the North Platte River (USGS, 1974). Analysis of 13 Canadian surface and groundwaters, including wells, showed copper at 20-860 μg/liter, the maximum in Lake Ontario (Procter & Gamble, 1974). Copper in excess of 100 μg/liter was reported in eight of 27 Illinois streams, with a maximum of 260 μg/liter (Ackerman, 1971). Where higher concentrations of copper are found in raw water, pollution from industrial sources can be suspected.

The effect of treatment and the pipe material in the distribution system can sometimes produce higher concentrations of copper in finished and tap water than found in the raw-water source. For example, copper tends to increase with the chlorination of water (Shapiro *et al.*, 1962). In Sweden, on the other hand, some water systems actually show a decrease in copper at the tap, compared with raw water (Bostrom and Wester, 1967). This may be a reflection of corrosion control or of the degree to which copper has replaced galvanized iron pipe in household plumbing in the United States since 1950. The survey of the 100 largest cities in the United States showed finished-water copper at less than 0.61–250 μg/liter, with a median of 83 μg/liter. In Denver (Barnett *et al.*, 1969), the metropolitan water system—five water plants with varying raw-water sources and treatment processes—showed a relationship between raw- versus finished-water copper concentration, in micrograms per liter, as follows: 25 and 7.6, 67 and 10.6, 4.8 and 4.2, 4.4 and 8.0, and 3.0 and 3.0. The process that almost doubled its copper content consisted of chlorination only. The copper concentration at the consumer tap averaged 0–12 μg/liter. In Washington County, Maryland, 669 copper determinations at the tap were made for both public and private water systems. Efforts were made to sample running water, rather than standing water in contact with plumbing systems overnight, because the latter has been shown to have greatly increased trace-metal concentrations in systems without corrosion control. The correlation coefficients of copper concentration with pH, with hardness, and with conductivity were −0.369, −0.162, and −0.173, respectively; all were significant to $p = 0.01$ (Oliver, 1974).

The principal anodic and cathodic reactions involving copper in fresh water are known (Camp, 1974). The cold-water corrosion rate of copper tubing as a function of pH is also known; corrosion decreases with increasing pH.

Copper in brass, pipe, and domestic utensils could provide a source of copper in water. Soft, low-pH water could raise the intake of copper by as much as 1,400 μg/day, whereas hard water would reduce the intake (Schroeder *et al.*, 1966).

The copper content of soils varies considerably with the parent rock, weathering, drainage, pH, and organic content. Copper uptake by plants depends on species and is generally quite low in highly organic alkaline soils. The copper concentration in commonly consumed vegetables and leafy plants seldom exceeds 25 ppm and usually is 10–15 ppm. Grains and seeds are good sources of copper, containing about 20–40 ppm. Oysters, clams, crustacea, and the liver and kidneys of animals may contain 200–400 ppm. The human intake of copper in food is estimated to be 2–5 mg/day.

CHEMICAL CHARACTERISTICS

Copper salts, such as the sulfates and chlorides, are highly soluble in water with a low pH, but hydrolyze and possibly precipitate copper in water of normal alkalinity. In the normal pH range of natural water containing carbon dioxide, copper might be precipitated as carbonate. This copper salt is soluble at 1.5 ppm in the absence of carbon dioxide. Copper hydroxide, $Cu(OH)_2$, is soluble to the extent of copper at about 1.9 ppm at 25°C. Copper is more soluble than ferric iron and more copper should remain in solution than ferric iron during the weathering and disintegration of rocks under oxidizing conditions. Copper, however, is dissolved and transported less readily than ferrous iron (USGS, 1959).

METABOLISM

Copper is recognized as an essential element for both plants and animals. It is a component of several enzymes that perform important physiologic functions. These involve the metabolism of iron and the rate of cell synthesis in the bone marrow.

Copper deficiency has been observed in both man and other animals. It is characterized by anemia, loss of hair pigment, reduced growth, and loss of arterial elasticity. Copper deficiency is not a problem in the United States. The absorption of copper, like all essential elements, from the gastrointestinal tract is limited. Of a daily intake of 2.5 mg, 32% is absorbed. The net absorption is about 5% after fecal and urine excretion. Storage of copper is highest in the liver, kidneys, and intestines.

HEALTH EFFECTS

Copper is a gastrointestinal tract irritant and can be highly toxic. There have been reports (Chuttani *et al.*, 1965) of suicide with gram quantities of $CuSO_4$. Less severe acute episodes have been reported from the ingestion of carbonated beverages that had been in contact with copper tubing or vessels (Hopper, 1958; Semple *et al.*, 1960; Wyllie, 1957; Nicholas, 1968). The doses were 40–50 mg of copper. There is a report of an infant fatality associated with the drinking of water that contained copper at 6.75 mg/liter for 14 months. Whether the child was genetically intolerant to copper is not known (Walker-Smith and Blomfield, 1973). Copper sulfate has been recommended as an emetic at doses (as $CuSO_4$) of 500 mg for adults and 37–50 mg for children (Karlson and Noren *et al.*, 1965). If vomiting does not occur, these doses are considered to be toxic in children (Holtzman and Haslam, 1968; Decker *et al.*, 1972).

The available evidence does not support chronic toxicity in normal human beings attributed to long-term intake of low ($<$1 mg) concentrations of copper by mouth (USFDA, 1975). Unlike most animals, sheep are especially sensitive to copper, and a chronic dietary intake of 20-80 ppm is known to be fatal (Todd, 1969; Adamson *et al.*, 1969; Doherty *et al.*, 1969).

The hazard to the general population from dietary copper up to 5 mg appears to be small. A few people are adversely affected by even normal amounts of copper in the diet. This disorder of copper metabolism, Wilson's disease, is inherited as an autosomal recessive trait and leads to hepatic cirrhosis and to necrosis and sclerosis of the corpus striatum

(Scheinbert and Sternlieb, 1965). Wilson's disease, formerly fatal within a few years, now can be arrested with chelating agents. There is some concern that any substantial increase in dietary copper intake will result in the conversion of latent cases to overt disease. In addition, there may be a few people who share with sheep the deficiency of glucose-6-phosphate dehydrogenase that is believed to cause hypersensitivity to copper (Salvido *et al.*, 1963).

The only teratogenic effects that may be attributed to copper in mammals are from a deficiency during pregnancy in sheep. It appears that a deficiency or excess of copper has significant consequences for developing embryos (Ferm, 1972).

The interim copper limit of 1 mg/liter of drinking water is based on consideration of taste, rather than toxicity. Depending on individual acuity, the threshold of taste varies from 1-5 mg/liter (Cohen *et al.*, 1974). The European standards for drinking-water are also set on the basis of taste and discoloration of fixtures: 0.05 mg/liter at the pumping station and 3 mg/liter after 16 h of contact with plumbing. The international standard sets 0.05 mg/liter as the acceptable limit, with a maximum of 1.5 mg/liter. The USSR also sets 0.05 mg/liter as the acceptable limit. This standard for copper in drinking water is only one-twentieth of the current interim standard. Only 81% of the systems surveyed in the 1975 *Interstate Carrier Water Supply System Analysis* could have met the 0.05 mg/liter international standard.

ANALYSIS

Copper content of fresh water can be determined by direct flame atomization, with a detection limit of 2 μg/liter. Copper is extracted with little difficulty by a wide variety of chelate-solvent systems. The U.S. Geological Survey (Brown *et al.*, 1970) uses the APDC-methylisobutylketone extraction of copper from samples at a pH of 2.8. Several other concentration procedures for fresh water have been described (USEPA, 1971; Paus, 1971; Traversy, 1971; Ichinose, 1974; Aldous *et al.*, 1975). Dethyldithiocarbamate can also be used as a chelating agent (Nix and Goodwin, 1970).

The graphite furnace has been used to increase sample atomization by Fernandez and Manning (1971), Paus (1971), Dolinsek and Stupar (1973), Barnard and Fishman (1973), and Surles *et al.* (1975) to implement the determination of copper in fresh water, with a detection limit of 0.05 μg/liter.

CONCLUSIONS AND RECOMMENDATIONS

At the copper levels found in several extensive water surveys, the potential for toxicity is virtually nonexistent for humans. The current recommended secondary interim standard of 1 mg/liter was only exceeded by 1.6% of 2,595 tap water samples taken in the Community Water Supply Study (USEPA, 1970). This value would appear adequate to protect the health of persons from toxicity due to copper in drinking water.

Lead

OCCURRENCE

The natural lead content of lake and river water worldwide has been estimated at 1-10 μg/liter (Livingstone, 1963). Kubota *et al.* (1974) studied concentrations of zinc, cadmium, lead, copper, and cobalt in rural streams in upstate New York as a model of their distribution under natural geochemical conditions and soil weathering. For lead, average distributions were as follows: soluble lead, 0.12 μg/liter (range, 0.05-0.93 μg/liter); lead in suspended particulate matter, 484 ppm; lead in soil, 7.0 ppm. These and other data suggest that much of the lead in natural water ends up in sedimentary deposits. There is, however, a distinct regional pattern of lead distribution in the United States.

A survey of the mineral content of finished water in the 100 largest cities in the United States was made by Shapiro (1962). For lead, the following values were found: maximum, 62 μg/liter; median, 3.7 μg/liter; minimum, not detectable. In another study of raw and finished water in the United States, covering the period 1962-1967, Kopp and Kroner (1967) reported the following data: frequency of detection, 18.1%; minimum, 1 μg/liter (minimum detectable amount); maximum, 139 μg/liter; mean, 33.9 μg/liter. The corresponding values for raw water were as follows: frequency of detection, 19.32%; minimum, 2 μg/liter; maximum, 140 μg/liter; mean, 23 μg/liter. The increment in the mean value for finished water suggests that lead is picked up from the plumbing system.

Water samples collected at the tap serviced by 969 water systems throughout the United States indicated an average lead concentration of 13.1 μg/liter (McCabe, 1970). Of the 2,595 samples, 1.4% contained more than the 1962 drinking-water standard of 50 μg/liter, with a maximum of 64 μg/liter.

Important local variations occur, apparently in relation to the use of soft "aggressive" water of slightly acidic pH and the use of lead pipe in service and domestic water lines. Craun and McCabe (1975) have used data from Seattle and Boston to illustrate the effect of "corrosive" water of slightly acidic pH. Both cities use impounded surface-water. Chlorination is the only treatment. Comparison between finished-water and tap-water samples showed that in Seattle 95% of the tap-water samples had higher concentrations, with 76% exceeding the limit of 50 μg/liter. In Boston, analyses similarly indicated that lead was being "picked up" in the distribution system; 65% of the tap-water samples exceeded the 50-μg/liter limit for lead. Karalekas *et al.* (1975) have made further studies in the metropolitan Boston area by collecting multiple water samples from 383 households in Boston, Cambridge, and Somerville, Massachusetts. These cities were selected for study mainly because of the wide use of lead pipe in service lines. Lead concentrations at the tap ranged from <13 to 1,510 μg/liter, with an overall mean of 30 μg/liter. Of the samples collected, 15.4% exceeded the EPA interim drinking-water standard of 50 μg/liter. In all cases, the lead content of drinking water was higher at the tap than at the treatment plant. Highest concentrations were found in early-morning samples, with the lowest mean concentrations in running water and intermediate values in standing water and in composite samples obtained throughout the day. The mean concentration for composite samples was 93 μg/liter; for this type of sample, 26.7% exceeded the standard of 50 μg/liter. The percentage of households exceeding the standard was greater in the Boston (25.5%) and Somerville (30%) areas than in Cambridge (14.5%). This was attributed to some differences in the overall composition of the different water-supply systems.

Available data generally indicate that the addition of lead to drinking water occurs chiefly in the distribution system, including household plumbing, and that this is most likely to occur in areas with soft "aggressive" water.

Craun and McCabe (1975) have reported that the average intake of lead from drinking-water by adults may be estimated at 26 μg/day, using the following assumptions: the average lead concentration in tap water is 13 μg/liter and the daily water consumption by adults is 2 liters. In children, water intake is related to caloric requirements, water absorbed from food, and the need to maintain a dilute urine. On the basis of body weight, water requirements are 2–3 times higher in children than in adults. If one assumes a heavy use of dehydrated powdered food and beverages for infant feeding, with reconstitution entirely with tap water, then lead intake from tap water in a 6-month-old infant may be as high as half the adult intake as estimated above, or 13 μg/day. Generally, for children under 3 yr of age who receive either a mixed diet or concentrated liquid formula, the amount of tap water used may be estimated at up to 500 ml/day, which would provide a lead intake of up to 6 μg/day, if one uses the average figure of 13 μg/liter of drinking water at the tap. For young children, this is small, in comparison with food lead.

For the general adult population, the lead content of foods is the major source of exposure. Kehoe (1961) estimated from fecal lead data in studies carried out primarily in men that daily dietary lead intake is approximately 300 μg/day. More recently, Tepper and Levin (1975) concluded that in women, 100 μg/day is a closer approximation of current dietary intake. For the adult, balance studies have indicated that absorption of dietary lead is approximately 5–10%.

Koybye *et al.* (1974) used "market basket" data and other information available to the FDA and estimated for 2-yr-old children that dietary intake is approximately 100 μg/day. Limited balance data (Alexander *et al.*, 1973) indicated an average intake of 9–10 μg/kg or 100–150 μg/day for 2–3-yr-old children. More important, these balance data in children are consistent with those in young growing animals and indicate that approximately 40–50% of dietary lead is absorbed and that 20–25% is retained. Although the distribution of retained lead between bone and soft tissue cannot be determined from these balance studies, autopsy data (Barry, 1975) show a steady increase in bone lead throughout the first 15–20 yr of life. For children, ingestion of soil and exposure to household dust in old houses are important additional sources of lead intake (Ter Haar and Aronow, 1975; Sayre *et al.*, 1974).

Residents near stationary point sources also constitute special lead-exposure groups (Landrigan *et al.*, 1975).

In summary, it appears that, at an average drinking-water-lead concentration of 13 μg/liter, lead intake from drinking water constitutes about one-tenth or less of that obtained from an ordinary diet.

CHEMICAL CHARACTERISTICS

Lead occurs in rocks primarily as the sulfide (galena) and in the form of oxides. It may replace some ions, such as calcium. Lead also occurs in potassium feldspar, where it replaces potassium. Lead carbonate is common in the oxidized zone of lead ores.

Lead sulfate is reported to be soluble in water to the extent of 31 ppm at 25°C. In natural water, this concentration is not approached, however, because a pH of less than 4.5 would probably be required to prevent the formation of lead hydroxide and carbonate. In natural water containing bicarbonate and carbonate alkalinity, the concentration of lead is usually limited by the solubility of lead carbonate. It has been reported that at 13°C water free of carbon dioxide will dissolve the equivalent of lead at 1.4 ppm; the solubility is increased nearly fourfold by the presence of carbon dioxide at 2.8 ppm. The presence of other ions may increase the solubility of lead. It is likely that lead is adsorbed by minerals in sediments and soils, so that the observed concentrations rarely reach the theoretical limit (USGS, 1959).

Lead may be dissolved from water pipes most readily by water that is low in hardness, bicarbonate, and pH and high in dissolved oxygen and nitrate.

The chemical forms and physical states in which lead and other trace metals occur in raw water are not well known. Recent reports (Guy and Chakrabarti, 1975a; Ramamoorthy and Kushner, 1975) suggested that the problem is complex and may well vary from one body of water to another. It has been demonstrated that some aquatic organisms can convert inorganic mercury and arsenic to alkyl compounds. Recent preliminary data (Wong *et al.*, 1975) suggested that under rather unnatural experimental conditions it is possible to alkylate lead. Wood (1976) has summarized basic conditions for the alkylation and reductive dealkylation of heavy metals in aquatic systems. He noted that the vitamin B_{12} found in microorganisms holds a unique position in aqueous systems for the alkylation of heavy metals. Conversely, cytochromes may be important in the reduction of metal ions to elemental form. These considerations are not cause for alarm, but they do indicate the need for research in this field. Progress may well depend on improved analytic techniques, if the total metal content is to be fractionated into its various constituents.

METABOLISM

The absorption of dietary lead is 5–10% in the adult (Kehoe, 1961) and 40–50% in children 2–3-years old (Alexander *et al.*, 1973). No data are available for very young infants, but animal data indicate that the percentage absorbed is age-related and may be higher in early infancy (NAS, 1976). Absorbed lead is excreted through both the kidneys and the intestinal tract. Long-term balance studies by Kehoe (1961) in adults suggested that adults are in balance. However, these data derived from a few people must be weighed against autopsy data, which indicate that, although soft-tissue lead concentrations remain stable in adults, bone lead content may increase with age, at least to the age of 40 or 50 yr (Barry, 1975; Gross *et al.*, 1975). Bone is the storage site for at least 90%

of the total lead body burden in adults and approximately 70% in growing children.

HEALTH EFFECTS

No beneficial effects of lead have yet been found. Acute lead poisoning is extremely rare, if it occurs at all in the general population. One child was estimated to have consumed approximately 1 g of lead per day in fruit juice during the 5 weeks immediately before his death (Klein *et al.*, 1970). In one adult, estimated to have consumed approximately 2 mg of lead per day, at least a year and a half elapsed before the onset of acute symptoms of plumbism (Harris and Elsea, 1967). Lead apparently does not cause gastrointestinal symptoms within a few hours, as is the case of acute poisoning due to ingestion of cadmium, iron, or other heavy metals and metalloids (such as arsenic).

The induction of renal tumors with lead has been demonstrated in rats but not in other species. Similarly, mutagenic and teratogenic effects have been reported in experimental systems (NAS, 1972). However, none of these effects have been documented in man. The main chronic adverse effects of lead are those produced in the hematopoietic system, central and peripheral nervous system, and kidneys. Although disturbance in heme synthesis is considered to be the critical or first adverse effect of lead (Nordberg, 1976), measures of comparable sensitivity for the detection of disturbances in nervous system metabolism are not available.

Zielhuis (1975a,b) has summarized available data on dose–response relationships for lead in man. Currently, the most sensitive effect is that on heme synthesis. There is a detectable and statistically significant increase in red-cell protoporphyrin in women and children, as blood-lead concentration increases above about 25–30 μg/dl (Roels, 1975; Zielhuis, 1975a,b). In men, increase in red-cell protoporphyrin apparently does not occur until blood-lead concentration exceeds about 35–40 μg/dl of whole blood. Zielhuis (1975a,b) and Albert *et al.* (1974) reviewed clinical data and suggested that the no-effect concentration of lead in the developing human nervous system is approximately 55–60 μg/dl of whole blood as judged by clinical outcome. However, animal data have suggested that this value may be lower (Brown, 1975; Carson *et al.*, 1974). In addition, Lancranjan *et al.* (1975) reported evidence of disturbance in reproductive function in occupationally exposed men with blood-lead concentrations in excess of about 50–60 μg/dl of whole blood. These disturbances included alterations in spermatogenesis (asthenospermia, hypospermia teratospermia) through a direct toxic effect of lead on the gonads. Comparable data for women are not available.

Preliminary clinical data from soft-water areas in Boston and in Scotland are now available and suggest a relationship between lead in tap water and blood-lead concentration. The consumption of soft water from the acidic moorlands of Scotland and northern England has been associated with clinical cases of lead poisoning (Bacon *et al.*, 1967; Beattie *et al.*, 1972). In these cases, it appears that soft well water or rainwater was not only conveyed in lead pipes, but also stored in lead-lined cisterns. In these clinical cases, the lead concentration in tap water ranged between 570 and 3,136 μg/liter. Such water had apparently been consumed over a number of years; those involved were adults. This led Moore *et al.* (1975) to make a more intensive study in Glasgow, Scotland. In a study of 23 Glasgow households, significant associations were found between water-lead content, length of lead piping, and use of a lead-lined storage tank.

Studies in Edinburgh, although showing a relationship between blood lead and tap-water lead, did not fully confirm the data from Glasgow. In Edinburgh, households with copper plumbing were compared with households with lead plumbing. The early-morning sample of water was drawn to clear the lines and then discarded, and a sample drawn later in the day was used. Water-lead concentration in homes with copper plumbing was less than that in homes with lead plumbing, and blood-lead content could be correlated with water-lead content.

In the Boston area, Craun and McCabe (1975) reported preliminary data indicating that, when household water-lead content in the sample obtained during the day exceeded 100 μg/liter and the data were controlled for proximity to traffic density, a significantly increased frequency of blood-lead concentrations in excess of 35 μg/dl was found. These human studies—although they involved a small number of subjects and were not controlled for sex, age, and smoking habits—suggested that drinking-water with a lead content greater than 100 μg/liter may be sufficient to raise and sustain blood-lead concentrations at above 25 μg/dl whole blood. This is the blood level that has been shown to be the apparent threshold for the increased red-cell protoporphyrin.

In a provocative retrospective study, Beattie *et al.* (1975) investigated 77 2–5-yr-old mentally retarded children and 77 nonretarded healthy control children, matched for age, sex, and geographic location in the city of Glasgow, Scotland. They did not have blood-lead data obtained at an earlier, more vulnerable period of development. They concluded that a child exposed during gestation and early infancy to a water-lead content greater than 800 μg/liter "is at least 1.7 times (and probably a much greater factor) more likely to be mentally defective than a child whose exposure to water-lead is completely unknown."

Experimental data strongly indicate that among human populations the fetus and young child, particularly under 3 yr old, are at increased risk of adverse effects due to lead. This is based on both a higher rate of intestinal absorption and a high rate of brain growth and maturation. Animal data further suggest that absorption and other dietary components play a very prominent role in this susceptibility (NAS, 1976). In addition, people with chronic renal insufficiency and metabolic disturbance in bone homeostasis and possibly those with zinc deficiency may be at increased risk. There are, however, no data on humans to substantiate these latter hypotheses.

ANALYSIS

The analysis of lead in biologic samples is fraught with difficulties. The great variations in comparisons between and within laboratories are well known (Lauwerys *et al.*, 1975).

The detection limit with direct flame atomization is 10 μg/liter. As for most trace metals in water, solvent extraction is the method of choice for concentration. The U.S. Geological Survey (Brown *et al.*, 1970) uses APDC-methylisobutylketone extraction at a pH of 2.8, and this procedure has been used by other investigators (Brooks *et al.*, 1967; USEPA, 1971; Paus, 1971; Traversy, 1971; APHA, 1971; Everson and Parker, 1974; Kinrade and Van Loon, 1974). Diethyldithiocarbamate has also been used to extract lead (Nix and Goodwin, 1970).

Specialized aspiration procedures may be used to improve lead detection limits. The sampling boat and Delves cup have a limit of 1 μg/liter (they use 1- and 0.1-ml samples, respectively) and have been applied to water analyses by Kerber and Fernandez (1971), Paus (1971), and Mains *et al.* (1975).

The graphite furnace will increase sample atomizaton and can be used to increase detection to as little as 0.05 μg/liter and has been used for fresh water analyses by Paus (1971), Fernandez and Manning (1971), Dolinsek and Stupar (1973), Barnard and Fishman (1973), Rattonetti (1974), and Surles *et al.* (1975).

CONCLUSIONS AND RECOMMENDATIONS

If one uses the critical toxic effect approach to preventive medicine, then a water-lead content of 100 μg/liter at the household tap is probably not acceptable. "The critical toxic effect is defined as the most sensitive and specific biological change which is outside of acceptable physiological variation" (Nordberg, 1976). Preliminary data suggest that the present limit of 50 μg/liter may not, in view of other sources of environmental exposure, provide a sufficient margin of safety, particularly for fetuses and young growing children. Although further studies will be necessary to arrive at a reasonable limit, it is suggested that the limit be lowered. This recommendation is made with the assumption that analytical methodology will be sufficient to detect this value above background.

1. A further elucidation of the neurochemical disturbance caused by lead is a basic research need, which should be worked out in appropriate animal models and followed with confirmatory clinical and epidemiologic studies, where possible. Much experimental evidence points to significant interactions between lead, copper, zinc, iron, calcium, and magnesium. These interactions are high-priority items, although their significance may pertain more to nutrition and genetic susceptibility than to drinking water itself.
2. Definitive studies in soft-water areas in relation to the influence of lead contents in the distribution system and measures for its control deserve the highest priority, insofar as drinking-water quality is concerned.
3. The question of whether or not lead can be alkylated by aquatic organisms in relation to drinking-water deserves high priority.
4. There are no data on illness of human infants between birth and 1 yr of age as related to lead. Dose-response data for this group, as well as for pregnant women, are urgently needed, to provide a base for estimating overall safe levels of lead exposure for these highly susceptible population groups. Dose-response data are also needed throughout the preschool years; there are very few data that satisfy both epidemiologic and toxicologic criteria for dose–response data in this group.
5. The needed data depend heavily on the availability of precise and accurate analytical measurements. Substantial improvements in methods are needed. Electrochemical approaches appear to be the most promising in this regard, including anodic stripping voltammetry and differential pulse polarography.

Magnesium

OCCURRENCE

In view of the geologic abundance, high solubility, and numerous industrial uses of magnesium, it is not surprising that seawater contains about 1,350 mg/liter. The average for natural fresh water is about 4 mg/liter. In a survey of finished water in public supplies of the 100 largest cities in the United States, Durfor and Becker (1964) reported a median concentration of 6.25 mg/liter, a maximum of 120 mg/liter, and a minimum of nil.

The USPHS drinking-water standards of 1925 included a maximum recommended magnesium concentration of 100 mg/liter. This limit was raised to 125 mg/liter in the 1942 and 1946 standards, but it was deleted in the 1962 standards. According to Stoefen (1973), the USSR has not set a limit on magnesium; however, the World Health Organization (WHO) has established European and International desirable limits ranging from 30 to 125 mg/liter, depending on the sulfate concentration. If the sulfate exceeds 250 mg/liter, the magnesium is limited to 30 mg/liter. The WHO specifies an absolute maximum of 150 mg/liter for magnesium in drinking water.

Several categories of foods are rich in magnesium—e.g., nuts, about 1,900 mg/kg; cereals, about 800 mg/kg; seafoods, about 350 mg/kg; meat, about 260 mg/kg; legumes, about 240 mg/kg; vegetables, about 170 mg/kg; and dairy products, about 150 mg/kg. Fruits, refined sugars, and fats are low in magnesium (Schroeder *et al.*, 1969).

CHEMICAL CHARACTERISTICS

Magnesium is one of the most common elements in ores, minerals, rocks, and soil. It constitutes about 2.1% of the earth's crust and ranks eighth among the elements in order of abundance. Because it is very active chemically, it is not found in the elemental state in nature. Most of its salts are very soluble; even the carbonate will dissolve to the extent of 100–300 mg/liter at 20°C. On the basis of the solubility product of magnesium hydroxide at 18°C, magnesium ions theoretically can be present in the following amounts: 28,000 g/liter at pH 7, 28.8 mg/liter at a pH of 10, and 0.288 mg/liter at a pH of 11. This solubility phenomenon is useful in treatment processes to remove magnesium from water; but, insofar as natural waters are concerned, it is described here merely to show that at common pH values magnesium ions may be present at concentrations of many grams per liter in dissolved form (McKee and Wolf, 1967).

METABOLISM

Magnesium is an essential element in human and animal nutrition and also in plants, where it is a component of all types of chlorophyll. It is the most abundant intracellular divalent cation in both plants and animals. It is an activator of many mammalian enzymes. Magnesium deficiency in humans and animals depends on many factors. It occurs in alcoholics, persons performing hard labor in hot climates, those with some endocrine disturbances, and patients using potent diuretics. Excessive magnesium in the body (hypermagnesemia) occurs in humans primarily as a result of severe kidney disease.

The average adult American ingests between 240-480 mg/day of magnesium in food and water. Magnesium intakes of 3.6–4.2 mg/kg/day are thought to be adequate to maintain magnesium balance in normal adults (Jones *et al.*, 1967). The recommended dietary allowances for magnesium are 300 mg/day for women, 350 mg/day for men, and 150 mg/day for children (Coussons, 1969). The nutritional value of magnesium supplements beyond these levels has not been established.

According to Szostak (1961), magnesium is one of the most important electrolytes in the body. In adults, the body content averages about 25 g (or about 350 mg/kg of body weight) and can vary from 21–28 g.

The tissues contain 98% of the body content of magnesium, with the other 2% found in extracellular fluids. The concentration of magnesium in plasma averages 21.6–25.2 mg/liter, with a normal range of 16.8–30 mg/liter. The greatest amount of magnesium is found in the skeleton, which contains more than half the magnesium stored in the body. For normal people on regular diets, the average daily absorption of available magnesium from the gastrointestinal tract is about 30–40%.

Aikawa *et al.* (1958) administered magnesium-28 orally to 26 human subjects. They found that fecal excretion within 120 h accounted for 59–88% of the administered dose. Less than 10% of the radioactivity was recovered in the urine within 72 h. The low renal excretion was thought to be due to poor gastrointestinal absorption.

Normally, the kidney is the major excretory pathway for magnesium, once it is absorbed. Hence, the kidney is the organ primarily responsible for regulating the total human body content of magnesium.

According to Consolazio *et al.* (1963), when men were exposed to desert temperatures for several days, 10–15% of the total output of magnesium occurred in perspiration. Under extreme conditions, sweat can account for 25% of the daily magnesium excretion; this could lead to hypomagnesemia.

HEALTH EFFECTS

Magnesium salts at levels over 700 mg/liter (especially magnesium sulfate) have a laxative effect, particularly on new users, although the human body can adapt to the effects of magnesium with time (McKee and Wolf, 1963). The most sensitive people are affected by $MgSO_4$ at about 400 mg/liter, and the average person, at about 1,000 mg/liter (Kehoe, 1953). Magnesium salts (principally magnesium hydroxide) are used extensively as antacids and laxatives. The usual therapeutic doses are 5–15 ml of a 7–8.5% solution of magnesium hydroxide and at least 250 mg of magnesium oxide (Goodman and Gilman, 1975).

Magnesium in water is not considered a public-health hazard, because the taste becomes quite unpleasant before toxic concentrations are reached (Negus, 1938). The taste threshold for magnesium has been reported by Lockhard *et al.* (1955) as 100 mg/liter in sensitive persons and about 500 mg/liter for the average person (Kehoe, 1953).

A thorough discussion of the role of magnesium in the human body is presented by Szostak (1961) but such detail is beyond the scope of this report. It is sufficient to note here that magnesium is an essential element in human nutrition, that most diets contain adequate amounts of magnesium, that hypomagnesemia occurs frequently in ruminant animals and occasionally in humans under stress, and that hypermagnesemia occurs in humans only as a result of kidney malfunction.

ANALYSIS

According to *Standard Methods* (APHA, 1971), three methods are used for the determination of magnesium in water. A gravimetric method can be used, but only after the removal of calcium salts.

Magnesism in water can also be determined by atomic-absorption spectrophotometry, with a sensitivity of 15 μg/liter, and by photometry with a sensitivity of 100 μg/liter.

CONCLUSIONS AND RECOMMENDATIONS

Magnesium is an essential element in human, animal, and plant nutrition. Excess magnesium in the diet is seldom harmful, for it is generally excreted in the feces. High concentrations of magnesium sulfate in drinking-water may have a cathartic effect on new users, but persons usually adapt to these levels with time. Excessive magnesium in body tissues and extracellular fluids occurs only as a result of severe kidney malfunction. Magnesium deficiency in humans may occur in alcoholics, persons performing hard labor in hot climates (because magnesium is excreted in sweat), those with some endrocrine disturbances, and patients using potent diuretics. Such deficiencies can best be overcome by oral administration of magnesium compounds.

The National Interim Primary Drinking Water Regulations contain no limit for magnesium, nor did the 1962 USPHS Drinking-Water Standards. The USSR has set no limit, but the WHO has recommended a maximum of 150 mg/liter. In view of the fact that concentrations of magnesium in drinking water less than that that impart astringent taste pose no health problem and are more likely to be beneficial, no limitation for reasons of health is needed.

Manganese

The NAS-NRC (1973) has reviewed the medical and biological effects of manganese; that work has been reviewed and evaluated for this report, and some sections are quoted here. The EPA has also discussed (1975) manganese, and portions of its review are cited.

OCCURRENCE

Durum and Haffty (1961) observed a maximum manganese concentration of 181–185 μg/liter in two different surface waters. The median for all samples was 20 μg/liter. Kopp and Kroner (1967) detected manganese in 51.4% of surface-water samples; the concentration ranged from 0.3–3230 μg/liter, with a mean of 59 μg/liter. A maximum of 1,200 μg/liter was detected in two different surface waters in 1974 (USGS, 1974).

CHEMICAL CHARACTERISTICS

In chemical behavior and occurrence in natural water, manganese resembles iron. However, manganese is much less abundant in rocks. As a result, the concentration of manganese in water generally is less than that of iron.

Manganese occurs in more than one oxidation state. The oxidation states of manganese to be expected in water are Mn^{+2} and Mn^{+4}. Manganese can also occur in more highly oxidized states (such as permanganate, MnO_4^-), but is not normally encountered in those forms in natural water. Under reducing conditions, manganese goes into solution in water containing carbon dioxide as manganous ion.

Manganous ion is more stable in water in the presence of oxygen than is ferrous ion under similar conditions. The presence of organic matter in water stabilizes manganous solutions, perhaps owing to formation of complex ions by organic compounds.

"Total" and "dissolved" manganese are reported separately in most water analyses. The difference between the two is likely to be less significant for manganese than for iron, but the same problem exists in determining actual conditions in the aquifer on the basis of "dissolved" manganese values. The "total" manganese values are better for determining these conditions, even though the manganese may be partly in the form of colloidal oxide and hydroxide by the time it is determined.

Manganese concentrations greater than 1 mg/liter may result where manganese-bearing minerals are attacked by water under reducing conditions or where some types of bacteria are active.

METABOLISM

The divalent manganese ion activates many enzyme reactions involved in carbohydrate breakdown and in the metabolism of organic acids, nitrogen, and phosphorus.

Manganese metabolism is regulated by the adrenal glands. Ingested manganese is absorbed through the intestine and is concentrated in the liver. Although manganese may be distributed to the tissues, most of the excess is discharged via the bile or by other gastrointestinal routes, thereby keeping the manganese concentration in various tissues relatively stable (USEPA, 1975). A small percentage of the manganese excreted into the intestines is reabsorbed and transported in the plasma in its trivalent form. Fast and slow components of the manganese disappearance curves have been identified that have respective half times of 4 days and 39 days in humans (USEPA, 1975). Inorganic manganese excretion is almost exclusively fecal. However, the organic form is excreted in both feces and urine (USEPA, 1975).

Manganese is found in minute concentrations in the cells of all living things and has been established as essential to a wide variety of organisms, including bacteria, plants, and mammals.

Manganese is widely distributed throughout the body; concentrations are characteristic for the various organs and vary little within or among species.

> Higher concentrations of manganese are generally associated with pigmented portions of the body including retina, pigmented conjunctiva, dark hair, and dark skin. The pituitary gland, pancreas, liver, kidney, and bones normally have higher concentrations of manganese, and skeletal muscle has a very low concentration . . . . The storage capacity of the liver for manganese is limited and offers a contrast in this regard with iron and copper . . . . Human livers from healthy people of all ages contain manganese at about 6–8 ppm (dry-weight basis). In contrast with many other trace metals, manganese does not accumulate significantly in the lungs with age, averaging about 0.22 ppm in aged man (NAS, 1973, pp. 80–81).

In foods consumed by humans, the highest concentrations of manganese are found in nuts, tea, and spices (USEPA, 1975). The average daily consumption of manganese for man is from 3 to 7 mg (NAS, 1973). Of the trace metals, manganese is third in the proportion of intake from water as compared to food (Craun and McCabe, 1975).

HEALTH EFFECTS

Manganese is an essential trace nutrient for microorganisms, plants, and animals, including all species of mammals and birds that have been investigated. Manganese deficiency has been observed in many mammalian species, both under field conditions and in the laboratory. It is therefore reasonable to conclude that man also has a nutritional requirement for manganese. The incidence of human manganese deficiency has not been investigated, nor has it been determined whether such a deficiency is a health hazard to man. Moreover, minimal human nutritional requirements have not been established. It will be necessary to determine such requirements if desirable limits of exposure to dietary and environmental manganese are to be established (NAS, 1973, p. 91).

Manganese is a coenzyme in many mitochondrial reactions. Examples of non-specific manganese-activated enzymes include hydrolases, kinases, decarboxylases, and transferases. Some enzymes such as succinic dehydrogenase have an absolute requirement for manganese (NAS, 1973).

Acute manganese poisoning is extremely rare. Chronic exposure is seldom fatal but may result in permanent crippling. Diagnosis is difficult unless a history of exposure of at least three months is present. The symptoms are sleepiness, muscular twitching, leg cramps, increased tendon reflexes, a peculiar characteristic spastic gait, emotional disturbances, and a fixed mask-like expression (USEPA, 1975, p. 6–1). The toxicity of specific manganese compounds appears to depend upon the type of manganese ion present and the oxidation state of the manganese; the divalent manganese cation is reported to be 2½–3 times more toxic than the trivalent cation (USEPA, 1975, p. 6–2).

Manganese has a very low order of acute oral toxicity. When rats are given 2,000 ppm in their diets growth is unaffected, and hens can tolerate 1,000 ppm without ill effects, but 4,800 ppm is toxic to young chickens (NAS, 1973).

Chronic manganese poisoning almost always is the result of inhaling high concentrations of manganese dust. The symptoms appear after several months and are often reversible if exposure is terminated. Even with an inhalation exposure there is some evidence that a large amount of manganese enters the body through intestinal absorption (EPA, 1975). Chronic manganese poisoning is characterized by progressive deterioration of the central nervous system; the effects are not completely reversible.

There is currently no evidence that human exposure to manganese at the levels commonly observed in the ambient atmosphere results in adverse health effects. The only human health effects attributable to manganese in ambient air were found in persons living in the immediate vicinity of two major point sources in Norway and Italy. Manganese pollution is presently a local problem, but the widespread use of manganese fuel additives would make man-made emissions more ubiquitous. There is no evidence that predicted manganese concentrations resulting from the use of methylcyclopentadienyl manganese tricarbonyl would result in adverse health effects; however, respiratory irritant effects from long-term or frequent exposure to low concentrations have not been thoroughly investigated. Most effects from manganese in humans appear to result from prolonged inhalation. Manganese pollution of water does not appear to be a problem except possibly in isolated cases of waste disposal. Atmospheric concentrations of manganese observed in urban areas can be attributed primarily to man-made sources. The principal source of atmospheric emissions is metallurgical processing (USEPA, 1975, p. 2–3).

Chronic exposures to high levels of manganese increase hemoglobin values and erythrocyte counts, which indicates that manganese stimulates production of erythrocytes, as does iron-deficiency anemia. Recovery from anemia caused by improper nutrition is much prompter following the administration of ferrous sulfate and manganese chloride than of ferrous sulfate alone, which demonstrates the relationship between the effect of manganese on erythrocyte production and the intestinal absorption of manganese in anemic individuals (USEPA, 1975, p. 6–2).

The neurologic manifestations of manganese poisoning appear to be caused mainly by inhalation of dust or fumes, with ingestion as an additional factor. An acute waterborne epidemic was reported in Japan in 1941.

An encephalitis-like disease occurred in six members of a family. All had the same symptoms, including loss of appetite, constipation, and a mask-like facial expression, with running saliva. Tonicity of muscles was decreased; the leg joints were painful and rigid; the arm muscles showed rigidity and tremors; there was temporary double vision; tendon reflexes were increased; and there was some mental disturbances, memory loss, and melancholia . . . . One victim had died, two were hospitalized, and three were up and about. Blood and spinal fluid samples were sterile, with normal cellular counts. Histologic examination of the autopsy material from brain and spinal cord showed no signs of encephalitis . . . .

Symptoms pointed strongly to some form of intoxication . . . . It was learned that the family maintained a bicycle-repair shop and that many old dry cells for bicycle lamps had been buried near a well that supplied water for the family. It was presumed that the intoxication was caused by manganese, which, with zinc, is a principal constitutent of the cells. [Well-water] analysis showed unusually high concentrations of manganese and zinc in the water from this and several other wells. Manganese and zinc were found in large quantities in the viscera of the autopsied victims and in the blood and urine of survivors. Ten more patients were discovered among the neighbors of the family; all had drunk the contaminated water (NAS, 1974, pp. 109–110).

Both acute and chronic effects of manganese poisoning are similar to Parkinson's disease. There appear to be some similarities between the clinical features of the extrapyramidal disease of manganism and those of Parkinsonism. There is some indirect evidence that chronic manganism and Parkinsonism may have similar biochemical abnormalities with respect to the extrapyramidal system.

It has been shown that levels of dopamine, one of the chemicals that functions in transmission of nervous impulses, are reduced in discrete areas of the brain in Parkinson's disease. L-Dopa, the precursor of dopamine, can cross the blood-brain barrier and be converted to dopamine in the brain. L-Dopa has proved to be quite beneficial in Parkinson's disease. It has has also been successfully used as therapy in persons with chronic manganism, which has been associated with decreased brain dopamine (NAS, 1974).

ANALYSIS

The manganese detection limit by direct flame atomization is 2 μg/liter. However, solvent extraction is used for many determinations. Analytic conditions are more critical for the extraction of manganese than for most other metals, because many manganese–chelate complexes are unstable in solution. With pH control and immediate analysis after extraction, accurate determinations are possible. The U.S. Geological Survey procedure (Brown *et al.*, 1970; Aldous *et al.*, 1975) uses the extraction of the manganese–APDC complex with methylisobutylketone at a pH of 6.0 with immediate aspiration of the extract. Yanagisawa *et al.* (1969) and Jenne and Ball (1972) have studied the stability of manganese chelates. When the graphite furnace is used to increase sample atomization, the detection limit is lowered to 0.01 μg/liter. Fernandez and Manning (1971), Barnard and Fishman (1973), Surles *et al.* (1975), and Shigematsu *et al.* (1975) have described its application to freshwater analysis.

CONCLUSIONS AND RECOMMENDATIONS

Manganese is an essential trace element for man. It plays an important role in many enzyme systems. Manganese toxicity has been associated with airborne exposure, but chronic toxicity from drinking water has not been reported. With surface water averaging less than 0.05 mg/liter in several surveys, the potential for harm from this source is virtually nonexistent.

The main problem with manganese in drinking water has to do with undesirable taste and discoloration of the water. The WHO (1970) suggests that such problems may arise at concentrations of manganese greater than 0.05 mg/liter, the same limit recommended by the USPHS (1962).

The manganese report from NAS (1973) suggested several research priorities for gaining a better understanding of manganese toxicity. Some of the questions which need answers include the following:

1. Is there individual human susceptibility to excessive or deficient concentrations of manganese? If so, how can it be detected, and how can it be predicted? Are the differences due to diet, genetic makeup, concomitant stress, variations in absorpton, disease, or interactions with drugs and chemicals? Are there also group differences?
2. What are the effects on pregnant women and infants of chronic excessive exposure to manganese? Is the fetus at risk?
3. What controls the metabolism and turnover of manganese?
4. What accounts for the time course of the symptoms in manganism? Why do the psychiatric symptoms precede the neurologic?
5. With few exceptions, manganese pollution does not occur in isolation from pollution from other substances. How do these pollutants interact? Are their effects merely additive, or do some combinations create special hazards to health?
6. Are the so-called lower oxidative states more toxic than the higher ones? This has often been reported but has not been proved. Indeed dose–response relations have not been established for any manganese compound. Does the toxicity of manganese depend on its physical form?
7. Further research is needed to determine the clinical value of present tests of blood, urine, and hair as indices of recent absorption of excessive manganese. Does increased manganese content of any of these samples correlate with later features of manganese toxicity? (NAS, 1973, pp. 137–138).

Mercury

OCCURRENCE

Mercury is one of the least abundant elements in the earth's crust, being seventy-fourth in a list of ninety. Greater than trace amounts are found in at least thirty ores, but in only one, the sulfide cinnabar, does the concentration justify commercial extraction.

A major use of mercury has been as a cathode in the electrolytic preparation of chlorine and caustic soda; this accounted for 33% of total demand in the United States in 1968. Electrical apparatus (lamps, arc rectifiers, and mercury battery cells) accounted for 27%, and industrial and control instruments (switches, thermometers, and barometers) and general laboratory applications accounted for 14% of demand. Use of mercury in antifouling and mildewproofing paints (12%) and mercury formulations used to control fungal diseases of seeds, bulbs, plants, and vegetation (5%) were other major sources of demand. The remainder (9%) was for dental amalgams, catalysts, pulp and paper manufacture, pharmaceuticals, and metallurgy and mining (Wallace *et al.*, 1971). Because of associated environmental hazards, the EPA in February 1976 canceled registrations for all pesticide products containing mercury used as bactericides and fungicides in paints and coatings, on turf, for seed treatment, and for any other use not specifically permitted (USEPA, 1976).

According to data published by the U. S. Geological Survey in 1970 (USGS, 1970), mercury concentrations in broad categories of rocks ranged from 0.01 to 20 ppm. Igneous rocks generally contain less than 0.2 ppm and sedimentary rocks generally average less than 0.10 ppm, except for organic rich shales, which may have concentrations of 10 ppm or more.

Seawater contains 0.03–2.0 μg/liter, depending on the sampled area, the depth, and the analyst. In a study of Pacific waters, mercury concentrations were found to increase from surface values of near 0.10 μg/liter to 0.15–0.27 μg/liter at greater depths. In an area seriously affected by pollution (Minamata Bay, Japan), values ranged from 1.6–3.6 μg/liter. Oceanic mercury is generally present as an anionic complex ($HgCl_3^-$), which does not have as pronounced a tendency to bind to particulate substances and then settle out as do mercury compounds found in fresh water (Wallace *et al.*, 1971).

Little attention was paid to mercury in water in the United States before 1970. A 5-yr summary (1962–1967) of trace metals in rivers and lakes of the United States prepared by the U.S. Department of the Interior, Federal Water Pollution Control Administration, did not include mercury among the trace elements reported (Kopp *et al.*, 1967). The Department of the Interior carried out a nationwide reconnaissance of mercury in U.S. waters in the summer and fall of 1970 (Jenne *et al.*, 1972). Of the samples from the industrial wastewater category, 30% contained mercury at greater than 10 μg/liter; nearly 0.5% of the samples in this group contained more than 1,000 μg/liter. Only 4% of the surface-water samples contained in excess of 10 μg/liter. The higher mercury concentrations were generally found in small streams. About half the 43 samples from the Mississippi River contained less than 0.1 μg/liter. The mercury content of lakes and reservoirs was between 0.1 and 1.8 μg/liter. With few exceptions, the mercury content of groundwater samples was below detection (0.1 μg/liter). In a survey done by the EPA Division of Water Hygiene, 273 community, recreational, and federal installation water supplies were examined. Of these 261 or 95.5% showed either no detectable mercury or less than 1.0 μg/liter in the raw and finished water. Eleven of the supplies had mercury concentrations of 1.0–4.8 μg/liter and one supply exceeded 5.0 μg/liter. When this one supply was extensively reexamined the mercury concentration was found to be less than 0.8 μg/liter (Hammerstrom *et al.*, 1972).

The combined effects of treatment and distribution on trace elements, including mercury, were investigated in the municipal water systems of three cities in Sweden. The concentration range for mercury was 0.09–0.4 μg/liter in raw water, and it remained unchanged in tap water in the three systems (Andelman, 1974).

All vegetable materials naturally contain traces of mercury, the actual amount depending on the locality from which the sample was taken, the species, and other factors. The mercury concentrations in plant materials generally range from 0.10 ppm down to 0.01 ppm or even less; but higher concentrations are found and may be caused by naturally high concentrations of mercury in the soil.

Background concentrations of mercury in animals are difficult to assess, particularly for terrestrial samples, because former agricultural uses of mercury products were so widespread and uncontaminated sources so rare. Data from the literature suggest that normal values for eggs and the flesh of birds and animals are generally less than 0.02 ppm. Marine fish have mercury concentrations usually below 0.10 ppm and nearly always below 0.15 ppm, but this depends very much on species as swordfish may contain more than 1 ppm. Concentrations of 0.20 ppm or less are assumed normal for freshwater fish, but once again this depends on species and region. The higher background concentrations in fish as compared to other animals, fruits, and vegetables are due to the marked ability of fish to accumulate methylmercury (Wallace *et al.*, 1971).

Of particular significance with regard to assessing the potential health hazard of mercury is the fact that the mercury in freshwater fish flesh is predominantly in the form of methylmercury compounds, despite the fact that most mercury released into rivers, lakes, and oceans is in the form of the inorganic salt or the metallic element (Goldwater and Clarkson, 1972). Methylmercury becomes available in the fish food chain through the transformation of inorganic mercury into the organic methylmercury form by microorganisms or other biologically derived alkylating systems present in the sediments of lakes, rivers, and estuaries. These systems are capable of forming methylmercury and dimethylmercury from inorganic mercury, under both aerobic and anaerobic conditions.

Although environmental mercury had been a matter of concern and under intensive investigation for many years elsewhere, notably in Sweden and Japan, it was not until 1970 that the problem received noteworthy attention in the United States. In March 1970, a Norwegian investigator working in Canada reported high concentrations of mercury in fish from Lake St. Clair. This triggered extensive investigations of mercury in fish from both Canada and the United States (Goldwater, 1971). The USFDA established a mercury concentration of 0.5 ppm in fish tissue as a guideline for evaluating results of the fish investigations. By September 1970, 18 states had taken specific actions, ranging from general warnings to closure of fishing in designated waters. Attention was focused on mercury-containing waste discharges from chlor-alkali plants. The operators of these plants took prompt action to reduce mercury discharges. The reductions were monitored by the Department of the Interior, which found that the overall extent of mercury emission dropped 86%, from 287 lb/day in July to 40 lb/day in September (Wallace *et al.*, 1971).

CHEMICAL CHARACTERISTICS

Metallic mercury is regarded as virtually insoluble in water. Mercury forms two series of salts, traditionally considered as being univalent and divalent. However, it has been shown that the "univalent" compounds contain the group Hg_2^{+2} (or $^+Hg{=}Hg^+$), with two mercury atoms covalently bound to each other, so this series is actually divalent. Univalent (mercurous) salts are mostly insoluble, and the divalent (mercuric) series is mostly soluble, except the iodide and sulfide. Mercury has a remarkable ability among metals to form compounds with organic radicals, normally linking covalently to a carbon atom. Organic mercury compounds can be conveniently classified into two types, RHgX and R_2Hg, where R is an organic radical and X an inorganic (radical) ion. RHgX compounds in general are crystalline solids whose properties depend on the nature of X. When X is chloride, bromide, iodide, cyanide, thiocyanide, or hydroxyl, the compound is a covalent nonpolar substance more soluble in organic liquids than in water. When X is a sulfate, nitrate, phosphate, or perchlorate radical, the substance is saltlike, that is, ionic. R_2Hg compounds are nonpolar, volatile, toxic liquids or low-melting-point solids. All are thermally unstable and light sensitive (Wallace *et al.*, 1971).

METABOLISM

Investigations of the metabolism of mercury and its various compounds, particularly the comprehensive studies in Japan and Sweden, have been reported on extensively. Takeuchi (1970) has summarized Japanese investigations of the biologic reactions and pathologic changes in human beings and animals caused by organic mercury contamination.

Specific data on human excretion of methylmercuric nitrate were derived from studies with orally administered labeled compound. Three male volunteers were given an oral dose of [^{203}Hg]methylmercuric nitrate. Over 90% was absorbed; maximum blood content was reached 3–6 h after ingestion. The liver contained 55% of the total radioactivity, with 12% in the head. The biologic half-life was determined to be 70–74 days (Ekman *et al.*, 1968; Aberg *et al.*, 1969; Falk *et al.*, 1971).

Methylmercury and other short-chain alkylmercury compounds exert their main toxicologic effects on the nervous system. In man, methylmercury concentrations in blood cells and hair provide the best index of exposure of the nervous system to methylmercury compounds. If exposure to other mercury compounds is minor, compared with exposure to methylmercury, analysis of total mercury may be used instead. Blood concentrations of mercury reflect more accurately the intake from recent exposure to methylmercury; hair concentrations reflect the average intake over a long period. The mercury concentrations in successive segments of hair over the period of its formation can indicate the degrees of past absorption of mercury compounds.

The factors that determine the biotransformation of mercurials, their passage through barriers in the body, and the ultimate action on cellular mechanisms are only beginning to be understood. The amount of a particular compound present in the body is the result of a balance between intake and excretion. When the same amount is taken in each day, the body content rises progressively to a plateau at which excretion equals intake. The time to reach a steady state in the body is determined by the half-time of excretion. Taking the half-time of excretion in man as 70 days, a steady state in a person will be reached in approximately a year. Once attained, the steady state concentration of mercury is proportional to the daily intake. Studies of methylmercury in humans support this conclusion (Goldwater *et al.*, 1972).

HEALTH EFFECTS

Exposure to metallic mercury via routes other than inhalation is infrequent. Oral doses of 100–500 g have been given to man with little effect, because of poor absorption, although they occasionally resulted in diarrhea. The comparative toxicity of inorganic mercury salts is related to their absorption. Thus, insoluble mercurous salts, such as calomel (mercurous chloride), are relatively nontoxic. In man, some data are available on accidental or intentional overdosage with mercuric chloride. The immediate effects of acute poisoning are due to irritation, coagulation, and superficial corrosion of exposed tissues. Chronic effects include kidney damage, as intestinal hemorrhage, and ulceration. Investigation of laboratory technicians subject to inhalation exposure to mercuric chloride (0.2–0.3 mg/m^3) showed high urinary concentrations of protein, considered suggestive of early renal tubular dysfunction. From these considerations, it appears that metallic mercury and inorganic mercury salts themselves are not significant contributors to the current problem concerning environmental contamination. The problem appears to be related mainly to methylmercury compounds in the environment, particularly in fish, and to accidental ingestion, either of treated seed grain or of meat from animals that had been fed grain treated with alkylmercury compounds (Lu *et al.*, 1972).

Two major outbreaks of environmentally related methylmercury intoxication have occurred in recent years in Japan—in the Minamata Bay area (1953–1961) and in Niigata (1964–1965). Of the 121 cases recorded in the Minamata Bay episode, there were 46 deaths. About half the adult victims, one-third of the children, and one-eighth of the fetal victims died. In Niigata, 30 cases, including five deaths, were reported in 1965. Thereafter, 17 cases, including one death and one fetal case, were reported from 1966–1970. In both outbreaks, industrial pollution of waters, with later contamination of fish and shellfish by mercury as methylmercury, was shown to be the cause (Berglund, 1971). There was no indication in the report that drinking water was considered as a possible contributor to the outbreaks.

There have been many reports of poisoning after accidental ingestion of methylmercury compounds. In Pakistan, in 1961, several families became ill after eating wheat seed treated with phenylmercuric acetate and ethylmercuric chloride, and 5 of 34 hospitalized patients died. A similar episode occurred in Guatemala in 1965, when there were 20 deaths among 45 people who displayed typical symptoms of mercury poisoning after eating wheat seed treated with methylmercury dicyandiamide. In Iraq, 331 cases of poisoning with 36 fatalities resulted between 1956 and 1960, owing to ingestion of seed treated with ethylmercuric-*p*-tolylsulfanilide. In Ghana, in 1967, 17 of 65 persons died after ingestion of stolen maize that had been treated with Merkuran, a product containing 2% ethylmercuric chloride (Lu *et al.*, 1972). Members of a family in Alamogordo, New Mexico, were victims of mercury intoxication in 1969 from eating meat from animals that had been fed grain treated with alkylmercury compounds. This episode is particularly significant, because it demonstrated the effects of methylmercury on the fetal nervous system: There was a case of mercury poisoning during a pregnancy. The patient's mother ate mercury-contaminated pork, probably during the second trimester of her pregnancy. The full-term boy who was born had severe tremors at birth, which persisted for several days. His urinary mercury concentration during the first day of life was 2.7 μg/liter, 100 times the quoted normal adult concentration. By 6 weeks of age, the infant was noted to be hypertonic and irritable; mercury could not be detected in his urine. By 8 months of age, he had myochonic seizures and was hypotonic, irritable, grossly retarded, and probably cortically blind. He had never been breast fed; this fact provided evidence that this was a case of intrauterine poisoning. The mother was asymptomatic, despite having documented increased urinary mercury concentrations during the third trimester of her pregnancy (Scanlon, 1975).

The frequency of occurrence of various symptoms and signs in Minamata disease (methylmercury poisoning) among adults, children, and infants as recorded in the Japanese studies is presented in Table V-11.

The amount of methylmercury needed to produce Minamata disease is

TABLE V-11 Frequency of Occurrence of Various Symptoms and Signs in Minamata Disease (%)

Symptoms	Infants[a]	Children	Adults
Mental disturbance	100	100	71
Ataxia	100	100	94
Impairment of the gait	100	100	82
Disturbance in speech	100	94	88
Hearing impairment	4.5	67	85
Constriction of visual fields		100?	100
Disturbance in chewing and swallowing	100	89	94
Brisk and increased tendon reflex	82	72	34
Pathological reflex	54	50	12
Involuntary movement	73	40	27–76
Primitive reflex	73	0	0
Impairment of superficial sensation	?	?	100
Salivation	72	56	24
Forced laughing	27	29	

(From Takeuchi, 1970)

[a]Exposed *in utero*.

not known, nor is there a specific biochemical test available as a diagnostic aid in mercury poisoning (Goldwater *et al.*, 1972). Establishment of exact relationships between the dose of a mercurial taken into the body and the health effects expected presents a number of difficulties. The nature of the mercury compound has a marked effect on absorption and metabolism, and therefore on toxicity. Data that refer only to the amount of elemental mercury are not of much help. Methods of analysis have not been very sensitive, so the effects of small doses continued over long periods cannot be followed accurately.

In a report issued in 1970, the Swedish Commission on Evaluating the Toxicity of Mercury in Fish set forth its recommendation related to allowable intakes of methylmercury (Berglund, 1971). It recommended the use of the "allowable daily intake" (ADI) as a method of warning consumers so they could restrict their intake of mercury-contaminated foods. On the basis of available information, they concluded that it appeared "justifiable" to assume that clinically manifest poisoning of adults sensitive to methylmercury may occur with a concentration in whole blood down to 0.2 μg/g, which seems to be reached on exposure to about 0.3 mg of mercury (as methylmercury) per day, or about 4 μg/kg/day. It was pointed out, however, that concentrations of 0.2 μg/g or higher in the blood cells had been measured in some 20 persons and concentrations exceeding 0.4 μg/g in four persons without any clinical symptoms of methylmercury poisoning in Sweden and Finland, and even concentrations of 50 μg/g or more in the hair of at least 130 persons in Japan who were not considered to be poisoned. They cited a number of elements of uncertainty that must be considered in further evaluation of these conclusions, including the acknowledgment that the data on prenatal poisoning are particularly limited. A safety factor of 10 was applied to the lowest mercury exposure that was assumed to cause the neurologic symptoms of clinically manifest intoxication. It was concluded that the "acceptable daily intake" of methylmercury through fish would correspond to about 0.03 mg of mercury (as methylmercury), or about 0.4 μg/kg of body weight.

ANALYSIS

Mercury in fresh water is below the detection limit of 250 μg/liter by conventional flame atomization. Issaq and Zielinski (1974) observed a 50-fold mercury signal enhancement when hydrogen peroxide was added to the aqueous mercury solution. Solvent extraction with APDC or dithizone may be used, but the preferred method of analysis is the cold-vapor technique of Hatch and Ott (1968). By this procedure, mercury vapor is formed by reduction of mercuric ions in solution by stannous chloride and passed through an absorption cell situated in the light path of a spectrophotometer. Detection limits better than 0.1 μg/liter are easily obtainable for water samples. Most other published procedures also use stannous chloride as the reducing agent (USEPA, 1971; Omang, 1971; Traversy, 1971; Baltisberger and Knudson, 1974).

Mercury in organic matter can be oxidized by persulfate; the resulting solution is analyzed for mercury by flameless atomic absorption (Alberts *et al.*, 1974; Feldman, 1974).

Methylmercury can be extracted with benzene and then subjected to flameless atomic-absorption analysis (Bisogni and Lawrence, 1974).

CONCLUSIONS AND RECOMMENDATIONS

The current problems concerning mercury contamination of the environment appear to be related mainly to methylmercury compounds. As far as humans are concerned, the presence of these compounds in foods (principally fish) and the accidental ingestion of treated seed grain or the ingestion of meat from animals that had been fed grain treated with alkylmercury compounds are the major problems. Drastic limitations imposed or being imposed by official agencies on the industrial discharge of mercury-containing wastes that contribute to methylmercury contamination of fish, on the allowable mercury content in fish used for human consumption, and on the use of mercurial fungicides should minimize the mercury hazard to man from these sources. There is no indication that mercury compounds in the concentrations and forms found in the ambient atmosphere or in drinking-water supplies contribute significantly to methylmercury intoxication in humans.

European drinking-water standards (WHO, 1970) do not contain a standard for mercury. The international standards for drinking water (WHO, 1971) recommend that the tentative upper limit for mercury in drinking-water be 1 μg/liter. The USSR has a standard of 5 μg/liter (inorganic compounds only) (Stofen, 1973). The EPA-proposed drinking-water standard for mercury is 2 μg/liter (total mercury). Drinking water containing mercury at this concentration will contribute a total of 4 μg to the daily intake. According to the EPA, only a small fraction of the mercury in drinking water is in alkyl form, and the contribution of methylmercury to the daily intake will be less than 4 ng (0.004 μg)—approximately 0.01% of the ADI for methylmercury recommended by the Swedish commission. At this level, the potential hazard to humans from mercury in U.S. water supplies is inconsequential, compared with the contribution from food.

In light of this and the fact that nearly all drinking-water supplies in the United States are already in compliance with the current interim regulation, there is serious question as to whether a standard is needed or serves any useful purpose. There is however, a lack of firm data on the ratio of organic mercury to total mercury in drinking water supplies, although it is generally accepted that mercury in drinking water is principally in inorganic form. Until it is demonstrated that this belief is universally applicable to water supplies, it appears desirable to limit the concentration of mercury in drinking water as if it were methylmercury.

There is a need for specific investigations to validate or modify the prevailing opinion that mercury in drinking water is principally in the inorganic form.

Molybdenum

OCCURRENCE

Molybdenum metal and its salts are used primarily in metallurgy and for electric and electronic apparatus. Other uses are in the glass and ceramics industries, for the production of pigments, and as a constituent of fertilizers for leguminous crops (McKee and Wolf, 1963; NAS, 1973; Davis, 1974). Molybdenum salts can reach surface and groundwater as a result of the mining of molybdenum sulfide. They are also by-products of the mining and milling of uranium. The burning of fossil fuels and natural weathering processes are other sources of molybdenum in the environment. Transport can be by air and water (Chappell, 1973).

Molybdenum is present in surface water and groundwater at very low concentrations. With emission spectroscopy, Durum and Haffty (1961) measured molybdenum in 59 samples of surface water from 15 rivers in the United States and Canada. The maximum concentration observed was 6.9 μg/liter, in the Colorado River at Yuma, Arizona. Kopp and Kroner (1967) noted the presence of molybdenum in 32.7% of their surface-water samples from the 15 major river basins of the coterminous United States, with concentrations ranging from 2.0 to 1,500 μg/liter. The overall mean was 60 μg/liter, and 26 stations had means greater than 50 μg/liter. Of the 4 stations recording the highest values, 3 were in Colorado and 1 was just across the border on a stream draining from Colorado (Chappell, 1973).

Chappell (1973) reported tap-water concentrations as high as 580 μg/liter. In the finished-water supplies of the 100 largest cities in the United States, Durfor and Becker (1964) reported the maximum molybdenum concentration as 68 μg/liter, the median as 1.4 μg/liter, and the minimal as not detectable. In a survey of 380 finished waters in the United States between 1 October 1962 and 30 September 1967, Kopp (1970) reported that 29.9% had measurable concentrations of molybdenum, with a maximum of 1,024 μg/liter, a minimum of 3 μg/liter, and a mean of 85.9 μg/liter. According to Hadjimarkos (1967), the mean drinking-water concentration was 8 μg/liter. Kehoe *et al.* (1944) reported that the concentrations of molybdenum ranged from nil to 270 μg/liter in groundwater and from 0.1 to 0.5 μg/liter in seawater. Wells used for watering livestock and irrigated forage at Canon City, Colorado, had up to 25,000 μg/liter and resulted in molybdenosis (Chappell, 1973).

Barnett *et al.* (1969) studied several trace metals in raw, treated, and tap water for the Denver municipal system. This system draws its supplies from three watersheds (one being Dillon Reservoir) and treats them in four filter plants, one of which is an old, slow sand filter. Distributed water was sampled at four carefully selected locations in residences. On 15 September 1966, water from Dillon Reservoir reached 530 μg/liter of molybdenum, but it was blended with water from the South Platte River before filtration.

Unlike copper and manganese, molybdenum is not removed significantly by treatment processes and not changed by distribution. At one tap, for example, a sample collected in May 1966 (when very little water from Dillon Reservoir was being used) contained 8 μg/liter; by 16 September 1966, the concentration in water from this tap was 190 μg/liter. Distribution and plumbing have very little, if any, measurable effect on molybdenum concentration.

The USSR has established a limit of 0.5 mg/liter for Mo^{+6} in surface water (Stoefen, 1973). Konovalov *et al.* (1966) reported the concentration of suspended and dissolved molybdenum in four major drainage basins of European USSR. In 32 samples, molybdenum was detected in only 4, with a maximum concentration of 14.8 μg/liter and a minimal concentration of 0.1 μg/liter. High concentrations occurred in rivers draining molybdenum mining and milling operations.

The atmospheric transport of molybdenum may be significant, but human ingestion of airborne molybdenum is unlikely to constitute a major pathway of intake. Kaakinen and Jorden (in Chappell, 1973) studied the fate of molybdenum in a coal-fired electric power plant in Colorado. Their results showed that molybdenum from coal is definitely enriched in fly ash leaving a coal-fired power plant in stack gases (even after treatment with electrostatic precipitators and wet scrubbers), but significantly decreased in bottom ash. Enrichment in fly ash appears to be related to the volatility of molybdenum and its adsorption on fine particles. Molybdenum that escapes in particulate matter in stack gases may be expected to settle to earth and enrich the soil, plants, and water, thereby possibly contributing to molybdenosis of livestock.

It is concluded that molybdenum in drinking-water, except possibly from highly contaminated molybdenum-mining wastewater, is not likely to constitute a significant portion of the total human daily intake of molybdenum. For example, according to Hadjimarkos (1967), the average drinking water provides only 1.6% of the daily human intake of molybdenum.

CHEMICAL CHARACTERISTICS

Molybdenum occurs in nature in a IV oxidation state in the sulfide molybdenite (the commercial source) and in a VI oxidation state in molybdate salts. It is uniformly distributed among igneous rocks, with a slight concentration in basaltic rocks. It makes up approximately 2 mg/kg of the continental crust (Davis, 1974). About 60% of the molybdenum mined in the United States is taken from the world's largest deposit of molybdenum sulfide, near Climax, Colorado (Chappell, 1973).

According to Asmangulyan (1965), molybdenum sulfide is sparingly soluble in water, but is fairly readily oxidized to form more soluble molydates (salts of molybdic acid), which are stable in water in the absence of a reducing agent. Organoleptic tests showed that ammonium molybdate imparted a slightly astringent taste to water, starting at a molybdenum concentration of 10 mg/liter. A concentration of 100 mg/liter produced a marked inhibitory effect on the biochemical oxygen demand (BOD) of water, but 10 mg/liter had no effect on the total number of bacteria in water.

METABOLISM

Schroeder *et al.* (1970) estimated that the daily intake of molybdenum was 390 μg. Hadjimarkos (1967) estimated the human intake of molybdenum in food at 1,000 μg/day. On the basis of very limited data, Tipton *et al.* (1966) calculated the total dietary intake of molybdenum by adults to be approximately 100 μg/day.

The mean daily dietary intake of molybdenum is so small (about 1 mg/day) and of such minor importance that its role in human nutrition and metabolism has been studied very little (Davis, 1974). Miller *et al.* (1959) did balance studies on 24 girls, 7–9 years old, who were fed molybdenum at an average of 75 mg/day; most of this appeared in the urine. The higher the protein intake, the less molybdenum was retained.

Molybdenum concentrations are normally very low in animal tissues. Davis (1974) presented the following concentrations for adult man:

Tissue	Molybdenum Concentration, mg/kg (dry weight)
Liver	3.2
Kidney	1.6
Spleen	0.20
Lung	0.15
Brain	0.14
Muscle	0.14

The molybdenum content of food varies greatly. In general, legumes, cereal grains, leafy vegetables, liver, and kidney are good sources; fruits, root and stem vegetables, muscle meats, and dairy products are among the poorest.

Molybdenum is excreted primarily in the urine, probably as molybdate anion (Davis, 1974).

According to Asmangulyan (1965), molybdenum is fairly rapidly eliminated from animals, but it has some slight cumulative properties, especially in the bones, kidneys, and liver.

HEALTH EFFECTS

Molybdenum is recognized as an essential mineral for both man and other animals. It is an integral part of at least two mammalian enzymes, xanthine oxidase and aldehyde oxidase (USFDA, 1975).

In man, molybdenum poisoning has rarely been observed. High intakes in Armenia (USSR) have been associated with high incidences of gout. In India, a bone-crippling disease occurs in areas where sorghum contains high amounts of molybdenum; it has been postulated that molybdenum increases the toxicity of fluoride in producing this disease. Both these human-related incidents are speculative and await more definitive information to establish cause-and-effect relationships (USFDA, 1975).

Although it is known that molybdenum is an essential trace element (Browning, 1961), excessive dosages in laboratory animals and in the forage of herbivores, such as cattle, have been deleterious. Molybdenum is picked up by forage crops from the soil moisture and concentrated in the foliage. Water-soluble molybdates in herbage cause cattle to scour severely—i.e., to have diarrhea—which sometimes results in death. Soil moisture from pastures in which cattle had scoured contained molybdenum at 20-100 mg/liter, whereas noninjurious fields contained less than 5 mg/liter. The herbage content of molybdenum varied with plant species on the same soil (McKee and Wolf, 1963, citing several references).

Animals vary greatly in their sensitivity to molybdenum. Cattle appear to be the most sensitive, with severe diarrhea occurring at intakes as low as about 20-100 mg/kg of forage. Pigs tolerate 1,000 mg/kg of diet without discernible ill effects. In young chickens, dietary supplements of 200, 2,000, and 4,000 mg/kg of food induced growth suppression and anemia. In rats being fed a copper-deficient diet, molybdenum at 10 mg/kg of food produced a reduction in the rate of weight gain, but if copper at 3 mg/kg of diet was present, no effect was observed when molybdenum was added at 100 mg/kg. High sulfate or sulfate-forming components, such as methionine, exacerbated the molybdenum toxicity (USFDA, 1975).

The toxicity of molybdenum in animals is related to a number of dietary factors, including copper, sulfate, endogenous sulfate-producing substances, and other trace metals that affect copper metabolism. The mechanisms by which these components ameliorate or intensify molybdenum toxicity are largely unknown, owing to the complexity of the interrelationships of these nutrients. Signs of toxicity in most species are similar to those of copper deficiency and often include reduced growth, loss of appetite, anemia, hair loss, bone defects, and loss of hair color (USFDA, 1975).

The daily food intake of animals is appreciably lower on molybdenum-containing diets than on control diets. Rejection of the diet may be a conditioned response caused by sensory detection of the presence of molybdate ion or its interaction with unidentified constituents of the diet (Monty, 1960).

Rats fed toxic dosages of molybdate showed a reduction in liver sulfide oxidase activity. Significantly, rats were unable to discriminate between the molybdate-containing diet and the control diet for the first 5 days after molybdate was added to the diet. If diets that had been "aged" for at least 5 days were offered to rats, they were able to discriminate against the molybdate-containing diet within 2 days. It has been postulated that molybdate interacts with some dietary constituent over a period of 5 days to produce a change that permits the rats to discriminate (Anon., 1962).

According to Asmangulyan (1965), who introduced various doses of molybdenum into the diets of young rabbits, chronic poisoning by molybdenum gives rise to marked functional changes, including an increase of sulfhydryl groups in the serum and liver and a decrease in vitamin C in the liver, at dosages as low as 0.5 mg/kg of diet. The fact that a rise in the content of biologically active sulfhydryl groups has been shown to be caused by molybdenum may assist in elucidating the mechanism of the "molybdenum gout" that is found in Armenia. The inactive dose of molybdenum for rabbits was 0.025 mg/kg of diet (or approximately 0.5 mg/liter in drinking-water). As a result, Asmangulyan recommended a maximum permissible concentration of molybdenum in open bodies of water of 0.5 mg/liter. This recommendation may well have been the evidence on which the USSR limit was based.

ANALYSIS

With atomic-absorption spectrophotometry, a detection limit of 20 μg/liter is attainable by direct aspiration into the flame, necessitating concentration for ordinary determinations. Chau and Lum-Shue-Chan (1969) have studied extraction systems for molybdenum and recommended an oxine–methylisobutylketone system, with extraction at a pH of 2–2.4. When the graphite furnace is used to increase sample atomization the detection limit is lowered to 0.5 μg/liter.

CONCLUSIONS AND RECOMMENDATIONS

Soluble molybdate ions are present in trace concentrations in many surface waters, primarily as a result of industrial waste, but also as a product of natural weathering of molybdenum-bearing soils. Both suspended insoluble molybdenum sulfide and soluble molybdates are present in streams that drain areas where molybdenum ore is mined and processed, especially in Colorado and New Mexico.

Typical diets contain molybdenum at around 100–1,000 μg/day, whereas typical surface water (except that draining mining areas) contains nil to about 100 μg/liter, with mean or median of about 10 μg/liter. Hence, it is evident that water is a minor factor in the total molybdenum intake in most locations.

In humans, molybdenum poisoning has rarely been observed. Although it has been implicated in gout in Armenia and in a bone-crippling disease in India, these involvements are speculative and await more definitive information to establish cause-and-effect relationships.

Molybdenosis in livestock, however, is a significant toxicologic problem in many areas. Consumption of molybdenum-rich forage by cattle and sheep causes severe diarrhea (scouring) that sometimes results in death. It can be prevented or ameliorated by the administration of copper, but the relationship of molybdenum, copper, and sulfate-forming compounds in animal metabolism needs further study.

The USSR has established a molybdenum limit of 0.5 mg/liter in open water, but the WHO has not yet promulgated a limit (Stoefen, 1973). The *National Primary Drinking Water Regulations* USEPA, 1975) do not set any limit for molybdenum.

Nickel

The National Academy of Sciences has recently completed an extensive review of the medical and biologic effects of nickel (1975). This section includes excerpts from that publication, *Nickel* (with appropriate page numbers shown).

OCCURRENCE

Kopp and Kroner reported that nickel was found in U.S. waters with a frequency of 16% and at an overall mean concentration of 19 μg/liter. The detection limit for nickel in water with total dissolved solids of 400 μg/liter was 20 μg/liter. If the dissolved solids amounted to 200 μg/liter, the detection limit would be 10 μg/liter (p. 9).

The Missouri River and Western Gulf basins had the lowest frequency of nickel detection and among the lowest mean concentrations, at 5 and 3 μg/liter, respectively. The highest mean concentration was 130 μg/liter, in the Cuyahoga River at Cleveland, Ohio (p. 9).

It was concluded that most of the nickel in surface water and groundwater originates from man's activities. This conclusion was strengthened by data on nickel concentrations determined by spectrographic analysis of evaporated residue of selected samples taken in 1962 of public water supplies of the 100 largest cities in the United States.

On the basis of analyses of nickel concentrations of 969 water supplies in the United States during 1969–1970, . . . the average concentration of nickel in water samples taken at the consumer's tap was 4.8 μg/liter. With an estimated daily intake of 2 liters of water, an adult would consume approximately 10 μg of nickel per day in drinking water (p. 11).

Man's exposure to nickel in food derives from the natural occurrence of nickel in food ingredients and from man-made sources, such as alloys, food-processing equipment, and fungicides, which may increase the amount of nickel in food substances beyond that naturally present . . . . With the exception of some preliminary studies in plants, nothing is known about the chemical form of nickel in foods. Detailed information of this type needs to be developed for consideration of possible differences in bioavailability and biotoxicity of nickel in foods. However, the available information indicates that the concentrations of nickel in foods are low and do not pose any toxicity problem (p. 51).

The usual oral intake of nickel by American adults [has been calculated] at 300–600 μg/day. Nickel ingestion may vary widely. [It has been calculated] that a person who ingests a 2,300-cal diet containing 100 g of protein, 250 g of carbohydrates, and 100 g of fat and who consumes meat, milk, fruit, refined white bread, wheatena, butter, and corn oil would take in 3–10 μg of nickel per day. At the other extreme, a diet that has the same calorie value and the same proportions of protein, carbohydrate, and fat might contain 700–900 μg of nickel per day, if the person consumes oysters, meat, milk, eggs, oats, whole-wheat or rye bread, some vegetables, potatoes, and legumes, with little added fat. The wide range of oral intake of nickel may also result from variable ingestion of beverages—such as tea, coffee, beer, and red wine—that contain more than 100 μg of nickel per 100 g (p. 62-63).

CHEMICAL CHARACTERISTICS

With the exception of carbonates, rocks low in silica are high in nickel, and those high in silica are relatively low in nickel. Farm soils of the world contain nickel at 0.0003–0.1%. The average farm soil in the United States contains nickel at more than 0.003%. Soils with less than 0.0003% are too acidic to support normal plant growth (p. 5).

The nickel content of seawater ranges from 0.1–0.5 μg/liter. In most groundwaters, nickel has not been identified; and in instances where it has been detected, analysts theorize that it is probably in colloidal form (p. 8).

It has been determined that, in the rock-weathering process, nickel goes into the insoluble minerals of the hydrolysates. Therefore, any nickel in surface or groundwaters is likely to be in small amounts, unless its presence is due to industrial pollution (p. 8).

METABOLISM

Most of the nickel that is ingested in food remains unabsorbed within the gastrointestinal tract and is excreted in the feces . . . . Fecal excretion of nickel by healthy human subjects [has been reported to be] 100 times greater than urinary excretion . . . . There appears to be a mechanism that limits the intestinal absorption of nickel in mammals, despite the relatively large amount of nickel present in their food (p. 63).

Inhalation from the atmosphere and tobacco smoke provides a mode of entry of nickel into the body:

The reported mean nickel content of cigarettes have ranged from 2.0–6.2 μg/cigarette. Analyses . . . have shown that 10–20% of the nickel in cigarettes is released into the mainstream smoke. Of that nickel 84% is in the gaseous phase and only 16% in the particulate phase. [There is suggestive evidence] that gaseous nickel in mainstream smoke occurs in the form of nickel carbonyl (pp. 178–179).

[It has been] calculated that a cigarette smoker would inhale a maximum of 14.8 μg of nickel per day from 40 cigarettes. [The estimated] actual retention of inhaled nickel within the body is probably only 75% of the calculated intake . . . (pp. 63-64).

There is wide variation in the average concentrations of nickel in urban atmospheres. Of urban areas of the United States that were surveyed during 1964 and 1966, the cleanest with respect to atmospheric nickel were Boise, Idaho; Albuquerque, New Mexico; and Moorhead, Minnesota. No nickel was detected in those three areas . . . . In comparison, the cities with the highest atmospheric concentrations of nickel were New York City (1966 average, 0.118 $\mu g/m^3$ of air) and East Chicago, Indiana (1964 average, 0.69 $\mu g/m^3$) . . . . The daily inhalation of nickel by residents of New York City and East Chicago [was estimated], assuming that 20 m^3 of air (24.1 kg) is inhaled daily, . . . at 2.36 μg of nickel per day and . . . 13.8 μg of nickel per day [for the two cities, respectively] (p. 63).

The metabolism of nickel that enters the body by the pulmonary route is similar to that of nickel compounds that are adminstered parenterally. Inhaled nickel carbonyl is excreted primarily in the urine and to a minor degree in the feces . . . . A correlation of atmospheric concentrations of nickel in a nickel smelting plant with the concentrations of nickel in the urine of exposed workmen [has been reported] (pp. 64-65).

It has also been shown that measurements of nickel in serum and urine can serve as biologic indexes of environmental exposure to nickel.

HEALTH EFFECTS

Man is not naturally exposed to the inhalation of atmospheric nickel, with the possible exception of nickel from volcanic emanations. The available evidence indicates that the natural concentrations of nickel in waters, soils, and foods do not constitute a biologic threat. Indeed, nickel may be an essential trace element for the nutrition of man and animals (p. 191).

Recent evidence suggests that nickel partially satisfies the criteria for essentiality of trace elements as micronutrients: presence of the element in the fetus or newborn, presence of homeostatic regulation of the metabolism of the element, demonstration of a metabolic pool of the element that is specifically influenced by hormonal substances or pathologic processes, demonstration of a metalloenzyme of which the element is an integral part, and demonstration of a deficiency syndrome that can be prevented or cured by trace amounts of the element (p. 89).

Nickel is probably essential for animal nutrition, but there has not yet been unequivocal demonstration that nickel deprivation produces consistent abnormalities in experimental animals that can be prevented or cured by the administration of nickel.

Toxicity studies have demonstrated that nickel and nickel salts have relatively low toxicity in various species of animals when administered orally. However, parenteral injections of nickel salts are much more toxic. Major signs of acute nickel toxicity consist of hyperglycemia and gastrointestinal and central nervous system effects. Ingested nickel is excreted primarily in the feces, whereas parenterally administered nickel is excreted mostly in the urine. Little informaion is available on animals relative to the acute effects of inhaled nickel compounds, except for nickel carbonyl, which is extraordinarily toxic . . . . Several nickel-containing substances—including nickel dust, nickel subsulfide, nickel oxide, nickel carbonyl, and nickel biscyclopentadiene—have been demonstrated to be carcinogenic in experimental animals after inhalation or parenteral administraion. There is no evidence that nickel compounds are carcinogenic in animals after oral or cutaneous exposure. There is very little information on the teratogenicity or mutagenicity of nickel compounds in experimental animals (p. 192).

Epidemiologic studies of workmen in nickel smelters and refineries have revealed a significantly increased incidence of cancers of the lungs and nasal cavities . . . . Respiratory cancers in nickel workers have usually developed after long latent periods, such as are typical of occupational cancers . . . . There is only scanty evidence of an increased incidence of respiratory cancers among workmen who have other types of occupational exposure to nickel, such as nickel electroplating and grinding.

Nickel is a common cause of chronic dermatitis in man, as a result of industrial and other exposures [and] use of nickel-containing alloys in jewelry, coinage, clothing fasteners, . . . utensils, [and] implanted therapeutic devices and prostheses . . . (p. 193).

Berg and Burbank (1972) found nickel in drinking water to be poorly correlated with mortality from oral or intestinal cancer. There was no correlation between nickel and mortality from nasal or pulmonary cancer, even though these are the types of cancer usually associated with industrial exposure to nickel.

ANALYSIS

Conventional flame atomization has a nickel detection limit of 2 μg/liter. Extraction procedures are usually used to concentrate the nickel before analysis. The APDC–methylisobutylketone extraction at a pH of 2.8 is used by the U.S. Geological Survey (Brown *et al.*, 1970). Others have used similar procedures for freshwater analysis (USEPA, 1971; Paus, 1971; Traversy, 1971; Kinrade and Van Loon, 1974; Aldous, 1975). Jenne and Ball (1972) have studied the stability of the nickel–APDC complex. Diethyldithiocarbamate has also been used as a chelating agent (Joyner *et al.*, 1967; Nix and Goodwin, 1970). Paus (1971) and Surles *et al.* (1975) have used the graphite furnace to increase sample atomization for freshwater analysis; this procedure has a nickel detection limit of 1 μg/liter with direct sampling into the furnace.

CONCLUSIONS AND RECOMMENDATIONS

Because of the low toxicity of nickel and nickel compounds in food and drinking water, the low concentrations present in drinking water, and the small daily intake of nickel in drinking water (compared with food), there is no present need to establish nationwide limits for nickel in drinking water. The USEPA *National Interim Primary Drinking Water Standards* and the WHO European standards for drinking water do not include standards for nickel.

There is no pressing need for research with regard to nickel in drinking water. In this regard, however, research to clarify the role of nickel in nutrition appears to be desirable, particularly as to its dietary essentiality.

Silver

OCCURRENCE

The intentional addition of silver to drinking water for disinfection is one possible source of silver in public water supplies. The silver ion has bactericidal characteristics at concentrations of 15–50 μg/liter (Von Nageli, 1893). As a result the Katadyn process and others have been promoted for treatment of drinking and swimming-pool water. The bactericidal action is slow, especially in cold water, and silver is neither viricidal nor cysticidal in the concentration used (Renn *et al.*, 1955). Dosages in excess of 150 μg/liter have been used in swimming pools, but, because of cost and the opalescence caused by colloidal silver chloride, the method is not practical or recommended for public supplies.

Data from 1,577 samples of well and surface water from 130 points in the United States showed detectable concentrations (0.1 μg/liter or more) of silver in only 104 samples. The concentration ranged from 0.1–38 μg/liter, with a median of 2.6 μg/liter (Kopp, 1969). The highest concentrations were noted in the St. Lawrence and Colorado Rivers (Durum and Hafty, 1961).

The examination of finished water in public supplies of the 100 largest cities in the United States revealed trace quantities of silver as high as 7 μg/liter, with a median of 2.3 μg/liter (Durfor and Becker, 1964). Another survey of finished water found silver in 6.1% of 380 samples, with concentrations of 0.3–5 μg/liter (mean, 2.2 μg/liter) (Kopp, 1973).

Chemical Analysis of Interstate Carrier Water Supply Systems (USEPA, 1975) reported nondetectable silver (<0.1 μg/liter) in 45% of the analyses; 99.5% of all determinations were equal to or less than 50 μg/liter, the interim standard. The community water-supply survey (McCabe, 1970) found that none of the 2,595 samples from household taps exceeded the standard. The maximum concentration was 30 μg/liter.

Unless lime softening in the water-treatment process results in a high pH, very little difference in silver concentration may be expected between raw and finished water. When water containing silver is used for culinary purposes, it is reasonable to assume that vegetables belonging to the family Brassicaceae—such as cabbage, turnips, cauliflower, and onions—would combine with the residual silver in the cooking water. The silver content of 2 or 4 liters of water could thus be ingested, but rarely by one person. Soil contains only small amounts, but humus from decaying plants may contain up to 5 ppm. Some foods, such as bran and wheat flour, contain trace quantities (less than 1 ppm), but mushrooms have unusually high concentrations—up to several hundred parts per million (Ramage, 1930).

CHEMICAL CHARACTERISTICS

Trace amounts of silver are found in natural and finished water originating from natural sources and from industrial waste. Silver is a rather rare element with a low solubility of 0.1–10 mg/liter, depending on pH and chloride concentration (Hem, 1970). Water-soluble silver compounds include the acetate, chlorate, nitrate and sulfate.

METABOLISM

For reasons still unknown, individuals and individual organs absorb silver selectively. Tissues of animals and humans do not often contain silver. About 10% of tissues and samples contain silver, and the concentrations rarely exceed 0.01 mg/100 grams (Kehoe *et al.,* 1940). The cases of generalized argyria prove that silver can be absorbed from the gastrointestional tract, by inhalation of dust, and after medication with silver compounds.

Excretion of silver is almost entirely in the feces, with only a trace to be found in the urine. There is little retention of silver in general, but, when it occurs the greatest concentrations are found in the reticuloendothelial organs. After intravenous injection in animals (Gammill, 1950), the order of silver concentration is spleen, liver, bone marrow, lungs, muscle, and skin. The balance between intake and elimination is inconclusive, but evidence suggests that ingested silver is only slightly stored.

HEALTH EFFECTS

Large single doses of colloidal silver can be fatal. A dose of 500 mg was lethal in a dog in 12 h (Shouse and Whipple, 1931); death was due to pulmonary edema and was preceded by anorexia and anemia.

In addition to hyperplasia of the bone marrow, repeated injection of silver has caused anemia (Shouse and Whipple, 1931). It was suggested that long-term feeding of animals with silver salts may cause vascular hypertension, hypertrophy of the right ventricle, and thickening of the glomerular membranes (Olcutt, 1950).

The chronic effects in man usually have taken the form of an unsightly permanent blue-gray discoloration of the skin, mucous membranes, and eyes known as "argyrosis" or "argyria." Although this is considered only a cosmetic defect, with no significant physiologic effect, some observers maintain that deposition in the kidney is associated with arteriosclerotic changes, and deposition in the eye, with poor night vision (Gettler, 1927; Velhagin, 1953).

Local and generalized argyria, rarely seen today, has been caused by medical use of silver by ingestion or injection. Topically applied silver ointments have been shown not to pass the dermal barrier; this ensures safety on contact with bathing water treated with silver preparations (Norgaard, 1954). Industrial poisoning is a more likely cause of argyria, which develops slowly after 2–25 yr of exposure. Estimates from industrial exposure show that the gradual accumulation of 1–5 g of silver will lead to generalized argyria (Hill and Pillsbury, 1939). The exact quantities of silver stored are not known. A safe assumption would be that 50% of the intake is retained in the body. Thus, the interim drinking-water level of 50 μg/liter would be equivalent to a retention of 50 μg of silver per day and would result in an accumulation of 1 g in 55 yr, to give a probable borderline argyria. However, the maximum measured silver concentration in drinking water was 30 μg/liter, which would mean 91 yr to retain the quantity believed to produce argyria. The usual silver concentrations in public water supplies are even lower—about 2–3 μg/liter. Some states have more stringent standards, such as California (10 μg/liter) and Illinois (0.5 μg/liter). The *Water Quality Criteria* (1972) concluded that, "Because silver in waters is rarely detected at levels above 1 μg/liter, a limit is not recommended for public water supply sources."

There is no evidence of any beneficial effect to be derived from the ingestion of silver in trace quantities.

ANALYSIS

Silver ions in solution are unstable under many conditions, but the addition of ethylenediaminetetraacetic acid to collected natural-water samples has been found to be an adequate preservative (West *et al.*, 1967). Nitric acid is used by the USEPA (1971) for stabilization.

With direct flame atomization, the detection limit for silver is 2 μg/liter. At the silver concentrations normally found in fresh water, some form of concentration is required for conventional atomization. An APDC–methylisobutylketone extraction at a pH of 2.8 is used by the U.S. Geological Survey (Brown *et al.*, 1970); similar procedures have been reported by others (Chao *et al.*, 1969; USEPA, 1971; Traversy, 1971; Kinrade and Van Loon, 1974).

When a graphite furnace is used to increase sample atomization the silver detection limit is lowered to 0.005 μg/liter with direct sampling. Rattonetti (1974) determined silver in fresh water with flameless atomic absorption. The sampling boat and Delves cup methods offer detection limits of 0.2 and 1 μg/liter, respectively.

CONCLUSIONS AND RECOMMENDATIONS

There seem to be no pressing research needs with regard to silver in drinking water. There seems to be little possibility that the addition of oligodynamic silver will have any place in public water supplies, and natural concentrations are so low that consideration should be given to taking silver off the list of substances included in primary drinking-water standards.

Tin

OCCURRENCE

Tin is seldom measured in natural water, in treated-water supplies, or at the tap. It is not indexed or mentioned in the NAS report on water-quality criteria in 1972 (USEPA, 1973), nor was it included by Durum *et al.* (1971) in their reconnaissance of selected minor elements in U.S. surface waters. It is not listed in the *National Interim Primary Drinking Water Regulations* (USEPA, 1975), nor in the USSR, European, or international drinking-water standards (Stoefen, 1973). Indeed, there are serious reservations about its valid determination, as noted below, and it is not included in *Standard Methods* (USEPA, 1976).

According to Beeson *et al.* (1976) public water supplies in 42 U.S. cities contained tin at 1.1–2.2 μg/liter, and water from 175 natural sources in west-central Arizona contained 0.8–30 μg/liter. Seawater contains 0.2–0.3 μg/liter. With emission spectrography, Durum and Haffty (1961) analyzed 59 samples of water from 15 rivers in the United States and Canada, of which 56 values were reported as zero, i.e., below the detection limit. The other three values were 1.3, 1.4, and 2.1 μg/liter.

Although tin is present in natural water only in traces, it may occur in industrial waste when water is stored for any length of time in tin-coated metal containers. Stannic and stannous chlorides are used as mordants for reviving colors and dyeing of fabrics, weighting of silk, and tinning of vessels. Stannic chromate is used in decorating porcelain. Stannic oxide is used in glassworks, in dye houses, and for fingernail polishes. Stannic sulfide is used in some lacquers and varnishes. Tin compounds are also used in fungicides, insecticides, and anthelmintics (McKee and Wolf, 1963). Finally, it should be noted that stannous fluoride is used in many toothpastes and consequently reaches municipal sewers. From various industrial processes and from municipal sewage, tin salts are bound to reach surface water or groundwater; but, because many of the salts are insoluble in water, it is unlikely that much of the tin will remain in solution or suspension.

The major source of human intake of tin is canned foods and beverages. It is usually present in canned foods and drinks at levels less than 100 mg/kg, but much higher concentrations (greater than 1,000 mg/kg) may be present in some products after prolonged storage in closed nonlacquered cans or after some days of storage in open cans (Monier-Williams, 1949).

Schroeder *et al.* (1964) reported that natural foods, many from garden soils, contained tin ranging from zero to 8.5 mg/kg on a fresh-weight basis or up to 40 mg/kg in dry material. These values are considerably lower than those observed for canned food and beverages, but both sets are three or more orders of magnitude greater than the concentrations in water.

Very little information is available on airborne tin, but there may be danger to industrial and agricultural workers from the inhalation of atmospheric organic tin compounds, e.g., triphenyltin acetate, used in fungicides and insecticides (Klimmer, 1968). Needless to say, the use of such pesticides increases the potential for intake of tin by ingestion of the pertinent crops as food. Dust sediments from industrial regions of Europe were reported by Morik and Morlin (1959) to contain tin at 10–10,000 mg/kg of dust.

CHEMICAL CHARACTERISTICS

In nature, tin is a decidedly minor rock component; it would not be expected to be found in natural water, except in very minor traces. Stannous hydroxide, $Sn(OH)_2$ is soluble in water at 25°C at about 1.6 ppm. At a pH considerably below that normally found in natural water, a much higher concentration may be possible; at a high pH, above the normal for natural water, tin may be part of an anion complex and dissolve in greater concentrations (USGS, 1959).

METABOLISM

According to the FDA (USFDA, 1975), "tin is poorly absorbed from the alimentary tract and most ingested tin is excreted via the feces. The tin that is absorbed is found mainly in the liver and lung with small traces in other tissues." In contrast, Kent and McCance (1941) found that at least half the dietary tin was excreted in urine. With a tin intake of 14.4 mg/day for 7 days, their subject excreted 7.2 mg/day in urine and 6.6 mg/day in feces. Hence, almost all the ingested tin was excreted.

It has been reported that the average human diet contains tin at 17.14 mg/day and that people can apparently tolerate 850-1000 mg/day (McKee and Wolf, 1963). In contrast, Schroeder *et al.* (1964) stated that the daily oral intake of tin by a man in the United States is between 1 and 30 mg/day, with typical intakes near 3–4 mg/day. Even the highest value (30 mg/day) is considerably lower than the 5–7 mg/kg of body weight at which toxic symptoms may appear (WHO, 1973). Tipton *et al.* (1969) reported that the daily intake of tin in the United States ranged from 0.10–100 mg, with an average of 5.8 mg. Again, such values are below those that might cause toxicity.

Higher concentrations of tin are found in tissue from people in wealthier countries, probably as a result of greater use of canned foods (Schroeder *et al.*, 1964).

HEALTH EFFECTS

There is no conclusive evidence that tin plays an essential biologic role in human nutrition (Browning, 1961). However, in rats maintained on purified amino-acid diets in trace elements, Schwarz *et al.* (1970) found that trimethyltinhydroxide, dibutyltinmaleate, stannic sulfate, and potassium stannate enhanced growth at tin dosages of 0.5–2.0 mg/kg of diet. Although the use of animal data to determine optimal intakes for people is subject to many possible errors, one might calculate that a 70-kg person would require tin at about 7.0 mg/day. Before tin can be conclusively considered as an essential trace element, effects should be demonstrated in several generations of various animals.

Inorganic tin is relatively nontoxic. DeGroot *et al.* (1973) fed inorganic tin compounds to rats for 13 weeks and found no toxic effects at tin concentrations of 450-650 mg/kg of diet. Indeed, some inorganic tin compounds had no effect on rats at three times that concentration.

Organic tin compounds, however, have demonstrated toxicities and have been used as fungicides, bactericides, insecticides, and anthelmintics (i.e., against intestinal worms). These compounds are generally of the type R_3SnX, where R is an alkyl group (especially ethyl or propyl) and X is an anion, such as chloride. The toxicities of organotin compounds have been reviewed by Barnes and Stoner (1959) and Poller (1970).

According to the FDA (USFDA), the "symptoms of acute tin toxicity" (to humans) "are nausea, abdominal cramping, diarrhea, and vomiting." These symptoms have often followed consumption of canned fruit juices containing 1,400 ppm tin, canned salmon containing 650 ppm tin, and vodka punch containing 2,000 ppm tin. The latter had been held in a tin can. Due to low intestinal absorption of tin, the acute toxic symptoms are probably due primarily to local irritation of the gastrointestinal tract.

"One hundred deaths in France resulted from capsules known as 'Stalinon,' used for treatment of staphylococcal skin infections. The capsules contained diethyltindiiodide (15 mg/capsule) and linoleic acid and were contaminated with mono- and triethyl tin." (USFDA, 1975)

ANALYSIS

Beeson *et al.* (1976) expressed serious reservations about the analytic determination of tin, especially at low concentrations. Many foreign substances in a sample interfere with the determination of tin by atomic absorption. Dry ashing is also subject to several errors, especially for most organotin compounds. As a result, many, or all, of the data reported on tin in water, food, and air can be accepted only with some reservations.

Direct flame atomization offers a tin detection limit of 10 μg/liter; however, tin can be determined to quite low concentrations by specialized atomization devices. With sodium borohydride as a reductant, Fernandez (1973) detected tin at 0.2 μg/liter in 20-ml sample. The acidity of the solution is critical and appears to be optimal near 0.2 N in hydrochloric acid. When the graphite furnace is used to increase sample atomization a detection limit of 0.1 μg/liter is possible (Everett *et al.*, 1974).

CONCLUSIONS AND RECOMMENDATIONS

Inorganic tin is relatively nontoxic, but organotin compounds can be toxic at very high concentrations. Indeed, they are used as fungicides, insecticides, and anthelmintics.

Tin has seldom been determined in natural or municipally treated water. The few available data generally show concentrations about 1 or 2 μg/liter. In contrast, tin is present in most natural foods, and especially in canned products, up to 30 mg/day. This is three or more orders of magnitude higher than the probable amount in a liter of tap water.

The EPA has not set a maximum containment level for tin in its *National Interim Primary Drinking Water Regulations.* No maximum containment level is recommended or needed.

Perhaps the foremost research need with respect to tin is the development of a rapid accurate method of determination at the low concentrations expected in drinking water. Until such a method is available, reliable data for natural or treated water cannot be expected.

Vanadium

The NAS has recently (1974) completed an extensive review on the medical and biologic effects of vanadium, which has been used in preparing this report.

OCCURRENCE

A high vanadium concentration of 6.7 μg/liter has been reported in the Sacramento River, Sacramento, California (Durum and Haffty, 1961). Kopp and Kroner (1967) observed detectable concentrations in 3.4% of the samples analyzed; the concentration ranged from 2 to 300 μg/liter, with an average of 40 μg/liter. One kind of pollution from vanadium must be noted when considering water. Residues from the milling and mining of vanadium are often heaped on the ground or used as landfills, thus being exposed to rainfall and groundwater drainage, which could result in water pollution for many miles around.

CHEMICAL CHARACTERISTICS

Vanadium does not occur naturally in highly concentrated forms. This is true despite the fact that it is as abundant in the earth's crust as zinc and nickel and occurs in at least 50 different mineral species. It usually occurs in some oxidized form usually as a metal vanadate. Vanadium can also be found in trace amounts in fossil fuels. The solubility in water of vanadium pentoxide and sodium metavanadate are 0.07 and 21.1 g/100 ml, respectively. Vanadium can also form covalent bonds with organic molecules to yield organometallic compounds (NAS, 1974).

METABOLISM

It has been reported that absorption of vanadium through the skin occurs from an approximately saturated (20%) solution of sodium metavanadate. Even with exposure to vanadium particles, the skin absorption appears to be of minor importance (NAS, 1974).

In an experimental study in which humans were exposed to vanadium oxide dust—with tests being run, before, during, and after exposure—the greatest amount of vanadium was found in the urine 3 days after exposure; none was detectable after a week. Fecal vanadium was at a maximum of 0.003 mg/g; none was detected after 2 weeks. All reactions to the exposure were respiratory. Coughing, mucus formation, rales, and expiratory wheezes were present, but did not last (NAS, 1974).

Vanadium concentrations in human tissues have been found to be less than 1 μg/g of ash, except in the lungs, where up to 108 mg/g (ashed material) has been reported after extremely high exposure. Vanadium pentoxide is readily absorbed from the lungs into the bloodstream (USEPA, 1975).

It would have to be concluded that absorption in the human body is extremely low; and it must be kept in mind that vanadium has not been proved to be essential to humans (Shakman, 1974).

Evidence seems to indicate that the excretion pathway of vanadium is through the kidney, regardless of the form administered. Rats, rabbits, and man all excrete sodium metavanadate via the urinary pathway. Man also excretes ammonium vanadyl tartrate in the urine (USEPA, 1975).

HEALTH ASPECTS

A relatively large amount of vanadium (some 30,000 metric tons/yr) enters the environment from man's activities, but no widespread detrimental effects have been identified. Presumably, man and other animals do not store or accumulate vanadium in hazardous amounts.

The degree of vanadium toxicity depends largely on the dispersion and solubility of vanadium aerosols in biologic media. Toxicity also depends on the valence; i.e., it increases with increasing valence, with pentavalent vanadium being most toxic. In addition, vanadium is toxic both as a cation and as an anion.

The oral LD_{50} of vanadium trioxide for albino mice is 130 mg/kg, while the LD_{50} for vanadium pentoxide and vanadium trichloride is 23 mg/kg (Roshchin *et al.*, 1965).

The major signs and symptoms of acute vanadium toxicity in man are primarily respiratory. Aside from its acute inflammatory effect on the lungs, it appears to act mainly on various enzyme systems.

Chronic respiratory exposure to vanadium may decrease cholesterol synthesis, uncouple oxidative phosphorylation in liver mitochondria, and decrease urinary excretion of 5-hydroxyindoleacetic acid, with transient bilirubinemia and albuminuria.

Another symptom is the appearance of scattered allergylike eczematous skin lesions. These are found, for the most part, on exposed skin. This allergic syndrome has been seen in workers and experimental animals. A persistent complication is a slight to moderate change in the mucous membranes of the upper respiratory tract, particularly the pharnyx; but no chronic bronchitis or changes in the lung have been reported. Permanent damage to the target organs, including the lungs, has never been conclusively established.

There is no evidence of chronic oral toxicity (NAS, 1974).

ANALYSIS

With a vanadium detection limit of 40 μg/liter, conventional flame atomization lacks sensitivity for direct determination in most samples. Crump-Wiesner and Purdy (1969) have studied various extraction systems and found that both vanadium (IV) and vanadium (V) are extracted from an aqueous solution at a pH of 3.8 with a cupferron–methylisobutylketone system. With direct sampling, the graphite furnace can be used to increase sample atomization with a detection limit of 5 μg/liter.

CONCLUSIONS AND RECOMMENDATIONS

A limit of 0.1 mg/liter has been suggested in the USSR as a maximum permissible limit for water basins (USEPA, 1975).

The lack of data on acute or chronic oral toxicity is not surprising because of the extremely low absorption of vanadium from the gastrointestinal tract. Inhaled vanadium can produce adverse health effects, but the available evidence does not indicate that vanadium in drinking water is a problem.

Zinc

Zinc is considered an essential trace element in human and animal nutrition. This topic has been recently reviewed in *Clinical Chemistry* (1975) in a special issue on trace elements, by Sandstead (1974), by Underwood (1971), and in *Toxicants Occurring Naturally in Foods* (NAS, 1972). The recommended daily dietary allowances for zinc recently recommended by the NAS (1974) are as follows: adults, 15 mg/day; growing children over a year old, 10 mg/day; and additional supplements during pregnancy and lactation. As far as human health in the general population is concerned, the major concern is not with toxicity, but rather with marginal or deficient zinc intake. The available data indicate that the contribution of drinking water to the daily nutritional requirement for zinc is negligible under most circumstances.

OCCURRENCE

In general, in streams and rivers, zinc is concentrated in sediments, but concentrations are quite low in running filtered water. It is reported that approximately 22,000 tons of zinc are used in fertilizers each year in the United States. The extent to which this may run off into rivers and streams is not known. Likewise, no significant body of data relative to the runoff into streams from dumps and metallurgic wastes has been found. Craun and McCabe's (1975) recent summary indicates that concentrations of zinc in finished water at the treatment plant are well below the 1962 drinking-water standard of 5 mg/liter. However, in areas of soft acidic water—in Seattle, Washington, and Boston, Massachusetts—pickup in the distribution system was noted in comparing water samples from the treatment plant with samples at the tap. In the Boston study, 35% of 108 samples showed pickup, but both mean and maximum concentrations in running water were well within the current limit (mean, 223 μg/liter; maximum, 1,625 μg/liter). In the more acidic water in Seattle, pickup of zinc was noted in 95% of samples, and 10% were in excess of the standard of 5 mg/liter. The maximum concentration found in the study was 5.46 mg/liter.

In rocks, zinc is most commonly present in the form of the sulfide sphalerite, which is the most important zinc ore. Zinc may replace iron or magnesium in certain minerals. It may be present in carbonate sediments. In the weathering process, soluble compounds of zinc are formed and the presence of at least traces of zinc in water probably is common. Concentrations of 40 ppm impart a strong astringent taste to water.

Food is the major source of zinc. This topic has been reviewed elsewhere (Sandstead, 1974; Underwood, 1971). Regarding industrial exposures, the acute metal fume fever generally attributed to zinc is a brief self-limited disease and is well known. In other types of industrial smelting operations, zinc, lead, and cadmium frequently occur together; the latter two are much more toxic than zinc. Where accidental discharge in water has been identified, it has been related to smelting and refining operations and has involved combined exposures to zinc, cadmium, and lead (Friberg *et al.*, 1974). Airborne zinc is generally not considered significant, as far as the general population is concerned.

CHEMICAL CHARACTERISTICS

Zinc chloride and sulfate are very soluble in water, but hydrolyze in solution and reduce the pH. If the pH is maintained by the presence of an excess of bicarbonates and other anions normally present in natural water, the solubility of zinc is likely to be controlled by the solubility of its carbonate and hydroxide. Zinc carbonate is soluble in pure water at 25°C to the extent of zinc at 107 mg/liter. The hydroxide is soluble only to the extent of zinc at 0.2 mg/liter. The pH at which zinc might precipitate as hydroxide is probably not reached in the presence of excess carbon dioxide in solution. At a very high pH, zinc may form anion complexes, but such conditions are not likely in natural water (USGS, 1959)

METABOLISM

An earlier NAS committee (Sandstead, 1974) identified zinc balance data in humans as an area needing much more research. In general, animal studies indicate that, although zinc is distributed throughout the body, including bone, there is a small labile pool with a rather rapid turnover. The urinary excretion of zinc is generally less than 1 mg/day.

HEALTH EFFECTS

Diets grossly deficient in zinc have been found in Iran and Egypt. These have been associated with growth failure, loss of taste, and, in the postpubertal male, hypogonadism and decreased fertility. It is likely that factors in addition to zinc may also be involved. With the exceptions of diminution of taste discrimination and appetite, such conditions have not been identified in the United States, although there is a suspicion that some segments of the population are marginally zinc-deficient. Of interest is the recent finding that patients with sickle-cell disease may be zinc-deficient, owing at least in part to an increased loss of zinc in the urine.

Acute adverse effects of zinc include acute metal fume fever by the inhalation of fumes. There appears, on the basis of animal studies, to be a rather wide margin of safety between tap-water zinc content and oral doses that will produce toxicity (NAS, 1973). There have been reports of human cases of zinc poisoning associated with the prolonged consumption of water from galvanized pipes. In two adults, irritability, muscular stiffness and pain, loss of appetite, and nausea were reported when the water contained zinc in a concentration of 40 mg/liter, which is well above the current secondary drinking-water standard of 5 mg/liter.

There is no evidence that zinc in excess is carcinogenic, mutagenic, or teratogenic.

Zinc interacts with other trace metals (Sandstead, 1974, 1976). It clearly has a protective action against cadmium and lead. Animal data suggest that the zinc:copper ratio in the diet may be important. As noted above, there may be an interaction between zinc and iron. If these experimental observations are, in fact, important for human health, then it is possible that the ratio of zinc to these other metals in drinking water may be of some importance. This problem has not been explored.

ANALYSIS

Most freshwater analyses may be made by using atomic-absorption spectrophotometry with direct aspiration, with a zinc detection limit of 1 μg/liter. The EPA (1971) and the U.S. Geological Survey (Brown *et al.*, 1970) procedures are typical. For low concentrations in fresh water, solvent extraction may be used. Mulford (1966), Paus (1971), Kinrade and Van Loon (1974), and Aldous *et al.* (1975) have found that the APDC–methylisobutylketone system extracts zinc at a pH of 2.6. Diethyldithiocarbamate (Joyner *et al.*, 1967; Nix and Goodwin, 1970), dithizone (Sachdev and West, 1969), and dibenzyldithiocarbamate (Ichinose, 1974) are among other chelating agents used for concentrating zinc. The Delves cup and sampling boat (Paus, 1971) have been used for zinc analysis, with detection limits of 50 and 30 μg/liter, respectively. Fernandez and Manning (1971) and Surles *et al.* (1975) have demonstrated the use of the graphite furnace to increase sample atomization for fresh-water analysis, with a zinc detection limit of 0.001 μg/liter. Background correction appears to be essential in atomic-absorption spectrophotometry. In recent years, since the introduction of background correction, normal plasma zinc concentrations have consistently decreased.

CONCLUSIONS AND RECOMMENDATIONS

Research needs have been proposed previously by an NAS committee (Sandstead, 1974). These are related primarily to the zinc content of foods, the need to determine whether a significant proportion of American diets are either deficient or marginal in zinc, and whether specific segments of the population are genetically susceptible to zinc deficiency. The recommendations include:

1. Assessment of the availability of zinc in food to man.
2. Determination of human zinc requirements in relation to age and physiologic state.
3. Evaluation of the possible implications of the zinc:cadmium ratio for health.
4. Determination of the zinc status of various well-defined populations and relation of these findings to other measures of nutritional status.
5. Assessment of the effect of zinc supplementation and enrichment on the health status of well-defined populations.

In addition, animal data suggest that zinc is also protective against lead toxicity. This possibly significant interaction needs further investigation. As far as drinking water is concerned, the present drinking-water standard, assuming an adult water consumption of 2 liters/day, would permit the intake from drinking water of up to 10 mg/day, which is less than the estimated adult dietary requirement for zinc. The available data on drinking water, however, suggest that the amounts in drinking water are far lower than this. Another area requiring further investigation is related to the zinc content in the presence of soft water and the use of galvanized pipes. The present recommended primary interim drinking-water standard of 5 mg/liter appears adequate for acceptable taste and appearance of drinking water.

Summary—Trace Metals

The Interim Primary Drinking Water Regulations list maximum allowable concentrations for six metallic elements—barium, cadmium, chromium, lead, mercury, and silver. Ten additional metals were reviewed in this study—beryllium, cobalt, copper, magnesium, manganese, molybdenum, nickel, tin, vanadium, and zinc. Sodium, which is also a metallic constituent, is considered in a separate section because the problems it poses are quite distinct from those associated with the other metallic substances.

Eight of these selected metals are known to be essential to human nutrition: chromium, cobalt, copper, magnesium, manganese, molybdenum, tin, and zinc. Nickel and vanadium probably are essential also, and it is possible that barium can be beneficial under certain conditions. The toxic metals, lead, mercury, and cadmium are believed not to be essential to humans. Beryllium and silver also are not known to be essential.

Elements that are beneficial in small quantities very often exhibit toxic properties when ingested in excessive amounts or concentrations. In assessment of the adverse health effects of such materials it is important not to overlook the deficiency problems that might be enountered if the substances were to be completely eliminated from water supplies.

Trace metals, usually in the form of ions, occur in water both as a result of natural processes and as a consequence of man's activities. Groundwaters, because of long contact with rocks and mineralized soils, usually contain greater concentrations of trace metals than surface waters. There is considerable temporal and spatial variation in concentrations of trace metals in surface waters. Generally, the trace metal concentrations of rivers tend to increase from source to mouth and to vary inversely with discharge, which dilutes the natural and industrial contaminations.

Of the 16 metals studied the relative contribution of man's activities to the concentrations found in water supplies can be rated roughly as follows: very great—cadmium, chromium, copper, mercury, lead, and zinc; high—silver, barium, molybdenum, tin; moderate—beryllium, cobalt, manganese, nickel, and vanadium; low—magnesium.

Other important sources of trace metals in drinking water are water treatment processes and pickup of metallic ions during storage and distribution. Although a large fraction of the United States continues to receive water from ground sources or from impounded upland sources without treatment other than disinfection, most large surface supplies are subjected to treatment that includes coagulation, sedimentation, filtration, and disinfection. Should trace metals occur in the raw-water supply, these normal water-treatment processes have either no effect or an uncertain one on removing the usual low level concentrations of these metals. Moreover, probable trace metal impurities in the technical-grade chemicals used may introduce additional concentrations into the treated water.

Control of the corrosive properties of the finished water is important to prevent increase in trace metal concentrations during storage and distribution. A wide variety of materials, including several metals, alloys, cements, plastics, and organic compounds, are used in the pumps, pipes, fittings, and reservoirs of distribution systems and home plumbing. Reactions, particularly of soft, low-pH waters, with materials of the distribution system very often have produced concentrations of iron, copper, zinc, lead, and cadmium at the tap much greater than those in the raw or treated waters at the plant.

The positive correlations between "hard" water supplies and reduced cardiovascular disease is discussed in detail elsewhere in this report.

Adverse health effects associated with trace metals depend upon the total intake from all sources—water, air, and food. As a general rule concentrations of trace metals in foodstuffs greatly exceed those found in drinking waters. Because the diet of most of the U.S. population is increasingly varied and comes from diverse geographical sources as a result of modern food distribution practices that counterbalance local excesses or deficiencies, the dietary intake of trace metals exhibits relatively small variation throughout the United States. This factor is helpful in evaluation of maximum no-adverse-health-effect concentrations for drinking water.

Airborne exposure to trace metals is largely occupational through the inhalation of industrial dusts or fumes, except for lead, to which there is more general exposure from motor exhaust fumes. Most evidence for acute and chronic health effects is derived from data on occupational exposures; caution must be observed in extrapolation of these data to the general public.

All of the trace metals studied are known to exhibit toxic effects at some level of intake. Many of these, however, are at levels greater than the maximum concentrations found in drinking water. To include such materials in primary drinking-water standards with a requirement for mandatory surveillance does not confer any health benefit. Adverse health effects from trace metals that are not found in excessive concentration in delivered water supplies can be avoided most readily by preventing the discharge of such contaminants into water in quantities that might increase concentrations to the maximum no-observed-adverse-health-effect level.

The following sections summarize the findings on individual trace metals.

Barium

It is rare to find barium in drinking water at a concentration in excess of 1 mg/liter because of the low solubility of barium sulfate. Natural and treated waters usually contain sufficient sulfate so that more than 1 to 1.5 mg/liter of barium cannot be maintained in solution.

Acid-soluble barium salts are very toxic, whereas insoluble compounds are benign. There has been no determination of the chronic effects of low levels of barium ingested over a long period of time. The chronic phase of poisoning is an occupational disability following prolonged exposure to barium dust.

It is recommended that animal studies involving long-term low-level ingestion of barium salts in water be carried out to determine possible health effects.

The Interim Primary Standard of 1 mg/liter for barium has been based on extrapolation from effects of industrial exposure to dusts of soluble barium salts. Insufficient data are available to estimate maximum no-adverse-health-effect levels on the basis of water intake. The limit of 4 mg/liter of the USSR is based on organoleptic factors. International and European standards of the World Health Organization do not list barium.

Beryllium

Beryllium is not likely to be found in natural waters in greater than trace amounts because of the relative insolubility of beryllium oxides and hydroxides in the usual pH range of drinking waters. The sulfate and chloride are very soluble, but they hydrolyze quickly to the insoluble hydroxide.

Beryllium produces acute or chronic toxicity in animals when ingested continuously as beryllium sulfate in food or water only at levels in excess of 10–20 mg/kg of body weight per day or at concentrations greater than 5 mg/liter. Soluble beryllium has been shown to be transported in the bloodstream to bone where it has been found to induce bone cancer in animals, but the data are insufficient to allow estimation of risk.

Prolonged inhalation of dusts containing beryllium is known to produce findings similar to pulmonary sarcoidosis. However, increased incidence of lung cancer among workers exposed to beryllium-containing dusts has not been found.

No maximal allowable concentration for beryllium has been listed in the Interim Primary Drinking Water Regulations, nor has the WHO recommended a maximum limit. The USSR, however, has set a limit of 0.2 μg/liter. Until now the maximum concentration of beryllium found in U.S. surface waters has been 1.2 μg/liter and in finished U.S. drinking waters has been 0.17 μg/liter. Only 1.7% of drinking-water supplies examined have been found to contain any detectable beryllium.

Additional studies of the frequency of occurrence and concentration levels of beryllium in natural waters are needed to determine the extent to which it presents a hazard to health.

Cadmium

Cadmium is not known to be an essential or beneficial element. It has been found in 2–3% of U.S. surface waters, generally in concentrations not exceeding a few milligrams per liter due to the low solubilities of cadmium carbonate and hydroxide at pH greater than 6. Only 0.2% of the supplies in the Community Water Supply Survey showed cadmium in excess of 0.01 mg/liter. In addition to its geological sources, cadmium enters water from the discharge of plating wastes and by the action of corrosive waters on distribution piping and home plumbing.

Food is the primary source of cadmium intake. Total daily intake from air, water, food, and tobacco ranges from 40 μg/day for the rural nonsmoker on a low cadimum diet to 190 μg/day for the urban smoker on a high cadmium diet. Drinking water conributes only a small fraction (<5%) to this total intake.

Chronic ingestion of cadmium at levels greater than 600 μg/day in combination with several other necessary predisposing factors was found to be responsible for the onset of Itai–Itai disease in Japan. Dietary intake of amounts in excess of a milligram per day is needed for appearance of acute toxicity. Major toxic effects are on the kidney; data indicate that the toxicity of cadmium is related to the zinc:cadmium ratio within the organs. Both zinc and calcium may be protective against cadmium toxicity. Persons deficient in these elements, and especially lactose-intolerant persons who are likely to be calcium-deficient, may constitute a high risk group toward cadmium. There have been some indications of carcinogenic and teratogenic effects of cadmium in animal studies, but dose–response relationships are unknown. Cadmium has also been implicated as a factor in hypertension.

Insufficient data are available for establishment of a maximum no-observed-adverse-health-effect value. It may be noted, however, that at a concentration level of 10 μg/liter in water, cadmium contributes only about 20% of the normal total daily adult intake with water consumption at 2 liters/day. Both the WHO and the USSR have set the maximum allowable limit for cadmium at 10 μg/liter.

Chromium

Microgram amounts of chromium, derived primarily from food, are essential for maintenance of normal glucose metabolism. Chromium (VI) is known to be toxic, principally on the basis of information from respiratory occupational exposures. Increased risk of lung cancer among those exposed occupationally to chromium (VI) has been established.

Although inhaled hexavalent chromium may cause cancer of the respiratory tract, the IARC working group concluded "there is no evidence that non-occupational exposure to chromium constitutes a cancer hazard."

Concentrations of chromium found in natural waters are limited by the low solubility of chromium (III) oxides. A study of more than 1,500 surface waters showed a maximum chromium content of 0.11 mg/liter, with a mean of 0.01 mg/liter.

Little information is available on average total daily intake of chromium in the United States, although it appears to be in the range of 60–280 μg/day. It has been suggested that diets containing mostly processed foods may be chromium-deficient. Tissue chromium in U.S. adults has been shown to decline with age.

In addition to the beneficial effect of chromium on glucose metabolism, there have been indications from animal studies that chromium deficiency may induce atherosclerosis.

Toxicity of chromium depends on the valence. No toxic effects were observed in rats when drinking water contained 25 mg/liter of trivalent chromium for a year or 5 mg/liter for life. Acutely toxic doses of trivalent chromium fall in the range of grams per kilogram of body weight. Hexavalent chromium was also tolerated at the 25 mg/liter level for a year by rats. Dogs showed no effects with 11 mg/liter over a 4-yr period. Higher doses are toxic, however, producing erosion of the gastrointestinal tract and kidney lesions.

The maximum limit of the Interim Primary Drinking Water Standards, 0.05 mg/liter, is only one-hundredth of the maximum no-observed-adverse-health effect concentration. The European standards of the WHO and Japanese standards give the same acceptable limit, but set it in terms of hexavalent chromium only. The USSR has limits of 0.1 mg/liter chromium (VI) and 0.5 mg/liter total chromium, based on organoleptic factors.

More information is needed on the carcinogenic potential of ingested chromium (VI) and chromium (III). If it becomes clear that highly toxic or carcinogenic effects occur only with chromium (VI) and a suitably sensitive analytical technique is available, then the standard might be set for chromium (VI) alone. In view of the U.S. trend toward dietary chromium deficiency and the suggestion that chromium protects against atherosclerosis, it seems advisable to investigate whether greater allowed concentrations are without adverse health effects, as some animal experiments suggest.

Cobalt

Cobalt is an essential element as a component of vitamin B_{12}. This is its only known nutritional function. Excessive intake of cobalt may be toxic with the most notable instance being the association of congestive heart failure with the consumption of beer containing about 1.5 mg/liter of cobalt.

Cobalt has been observed in natural waters only in trace amounts. Most waters have no detectable cobalt and values greater than 10 μg/liter are rare. The maximum recorded value in any of several broad studies was 99 μg/liter.

The major source of cobalt is food; concentration in green, leafy vegetables may be as great as 0.5 mg/kg dry weight. Normally, less than 1% of total intake of cobalt is derived from aqueous sources.

Acute toxic effects in animals have been observed only with daily cobalt doses greater than several mg/kg of body weight. Chronic cobalt toxicity has been observed in children taking cobalt preparations to correct anemia at daily doses of 1–6 mg/kg body weight.

The Interim Primary Drinking Water Standards do not list cobalt, nor has the WHO recommended a limit in its International or European standards. The USSR has set a limit of 1.0 mg/liter.

Because the maximum no-observed-adverse-health-effect level is more than an order of magnitude greater than the concentration found in any natural-water or drinking-water supply, there appears to be no reason at present to regulate the concentration of cobalt in drinking water.

Copper

Copper is an essential element for both plants and animals; it is a component of several enzymes that perform important physiological functions.

Copper is a minor constituent of natural waters, the concentration ranging from 1 to 280 μg/liter in a survey of 1,600 surface waters of the United States. Concentrations may be increased in drinking waters to several mg/liter by corrosion of copper piping in distribution systems, particularly with soft, nonalkaline waters. Copper may also be released into water in industrial discharges and has been used for algal control in reservoirs at concentrations of a few tenths of a milligram per liter.

Average total intake of copper is about 2.5 mg/day, so that when water contains more than 1 mg/liter of copper, the intake from water may equal or exceed that from food.

The general health hazard from excess copper intake at a level of a few milligrams per liter appears to be small, but few people are adversely affected by ingestion of even trace amounts of copper. This disorder of copper metabolism, called Wilson's disease, can be arrested by the use of chelating agents. Individuals with deficiency of glucose-6-phosphate dehydrogenase may be sensitive to copper.

The USPHS Drinking Water Standards (1962) recommended a limit for copper of 1 mg/liter based on organoleptic rather than health effects. Because no general adverse-health-effects have been observed at the organoleptic limit and because the few individuals with metabolic deficiency are at the mercy of total copper intake rather than copper in water, there is no hygienic reason to impose a limit lower than the presently accepted secondary standard.

Lead

No beneficial effects of lead on human or animal development have yet been found. Although acute lead poisoning is rare, chronic lead toxicity is severe and occurs even with low daily intake of lead (<1 mg) because of its accumulation in bone and tissue.

The natural lead content of surface waters is generally small. In a survey of nearly 1,600 raw surface waters 20% were found to contain detectable concentrations of lead and these had a mean concentration equal to 0.023 mg/liter. The lead concentration in municipal supplies at the tap may be much greater, however, for soft, low pH (agressive) waters will dissolve lead from service connections, lead-lined household piping or soldered joints. Lead concentrations in excess of the interim standard of 0.05 mg/liter were found in 1.4% of the water systems tested in the Community Water Supply Survey. The maximum value was 0.64 mg/liter.

The mean concentration of lead in U.S. drinking waters has been estimated to be 0.013 mg/liter. Consumption of 2 liters/day per capita gives a mean daily intake of 26 μg.

Lead intake from food varies greatly with mean daily values estimated at 100–300 μg per capita for adults. Average water intake is considerably less than that from food, but when the concentration in water is close to or exceeds the interim standard of 0.05 mg/liter, water intake approaches that from food.

Absorption of lead from dietary sources, either food or water, is estimated to be about 10% for adults. Daily lead absorption from food is, then, 10–30 μg, while absorption from water ranges from an average of 3 μg to 10 μg or more, when water having a lead concentration of 0.05 mg/liter or greater is ingested at 2 liters/day.

The daily intake from air also ranges widely, and is greatest among city dwellers. For a daily inspiration volume of 20 m^3 for adults and a lead concentration of 3 $\mu g/m^3$ in urban air, the per capita daily intake is 60 μg. The absorption percentage from air is about 40%, however, so that the daily quantity absorbed is 24 μg, a value comparable with the dietary absorption.

The sum of the estimated absorptions from the various routes, 50–60 μg/day, is already at the maximum no-observed-adverse-health-effect values of 50–60 μg/day.

Children, and especially inner-city urban children, are a special risk group with regard to lead toxicity. A primary reason is that absorption of lead from food and water is 40–50% for 2–3-yr-old children, rather than the 5 to 10% characteristic of adults. Also, water intake per kilogram of body weight is considerably greater for young children than for adults. Moreover, lead concentrations in urban air increase with proximity to the ground, so that urban children tend to have increased intake from this source. Young children also have the added risk of ingestion of flaking lead-based paints especially in depressed, older, urban areas.

Dietary lead intake for a 2-yr-old child (12 kg) has been estimated to be 100 μg/day (8.3 μg/kg/day); with water at the present 0.05 mg/liter limit and a consumption of 1.4 liter/day, and with air intake about 18 μg/day, the estimated total intake for a 2-yr-old would be close to 190 μg/day, not including other possible sources. If the water contains 0.1 mg/liter of lead, the present allowable limits of the WHO European standards and of the USSR, then an intake of nearly 260 μg lead/day for a 2-yr-old child can be estimated. With this intake an overall absorption close to 100 μg/day can be estimated, a value suggesting that the allowable concentrations of the WHO European standards and the USSR may fail to provide adequate protection for children.

Major chronic adverse effects of lead are produced in the hematopoietic system, central and peripheral nervous systems, and kidneys. Disturbance in heme synthesis is considered to be the most sensitive effect. There is a detectable increase in red-cell protoporphyrin in women and children with blood lead concentrations greater than about 25–30 μg/dl. For men occupationally exposed, the maximum no-observed-adverse-health-effect level appears to be somewhat greater at 50–60 μg/dl.

Results of studies in the Boston area indicate that increased blood levels of lead will occur in children when the water supply contains 0.05–0.1 mg/liter of lead. Thus, the interim limit of 0.05 mg/liter may not provide the margin of safety to safeguard the high-risk population in urban areas. Although satisfactory for a 70-kg adult, the WHO recommendation of 5 μg of lead per kg/day as a safe total daily intake cannot be met for a 12-kg child when the water supply contains as much as 0.05 mg/liter. It is concluded that the no-observed-adverse-health-effect level cannot be set with assurance at any value greater than 0.025 mg/liter.

Magnesium

Magnesium is an essential element in human, animal, and plant nutrition. It is geologically ubiquitous and the industrial uses of its salts are legion. The average U.S. adult ingests between 240 and 480 mg of magnesium per day. Magnesium intake from 3.6–4.2 mg/kg of body weight are believed to be adequate to maintain magnesium balance, which is closely regulated by normal kidneys. The median concentration of magnesium in the water of the 100 largest U.S. cities was reported at 6.26 mg/liter with a maximum of 120 mg/liter. It can be higher, especially in arid western states.

An excess of magnesium in the diet is seldom harmful, for it is generally excreted promptly in feces. High concentrations of magnesium sulfate in drinking water have a cathartic effect on new users, but a tolerance is soon acquired. Excessive magnesium in body tissues and extracellular fluids occurs only as a result of severe kidney malfunction. Magnesium deficiency in humans may occur in alcoholics, persons performing hard labor in hot climates (because magnesium is excreted in perspiration), those with certain endrocrine disturbances, and patients using potent diuretics. Such deficiencies can best be overcome by oral administration of magnesium compounds.

The National Interim Primary Drinking Water Regulations do not contain a limit for magnesium, nor did the 1962 USPHS drinking water standards. The USSR has set no limit, but the WHO has recommended a maximum of 150 mg/liter. In view of the fact that concentrations of magnesium in drinking water less than those that impart astringent taste pose no health problem and are more likely to be beneficial, no limitation for reasons of health appears needed.

Manganese

Manganese resembles iron in its chemical behavior and occurrence in natural waters, but is found less frequently and usually at lower concentrations than iron. Manganese, like iron, is an essential trace nutrient for plants and animals. It is not known whether human manganese deficiency occurs in the United States. The solubility of the several oxidation states of manganese (II, III, and IV) depends upon the pH, dissolved oxygen, and presence of complexing agents. Occasionally, deep lakes or impounding reservoirs that contain organic sediments under anerobic reducing conditions can distribute several mg/liter of Mn^{+2} throughout the water body during "turnover" mixing. Normally, however, manganese in natural surface waters is less than 20 μg/liter.

Manganese can be absorbed by inhalation, ingestion, and through the skin; the consequences of this have been recently reviewed in depth by the National Academy of Sciences. It has been known that the occupational inhalation of manganese dusts results in a disease of the central nervous system resembling Parkinsonism and a form of pneumonia.

Ingestion of manganese in moderate excess of the normal dietary level of 3–7 mg/day is not considered harmful. A reported outbreak of manganism in Japan was attributed to drinking well water containing about 14 mg/liter of manganese.

The maximum concentration of manganese found in the 1975 Survey of Interstate Water Supply Systems was 0.4 mg/liter except for samples from two Alaskan airports which showed 1.0 and 1.1 mg/liter. A total of 669 supplies were examined. Similarly the maximum concentration found in the 1969 Community Water Supply Survey was 1.3 mg/liter from 969 supplies. Both these maximum concentrations are an order of magnitude less than minimum concentrations at which adverse health effects are observed. Moreover, even with manganese at 0.4 mg/liter the intake of manganese from water would be only about 15% of the normal total dietary intake of manganese.

Because concentrations of manganese found in water supplies are much less than those at which adverse health effects have been observed and because the regulation of manganese for esthetic and economic reasons is also far more stringent than would be required for reasons of health, there seems little need to establish a maximum no-observed-adverse-health-effect value.

Mercury

Mercury is a comparatively rare element. It is relatively insoluble in the inorganic form and can exist only in extremely small quantities under natural conditions. Recent measurements show that only 4% of water supplies contain mercury at concentrations greater than 1 μg/liter. Industrial use has resulted in increased environmental contamination. The health effects of populations occupationally exposed to mercury and mercury compounds has long been recognized, but the problem of contamination of the general environment is of recent origin.

Inorganic mercury in bottom sediments can be transformed biochemically to injurious methylmercury or other organic mercurial compounds. The organic form readily enters the food chain with concentration factors as great as 3,000 in fish.

Several investigators have estimated the blood levels of mercury at which the identifiable symptoms of mercury intoxication occur. These levels may be obtained with a steady mercury intake of from 4–14 μg/kg/day. This would be 240–840 μg/day for adults and 80–280 μg/day for children. It is estimated that the normal diet will contribute about 10 μg/day of mercury. With daily intake of 10 μg from food and 4 μg from water it appears that there is considerable margin of safety. However, those individuals regularly consuming fish from contaminated areas may exceed the normal intake by a factor of three or more and thus constitute a high-risk population.

There is no indication that concentrations of mercury in drinking water or air have contributed in any significant way to methylmercury intoxication of the general population. The interim standard limits the daily intake to 3–4 μg/day. Nearly all public water supplies in the United States contain less than 2 μg/liter of mercury. The WHO has set no limit and the USSR has a maximum permissible concentration of 5 μg/liter.

Molybdenum

Soluble molybdate ions are present in trace concentrations in many surface waters, primarily as a result of discharge of industrial wastes but also as a product of natural weathering of molybdenum-bearing soils. Both suspended insoluble molybdenum disulfide and soluble molybdates are present in streams draining areas where molybdenum ore is mined and processed, especially in Colorado and New Mexico.

Typical diets contain on the order of 100–1,000 μg/kg, whereas typical surface waters (except those draining mining areas) contain less than 100 μg/liter, with median values about 10 μg/liter. Hence, water is a minor factor in the total molybdenum intake in most locations. Since some finished waters have been reported to contain as much as 1 mg/liter, some water intake may provide as much as 2,000 μg/day of molybdenum. More information is needed about adverse effects of molybdenum at these levels to deal properly with such supplies.

Molybdenum poisoning has rarely been observed in humans. Although it has been implicated for gout in Armenia and for a bone-crippling disease in India, more information is needed to establish cause-and-effect relationships.

Molybdenosis in livestock is a significant toxicological problem in many areas of the world. Consumption of molybdenum-rich forage by cattle and sheep causes severe diarrhea (scouring) that sometimes results in death. It can be prevented or ameliorated by the administration of copper, but the relationship of molybdenum, copper, and sulfate-forming compounds in animal metabolism needs further study.

The USSR has established a limit for molybdenum of 0.5 mg/liter in open waters, but the WHO has not promulgated a limit.

Nickel

Nickel may occur in water from trace amounts of a few micrograms per liter to a maximum of 100 μg/liter. At these levels the daily intake of nickel from water ranges from less than 10 μg/day to a maximum of 200 μg/day, as compared to a normal food intake of 300–600 μg/day. Available information indicates that nickel does not pose a toxicity problem because the absorption from food or water is low. The principle reason for considering nickel stems from epidemiological evidence that occupational exposure to nickel compounds through the respiratory tract increases the risk of lung cancer and nasal-cavity cancer. There is difficulty in separating the effect of nickel from the simultaneous inhalation of other carcinogens including arsenic and chromium.

Because of the generally low concentration of nickel in drinking water and its reported low oral toxicity, there is no present need to set primary health effect limits for nickel in water. WHO and the USSR have set no standards for nickel in drinking water.

Silver

Trace amounts of silver are found in some natural waters and in a few community water supplies. It has not been detected at levels exceeding the interim standard of 50 μg/liter. Colloidal siver consumed in large doses—several hundred mg/kg of body weight—can cause anemia and possibly death. The main chronic effect in man is "argyria." Argyria is a cosmetic defect once caused through medical or occupational exposure to silver preparations. It is rarely encountered now. Dosages of from 1 to 5 g of silver are sufficient to produce this syndrome.

On the assumption of 50% absorption of silver, consumption of 2 liters/day of water containing 0.005 mg/liter of silver would result in an accumulation of 1 g of silver over 55 yr.

Since silver ion has not been detected in water supplies in concentrations greater than half the no-observed-adverse-health-effect level, regulation of its concentration as a primary standard would appear to be unnecessary.

Tin

There is some indication that tin may be a beneficial micronutrient, although it has not been conclusively demonstrated that tin is an essential trace element in human nutrition. Inorganic tin is relatively nontoxic, but organotin compounds can be toxic at high concentrations. Indeed, they are used an fungicides, insecticides, and antihelminthics.

Tin has seldom been determined in natural or municipally treated water. The few available data generally show concentrations of the order of one or two μg/liter. In contrast, tin is present in most natural foods, and especially in canned products, to the extent that the normal human ingestion varies from 1–30 mg/day, which is three or more orders of magnitude higher than the probable concentration in a liter of tap water.

EPA has not set a limit for tin in its National Interim Primary Drinking Water Regulations. In view of the foregoing considerations, no regulation seems necessary.

Vanadium

Vanadium is a trace metal that has been introduced into the environment in large quantities. Fresh surface waters show concentrations in the 2–300 μg/liter range, but with low frequency of detection. The data are limited on levels in finished drinking waters, but vanadium concentrations up to 19 μg/liter have been reported.

Occupational exposure to pentoxides and trioxides of vanadium leads to ear, nose and throat irritation and generally impaired health. The consequences of exposure to vanadium in air, water and food have been reviewed recently. There is no evidence of chronic oral toxicity.

Vanadium is considered a beneficial nutrient at μg/liter levels, having been suggested as protective against atherosclerosis.

Zinc

Concentrations of zinc in surface water are correlated with man's activities and with urban and industrial runoff. The solubility of zinc is variable, depending upon the pH of the water. In the same manner as lead and cadmium, zinc is dissolved in concentrations as great as several mg/liter from galvanized pipes and tanks in soft-water systems. Concentrations ranging from 2–1,200 μg/liter were detected in 77% of 1,577 surface water samples and 3–2,000 μg/liter in 380 drinking waters.

Zinc is relatively nontoxic and is an essential trace element with recommended minimum intake levels of 15 mg/day for adults and 10 mg/day for children over 1 yr of age. A wide margin of safety exists between normal intake from the diet and those likely to cause oral toxicity. Concentrations of 30 mg/liter or more impart a strong astringent taste and milky appearance to water. Some acute adverse effects have been reported from consumption of water containing zinc at 40–50 μg/liter. There are no known chronic adverse effects of low-level zinc intake in diet, but human zinc deficiency has been identified.

The presently established standard (USPHS) for zinc in drinking water is a "recommended" or secondary standard based on the threshold of the metallic taste at about 5 mg/liter. The WHO recommends the same limit; however, the USSR has established a limit for zinc at 1 mg/liter for other than health reasons.

OTHER INORGANIC CONSTITUENTS

Arsenic

OCCURRENCE

Arsenic is widely distributed in low concentrations in the waters of the United States (Durum, 1974). In one study of selected minor elements in

TABLE V-12 Regional Summary of Arsenic in U.S. Surface Waters

Region	Maximum, μg/liter	Minimum, μg/liter	Median, μg/liter	Proportion, <10 μg/liter, %	Proportion, >10 μg/liter, %
New England and Northeast	60	<10	<10	80	20
Southeast	1,110	<10	<10	70	30
Central	140	<10	<10	75	25
Southwest	10	<10	<10	87	13
Northwest	30	<10	<10	86	14

(From Durum *et al.*, 1971)

728 samples of U.S. surface waters, the concentration of arsenic ranged from less than 10 to 1,100 μg/liter (10-1,100 ppb). A study by the U.S. Geological Survey (USGS, 1970) of river waters revealed that the median concentration of arsenic was less than 10 μg/liter, the lower limit of detection, but 22% of the samples had concentrations of 10–20 μg/liter (Table V-12). In this survey, except for local anomalies where arsenic concentrations could be traced to urban waters or to industrial sources, no major regional differences could be detected in average values or in percentage of contaminated samples.

The distribution of arsenic in waters and sediments of the Puget Sound region (Washington) has been studied by Crecelius and Carpenter (1974). A large copper smelter in the area releases about 300 tons of arsenic per year into the atmosphere in stack dust and about the same amount in liquid effluent directly into Puget Sound.

The concentrations of arsenic in Puget Sound waters are 1.5–2.0 μg/liter, except for surface waters within a few miles of the smelter, where they may reach 1,000 μg/liter. Away from the immediate smelter area, the concentrations of arsenic in the Sound are not likely to rise above 1–2 μg/liter because of the 1/2-yr replacement time for waters in Puget Sound.

There have been a number of reports of isolated instances of higher than usual concentrations of arsenic in well waters. Lassen County, California (Goldsmith *et al.*, 1972), was one such area. It was examined because of arsenic in well water ranging from 0.1 mg/liter or less to 1.4 mg/liter—well above maximal allowable standards. This compares with the 0.05 mg/liter recommended by the U.S. Public Health Service as well as the WHO in its International and European drinking-water standards. The Lassen County study indicated that when the arsenic concentration in water was above 0.05 mg/liter, storage in hair increased, but there was no evidence of specific illness associated with concentrations up to 1.4 mg/liter.

In Perham, Minnesota, a newly bored well was associated with illness in 13 people whose hair samples contained arsenic at 37–1,680 μg/g. The well water serving these patients contained arsenic from 11,800 to 21,000 μg/liter; this was later determined to come from ground contamination by residual arsenical grasshopper bait (Feinglass, 1973).

Antofagasta, a city of 130,000 in Chile, had a water supply containing high quantities of arsenic (800 ppb) between 1958 and 1970. The source of the high arsenic content was the Toconce River, whose waters come from the Andes Mountains at an altitude of 3,000 m and were brought 300 km to Antofagasta (Borgono and Greiber, 1972). At the begining of the 1960's, the first cutaneous manifestations were noted in children. There were several severe cases, including a few fatal ones, of arsenism at the Calvo Mackenna Hospital in Santiago. The principal finding was the close relation between the prevalence of cutaneous lesions (over 30% of the population) and the exposure to drinking water with a high arsenic content. The arsenic content of the hair and water supplies decreased markedly after action was initiated to clean up the water supply by opening a new water-treatment plant.

Natural sources, including the erosion of surface rocks, probably account for a significant portion of arsenic found in surface water and groundwater. Fleisher (1973) noted that fumarolic gases associated with volcanism have been reported to contain arsenic at up to 700 ppb, and waters of hot springs contain up to 13,700 ppb. Otherwise, scattered data for arsenic in groundwater indicate low concentrations, often below the limit of detection and perhaps averaging around 1 μg/liter (1 ppb). Isolated instances of arsenic in such concentrations which warrant surveillance have been reported.

Arsenic is found in many foods; it occurs naturally in some and is introduced into others by way of feeds and pesticides. Crustaceans and other shellfish may contain up to 170 ppm (Frost, 1967). Apples that have been sprayed with lead arsenate to control codling moths might contain as much as 2 mg of residue. Wine and cider may contain arsenic, but it is usually removed during processing. Wine yeasts have been shown to contain arsenic in amounts up to 180 ppm, and baker's yeast up to 17 ppm. Meat may contain traces of arsanilic acid that has been used as a growth additive in cattle and poultry feeds. Theoretically, these additives are discontinued several days before marketing, and, in fact, the FDA allows an animal tissue arsenic content of 2.65 μg/g. There has been considerable speculation about the addition of any arsenic to the diet of animals. Arsenic was found in 3.2% of samples of food items examined in the United States during a market-basket survey; residues ranged between 0.1 and 4.7 mg/kg (Cummings, 1966). The daily intake in the United States is calculated to be 0.137–0.330 mg (Duggan and Lipscomb, 1969).

Arsenic occurs in the earth's crust in concentrations averaging 2 ppm (Fleischer, 1973). It is concentrated in shales, clays, phosphorites, coals, sedimentary iron ore, and manganese ores. In the United States, arsenic is produced (and distributed into the environment) largely as a result of smelting nonferrous-metal ores, particularly copper. Recent analyses of petroleum show a median arsenic concentration of 90 ppb, but there are few data. Superphosphate fertilizer made by treatment of phosphorite with sulfuric acid has been reported to contain as much as 0.1% arsenic.

METABOLISM

The metabolism of arsenicals by mammalian systems has been reviewed in detail by Frost (1967), Lisella *et al.* (1972), Harvey (1975), and others. The present discussion summarizes the available information.

Absorption

Water-soluble arsenicals are readily absorbed through the gastrointestinal tract, lungs, and skin; some nonpolar organic forms are also absorbed from the intestine and skin (Hwang and Schanker, 1973; Tarrant and Allard, 1972). Arsenic trioxide is only slightly soluble in water and is not well absorbed. Pentavalent arsenic, As(+V), whether inorganic or organic, is better absorbed than the trivalent form, because As(+V) is less reactive with membranes of the gastrointestinal tract. Arsenites are generally better absorbed through skin than arsenates, and absorption depends heavily on lipid solubility of the compound.

Some of the selective toxicity of arsenic is explained by arsenates penetration of insect cuticle more rapidly than of human skin. Arsenite is more toxic to humans than arsenate and is more readily absorbed through human skin (Harvey, 1975).

Distribution

Arsenic is distributed primarily to the liver, kidneys, intestinal wall, spleen and lungs. The extent to which arsenic is taken up by these tissues depends on the rate of exposure and the chemical form.

In guinea pigs, rabbits, apes, and humans, radioarsenite (^{74}As) injected subcutaneously was distributed to muscles and other tissues (Hunter *et al.*, 1942). Sodium arsenite (^{76}As) that was injected intramuscularly to rabbits was found mainly in liver, kidneys, and lungs (Ducoff *et al.*, 1948).

Arsenic is immobilized by binding to sulfhydryl groups in the keratin of hair and nails. Deposition begins within 2 weeks after administration, and the arsenic deposited may remain for the lifetime of the hair or nail. In this way deposition also serves as an excretory mechanism.

Excretion

There is a great deal of confusion in the literature regarding accumulation of arsenic. Rats (and possibly cats) appear unique, for they accumulate arsenic in the blood, bound to hemoglobin, whereas in other species there is no accumulation (Lanz *et al.*, 1950; Hove *et al.*, 1938; Peoples, 1964).

Arsenate is rapidly excreted in the urine (Lanz *et al.*, 1950; Ginsburg, 1965). Arsenate, however, can be reabsorbed by the proximal tubule in the dog kidney and re-excreted as arsenite (Ginsburg, 1965). Arsenite is excreted slowly in the urine, and it can take up to 10 days to completely excrete a single dose of parenterally administered trivalent arsenic (Hunter *et al.*, 1942). It appears that arsenite is slowly oxidized to arsenate in the body and filtered into the urine in the pentavalent form.

Mealy *et al.* (1959) suggested that arsenite is excreted by humans in three phases. More than 99% of radioactive sodium arsenite (^{74}As) injected intravenously into five human volunteers was excreted in the first 15 h after administration, most of the balance was excreted at a constant low rate over the next 155 h, and the remainder was excreted at an even lower rate. An alternative explanation for this observation is that the three phases are artifacts of the sampling time.

Administration of arsenic to cows does not appear to influence arsenic concentrations in milk, although tissue concentrations increased (Peoples, 1964). Arsenic acid (Peoples, 1964), lead arsenate (Marshall *et al.*, 1963), and arsenic trioxide (Fitch *et al.*, 1939) given to cows are readily excreted as pentavalent arsenic in the urine.

Transformation

Little is known about the biotransformation of arsenic in man in spite of the long use of arsenicals as pharmaceuticals and pesticides.

Arsenic inhibits the activity of many enzymes by reacting with sulfhydryl groups. In most cases the arsenical is converted to the trivalent form as an arsenite or arsenoxide (R – As = 0). This active form of arsenic then combines with two sulfhydryl groups (often from two protein molecules) to form such products as R – As – (S-protein)$_2$ (Harvey, 1975). Intramolecular reactions also occur when arsenic combines with both sulfhydryl groups of α-lipoic (thioctic) acid to form a six-membered ring compound. Such reactions are considered responsible for much of the toxic action of arsenicals.

HEALTH EFFECTS

The toxicity of various arsenic compounds is extremely variable and depends on the species exposed, the formulation of the arsenical, the route of exposure, and the rate and duration of exposure. An assumption that all arsenic compounds are equally toxic is incorrect. Although man and other animals are susceptible to arsenic poisoning, there is a wide variation among species in susceptibility to a specific arsenic compound.

Similarly, there is a wide variation in toxicity of the various arsenical formulations to a given species. Because of the many factors influencing the toxicity of arsenic, there is little point in attempting to state its toxicity in terms of milligrams per kilogram of body weight. It may be said, however, that the lethal oral dose of the more toxic arsenic compounds in most species appears to be 1–25 mg/kg of body weight, whereas the lethal dose for the less toxic compounds may range from 10–400 times this amount (Buck *et al.*, 1973; Penrose, 1974).

Groups of arsenic compounds can be listed as follows in decreasing order of toxicity (Penrose, 1974):

Arsines (trivalent, inorganic or organic)
Arsenite (inorganic)
Arsenoxides (trivalent with two bonds to oxygen)
Arsenate (inorganic)
Pentavalent arsenicals, such as arsonic acids
Arsonium compounds (four organic groups with a positive charge on arsenic)
Metallic arsenic

Arsine gas is an indirect hemolytic agent due to its inhibition of red-cell catalase, which leads to accumulation of hydrogen peroxide which in turn destroys the red-cell membrane (Moeschlin, 1965).

Inorganic arsenite or its anhydride, arsenous oxide, are the most common commercial forms of arsenic. Their acute toxic effects follow a short latent period and include rapid collapse, shock, and death.

Arsenoxides and inorganic pentavalent arsenicals vary considerably in their toxicity. Although they are usually less toxic than the arsenites, their effects on biologic systems appear to be the same.

In general, the phenylarsonic compounds are less hazardous for mammals than other arsenical compounds. The toxic effects of these compounds are manifested by incoordination, inability to control body and limb movements, and ataxia resulting from demyelination of the peripheral nerves (Ledet, 1973).

Arsonium compounds and metallic arsenic are quite stable and have relatively low toxicity (Schroeder and Balassa, 1966; Penrose, 1974).

Toxic Effects In Humans

Human exposure to arsenic sufficient to cause severe toxicosis usually occurs through ingestion of contaminated food or drink. The signs and symptoms are variable in degree and timing and depend on the form and amount of arsenic, the age of the patient, and other factors (Willcox, 1922). The major characteristics of acute arsenic poisoning are profound gastrointestinal damage and cardiac abnormalities.

Symptoms may appear within 8 min if the arsenic is in solution, but may be delayed up to 10 h if it is solid and taken with a meal. The signs include excruciating abdominal pain, forceful vomiting, cramps in the legs, restlessness, and spasms. "A feeble, frequent, and irregular pulse ushers in the other symptoms of collapse, the livid and anxious face, sunken eyes, cold and clammy skin. . . . A small proportion of the cases are classed as nervous or cerebral because . . . the . . . conspicuous . . . phenomena are . . . prostration, stupor, convulsions, paralysis, collapse, and death in coma" (Holland, 1904). Only a small fraction of patients will develop any kind of skin reaction secondary to acute arsenic poisoning. Presumably, the arsenic is absorbed from the damaged gut and finds its way to the skin. The usual reaction in these circumstances is acute exfoliative erythroderma, probably reflecting the fact that arsenic is a capillary poison (Harvey, 1965).

Exposure to amounts of arsenic sufficient to cause symptoms is probably more common than that sufficient to produce systemic collapse. The patient may go for weeks with gradually increasing or variable signs and symptoms related to several organ systems and with the appearance of a progressive chronic disease. If death occurs, it may appear to have been the consequence of an obscure "natural" disease. Skin manifestations of such victims are particularly prominent.

In 1901, over 500 beer-drinkers afflicted with an unusual poisoning attributed to arsenic in one of the ingredients were studied by Reynolds (1901). The symptoms appeared after many months of drinking 2–16 pints per day of beer which contained a fraction of "the quantity of arsenic which (would be prescribed for) an epileptic." Although Frost (1970) has refuted his conclusions and provided evidence that selenium may have been the contaminant, the clinical manifestations described were compatible with those produced by arsenic. The first symptoms to appear were digestive, especially vomiting and diarrhea. Within a few weeks, catarrhal symptoms appeared—such as conjunctivitis, rhinitis, laryngitis, bronchitis—as well as various skin eruptions. Hoarseness due to thickening of the vocal chords and hemoptysis were also mentioned. Insidious development of neurologic signs and symptoms began before the appearance of the classical skin lesions, but sometimes were so vague as to go undiagnosed for many weeks. Involvement of the nervous system began with sensory changes, including paresthesias, hyperesthesias, and neuralgias. There was marked muscle tenderness: motor weakness of all degrees (including paralysis with muscle atrophy, progressing from distal to proximal groups) was a frequent observation. Left-side heart failure with severe peripheral edema was observed in one-fourth of the patients, and the 13 deaths in this series were all due to congestive heart failure. Reynolds also described the nail changes of subacute arsenic poisoning, observable some weeks after the intake of the poison was stopped. When normal nail grew out, it revealed "transverse white ridge across the nail; proximal to this the nail is normal, but distal to it the nail is whiter, cracked, thin, and towards the tip also papery and much flattened. In some cases there have been a series of parallel transverse ridges on the nail almost suggesting a series of weekend drinking bouts." This feature of arsenic exposure, commonly called "Mees lines" on the basis of a later description, has also been described by Aldrich (1904).

Mitzuta *et al.* (1956) reported on 220 patients of all ages who had been poisoned by contaminated soy sauce, with an average estimated ingestion of roughly 3 mg of arsenic (probably as calcium arsenate) daily for 2–3 weeks. In this group, 85% had facial edema and anorexia; fewer than 10% had exanthemata, desquamation, and hyperpigmentation; and about 20% had peripheral neuropathy. Except for headaches and fever, the findings in these patients appeared to be very similar to those reported by Reynolds (1901). The Japanese report offered additional information based upon modern diagnostic techniques. Although the majority of patients' livers were enlarged, relatively few abnormalities were found in liver-function tests; and the histopathologic description of five liver biopsies did not reveal severe degenerative changes. There were no findings suggestive of congestive failure, but electrocardiograms were abnormal in 16 of 20 patients, and this confirmed the reports of Josephson *et al.* (1951) and Nagai *et al.* (1956). The Japanese patients' symptoms tended to diminish after 5 or 6 days, despite continued intake of arsenic, and neurologic symptoms became prominent as much as 2 weeks after arsenic ingestion was discontinued, at which time urinary arsenic content remained high. Hair was found to contain arsenic at 2.8–13.0 ppm near the root, compared with 0–1.5 ppm near the end and 0.4–2.8 ppm in hair from control patients.

In the early 1960's, physicians in Antofagasta, Chile, noted dermatologic manifestations and some deaths, particularly among children, that were traced to a water supply containing arsenic at 800 ppb. This water supply had been in operation only since 1958. In 1971, Borgono and Greiber (1972) reported on a series of studies of the inhabitants of this city. They compared 180 inhabitants of Antofasgasta with 98 people who lived in a city (Iquique) with a normal water supply. Most of the people studied were less than 10 yr old. Among the residents of Antofagasta the primary symptoms reported were abnormal skin pigmentation (80%);

chronic coryza (60%); hyperkeratosis (36%); various cardiovascular manifestations, i.e., Raynaud's syndrome (30%); acrocyanosis (27%); abdominal pain (39%); chronic diarrhea (7%); and lip herpes (13%). The incidence of these symptoms in the control population was substantially lower or nonexistent.

Two additional reports on the Antofagasta studies are worthy of note. Zaldivar (1974) further described a study on a total of 457 patients (208 males, 249 females) bearing cutaneous lesions (leukoderma, melanoderma, hyperkeratosis, squamous-cell carcinoma). Children (0–15 yr of age) accounted for 69.2% of male cases, and for 77.5% of female cases. These patients exhibited high arsenic content in the hair. The mean concentration of arsenic in drinking water in the period 1968–1969 was 580 ppb versus 80 ppb in 1971, differing by a factor of 7.2. Such difference was attributed to a new filter plant, which started operation in May 1970. The average incidence rates per 100,000 population for cases with cutaneous lesions in 1968–1969 were 145.5 for males and 168.0 for females. The incidence rates decreased in 1971 to 9.1 for males and 10.0 for females.

Among the 337 registered children, 5 died showing thrombosis of brain arteries, thrombosis of mesenteric artery, restriction of lumen of coronary arteries, and/or myorcardial infarction. Of the 64 registered adult males, 2 developed multiple skin carcinomata with lymph node metastases.

A number of questions are raised regarding this report. For example, the decrease in cutaneous lesions seemed to be too rapid, following installation of the water-treatment plant, suggesting other factors were involved. Protection of the 8–10-yr-old age group showed up in three years and adults exposed for more than 15 yr also had a decrease in incidence rate of cutaneous lesions.

In a follow-up study, Borgono *et al.* (1976) investigated clinical and epidemiologic aspects of the cases first reported in 1971. The study was carried out through the examination of arsenic content in hair and nail clipping samples of the inhabitants of Antofagasta and the determination of this element in cultivated vegetables and carbonated beverages. Also a clinical study was made in school children, looking for cutaneous lesions attributed to arsenicism. Six years after the water treatment plant started to operate the problem had diminished considerably. Arsenic determination of hair and nails of children 6 yr of age or less, born since the water treatment plant went into operation, indicated no cutaneous lesions in this age group. However, those over 6 yr of age still had significant arsenic residues in hair and nails. Although the clinical manifestations have improved, arsenic content of water, soft drinks, and in some foods are still considerably above safe levels and require additional sanitary engineering improvements.

The Raynaud's phenomenon and acrocyanosis in this population are reminiscent of the report from Taiwan by Tseng *et al.* (1968), suggesting that chronic arsenism affects the vasculature in a way similar to the more acute phenomena described by Reynolds and others as erythromelalgia and acrocyanosis. Tseng *et al.* surveyed a group of 40,421 (from a population "at risk" of 103,154) and found hyperpigmentation in 18.4%, keratotic lesions in 7.1%, and blackfoot disease (apparently secondary to arterial spasm in the legs) in 0.9%. All these phenomena were shown to increase with increasing arsenic concentration in the well water of the 37 villages studied. They also increased with age, but the earliest ages noted for specific findings were 3 yr for the characteristic hyperpigmentation and 4 yr for keratoses. The concentration of arsenic in the wells ranged from 17 to 1097 ppb. No cases of melanosis or keratosis were found in a group of 2,552 people living in an area where the wells contained almost no arsenic.

Feinglass (1973) reported on 13 persons exposed for 2.5 months to well water contaminated with buried arsenical insecticide. Most patients were seen only once, and the most prominent features were intermittent gastrointestinal symptoms related to water ingestion. Two of the 13 had nail changes, and 6 to 8 had increased arsenic content of the scalp hair. The author did not mention edema, exanthema, hyperpigmentation, or hyperkeratosis.

There are many scattered case reports of subacute to chronic arsenic poisoning in the literature. Silver and Wainman (1952) described a patient who ingested approximately 8.8 mg of arsenic trioxide as Fowler's solution daily for a total period of 28 months, as a remedy for asthma. Signs of arsenic poisoning, manifested as increased freckling and as darkening of the nipples, first appeared in association with gastrointestinal symptoms after 13 months; redness and puffiness about the eyes and hyperkeratoses developed at approximately 1.5 yr. Neurologic symptoms in the form of paresthesias and weakness were the last to be noted, occurring after 2 yr. When the arsenic intake was stopped, the pigmentation lightened, but the hyperkeratoses remained, and the asthma became more difficult to control.

Perry *et al.* (1948) noted that all of a group of chemical workers handling inorganic arsenic compounds had pigmentary changes and that one-third of them had "warts," although these were not well described. They reported that the cutaneous "changes were so evident that [the examiner] could readily tell whether the man . . . was a chemical worker." All these workers had increased urinary arsenic compatible in degree with the extent of exposure; this indicates systemic absorption of the arsenic from dust, probably through the lungs and skin.

Some clinical and experimental evidence suggests that arsenic has the capacity to suppress the immune response selectively. For many medical conditions for which arsenic was most popular, steroid drugs are now the treatment of choice. The high incidence of herpes zoster and herpes simplex in cases of subacute arsenic poisoning is reminiscent of patients who were deliberately immunosuppressed to receive kidney transplants. Recurrent pulmonary infections in children in the Antofagasta episode is reminiscent of children with congenital immunodeficiency syndromes. Arsenic is reputed to reduce the lymphocyte count in leukemia which may reflect a selective sensitivity of this cell type, which again is analogous to the effects of steroids (Borgono and Greiber, 1972).

Carcinogenicity A number of studies in man have linked the appearance of cancer to exposure to inorganic arsenic compounds. Evidence has come from the use of arsenicals as drugs, from geographic areas with high concentrations of arsenic in drinking water, and from arsenic-exposed industrial groups, such as miners and smelters, workers in factories manufacturing arsenic-containing pesticides, and vineyard workers. However, the association of cancer with a history of exposure to arsenic in one form or another must be carefully evaluated before arsenic is incriminated as the causative agent (NAS, 1976).

Evidence of the carcinogenicity of arsenic in man is based almost entirely on descriptive, retrospective, epidemiologic studies. Thus, a change in the rate for cancer in various population groups has been identified, suggesting the influence of carcinogens in the environment of the groups. Although case histories of persons in the afflicted groups have shown exposure to an arsenical, the many variables to which man is subject cannot be controlled in retrospective studies. In none of the human studies was there satisfactory control of exposure to known carcinogens (including cigarette smoke, asbestos, ionizing radiation, polycyclic hydrocarbons, pesticides, and ultraviolet light) or other unknown carcinogens in the environment.

The clinical association of skin cancer with the therapeutic administration of arsenic compounds began with a report by Hutchinson (1888). Six patients in whom skin cancer occurred had suffered for very long periods from diseases of the skin (five with psoriasis, one with pemphigus). In five of the cases, arsenic was known to have been used for a long time. Neubauer (1947) summarized 143 published cases of therapeutic arsenical epitheliomas. Only a small, but undetermined, proportion of people treated with arsenicals developed cancers. Of the 143 patients, about 70% received arsenicals for skin disease; of these, half had psoriasis. Nearly all the 143 patients received arsenic in the inorganic trivalent form, the most common drug being potassium arsenite as Fowler's solution. Multiple horn keratoses, especially of the punctate or warty form on the palms and soles, were commonly reported in patients who had received Fowler's solution. Keratoses occurred in about 90% of the cases of cancer ascribed to treatment with Fowler's solution; about half the skin cancers were squamous carcinomas arising in keratotic areas of the hands, heels, and toes. The rest were multiple superficial epitheliomas of the basal-cell variety localized on the trunk and proximal parts of the extremities. Only a few of the 143 cases arose in psoriatic patches. There was a substantial frequency of mixed types of epitheliomas. Of the 143 patients, 70% had multiple lesions, with an average of two per case. The elapsed time from the beginning of administration of the arsenical drug to the beginning of the epitheliomatous growth was variable, but averaged 18 yr, regardless of the type of lesion. The latent period for the onset of keratosis was about 9 yr. In spite of the long latent period, skin cancers started when the patients were relatively young, 30% when they were 40 or younger and 70% when they were 50 or younger.

There have been numerous reports of arsenic-related occupational cancer, such as those of lung-cancer mortality among Southern Rhodesian gold miners (Osburn, 1957) and of concurrent lung and liver cancer and clinical arsenism among German vineyard workers exposed to lead arsenate dust (Braun, 1958; Roth, 1957). The association of cancer with arsenic has sometimes been based on the existence of palmar or plantar keratoses (Sommers and McManus, 1953). However, because of the increased concentration of arsenic in the lesions of Bowen's disease, arsenic has been considered as a possible cause of the disease and accompanying visceral tumors, without prior exposure to arsenicals (Graham *et al.*, 1961).

Hill and Faning (1948) compared the death records of workers in a British sheep-dip factory with those of other workers in the same district. Of the 75 factory-workers deaths, 22 (29%) were due to cancer; of the 1,216 other deaths, 157 (13%) were due to cancer. The sites of cancer were primarily the respiratory system and the skin in the factory workers, and there was a considerable incidence of cancer of digestive and abdominal organs in both factory workers and other occupational groups. The median air arsenic content for the chemical workers at the various operations ranged from 254 to 696 $\mu g/m^3$. As an upper limit, this represented inhalation of about 1 g of arsenic per year. The excretion of arsenic in the urine of 127 current employees was determined and varied widely. Some exposed workers excreted from 1 to nearly 2 mg/day, whereas many excreted less than 0.1 mg/day. A few of the persons in the control group had very high excretion rates, for no explained reason. It is important to note that 20 of 31 current factory workers had been exposed to airborne sodium arsenite for more than 10 yr, and 5 of them for 40–50 yr. Furthermore, the median age of the 31 exposed workers was 52 yr. None of these men's lungs had pathologic signs attributable to their exposure to sodium arsenite (radiographs, vital capacity, and exercise capacity were studied). The authors concluded that the study of factory workers had produced no concrete evidence to confirm the association of arsenic exposure to death from cancer.

Lee and Fraumeni (1969) compared the mortality experience of 8,047 white male smelter workers exposed to arsenic trioxide and sulfur dioxide during 1938–1963 with that of the white population in the same state. There was a threefold greater total mortality from respiratory cancer in smelter workers, many of whom were also exposed to silica, ferromanganese dust, and and other fumes.

Snegireff and Lombard (1951) made a substantial study of cancer mortality in a metallurgic plant in which arsenic was handled and in a control plant in which "working conditions approximate those of Plant A except that no arsenic is handled." The authors stated that total cancer mortality in the two plants was not significantly different from the figures for the state as a whole, and they concluded that handling of arsenic trioxide did not cause a significant change in cancer mortality. Their data demonstrated, however, evidence of a respiratory system carcinogen among workers of both plants, but arsenic may not have been involved.

A study at the Dow Chemical Company was carried out to examine the incidence of respiratory cancer among 173 workers who were exposed primarily to lead arsenate and calcium arsenate and 1,890 workers who worked in the same plant but were not exposed to arsenic (Ott *et al.*, 1974). Data were presented on the relationship between cumulative arsenic exposure and the ratio of observed to expected deaths from lung cancer. The average exposure of each worker was calculated on the basis of records of job assignments and data on the arsenic content of the air in various parts of the plant. Deaths from respiratory malignancy were 6–7 times greater than expected for total inhaled quantities of 10.3 mg and 2–4 times greater for 4.84–8.17 mg. There was no association between the extent of exposure and the time from beginning of exposure to death; most of the respiratory cancers occurred 20–40 yr after initial exposure, regardless of total exposure.

In contrast with the Dow Chemical Company workers, orchard workers who used lead arsenate had no evidence of increased cancer (Nelson *et al.*, 1973). A mortality study involving a cohort of 1,231 workers in Wenatchee, Washington, who had participated in a 1938 morbidity survey of the effects of exposure to lead arsenate insecticide spray was conducted in 1968–1969. Air concentrations of arsenic during spraying averaged 0.14 mg/m³. The workers were grouped in three categories according to exposure and compared in terms of standardized mortality ratios with the mortality experience of the State of Washington. There was no evidence of increased mortality from cancer, heart disease, or vascular lesions.

High incidences of skin cancer have been reported in several groups exposed to high concentrations of arsenic in drinking water, including people in the district of Reichenstein in Silesia (Geyer, 1898), Cordoba Province in Argentina (Bergoglio, 1964), and Taiwan (Tseng *et al.*, 1968).

The existence of arsenic in waters in an eastern area of the province of Cordoba, Argentina, has been known for many decades; it has been associated with the occurrence of hyperpigmentation, keratosis, and skin cancer. A study made in 1949–1959 indicated a higher proportion of deaths from cancer in the arsenical region than in the rest of the province—23.8% vs. 15.3% (Bergoglio, 1964). The excess was due mainly to cancer of the respiratory and digestive tracts in both men and women and was unrelated to socioeconomic differences.

A study by Tseng *et al.* (1968) was done on the southwest coast of Taiwan, where there were artesian wells that had been used for more than 45 yr with high concentrations of arsenic. Most of the well water in the endemic area had an arsenic content of around 0.5 ppm. The total population of the area was approximately 100,000, and the survey encompassed the 40,421 inhabitants of 37 villages. The overall prevalence rates for skin cancer, hyperpigmentation, and keratosis were 10.6/1,000, 183.5/1,000, and 71.0/1,000, respectively. The male:female ratios were 2.9:1 for skin cancer and 1.1:1 for hyperpigmentation and keratosis. The prevalence of each of the three conditions increased steadily with age, although there was a decline for cancer and hyperpigmentation in women above 69. The prevalence rate for each condition varied directly with the arsenic content of the well water.

In a continuing survey and follow-up in some villages of Taiwan, Tseng (1976) confirmed that the prevalence rates for skin cancer and blackfoot disease showed an ascending gradient according to the arsenic content of well water, i.e., the higher the arsenic content, the more patients with skin cancer and blackfoot disease. A dose–response relationship between blackfoot disease and the duration of water intake was also noted. Furthermore, the degree of permanent impairment of a patient was noted to be directly related to duration of intake of arsenical water and alternatively to duration of such intake at the time of onset. The most common cause of death in the patients with skin cancer and blackfoot disease was carcinoma of various sites. The 5-yr survival rate after blackfoot onset was 76.3%; 10-yr survival rate, 63.3%; and 15-yr survival rate, 52.2%. The 50% survival point was 16 yr after onset of the disease.

The more recent observations from Chile and from Taiwan emphasize the public health problems associated with arsenic in specific geographic areas.

Recent reports from Sweden (Pershagen *et al.*, 1976) are of interest. The study concerns mortality in an area surrounding an arsenic emitting plant. A metallurgic plant, founded in 1928, processed mainly nonferrous metals. Since the starting of operations it has been using ore with a high arsenic content that has resulted in environmental pollution of air and water with arsenic, as well as other metals and sulphur dioxide.

The causes of death for the population of two parishes in the vicinity of the plant were listed from the National Swedish Register on Death Causes. A reference area in the same part of Sweden with similar degree of urbanization, occupational profile, and age distribution was chosen. The causes of death for the two populations were followed during a period of 14 yr. A markedly higher mortality rate for lung cancer was noted in men in the exposed area. Also when the occupationally exposed were excluded there remained indications of an increased mortality in men due to primary respiratory cancer.

A continuation of this investigation in the form of a cohort study will consider both the mortality and cancer incidence.

Tsuchiya (1976) has recently reported from Japan a number of incidents of arsenic poisoning associated with a variety of vehicles including powdered milk, soy sauce, well water, mines, and smelters. Effects varied according to the dose, duration, and route of exposure. In the milk incident, infants were exposed to relatively high doses of arsenic in powdered milk and the victims developed acute symptoms of the gastrointestinal tract; in some cases, symptoms of the central nervous system, anemia, neuropathy, cardiovascular and skin changes, but no neoplasms. It is not clear whether the symptoms of the central nervous system were due to the stimulation of the cerebral membrane or to organic changes of the cerebral parenchyma. It is important to note that the development of some possible changes of the brain as indicated by EEG and possibly by the higher incidence of epilepsy occurred at a later stage—as late as 15 yr after clinical changes had disappeared. No other study has reported the development of chronic encephalopathy among heavily exposed children or adults.

Another important question after having reviewed these episodes is whether arsenic is related to the production of liver cirrhosis. In incidents reported in Japan, there is no increased prevalence of liver cirrhosis among those exposed to arsenic. In the well water incident, the married couple who had been drinking water containing 0.125 ppm arsenic showed liver cirrhosis (the husband) and Banti syndrome (the wife). However, since no cases of either disease have been observed among those who suffered heavier exposure, the relationship between these diseases and arsenic is still open to question.

In the soy sauce incident, it was noted that the symptoms improved even while the ingestion of the contaminated soy sauce was still in progress. The mechanism of this phenomenon should be further investigated.

The report on the increased prevalence of abnormal EMG findings is also of interest since prolongation of electric conduction velocity has been reported in persons whose blood lead level was lower than 70 μg/100 ml.

Since there have been no other reports on the increased risk of lung cancer due to arsenic among occupationally exposed workers in Japan, and also since the induction of lung cancer by arsenic in animal experiments has not been successful, the direct relationship between arsenic and lung cancer is still open to question. In the Saganoseki copper smelter incident, attention was drawn to the fact that smelter workers had also been exposed rather heavily to substances other than arsenic, including polynuclear organic substances, sulfur dioxide and possibly to other chemical substances.

Mutagenicity Petres and Berger (1972) and Petres and Hundeiker (1968) have reported chromosomal breakage in human leukocyte cultures after short-term *in vitro* exposure to sodium arsenate and in cultures obtained after long-term exposure to arsenical compounds *in vivo*. The cytotoxic and mutagenic effects of sodium arsenate were tested *in vitro* on phytohemagglutinin-stimulated lymphocyte cultures in concentrations of 0.05–30 μg/ml of culture medium. It was reported that 33% of metaphase plates were disrupted at 0.1 μg/ml and 80–100% at 2 μg/ml or greater. The "mitosis index" and the "(^{3}H) thymidine labeling index" were decreased.

Petres *et al.* (1976) did chromosome analyses of lymphocytes from patients who had been exposed to arsenic. They showed frequent structural and numerical aberrations even following an interval of decades since the last exposure.

The *in vitro* addition of sodium arsenate induced the same chromosome changes in lymphocyte cultures from healthy subjects. Radioactive incorporation studies showed that arsenate was able to inhibit dose-dependently the incorporation of radioactively-labeled nucleotide in

RNA and DNA. Beyond that, arsenic blocked the cells in the S- and G-phase.

A general explanation for the inhibitory effect of inorganic arsenic on cell metabolism is the known strong affinity of arsenic to enzymes, especially to those containing sulfhydryl groups. These studies require attention and further investigation.

The overall significance of these chromosomal studies is difficult to assess, because many unrelated compounds may cause similar effects. The fact that arsenic compounds have caused chromosomal damage in a number of biologic systems, however, should alert toxicologists to a possible role of arsenic in chemically induced mutagenesis.

In vivo studies were made on 34 patients at the University of Freiburg skin clinic (Petres *et al.*, 1970). Thirteen of these patients had had intensive arsenic therapy for psoriasis, some more than 20 yr before the experiment. The control group (21 patients) consisted of 14 psoriasis patients and 7 with eczema, none of whom had had arsenic treatment. Phytohemagglutinin-stimulated lymphocyte cultures were prepared from each patient for evaluation of chromosomal aberrations. The incidence of aberrations was remarkably greater in the cultures of patients who had been treated with arsenic.

Paton and Allison (1972) investigated the effect of sodium arsenate, sodium arsenite, and acetylarsan on chromosomes in cultures of human leukocytes and diploid fibroblasts. Sublethal doses of the arsenicals were added to leukocyte and fibroblast cultures at varous times between 2 and 48 h before fixation. In leukocyte cultures treated with sodium arsenite at $0.29–1.8 \times 10^{-8}$ *M* for the last 48 h of the culture period, 60% of 148 metaphases examined were found to have chromatid breaks. No significant number of breaks were found in cultures treated with sodium arsenate at 0.58×10^{-8} *M*, the highest nontoxic concentration. Chromosomal damage was observed in diploid fibroblasts to which sodium arsenite was added to the medium for the last 24 h of culture; chromatid breaks were found in 20% of 459 metaphases examined. However, treatment with acetylarsan at 6.0×10^{-8} *M* resulted in 20% chromatid breaks in 50 metaphases examined.

Environmental exposure to arsenicals has been correlated with a high skin cancer risk among populations exposed to sunlight. These observations suggest that arsenic might interfere with the repair of damage to DNA (mostly thymine dimers) resulting from the ultraviolet rays in sunlight. To test this hypothesis Rossman *et al.* (1976) have used strains of *E. coli*, differing from each other only in one or more repair fuctions, to study the interactions. Cultures of *E. coli* were exposed to UV light and then plated in the presence or absence of sodium arsenite. Survival after irradiation of wild-type *E. coli* (WP) was significantly decreased by 0.5 m*M* arsenite. This effect was also seen in strains unable to carry out excision repair, suggesting that arsenite inhibits one or more steps in the postreplication repair pathways. This was confirmed by the finding that arsenite has no effect on the postirradiation survival of a *recA* mutant, which does not carry out postreplication repair.

Mutagenesis after UV-irradiation depends on the *recA*$^+$ and *lex*$^+$ genes. Arsenite decreases mutagenesis in strains containing these genes. In order to determine its mechanism of action, Rossman *et al.* studied dose–response relationships of arsenite on a number of cellular functions. The most sensitive cellular functions found were the induction of β-galactosidase and the synthesis of RNA. Since error-prone repair in *E. coli* is an inducible process, the inhibition of mutagenesis after UV irradiation may be the result of inhibition of messenger RNA.

Since arsenite inhibits DNA repair in *E. coli*, specifically postreplication repair, this may be a possible mechanism through which it influences the induction of cancer.

Toxic Effects in Animals

Arsenic appears to be second only to lead in importance as a toxicant in farm and household animals (Buck *et al.*, 1973; Hatch and Funnell, 1969). Some of the more common sources of arsenic poisoning include grass clippings from lawns that have been treated with arsenical crabgrass control preparations; grass, weeds, shrubbery, and other foliage that have been sprayed with arsenical herbicides (Buck, 1969); dipping of animals in vats that even years before had been charged with arsenic trioxide; and soils heavily contaminated with arsenic, either from the burning of arsenic formulations in rubbage piles or through the application of arsenical pesticides to orchards and truck gardens (Clarke and Clarke, 1967; Radeleff, 1970). Arsenical compounds dissolved in water are much more readily absorbed, and thus more toxic than when incorporated into feed (Buck *et al.* 1973).

In practice, the most dangerous arsenical preparations are dips, herbicides, and defoliants, in which the arsenic is in a highly soluble trivalent form, usually arsenite. Animals often seek out and eat such materials as insulation, rodent bait, and dirt and foliage that have been contaminated with arsenic (Buck, *et al.*, 1973).

Animals that are weak, debilitated, and dehydrated are much more susceptible to arsenic poisoning than normal animals, probably because renal excretion is reduced.

Arsenic poisoning in most animals is usually manifested by an acute or subacute syndrome. Arsenic affects tissues that are rich in oxidative systems, primarily the alimentary tract, kidneys, liver, lungs, and skin. It is a potent capillary poison; although all capillary beds may be involved, the splanchnic area is most commonly affected. Capillary damage and dilatation result from transudation of plasma into the intestinal tract and from sharply reduced blood volume. The capillary transudation of plasma results in the formation of vesicles and edema of the gastrointestinal mucosa, which eventually lead to epithelial sloughing and discharge of the plasma into the gastrointestinal tract. (Radeleff, 1970). Blood pressure usually falls to the point of shock, and cardiac muscle becomes weakened; these effects contribute to circulatory failure.

Toxic arsenic nephrosis is more commonly seen in small animals and man than in farm animals. Glomerular capillaries dilate, allowing the escape of plasma; this results from the loss of fluid through other capillary beds, and the low blood pressure contributes to the oliguria that is characteristic of arsenic poisoning. The urine usually contains protein, red blood cells, and casts (Buck *et al.*, 1973).

After percutaneous exposure, capillary dilatation and degeneration may result in blistering and edema, after which the skin may become dry and papery. The skin may then crack and bleed, providing a choice site for secondary bacterial invaders (Radeleff, 1970).

In subacute arsenic poisoning, animals may live for several days and show depression, anorexia, watery diarrhea, and increased urination followed by anuria, dehydration, thirst, partial paralysis of the rear limbs, trembling, stupor, coldness of extremities, and subnormal temperature. The stools may contain shreds of intestinal mucosa and blood.

Characteristic gross effects associated with inorganic, aliphatic, and aromatic trivalent arsenic poisoning include localized or general reddening of the gastric mucosa, reddening of the small-intestinal mucosa (especially the first few feet of the duodenum), fluid and often foul-smelling gastrointestinal contents, a soft yellow liver, and red edematous lungs. Occasionally, in acute poisoning, no gross changes are noted post mortem. The inflammation is usually followed by edema, rupture of the blood vessels, and necrosis of the mucosa and submucosa. This necrosis sometimes progresses to perforation of the stomach or intestine. The gastrointestinal contents may include blood and shreds of mucosa. There may occasionally be hemorrhages on all surfaces of the heart and on the peritoneum (Clarke and Clarke, 1967).

Histopathologic changes include edema of the gastrointestinal mucosa and submucosa, necrosis and sloughing of mucosal epithelium, renal tubular degeneration, hepatic fatty changes and necrosis, and capillary degeneration in vascular beds of the gastrointestinal tract, skin, and other organs (Buck *et al.*, 1973; Radeleff, 1970).

The work of Schroeder *et al.* (1968) and Peoples (1964) indicates that the rat may be unique in its susceptibility to and metabolism of arsenic compounds. Schroeder *et al.* noted that, although rats consuming water containing arsenite at 5 ppm accumulated arsenic at 27-47 ppm in their body tissues, they developed no signs of toxicosis and survived a normal 3.5-yr life span. Peoples showed that the rat is unique in its low rate of excretion of arsenic. Both reported that the blood of rats tended to accumulate high concentrations (100–300 ppm) of arsenic. This is not observed in humans. The low rate of arsenic excretion by the rat is probably due to fixation of 80–90% in the hemoglobin, which must break down before arsenic is released. These experiments are sufficient to cast doubt on the extrapolation of data from arsenic experiments involving rats to man.

Several phenylarsonic formulations have been used as feed additives for disease control and improvement of weight gain in swine and poultry since the mid-1940's. These phenylarsonic acids and their salts include arsanilic acid, 3-nitro-4-hydroxyphenylarsonic acid, 4-nitro-phenylarsonic acid, and 4-ureido-1-phenylarsonic acid.

There remains considerable controversy regarding the mode of action of the phenylarsonic compounds. However, they seem to have an action different from that of inorganic, aliphatic, and aromatic trivalent arsenic compounds. The arsenic incorporated in the feed additives is in the pentavalent form, and it is likely that the phenylarsonic compounds have their primary action as pentavalent arsenicals; this may account for their distinctive effects in birds and animals. Some workers have suggested that both the toxicity and the efficiency of these compounds are due to their degradation and reduction to inorganic trivalent forms (Eagle and Doak, 1951; Harvey, 1965; and Voegtlin and Thompson, 1923). Others have clearly established that these compounds are excreted unchanged by chickens and that there is no evidence that they are converted to inorganic arsenic (Moody and Williams, 1964a; Moody and Williams, 1964b; Overby and Fredrickson, 1963, 1965; and Overby and Straube, 1965). Similar experiments by other workers with rats, rabbits, and swine indicate that the phenylarsonic compounds are for the most part excreted unchanged by the kidneys, although some apparently undergo a limited biotransformation (Moody and Williams, 1964b).

Because pentavalent arsenic compounds do not readily react with sulfhydryl groups and because the phenylarsonic acids are apparently excreted unchanged, one must conclude that the mechanism of their action is something other than interaction with sulfhydryl containing enzymes and proteins.

Clinical signs of phenylarsonic toxicosis in swine and poultry include incoordination, inability to control body and limb movements, and ataxia. After a few days, swine and poultry may become paralyzed, but will continue to eat and drink. Arsanilic acid and its sodium salt may produce blindness but this is rarely seen when it is used as one of the most common feed additives. Erythema of the skin, especially in white animals, and sensitivity to sunlight may be present. The clinical signs are reversible up to a point. Removing the excess arsenical will result in recovery within a few days, unless the clinical signs have progressed to partial or complete paralysis due to irreversible peripheral nerve degeneration (Buck, 1969b; Oliver and Roe, 1957).

Chronic arsenic toxicosis has not been encountered significantly in animals.

Gainer and Pry (1972) reported that virus-infected mice treated subcutaneously with large doses of arsenicals had higher mortality rates than unexposed controls. Viral diseases so affected by arsenic were pseudorabies, encephalomyocarditis, and St. Louis encephalitis. The effects were similar when 3-nitro-4-hydroxyphenylarsonic salt (75–100 ppm) was added to drinking water. Gainer (1972) reported that sodium arsenite inhibited the induction of interferon in rabbit kidney cell cultures. It was found, however, that, although high concentrations of arsenite inhibited the action of exogenous mouse interferon added to cultures of mouse embryo cells, low concentrations of arsenite increased the antiviral activity of low concentrations of interferon.

Carcinogenicity Animal studies have not demonstrated carcinogenicity of arsenic compounds even when administered at near the maximal tolerated dosage for long periods. There are two exceptions, however. Halver (1962) reported the occurrence of hepatomas in trout fed a synthetic diet containing carbarsone at 480 mg/100 g of diet. The data were reviewed by Kraybill and Shimkin (1964). Of 50 trout exposed to carbarsone, 5 developed hepatomas. There were no hepatomas in a large control group fed the synthetic diet without carbarsone. Osswald and Goerttler (1971) reported that subcutaneous injections of sodium arsenate in pregnant Swiss mice caused a considerable increase in the incidence of leukemia in both the mothers and their offspring. A 0.005% aqueous sodium arsenate solution was injected daily during pregnancy for a total of 20 injections, each containing arsenic at 0.5 mg/kg of body weight. Some groups of offspring from the arsenic-treated females were given an additional 20 subcutaneous injections of sodium arsenate (arsenic equivalent 0.5 mg/kg) at weekly intervals. Leukemia occurred in 11 of 24 mothers (46%), 7 of 34 male offspring (21%), and 6 of 37 female offspring (16%). In the offspring given the additional 20 injections, 17 of 41 males (41%) and 24 of 50 females (48%) developed leukemia. Leukemia developed in only three of 35 male (9%) and in none of 20 female offspring of untreated control mice. Furthermore, 11 of 19 mice (58%) developed lymphoma after 20 weekly intravenous injections, each containing 0.5 mg/kg of arsenic as sodium arsenate.

Long-term studies of effects of arsanilic acid on chickens, pigs, and rats were reported by Frost *et al.* (1967). No adverse effects were seen in the chickens and pigs after 4 yr of feeding, nor in pigs fed 0.01% arsanilic acid in their diets for three generations. Male and female weanling rats from the F_2 generation of a six-generation breeding study in which 0.01% and 0.05% arsanilic acid was fed were held on the 0.01% arsanilic acid diet or on the control diet for 116 weeks. The overall tumor incidence was the same in all groups and resembled the historical incidence of tumors in the colony, 35–45%.

Boutwell (1963) used female mice known to be highly susceptible to skin tumors in a test for cocarcinogenicity of potassium arsenite. It was tested as an initiator, both orally by stomach tube (a total of 2.4 mg in 5 days) and dermally (a total of 1.2 mg in eight applications during 5 days). The initiating exposure was followed by topical application of croton oil twice a week for 18 weeks. He also tested potassium arsenite as a promoter by daily applications (a total of 2.3 mg/week) after a single 75-μg dose of dimethylbenzanthracene (DMBA). The prolonged skin applications of potassium arsenite were hyperkeratotic and ulcerogenic. Other experiments were done to determine whether arsenic would increase the yield of skin cancers caused by a suboptimal regimen of DMBA plus croton oil given either at the time of DMBA initiation or during the 24-week period of croton oil promotion. Under the latter condition, the mice were fed potassium arsenite at 169 mg/kg of food. In no case was there an effect of arsenite on skin carcinogenesis in these experiments. Many tumors developed in the positive control mice, beginning as early as 6 weeks after treatment began.

Baroni *et al.* (1963) conducted similar studies with male and female Swiss mice, testing the oral effects of potassium arsenite (100 ppm in drinking water) as an initiator with croton oil promotion and as a promoter for DMBA and urethane initiation. Local skin applications of sodium arsenate were tested as a promoter after initiation with DMBA or urethane. The arsenicals had no effect on carcinogenesis, and only a very slight degree of keratosis was observed.

Milner (1969) used three strains of mice that differed in susceptibility to the induction of skin tumors with the application of methycholanthrene-impregnated paraffin disks to the skin for 2–3 weeks. The treated site was transplanted syngeneically and observed for 8 weeks for tumor formation. Arsenic trioxide (100 ppm in drinking water) was administered either during methylcholanthrene exposure, after transplantation, or both. Arsenic exposure was associated with a small increase in papillomas in the low-susceptibility strain, a small decrease in the high-susceptibility strain, and no effect in the intermediate-susceptibility strain.

Byron *et al.* (1967) fed sodium arsenite at 15–250 ppm and sodium arsenate at 30–400 ppm to Osborne–Mendel rats in a 2-yr study. No carcinogenic activity of either material was found. These investigators also did a 2-yr arsenic feeding experiment on dogs, with negative results. This length of time, however, is not adequate for studying carcinogenesis in dogs.

Hueper and Payne (1962) incorporated arsenic trioxide in the drinking water (either plain or with 12% ethanol) of rats and mice. The initial concentration of 4 mg/liter was increased by 2 mg/liter each month, to a maximum of 34 mg/liter at 15 months. Thus, the daily intake of arsenic trioxide ranged from 0.1–0.8 mg. The administration of arsenic trioxide was continued for 24 months. Neither the rats nor the mice developed any cancers in suspected target organs—skin, lungs, and liver.

Kanisawa and Schroeder (1967) and Schroeder *et al.* (1968) found no carcinogenic effects of potassium arsenite at 5 ppm in drinking water in mice or rats exposed from weaning to senescence.

Kroes *et al.* (1974) studied the carcinogenicity of lead arsenate and sodium arsenate with SPF-Wistar-derived male and female rats. In addition, some groups were intubated with a subcarcinogenic dose of diethylnitrosamine to determine synergistic action leading to lung tumors. Food intake and body weights were recorded, and complete gross and microscopic examinations were made on all animals. Lead arsenate that was incorporated in the diet at 1,850 ppm was toxic and caused increased mortality; one adenoma of the renal cortex and one bile duct carcinoma were found in this group. No carcinogenicity was associated with the feeding of lead arsenate at 463 ppm or sodium arsenate at 416 ppm. No synergism with the nitrosamine was observed.

In summary, there is epidemiologic evidence of the carcinogenic action of arsenic on the skin and lungs of humans, on the basis of experience with the medicinal use of inorganic trivalent arsenic, occupational groups exposed to inorganic trivalent or pentavalent arsenic dusts, and populations exposed to high concentrations of arsenic in drinking water. In most instances, however, the exposures to arsenic have been concurrent with exposures to other agents, and the available data do not exclude the possibility that cofactors are important in the carcinogenic response to arsenic. Differences in the type and distribution of tumors, attributed to the ingestion of arsenic, raise serious questions with respect to a simple etiologic relation of arsenic to the various findings. There is no established procedure to demonstrate carcinogenicity of arsenic in experimental animals. This phenomenon remains an enigma. One must conclude either that arsenic is not a carcinogen for animals or that circumstances not yet understood are essential to demonstrate a role for arsenic in experimental carcinogenesis.

Mutagenicity Most of the research on mutagenesis of arsenic has centered on chromosomal reactions to sodium arsenate. There are no data based on the host-mediated assay or the dominant-lethal technique.

Levan (1945) treated root meristem cultures of *Allium cepa* for 4 h with an unspecified arsenic salt at 10 concentrations, from lethal to no-effect. Chromosomal changes were observed, including spindle disturbances and metaphase arrests. Similar effects were observed after treatment with salts of 24 other metals.

Arsenate has also been found to increase the total frequency of exchanged chromosomes in *Drosophila melanogaster* treated with selenocystine (Walker and Bradly, 1969), and several organic arsenicals have a synergistic effect on the number of abnormalities in barley chromosomes caused by ethylmethane sulfonate (Moutschen and Degraeve, 1965).

Teratogenicity Franke *et al.* (1936) performed what might be called the first teratogenic study of an arsenic compound, when they tested the effect of sodium arsenite on the development of chick embryos. Injection of sublethal concentrations of arsenic into the eggs produced ectopic conditions, but no monstrosities, as are produced by selenium.

Ridgway and Karnofsky (1952) found that injection of sodium arsenate into embryonate chicken eggs at 4 days in doses of 0.20 mg/egg caused no specific gross abnormalities in the resulting embryos 14 days later. Growth retardation, impaired feather growth, and abdominal swelling were noted.

Recent studies have demonstrated teratogenic effects of intravenous administration of sodium arsenate in mice and hamsters (Ferm and Carpenter, 1968; Ferm *et al.*, 1971). Single doses (15–20 mg/kg) were administered on the eighth day of gestation, and the results were observed on the fifteenth day: there was a high incidence of anencephaly and other defects. Up to 80% of the embryos had anencephaly; up to 65%, rib malformations; up to 30%, exencephaly; and approximately

20%, genitourinary malformations. Incidences of renal agenesis and cleft lip and palate were lower. Further analysis of the teratogenic consequences of sodium arsenate by Holmberg and Ferm (1969) showed that sodium selenite injected at 2 mg/kg simultaneously with a teratogenic dose of sodium arsenate decreased the number of fetal resorptions and congenital malformations caused by the arsenical.

In mouse studies, Hood and Bishop (1972) administered a single dose of sodium arsenate or arsenite by intraperitoneal injection on a specific day from the sixth to the twelfth day of gestation and observed the results on the eighteenth day. The injections given on the ninth day were most teratogenic; 60% of 96 implantations were resorbed or dead, and 63% were grossly malformed. The defects included exencephaly, micrognathia, protruding tongue, agnathia, open eye, cleft lip, fused vertebrae, and forked ribs. Mice that received injections of distilled water served as controls. Although teratogenic effects were seen at 45 mg/kg, 25 mg/kg was without effect. Sodium arsenite was more effective, which indicated that the extent of fetal anomalies caused by sodium arsenite at 10 mg/kg was comparable with that caused by sodium arsenate at 45 mg/kg. Hood and Pike (1972) reported that BAL, when administered to mice at 50 mg/kg by intraperitoneal injection within 4 h of sodium arsenate at 40 mg/kg, prevented the arsenic-induced teratogenesis.

Potassium arsenate was fed to four pregnant ewes at 0.5 mg/kg during most of pregnancy without effect (James *et al.* 1966).

Interactions Moxon (1938) first reported the protective effect of arsenic against selenium poisoning when he found that sodium arsenite (5 ppm) in drinking water reduced liver damage in rats on a diet containing selenium at 15 ppm in seleniferous wheat. Moxon and DuBois (1939) demonstrated that arsenic was unique in its ability to prevent selenium toxicity. The protective effect of arsenic against dietary selenium was not seen when the arsenic was added to the diet, instead of the drinking water (Ganther and Baumann, 1962). Frost (1967) reported that selenium and arsenic are additive in toxicity if both are added to the drinking water.

Ganther and Bauman (1962) reported that excretion of selenium into the gastrointestinal tract was markedly stimulated by arsenic when both elements were injected parenterally. Levander and Bauman (1966a,b) showed that this increased selenium excretion occurred through the bile.

Sodium arsenite is the most effective in enhancing biliary excretion of selenium, but arsenate and the phenylarsonates were also somewhat effective. This leads one to question the role of phenylarsonic feed additives in exacerbation of selenium deficiency in animals. Surprisingly, Muth *et al.* (1971) reported that sodium arsenate (1 ppm) added to a selenium-deficient diet significantly reduced the incidence of myopathy in lambs. This work has not been confirmed.

Beneficial Effects A number of older publications suggested that small amounts of arsenic may have beneficial effects in human and animal health (Underwood, 1971). Until recently, however, there has been no proof of the essentiality of arsenic in mammals. Hove *et al.* (1938) concluded that, if arsenic were essential to the rat, the requirement must be somewhere below 2 μg daily. Schroeder and Balassa (1966) reported that rats and mice grew well when they received only 0.26 μg of arsenic per 100 g of body weight per day in food (0.026 mg/kg). In a recent preliminary report, Nielsen *et al.* (1975) presented evidence that rats require arsenic at about 30 ppb in a synthetic diet. The deficiency signs were rough hair coat, retarded growth, splenomegaly, reduced hematocrit, and increased red-cell fragility.

The phenylarsonic compounds have been used as feed additives for disease control and improvement of weight gain in swine and poultry since the mid-1940's (Bird *et al.*, 1949; Frost, 1967; Morehouse, 1949).

ANALYSIS

Much difficulty has been experienced with chemical analyses for arsenic, especially in biologic samples. Improvements in instrumentation, especially atomic-absorption spectrophotometers, have facilitated such analyses somewhat. In most cases, arsenic determinations on drinking-water samples are less complicated than those on biologic samples.

Determination of Arsenic in Drinking Water

The current National Interim Primary Drinking Water Regulation for arsenic, 50 μg/liter, is 5 times as great as that for selenium. As was the case for selenium, the *1975 Chemical Analysis of Interstate Carrier Water Supply Systems* (USEPA, 1975) indicated that the maximal allowable concentration was seldom exceeded, although in a few instances the method of analysis had a minimal detection limit higher than the standard.

One of the most sensitive methods for arsenic analysis in water is the atomic-absorption procedure of Fernandez (1973). The method has an absolute detection limit of 10 ng, which, for a 20-ml sample, provides a solution detection limit of 0.5 μg/liter—a hundred times less than the drinking-water standard of 50 μg/liter. The sensitivity can be increased by using an electrodeless discharge lamp, giving an absolute detection limit of 3 ng and a concentration detection limit of 0.15 μg/liter. The method applies to both inorganic and organic arsenic. There are few interference problems with drinking-water samples.

Determination of Arsenic in Biologic Samples

A modification of the Fernandez (1973) atomic-absorption method has been adopted by the National Institute for Occupational Safety and Health (1974) for urine and hair samples. The samples are digested in acid: after acid removal, the arsenic is converted to arsine with metallic zinc or sodium borohydride, $NaBH_4$. The arsine is flushed into the burner of the atomic-absorption spectrophotometer for measurement. As little as 1 μg of arsenic per liter of urine can be detected by this method.

Colorimetric methods can detect as little as 10 μg/liter of arsenic in urine (National Institute for Occupational Safety and Health, 1974; Horwitz, 1970). The samples are digested as stated above, and the arsine generated reacts with ammonium molybdate, sulfuric acid, and hydrazine sulfate, to develop a chromophore with an absorption peak at 845 nm; or the arsine reacts with silver diethyldithiocarbamate, and the chromophore concentration is determined at 522 nm. (If pyridine is present, an altered chromophore is measured at 560 nm.) At concentrations approaching the arsenic concentration, antimony will interfere with the colorimetric assays.

CONCLUSIONS AND RECOMMENDATIONS

The evidence for an association between arsenic and disease in some human populations has been further strengthened by recent epidemiological studies such as those conducted in the waters of Puget Sound, in local water supplies such as those in Lassen County, California; Perham, Minnesota; Lane County, Oregon; Antofagasta, Chile; and on the southwest coast of Taiwan. Skin lesions, including cancer, and a circulatory disorder referred to as "blackfoot" are major clinical problems where chronic exposure to arsenic exists. Human disease associated with arsenic is not exactly duplicated in animals, although misuse of arsenicals results in disease in dogs and in cattle. There is no animal model for study of arsenic-induced cancer. Arsenic causes fetal death at high doses and malformations at lower exposure in hamsters, mice, and rats. Bacterial systems have revealed that arsenic interferes with DNA repair. The different forms of arsenic that exist in the environment may account for differences in clinical manifestations between different localities.

Environmental sources of arsenic, aside from those listed above include some coal-fired power plants and nonferrous smelting operations. Natural sources include volcanoes and hot springs.

Although various analytical techniques are available for speciation of some arsenicals in air and water, others require better methods for accurate analysis at low concentrations. A system for interlaboratory cross-checking for analytic accuracy is needed. Several factors impinge on attempts to evaluate analytical data from human populations such as media being examined (blood, urine, hair, nails), route and dose level, and a requirement for analytical methods capable of measuring total arsenic absorption from all routes of exposure.

There are very little data on kinetics and metabolism of arsenic and its compounds, although it appears that much of a dose is excreted via the urine; some is degraded and some may be excreted without metabolic degradation. Arsenic trioxide and pentoxide, in humans, appears to be excreted mainly in the methylated form.

There is some epidemiological evidence that high concentrations of arsenic in drinking water are associated with skin cancer. When the level was reduced by water treatment to 80 μg/liter, the incidence was reduced but still detectable. The existence of other cocarcinogens in these water supplies has not been extensively studied. If the time factors for the development of cancer are shown to be reasonable, then the current interim standard of 50 μg/liter may not provide an adequate margin of safety.

RECOMMENDATIONS FOR RESEARCH

1. Improvement and standardization of speciation techniques for analyses and application to various biological materials.
2. Interlaboratory cross-checking of the accuracy of the many methods using different matrices.
3. More accurate determination of quantities of environmental arsenic, their sources and fate.
4. Studies about metabolism in man and animals; rates and mechanisms of methylation–demethylation in man, animals, and ecosystems. Transfer of arsenic species across tissue barriers, absorption, distribution, and excretion.
5. Investigations about interactions of arsenic and other environmental factors that may account for difference in human clinical observations, and effects of diet, race, and climate.
6. Development of an animal model for carcinogenicity studies with particular reference to arsenic trioxide and pentoxide.

7. Studies about different responses to arsenic by individuals and species, particularly long-term, low-level exposure.

8. Further studies on the effect of arsenic on cellular mechanisms, as well as teratology and mutagenicity studies.

9. More uniform and improved methods for epidemiologic studies, coordinated by an international agency.

Selenium

OCCURRENCE

Selenium is obtained industrially, primarily in conjunction with electrolytic copper refining. Selenium is used in manufacture of electronics equipment (rectifiers, photocells, and xerography), steel (for machinability and porosity control), pigments, glass (for decolorization and pigmentation), and ceramics (for colored glazes). It is used principally in elemental form and in such compounds as selenium dioxide, sodium selenite, sodium selenate, and iron selenate (Cooper, 1967).

Selenium has a profound effect on animals, and either a deficiency or an excess can result in adverse biologic responses. There is a relatively narrow margin of safety for many species, and it is conceivable that an excess of selenium in drinking water can constitute a potential danger. Until recently, selenium was included in a list of carcinogic agents by the Food and Drug Administration (FDA), because of reports of animal research in the United States and Russia (Frost, 1960; Frost, 1972; Tscherkes *et al.*, 1963; Volgarev and Tscherkes, 1967). The evidence of carcinogenicity of selenium in these studies was tenuous and widely debated. The FDA now permits the addition of selenium to the feeds of turkeys, chickens, and swine, and, because these feeds are mixed in commercial milling operations, the distribution of selenium may become wider than is now anticipated. Selenium can reach toxic concentrations in water from wells drilled through seleniferous shales rich in soluble selenium, and other sources of water contamination are known. Therefore, a better understanding of sources, distribution, metabolism, and health effects is required.

Water-soluble selenium has been identified in soils (Olson *et al.*, 1942) and in some salt deposits (Byers *et al.*, 1938), and the presence of selenium in other geologic materials has also been documented (Beath, 1946). There is a wide variation in concentration of selenium, depending on geologic location. Thus, groundwaters and surface waters may contain significant amounts of selenium, particularly in areas where there is an

TABLE V-13 Selenium in the Natural Environment

Material	Selenium Concentration, ppm	
	Average	Range
Igneous rock	0.05	—
Shale	0.60	—
Sandstone	0.05	—
Limestone	0.08	—
Coal (ash)	3.3	0.46–10.6
Phosphate rock	19.0	—
Soil	0.1–2.0	<0.4–1,200
Surface water	0.0002	0.0001–0.4
Forage grasses	0.26	<0.01–9.0
Forage legumes	0.2	0.075–0.7
Vegetables and fruits	0.05	0.01–0.20

(From Cannon, 1974)

excess of selenium in rocks and soils; in other areas, there may be little (if any) detectable selenium in the water.

There is little in the literature to indicate that surface waters contain toxic amounts of selenium; in fact (Table V-13), it is likely that there is an insufficient amount of selenium in the water alone to provide the nutrient requirements of most animals (Cannon, 1974), but concentrations may vary in different places. An extensive study by the Department of Health, Education, and Welfare involving analyses of 535 samples of water from major U.S. watersheds indicated that over a 4-yr period only two samples contained selenium at more than 10 μg/liter of water, the U.S. drinking-water standard (Lakin and Davidson, 1967). In another study, over a 2-yr period, it was reported that there was a maximum of 10 and a mean of 8 μg/liter in 194 public finished water supplies (Taylor, 1963). In a study in Oregon, the majority of farm samples of water had less than 1 μg/liter (Hadjimarkos and Bonhorst, 1961). This study extended over a 2-yr period and included samples from three counties. In Germany and in Australia, village water supplies have been reported to contain from less than 1 to 5.3 μg/liter (Oelschager and Menke, 1969; Edmond, 1967). River water may contain high concentrations of selenium where irrigation drainage from seleniferous soils empties into it; values of 2,000 μg/liter have been reported (Williams and Byers, 1935).

The water from some springs and shallow wells contains selenium at more than 100 μg/liter (Byers *et al.*, 1938; Miller and Byers, 1935; Morette and Diven, 1965), but deep wells may contain only a few micrograms per liter. Water from some Wyoming wells contains enough selenium to be poisonous to man and livestock (Beath, 1962a), but these are in seleniferous areas. In another report from Wyoming, a high concentration of selenate in well water on an Indian reservation was associated with the loss of hair and nails in children (Beath, 1962).

Another source of selenium is the effluent from sewage plants which may contribute as much as 280 μg/liter in raw sewage, 45 μg/liter in primary effluent, and 5 μg/liter in secondary effluent (Baird *et al.*, 1972).

Of 418 samples obtained from interstate carrier systems, only one failed to meet the mandatory drinking-water standard (Chemical Analysis of Interstate Carrier Water Supply Systems, USEPA, 1975).

It appears from a large number of reports that the selenium content of ocean water is very low. This is attributed primarily to the precipitation of selenite by oxides of iron and manganese (Goldschmidt and Strock, 1935; Ishibashi *et al.*, 1953; Strock, 1935).

In areas where the selenium content of the soil is high, the water in lakes may vary widely in selenium content (Abu-Erreish, 1967). Although the hypothesis that precipitation of selenium by various means results in low concentration in some cases, this has not been documented. Emerging data indicate that the microbial environment of lake-bottom sediment may influence selenium concentrations in the lake water (Chau *et al.*, 1976).

Available reports indicate little danger of toxicity from amounts of selenium in finished waters, but wells drilled through seleniferous shale containing soluble selenium may have concentrations of selenium high enough to be of concern. Furthermore, finished water for domestic consumption usually is not analyzed for selenium, and, although it appears that most waters have relatively low concentrations, in some cases the selenium may approach toxic concentrations. Recent studies by the U.S. Geological Survey reported that some farms near Denver, Colorado, had high selenium concentrations in their water supplies. Some of the water on a South Dakota Indian reservation contained as much as 210 μg/liter (U.S. Public Health Drinking Water Standards, 1972).

Water that is consumed by human populations rarely constitutes a significant source of selenium. Even with the very low concentrations of selenium found in rivers, there is a significant transport of the element into oceans. This has been estimated at as much as 8,000 tons of selenium per year discharged into the oceans from rivers (Bertine, 1971). For this reason, aside from quality, water is important in leaching and transporting the element under some conditions.

Selenium occurs naturally in the following oxidation states: selenide (-II), elemental selenium (0), selenite (+IV), and selenate (+VI). Recent published literature indicates that problems of environmental contamination are very likely minimized because nearly all organic selenium is in the -II oxidation state; this decomposes to elemental selenium, very little of which is absorbed (Klayman and Gunther, 1973; Okamota and Gunther, 1972). Compounds of major concern to environmental toxicologists are selenite (+IV) and selenate (+VI). These are the forms that occur most often in water. The +II oxidation state has not been reported to occur naturally.

Selenate (+VI) is taken up from water or soil by plants and may reach toxic concentrations (Moxon *et al.*, 1939). Selenite (+IV) salts are less soluble than the corresponding selenates. Of special interest is the low solubility of the ferric selenites (Geering *et al.*, 1968). It is also of considerable importance that selenite is rapidly reduced to elemental selenium under acid conditions by mild reducing agents, such as ascorbic acid. It is likely that selenite will either form insoluble compounds with ferric oxide or be reduced to insoluble elemental selenium, either of which would minimize the potential hazard in water.

Because elemental selenium is practically insoluble and may be derived by high-temperature decomposition of some natural materials, a buffer of safety for water and other environmental sources is provided. For example, in the combustion of fossil fuels or organic materials, selenium dioxide, which is formed from elemental selenium, is reduced to elemental selenium by the sulfur dioxide that is formed during the combustion of these materials (Weiss *et al.*, 1971). The amount of sulfur dioxide formed during such combustion is always greatly in excess of the amount required for the reduction of the selenium dioxide. For these reasons, elemental selenium appears to be a major inert form that provides a wide margin of safety by serving as a sink for selenium introduced into the environment.

Selenide (-II) occurs as hydrogen selenide, which is a volatile acid with toxic fumes. Hydrogen selenide, however, decomposes rapidly in air to form elemental selenium and water, thus eliminating the hazard from this compound for most people, except those involved in industrial installations. It appears that a large amount of insoluble selenide and possibly elemental selenium pass through most animals without appreciable absorption; this is particularly so in ruminants (Peterson and Spedding, 1963).

The geochemical behavior of selenium in water resembles that of sulfur. Both are volatile and are emitted as gases during the natural course of volcanic eruption, during the smelting of sulfide ores, and in the burning of coal. It is only where the water-soluble selenate ion occurs in soils that plants can take up significant amounts of it. For this reason, cretaceous shales of a relatively low selenium content produce toxic vegetation, whereas soils that have a much higher selenium content (e.g., in Hawaii and Puerto Rico) do not produce toxic amounts in plants, because the selenium occurs as selenite bound to ferric oxide (Lakin, 1972; Cannon, 1974).

In the +IV state, selenium occurs as organic selenite. Soluble selenites are highly toxic. Selenite binds easily to iron and aluminum, with which it forms stable absorption complexes.

Alkaline water conditions favor the formation of the +VI form, selenate. Selenates are quite soluble, highly toxic, not tightly complexed by sesquioxides, easily leached from soils, and available to plants.

In general, one would expect to find higher amounts of selenium in foods and water in areas that have been designated as seleniferous. The data in a number of reports suggest that feeds that are highest in protein usually are highest in selenium content (Scott and Thompson, 1971). It may be concluded, however, that the selenium concentration in plants depends largely on the concentration and availability of selenium in the soil where the plants are grown. For example, in South Dakota whole milk may contain 1.2 ppm, whole eggs as much as 10 ppm, and vegetables (string beans, lettuce, turnip leaves, and cabbage) from 2 to 100 ppm; the concentrations in the milk and eggs probably reflect that in the feed. A number of investigators have found samples of wheat and wheat products that contain selenium at 1-4 ppm (Lakin and Byers, 1941; Robinson, 1936). Selenium concentrations in the gluten fractions are usually 4–5 times greater than that in the whole wheat.

Foods from nonseleniferous areas contribute little to the overall

TABLE V-14 Selenium Content of Some Foods in the American Diet

Food	Average Selenium Content, ppm (wet wt.)
Vegetables, canned and fresh	0.010 (0.004–0.039)
Fresh garlic	0.249
Mushrooms, canned and fresh	0.118
Fruits, canned and fresh	0.006 (<0.002–0.013)
Cereal products	0.38 (0.026–0.665)
Egg white	0.051
Egg yolk	0.183
Brown sugar	0.11
White sugar	0.003
Cheeses	0.082 (0.052–0.105)
Table cream	0.006
Whole milk	0.012
Meat (excluding kidney)	0.224 (0.116–0.432)
Seafood	0.532 (0.337–0.658)

TABLE V-15 Estimated Selenium Emission Factors[a]

Source	Estimated Selenium Emission Factors
Mining and milling	
Copper	0.015 lb/thousand tons of ore mined
Lead	0.047 Do.
Zinc	0.032 Do.
Phosphate (western)	0.350 Do.
Uranium	0.350 Do.
Smelting and refining	
Copper	0.25 lb/ton of copper produced
Lead	0.05 lb/ton of lead produced
zinc	0.04 lb/ton of zinc produced
Selenium refining	
Primary (from copper by-products)	277 lb/ton of selenium recovered
Secondary	100 Do.
End product manufacturing	
Glass and ceramics	700 lb/ton of selenium consumed
Electronics and electric	2 Do.
Duplicating	2 Do.
Pigments	15 Do.
Iron and steel alloys	1,000 Do.
Other	10 Do.
Other	
Coal	2.90 lb/1,000 tons of coal burned
Oil	0.21 lb/1,000 barrels of oil burned
Incineration	0.02 lb/1,000 tons of refuse burned

[a]Derived from Davis (1972).

dietary intake of selenium. Eggs and milk, fish, various types of meat, poultry, coffee, and tea all vary somewhat in their selenium content, but in general contribute minimally to the dietary intake. Table V-14 lists the selenium content of staple foods of the American diet (Morris and Levander, 1970).

There are occasional cases of industrial exposure to selenium when it is used in relatively high concentrations; the most notable is in copper refining, where selenium is a by-product. Potential industrial sources of exposure to selenium have been reviewed (Davis, 1972; Dudley, 1938). Table V-15 (derived from Davis, 1972) provides estimates of selenium emission factors.

Selenium is not normally used in agriculture, so it is unlikely that agriculture itself will contribute a significant amount to the water supplies. However, now that selenium is being added to the feeds of turkeys, chickens, and swine, some slight increase in soil concentrations may take place; if this occurs, runoff water might increase the selenium content of lakes and streams to a small degree.

METABOLISM

The absorption, distribution, biotransformation, and excretion of selenium in microorganisms, plants, animals, and humans have recently been reviewed in detail (NAS, 1976). The present discussion is focused on selenium metabolism in animals and humans.

Absorption

Both inorganic and organic forms of selenium can be readily absorbed from the gastrointestinal tract. Although little is known about the uptake of ingested selenates, selenites are passively absorbed from mammalian intestine (McConnell and Cho, 1965; Brown *et al.*, 1972). Selenite is absorbed more rapidly by monogastric animals than in ruminant animals, perhaps owing to bacterial reduction of selenite to elemental selenium or other insoluble forms in the ruminant gastrointestinal tract (Wright and Bell, 1966).

Selenocystine is passively absorbed from the intestine, but in the hamster selenomethionine can be absorbed against a concentration gradient; the active absorption of selenomethionine is inhibited by low concentrations of S-methionine (Spencer and Blau, 1962; McConnell and Cho, 1965). Absorption of sodium selenite through rat skin has been reported (Dutkiewicz *et al.*, 1971).

Distribution

In the dog, as selenate is absorbed it binds to plasma albumin, gradually shifts to globulins, and finally becomes associated with red cells (McConnell, 1941; McConnell *et al.*, 1960). The uptake of selenium by red cells varies inversely with dietary concentration (Wright and Bell, 1963), and this relationship has been proposed for several groups of animals and humans (Weswig *et al.*, 1966; Burk *et al.*, 1967; Lopex *et al.*, 1968).

Selenite and selenate, after single subacute administration to rats (McConnell, 1941) and mice (Heinrich and Kelsey, 1955) are distributed largely to the liver, kidneys, muscle mass, gastrointestinal tract, and blood. In rats, selenite distribution to the liver appears to be unaffected by the concentration of selenium in the maintenance diet (0.04–5.04 ppm), but a greater percentage of administered selenite goes to the kidney, blood, and muscles in rats on low-selenium diets, compared with animals maintained at higher selenium concentrations (Hopkins *et al.*, 1966). With chronic administration, selenium is also distributed to the testes (Broyer *et al.*, 1966; Burk *et al.*, 1972).

Selenite distribution within the liver cell has been determined. More than half is in the cytosol and, depending on dose and diet, the rest is variably distributed in other fractions; injected selenite is found more in the mitochondria than in microsomes or nuclei (McConnell and Roth, 1962), whereas, in rats fed a selenium-deficient diet, nuclei and microsomes have about equal amounts of selenium and much more than mitochrondria (Brown and Burk, 1973). Selenium in the liver turns over rapidly.

Selenoamino acids and inorganic selenium are distributed similarly, except that selenomethionine and selenocystine accumulate in the pancreas to a greater extent than selenite (Jacobsson, 1966). When mice are fed alfalfa grown on selenium-75 selenious acid, the radiolabel is found more in kidneys than in liver or pancreas and to a much lesser extent in lungs, heart, spleen, skin, and brain (Jones and Godwin, 1962, 1963).

Studies on selenium distribution in pregnant ewes have demonstrated a placental barrier. The maternal fetal plasma ratio of selenium concentrations sheep was 12:1 for a single fetus and 22:1 in the case of double fetuses (Wright and Bell, 1964). Selenium transfer across the placenta was slow but continuous.

In many instances, the distribution of selenium to tissues and cells depends on the animal's nutritional status regarding selenium; the time after administration is also important, in that selenium distributions shift with time (Wright, 1967).

Excretion

The principal route of excretion of selenium is via the urine. Approximately 40% of the selenate administered to rats is excreted in the urine in the first 24 h, and the rate of excretion is much lower after that (McConnell, 1941). The dietary concentration of selenium has a pronounced effect on excretion; rats maintained on low-selenium diets (0.004 ppm) excreted 6% of a dose of radioselenium in the urine in 10 days, and animals on high-selenium diets (1 ppm) excreted 67% of an equal dose of radioselenium in the same time (Burk *et al.*, 1972). Whether this represents an ability to conserve selenium when intake is low or an increased ability to excrete selenium when intake is high is not clear.

Fecal excretion of selenium by rats is small in most situations other than poisoning (Burk *et al.*, 1972). In swine, fecal excretion of selenium was about 5 times greater when sodium selenite was administered orally than when it was administered intravenously, although the total excretion was the same, regardless of route of administration (Wright and Bell, 1966). Fecal excretion of selenium by sheep was approximately the same as in swine after intravenous injection of sodium selenite, but increased 13-fold after oral administration. Swine absorb selenium better than sheep, and the greater fecal excretion by sheep may be due to bacterial reduction of selenite to insoluble elemental selenium.

Pulmonary excretion of selenium is important only in subacute poisoning and depends on the dietary concentrations of protein, methionine, and selenium (Olson *et al.*, 1963).

Storage

Selenium binds to cystine-rich keratin and consequently is found in hair and nails (McConnell and Kreamer, 1960). When wool is chemically reduced and treated with selenium dioxide, the selenium forms a selenodithio bridge between two cysteine units (R—S—Se—S—R) (Holker and Speakman, 1958).

Radioselenium injected into dogs was retained in hair for as long as 316 days (McConnell and Kreamer, 1960). The effect of diet on the long-term rate of loss of selenium has been studied in rats; increasing the dietary selenium content decreases selenium retention (Burk *et al.*, 1972, 1973). Cattle, sheep, and swine fed inorganic selenium for several weeks take 10–20 weeks to return to baseline tissue selenium concentrations when put on depletion diets; if the animals are fed organic forms of selenium, it takes even longer for tissue concentrations to return to baseline (Kuttler *et al.*, 1961; Hidiroglou *et al.*, 1971; Ku *et al.*, 1972).

Biotransformation

Little is known about the biochemistry of selenium in mammalian systems. At concentrations required nutritionally, selenium is incorporated into specific functional proteins; at higher concentrations, it is incorporated into molecules normally served by sulfur. Selenium analogs are often less stable than sulfur compounds, and this lability may be the basis of toxicity. Selenium biochemistry has been the subject of recent reviews (Stadtman, 1974; NAS, 1976).

By the mechanism used for sulfate ion, microorganisms are capable of activating selenate with adenosine triphosphate (Wilson and Bandurski, 1956), but it is not clear that appreciable amounts of activated selenate (APSe) are reduced to selenite via 3′-phosphoadenosine-5′-phosphoselenate (PAPSe), which would be directly analogous to the recognized reduction of activated sulfate (APS) to sulfite by phosphoadenosine phosphosulfate (PAPS). In animals, PAPS is important in the formation of sulfate esters in the detoxication of foreign compounds and the metabolism of steroids and other indigenous compounds (Lipmann, 1958); the activity of PAPSe, if formed, in formation of selenate esters is not known. Although selenate and selenite ions are absorbed and incorporated into organic molecules as selenide, it is not fully known how the reduction of selenium is accomplished (Stadtman, 1974).

Selenite is methylated by mammalian tissues in an apparent detoxication process. Mouse liver and kidneys use S-adenosylmethionine and reduced glutathione to form dimethylselenide from selenite (Ganther, 1966); the lungs are also active in the methylation, but muscle, spleen, and heart have little activity. Dimethylselenide is less toxic than sodium selenite (McConnell and Portman, 1952a). Sodium selenate is also reduced and converted to dimethylselenide in rats (McConnell and Portman, 1952b).

Selenite and selenate are metabolized to trimethylselenonium ion, $(CH_3)_3Se^+$, which is the principal excretory product of selenium in urine (30–50% of the urinary selenium) (Byard, 1968; Palmer *et al.*, 1969, 1974). Again, trimethylselenonium ion is less toxic than selenite or selenate ion (Obermeyer *et al.*, 1971). Although these methylated products are less toxic than the parent selenium compounds, they are involved by unknown mechanisms in synergistic toxicity; dimethylselenide and mercury toxicities are synergistic (Parizek *et al.*, 1971), as are those of trimethylselenonium ion and arsenic (Obermeyer *et al.* (1971).

In mammalian systems, inorganic selenium usually is not incorporated into amino acids (Cummins and Martin, 1967), although there is some evidence of the incorporation of selenium from sodium selenite into a rabbit protein (Godwin and Fuss, 1972). The matter is confusing, because inorganic selenium can be reduced to complex with disulfides to give selenodisulfides (R—S—Se—S—R), as is the case with two molecules of cysteine (Painter, 1941; Ganther, 1968) or reduced glutathione (Ganther, 1971).

Selenium appears to serve as an essential element in some oxidation-reduction processes in mammals. Sheep skeletal muscles contain a small (mol. wt., 10,000) selenoprotein that has a heme group. Although the selenium appears to be an integral part of the protein, its position and function in the protein are not known (Pedersen *et al.*, 1973).

A second selenoprotein is known: glutathione peroxidase, an enzyme, catalyzes the reduction of hydrogen peroxide. The activity of glutathione peroxidase in red cells of selenium-deficient animals is low, but may be restored specifically by selenium administration (Roturck *et al.*, 1973). The enzyme has a molecular weight of 84,000 and is composed of four subunits of molecular weight 21,000 each; each subunit contains one atom of selenium (Flohe *et al.*, 1973).

HEALTH EFFECTS

Although the essentiality of selenium as a nutrient for domestic and laboratory animals was established only fairly recently, its toxicity in animals has been known for more than a century. As a toxic element, selenium may produce a variety of clinical and toxicological syndromes, depending on the animal species, the dose, and the duration of exposure.

Toxic Effects in Humans

Reviews of selenium toxicity in humans include papers by Cooper (1967), Cerwenka and Cooper (1961), and Amor and Pringle (1945) and a monograph by the NRC Subcommittee on Selenium (NAS, 1976).

Elemental selenium is relatively nontoxic, but some compounds such as soluble salts of selenium dioxide, selenium trioxide, and some halogen compounds are toxic in humans with hydrogen selenide, one of the most toxic and irritating selenium compounds. The toxic vapors and soluble salts are readily absorbed by the tissues of the lungs and alimentary canal and perhaps by the skin.

Exposure of humans to selenium in most industrial situations is through the skin and lungs by exposure to dust or fumes. Selenium fumes in sufficient concentration can produce an acute respiratory distress syndrome in exposed humans. Most acute exposures to selenium and its compounds result in such symptoms as irritation of eyes and mucous membranes, sneezing, coughing, dizziness, dyspnea, dermatitis, headaches, pulmonary edema, nausea and garlic breath odor. Prolonged exposure can result in death (Clinton, 1947; Glover, 1954, 1970; Middleton, 1947; Dudley, 1938; Buchan, 1947; Dudley and Miller, 1941; Carter, 1966).

Chronic exposure of humans to selenium by ingestion or via the lungs (by inhalation of dusts and fumes) produced a set of signs and symptoms that included depression, nervousness, occasional dermatitis, gastrointestinal disturbance, giddiness, and garlic odor of the breath and sweat

(Cooper, 1967; Lemley and Merryman, 1941). Amor and Pringle (1945) and Glover (1970) considered the presence of a garlic breath odor to be the earliest and most characteristic sign of selenium absorption. However, the garlic odor is not specific for selenium, inasmuch as it is observed after absorption of tellurium. Garlic odor after selenium absorption is apparently due to formation of dimethyl selenium (Glover, 1970; Carter, 1966). Motley *et al.* (1937) suggested that the elimination of dimethyl selenium in the breath may give rise to sore throats and pneumonitis.

Selenium has been implicated as having an influence on the incidence of dental caries. Epidemiologic studies of children indicated that the small amounts of selenium present in foodstuffs in some regions were significant in increasing the incidence of dental caries if consumed during the period of the development of the teeth (Hadjimarkos and Bonhorst, 1958; Tank and Storvick, 1960). Studies in rats indicate a cariogenic role for selenium: Buttner (1963) reported that the addition of selenium at 2.3 and 4.6 ppm as sodium selenite to the drinking water of pregnant rats and to their offspring increased the incidence of caries in proportion to the amount of selenium present and also reduced the number of young born.

Nagai (1959) described signs of poisoning in Japan among workers in the manufacture of selenium rectifiers. Long employment was followed by hypochromic anemia and leukopenia. Female workers had irregular menses or menostasis.

Smith and Westfall (1937), in a detailed study of correlate symptomatology with selenium excretion and selenium intake in the diet in humans in a highly seleniferous area, found that the most frequent symptoms were gastrointestinal disturbances, bad teeth, icteroid discoloration of the skin, and sallow and pallid skin color in younger people. None of the symptoms were regarded as specific effects of selenium intake, and it was not certain that any resulted directly from continual ingestion of selenium.

Therapeutic Uses

Selenium sulfide combined with bentonite and mixed with detergent is marketed under the trade name Selsun as a shampoo. The combination of selenium sulfide and detergent has been used in the treatment of seborrheic dermatitis and of tinea versicolor. The literature dealing with the therapeutic effects of selenium in seborrheic dermatitis was reviewed by Matson (1956). Cohen (1954) and Fritz (1955) reported that the selenium sulfide suspension was effective in the treatment of granulated eyelids (blepharitis marginalis). Eisenberg (1955) and Grover (1956) reported unfavorable reactions such as loss of hair and local skin irritation after the use of Selsun as a therapeutic agent. Albright and Hitch (1966), Giordano (1963), Levan (1957), and Robinson and Yaffee (1957) used selenium sulfide in the treatment of tinea versicolor. How useful the treatment with selenium has been has not been established by adequate followup studies. Ransone *et al.* (1961) described a case of systemic selenium toxicity in a woman with open scalp lesions who had used the shampoo two or three times a week for 8 months.

Diagnostic Uses

Blau and Manshe (1961) found by the use of [^{75}Se]selenomethionine in dogs that the compound had sufficient specificity for localization in the pancreas that it could be used for visualization of the pancreas by isotope scanning methods. There are no known precautions or contraindications to the use of [^{75}Se]selenomethionine for scanning of human pancreas as the total selenium required is approximately 50 μg (Rosenfeld and Beath, 1964). Herrera *et al.* (1965) reported that [^{75}Se]selenonmethionine given intravenously for scanning of the pancreas was incorporated sufficiently into cells of lymphomas to allow detection of these tumors.

Potchen (1963), DiGiulio and Beirwaltes (1964), and Haynie *et al.* (1964) have reported that the localization of [^{75}Se]selenomethionine was sufficiently higher in the parathyroid gland than in the thyroid gland and other surrounding tissues to make it usable for localization of parathyroid gland adenoma.

Garrow and Douglas (1968) suggested the use of [^{75}Se]selenomethionine for the measurement of placental competence. Douglas (1969) assessed the possible dangers and found that the test cannot be considered dangerous, because the radiation dose is too low to be considered harmful to a fetus. Lee and Garrow (1970) found no adverse reactions after its use in 467 patients.

Toxic Effects on Animals

Domestic Animals Selenium toxicity in domestic animals has been the subject of several reviews (Anderson *et al.*, 1961; Harr and Muth, 1972; Rosenfeld and Beath, 1964; Muth and Binns, 1964). Toxicity syndromes may be acute or chronic. The acute form results from the ingestion or injection of large quantities of selenium. Chronic selenosis is due to consumption of small amounts of selenium compounds over weeks or months. In some studies in domestic animals with inorganic forms of selenium, chronic administration eventually resulted in an acute syndrome followed within a short period by death.

Shortridge *et al.* (1971) described an accidental occurrence of acute selenium poisoning in calves. The animals were to receive prophylactic subcutaneous injections of a sodium selenite solution; owing to an error in the preparation of the solution, they received 100 mg of selenium (approximately 0.5 mg/kg of body weight) instead of the intended 12 mg. The calves were depressed and salivating and had respiratory distress within 2 h of injection. Within 5 weeks, 67% had died. Dyspnea was the most noticeable clinical sign in the calves that died.

A few reports detail the acute toxic signs and lesions in sheep caused by selenium poisoning, including papers by Caravaggi *et al.* (1970), Gabbedy and Dickson (1969), Morrow (1968), and Lambourne and Mason (1969). In the accidental poisoning cases described by Morrow (1968), young lambs were given 10 mg of sodium selenite orally. Seven died within 10-16 h; eight others developed diarrhea, but recovered; and five were unaffected.

Herigstad *et al.* (1973) studied the toxicosis produced by sodium selenite (inorganic) and selenomethionine (organic) in young swine. Concentration in the ration varied from 0.1 to 600 ppm. At higher doses, survival varied from 1 to 10 days. A dose of 3 mg of selenium produced fatal selenium toxicosis within 2.5–14 h.

Laboratory Animals Franke and Potter (1936) found that the minimal fatal dose (the smallest dose that killed 75% or more of the animals in 48 h) of selenium as sodium selenite injected intraperitoneally was 7.3 mg/kg of body weight. Smith *et al.* (1937) reported the intravenous LD_{50} of selenium as both selenite and selenate to be 3 mg/kg of body weight.

Hopkins *et al.* (1966) reported poor growth in weanling rats fed various semipurified diets containing selenium at 5 ppm as selenite for 2 weeks when the ration was composed of natural feedstuffs.

Halverson *et al.* (1966) fed selenium as sodium selenite and as seleniferous wheat to young rats at concentrations of 1.6, 3.2, 4.8. 6.4, 8.0, 9.6, and 11.2 ppm in a wheat diet. Growth depression occurred when the diet contained 6.4 ppm selenium or more. Mortality occurred after the fourth week of feeding at selenium concentrations of 8 ppm or more. A concentration of 8 ppm resulted in enlargement of the pancreas, reduction of hemoglobin content, and increased serum bilirubin.

Palmer and Olson (1974) administered several concentrations of sodium selenite or sodium selenate in the drinking water to weanling rats. Selenium at concentrations of 2 or 3 ppm produced only a small reduction in weight gain and no mortality. Rats given water containing either form of selenium at 6 or 9 ppm had increased mortality. Smith *et al.* (1937) found that the toxicity of the selenite and selenate ions was similar when given intravenously and intraperitoneal. Franke and Moxon (1936) reported that rats fed seleniferous grains reduced their feed intake, lost weight or gained weight slowly, developed a hunched back, and had yellow staining of fur about the genitals. Necropsy findings included general visceral congestion, anemia, and cirrhosis of the liver.

Morss and Olcott (1967) administered selenium to rats orally at 10–15 mg/kg of body weight. The rats lost weight, and many developed diarrhea and had bleeding from the nose, lacrimation, and depression. The LD_{50} was approximately 12.5 mg/kg.

Halverson *et al.* (1970) reported that the anemia produced in rats by feeding of sodium selenite at 5-15 ppm was due to hemolysis. The synthesis of new red cells appeared unaffected.

Campo and Bieln (1971) found histologic changes of the epiphyseal plate in rats given selenium at 4–88 mg/kg of body weight intraperitoneally as sodium selenate for 13 days. Changes included blurring of the cellular and lacunar outlines, decrease in basophilia, disruption of cell columnation, and increase in widths of zones of proliferating and maturing chondrocytes.

McConnell and Portman (1952a) found that dimethyl selenide had a low degree of toxicity in mice; LD_{50} was 1.3 g/kg by intraperitoneal injection. A state of hyperpnea lasted for 2–3 h, and the breath had a garlic odor. Convulsions were followed by death within a few hours of administration in most mice, but a few lived for 36 h. Mautner and Jaffee (1958) reported that the LD_{50} of 6-selenopurine by intraperitoneal injection was 160 ± 37 mg/kg of body weight.

Hadjimarkos (1970) gave male hamsters selenium as sodium selenite in their drinking water at 6, 9, and 12 ppm. Signs of toxicity were not observed at 6 ppm, but concentrations of 9 and 12 ppm caused a reduction in weight gain. These groups also consumed less water—45% less than controls.

Smith *et al.* (1937) studied selenium toxicity in cats and reported that the minimal lethal dose of selenium as sodium selenate or selenite was about 1.5–3.0 mg/kg of body weight, regardless of the route of administration; subcutaneous, intraperitoneal, and intravenous routes were investigated.

Rhian and Moxon (1943) compared the toxic effects of seleniferous grain and inorganic selenium as sodium selenite in dogs. Manifestations of selenium intoxication were similar to those in other laboratory animals. Signs appeared when the diet contained selenium at 7.2 ppm as seleniferous grain and at 10 ppm as selenite. A selenium concentration of 20 ppm caused anorexia and death within a short time.

Schroeder and Mitchener (1971a) administered selenate and selenite to rats in the drinking water at 2 ppm for a year and then at 3 ppm for another year. Selenate at these intakes was not toxic, with respect to growth, survival, and longevity. Rosenfeld and Beath (1947), Smith *et al.* (1937), and Smith (1941) described the signs and lesions in rats undergoing chronic selenium poisoning: marked loss of body weight to cachexia, often accompanied by ascites and hydrothorax; hunched backs; coarse, disheveled pelage; and anemia.

Schroeder and Mitchener (1972) gave selenium as sodium selenite and sodium selenate to mice in the drinking water at 3 ppm for life. The two forms of selenium did not produce signs of toxicity with respect to growth, survival, or longevity in males; longevity in females was decreased. The incidence of spontaneous tumors was not affected. Schroeder and Mitchener (1971b) reported that selenate fed to pregnant mice in successive generations was very toxic at doses tolerated in weanling and nonpregnant adult mice. The results were death, failure to breed, and production of stunted mice.

Animal experiments indicate that the young are more susceptible than adults of the same species. Franke and Potter (1936) reported that the tolerance of rats to seleniferous diets increases markedly between the ages of 21 and 42 days.

Carcinogenicity Nelson *et al.* (1943) reported the induction of cirrhosis and tumors in the livers of male Osborne–Mendel rats fed either seleniferous grain or a solution of ammonium potassium sulfide and ammonium potassium selenide. The protein concentration of the diets was 12% and selenium concentrations were 5, 7, and 10 ppm. Of 53 rats surviving for 18 months, 11 developed tumors in cirrhotic livers and the other 42 contained focal hyperplasias. No metastatic growths were observed, and no tumors occurred in livers of rats not surviving for 18 months. The hepatic tumors were composed of regular or irregular cords of large hepatocytes without prominent cellular atypism.

Tscherkes and co-workers (1963) fed male rats a 12% protein diet containing selenium at 0.43 mg/100 g of diet. Of 23 rats surviving for 18 months, 10 had tumors: 3 had malignant hepatic tumors, and 2 of these had lung metastases; 4 had sarcomas; and 3 had hepatic adenomas. Three of 40 rats fed selenium at 0.86 mg/100 g of diet had sarcomas in the mediastinal and retroperitoneal lymph nodes. In a later study by Volgarev and Tscherkes (1967), the incidence of tumors designated "carcinoma" was reduced when protein in the diet was increased from 12 to 30%. The tumor incidence was 8.5% in 200 rats. The incidence of tumors was 35% in rats fed a diet with selenium at 0.43 mg/100 g and 12% casein; 8.5% in rats fed selenium at 0.86 mg/100 g and 30% casein; and 0% in a group fed selenium at 0.43 mg/100 g, 12% casein, and dietary additives.

Harr *et al.* (1967) fed female Wistar rats commercial and semipurified diets containing selenium at several concentrations, including 2 ppm with 12% casein; 2, 6 and 8 ppm with 22% casein; and 4, 6, and 8 ppm with methionine and 12% casein. The hepatic lesions were designated acute and chronic hepatitis and focal hyperplasia with marked cellular atypism. None of the rats had hepatic cirrhosis. Hyperplasias were most numerous in rats fed a control diet for 50–250 days after an 84-day period of selenium feeding and rats fed selenium and control diets in alternate weeks. Fewer toxic and hyperplastic lesions were found in rats fed selenium-supplemented commercial diets than in rats fed the purified diets with added selenium. They concluded that selenium as selenite and selenate was not carcinogenic in the rat.

Schroeder and Mitchener (1971a) reported tumor incidences of 38% in older male rats fed selenite at 3 ppm and 75% in older female rats. Of the tumors, 14% of those in the males and 52% of those in the females were considered malignant. The rate of metastastic lesions was high. In a later study by Schroeder and Mitchener (1972), in which rats were given selenium at 2 ppm as sodium selenite and sodium selenate for a year and then changed to selenium at 3 ppm, the incidence of tumors in the selenate group was 62.5% (control, 31%) and the incidence of malignant tumors was 42% (control, 17%).

The "positive" studies do not establish selenium as a carcinogen in that there were several deficiencies in the experimental design and the interpretation of the lesions:

1. It is possible and probable that some of the "low-grade carcinomas" described by Nelson and colleagues (1943) were degenerative lesions in the cirrhotic livers, rather than tumors.
2. It seems likely that acetaminophenyl selenium dehydroxide has an inherent goitrogenic activity apart from its selenium content, and there are no other reports that selenium is tumorigenic for the thyroid.
3. The low incidence of "spontaneous" tumors occurring in rats not receiving selenium and variations observed by several investigators can be due in part to age, sex, strain, diet, and contamination of diets with other carcinogens.
4. The reports of Schroeder and Mitchener (1971a) have not been confirmed or sufficiently documented.

5. Epidemiologic and demographic studies do not suggest that selenium is carcinogenic. Some regions of the world, including the north central and Rocky Mountain regions of the United States, are geologically rich in selenium. The incidence of cancer in humans is lower in these regions than in nonseleniferous regions (Shamberger, 1970).

6. Selenium is not carcinogenic in the mouse (Schroeder and Mitchener, 1972).

Mutagenicity No reports of mutagenicity by selenium compounds were found.

Teratogenicity The chick embryo is extremely sensitive to low concentrations of selenium. Concentrations in feeds too low to produce signs of poisoning in adult poultry and other farm animals have reduced hatchability and produced deformities in chicks. Poor hatchability of eggs due to deformities in the chicks was found by Franke and Tully (1935) to occur in areas where toxic feedstuffs were produced.

Holmberg and Ferm (1969) found that selenium as sodium selenite at 2 mg/kg of body weight was not teratogenic in hamsters when injected intravenously on the eighth day of pregnancy.

Reproduction Franke and Potter (1936) fed seleniferous-wheat diets to rats at ages of 21–186 days. Rats that survived the toxic diets for relatively long periods had subnormal growth and reduced reproductive capacity. Matings between animals that were fed the selenium diets were infertile. Matings in which one animal was fed the normal diet and the other a toxic diet were sometimes fertile, but poisoned females were unable to raise their young. Rosenfeld and Beath (1954) provided pregnant rats with water containing selenium at 1.5, 2.5, and 7.5 ppm as potassium selenate. Normal litters were obtained from females given the seleniferous water at 1.5 and 2.5 ppm. The second generation of selenium-dosed rats had normal litters, but the number of weaned pups was decreased by about 50%. In the group of females given the water with selenium at 7.5 ppm, fertility was reduced, the number of survivors was decreased, and growth of the young was reduced. When water containing 7.5 ppm selenium was provided on days 5–8 before parturition, the rats had normal litters, but the number of pups weaned was reduced with the continued intake of selenium. By mating of normal with selenium-exposed animals, it was determined that failure of reproduction in the rats was due to the effect of selenium on the female. Schroeder and Mitchener (1971b) gave mice selenium in the drinking water from weaning through several generations. Normal litters were produced until the third generation, which contained fewer and smaller litters with runts. Failure to breed and excessive deaths before weaning were also observed.

Interactions Interrelationships of selenium toxicity with arsenic, mercury, cadmium, silver, and thallium have been described (Diplock, 1976).

Moxon (1938) established that acute and chronic toxicity produced by feeding of seleniferous grains containing selenium at 15 ppm could be alleviated or prevented by administration of arsenic at 5 ppm as sodium arsenate in the drinking water. Ganther and Baumann (1962) used subacute dosages of arsenic and selenium and found that excretion of selenium into the gastrointestinal tract was stimulated by arsenic. Levander and Baumann (1966) demonstrated that bile was the route of excretion for selenium in arsenic-treated animals. A tenfold increase in the amount of selenium excreted into the bile of rats prepared with acute biliary fistulas was found. Levander (1972) suggested that arsenic protection against selenium toxicity may be mediated by combination of arsenic with selenium in the liver through reaction to selenol compounds to form a detoxication conjugate readily passed into the bile.

Levander and Argrett (1969) described the effect of mercuric salts on the metabolism of selenium. Mercury increased the retention of selenium in the blood, kidneys, and spleen. Parizek *et al.* (1974) reported that selenium compounds protected against the toxicity of mercury. The renal and intestinal lesions produced by mercuric chloride at 20 μmol/kg of body weight were abolished by the same dose of selenium as sodium selenite when given 1 h after mercuric chloride. Rats given lethal doses of mercuric chloride with selenium survived, and there were few gross lesions. The excretion of mercury was decreased by selenium. Parizek *et al.* (1971) found that the transport of mercury across the placenta in pregnant rats was decreased by selenium, and less mercury was secreted into the milk. The bioavailability of selenium was much lower in the rats treated with mercury. Ganther *et al.* (1972) reported that survival of Japanese quail given mercury at 20 ppm as methylmercury in diets containing 17% tuna was considerably longer than survival of quail exposed to the same concentration of methylmercury in a corn-soya diet. A striking correlation was found between the concentrations of selenium and mercury in the batches of tuna; batches that had little selenium contained low concentrations of mercury, and, when the concentration of mercury was high, the selenium concentration was also high (selenium:mercury, 2.91:2.97 ppm). The selenium in the tuna lowered the toxicity in the quail of the methylmercury added at 20 ppm. In an experiment with rats fed a basal diet containing 20% casein with and without the addition of selenium at 0.5 ppm as sodium selenite, it was found that mercury at 10 ppm as methylmercury produced 100% mortality after 6 weeks of feeding, but selenium was completely effective in preventing mortality.

Parizek and Zahor (1956) reported that the administration of cadmium at subtoxic concentrations by subcutaneous-injection-produced necrosis of the testes of rats. Kar *et al.* (1960) found that the cadmium-induced lesions in the testes could be prevented by the administration of selenium. Mason and Young (1967) reported that the testicular injury produced by single subcutaneous injections of 0.45 mg of cadmium chloride in rats was protected against by half-equimolar selenium dioxide injected at the same time as cadmium. Protection was also provided by daily subcutaneous injections of half-equimolar selenium dioxide given over 6 successive days before cadmium. Parizek *et al.* (1968) and Gunn *et al.* (1968) found that mortality of rats given lethal doses of cadmium was much reduced by administration of selenium. Holmberg and Ferm (1969) found that the teratogenicity of cadmium was considerably reduced by selenium. Kar *et al.* (1959) and Parizek *et al.* (1968) found that cadmium would selectively damage the nonovulating ovary in the rat and that this damage was prevented by administration of selenium. Parizek *et al.* (1968) and Parizek (1964) found that cadmium produced necrosis and destruction of the placenta and that these changes could be prevented by the administration of selenium. Similarly, the "toxemia of pregnancy" induced by cadmium could be prevented by selenium (Parizek, 1965).

Diplock *et al.* (1967) and Grasso *et al.* (1969) reported that 0.15% dietary silver acetate produced toxicity in rats and chicks deficient in vitamin E. When the diets were adequate in vitamin E and selenium, the silver was not toxic. The removal of the vitamin E resulted in 100% mortality within 49–64 days. The addition of selenium to the diet at 1.0 ppm produced a protection of 55% against toxic effects of silver. Grasso *et al.* (1969) studied the lesions produced in the liver by silver and the lesions caused by dietary deprivation of vitamin E and selenium. The lesions were similar.

Hollo and Zlatarov (1960) reported that mortality induced by thallium poisoning could be prevented by the parenteral administration of selenate. Rusiecki and Brzezinski (1966) found that oral administration of selenate prevented the toxicity of thallium and that the content of thallium in liver, kidneys, and bones was increased by the selenate. Levander and Argrett (1969) observed that the subcutaneous injection of thallium acetate increased the retention of selenium in the liver and kidneys and decreased the pulmonary and urinary excretion of selenium.

Levander and Morris (1970) used a peanut-meal diet and found that neither methionine nor vitamin E alone gave much protection against hepatic damage produced by excessive selenium. Combinations of methionine and vitamin E were effective, and the degree of protection was approximately proportional to the concentration of vitamin E added to the diet. Selenium concentrations of the liver and kidneys from rats fed the diets supplemented with methionine and vitamin E were less than those of the same organs from rats fed either methionine or vitamin E alone or no supplement. The results were compatible with the hypothesis that methionine detoxifies selenium by forming methylated derivatives of the element that are eliminated via the breath and the urine. Vitamin E and some fat-soluble antioxidants increase the availability of the methyl group of methionine for this process.

Moxon and DuBois (1939) reported that the combined administration of fluoride and selenium to rats increased the toxicity of selenium. They added fluoride at 5 ppm to the drinking water of young rats fed a diet containing selenium at 11 ppm as seleniferous wheat. Mortality was increased, and weight gains were decreased, as were feed intake and water intake. Hadjimarkos (1969) gave rats selenium at 3 ppm as sodium selenite and fluoride at 50 ppm as sodium fluoride. A second group received water with selenium at 3 ppm. The growth and mortality data indicated that the combined administration of selenium and fluoride did not increase the severity of signs of selenium toxicity.

Beneficial Effects

Diplock (1976) recently reviewed the multitude of studies concerned with the nutritional roles of selenium in laboratory and domestic animals and poultry. Selenium, the factor 3 of baker's yeast, was effective in preventing hepatic necrosis in rats; exudative diathesis in chicks and turkey poults; skeletal muscle degeneration and necrosis in poultry, domestic animals (such as lambs, calves, and swine), and laboratory rodents; hepatitis dietetica in swine, and cardiac myopathy in turkeys, swine, sheep, and cattle. Other selenium-deficiency diseases include reduced fertility, embryonic mortality, and unthriftiness in sheep and smooth muscle (gizzard) myopathy in turkey poults. Degeneration and necrosis of pancreatic acinar epithelium followed by fibrosis have been produced in chicks by selenium deficiency in the presence of adequate polyunsaturated fatty acids and vitamin E (Thompson and Scott, 1962).

Several reports have indicated that selenium has antitumor activity in some animal model systems, and these were reviewed by Shapiro (1972). Clayton and Baumann (1949) reported that the incidence of hepatic tumors induced by feeding of dimethylaminoazobenzene was decreased by about half by a diet containing selenium at 5 ppm. Shamberger (1970) found that selenium as sodium selenide greatly reduced the number of tumors in mice when administered concomitantly with croton oil to mouse skin treated with dimethylbenz[*a*]anthracene (DMBA). Shamberger (1970), in a study in which DMBA was applied to the shaved skin of ICR mice, found that sodium selenide (0.0005%) applied after DMBA reduced the incidence of papillomas. Sodium selenide applied concomitantly with 0.01% methylcholanthrene reduced the total numbers of papillomas and cancers, compared with controls. Dietary sodium selenite at 1 ppm markedly reduced the number of papillomas induced by the combination of DMBA-croton oil and by benzo[*a*]pyrene.

Mautner and Jaffe (1958) used experimental mouse tumor systems and reported that equimolar amounts of 6-selenopurine and 6-mercaptopurine produced similar degrees of inhibition of the growth of L1210 leukemia cells. 6-Selenopurine was somewhat more toxic than 6-mercaptopurine at doses required to cause 50% (or greater) reduction in tumor size. Activity of 6-selenopurine against leukemia L5178-Y and sarcoma S-180 was less than that of 6-mercaptopurine, and the highest dose that caused a significant inhibition of tumor growth was markedly toxic. Mautner *et al.* (1963) found that intraperitoneal and subcutaneous injections of selenoguanine inhibited the growth of L5178-Y lymphoma in mice. Riley (1968) studied the relationship between subcutaneous mast cell populations and papilloma induction and found that topical selenium decreased the incidence of papilloma and prevented the accumulation of mast cells at the base of the tumors in mice treated with carcinogen.

ANALYSIS

In the last 20 yr, much effort has been given to development of quantitative methods of analysis for nanogram amounts of selenium in a variety of materials. Methods include titrimetry, colorimetry, fluorometry, atomic absorption, polarograpy, and neutron activation. For samples containing large (microgram or milligram) amounts of selenium, titrimetry and colorimetry are usually satisfactory. Good microanalytic methods include fluorescence and atomic-absorption spectroscopy. Olson *et al.* (1973) and Watkinson (1967) have reviewed methods for determination of selenium.

Water

The current U.S. Public Health Service drinking water standard for selenium is 10 μg/liter (as total selenium); according to the 1975 *Chemical Analysis of Interstate Carrier Water Supply Systems* published by the EPA (1975), this concentration is rarely exceeded. Methods with sensitivities better than 10 ppb (10 μg/liter) are required for determinations in most drinking water.

The atomic-absorption method of Fernandez (1973) offers a highly sensitive and simple method of detecting nanogram quantities of selenium (and arsenic). The selenium in the water sample is reduced to gaseous hydride with sodium borohydride ($NaBH_4$). The hydride is carried into an argon-hydrogen-entrained air flame with argon carrier gas. An atomic-absorption spectrophotometer with an electrodeless discharge lamp can have an absolute detection limit of 15 ppb based on a 20-ml sample volume. With a hollow-cathode lamp, the solution detection limit is 0.25 ppb (μg/liter). With either lamp, the method offers a precision (coefficient of variation) of 3%. The method detects both inorganic and organic selenium, and drinking-water samples offer few interfering compounds.

Polarographic procedures have been developed for selenium, but do not have the sensitivity and specificity of atomic-absorption methods.

Lambert *et al.* (1951) developed a colorimetric method for water analysis based on conversion of inorganic and organic selenium to selenious acid, which was then used to oxidize iodide quantitatively to elemental iodine; the iodine was determined colorimetrically. The method was subject to several interferences and could reliably detect selenium in water only at concentrations of 0.1 ppm (100 μg/liter) or more.

Greater sensitivity (by a factor of 10) is obtained with fluorometric methods of analysis. Selenium, as selenious acid, is complexed with 3,3-diaminobenzidine (Cousins, 1960) or 2,3-diaminonaphthalene (Parker and Harvey, 1961). Watkinsin (1960) reported measuring less than 10 ng of selenium with a standard deviation of 0.5 ng, using 2,3-diaminonaphthalene fluorometric analysis. Iron and copper interfere with the analysis, and the technique is considerably more involved than the atomic-absorption method.

Biological Samples

The atomic-absorption method described above for drinking water can be applied to acid digests of biologic samples. Fluorescence methods are also widely used. The *Official Methods of Analysis of the Association of Official Analytical Chemists* (Horwitz, 1970) lists a 2,3-diaminonaphthalene fluorometric method for plant specimens containing selenium at less than 4 ppm; the analysis takes several hours to complete. For plants containing larger concentrations of selenium, the AOAC uses a colorimetric method, precipitating the distilled selenium with hydroxylamine hydrochloride and measuring the selenium concentration against prepared standards with a color comparator. For seleniferous plants in which the selenium concentration exceeds 100 ppm, a gravimetric method is listed by the AOAC.

For food samples, the official AOAC final action method is an acid digestion in the presence of a mercuric oxide fixate. The selenium is distilled as the bromide and reduced to elemental selenium with sulfur dioxide, and its concentration is determined as selenious acid, H_2SeO_3, by titration with sodium thiosulfate and iodine.

Neutron-activation analysis has been used successfully to measure selenium in biological samples. Irradiation of the sample with neutrons in a nuclear reactor produces many radioactive elements, including selenium. Three radionuclides of selenium are produced at sufficiently high specific activity to be useful for determinations in biologic samples. The half-lives of these radionuclides are 120 days for selenium-75, 17.5 for selenium-77, and 18.6 min for selenium-81; the first two are gamma emitters and selenium-81 is a beta-emitter (Bowen and Cawse, 1963). Isolation of a specific radionuclide can require much time and effort and is generally limited to waiting several weeks for the short-lived elements to decay, spectrometrically analyzing for gamma-emission peaks at 121 + 136 and 265 + 280 keV (Grant *et al.*, 1961), distilling the selenium with hydrogen bromide or extracting into an organic solvent the selenium complex of diaminobenzidene or diaminonaphthalene (Betteridge, 1965). Such techniques are reported to detect as little as 10 ng of selenium per sample.

Reliability

Before 1960, most water samples were analyzed by colorimetric or titrimetric methods for selenium, and these methods are of low sensitivity by today's standards. In fact, the minimal detectable concentrations by these methods are higher than the drinking-water standard of 10 μg/liter. Water analyses completed before 1960 are likely to contain false-negative results, that is, reporting no detectable selenium when, in fact, the drinking-water standard of 1962 may have been exceeded.

Methods requiring prolonged air drying of the sample, especially at temperatures above 60°C, or requiring distillation are subject to loss of selenium which results in underestimation of the selenium content. Many compounds have the potential of interfering with selenium determinations; iron, copper, and arsenic seem to offer the most problems in water analysis, but are well accounted for in the colorimetric method of Lambert *et al.* (1951) and its modifications.

CONCLUSIONS AND RECOMMENDATIONS

The determination of a "no-adverse-effect" concentration of selenium is complicated by numerous experimental variables. The toxic effect of selenium depends on the type of selenium compound administered, whether it is organic or inorganic, the valence state of the selenium ion, the species and sex of the laboratory animal used, the age of the animal, the conditions and duration of the test, and the diet—whether natural or semipurified ingredients, the protein content, the caloric intake, the type of protein, and the presence and concentrations of other elements, such as arsenic, mercury, thallium, and fluorine. The criterion of toxicity used is also important in establishing a no-effect concentration and growth may be the best indicator of toxicity.

Harr and Muth (1972) used a semipurified diet in rats and reported that the minimal toxic concentration for induction of hepatic lesions was 0.25 ppm. A concentration of 0.75 ppm was considered the minimal concentration, with respect to longevity and development of cardiac, renal, and splenic lesions. However, rats fed selenium at 0.5 ppm grew as well as control rats. Halverson *et al.* (1966), in a study of rats and wheat diets, found that selenium at 3.2 ppm as sodium selenite did not affect growth over the feeding period of 6 weeks. Thapar *et al.* (1969) reported that a dietary selenite concentration of 2 ppm had no detrimental effect on chickens fed over a life cycle. Although there is now general agreement that selenium is an essential element for man as it is for domestic animals, virtually nothing is known about the forms and quantities of selenium consumed by man, in part because of inadequate methodology for collecting material and for accurate analysis. This must be corrected before the environment (water, air, food) can be satisfactorily monitored.

Metabolism and kinetics of the various forms of selenium require intense research efforts. Molecular transformations must be determined in mammalian systems and the interactions between selenium and other environmental materials, particularly mercury, cadmium, and arsenic.

Little information is available as to effects of long-term exposure to relatively low levels of selenium. Although selenium is toxic to man and animals in high doses, these are usually a result of accidental exposure. Rather than concern for toxicity the literature indicates that there is a greater potential for a deficiency. Consideration should be given to raising current permitted levels in waters of the United States.

The paucity of definitive data on selenium and human health requires a number of approaches toward elucidating the role of selenium in the mammalian system. The following recommendations are suggested:

1. There is a critical need for more rapid, accurate, and reproducible analytic methods that will permit both qualitative and quantitative assays. Information on chemical forms, oxidation states, and solubility in water is needed. This is probably the most limiting need for progress over a broad front in selenium research.
2. Systems for monitoring the environment (water, air, food) should be improved.
3. Basic research should be conducted to define molecular transformations in the mammalian system.
4. Effects of selenium on the toxicity of mercury, cadmium and arsenic should be studied.
5. Natural and industrial emission and cycling of selenium in the environment should be investigated.
6. The effects on animal systems of long-term low concentrations of selenium in combination with other trace elements in the environment should be determined.
7. Baseline data on selenium concentrations in humans in health and disease are needed.
8. The effects of selenium deficiency and excess on induced and spontaneous animal tumors should be determined.

Fluoride

OCCURRENCE

Fluorine is the most electronegative of all elements, existing naturally in the form of fluoride. It is the 17th most abundant element in the earth's crust, occurring principally as fluorite, CaF_2, and fluoroapatite, $Ca_{10}(PO_4)_6F_2$. It is present in small amounts in most soils except those that have been strongly leached. The concentration of fluoride in natural waters depends principally on the solubility of the fluoride-containing rocks with which the water is in contact.

In 1969 the general Community Water Supply Survey of the Public Health Service sampled 969 water supplies and found fluoride ranging from less than 0.2 up to 4.40 mg/liter. Fifty-two systems had fluoride concentrations greater than the then-recommended limits for this constituent.

A more extensive survey in the same year by the Dental Health Division of the Public Health Service (1970) showed that 8.1 million people in 2,630 communities in 44 states were consuming water with more than 0.7 mg/liter of naturally occurring fluoride. Nearly 1 million people in 524 communities were receiving water with more than 2 mg/liter of naturally occurring fluoride.

Most of the communities with more than 0.7 mg/liter natural fluoride were in: Arizona, Colorado, Illinois, Iowa, New Mexico, Ohio, Oklahoma, South Dakota, and Texas. There were no reports of community water supplies with as much as 0.7 mg/liter fluoride from Delaware, Hawaii, Massachusetts, Pennsylvania, Tennessee, or Vermont.

The WHO monograph, "Fluorides and Human Health" (1970, pp. 17–59), notes that high concentrations of fluoride are found in areas of every continent and that dental fluorosis is a problem from Finland to South Africa and from England to Japan.

Fluoride in Water Treatment

Conventional procedures of water treatment, i.e., clarification, filtration, softening, and disinfection, have little or no effect on the fluoride concentration in water. However, it was noted in Ohio in the 1930's that if the pH was increased during softening operations to a value high enough to precipitate magnesium hydroxide, some removal of fluoride was accomplished (Scott *et al.*, 1937). In most full-scale plants the removal of fluoride was less than 50 percent.

Two special processes have been used for fluoride removal, both based on the adsorption of fluoride on granular media, either activated alumina or bone char (Maier, 1963). The water containing fluoride is passed through a bed of the medium until the effluent concentration exceeds an acceptable value. The medium is then regenerated with a solution of sodium hydroxide to remove adsorbed fluoride. Costs of this type of treatment are such that few communities have undertaken voluntarily to remove fluoride from their supplies.

Addition of Fluoride to Water Supplies

For more than 30 yr, the practice of adding fluoride to drinking water has been practiced in the United States for reduction of dental caries. The principal chemicals used for this purpose are sodium fluoride, sodium silicofluoride, hydroflurosilicic acid, and ammonium silicofluoride (Maier, 1963). These chemicals require care in handling and must be dispensed with properly designed chemical feeding systems, but these are readily available. The usual dosage has been in the range of 1 mg/liter.

When any one of these chemicals is dispersed in water at the 1 mg/liter range, it dissociates almost completely.

Other Sources of Fluoride

Food Fluoride is present to some extent in nearly all foods, but the concentrations vary widely. Studies of the fluoride contents of foodstuffs reported in the WHO Monograph (1970) have been reviewed by Muhlar (1970). Prival and Fisher (1973) have made a more recent compilation of these fluoride contents.

Among the foodstuffs notably high in fluoride are fish, particularly those, such as sardines, that are eaten with the bones. Fish-meal flour, which is produced from the whole fish, is also high in fluoride. Tea is unusually rich in fluoride. Milk and most fruits are generally low in fluoride. Vegetables vary greatly in fluoride content.

Hodge and Smith (1965) computed the total fluoride intake from food at 0.5–1.5 mg/day for areas with nonfluoridated water. Marier and Rose (1966) showed that use of fluoridated water in canneries increased the fluoride content of canned food by 0.5 mg/liter and converted this to 0.5 mg/day in the diet. The proposed total intake from the diet then became 1.0–2.0 mg/day.

However, the Hodge and Smith estimate came from Machle and Largent (1943), whose values were based erroneously on earlier work (Machle *et al.*, 1942). In this earlier work the average total fluoride intake per day for 20 weeks was just under 0.5 mg with only 0.16 mg of the intake from food as such. In a more recent review Hodge and Smith (1970) have lowered their estimate to 0.3–0.8 mg fluoride daily from the diet.

Recent studies indicate that the total intake of fluoride is as high as 3 mg/day rather than the earlier figure of 1.5 mg/day, primarily because of increases in the estimated levels of fluoride in foods (Spencer *et al.*, 1970). Balance data presented by Spencer also suggest a higher retention by bone, nearly 2 mg/day rather than the 0.2 mg/day indicated earlier.

Two recent articles from Spencer's group (Kramer *et al.*, 1974; Dace *et al.*, 1974) appear to support a higher estimate for dietary fluoride intake. The first is based on hospital-prepared food from 16 U.S. cities. The fluoride intake from food in the fluoridated communities was found to range from 1.6–3.4 mg/day (av. 2.6) while that from nonfluoridated cities was 0.8–1.0 mg (av. 0.9). The very high values and the marked difference between fluoridated and nonfluoridated cities can be explained in part by the inclusion of coffee and other water-based beverages as dietary intake, a classification not usually followed by other investigators. The second article reports average fluoride intake from diets used in balance studies in a fluoridated city over a 6-yr period as 2.0 mg/day.

These findings are important because, if valid, they might represent a shift in intake that could lead to dental fluorosis in fluoridated communities. Also, a retention of 2 mg/day would mean that an average individual would experience skeletal fluorosis after 40 yr, based on an accumulation of 10,000 ppm fluoride in bone ash. However, these new estimates for fluoride in food are questionable; consequently, so are their implications. The values are suspect because of analytical problems. The diffusion method of Singer and Armstrong (1969a) was used with a colorimetric reagent and false high values are obtained with this technique (Taves, 1966).

A study more limited in scope, because it was restricted to 16- to 19-yr old males, found 2.0–2.3 mg/day total fluoride intake (San Filippo and Battistone, 1971). The increase over earlier values may reflect the fact that the food portions were large for the test group.

Data from balance studies in children tend to support the lower values. The dietary fluoride intake for nine children aged 4 to 18 years averaged 0.3 mg/day (Forbes *et al.*, 1973).

The quickest and most reliable method of checking whether there has been a shift in total intake of fluoride in the past 20–30 yr is through surveys of the urinary and bone fluoride concentrations occurring in people in fluoridated communities. There has been no question about the analytical techniques used in these earlier data on urine and bone because the concentrations involved were relatively high. A recent (Parkins, 1974) bone survey in Iowa done at autopsies showed bone fluoride levels higher than those in earlier publications, particularly when taking into account that they are for unashed bone, which means that the concentrations need to be approximately doubled to compare them to values for ashed bone. Detailed comparison of the method he used has shown no systematic error, but other bone fluoride values found in Rochester, New York, show concentrations which match earlier values almost exactly (Charen *et al.*, in preparation, 1976).

Private communication with Parkins has not clarified the discrepancy, but he has indicated that the usual fluoride concentration in the urine is about 50 μM, which is the same as earlier reports as well as the values found in a few samples analyzed from Rochester residents. Obviously additional work is desirable to clarify these questions, but earlier values for average fluoride intake and balance still appear to be valid.

Industrial exposure Industrial exposure to fluoride-containing dusts and gases has been a serious problem in many parts of the world. A committee of the National Academy of Sciences on the Biological Effects of Atmospheric Pollutants (1971) reported on fluoride as an atmospheric pollutant both in the work place and in the ambient air.

Operations that introduce fluoride dusts and gases into the atmosphere include: grinding, drying, and calcining of fluoride-containing minerals; acidulation of the minerals; smelting; electrochemical reduction of metals with fluoride fluxes or melts as in the aluminum and steel industry; kiln firing of brick and other clay products and the combustion of coal.

Generally speaking, good progress has been made in reducing fluoride exposure to industrial workers by ventilation and emission control practices.

Air Air pollution by fluoride dusts and gases has done substantial damage to vegetation and to animals in the vicinity of industrial fluoride sources. However, the contribution of ambient air to human fluoride intake is only a few hundredths of a milligram per day (NAS, 1971), an amount that is insignificant in comparison with other sources of fluoride.

METABOLISM

Radiofluoride studies show metabolism of fluoride in the body to be simple. Hence, fluoride is unlikely to give rise to intolerance by reason of disease or genetics. Accumulation has been found to occur only in the kidneys and calcified tissues. The reabsorption of water without the reabsorption of fluoride in the kidneys explains the increased concentration in the kidneys. The isomorphism of the fluoride ion for the hydroxyl ion in hydroxyapatite explains the increased concentration of fluoride in calcified tissues. Some of the fluoride ingested is retained in the calcified tissues; however, the rate of such retention decreases with age, so adults are nearly in balance (Hodge, 1961).

There has long been confusion about the relationship of serum fluoride concentration to intake, confusion that carries over to recent reviews. Some 24 yr ago, Smith, Gardner, and Hodge found a 2–3-fold increase in the average serum fluoride concentration of people living in a fluoridated community, compared to those in a nonfluoridated community (0.7 vs. 1.8 μM, or 0.014 vs. 0.036 ppm) (Smith *et al.*, 1950; see Taves, 1966, for revised values). Such a relationship would be expected, if about 0.5 mg of fluoride per day were coming from food in the nonfluoridated community and 1.5 mg from food and water in the fluoridated area.

This work was ignored by Singer and Armstrong (1960) when they developed what appeared to be improved analytic techniques. They found more fluoride in the serum (7.5 μM, or 0.15 ppm), but found no differences related to intake, although concentrations in the drinking water varied from 0 to 2.5 ppm. No adequate explanation was offered as to how the urinary and bone concentrations could be directly related to the intake of fluoride, while serum concentrations remained constant. Threshold phenomena in both kidney and bone would have to be present to maintain a constant serum concentration, but there was no reason to think that a threshold existed in either case. The exchange and uptake into the bone compartments cause a buffering of the serum fluoride concentration, both short-term (days) and long-term (years). However, this does not explain why the average serum fluoride concentration would be the same in different communities. Even though buffering would tend to diminish the surges of serum fluoride due to ingestion, the mean value should be an integrated reflection of the average intake and bone fluoride stores.

The explanation for the confusion is to be found in the presence of two forms of fluoride in human serum, one of which can be shown to exchange with added radioactive fluoride and one which cannot (Taves, 1968a,b). The exchangeable fraction is smaller and is the same as ionic fluoride. Ionic fluoride can be measured directly with a fluoride electrode reasonably well, and even more accurately after diffusion or ultrafiltration. It can also be measured with a fluorometric reagent. The renal clearance of this fraction coincides with the renal clearance of radioactive fluoride (Taves, 1967), and also varies with the fluoride concentration in the water supply (Guy *et al.*, 1976).

With fluoride content of water at 1 ppm, the serum inorganic fluoride content is on the average less than 1 μM, or 0.02 ppm (Taves, 1966; Singer and Armstrong, 1973; Hanjijarvi *et al.*, 1972). This contrasts with the average value of 0.15 ppm found by Singer and Armstrong after ashing and distillation, a value that should now be labeled "total" fluoride. In other words, variations in serum inorganic fluoride were hidden by a larger fraction of organic fluoride, which was being measured along with inorganic fluoride when ashing was employed.

Guy *et al.* (1976) reported the isolation of an 8-carbon perfluorinated compound from human plasma. If the second form of fluoride proves to represent only chemicals of this type with no relation to fluoridation, the case for the safety of fluoridation will have been strengthened, in that the behavior of inorganic fluoride in the body will have become simple and understandable. Whether food is the source of this second form of fluoride is unclear, in part because the reports of organic fluoride in food have not been confirmed (Weinstein *et al.*, 1972). There is heavy use of fluorocompounds industrially and in homes (Bryce, 1964). This may explain its presence in humans.

Under steady-state conditions, at least 99% of the fluoride present in the body is sequestered in calcified tissues. Most of the remainder is present in plasma and is thus available for excretion. Hodge (1961) has emphasized that skeletal sequestration and renal excretion are the two major means by which the body prevents the accumulation of toxic amounts of fluoride ion. Chen *et al.* (1956) measured the renal clearance of fluoride in female dogs. After showing that fluoride was completely ultrafiltrable in dog plasma, they used routine clearance procedures in animals drinking tap water containing fluoride at 1 ppm (artificially fluoridated). The average normal renal fluoride clearance was 2.7 ml/min, and the fluoride:chloride clearance ratio was 19:1. During mannitol diuresis, fluoride clearance varied directly with the urinary flow rate. Hypertonic sodium chloride infusion also increased the clearance of fluoride. Although the authors claimed that the intravenous administration of sodium nitrate or sodium sulfate did not affect fluoride excretion, their data did not establish that point. Plasma fluoride concentrations in their experiments ranged from 12 to 61 μg/100 ml (6.3-33 μM).

Carlson *et al.* (1960a) studied the renal excretion and clearance of radiofluoride in dogs. Reabsorption ranged from 14 to 92% of the filtered load and was consistently less than reabsorption of chloride. Renal clearance of fluoride varied directly with urinary flow rate. There was no indication that renal tubular secretion occurred.

In a later study, Carlson *et al.* (1960b) fed 1 mg of radiofluoride to each of two adult humans. Fluoride clearance always exceeded chloride clearance and increased with urinary flow rate. Fluoride clearance was always smaller than creatinine clearance. Although less than 10% of the ingested radioisotope was present in the plasma volume at any time, about one-third of the ingested dose appeared in the urine within 4 h. Chlorothiazide, a benzothiadiazine diuretic, increased the clearance and excretion of fluoride. Plasma contained 72% of the whole-blood fluoride. This differential distribution between plasma and red cells was also observed in dogs (Carlson *et al.*, 1960c).

More recently Whitford *et al.* (1976) have demonstrated that the renal clearance of fluoride is inversely related to tubular fluid pH. They showed that urine flow rate and chloride clearance, which were previously thought to be the main determinants of fluoride clearance, were not strongly associated with fluoride clearance.

Walser and Rahill (1965) have shown that the renal tubular reabsorption of iodide, bromide, and fluoride is related to the simultaneous reabsorption of chloride. The results indicate that all the halides are reabsorbed predominately by the same mechanisms. If reabsorption of fluoride is achieved by utilization of renal chloride-transporting systems, chloride must be the preferred substrate because the clearance of fluoride is generally much greater than the simultaneous clearance of chloride.

A summary of the findings from these studies on renal handling of fluoride is:

1. Virtually all the fluoride in plasma (human or dog) is ultrafiltrable.
2. Renal excretion of radiofluoride depends on glomerular filtration and variable tubular reabsorption.
3 Probably, reabsorption is largely passive, with fluoride being less permeable than chloride.
4. Fluoride excretion increases when the plasma concentration is increased.
5. Procedures that increase urinary flow rate (e.g., administration of osmotic diuretics, hypertonic saline, or diuretic drugs) increase the clearance of fluoride.

HEALTH ASPECTS

Acute Effects

Acute toxicity from fluoride is quite rare and occurrs principally as a result of suicide or accidental poisoning. The lethal dose of sodium fluoride for man is about 5 g, but there are reports of recovery from amounts much greater as well as deaths from smaller quantities (Goodman and Gilman, 1975).

Initial symptoms of toxicity are a result of the local action of fluoride on the mucosa of the gastrointestinal tract. Vomiting, abdominal pain, nausea, and diarrhea are followed by paresthesias, hyperactive reflexes and tonic and clonic convulsions. No system of the body can be considered exempt, and death is usually due to respiratory paralysis or cardiac failure. Many of the signs and symptoms of acute fluoride toxicity are a result of the calcium-binding effects of fluoride (Goodman and Gilman, 1975; WHO, 1970).

2, Chronic Effects

Chronic toxicological studies indicate that teeth and bone are the most fluoride-sensitive tissues. The margin of safety with fluoridated water (assuming an intake of 1 mg/day) has beeen estimated to be 2-8-fold for dental mottling. Years of experience with fluoridation without apparent objectionable mottling (see below for possible exceptions) attest to the adequacy of this low margin of safety. Crippling skeletal fluorosis has a 20- to 40-fold margin of safety for the average person, again assuming an intake of only 1 mg/day (Hodge, 1961 and 1962).

Epidemiological studies where the water is naturally high in fluoride have reported no adverse effects, except in rare cases, until the concentration is many times that recommended for artificial fluoridation (Hagen *et al.*, 1954; Leone *et al.*, 1954; AMA, 1957). Indeed, there is a suggestion that 1–5 ppm may prevent bone loss to some degree and decrease the amount of soft tissue calcification in older people (Bernstein *et al.*, 1966).

Controlled studies with recommended levels of added fluoride, such as in Kingston–Newburg, have reported no evidence of adverse effects (Ast *et al.*, 1956).

a) Mongolism

The possibility that mongolism is caused by fluoride in the drinking water stems from a report by Rappaport (1959), in which he observed a dose-related association between the number of cases of mongolism registered in institutions and the concentrations of fluoride in the water. From the towns with less than 0.1 ppm to those with 1.0–2.6 ppm, the increase was nearly 3-fold. This study has been criticized because the case rates were less than half those found in intensive case-finding studies (Royal College of Physicians, 1976).

Three intensive case-finding studies in Britain (Berry, 1958, and two unpublished ones cited by the Royal College of Physicians, 1976) with different fluoride concentrations in the water have not shown such an association. Heavy tea drinking in England (Cook, 1970) might obscure differences in the British studies. However, the absolute rates were similar to those in a recent intensive case-finding study in Massachusetts (Needleman *et al.*, 1974), in which no difference was noted between fluoridated and nonfluoridated communities. Therefore, for Rappaport's hypothesis to be maintained, an explanation as to why the British rate did not reflect increased consumption of fluoride from tea drinking would be necessary. Needleman estimated that he could have detected an increase of as little as 20% at the 95% confidence level. He admitted that his evidence was not adequate to rule out an effect where fluoridation had been present for the lifetime of the mother, because his data involved a relatively short period of fluoridation.

Sensitivity to Fluoride

A recent report (Grimbergen, 1974) suggests confirmation of the earlier claims by Waldbott (1962) that some people are very sensitive to fluoride. Waldbott's claims have been dismissed on two grounds: that he was the only one to report such effects, and that sensitivity of this type has not been reported among the billions of tea drinkers in the world who would be ingesting extra fluoride (WHO, 1970, p. 15).

Grimbergen's report was a preliminay methodological paper and is not convincing. Two aspects of the methodology seem weak and could lead to erroneous conclusions. First, when large numbers of double-blind tests are done, it is to be expected that control patients will occasionally have symptoms that correspond to those associated with the administration of fluoride; the investigator should indicate the rate of positive responses and the results of retesting. Second, the patients selected themselves for inclusion in the study based on their beliefs that they were already sensitive to fluoride. Waldbott's case reports (1962) are more completely documented and he used concentrations that were probably too low to be identified by taste. He reported 29 positive responders among 48 people tested. The Royal College of Physicians (1976, p. 63) review stated that sodium fluoride at 1 mg/15 ml of distilled water has a distinctive taste. However, Taves (unpublished, 1976) found that four people out of five could not tell the difference at 1 mg/15 ml.

Waldbott and Grimberger are not the only ones who have described patients with syndromes that they explained as intolerance to fluoride. Douglas (1947) tested 32 patients in a group of 133 with histories suggestive of sensitivity to fluoride-containing dentifrices. He implied that none were able to complete a series of six alternating trials using fluoride and nonfluoride toothpastes, because of intolerance, mainly in the form of ulcerations of the mouth. Feltman and Kosel claimed that, among pregnant mothers and their children, 1% (at least four of them) reacted adversely to 1 mg fluoride tablets. They stated that they established (by means of placebos) that it was the fluoride, rather than the binder, that caused the adverse effect (Feltman, 1956; Feltman and Kosel, 1961). Shea, Gillespie, and Waldbott (1967) reported on seven cases of patient improvement after discontinuing vitamin drops or toothpaste containing fluoride. They subjected one case to a double-blind study with sodium fluoride. In the cases involving toothpaste, the associated cation is not stated. Stannous fluoride is commonly used in toothpaste; therefore, sensitivity to tin, rather than to fluoride, cannot be ruled out. Petraborg (1974) reported on seven case histories of what seemed to be fluoride sensitivity, but the patients were not subjected to objective tests, so the evidence is weak.

The quantities of fluoride involved are clearly relevant to the question of the safety of fluoridation. But, if Feltman and Kosel's estimate of 1% intolerant people is correct, there should have been more reports of adverse effects in the studies in which fluoride tablets were given to schoolchildren (at least 10,000 children by 1967, mainly in Switzerland) (O'Meara, 1968). Also, as methoxyflurane anesthesia for surgery typically causes serum fluoride content to increase to 30–50 times normal (Fry *et al.*, 1973), there should have been striking cases of such intolerance in an estimated 12 million patients who have recieved methoxyflurane (NAS–NRC, 1971). Moreover, cases of intolerance to fluoride (20–100 mg/day) for osteoporosis have been associated with very few symptoms of the type reported by Waldbott. There have not been reports of intolerance from people who move into and out of numerous towns with naturally high fluoridated water supplies. Opportunities for such discovery existed before any bias for or against fluoridation.

So, although sensitivity to fluoride has not been demonstrated firmly, a possibility of sensitivity or idiosyncratic reaction to fluoride should be kept in mind. Clarification might come from two kinds of study. Studies on the administration of fluoride drops or tablets for prevention of dental caries should include consideration of possible intolerance and definite statements should be made about any findings in this regard; in most such reports, no comments are made about a search for intolerance. Quissell and Suttie (1972) have demonstrated an ability of fluoride-resistant cells to remove or exclude fluoride from their interiors *in vitro*. Humans or animals receiving fluoride for long periods should be studied to see whether a cellular resistance develops *in vivo*. If this could be demonstrated, the metabolic consequences of resistance or its absence might shed light on how intolerance could occur.

Renal Patients

The effect of impaired renal function on the handling of fluoride could not be adequately studied until accurate measurements of serum ionic fluoride could be made. Evidence that was thought to carry some weight in the past, such as the lack of observed increase in serum concentration and the similarity of urinary fluoride concentrations in patients with renal disease, is faulty. Difficulties with serum fluoride values have already been discussed. Urinary concentrations will reflect impaired renal ability to excrete fluoride only if there has not been sufficient time for equilibrium with fluoride intake to be reached.

Three reports confirm the belief that renal patients have a lower margin of safety than the average person. Hanhijari *et al.* (1972) noted that serum fluoride concentrations in patients with renal disease were as much as 5 times greater than in normal people. The increase can be explained on the basis of decreased renal clearnace of inorganic fluoride (Berman and Taves, 1973). One case of symptomatic skeletal fluorosis (radiculomyelopathy) has been reported from an area in Texas with natural fluoride at 2.3–3.5 ppm in the water. (Sauerbrunn *et al.*, 1965). There have been two cases of suspected skeletal fluorosis (based on X-ray evidence) in the United States with fluoride at 2–3 ppm in the drinking water (Juncos and Donadio, 1972). The combination of renal impairment and very high water intake was thought to account for these findings.

The best available information on the implications of increased serum fluoride concentration in renal patients is from studies on patients requiring renal dialysis. In these patients, serum fluoride during dialysis rises to about 25-30 μM; consequently, any effects should appear earlier than in renal patients not on dialysis. A double-blind study of the effect of fluoridated dialysate in long-term hemodialysis has been conducted by deionizing the water and adding fluoride or chloride via coded ampules to the dialyzing water of the artificial-kidney machine. Twenty patients were investigated for over a year (average, 20 months). Patients on fluoride showed no differences, when compared with the control group, except for the histologic observation of increased thickness of trabecular bone (Oreopoulos *et al.*, 1974).

The question of effects on patients who are maintained on dialysis for longer periods, or who are not yet adults, is certainly not settled. The fasting (5–10 μM) and maximal (25–30 μM) serum fluoride concentrations in hemodialysis patients are almost identical with concentrations in patients being treated with fluoride for various bone diseases (Taves, unpublished data); hence, some effect is possible.

The implications, however, of bone effect (fluorosis) from excess fluoride are not clear, unless a limitation of joint movement or compression of exit of the spinal nerves occurs. Fluoride is being used deliberately to produce increased bone density in patients with bone disease; therefore, it may be that small increases in bone density in renal patients may be advantageous, rather than harmful. Whether treatment with fluoride will result in improved bone density may be determined by the interrelated metabolism of calcium and vitamin D (Jowsey *et al.*,

1968). Because calcium metabolism is altered in patients with renal disease, a beneficial effect of long-term fluoridated-water hemodialysis may not be automatic, even if fluoride proves to be beneficial in other bone diseases or in preventing fractures due to osteoporosis.

The possibility of adverse effects in renal patients still dependent on their own kidneys cannot be entirely ruled out by a demonstration of benefit to those on dialysis. The possibility of adverse effects of fluoride on marginally functional kidneys has to be considered for patients with renal failure, but certain lines of evidence make adverse effects unlikely. Considerable information has been collected on serum concentrations that will cause functional renal changes. This was the result of evidence that inorganic fluoride from the metabolism of methoxyflurane was the cause of the polyuria occasionally seen after the use of that anesthetic. The serum concentrations of inorganic fluoride necessary to cause polyuria were found to start at about 40–50 μM, and severe effects required 150 μM. The immediate cause of the polyuria is the loss of the electrolyte concentration gradient from the cortex to the papilla (Whitford and Taves, 1973).

Cancer

Early in 1975 it was claimed by Yamouyiannis that there is a linkage between fluoridation of water and increased cancer rates. The initial data presented and shown in Table V-16 are the sum of rates for nine specific

TABLE V-16 Selected Cancer Mortality Rates for the Largest Cities with Fluoridated and Nonfluoridated Water (per 100,000)

Fluoridated		Nonfluoridated	
Chicago	121.0	Los Angeles	94.3
Philadelphia	124.6	Houston	82.7
Baltimore	119.2	Boston	123.1
Washington	113.1	New Orleans	104.1
Cleveland	121.9	San Antonio	84.2
San Francisco	119.9	San Diego	85.6
Milwaukee	125.9	Seattle	96.7
St. Louis	119.3	Cincinnati	115.2
Pittsburgh	112.1	Memphis	83.4
Buffalo	121.6	Atlanta	85.8
Mean	119.9		95.5

(From Yiamouyiannis, 1975)

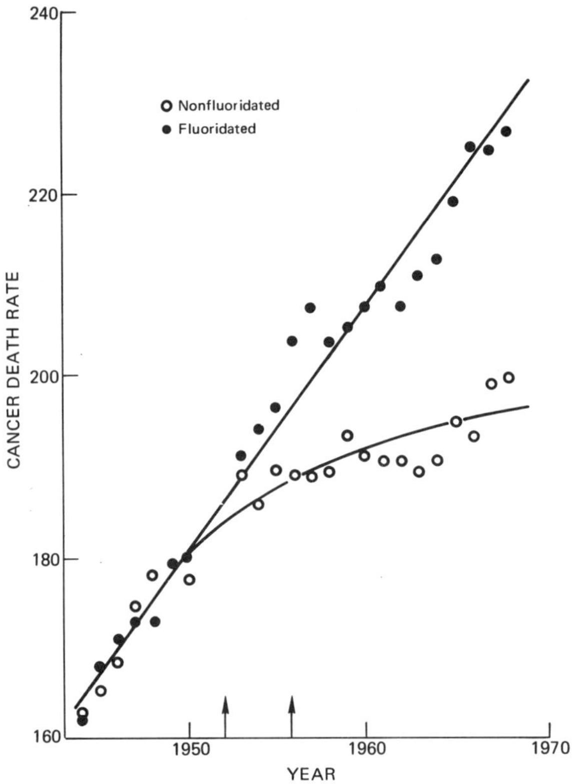

FIGURE V-1 Average crude cancer death rates for the 10 fluoridated cities from Table V-16 and 10 nonfluoridated cities selected from the 15 largest ones to match the pre-fluoridation period, 1944–1950. The two arrows mark the time when fluoridation was instituted in these cities. Reprinted, with permission, from Yiamouyiannis and Burk, 1975.

cancer sites (seven for white males and two for white females) for the 10 largest cities with fluoridated water supplies for more than 12 yr prior to 1970 and for the 10 largest nonfluoridated U.S. cities. The source of the data was the age-specific cancer rates for a 20-yr period by site and county compiled by the National Cancer Institute (NCI) and published by the Department of Health, Education, and Welfare (HEW) in 1974. There is clearly a difference between the two groups of cities, with the fluoridated ones having about 25/100,000 more cancer deaths than the nonfluoridated ones.

Later, in September 1975, Yamouyiannis and Burk submitted data to NCI suggesting that there had been a change in cancer rates with time for fluoridated cities as compared with nonfluoridated ones. A later version of the same data is shown in Figure V-1, where average annual crude cancer mortality rates have been plotted as a function of time for the 10 largest fluoridated cities and for 10 control cities, selected from among the largest nonfluoridated cities giving the same average crude death rates prior to 1952, for both groups. As can be seen, the average crude mortality rates diverge markedly after 1952, when the one group of cities initiated fluoridation.

In considering this evidence the National Cancer Institute found that Yamouyiannis and Burk had failed to take into account differing demographic factors and age distributions that affect cancer rates. When the NCI used 1950 rates for the U.S. population as a whole to adjust the crude mortality rates of Figure V-1 for sex, race, and age and expressed the results as the ratio of observed deaths to expected deaths (standard mortality ratios, SMR) the time trends are eliminated as shown in Figure V-2.

The SMR's are greater than unity for both sets of cities and greater in

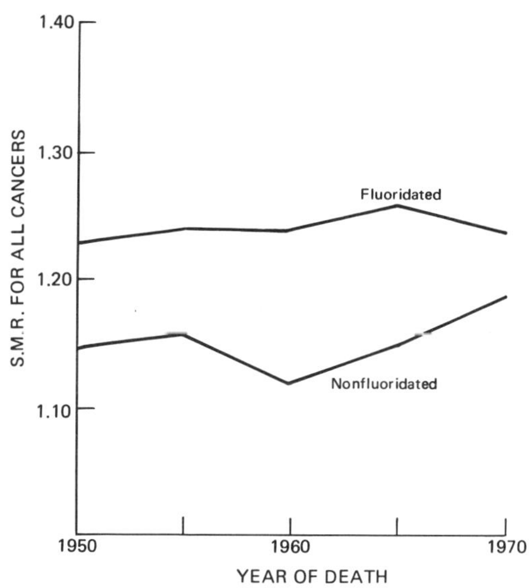

FIGURE V-2 Standard mortality ratios for all cancers for the cities of Figure V-1. Reprinted, with permission, from Hoover, 1976.

the fluoridated than in the nonfluoridated ones, but there is no change in these ratios with time from 1950 to 1970 (Hoover, 1976).

In supplementary studies, NCI (1975) investigated the absolute differences in cancer rates in fluoridated and nonfluoridated areas. One study, results of which are shown in Table V-17, dealt with reasons for the differences shown in Table V-16. Regression analyses were conducted for each of the nine cancer sites and the counties of the cities listed in Table V-16 using fluoridation as an independent variable alone and then after correction for a number of demographic variables. As shown in Table V-17, columns 3 and 4, the slopes of the regression lines (β) are generally positive and the F values are generally greater than 6 when only fluoridation status is considered, in agreement with the claim of

TABLE V-17 Regression Coefficients (β) and F Values Associated with a Fluoride Variable Entered into a Regression Analysis to Predict Sex and Site-Specific Cancer Mortality Rates in 20 Counties with and without Control for Demographic Risk Factors

	Without Control			With Control	
	Sex	β	F	β	F
Mouth and throat	M	1.14	2.6	−0.78	0.8
	F	−0.16	1.9	−0.13	0.9
Esophagus	M	2.55	25.0	0.57	1.2
	F	−0.08	0.5	−0.29	2.6
Stomach	M	5.02	19.7	2.31	11.6
	F	2.22	11.1	0.79	7.4
Colon	M	5.47	23.1	0.64	0.3
	F	3.57	13.3	−0.31	0.1
Rectum	M	3.72	21.5	1.12	1.1
	F	1.50	17.5	0.22	0.2
Breast	F	3.85	16.1	0.76	0.2
Ovary	F	1.18	9.8	0.69	2.3
Kidney	M	0.44	7.2	0.11	0.2
	F	0.21	8.2	0.07	0.7
Bladder	M	1.49	13.1	0.84	1.3
	F	0.36	8.9	0.26	2.2

(From Hoover, 1976)

Yiamouyiannis. When demographic variables are taken into account, however, the F values, given in the last column, become insignificant except for stomach cancer. Further regression analysis, allowing also for control of the specific high-risk ethnic groups for cancer, yielded a nonsignificant F value of 0.02 for females with only the F value for males, 6.9 remaining greater than the 95% confidence level. Since one positive correlation of this sort occurs by chance in 5% of cases examined and 16 cases were examined in this instance, this result cannot be regarded as strong evidence of a linkage between fluoridation and cancer.

Some linkage may not be unreasonable, however, for fluoride will exist primarily as hydrofluoric acid, a highly penetrating and irritating chemical, in the acidic stomach. Hydrofluoric acid is also a possible mutagen in plants (Mohamed, 1969) and drosophila (Mohamed and Kemmer, 1970). This will be considered more fully in a later section.

Two other studies by NCI (1975) give additional information on a possible linkage of fluorides to stomach cancer. In the first of these, cancer data for all the U.S. counties in which at least two-thirds of the population was first fluoridated between 1950 and 1965 were grouped into 5-yr intervals in order to study changes with time. Results are shown in Table V-18 in terms of standard mortality ratios at some particular sites. The bone and kidney are of special interest because fluoride is concentrated in those tissues.

None of the specific sites give any indication of an increase in cancer following fluoridation; rather a possible decrease is suggested. The "other" category is of interest as the only grouping which suggested a possible increase for both sexes.

The other study compared naturally fluoridated and nonfluoridated counties in Texas on the same basis as in the previous one. Results are shown in Table V-19. The SMR's are more variable because of the smaller numbers involved, but there are no consistent trends with increasing fluoride content except for a possible decrease in the "other" category.

Thus, there is no confirmation of the hypothesis that fluorides or fluoridation causes cancer. Moreover, epidemiological studies in England fail to support the hypothesis that stomach or any other cancer is associated with fluoride intake (Kinlen, 1975; Royal College of Physicians, 1976).

An independent evaluation of the data presented by Yiamouyiannis and Burk was carried out by Taves (1976) using the same basic statistics as those used by NCI (U.S. Census and Vital Statistics). To gain more precision, the cancer mortalities observed in the year prior to the census year have been averaged with the figures for the census year.

TABLE V-18 SMR's and Number of Deaths[a] from Cancer in 5-yr Intervals before and after Fluoridation of Water Supply

Site:	Stomach		Kidney	
Sex:	Men	Women	Men	Women
Prior to fluoridation				
10 yr	1.0 (352)	0.9 (205)	1.1 (76)	1.2 (44)
5 yr	1.3 (4,509)	1.2 (2,630)	1.1 (785)	1.3 (517)
Pentad of fluoridation				
	1.2 (8,053)	1.2 (5,143)	1.2 (1,796)	1.1 (991)
After fluoridation				
5 yr	1.2 (6,971)	1.1 (4,340)	1.2 (1,946)	1.1 (1,142)
10 yr	1.2 (5,597)	1.1 (3,655)	1.1 (1,889)	1.0 (1,072)
15 yr	1.0 (2,454)	1.0 (1,671)	1.1 (1,009)	1.0 (633)

Site:	Bone		Other	
Sex:	Men	Women	Men	Women
Prior to fluoridation				
10 yr	0.9 (28)	1.1 (23)	1.0 (203)	0.8 (184)
5 yr	1.2 (351)	1.1 (216)	0.9 (1,923)	0.9 (2,042)
Pentad of fluoridation				
	1.1 (642)	1.0 (438)	1.0 (4,436)	1.0 (4,844)
After fluoridation				
5 yr	1.1 (597)	1.1 (413)	1.0 (4,682)	1.0 (4,871)
10 yr	1.1 (499)	1.1 (358)	1.1 (5,173)	1.1 (5,383)
15 yr	1.0 (269)	1.0 (173)	1.2 (3,400)	1.2 (3,678)

[a]Number of deaths in parentheses.
(From Hoover, 1976)

During evaluation of the data, it was noted that only 1 of the fluoridated cities had gained in population from 1950 to 1970, whereas 7 of the 10 nonfluoridated cities had gained. Accordingly, the next 10 largest fluoridated cities, 7 of which had gained in population over the 20 yr, were also evaluated. In addition, data were also compiled on the 5 large nonfluoridated cities that had been omitted from the original control group.

Results are shown in Figure V-3 and in Table V-20. In no case is there a significantly different time trend; thus, the assertion that fluoridation has caused an increase in cancer rates does not hold up. The rates in fluoridated cities are higher only for a particular set of cities and the higher rates in these cities were present before fluoridation. When the data for all 20 fluoridated cities and all 15 nonfluoridated cities are combined as shown in Table V-20, the standard mortality ratios for the fluoridated cities are remarkably constant.

For negative results like those described in the preceding section it is important to assess the magnitude of the effect that would escape detection. Statistically, such evaluations are known as estimations of error of the second kind, beta error or power of the test (Dixon and Massey, 1969). For the Taves study, for example, it was computed that a 1.5% increase in cancer death rates would have been detected with 95% confidence. The results of the large NCI study by 5-yr periods have a similar detection limit with about a 10% detection limit for increase in cancer at specific sites (Taves, 1977).

Other observations of possible positive correlations between fluoride intake and cancer, although not conclusive, deserve attention and further investigation. Okamura and Matsuhisa (1963) showed a correlation between stomach cancer and the fluoride content of rice and "miso." The fluoride values reported for food by Okamura are many times those expected in this country and are based on analytic methods that would not distinguish between organic and inorganic fluoride. So, even if the correlation is causal, it is not clear that fluoride ion is involved. Hirayama (1977) reported that stomach cancer rates in Japan were positively correlated with the amounts of hot tea and fish consumed and negatively

TABLE V-19 Site and Sex Specific SMR's and Observed Number of Cancer Deaths[a] (1950–1969) in Counties in Texas Grouped According to Natural Fluoride Levels

		Levels of Natural Fluoride			
Site	Sex	Control	Low	Intermediate	High
Stomach	Men	1.0 (375)	1.0 (914)	1.1 (239)	1.1 (112)
	Women	1.0 (236)	1.0 (583)	1.0 (122)	1.0 (55)
Kidney	Men	1.1 (121)	1.0 (235)	1.2 (84)	0.6 (19)
	Women	1.0 (68)	1.0 (163)	1.0 (46)	1.2 (23)
Bone	Men	1.0 (40)	1.0 (118)	1.2 (39)	0.6 (8)
	Women	0.9 (27)	1.1 (70)	0.9 (14)	0.8 (5)
Other and unspecified	Men	1.0 (319)	1.0 (774)	1.0 (211)	0.9 (83)
	Women	1.0 (318)	1.0 (854)	0.9 (170)	0.9 (73)

[a]Number of deaths in parentheses.
(From Hoover, 1976)

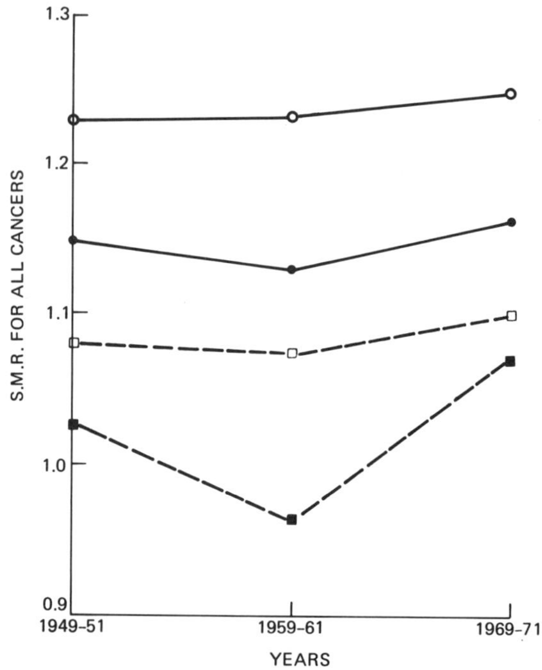

FIGURE V-3 Standard mortality ratios for all cancers using average of 2 yr observed mortality. Fluoridated cities of Figure V-1, open circles; nonfluoridated cities of Figure V-1, closed circles. Next 10 largest fluoridated cities, open squares; the closed squares are the 5 nonfluoridated cities omitted from 15 largest nonfluoridated shown in Figure V-1.

correlated with the amount of milk drunk. Tea and fish have been reported to have higher levels of fluoride than other foods, and milk would be expected to act as a binding agent and buffer to reduce effective concentrations of hydrogen fluoride (HF) in the stomach.

There was an observation in the Kingston–Newburgh (Ast *et al.*, 1956) study that was considered spurious and has never been followed up. There was a 13.5% incidence of cortical defects in bone in the fluoridated community but only 7.5% in the nonfluoridated community. With 474 and 375 children in the respective groups, the *t* value was 2.85, which is statistically significant (Schlesinger, 1956). Caffey (1955) noted that the age, sex, and anatomical distribution of these bone defects are "strikingly" similar to that of osteogenic sarcoma. While progression of cortical defects to malignancies has not been observed clinically, it would be important to have direct evidence that osteogenic sarcoma rates in males under 30 have not increased with fluoridation. The overall bone cancer rates do not appear to have been affected by fluoridation. However, bone cancer rates are dominated by the older age groups, which could obscure a difference in the younger ages.

Taylor and Taylor (1964, 1965) concluded that low concentrations of fluoride increase the rate of tumor growth in animals or eggs. Their studies are not convincing because they show no dose-response effect over a very wide range of doses. Such findings generally indicate inadequate controls or the presence of bias. The use of distilled water for control, rather than an equivalent amount of sodium chloride, might be a cause of inadequacy in the controls. Distilled water tends to pick up metal ions to a greater extent than does a solution. The data of Flemming (1953) suggested a beneficial effect from fluoride at 20 ppm in the drinking water of mice with implanted tumors. An abstract by Bittner and Armstrong (1952) indicated no carcinogenic effect from 5 to 20 ppm fluoride in the drinking water on the survival of the ZBC-strain mice.

In summary, the available evidence does not suggest that fluoridation has increased the overall cancer mortality rates. The margin of possible error is very low, approaching 3/100,000. This is the theoretical effect that could have been missed with present statistical techniques. The NCI studies probably lowered the margin of error by a factor of 5 from the best previous study (Hagen *et al.*, 1954).

Mutagenesis, Teratogenesis, Birth Defects

There are a number of papers suggesting or claiming that fluoride is mutagenic, but relatively little attention has been paid to them. This lack of attention probably stems from the fact that the published evidence has

TABLE V-20 Standard Mortality Ratios (SMR) for All Cities, Expected Deaths Based on U.S. Rates for 1950

	Nonfluoridated (15)		Fluoridated (20)	
Time, 2 yr	Observed Deaths	SMR	Observed Deaths	SMR
1949–1951	26,952	1.1272	53,908	1.1961
1959–1961	33,377	1.0899	60,185	1.1958
1969–1971	38,825	1.1390	61,938	1.2116

been in plants and *Drosophila,* primarily with high doses of HF rather than fluoride ion. As noted above, the possibility of mutagenesis due to HF is potentially important in cancer of the stomach. Ingested fluoride ion can become HF in the stomach because the pK of HF is 3.18 and the pH of the stomach without food is generally about 1. Although stomach cancer rates show no consistent indication of a relationship to fluoridation in the United States, the much higher stomach cancer rates in Japan are related to intake patterns that are compatible with a hypothesis that fluoride is the crucial factor involved (Taves, 1977). Therefore, the work in plants with HF will be reviewed after consideration of the recent work of Mohamed and Chandler (1976), in which 1 ppm NaF (presumably 0.5 ppm fluoride) reportedly caused permanent damage to the chromosomes of bone-marrow cells and spermatocytes in mice. Increased rates of congenital malformations and decreased rates of reproduction can also be consequences of mutation. Hence, the available evidence on these topics as related to fluoride ingestion is also part of this section.

Mohamed and Chandler's experiment consisted of feeding mice a low-fluoride diet together with varying concentrations of sodium fluoride in distilled water for two time periods, 3 and 6 weeks. The concentrations of sodium fluoride were 0, 1, 10, 50, 100, and 200 ppm. Sixty-four mice, plus eight baseline controls, were put on a low-fluoride diet and given distilled water to drink for 1 week prior to the start of the experiment. The data consisted of food intake, water consumption, fluoride concentration of the bone ash, and cytological examination of chromosomes from bone-marrow cells and spermatocytes.

The frequency distribution of chromosomal changes in bone-marrow cells was given as a percentage. Two things are of note that are not commented on by the authors. One is the fact that the numbers of cells examined are not consistent with the number of animals in the groups, four to each treatment group and eight to each control group, and vary markedly, 737–1,345 for the groups with the same number of animals. The lack of twice the number of observations in the larger groups raises the question of how animals or slides were selected. Was each animal represented with the same intensity of searching, and, if not, what determined the intensity of the search? The second point of note is that the largest change in frequency of abnormality occurs between 0 and 1 ppm NaF. This is odd because there is little or no difference in the bone fluoride concentrations with these two dose levels. A possible difference between the controls and the rest of the animals is that the distilled water dissolved more metal ions than the distilled water with NaF and that this difference in intake was important in the marginally iron-deficient diet (Tao and Suttie, 1976). This type of response makes the claim of an effect down to the 1-ppm level uncertain. Using the 1-ppm NaF animals as the controls, rather than those receiving distilled water, would make the changes in chromosomal fragments unimpressive. There is still, however, a doubling of "ball metaphase" rings and bridges that is recorded. Ball metaphase is not commonly recognized by cytologists and was not noted by Temple and Weinstein (personal communication) when they repeated the work of Mohamed *et al.* (1966a) on onion root tip with $10^{-2}M$ fluoride.

The spermatocyte changes also show things of note which were not commented on by the authors. In this case, the numbers of cells examined are again very irregular. However, the total for the control groups is approximately double, properly reflecting the group sizes. The serious discrepancy, however, is that there is no way that the percentages given for the frequency of abnormalities can be derived from the number of cells examined. The cells examined are scored as having either breaks, fragments, or both for the first meiotic anaphase and telophase and for the second anaphase and telophase. If each number of cells listed to the left of these two sets of frequencies is divided into 1, 2, 3, etc., to the 4th decimal place, multiplied by 100, and then compared to the percentages listed, only 27 of 90 can be rationalized on the basis of rounding errors. It is, therefore, clear that the listed sets and number of cells are not the numbers from which the corresponding percentages were derived. It is possible that the authors meant that the number of cells was the sum of two denominators. However, there are several frequencies listed for a given exposure of cells examined would have to have been considerably larger than the total as given.

Mohamed's earlier work in onion root tips (Mohamed *et al.*, 1966a) and tomatoes (Mohamed *et al.*, 1966b) was done without the use of random numbers to code the slides, but his work in corn (Mohamed, 1970) was done by random assignment of the slide numbers prior to reading, even though this is not mentioned in the paper (phone conversation to D. R. T.) There is apparently no published confirmation of any of this work. An unpublished study (Temple and Weinstein, 1976) was able to confirm increased bridges and fragments of chromosomes in onion root tips when grown in $10^{-2}M$ fluoride, but they did not confirm the observation of ball metaphase.

The only published second generation study to provide direct evidence of mutation was done by Mohamed (1968). In this study he exposed tomato plants to HF. The summary gives the concentration as 3 mg/m^3, but this should read 3 μg/m^3 (phone conversation to D. R. T.) The dose or time of parental exposure is not given in the body of the paper. A phone conversation revealed that the seeds came from plants exposed in a previous study (Mohamed *et al.*, 1966b) in which all flower buds past the stage used for the chromosome smears were destroyed so that the fruit grown from the recovered plants would not have been exposed to HF subsequent to the formation of flowers. If the exposure had continued beyond this point, abnormal numbers of cotyledons would not necessarily indicate genetic damage. Abnormal numbers and shapes of the cotyledons occurred in the treated groups about 3 times more often than the 4.7% of the controls. Fasciated petioles, wiry plants, and plumuless plants were noted only in the treated plants, but the frequency was irregularly related to the duration of exposure. Dwarf plants and double stalks increased from 0.8% in the controls to 5% in the treated plants with uniform increases in four of the five exposure periods of increasing length. These descriptions of damage sound arbitrary, and no criteria are listed; hence, the lack of blind reading leaves the data unconvincing. The article stated that work is in progress to determine whether the effect was due to minute chromosomal changes or to changes within the gene. However, there have been no citations of this article through the June 1976 issue of *Citation Index,* suggesting that the findings have not been confirmed. Temple and Weinstein (1976) were unable to confirm these findings with the same or a different strain of tomato. The negative results with the same strain are limited however, because of the low rate of seed germination under the conditions used.

There has been work on *Drosophila* by several different laboratories with a variety of conclusions. Mohamed (1971) claims to have proven that HF in concentrations too low to cause death is mutagenic in *Drosophila melanogaster.* The basis for his claim is genetic analysis of the progeny of flies exposed for 6–12 hr to air which had been bubbled through 2.5% HF.

The analysis involved looking at the ratio of the homozygous to heterozygous offspring from F_1 generation sib matings. The tester females were heterozygous for a recessive lethal so that F_2 generations could only be homozygous for the paternal chromosomes in question; i.e., 33% would be expected. These F_1 sibs were selected on the bases of marker genes to have the same paternal gene. The control groups showed 34.69 ± 0.86% homozygous and the treated groups showed 26.84 ± 0.09 to 25.52 ± 1.54% homozygous, a clearly significant difference. The author claims a statistically significant difference between the exposed groups, but this is true only if the data in his tables are in error and the ± are standard deviations rather than standard errors, as listed. The small dose effect may be due to having discontinued the introduction of the HF after 1 h and erroneously assuming that the concentration stayed constant for the remaining time of the exposure period. In the previous paper (Mohamed and Kemmer, 1970), continuous exposure to air bubbled through 5% HF resulted in only three males being left to test, which suggests that the use of a 2.5% solution in the 1971 study is quite high. In order to prove the contention of mutagenicity, the males should have been mated prior to treatment to show that their genes were in fact normal before exposure to HF.

Mukherjee and Sobels (1968) reported that injection of 1 m*M* NaF (unstated amount), as compared to injection of 1 m*M* NaCl increased the percent lethals produced by 2,000 R radiation. The percent lethals in the NaCl groups was about 5% in four experiments, while it was 6 to 10% in the NaF groups.

Vogel (1973) stated that 1 m*M* fluoride in 5% glucose fed to *Drosophila* larva was a weak mutagen but acted as a powerful antimutagen in combination with a strong mutagen. The evidence for a weak mutagen effect is slim. In one of three experiments, there were three lethals compared to one in the controls and one in each of two exposure groups. With only fluoride exposure, the egg-laying capacity was clearly depressed in most experiments and the hatchability was generally, but not always lower. Hence, he concluded that fluoride had a sterilizing effect. Treatment with the trialkylating agent Trenimon alone showed 13.1% lethals but in combination with 12 m*M* F, 3.4% lethals without a consistent difference in the number of eggs laid or their hatchability. A second experiment showed 8.6 and 1.3%, respectively. Since at least 350 chromosomes were tested for each group in each experiment, these differences are clearly statistically significant.

Herskowitz and Norton (1963) showed a marked increase in the incidence of melanotic tumors in two strains of *Drosophila*. The controls were 0.0% and 7.1%, while the treatment of the larvae with 1 to 30 m*M* fluoride caused a smooth dose response up to nearly 100% occurrence. The group sizes were 1,500 so the numbers are highly significant statistically.

Obe and Slacik-Erben (1973) reported a 25–50% decrease in the total breaking events of chromosomes of human cells *in vitro* with three separate strong mutagens in combination with 1 m*M* fluoride. Slacik-Erben and Obe's further work (1976) attempting to clarify the role of sodium fluoride and antimutagenic effects with Trenimon gives control data which show no effect from 1 m*M* fluoride alone. The human cells in this case were lymphocytes stimulated with phytohaemagglutinin in which nucleotide incorporation and mitotic index were followed for over 2 days. The data curves for two experiments were averaged and plotted; hence, only a visual judgement of no-effect can be made and no estimate of the power of the test is given.

Jagiello and Ja-Shein (1974) exposed mammalian eggs to NaF and concluded that some changes were taking pace. The earliest effect noted was clumping of the chromosomes at meiosis in cow oocytes exposed to 10 ppm (500 μM). This was the lowest concentration used. There is no indication of blind reading of the smears.

There is some evidence of decreased fertility or reproduction with doses of fluoride below obvious toxic levels, which might be related to mutation and is of interest even if it is not related. Gerdes *et al.*, 1971 found a 5–10% reduction in male *Drosophila* fertility, a 30% reduction of female fecundity, and a 20% reduction of egg hatchability from the second generation with 6 weeks exposure to 2.9 ppm HF. These changes in the second generation (C_1) were attributed to genetic effects rather than to direct effects on the eggs. This claim is not convincing, since the eggs giving rise to the first generation would also have been exposed for some hours to the HF.

Rensburg and Vos (1966) concluded that for normal reproduction in Afrikaner heifers under ordinary ranching conditions, the fluoride concentration should be less than 5 ppm. They found that the number of calves produced by the animals on 12 ppm water was decreased by about one-half as compared to those drinking 5 ppm. They speculate that there are functional disturbances of the ovaries due to fluoride under range conditions, which are marginal for several months each year.

If fluoride were an important mutagen for humans, there would be real concern that cancer rates and congenital malformations might increase. There is a new set of data on each of these possibilities. (See Report of The Royal College of Physicians, 1976, for a review of the largely unpublished earlier data.) In the case of human cancer, the data can rule out an effect larger than 2% (Taves, 1977). Congenital malformation rates, relative to fluoridation, were collected by Erickson *et al.* (1976) in the counties around Atlanta. The overall rates were 292.6 abnormalties per 10,000 live births for the fluoridated and 270 per 10,000 for the nonfluoridated populations. The Chi square was 3.58, and 3.84 is needed to be significant at the 0.05 level. While the difference is not statistically significant, an increase of 10% certainly can not be ruled out. About half of the population of the county (Fulton County, which contains Atlanta) was represented in both the fluoridated and nonfluoridated populations, because fluoridation was introduced in the middle of the time when the data were being collected; consequently, the period of exposure was generally short. A second part of this study, however, used data from a 10-yr exposure period and shows the opposite relationship; i.e., a statistically significant lower rate in the population exposed to fluoridation. The difficulty in relying too heavily on later data is that the rates are about one-third of the Atlanta data, a fact that suggests serious under-reporting. Since a similar degree of apparent under-reporting has been cited to discredit Rapaport's findings on mongolism (Royal College of Physicians, 1976; Needleman *et al.*, 1975), it is inconsistent to place great faith in this negative study even though it is about 10 times larger than Rapaport's.

The above evidence will not convince most scientists that fluoride is mutagenic for any species, but it certainly does not rule out that possibility, particularly for *Drosophila.* However, even if fluoride is shown to be mutagenic for species other than man, its relevance to man would be questionable in the face of the available human data.

Mottling

The WHO report (1970, p. 299) includes a figure showing the relationship of the community fluorosis (mottling) index (as a function of water fluoride concentrations) to the mean annual temperature. The figure indicates that fluoride should be removed from water when its concentration is greater than 0.8–1.6 mg/liter, depending on temperature, in order to avoid objectionable dental mottling. More recently collected data by Richards *et al.* (1967) led them to conclude that 0.7–1.3 mg/liter would be appropriate maximum concentrations to recommend, again depending on average temperature. These values overlap the WHO values and represent good agreement. Richards *et al.* preferred average maximum temperature to mean annual temperature as a basis for the recommendations. No recent U.S. surveys or studies of communities have been found on which a sound decision could be made that greater concentrations are without objectionable effect. A report from Sweden by Ericsson and Ribelius (1971) suggests more mottling at 1.2 ppm than would be acceptable to many. They indicate that only 1 of 92 children had objectionable mottling, but their graph showed 9 graded at 3.0, which was defined as the "whole surface affected, often brown discoloration." They note that this was a higher incidence than previously reported for the same degree of intake. Whether this related to some peculiarity, such as high fish consumption, which would not be applicable to U.S. communities, is not clear.

Recent work in England has confirmed the view that considerable dental mottling is not due to fluoride and that the optimal concentration of fluoride may, in fact, decrease the amount of dental mottling (Al-

Alousi *et al.*, 1975; Jackson *et al.*, 1975). The presence of discolored (brown) areas in a few teeth even in the low-fluoride area suggests that better methods of ascribing etiology need to be developed and the question of objectionable mottling reevaluated.

Two cases of dental mottling in children with diabetes insipidus living in fluoridated communities have been reported (Greenberg *et al.*, 1974). The Royal College of Physicians (1976) report tended to dismiss the possibility that the dental mottling was due to fluoride on the grounds that other conditions might have caused it and that similar observations were lacking in a center for children with renal disease. The fluid intake was estimated to be 2.5–6 times normal; however, it was also stated that the urinary volume was as much as 9 liters/day. Such volume would require an intake 18 times normal (Greenberg *et al.*, 1974). With such unusual intakes, it would not be unreasonable to find dental fluorosis; perhaps the more pertinent question is, "Why is it not noted more often?"

It is possible that objectionable mottling is being avoided in naturally high-fluoride areas in the United States by the practice of drinking bottled water or beverages and by the use of air conditioning, which would decrease the fluid intake. Those who do not have these amenities may be either too transient or too nonvocal to be noted. The "moderate" dental fluorosis shown by Hodge and Smith (1965, p. 443) in a community with "about 2 ppm" would be objectionable to most, if not all, parents, although there seems to be little consumer research on the matter.

Recently one of the authors (D. R. T.) visited several areas in Texas (Lubbock and Amarillo) that have high natural fluoride concentrations in their drinking water. Several health officials reviewed for him their observations concerning renal dialysis and dental mottling with respect to fluoride. Their experience has been that there seems to be less bone disease in patients who come to dialysis centers from high fluoride areas. While Lubbock and Amarillo have in recent years decreased the fluoride content of their drinking water supplies, the neighboring towns generally have not changed. The health officials in the surrounding areas have observed a decrease in dental mottling, as well as a decrease in rampant caries. In light of these recent observations, it is suggested that such communities be extensively resurveyed before any changes are made in fluoride standards for public water supplies.

In light of the ability of anyone to observe and object to dental mottling, it seems presumptuous for experts to recommend acceptable fluoride concentrations without direct evidence on the levels of fluoride that may be causing difficulty.

General Epidemiological Studies

The largest study of overall mortality rates in high-fluoride (0.4–4.0 ppm) vs. low-fluoride (<0.25 ppm) areas considered 32 paired cities (Hagen *et al.*, 1954). The average mortality in the high-fluoride areas was 1,010.6/100,000, which was 5.6/100,000 higher than in the control cities. This difference is not statistically significant, because the standard error of the difference is 27/100,000. Conversely, the smallest real difference that the study can be 95% sure of ruling out is 51/100,000, which is 1.69 (the one-tailed critical value for 31 degrees of freedom) times the standard error of the mean plus 5 (the actual difference). In other works, the study would be expected to have this small a difference (or less) only one-twentieth of the times even if there were a real difference of 51/100,000. Considering that the populations studied probably were not very stable, even greater differences cannot be ruled out.

One alternative to increasing the size of the study population is to consider populations exposed to much higher concentrations in the water. The Bartlett–Cameron study (Leone *et al.*, 1954) is an example: fluoride concentrations in the water supplies were 8 and 0.7 mg/liter, respectively. People were selected who had resided for over 15 yr in either area, but no information was given about whether they drank community or bottled water. The same people were studied 10 yr later. The authors concluded that there was no statistically significant difference between the two groups taken as a whole. There were however, five of forty tests which showed statistically significant differences, some favoring the high fluoride group. Since several such individual differences would be expected to appear statistically significant by chance with so many tests these differences do not force rejection of the null hypothesis. The authors of the report conclude that there was not a statistically significant difference between the numbers of deaths. They do not give the age and sex-adjusted values, but these were over twice as high in the high-fluoride area. The AMA committee (1956) that reviewed the data concluded that the difference was just barely statistically significant (0.045). The AMA committee minimized the importance of this difference by quoting Roholm's statement that he had not observed an increase in mortality among crysolite workers whose fluoride intake was presumably even higher. Roholm, however, also concluded that he could not rule out an increase in mortality. He had only 12 autopsy cases available, and they were not in a controlled study.

It is clear that the studies discussed leave a considerable area of uncertainty. This could be reduced relatively easily. Fluoridation was introduced into many large cities in the early 1950's and into only a few cities since then, so there is a basis for an unusually large study for which the data have been collected but not examined for detrimental or beneficial effects. The positive effects might occur from better nutrition with less caries and tooth loss or from decreased soft tissue calcification. The cancer mortality studies of the NCI involved populations 10–50 times larger than those from the 32 paired cities, and the accumulating data will have an even larger potential. The data presumably are available within the federal agencies and could be run through the same basic programs as set up by the NCI for cancer mortality, to look at total as well as other separate categories of death.

The lack of such studies on the continuing evaluation of fluoridation probably stems from the failure of scientists to ask what the no-effect limits are. Without statements about the power of the tests, the implication of finding no-effect is construed to be that no effect exists. Such implication leaves little incentive to do a better study. Currently, the only motivation for such studies is an interest in checking allegations as they arise.

SUMMARY AND CONCLUSIONS

In summary, there is no generally accepted evidence that anyone has been harmed by drinking water with fluoride concentrations considered optimal for the annual mean temperatures in the temperate zones. It seems likely, however, that objectionable dental fluorosis occurred in two children with diabetes insipidus. Bone changes, possibly desirable, have been noted in patients being dialyzed against large volumes of fluoridated water. Similar changes can be expected in the rare renal patient with a long history of renal insufficiency and a high fluid intake that includes large amounts of tea. With this particular combination of circumstances, the lowest drinking-water concentration of fluoride associated with symptomatic skeletal fluorosis that has been reported to date is 3 ppm, outside of countries such as India. It should be possible for the medical profession to avoid the possible adverse effects of fluoride under the conditions described above, thereby making it unnecessary to limit the concentrations of fluoride in order to protect these rare patients. On the basis of studies done more than 15 yr ago, occasional objectionable mottling would be expected to occur in communities in the hotter regions of the United States with water that contains fluoride at 1 ppm or higher and in any community with water that contains fluoride at 2 ppm or higher. However, this may not be the case today; more liberal provisional limits seem appropriate while studies are conducted to clarify the subject.

The possibility of fluoride causing other adverse effects (allergic responses, monogolism, and cancer) or beneficial effects other than decreased dental caries has not been adequately documented to carry weight in the practical decision about the desirable levels of fluoride. The questions of monogolism and cancer have been raised on the basis of epidemiological data for which there is contrary evidence and the risk factors involved in any case are too low to establish a causal association. The allergic responses claimed by some reports are based on clinical observations and in some case double blind tests. The reservation in accepting these at face value is the lack of similar reports in much larger numbers of people who have been exposed to considerably more fluoride than was involved in the original observations. From a scientific point of view none of these effects can be ruled out, but the available data are rather limited or easily improved so further study is indicated.

RESEARCH RECOMMENDATIONS

1. Better criteria should be developed for diagnosing dental fluorosis, as distinct from dental mottling.
2. The present rate of dental fluorosis (particularly staining) in communities with fluoride at more than 1 ppm in the water supply should be determined.
3. Bone and blood fluoride concentrations of patients with chronic renal disease in communities with fluoride at 2 ppm or more should be compared with those of similar patients in low-fluoride areas, to see whether there is a difference radiologically, histologically, or clinically, particularly with regard to bone pain and fracture rates.
4. The inorganic fluoride content of food, as distinct from the total fluoride content, should be determined, to settle the issue of whether there has been an increase.
5. Rappaport's study on mongolism should be repeated with the same cities; if there is still an association, intensive case-finding should be carried out, to check whether the lack of case-finding was important in his results.
6. Mortality ratios should be evaluated by cause of death in the fluoridated vs. nonfluoridated areas.
7. There should be *in vivo* studies on the possibility of the development of cellular tolerance or intolerance to fluoride.
8. The nonhuman-primate study of Manocha *et al.* (1975) should be repeated with 5 ppm water and better controls, to check the reported renal enzyme changes.
9. Chromosomal studies of mice drinking water with low F concentra-

tions should be repeated to determine if chromosome abnormalities are induced.

10. Dominant lethal studies should be done in rats and mice by feeding the males various dose levels of fluoride and mating to tester females on a normal diet. This is easier to do and would confirm item 9, if positive, but not necessarily be inconsistent, if negative.

11. Further evaluation of cancer death rates and congenital malformation rates in large fluoridated cities as compared to nonfluoridated cities should be made.

Sodium

OCCURRENCE

Sodium ion is an ubiquitous constituent of natural waters. It is derived geologically from the leaching of surface and underground deposits of salts such as sodium chloride, from the decomposition of sodium aluminum silicates and similar minerals, from the incorporation of evaporated ocean spray particles into rainfall, and from the intrusion of seawater into freshwater aquifers. Salt spray from the sea is often the largest contributor of sodium ions within 50–100 miles of seacoasts. Some soils exhibit the property of ion exchange in which calcium ions in the water are replaced by sodium ions during normal leaching.

Human activities also contribute sodium ions to natural waters. The sodium chloride used as a deicing agent on roads enters water supplies in runoff from both roads and storage depots. The quantity of sodium ion from this source has increased progressively since 1947 from about 0.5

TABLE V-21 Sodium Ion Concentration in Drinking Water

Sodium Ion Concentration, mg/liter	No. of Samples	Percent of Samples
0–19.9	1,194	58.2
20–49.9	391	19.0
50–99.9	190	9.3
100–249.9	178	8.7
250–399.9	74	3.6
400–499.9	10	0.5
500–999.9	14	0.7
1,000 or higher	2	0.1
Total	2,053	100.1

(From White *et al.*, 1967)

million tons to 9 million tons in 1970 (USEPA, 1971). This added sodium chloride is distributed throughout the snow belt of the northern United States and is most heavily concentrated around metropolitan areas. (American Public Works Association, 1969; Hanes *et al.*, 1970; Hutchinson, 1971; Bubeck *et al.*, 1971).

Municipal use of water typically results in the addition of 20–50 mg/liter of sodium ion, primarily from urine and washing products. Procedures for water treatment often produce a finished water with greater sodium-ion concentration than the raw water from which it was derived. Sources of sodium ion in the treatment of water include sodium hypochlorite, sodium hydroxide, sodium carbonate, and sodium silicate.

A survey of 2,100 water supplies, covering approximately 50% of the population of the United States, was carried out in 1963–1966 by the Heart Disease Control Program, Division of Chronic Diseases and the Water Supply Section, Division of Environmental Engineering, both of the U.S. Public Health Service. The distribution of sodium ion found in this survey ranged from 0.4 to 1,900 mg/liter as shown in Table V-21. Some 42% of the supplies had sodium ion concentrations in excess of 20 mg/liter and nearly 5% had concentrations greater than 250 mg/liter.

Similar results were shown in the 1975 report, of *Chemical Analysis of Interstate Carrier Water Supply Systems.* For 630 systems the range of sodium ion concentrations was from <1 to 402 mg/liter. A total of 42% had concentrations greater than 20 mg/liter and 3% had concentrations greater than 200 mg/liter.

Daily Intake of Sodium Ion

Few studies of habitual sodium-ion intake in healthy adults have been reported. Such data as have been reported are based on measurement of sodium excretion in 24-h or 12-h urine collections. Since ingested sodium is mostly excreted in urine, these figures give an acceptable estimate of sodium intake for the period immediately preceding and embracing the time of urine collection. Wide variations occur among individuals and in the same individual from day to day (Dawber *et al.*, 1967). Dahl (1958) reported a mean 24-h excretion of 4,100 mg with a range from 1,600 to 9,600 mg in 71 working adult males in New York. Langford *et al.* (in press) reported a mean sodium excretion of 2,822 mg per 24 h in 171 black women ranging in age from 35–44 yr. A recent estimate for infants is 69–92 mg/kg/day (American Academy of Pediatrics, 1974). Sodium chloride is added to many foods during processing, such as baby foods. Additional sodium chloride is often added during cooking and again at the table.

Habitual intake of sodium bears no relationship to physiological need. Estimated daily losses of sodium in urine, stool, skin, and insensible perspiration in subjects on markedly restricted sodium intake total 40–185 mg/day (Dahl, 1958). Additional losses occur during sweating; however, sodium content of sweat is adjusted during sodium deprivation by adrenocortical influences. Healthy individuals have been shown to maintain sodium balance on a sodium intake of less than 2,000 mg/24 h while sweating 9 liters/day (Conn, 1949). A variety of preindustrial societies, in widely divergent habitats (tropical jungle, desert, arctic, etc.) subsist for generations on sodium intake less than 1,000 mg/day and show no evidence of sodium deprivation (Dahl, 1958; Page, *et al.*, 1974). Total body sodium content is about 130,000 mg for a 70-kg man (Widdowson *et al.*, 1951). Requirements for sodium in growing infants and children are estimated at less than 200 mg/day (American Academy of Pediatrics, 1974).

It thus appears that habitual intake of sodium in adults in the United States often exceeds body need by 10-fold or more. Evidence that this excessive intake may have harmful consequences is summarized elsewhere in this report.

Since adult fluid intake averages 1.5–3 liters/day, sodium intake from drinking water represents less than 10% of the habitual total intake of 3,000–4,000 mg as long as the sodium content of the water does not exceed 200 mg/liter. Adverse health effects may be anticipated with sodium concentrations greater than 20 mg/liter, however, for that special risk group restricted to total sodium intake of 500 mg/day, for intake from food cannot feasibly be reduced to less than about 440 mg/day (White *et al.*, 1967). For this group, whose diets must be medically supervised in a careful manner, knowledge of the sodium-ion concentration of the drinking water permits prescription of low-sodium water when necessary.

METABOLISM

A full description of the physiologic mechanisms governing sodium metabolism is beyond the scope of this report; excellent summaries are available elsewhere (DeWardener, 1973; Early, 1972; Burg, 1976). Sodium is rapidly and almost quantitatively absorbed from the gastrointestinal tract. It is distributed as the most abundant cation of plasma and extracellular fluid in man and all other vertebrates. It is present in bone and (in low concentrations) in cells of most tissues, except adipose tissue, from which it is virtually absent. The concentration of sodium in extracellular fluid is maintained within narrow limits through regulation of the excretion of water by the kidney, under the influence of endocrine, cardiovascular, and autonomic regulatory mechanisms. The total amount of sodium in extracellular fluid thus determines the volume of these fluids. The volume of plasma and of extracellular fluid is in turn governed by regulatory mechanisms involving the endocrine, cardiovascular, and autonomic nervous systems, which regulate volume primarily by influencing renal excretion of sodium. Arterial blood pressure influences and is influenced by variations in plasma volume.

HEALTH EFFECTS

Acute Effects

Acute adverse effects of sodium in the healthy population are probably confined to neonates and young infants and will be discussed later.

Chronic Effects

An impressive amount of evidence has accumulated over the last several decades that sodium taken in excess of physiologic need is important in inducing an age-related increase in blood pressure that culminates in hypertension in genetically susceptible people.

The prevalence of hypertension in the adult population of United States is 15–20% among Caucasians (U.S. National Center for Health Statistics, 1964) and substantially higher among blacks (Stamler *et al.*, 1960). Thus some 30–40 million Americans are afflicted with this disease.

Evidence both in animals (Dahl *et al.*, 1962) and in man (Ostfield and Paul, 1963; Thomas, 1973) indicates that a genetic factor operates to make some people susceptible to hypertension. One or more environmental factors may then induce the development of hypertension in these people. A wide variety of environmental factors have been implicated in the induction of hypertension, including sodium ion, obesity, trace minerals, and psychosocial stress factors. Evidence that sodium ion is involved as a causative agent in hypertension has three main sources: animal experiments, clinical observations, and epidemiologic studies. The salient features of this evidence are summarized briefly in the following paragraphs.

Animal Experiments Observations (Meneely and Dahl, 1961; Dahl, 1960, 1972) extending over a period of 20 yr have repeatedly shown that sodium ion induces hypertension in genetically susceptible rats. Rats given sodium chloride at 2.8–9.8% in diet rations develop hypertension within a few weeks or months. When unselected rats are used in such experiments, the incidence and severity of hypertension vary directly with the sodium chloride concentration in the diet (Meneely and Dahl, 1961). Approximately 80% of animals eventually develop some degree of elevated blood pressure (Dahl, 1960). In selective breeding experiments, "sodium-sensitive" and "sodium-resistent" strains can be produced by inbreeding separately rats that do and rats that do not develop hypertension in response to sodium chloride (Dahl, 1972). Among genetically sodium-sensitive rats, young animals are more sensitive to the effects of sodium than adults (Meneely and Dahl, 1961). When hypertension becomes established in these animals, it is not corrected by reducing sodium intake (Tobian *et al.*, 1969). Despite many generations of inbreeding, the sodium-sensitive animals will maintain normal blood pressure throughout life if they are never exposed to excessive intake of sodium (Dahl, 1972).

Although there is not general agreement as to the exact mechanism by which excess sodium ion induces hypertension, considerable evidence has accumulated in the last few years that it involves the regulatory mechanisms governing the renal excretion of sodium. Transplantation of kidneys between sodium-resistant and sodium-sensitive rats results in a blood-pressure increase in the rat that receives the sodium-sensitive kidney and a decrease in the rat that receives the sodium-resistant kidney (Dahl *et al.*, 1974).

An important determinant of sodium excretion by the normal kidney is the arterial perfusion pressure (Guyton *et al.*, 1972). Recent studies have shown that the relationship between perfusion pressure and sodium excretion is altered in sodium-sensitive animals in which hypertension has been induced by sodium feeding. Higher arterial pressure is required to excrete the same quantity of sodium in the hypertensive animals than in pair-matched control animals of the same strain whose blood pressure remains normal on high sodium intake (Tobian, 1975).

Correlative data from several other types of experiments support the importance of sodium excretion as a central determinant of arterial blood pressure in all forms of hypertension, and in normal animals as well.

In recently developed strains of "spontaneously hypertensive rats" (highly inbred animals), hypertension develops spontaneously and does not require induction by sodium ion or other identifiable environmental factors (Okamoto, 1969). Hypertension in these animals is corrected by transplanting into them kidneys from normal animals (Bianchi *et al.*, 1973). From these and other data, it has been suggested that hypertension in the spontaneously hypertensive rat is related to a genetically determined alteration in renal sodium excretion similar to that induced by sodium loading in the sodium-sensitive rat (Coleman *et al.*, 1975).

In animals made hypertensive by constricting one or both renal arteries, hypertension is due primarily to release of renin by the ischemic kidney (Gross, 1971). In recent studies of this form of hypertension, a one-kidney model (one kidney constricted, the other excised) and a two-kidney model (one kidney constricted, the other intact) have been used for examining interrelations among blood pressure, sodium ion, and renin (Gavras *et al.*, 1973). Experiments with these models and with inhibitors of the renin–angiotensin system have revealed that, when sodium ion is depleted, arterial blood pressure becomes dependent on the renin–angiotensin system, and that, during sodium loading, the renin-angiotensin system is depressed and arterial pressure depends on sodium ion (i.e., plasma volume). Studies in normotensive animals strongly suggest that this interaction between sodium and the renin–angiotensin system is a primary determinant of blood pressure in normal animals as well (Gavras *et al.*, 1973).

Hypertension may be developed in rats by giving mineralcorticoids, such as desoxycorticosterone (DOC) (Selye *et al.*, 1943). However, if the animals are maintained on a low-sodium diet, hypertension does not develop (Gross, 1960). It appears that the mechanism by which these animals become hypertensive is related to the sodium-retaining action of DOC on the renal tubule.

Nephrectomized animals become hypertensive (renoprival hypertension) on ordinary rations. However, if sodium and water intake are restricted, or if plasma volume is maintained by filtration and dialysis, hypertension is prevented or, if established, is corrected and controlled (Braun-Menendez and Covian, 1948).

During the last decade, sophisticated computer models of the circulation have been devised that include all known physiologic control loops. Studies with such models have demonstrated that some alteration in renal excretion of sodium is necessary to produce permanent hypertension (Guyton *et al.*, 1972).

Clinical Studies in Hypertensive Human Subjects One of the earliest modes of effective treatment for human hypertension was the "rice diet," consisting of rice and fresh fruit and little else (Kempner, 1948). This diet has repeatedly been shown to be effective in lowering blood pressure in approximately 70% of patients with hypertension. The rice diet provides approximately 200 mg of sodium per day. It has been shown that it is the sodium restriction that is responsible for the lowering of blood pressure (Dole *et al.*, 1950; Dahl, 1972). Smaller degrees of sodium restriction do not consistently lower blood pressure in established hypertension (Hatch *et al.*, 1954). Conversely, a very high dietary intake of sodium raises blood pressure in patients with hypertension (Perera and Blood, 1947).

Removal of sodium by regular daily use of diuretic medications is a well-established principle of modern antihypertensive therapy (Page and Sidd, 1973). Use of diuretics alone is effective in significantly reducing blood pressure in 40–66% of patients with hypertension (Conway and Lauwers, 1960; Brest, 1960). A continuing reduction in plasma volume resulting from diuretic therapy occurs in patients who respond to these medications with a reduction in blood pressure (Tarazi *et al.*, 1970) and is thought by many investigators to be responsible for their effectiveness.

In most patients with kidney failure, there is a direct relationship between sodium intake and blood pressure (Ulvila *et al.*, 1972). In such patients, blood pressure is controlled by reducing sodium intake or by reducing plasma and extracellular fluid volume with diuretics, dialysis, or filtration procedures (Vertes *et al.*, 1969; Ulvila *et al.*, 1972). Patients who fail to respond to sodium (volume) depletion can be shown to have renin-dependent hypertension and respond to volume depletion after bilateral nephrectomy (Vertes *et al.*, 1969).

In normal subjects, large loads of sodium do not consistently influence arterial blood pressure in short-term experiments (Kirkendall *et al.*, 1972). No carefully controlled long-term study has been done to assess the effects of chronic salt loading in normal subjects.

Epidemiologic Studies Long-term longitudinal studies of U.S. population samples (Kannel *et al.*; 1969, Kannel *et al.*, 1969a; Chiang *et al.*, 1970) have demonstrated beyond doubt that increased blood pressure, of whatever degree, conveys an important risk of cardiovascular disease.

Epidemiologic data bearing on the possibility of preventing hypertension have been reviewed recently (Page, 1976). It is universally agreed that a genetic factor is important in determining susceptibility to hypertension (Ostfeld and Paul, 1963). The exact mode of inheritance has not been clearly established (Thomas, 1973). However, most studies favor the interpretation that a polygenic, rather than single-gene, mode of inheritance best explains the existing data on familial occurrence (Pickering, 1965; Miall and Chinn, 1973; Ostfeld and Paul, 1963).

Both systolic blood pressure and diastolic blood pressure tend to rise with age in the United States (U.S. Center for Health Statistics, 1964) and most other industrialized countries (Hamilton *et al.*, 1954; Miall and Chinn, 1973; Kahn *et al.*, 1972). Although hypertension is most commonly recognized in the fourth and fifth decades of life, recent studies have shown that an upward trend in blood pressure is present in childhood (Zinner *et al.*, 1971, Buck 1973) and that the children of hypertensive parents have higher blood pressure and a stronger upward trend than the children of normotensive parents. These trends are detectable as early as the age of 2 yr (Zinner *et al.*, 1971).

Although long-term prospective studies on the children of hypertensives are still incomplete, available data strongly suggest that early trends in blood pressure presage later expression of hypertension and that efforts to prevent hypertension might best be directed toward infants and young children who are beginning to show age-related upward blood-pressure trends (Buck, 1973).

Population studies in many parts of the world show blood pressure rising with age and prevalences of hypertension comparable with those seen in the United States. Nevertheless, studies of a substantial number of societies that are outside the major Western culture disclose an absence of hypertension and little or no tendency of blood pressure to increase with age. These low-blood-pressure populations represent many different racial groups, climates, customs, and modes of subsistence. When comparisons are made between these populations and people of similar origin who have been assimilated into Western civilization, the acculturated groups show blood pressure rising with age. Thus, low-blood-pressure populations are not genetically protected from rising arterial pressure. Explanation must be sought among environmental factors.

Low-blood-pressure populations include Chinese aborigines (Morse and Beh, 1937); Greenland Eskimos (Thomas, 1927); Melanesian tribes from several areas in New Guinea (Whyte, 1958; Maddocks, 1967) and the Solomon Islands (Page *et al.*, 1974); Polynesians from isolated islands in the Fiji (Maddocks, 1961), Cook (Prior *et al.*, 1968), Caroline (Murrill, 1949), and Tokelau (Prior *et al.*, 1974) groups; Easter Islanders (Cruz-Coke *et al.*, 1964); Australian aborigines (Abbie and Schroder, 1960); nomadic tribes in Kenya (Shaper *et al.*, 1969); Congo pygmies (Mann *et al.*, 1962); bushmen of the Kalahari Desert (Truswell *et al.*, 1972); Masai from Tanzania (Mann *et al.*, 1964); West Malaysians (Burns-Cox, 1970); and South and Central American Indians from Chile (Cruz-Coke, *et al.*, 1973), Brazil (Lowenstein, 1961), Surinam (Glanville and Geerdink, 1972), and Guatemala (Hoobler *et al.*, 1965). By contrast, rising blood pressure with age and clinical hypertension have been seen in acculturated town-dwelling persons of nearly all these diverse populations.

Acculturation, or the assimilation into the dominant culture of persons from traditionally oriented preindustrial societies, affects nearly every aspect of life. Most often, the multiplicity of forces acting simultaneously makes it impossible to determine the effect of a single factor on biologic changes, such as blood-pressure trends, within populations. Obviously, such factors as general health and nutrition, weight, psychosocial stresses, and the totality of changes involved in acculturation must be considered in interpreting such changes. Low-blood-pressure populations with markedly different diets have been described (Page, 1976). Change toward a more Westernized diet is a universal feature of acculturation. For example, salt, canned meat and fish, rice, wheat, flour, and sugar progressively supplant traditional dietary items (Page, 1976).

In long-term population studies in many countries, weight gain has been the most consistent factor in predicting hypertension (Epstein and Eckoff, 1967; Kahn *et al.*, 1972). The tendency toward rising weight and blood pressure is complex and may be partly genetically linked (Thomas, 1973). Whereas mean weight in industrialized societies tends to rise with age, this is not true in many preindustrial societies (Page, 1976). However, acculturation is often associated with rising weight, and it is difficult to separate this change from other effects of changed diet and activity.

Among low-blood-pressure populations, low sodium intake has been an invariable feature of habitual dietary patterns (Shaper, 1972; Page, 1976). Where quantitative data are available, sodium intake among low-blood-pressure populations averages less than 2,000 mg/day (Dahl, 1972; Page *et al.*, 1974). Upper limits have not been established. Statements to the contrary have been unsupported by data and appear to be based on an assumption that availability of salt, as in coastal peoples or inhabitants of small islands, is necessarily associated with high sodium intake. The available evidence fails to support this assumption (Page, 1976).

In a detailed analysis of six Solomon Islands societies (Page *et al.*, 1974), blood pressure was found to be rising with age in females of the three more acculturated populations, but not in the three less acculturated. All six societies were relatively unacculturated by Western standards, and weight decreased with age in all. Blood-pressure trends were correlated best with sodium intake. The highest blood pressures were found among a group (third out of six in acculturation rank) who had by far the highest sodium intake. A similar relationship between blood pressure and sodium intake has been reported among Polynesians (Prior *et al.*, 1968) and Indians in Brazil (Lowenstein, 1961) and the southwestern United States (Strotz and Shorr, 1973).

Dahl (1960) reported a rough correlation between sodium intake and prevalence of hypertension among populations. Examples of populations with very high sodium intake and high prevalence of hypertension include northern Honshu, Japan (Dahl, 1960) and coastal fishing villages of Newfoundland (Fodor *et al.*, 1973).

With some exceptions, studies of blood pressure and sodium excretion have failed to show clear-cut correlations between these variables in either black or white populations in the United States (Dawber *et al.*, 1967; Langford and Watson, 1975). Lack of significant correlation in intrapopulation studies has been interpreted as evidence against an important etiologic role for sodium in human hypertension. However, the lack of correlation can be equally well explained by the presence of widely variable genetic susceptibility to the effects of sodium on blood pressure plus a high average sodium intake in the population in question. In these circumstances, variation in blood pressure may be related more to the genetic factor than to sodium intake.

In the United States, blood-pressure averages are higher, and the prevalence of hypertension is greater among blacks than among Caucasians (Stamler *et al.*, 1960). In addition, socioeconomic and urban–rural trends have been identified in both whites and blacks with higher arterial pressure in the lower socioeconomic and the more rural populations (Langford *et al.*, 1968). Differences in urinary sodium excretion are not correlated with these trends. However, higher sodium:potassium and sodium:calcium ratios are found in the groups with higher arterial pressure (Langford and Watson, 1971). More research in these areas should be encouraged.

Especially Susceptible Segments of the Population Data from British studies suggest that a significant number of "crib deaths" (sudden unexpected deaths between the ages of 2 weeks and 2 yr) may be due to hypernatremia, and that some infants who do not die may sustain permanent brain damage from hypernatremia. A number of such deaths have been attributed to the use of dry feeding formulas reconstituted with water that is high in sodium (Robertson, 1975).

Adult Patients Requiring Low-Sodium Diets The National Center for Health Statistics, on the basis of a representative survey sample of 15,778 subjects aged 12–74 yr, estimated that 2.8%, or approximately 6.2 million Americans, are currently on low-sodium diets prescribed for reasons of illness. The low-sodium diets most commonly prescribed limit the patient to either 2.0, 1.0, or 0.5 g of sodium for 24 h. Where water supplies contain more than 20 mg/liter, dietary sodium restriction to less than 1.0 g/day is difficult to achieve and maintain. White *et al.* (1967) concluded that 40% of municipal water supplies sampled are unsatisfactory for use with diets that limit sodium strictly.

ANALYSIS

Quantitative analysis of sodium in water poses no serious technologic or methodologic difficulty. Flame-emission spectrophotometry is the method for determining sodium ion in solution. It measures the light energy emitted by the sodium ions in aqueous solution after excitation of the sodium atom by passage into a flame. Flame-emission spectrophotometry has advantages of simplicity, speed, and sensitivity, with precision comparable with that of the older and more difficult gravimetric method.

SUMMARY AND RECOMMENDATIONS

The healthy population includes a large segment (15–20%) who are at risk of developing hypertension. There is evidence linking excessive sodium intake to hypertension, but for man the evidence is largely indirect. The risk of hypertension depends on genetic susceptibility and is influenced by other factors in addition to sodium intake. The development of hypertension is characterized by long latency and slowly rising blood pressure, entering the hypertensive range in middle life. People at greatest risk cannot be identified with certainty in advance. For most people, the contribution of drinking water to sodium intake is small in relation to total dietary intake.

Because drinking water is an obligatory dietary ingredient, concentrations should be maintained at the lowest practicable levels, and trends toward increasing concentrations of sodium in water supplies as a result of deicing and water-softening procedures should be discouraged. Optimal concentrations of sodium should be regarded as the lowest feasible.

Specification of a "no-observed-adverse-health-effect" level in water for a substance like sodium for which the effect is associated with total dietary intake and for which usual food intake is already greater than a desirable level is impossible.

The defining of upper allowable limits is inevitably arbitrary. Reduction in hypertension for a small segment of the U.S. population who are on severely restricted diets requires a total intake of sodium less than 500 mg/day. These persons need water containing less than 20 mg/liter sodium ion.

A larger proportion of the population, about 3%, is on sodium-restricted diets calling for sodium intake of less than 2,000 mg/day. The fraction of this that can be allocated to water varies, depending on medical judgment for individual instances. Knowledge of the sodium ion content of the water supply and maintenance of it at the lowest practicable concentration is clearly helpful in arranging diets with suitable sodium intake.

It appears that at least 40% of the total population would benefit if total sodium ion intake were maintained not greater than 2,000 mg/day. With sodium ion concentration in the water supply not more than 100 mg/liter, the contribution of water to the desired total intake of sodium would be 10% or less for a daily consumption of two liters.

Research Needs

1. A large and impressive body of data has been accumulated that relates excessive sodium intake to the development of hypertension. Nevertheless, the role of sodium in hypertension remains controversial. Genetic factors, hormones, other dietary factors, and psychosocial stresses also influence blood pressure in important ways. Research should be encouraged to clarify the relative roles and interactions of these influences and the mechanisms by which blood pressure is affected at the physiologic and cellular levels.
2. More information is needed on the average daily intake of sodium, potassium, calcium, and trace metals by different segments of the U.S. population and on the relative contributions of water and other dietary sources to intake.
3. Also more information is needed on day-to-day and seasonal variations in the composition of water supplies and on the variation in water intake in different segments of the population.
4. Removal of sodium from water by methods currently available is expensive and inefficient. Research directed to developing efficient methods for bulk desalinization of water should be encouraged.
5. Use of sodium chloride for deicing roads results in an increase of the sodium content of public water supplies. Research should be continued toward alternative methods of highway ice control.

Nitrate

OCCURRENCE

Nitrate ion is the thermodynamically stable form of combined nitrogen for terrestrial, oxygenated aqueous systems. Accordingly, there is a tendency for all nitrogenous materials in natural waters to be converted into nitrate. All sources of combined nitrogen must, therefore, be regarded as potential sources of nitrate.

Major point sources of combined nitrogen are municipal and industrial

TABLE V-22 Well Depth and Nitrate Content of Water

		Concentration of Nitrate (as Nitrogen)[a]			
Depth Well, m	No. Analyses	0.2 mg/liter	2 mg/liter	10 mg/liter	20 mg/liter
0.8	480	87	56	28	13
9–15	926	80	40	20	10
16–30	1,568	64	18	5	1.8
31–60	2,042	61	11	3	0.7
Over 60	3,828	55	5	0.6	0.1

(From Larson and Henley, 1966)

[a]Percentages of analyses having nitrate equal to or greater than each of the four concentrations shown.

wastewaters, refuse dumps, animal feed lots, and septic tanks. Diffuse sources include runoff or leachate from manured or fertilized agricultural lands, urban drainage, and biochemical nitrogen fixation. Some tenths of a milligram per liter of combined nitrogen occurs in rainfall from solution of atmospheric ammonia and oxides of nitrogen.

In the Community Water Supply Survey of the Bureau of Water Hygiene in 1969, the range of nitrate concentrations found was 0.0–127 mg/liter. Nineteen systems, about 3% of those examined for nitrate, had concentrations in excess of the recommended limit of 45 mg/liter.

Groundwaters from shallow wells often have large concentrations of nitrate. Statewide records in Illinois (Table V-22) show high nitrate to be more common in wells less than 50 feet deep (Larson and Henley, 1966). For example, 81% of 221 dug wells and 34% of drilled wells in Washington County, Illinois, contained more than 10 mg/liter of nitrate-N. Farm ponds had less than 3 mg/liter nitrate-N (Dickey *et al.*, 1972). Analyses of over 5,000 waters in Missouri showed that 27% of the waters contained nitrate-N in excess of 10 mg/liter (Smith, 1970). Concentrations of nitrate in farm ponds were much less, similar to those found in Illinois. In Wisconsin, 45% of 250 wells that were examined twice monthly for more than a year consistently yielded water containing more than 10 mg/liter nitrate-N and 71% of the well waters exceeded this level at least once (Crabtree, 1970).

In Nassau County, New York, 370 wells supply 1.5 million people. In 1969, water from 20 of these wells showed more than 10 mg/liter nitrate-N (Smith and Baier, 1969). In Southern California, certain public water supplies have exceeded 10 mg/liter nitrate-N since 1935.

In Hall County, Nebraska (Piskin, 1973), nitrate concentrations in well-water samples were related to characteristics of the unsaturated zone. Hydraulic conductivity of the unsaturated zone permitted excessive water and nitrate of the surface to reach the aquifer at 10–100-ft depth (Table V-23).

Observations on fertilized soils in Illinois showed no signs of nitrate percolation to groundwater. No observations were made on sandy soils.

The U.S. Geological Survey has records on nitrate concentrations in six major rivers from 1950 to 1970. Trends toward increasing concentration were indicated for the Delaware, San Joaquin, and Ohio Rivers. No distinct trend was observed in the Colorado River, and trends to decreased values were noted for the Missouri at Nebraska City and the Brazos River. Overall concentrations ranged from 0.6–1.5 mg/liter nitrate-N.

Analyses by the Illinois State Water Survey since 1945 show trends toward increased nitrate for the Wabash, Ohio and Mississippi Rivers (Harmeson *et al.*, 1973). For other streams within Illinois the trends to greater concentrations were sharper than those of the major rivers. Characteristically, the highest levels occurred during the spring rainy season in the smallest watersheds, where intensive cultivation of row crops necessitated high fertilization and tile drainage (Harmeson, *et al.*, 1971). In 1897–1899, the load from the Illinois River at Kampsville was calculated to be 2.33 kg nitrate–nitrogen/ha/yr, and in 1900–1902, the load was still 2.33 kg/ha/yr (Palmer, 1903). In 1956–1961, at nearby Peoria, the load was 8.6 kg/ha/yr; in 1961–1966, it was 13.6 kg/ha/yr; and in 1966–1971, it was 16.7 kg/ha/yr (Harmeson *et al.*, 1973).

When downstream concentrations in surface waters are examined, it must be realized that nitrate levels may decrease by dilution, and by rapid assimilation of nitrate into aquatic plants. Also, when trends are examined it should be recognized that the rate of application of nitrogenous fertilizers increased only gradually from 1945 to 1960, but

TABLE V-23 Nitrate Concentration in Water Samples and Sand; Percentage in the Unsaturated Zone in Hall County, Nebraska

Fraction of Sand in Unsaturated Zone, %	Nitrate concentration, mg/liter					
	<10		>10		>45	
	No.	%	No.	%	No.	%
<25	63	77.8	18	22.2	7	8.6
25–50	45	73.8	16	26.2	1	1.6
50–75	69	47.6	76	54.2	3	15.9
>75	99	44.2	125	55.8	34	15.2
Total wells	276	—	235	—	65	—

(From Piskin, 1973)

TABLE V-24 Estimated Average Daily Ingestion of Nitrate and Nitrite in the United States

Source	Nitrate		Nitrite	
	mg	%	mg	%
Vegetables	86.1	86.3	0.20	1.8
Fruits, juices	1.4	1.4	0.00	0.0
Milk and products	0.2	0.2	0.00	0.0
Bread	2.0	2.0	0.02	0.2
Water	0.7	0.7	0.0	0.0
Cured meats	9.4	9.4	2.38	21.2
Saliva	30.0[a]		8.62	76.8
Total	99.8	100	11.22	100

[a]Not included in total.
(From J. White, Jr., *Journal of Agricultural and Food Chemistry*, 23:886, 1975)

increased fivefold from 1960 to 1967 and then leveled off with only a gradual increase to the present.

Nitrate may be biochemically assimilated from water by growing plants or may be converted to gaseous nitrogen in anoxic situations. In oxygenated waters, it is quite stable and not easy to remove. Denitrification to nitrogen gas and ion exchange are technically feasible processes for nitrate removal, but they have not been extensively developed on a municipal scale. So, concentrations in finished drinking waters at the tap are usually the same as those in the source waters.

Other Sources of Nitrate

Ordinarily, the major human intake of nitrate is from food rather than from water. The mean food intake for nitrate plus nitrite in the United States has been estimated to be nearly 120 mg/day (White, 1975), most of it coming from vegetables such as celery, potatoes, lettuce, melons, cabbage, spinach and root vegetables, some of which may contain several thousand parts per million of nitrate (Table V-24).

Nitrate is secreted in the saliva, the mean value being about 40 mg/day, of which about 10 mg/day is reduced to nitrite and found in that form. These quantities, although internally derived, also represent inputs to the gastric system.

The variability from individual to individual must be very high, because different classes of foods vary significantly in nitrate content from near zero for fruits, milk, and cereal products to thousands of parts per million for certain vegetables. Aside from vegetables, the next largest contribution comes from cured meats. The history of use of nitrate and nitrite for meat-curing has recently been reviewed (Binkerd and Kolari, 1975). The amounts of nitrate and nitrite used in meat-curing have been on the decline for many years, and regulations expected to be promulgated in the near future will decrease their use even further. Thus, it is likely that vegetables will continue to supply the bulk of dietary nitrate.

Man's exposure to nitrite is also summarized in Table V-24. Most is a result of reduction of nitrate in saliva (Tannenbaum *et al.*, 1974) to nitrite. However, other routes of reduction may occur.

METABOLISM

Little is known of nitrate metabolism in man. It is generally assumed that absorption takes place in the upper portion of the small intestine and that excretion is primarily, if not exclusively, through the kidney (Sollman, 1957).

It is well known that nitrate is absorbed in the upper gastrointestinal tract (Sollman, 1957) and concentrated from the plasma into saliva by the salivary glands (Burgen and Emmelin, 1961). Although the rate of clearance of salivary constituents is highly variable, the cleansing of mucosal surfaces is quite efficient, and clearance is rapid (Gibbons and van Houte, 1975). A great deal of effort has gone into the study of iodide distribution in man, but very little into the study of nitrate distribution. However, Burgen and Emmelin (1961) summarized a number of studies that suggested that nitrate is transported by the same ion-transport system as iodide, perchlorate, and thiocyanate. Furthermore, the transport system operates in the thyroid, gastric mucosa, and mammary glands, as well as in the salivary ducts.

It is of considerable significance that major differences occur among mammalian species in their ability to concentrate nitrate from plasma into saliva (Cohen and Myant, 1959). Large interspecies differences have also been shown to occur in the elimination kinetics of nitrate (Schneider and Yeary, 1975). Preliminary observations on a number of species have shown that not all animals reduce nitrate to nitrite in saliva (P. M. Newberne, personal communication). Thus, nitrate metabolism in man cannot be readily predicted from animal data.

Several studies have suggested that large differences in nitrate metabolism may occur between individuals. These differences can span about three orders of magnitude when all the available data, including diet and physiological status, are taken into consideration.

Earlier investigations did not consider the effects of conversion of nitrate to nitrite in saliva. Recent studies (Tannenbaum *et al.*, 1976a) have demonstrated that high nitrate intake can lead to large increases in the concentration of salivary nitrite. Although the pattern and extent of nitrite concentration vary from individual to individual, all persons tested had very large increases in nitrite concentration after consumption of even a small quantity (50 ml) of celery juice containing sodium nitrate at 1,200 mg/liter.

Salivary nitrite concentrations observed after consumption of celery juice are different from those reported by investigators using different foods as nitrate sources. Harada *et al.* (1975) found nitrate at 600 mg/liter or higher in saliva after ingestion of salted Chinese cabbage. The nitrite observed under these conditions reached about 100 mg/liter. These studies were performed on only a few people. Stephany and Schuller (1974) fed people several vegetables under a variety of conditions and observed increases in nitrite. In one experiment, a cooked onionlike vegetable (postelein) caused an increase in nitrite to about 200 mg/liter in 2 h; it reached 300 mg/liter in 17 h and declined slowly thereafter. In the work of Spiegelhalder *et al.* (1970), beet juice was the source of nitrate, and maximum nitrite concentration of about 150 mg/liter was observed.

There does not appear to be any significant discrepancy among these observations. Two major factors other than nitrate intake determine the salivary nitrite content: the subject's oral microflora and other constituents in the nitrate-containing food.

It is not yet possible to construct a complete pharmacokinetic model of nitrate metabolism, but such a model will have to incorporate the following salient points (Tannenbaum *et al.*, in press):

1. The half-life for clearance of nitrate, and consequently nitrite, is about 12 h.
2. The maximal concentration of nitrite in saliva depends primarily on nitrate intake up to approximately 100 mg of sodium nitrate and increases relatively little with intake greater than 100 mg.
3. The nitrate source is as important in determining salivary nitrite concentration as the amount of nitrate consumed.
4. The conversion of nitrate to nitrite depends on the oral microflora.

HEALTH ASPECTS

Two health hazards are related to the consumption of water containing large concentrations of nitrate (or nitrite): induction of methemoglobinemia, particularly in infants, and potential formation of carcinogenic nitrosamines.

Acute toxicity of nitrate occurs as a result of reduction to nitrite, a process that can occur under specific conditions in the stomach, as well as in the saliva. Nitrite acts in the blood to oxidize the hemoglobin to methemoglobin, which does not perform as an oxygen carrier to the tissues. Consequently, anoxia and death may ensue.

Healthy adults are reported to be able to consume large quantities of nitrate in drinking water with relatively little, if any, effect (Bosch *et al.*, 1950; Oregeron *et al.*, 1957). Acute nitrate toxicity is almost always seen in infants rather than adults. This increased susceptibility of infants has been attributed to high intake per unit weight, to the presence of nitrate-reducing bacteria in the upper gastrointestinal tract, to the condition of the mucosa, and to greater ease of oxidation of fetal hemoglobin (Walton, 1951).

Gastric pH greater than 4 is conducive to the growth of nitrate-reducing bacteria. Such gastric conditions are likely to occur with infants, who are prone to upset stomachs and achlorhydria (Comly, 1945).

Assessment of maximum nitrate levels in water exhibiting no adverse health effects has been based principally on a study of known cases of methemoglobinemia. The early survey of Walton showed that no cases on methemoglobinemia were reported when the water contained less than 10 mg/liter nitrate as nitrogen. Later, Sattelmacher (1962) found 3% of 467 cases in which the nitrate concentration of the water supply was less than 9 mg/liter as nitrogen and Simon *et al.* (1964) found 4.4% of 249 cases in which the recorded concentration of nitrate as nitrogen was less than 11 mg/liter.

Acceptance of these results as definitive is complicated by several factors:

1. Poor analytical methods.
2. Nitrate analyses frequently were performed some time after the case had occurred and so the concentration at the time of the illness is not really known.
3. Boiling of the water prior to feeding would have concentrated the nitrate over that in the raw water.
4. Incidence of toxicity should be related to total intake of nitrate, not just water concentration. Concurrent ingestion of vegetable puree or juice could have provided much enhanced nitrate intake in some cases.
5. Only one of the U.S. cases has been associated with a *public* water supply, regardless of nitrate content. It is known that many infants have drunk water in which nitrate as N was greater than 10 mg/liter without developing methemoglobinemia.

Studies supplementary to the previous ones in which levels of methemoglobin in the blood of infants were related to concentrations of nitrate in the water being fed have been reported by Winton (1971) and by Shuval and Gruener (1975). Both studies showed detectable enhancement of methemoglobin levels in infants being supplied with water containing nitrate as nitrogen only slightly in excess of 10 mg/liter. Although the full significance to health of increases in sub-clinical levels of methemoglobin is unclear, they presumably represent an onset of the toxicity leading to methemoglobinemia and therefore refer to a maximum level of nitrate for no-adverse-health effects.

Normally less than 2% of total hemoglobin is present as methemoglobin (Ferrant, 1946; Gross, 1964; Jaffe and Heller, 1964). No external signs or symptoms are noted generally as long as the methemoglobin is less than 5%. Between 5 and 10% methemoglobin the first signs of cyanosis can be seen (Knotek and Schmidt, 1964). In trained subjects undergoing work tests, 10–20% methemoglobin was found to result in impaired oxygenation of muscles. A Russian study of 800 children in day nurseries (Subbotin, 1961) found that over 90% of them who ingested water with 20–40 mg/liter of nitrate had elevated levels of blood methemoglobin and 50% showed levels in excess of 5%. On the other hand, there was no elevation of methemoglobin level with 9 mg/liter of nitrate in the water.

It can be concluded that, from the viewpoint of induction of methemoglobinemia, the maximum concentration of nitrate in water exhibiting no-observed-adverse-health effect is close to the interim standard of 10 mg/liter as nitrogen. However, there appears to be little margin of safety for some infants with the standard at this concentration.

There appear to be five possible conditions for poisoning of man or animals:

1. The presence of microorganisms in the rumen of cattle causes reduction of nitrate to nitrite. Absorption of the nitrite ion can result in toxicity to cattle (Bradley *et al.*, 1939). The enlarged cecum and colon of horses also provide a location for microbial reduction of nitrate (Bradley *et al.*, 1940; Knotek and Schmidt, 1964).

2. The more alkaline stomach of infants younger than 4 months old allows growth of microorganisms that can reduce nitrate to nitrite: therefore, high-nitrate water can be toxic to the very young (Knotek and Schmidt, 1964; Richards and Knowles, 1969; Schuphan, 1965).

3. When processed or unprocessed spinach is stored under conditions permitting growth of microorganisms, nitrate can be reduced to nitrite. Spinach left at room temperature for some time after cooking or after a jar of baby food has been opened has caused toxicity in babies. Other

vegetables or prepared foods high in nitrate can also cause problems (Schuphan 1965; Simon, 1966; Sinios and Wodsak, 1965).

4. Nitrite has occurred in damp forage materals that were high in nitrate. Ingestion by livestock proved toxic (Olson and Moxon, 1942).

5. There have been cases of outright nitrite poisoning where the legal limit for food additives has been exceeded by a factor of 10 or where nitrite has been mistaken for common salt.

A summary of studies on direct acute toxic effects of ingestion of nitrate and nitrite by different species of animals, including man, has recently been published (Ridder and Oehme, 1974). Excerpts from their report are presented in the following paragraphs:

Monogastric animals are more tolerant to excessive levels of nitrate in their diet than are ruminants. Dogs have been fed up to 2% (20,000 ppm) nitrate in their diet without any adverse health effects (Olson *et al.*, 1972; USPHS, 1962). Rats have been fed approximately 1% (10,000 ppm) nitrate for a lifetime without adverse effects (USPHS, 1962). Healthy human adults are reported to be able to consume large quantities of nitrate in drinking water with relatively little, if any, effects (Bosch *et al.*, 1950; Oregeron *et al.*, 1957).

However, the physiological effects noted with ingestion of nitrate in food and water are variable. This may be explained by the metabolic and physiologic differences existing between animals. Toxicity usually results when nitrate in the food is reduced to nitrite prior to ingestion. Under specific conditions, this reduction can occur in the stomach. Some tissues of all animals are able to reduce nitrate to nitrite.

In swine, larger doses of nitrites are required to produce the methemoglobin levels necessary for acute toxicity (Curtin and London, 1966). The pig was found to have the slowest rates of methemoglobin formation and methemoglobin reduction (Smith and Beutler, 1966). A relative lack in response to treatment with methylene blue was also noted.

Swine are only susceptible to nitrite when the nitrite is pre-formed (Blood and Henderson, 1968). The toxic level of nitrites for pigs is listed as 88 mg/kg.

Some of the clinical signs of chronic nitrate toxicity in swine are vitamin A deficiency, thyroid dysfunction, decreased rate of gain, arthritic conditions, and abortions. Lymphocytic leukocytosis and erythrocytosis have also been reported (Curtin and London, 1966).

Nitrate, when given orally to dogs was reduced to nitrite, but the amount reduced varied from practically none to a quantity sufficient to bring about methemoglobinemia (Singer, 1968). When given orally or intravenously, the nitrate ion caused over-excretion of chloride, resulting in hypochloremia, alkalosis, and digestive disturbances (Green and Hiatt, 1954). Dehydration occurred due to the diuretic effect of nitrates (Green and Hiatt, 1955).

The physiologic effects of nitrate toxicity in humans are largely unknown. Acute nitrate toxicity is almost always seen in infants rather than adults, and results from ingestion of well waters and vegetables high in nitrates. Comly (1945) deduced that infants were prone to upset stomachs and achlorhydria. As a result, the stomach pH increased in alkalinity allowing nitrate-reducing organisms to enter and to reduce nitrates to nitrites.

A gastric pH above 4 supports nitrate-reducing organisms (Bosch *et al.*, 1950; American Academy of Pediatrics Committee on Nutrition, 1970). Digestive disorders causing injury to the gastrointestnal mucosa and the resulting increased absorption was evident in several cases of infant methemoglobinemia reported in Minnesota (Bosch *et al.*, 1950).

Immature enzyme systems may also be of importance (Comly, 1945). Methemoglobin formation rate in human adults is close to the rate observed in cattle. However, in man, the rate of methemoglobin reduction occurred the fastest of all species studied (Smith and Beutler, 1966). Approximately 1% of the adult hemoglobin is present as methemoglobin (Jaffe and Heller, 1964). This constant concentration exists as a result of the balance between the oxidation of hemoglobin and the reduction of methemoglobin. Fetal hemoglobin (hemoglobin F) is oxidized by nitrite to methemoglobin at a rate twice as rapid as adult hemoglobin (hemoglobin A). Furthermore, the enzymatic capacity of the erythrocytes of newborn infants to reduce methemoglobin to hemoglobin appears less than that of adults (Jaffe and Heller, 1964). The difference is probably due to a developmental deficiency in the activity of DPNH-methemoglobin reductase (diphosphopyridine nucleotide) (Jaffe and Heller, 1964). As opposed to adults, several clinical, physiologic, and metabolic factors predispose infants to development of methemoglobinemia and acute nitrate poisoning.

Several studies have been conducted on long-term chronic feeding of nitrite to rats. In one study (Druckrey *et al.*, 1963), rats received sodium nitrite at 100 mg/kg in drinking water daily during their entire life span over three generations; no evidence of chronic toxicity, carcinogenicity, or teratogenicity was found. A second investigation (Greenblatt *et al.*, 1973) involved feeding sodium nitrite alone or with amino acids to rats for 67 weeks, for a total dose of 3.35 g of sodium nitrite per rat; no effect was seen in any of the animals receiving nitrite. A third study (Van Logten *et al.*, 1972) involved feeding rats canned meat processed with sodium nitrite at 5,000 ppm over a lifetime; no effect was seen in any of a large variety of chemical, biochemical or histopatho- logic indexes in the test animals.

However, in other laboratory studies (Shuval and Gruener, 1972) chronic exposure of rats to sodium nitrite at 2,000 and 3,000 mg/liter in drinking water for 2 yr was associated with distinct pathologic changes in heart and lung tissues. Also, mice chronically exposed to sodium nitrite at 1,000 and 2,000 mg/liter in drinking water showed reduced motor activity. EEG recordings from implanted electrodes revealed major changes in brain electric activity in rats receiving nitrite at 100–2,000 mg/liter. These changes persisted after exposure to nitrite ceased.

Gruener *et al.* (1973) showed that transplacental passage of nitrite occurred in pregnant rats given doses at 2.5–50 mg/kg orally or interperitoneally with production of methemoglobinemia in the fetuses. The concentrations of nitrite and methemoglobin reached in the fetal blood were lower than those in the maternal blood. Fetal rats were found to have methemoglobin reductase activity approximately 10 times higher than that of adult rats. In contrast, human adult blood exhibited methemoglobin reductase activity 1.5 times higher than did human cord blood (Gruener *et al.*, 1973). Rats born of dams exposed to nitrite during gestation had high mortality rates and poor growth and development.

The other health hazard proposed for nitrate in water, that it may act as a procarcinogen, is much more speculative. A series of reactions is involved by which it is proposed that nitrate in water may be converted to N-nitroso compounds that are the direct carcinogenic agent. The steps in the reaction sequence are:

1. Reduction of nitrate to nitrite.
2. Reaction of nitrite with secondary amines or amides in food or water to form N-nitroso compounds.
3. Carcinogenic reaction of N-nitroso compound.

To the extent that this series of processes actually operates in the human body, nitrate has a capacity to become a procarcinogen. In this event, potential carcinogenesis will be the major hazard involved in the ingestion of nitrate. The full series of reactions has not yet been demonstrated, however, so that the problem is a prospective rather than a realized one. The possible role of nitrate in water in contrast to the role of the normally much greater ingestion in foods has also not been determined.

More than one hundred N-nitroso compounds have been tested for carcinogenicity and about 75–80% have been found to cause cancer in animals (Magee and Barnes, 1967; Druckrey *et al.*, 1967; Shank, 1975; Mirvish, 1975a). Although there is no definite evidence that nitrosamines or other N-nitroso compounds have induced cancer in man, several suggestive epidemiological correlations have been reported (Clifford, 1970; Fong and Chan, 1973; Burrell *et al.*, 1966; Mirvish, 1972; Gregor, 1974) and there is no reason to suppose that man is not susceptible.

Reaction of nitrites and secondary amines or amides occurs readily in acidic solution and particularly at the normal pH range of 1–5 characteristic of gastric contents after a meal (Mirvish, 1975a, 1975b). Moreover, simultaneous feeding of nitrite and amines to mammals results in the formation of nitrosamines in the stomach and the producton of gastric tumors (Sander *et al.*, 1968; Greenblatt *et al.*, 1971; Sander and Schweinsberg, 1972; Mirvish, 1975b; Newberne and Shank, 1973). On the other hand, cancers were not observed when nitrate and amine were administered together to mice, indicating little reduction of nitrate to nitrite in the mouse stomach.

The relation of nitrate concentrations in water supplies to the first step in the reaction sequence for man is still more problematic, however. The major source of nitrite to the stomach, at least for healthy individuals, is the saliva, normally containing 6–15 mg/liter of nitrite (Tannenbaum *et al.*, 1974). The ingestion of foods, such as vegetables or vegetable juices containing nitrate at hundreds or thousands of milligrams per liter, can lead to much greater salivary concentrations of nitrite, in the range of hundreds of milligrams per liter (Tannenbaum, *et al.*, 1976a,b). However, the effect of concentration of nitrate in drinking water on salivary nitrite concentration is not known.

Nitrite may be formed from nitrate in the stomach by bacterial reduction, as discussed in connection with the induction of methemoglobinemia. Little reduction occurs in man, however, unless the gastric pH is greater than 4.6 (Mucha *et al.*, 1965; Sander and Schweinsburg, 1968). Thus, the pH condition for formation of nitrite is quite different from the pH range for ready formation of N-nitroso compounds, pH 3.5 or less.

Other organs of interest in connection with nitrate reduction and N-nitroso compound formation are the infected urinary bladder, the large intestine and the mouth itself (Mirvish, 1975b). Brooks *et al.* (1972), for example, found dimethylnitrosamine in the urine of two people having *Proteus mirabilis* infections of the bladder.

Epidemiologically, correlations have been shown to occur between incidence of gastric cancer and concentration of nitrate in the drinking water. For example, Hill *et al.* (1973) pointed out that the town of Worksop, England, with 90 mg/liter nitrate in the drinking water for many years, had an incidence of gastric cancer 25% greater (100% greater for those 75 and over) than that of similar control towns. In the control towns, the weekly nitrate intake was about 400 mg (100 mg from meat, 200 mg from vegetables, 100 mg from water) whereas in Worksop the total intake was 900 mg/week, with 600 mg from water.

Similarly, it has been shown that the unusually high incidence of stomach cancer in certain mountainous areas of Colombia (Hawksworth *et al.*, 1975; Correa *et al.*, 1975) is associated with high concentration of nitrate in the drinking water. In the area of high cancer incidence, there is 110 mg/liter nitrate in the drinking water compared to much lower values in control low-incidence areas. As much as 180 mg/liter nitrate was found in the urine of persons in the high-incidence area, but never more than 45 mg/liter in the low-incidence regions.

Findings such as these are preliminary and suggestive. They provide no firm evidence of a causal link between incidence of cancer and high intake of nitrate. They do indicate a need for caution in assessment of lack of adverse health effects even at the 10 mg/liter concentration level for nitrate as nitrogen and a need for continued intensive study on the metabolism and effects of nitrate in man.

ANALYSIS

A variety of methods for determination of nitrate exists, but none is particularly precise, accurate or sensitive in the milligram per liter concentration range (Schuller and Veen, 1967; Boltz, 1973). Further development and standardization of analytical methodology will be required if standard routine determinations are to be considered reliable within the range required for proper control and assessment of health effects.

Most standard procedures for nitrate determination in the mg/liter range are spectrophotometric. Traditionally, three types of reaction of nitrate have been used as bases: nitration of a phenolic substance to a colored derivative; oxidation of an organic substance to a colored product; and reduction of the nitrate to nitrite or ammonia, followed by reaction of the reduced nitrogenous materials to give colored substances. In addition, direct spectrophotometric determination based on ultraviolet absorption of nitrate at 273 nm is possible and becoming established. Electrochemical determination with the use of a nitrate electrode may also be feasible, but is subject to numerous interferences (Usher and Telling, 1975; Milham *et al.*, 1970; Morie *et al.*, 1972).

With all these techniques there has been a consistent problem of reproducibility. Analyses of samples containing water-soluble organic matter and low concentrations of nitrate tend to give erratic values. These erratic values have been attributed to: reduction of nitrate by organic matter in the presence of strong acids; considerable charring, which contributes color that is measured as nitrate in some procedures; and organic anions, which are often co-extracted and interfere in the determination of nitrate.

In oxidation methods, e.g., using brucine, the color developed does not always obey Beer's law, and continual calibration of the standard curve is necessary (Usher and Telling, 1975). Interference from nitrite, chloride, and carbohydrate has been reported (Usher and Telling, 1975).

Reduction of nitrate to nitrite can be accomplished by the use of various reagents, such as copper, zinc, hydrazine sulfate, cadmium powder, and spongy cadmium (Usher and Telling, 1975). The reducing agents are not sufficiently specific and most of them give either incomplete reduction or further reduction of nitrite to ammonia. Since nitrite is ultimately determined, both defects tend to give low results. Likewise, reduction of nitrate to ammonia with zinc or any one of a number of alloys or amalgams tends to be incomplete at the concentration levels common in water samples.

Because of these analytical problems determinations of nitrate in water samples should not be regarded as valid to better than 10% or 1 mg/liter. If suitable methods for the elimination of background interference are developed, then the direct ultraviolet spectrophotometric method may provide greater precision, accuracy and sensitivity.

In contrast to the determination of nitrate that of nitrite is highly sensitive to 1 μg/liter and generally convenient and accurate. The methods are based on reaction with a primary aromatic amine in acid solution to form a diazonium salt followed by coupling with a second phenol or aromatic amine to give an intensely colored azo dye.

CONCLUSIONS AND RECOMMENDATIONS

Nitrate in water at concentrations less than a thousand milligrams per liter is not of serious concern as a direct toxicant. It is a health hazard because of its conversion to nitrite. Nitrite is directly toxic by reaction with hemoglobin to form methemoglobin and cause methemoglobinemia. It also reacts readily under appropriate conditions with secondary amines and similar nitrogenous compounds to form N-nitroso compounds, many of which are potent carcinogens.

Epidemiological evidence on the occurrence of methemoglobinemia in infants tends to confirm a value near 10 mg/liter nitrate as nitrogen as a maximum concentration level for water with no observed adverse health effects, but there is little margin of safety in this value.

The highly sporadic incidence of methemoglobinemia when drinking water that contains much greater concentration of nitrate is used suggests, however, that factors other than nitrate intake are important in connection with development of the disease. For example, no cases of clinical methemoglobinemia could be found in two recent studies of communities in Southern California and central Illinois, where the water supplies were on occasion found to contain as much as 20 mg/liter of nitrate as N (Shearer, *et al.*, 1972; Winton, *et al.*, 1970). More research is needed on the metabolism of nitrate and on factors that affect the rate of extent of reduction to nitrite, as well as on those that influence subsequent reaction of nitrite to form methemoglobin.

Each link in the chain of reactions from nitrate to N-nitroso compound has been shown to occur in some conditions in man or other animals. The extent of operation of the overall reaction chain in man has not been shown however, nor is there knowledge of the ways in which other environmental or internal factors may affect potential formation of N-nitroso compounds. In particular, relative effects of salivary nitrate as compared with nitrate in imbibed water have not been elucidated. There is thus little scientific basis to support conclusions on the safety of any concentration of nitrate in water with regard to carcinogenic potential.

Sulfate

OCCURRENCE

Sulfate is found almost universally in natural waters in concentrations ranging from a few tenths of a milligram/liter up to several thousand milligrams/liter. It occurs frequently in rainfall, particularly from air masses that have encountered metropolitan areas, sometimes at concentrations greater than 10 mg/liter.

One of the most important terrestrial sources is evaporite sediment, from which magnesium, sodium and especially calcium sulfate may be leached. Metallic sulfides, such as iron pyrites, occur in both igneous and sedimentary rocks; they are oxidized to sulfate by moist oxygen during weathering processes. Some sulfate is formed during oxidative decay of organic matter.

Sulfate may also enter water courses through waste discharges. Household wastes, including detergents, add 10 or more mg/liter of sulfate to sewage. Tanneries, steel mills, sulfate-pulp mills and textile plants are all important industrial sources of sulfate.

In the 1970 survey of drinking water supplies the range of sulfate concentrations for the 969 samples was from less than 1 mg/liter up to 770 mg/liter with a median of 46 mg/liter. Twenty-five supplies, about 3% of those tested, showed sulfate in excess of the maximum recommended value in the 1962 U.S. Public Health Service Drinking Water Standards (250 mg/liter). Similar results were obtained in the Interstate Water Carrier Analyses of 1975 (USEPA, 1975). Of 625 supplies analyzed, 21 or 3.4% were found to contain sulfate greater than 250 mg/liter, the greatest concentration being 978 mg/liter.

Once sulfate has been dissolved in water, it becomes a permanent solute except when it is anaerobically reduced to sulfide and precipitated in sediments, released to the atmosphere as H_2S, or incorporated in living organic matter. Most inorganic sulfates are quite soluble except for the lead and barium salts. Sulfate is not removed from water by any of the common treatment processes. Desalination techniques such as ion exchange, reverse osmosis or membrane electrodialysis must be employed.

HEALTH ASPECTS

The major observed health effect of sulfate is its laxative action. Peterson (1951) observed that when the laxative doses of Glauber's salt, Na_2SO_4, and Epsom salt, $MgSO_4$, were translated into water concentrations based on a 2-liter daily supply, the laxative concentrations should be 300 mg/liter for Na_2SO_4 and 390 mg/liter for $MgSO_4$.

Results of a survey on the reactions of water consumers by the North Dakota State Department of Health (Peterson, 1951) indicated that a laxative effect was perceived at 750 mg/liter, but not at 600 mg/liter or less. The presence of Mg^{+2} at a concentration about equivalent to that of sulfate made the laxative effect manifest at lesser sulfate concentrations.

A more detailed analysis of the data by Moore (1952) led to the conclusion that most people experienced a laxative effect when sulfate plus magnesium exceeded 1,000 mg/liter. Moore's tabulation of the data is shown in Table V-25.

An *et al.* (1967) reported that concentrations of sulfate in water between 500 and 1,000 mg/liter caused slight, but significant, decrease in acidity

TABLE V-25 Laxative Effect of Well Water Containing Magnesium and Sulfate

Substance in Water	Concentration, mg/liter	No. Wells	Laxative Effects Yes	Laxative Effects No	Effects Not Stated	Percent of "Yes" Answers
Magnesium plus sulfate	0–200	51	9	34	8	21
	200–500	45	7	27	11	21
	500–1,000	56	11	28	17	28
	1,000–1,500	36	18	10	8	64
	1,500–2,000	14	6	4	4	60
	2,000–3,000	21	13	3	5	81
	Over 3,000	14	5	1	8	83
Sulfate	0–200	56	10	36	10	22
	200–500	47	9	28	10	24
	500–1,000	56	13	26	17	33
	1,000–1,500	34	16	10	8	62
	1,500–2,000	16	9	4	3	69
	2,000–3,000	20	9	3	8	75
	Over 3,000	8	3	0	5	100

[a]Based only on total of "yes" and "no" answers. It is probable that a large proportion of the wells for which no statements were made were not regularly used as water supplies.
(From Moore, 1952)

TABLE V-26 Influence of Sulfates on the Taste of Water and Coffee

	Threshold Concentration, mg/liter					
	Median		Range		Average	
Compound	Salt	Anion	Salt	Anion	Salt	Anion
Na_2SO_4	350	327	250–550	169–372	—	—
$CaSO_4$	525	340	250–900	177–635	—	—
$MgSO_4$	525	419	400–600	320–479	500	400

(From Lockhart *et al.*, 1955)

of gastric juice. Also, persons living at Shumilova Settlement (USSR) experienced diarrhea and taste deterioration when the concentration of sulfate increased from 571–1,235 mg/liter. Korotchenok (1946), however, reported that there were no acute toxic effects noted in Western Turkmenia (USSR) from the consumption of water with as much as 1,295 mg/liter of sulfate.

Macfayden (1953) reported on one village in British Somaliland that was using a water containing sulfate at a concentration about 4,400 mg/liter.

Studies by Digesti and Weeth (1973) gave results indicating that growing cattle can tolerate water containing sulfate at 2,500 mg/liter without ill effect. They concluded, moreover, that this value was nearly the maximum safe concentration.

The taste threshold for sulfate in water has been reported to lie between 300 and 400 mg/liter (Whipple, 1907; Lockhart *et al.*, 1955). Table V-26 shows a summary of the data.

The 1962 Drinking Water Standards of the U.S. Public Health Service recommended that sulfate in water should not exceed 250 mg/liter, except when no more suitable supplies are or can be made available. The World Health Organization, in its European Standards For Drinking Water, set a sulfate limit of 250 mg/liter (WHO, 1970).

OTHER ASPECTS

Ingleson *et al.* (1949) state that sulfate appears not to increase the corrosion of brass fittings in domestic water systems. Holl (1935) found that concentrations of sulfate less than 200 mg/liter do not increase the plumbosolvency of water.

Kellam (1933) has reported that sulfate at concentration less than 25 mg/liter has little effect on the corrosiveness of water toward concrete, but Hammerton (1945) claims that concentrations greater than 1,000 mg/liter cause rapid corrosive attack.

Great concentrations of sulfate may be toxic to plants. According to Schofield (1936) water containing more than 960 mg/liter of sulfate is unsuitable for irrigation.

ANALYSIS

The preferred standard technique for determination of sulfate is precipitation of barium sulfate followed by ignition of the collected precipitate. Results for concentrations in the range of 100 mg/liter have shown standard deviations near 5%; the sensitivity is about 1 mg/liter (American Public Health Association, 1976).

Routine determinations can be performed more conveniently with only slight decrease in precision by collecting and drying the barium sulfate on a fritted glass or membrane filter, rather than igniting it.

Turbidimetric measurement of precipitated barium sulfate is rapid and particularly suitable for concentrations of sulfate less than 100 mg/liter. The limiting sensitivity remains nearly 1 mg/liter, however.

CONCLUSIONS AND RECOMMENDATIONS

No adverse health effects have been noted for concentrations of sulfate in water less than about 500 mg/liter. The only observed physiological effect at greater concentrations to more than 1,000 mg/liter has been the induction of diarrhea.

The taste threshold for sulfate in water lies between 300 and 400 mg/liter for most persons, but some individuals are able to detect as little as 200 mg/liter.

Summary—Other Inorganic Constituents

ARSENIC

Arsenic is widely distributed in the waters of the United States but generally in low concentration. In 728 samples of surface water, the concentration of arsenic ranged from less than 10 μg to a maximum of 1,200 μg/liter. The median value for arsenic in river waters was less than 10 μg/liter. High levels of arsenic in well waters have also been reported; occasionally exceeding 1 mg/liter.

Waters may be contaminated with many different forms of arsenic, each of which has different toxicological properties. Arsenic occurs in many different forms which vary in their solubility and other physical and chemical properties. Those of most concern are water-soluble compounds.

Arsenic is found in pork, poultry and shellfish; the last may contain up to 170 ppm. The daily median intake of arsenic in the United States from all sources has been estimated to be 137–330 μg.

A major problem in understanding the metabolism and toxicity of arsenic has been the difficulty in finding a suitable animal model.

The relative toxicity of different forms of arsenic can be explained, in part, by the fact that the more toxic trivalent compounds are retained in the tissues in greater amounts and are excreted more slowly than the less toxic.

Arsenic affects tissues that are rich in oxidative systems primarily the alimentary tract, kidneys, liver, lungs and epidermis. It is very damaging to capillaries and this results in hemorrhage into the gastrointestinal tract, sloughing of mucosal epithelium, renal tubular degeneration, hepatic fatty changes and necrosis.

The major characteristics of acute arsenic poisoning in humans are profound gastrointestinal damage and cardiac abnormalities. Subacute exposure results in vomiting, diarrhea, conjunctivitis, rhinitis, laryngitis, bronchitis, skin eruptions, neurologic signs and symptoms, muscle tenderness, and transverse white ridge on the finger nails (Mees lines).

Chronic arsenic toxicosis has not been encountered to any significant extent in animals; effects in man include cancer of the skin and lungs. In most human exposure, concomitant exposures to other agents confound interpretation of observations.

Although there appears to be some doubt regarding the carcinogenicity of arsenic compounds, there is epidemiological evidence that cutaneous lesions (leukoderma, melanoderma, hyperkeratosis, squamous-cell carcinoma) are associated with drinking water with higher than normal arsenic concentration. The city of Antofagosta, Chile, is a remarkable example of cause and effect. A city of 100,000 population drinking for decades a water containing a weighted average arsenic of 598 μg/liter resulted in an incidence of cutaneous skin lesions of 313/100,000 per year. After the water-treatment plant was completed, which reduced the arsenic level to 80 μg/liter, the incidence of cutaneous lesions dropped to 19/100,000 per year. This finding suggests that even 80 μg/liter exceeds the acceptable level for a public water supply.

Animal studies have failed to demonstrate carcinogenicity for arsenic compounds; mutagenicity and teratogenicity studies have yielded variable results.

In conclusion, there is some epidemiological evidence that high concentrations of arsenic in drinking water are associated with skin cancer. When the level was reduced by water treatment to 80 μg/liter, the incidence was reduced but still detectable. The existence of other cocarcinogens in these water supplies has not been extensively studied. If the time factors for the development of cancer are shown to be reasonable, then the current interim standard of 50 μg/liter may not provide an adequate margin of safety.

Research Needs

1. Improvement of analytical techniques and methodology for better adaptability to water and foods; definition of chemical form is required.
2. Epidemiologic and analytical studies to determine extent of the various forms of arsenic at low concentrations in the environment and their relation to disease patterns.
3. Development of a suitable animal model for a study of low-level long-term studies.
4. Intensive studies into the metabolism of arsenic in mammalian systems.
5. Studies about interaction of arsenic, with other trace elements in the environment (Se, Cu, Zn, etc.).

SELENIUM

Selenium is found in water principally as a result of leaching from rocks and soils that are high in selenium content. Most toxicity from selenium is a result of drinking water from wells drilled through seleniferous shales rich in soluble selenium. There is an insufficient amount of selenium in water alone to provide even the nutrient requirements of most animals, but concentrations vary in different places. Analyses of 535 samples of water from major U.S. watersheds indicated that over a 4-yr period only two samples contained selenium at more than 10 μg/liter of water, the current U.S. interim drinking water standard.

In another study, a maximum of 10 and a mean of 8 μg/liter in 194 public finished water supplies in the U.S. has been reported. In Germany and in Australia, village water supplies have been reported to contain from 1 to 5.3 μg/liter. Shallow or deep wells contain varying concentrations of selenium. For example, deep wells in Wyoming may contain only a few micrograms per liter while other wells contain enough selenium to be poisonous to man and livestock; some of these have been associated with the loss of hair and nails in children. Foods from nonseleniferous areas contribute very little to the overall dietary intake of selenium. Eggs and milk, fish, various types of meat, poultry, coffee, and tea all vary somewhat in their selenium content, but in general contribute minimally to the dietary intake.

Inorganic and organic forms of selenium are readily absorbed from the gastrointestinal tract of animals. Selenite is absorbed more rapidly by monogastric animals compared to ruminant animals, perhaps due to bacterial reduction of selenite to elemental selenium or other insoluble forms in the ruminant gastrointestinal tract.

Selenite and selenate are distributed largely to the liver, kidneys, muscle mass, gastrointestinal tract, and blood. Chronic administration of selenium results in increased concentration in the testes. The principal route of excretion of selenium is via the urine.

At higher exposure levels, selenium is incorporated into molecules normally served by sulfur; it is methylated by mammalian tissues in an apparent detoxication process. Selenite and selenate are metabolized to trimethyl-selenonium ion, which is the principal excretory product for selenium in urine.

The toxicity of selenium can be altered extensively by interactions with sulfate, methionine, cystine, mercury, lead, zinc, cadmium, copper, arsenic, and vitamin E, but little is known about these interactions.

Selenium is essential for domestic animals but the margin of safety is relatively narrow. A low level of selenium is essential to prevent myopathies, liver injury, and congenital abnormalities in domestic and laboratory animals and poultry, and there is little reason to believe that humans differ appreciably in this regard; however, data are lacking. High dietary selenium is toxic to animals and a defined set of signs and lesions have been established for acute, and subchronic exposure to toxic concentrations in several species. Chronic, long-term studies have been limited primarily to feeding studies in the rat and those have involved relatively high concentrations of the element.

With the exception of a limited number of reports of acute exposures to toxic levels under industrial circumstances, or other accidental exposure, an indication for health effects on human populations must be extrapolated from animal data. Inhalation causes acute respiratory distress, and skin exposure causes severe local irritation and dermatitis. The severity of response will depend on the chemical form of selenium.

In animals, acute exposure to selenium causes respiratory distress, diarrhea, pulmonary edma, hemorrhage, liver, and renal necrosis. Chronic exposure results in death from gastroenteritis, myocardial damage, hydrothorax, pulmonary edema, renal and liver damage. Sodium selenite is toxic to rats at concentrations of 6–9 mg/liter in drinking water; concentrations of 1 mg/liter are without observed toxic effect.

Chronic exposure of humans to selenium by inhalation or by ingestion results in central nervous system and gastrointestinal disturbances, and dermatitis.

The high selenium content of diet and water in areas of seleniferous soils has been associated with "alkali disease" in cattle. Human populations living in these areas are not similarly affected. This is believed to be due to the wide geographical sources of food consumed and the loss of selenium during processing. Where feed is low in selenium, water containing 400–500 μg/liter is too low to cause poisoning in the cattle. For livestock water the maximum recommended concentration is 50 μg/liter.

The only documentation of human toxicity from drinking water involved a family consuming well water which contained selenium at 9,000 μg/liter. In 1942, the USPHS drinking water standard listed selenium for the first time along with fluoride and arsenic. The level set was 50 μg/liter and easily met by public water supplies.

The interim standard of 10 μg/liter was recommended in 1962 because of evidence that selenium was carcinogenic in animal studies. The current literature review of animal studies does not support this contention nor is there any epidemiological evidence implicating a higher than normal cancer incidence among those having higher than normal daily intake of selenium.

The established requirement for selenium in most animal species indicates a need for more data on potential or real deficits or excesses in human populations. The concentration of selenium in waters of the United States varies widely and currently there is no evidence to suggest a problem. The totality of evidence indicates that there is greater overall potential for selenium deficiency than for selenium toxicity with current intake levels of selenium. The maximum no-observed-adverse health effect level for selenium in water is not less than 100 μg/liter and appears to be as great as 500 μg/liter. A concentration of 20 μg/liter just barely provides a minimum nutritional amount of selenium with a consumption of 2 liters a day.

In conclusion, there is evidence that selenium may be an essential trace element for humans. The current interim standard of 0.01 μg/liter was established because there was some concern that selenium was a carcinogen. This claim cannot be supported by a review of the current literature. To this end these effects must be investigated and the current interim standard re-evaluated.

The paucity of definitive data on selenium and human health requires a number of research approaches to elucidate the role of selenium in the mammalian system. The following research needs are suggested:

1. Techniques need to be developed for more rapid, accurate and reproducible analytical methods which will permit both qualitative and quantitative assays of chemical forms, oxidation state, and solubility in water.
2. Improved systems for monitoring selenium in the environment (water, air, food).
3. Research to define molecular transformations in the mammalian system.
4. Programs to study interactions between selenium, mercury, cadmium, arsenic, and other trace elements and heavy metals in the biosphere and in animal organisms.
5. A determination of natural and industrial emissions and cycling of selenium in the environment.
6. Effects in animal system of long-term, low levels of selenium singly and in combination with other trace elements in the environment.
7. Baseline data on selenium levels in humans in health and disease.
8. Effects of deficiency or an excess of selenium on the development of animal tumors.
9. Determine whether some segments of the human population of the United States require additional selenium for optimum health.

FLUORIDE

Fluoride is found widely in water supplies, but the concentration is usually not great enough to be undesirable. The maximum concentration found for the 969 supplies studies in the 1969 Community Water Supply Survey was 4.4 mg/liter. Most supplies not fluoridated had fluoride concentrations less than 0.3 mg/liter.

A more extensive survey by the Dental Health Division of the U.S. Public Health Service showed more than 2,600 communities with a population of 8 million people had water supplies with more than 0.7 mg/liter of naturally occurring fluoride. Most of these communities are in Arizona, Colorado, Illinois, Iowa, New Mexico, Ohio, Oklahoma, South Dakota, and Texas. Of these, 524 communities representing 1 million people had fluoride concentrations more than 2 mg/liter, which is an upper limit not known to produce objectionable mottling even with high temperatures.

Small amounts of fluoride, of the order of 1 mg/liter, depending on the environmental temperature, in ingested water and beverages, are generally conceded to have a beneficial effect on prevention of dental caries, particularly among children. This review did not systematically review the evidence for the beneficial effects of fluoride.

Two forms of chronic toxic effects are recognized generally as being caused by excess intake of fluoride over long periods of time. These are mottling of tooth enamel or dental fluorosis, and skeletal fluorosis. In both cases, it is necessary to consider the severity since the very mild forms are considered beneficial by some. The most sensitive of these effects is the mottling of tooth enamel, which, depending on the temperature, may occur to an objectionable degree with fluoride concentrations in drinking water of only 0.8–1.6 mg/liter. Apparently there has been little systematic investigation of the degree to which consumers of drinking water with several mg/liter of fluoride regard the resultant mottling as an adverse health effect.

Skeletal fluorosis has been observed with use of water containing more than 3 mg/liter. It now appears that long-term consumption of water containing fluoride in excess of 1 mg/liter runs into a fair probability of objectionable dental mottling and increased bone density in patients with long-standing renal disease or polydipsia. Increased bone density, however, has often been regarded as a beneficial rather than an adverse effect.

Intake of fluoride for long periods in amounts greater than 20–40 mg/day may result in crippling skeletal fluorosis.

Other reported adverse health effects of intake of milligram per liter levels of fluoride in drinking water, including mongolism, cancer mortality, mutagenic or birth effects, and sensitivity have either been unconfirmed or found lacking in substance. There is also no evidence that there is any difference between the effects of naturally occurring or intentionally added fluoride.

Epidemiological studies where the water is naturally high in fluoride have found no adverse effects except in rare cases, until the concentration is many times that recommended for added fluoride. Controlled studies with fluoridiation at the 1 mg/liter level have reported no instances of adverse effects. Available evidence does not suggest that fluoridation has increased or decreased cancer mortality rates; the margin of error is very low, approaching 2 per 100,000. This is the theoretical effect that could have been missed with present statistical techniques.

Additional studies of mottling and skeletal fluorosis need to be done in communities with several mg/liter fluoride in their water supplies to ascertain whether the no-adverse-health effect level for fluoride is greater or less than 1 mg/liter. In addition sociological studies are needed to ascertain the extent to which dental mottling is regarded as an adverse effect.

SODIUM

Sodium ion is an ubiquitous constituent of natural waters. It is derived geologically from the leaching of surface and underground deposits of salts such as sodium chloride, from the decomposition of sodium aluminum silicates and similar minerals, from the incorporation of evaporated ocean spray particles into rainfall and from the intrusion of seawater into freshwater aquifers. The sodium chloride used as a deicing agent on roads enters water supplies in runoff from both roads and storage depots. This added sodium chloride amounting to 9 million tons in 1970 is distributed throughout the snow belt of the northern United States and is most heavily concentrated around metropolitan areas.

A survey of 2,100 supplies, covering approximately 50% of the population of the United States, was carried out in 1963–1966. The distribution of sodium ion found in this survey ranged from 0.4–1900 mg/liter. Some 42% of the supplies had sodium ion concentrations in excess of 20 mg/liter and nearly 5% had concentrations greater than 250 mg/liter.

Few studies of habitual sodium-ion intake for healthy adults in the United States have been reported. Such data as have been reported are based on measurement of sodium excretion in 12- or 24-h urine collections. Wide variations occur among individuals and in the same individual from day to day. One study reported a mean 24-h excretion of 4,100 mg with a range from 1,600–9,600 mg in 71 working adult males in New York. Another reported a mean sodium excretion near 2,800 per 24 h in 171 black women ranging in age from 35 to 44 yr. A recent estimate for infants is 69–92 mg/kg/day.

Sodium chloride is added to many foods during processing. Additional sodium chloride is often added during cooking, and again at the table. None of this is essential, for habitual intake of sodium bears no relationship to physiological need. Healthy individuals have been shown to maintain sodium balance on a sodium intake of less than 2,000 mg/24 h while sweating 9 liters/day. A variety of preindustrial societies, in widely divergent habitats (tropical jungle, desert, arctic, etc.) subsist for generations on sodium intake less than 1,000 mg/day and show no evidence of sodium deprivation. Requirements for sodium in growing infants and children are estimated at less than 200 mg/day.

It thus appears that habitual intake of sodium in adults in the United States often exceeds body need by 10-fold or more. Evidence that this excessive intake may have harmful consequences is summarized in the detailed report.

Specification of a "no-observed-adverse-health-effect" level in water for a substance like sodium, for which the effect is associated with total dietary intake and for which usual food intake is already greater than a desirable level, is impossible.

Since adult fluid intake averages 1.5–3 liters/day, sodium intake from drinking water represents less than 10% of the habitual total intake of 3,000-4,000 mg as long as the sodium content of the water does not exceed 200 mg/liter. Adverse health effects may be anticipated with sodium concentrations in water greater than 20 mg/liter only for that special risk group restricted to total sodium intake of 500 mg/day, because intake from food cannot be reduced feasibly to less than 440 mg/day. For this group, whose diets must be medically supervised in a careful manner, knowledge of the sodium ion concentration of the drinking water permits prescription of bottled water low in sodium when necessary.

A larger proportion of the population, about 3%, is on sodium-restricted diets calling for sodium intake of less than 2,000 mg/day. The fraction of this that can be allocated to water varies, depending on medical judgment for individual instances. Knowledge of the sodium-ion content of the water supply and maintenance of it at the lowest practicable concentration is clearly helpful in arranging diets with suitable sodium intake. In many diets allowance is made for water to contain 100 mg/liter of sodium.

It appears that at least 40% of the total population would benefit if total sodium-ion intake were maintained at not greater than 2,000 mg/day. With sodium-ion concentration in the water supply not more than 100 mg/liter, the contribution of water to the desired total intake of sodium would be 10% or less for a daily consumption of 2 liters.

NITRATE

All sources of combined nitrogen must be regarded as potential sources of nitrate, for there is a tendency for all nitrogenous materials in natural waters to be converted into nitrate. Major point sources of combined nitrogen in water are municipal and industrial wastewaters, refuse dumps, animal feed lots and septic tanks. Diffuse sources include runoff or leachate from manured or fertilized agricultural lands, urban drainage and biochemical nitrogen fixation. Some tenths of a milligram/liter of combined nitrogen occurs in rainfall from solution of atmospheric ammonia and oxides of nitrogen.

In the Community Water Supply Survey of the Bureau of Water Hygiene in 1969, the range of nitrate concentrations found was 0–127 mg/liter. Nineteen systems, about 3% of those examined for nitrate, had concentrations in excess of the recommended limit of 45 mg/liter as nitrate.

Ordinarily, the major human intake of nitrate is from food rather than from water. The mean food intake in the United States has been estimated to be nearly 100 mg/day, most of it coming from vegetables such as spinach, lettuce, and root vegetables, which may contain several thousand parts per million of nitrate.

Nitrate is secreted in the saliva, the mean value being about 40 mg/day, of which about 10 mg/day is reduced to nitrite and found in that form. These quantities, although internally derived, also represent inputs to the gastric system.

Two health hazards are related to the consumption of water containing large concentrations of nitrate (or nitrite): induction of methemoglobinemia, particularly in infants, and possible formation of carcinogenic nitrosamines.

Acute toxicity of nitrate occurs as a result of reduction to nitrite, a process that can occur under specific conditions in the stomach, as well as in the saliva. Nitrite acts in the blood to oxidize the hemoglobin to methemoglobin, which does not perform as an oxygen carrier to the tissues. Consequently, anoxia and death may ensue.

Healthy adults are reported to be able to consume large quantities of nitrate in drinking water with relatively little, if any, effects. Acute nitrate toxicity is almost always seen in infants rather than adults. This increased susceptibility of infants has been attributed to high intake per unit weight, to the presence of nitrate-reducing bacteria in the upper gastrointestinal tract, to the condition of the mucosa and to greater ease of oxidation of fetal hemoglobin.

Assessment of maximum nitrate levels in water exhibiting no adverse health effects has been based principally on a study of known cases of methemoglobinemia. No cases of methemoglobinemia have been reported when the water contained less than 10 mg/liter nitrate as nitrogen. Later, a small percentage of cases were found in which the nitrate concentration of the drinking water was somewhat less. Only one U.S. case has been associated with a *public* water supply regardless of nitrate content.

Studies supplementary to the previous ones in which levels of methemoglobin in the blood of infants were related to concentrations of nitrate in the water being fed showed detectable enhancement of methemoglobin levels in infants being supplied with water containing nitrate as nitrogen only slightly in excess of 10 mg/liter.

It can be concluded that, from the viewpoint of induction of methemoglobinemia, the maximum concentration of nitrate in water exhibiting no significant adverse health effects is close to the interim standard of 10 mg/liter as nitrogen. However, there appears to be little margin of safety for some infants with the standard at this concentration.

The other health hazard proposed for nitrate in water, that it may act as a procarcinogen, is more speculative. A series of reactions is involved by which it is proposed that nitrate in water may be converted to N-nitroso compounds that are carcinogenic agents. The steps in the reaction sequence are:

1. Reduction of nitrate to nitrite.
2. Reaction of nitrite with secondary amines or amides in food or water to form N-nitroso compounds.
3. Carcinogenic reaction of N-nitroso compound.

Reaction of nitrites and secondary amines or amides to form N-nitroso compounds occurs readily in acidic solution and particularly at the normal pH range of 1 to 5 characteristic of gastric contents after a meal.

However, the relation of nitrate concentrations in water supplies to the presence of nitrite in the digestive tract is much more problematic. The major source of nitrite to the stomach, at least for healthy individuals, is the saliva, normally containing 6–15 mg/liter of nitrite. Little reduction of nitrate to nitrite occurs in the human stomach unless the gastric pH is greater than 4.6. Thus the pH condition for formation of nitrite is quite different from the pH range for ready formation of N-nitroso compounds, pH 3.5 or less.

Epidemiologically, correlations have been shown to occur between incidence of gastric cancer and concentration of nitrate in the drinking water. An unusually high incidence of stomach cancer in certain mountainous areas of Colombia is associated with high concentration of nitrate in the drinking water.

The findings, however, are preliminary and only suggestive. They provide no firm evidence of a causal link between incidence of cancer and high intake of nitrate. They do indicate a need for caution in assessment of lack of adverse health effects even at the 10 mg/liter concentration level for nitrate as nitrogen and a need for continued intensive study on the metabolism and effects of nitrate in man.

In conclusion, epidemiological evidence on the occurrence of methemoglobinemia in infants tends to confirm a value near 10 mg/liter nitrate as nitrogen as a maximum concentration level for water with no-observed-adverse-health effects, but there is little margin of safety in this value. There is little scientific basis to support conclusions on the hazard of any concentration of nitrate in water with regard to carcinogenic potential.

SULFATE

No adverse health effects have been noted for concentrations of sulfate in water less than about 500 mg/liter. The only observed physiological effect at concentrations greater than 1000 mg/liter has been the induction of diarrhea.

The taste threshold for sulfate in water lies between 300 and 400 mg/liter for most persons, but some individuals are able to detect as little as 200 mg/liter.

WATER HARDNESS AND HEALTH

Introduction

The principal focus of *Drinking Water and Health* is on possible adverse health effects from contaminants in drinking water. However, certain inorganic or mineral constituents of drinking water that, by usual definition, are not considered to be "contaminants" have been recently reported to be of public health importance. These are constituents that are associated with the level of "hardness" of the water and that occur naturally or that are picked up from water-treatment or distribution systems.

Hardness may be defined as the sum of the polyvalent cations present in water. The most common such cations are calcium and magnesium. Hardness usually is expressed in terms of the equivalent quantity of calcium carbonate ($CaCO_3$). There are no distinctly defined levels for what constitutes a hard or a soft water supply. Generally, water with less than 75 mg/liter (ppm) of $CaCO_3$ is considered soft and above this concentration as hard.

There has been a great deal of interest in the relationship between the hardness of drinking water and morbidity and mortality since the studies, almost 20 yr ago, of Kobayashi in Japan (1957) and Schroeder (1960) in the United States. Subsequently, numerous other studies have been carried out throughout the world which indicate some water factor(s) are statistically correlated with pathologic effects, particularly various cardiovascular diseases. As a result, a voluminous body of literature on these studies has developed and the problem has been the subject of several comprehensive reviews. The Subcommittee on Morbidity and Mortality, in preparing this report, has relied heavily on several of these reviews, notably those by Craun and McCabe (1975), Heyden (1976), Neri *et al.* (1974), Sauer (1974), Sharrett and Feinleib (1975), Schroeder and Kraemer (1974), and Winton and McCabe (1970). These reviews have been abstracted and summarized rather than reprinting the same material or attempting another review.

It should be noted, also, that the World Health Organization and the International Atomic Energy Agency consider that there is sufficient evidence for the involvement of trace elements in the pathogenesis of cardiovascular diseases to warrant international collaborative studies on the problem (IAEA, 1973; WHO, 1973). The possible causal association between water hardness and cardiovascular disease has been recognized in Great Britain to be of enough potential public health importance to have resulted in official governmental expert review of the problem (MRC, 1970; COMA, 1974).

More than 50 studies in nine countries have been carried out on possible relationship of water hardness and health. Most of the investigations were in the United Kingdom, United States, and Canada; they reveal a consistent trend of significant statistical associations between the hardness characteristics of drinking water and the incidence of cardiovascular problems (heart disease, hypertension, and stroke) and, to a lesser extent, other diseases. Generally, reports have shown an inverse correlation between the the incidence of cardiovascular disease and the amount of hardness of drinking water, or, conversely, a positive correlation with the degree of softness. Studies in the United States and Canada have shown that age-adjusted cardiovascular mortality rates among populations using very soft water may be as much as 15–20% higher than among populations using hard water. The differential reported for the United Kingdom may be as high as 40%.

Cardiovascular diseases are the leading cause of death in the United States, where they account for more than 50% of all causes of death, or roughly 1 million deaths each year, and death rates from coronary heart disease have been steadily increasing over the past few decades.

It is evident, therefore, that if water factors are ultimately proven to be involved causally in the pathogenesis of cardiovascular disease, then we are confronted with a major public health problem and current water treatment practices will have to be greatly modified.

The credibility of these water-factor studies depend more on the consistent trend of the findings than their biological plausibility or the size of the correlation coefficients or the actual significance levels.

However, there is some scientific justification for the biological plausibility of these associations. There has been increasing evidence that certain trace elements play an important role in a number of biological processes through their action as activators or inhibitors of enzymatic reactions, by competing with other elements and proteins for binding sites, by influencing the permeability of cell membranes, or through other mechanisms. It is assumed that these elements can also directly or indirectly exert an action on cardiac cells, the blood vessel walls, on blood pressure, or other systems related to cardiovascular function, such as lipid and carbohydrate metabolism. It is assumed further that water quality can affect man's trace element or mineral balance and, consequently, cardiovascular function.

As previously noted, the preponderance of reported evidence indicates statistically significant correlations between some drinking water factor(s) and the incidence of cardiovascular diseases resulting in a general impression that inorganic substances in water may be causally implicated. It must be emphasized, however, that there is considerable disagreement among various investigators concerning the magnitude or even the existence of a "water factor" risk, the identity of the water factor(s), the mode of action, and the specific pathologic effects.

Theories on Risk Factors

Several hypotheses have been offered on how components of drinking water may affect cardiovascular function and disease; these generally fall into one of the following classes:

1. That one or more of the principal "bulk" constituents of hardness in tap water are protective.
2. That one or more of the trace elements that tend to be present in hard water are protective.
3. That harmful metals are present in soft water, possibly having been picked up by leaching from the distribution system.
4. That other factors are involved. Each class of hypotheses is briefly reviewed below.

PROTECTIVE EFFECT FROM BULK CONSTITUENTS OF HARD WATER

Hardness is not a specific constituent of water, but is a complex and variable mixture of cations and anions. Several investigators have attributed the disease-protective effect of hard water to the presence of calcium and magnesium, which are the principal cations found in hard water. Calcium, magnesium, and hardness generally correlate well with one another. In a few studies, however, it was possible to discriminate between the two elements and treat them as separate variables. When calcium and magnesium are separately correlated with cardiovascular disease rates, calcium appears to correlate with greater significance in the United Kingdom, whereas in the United States the correlations are about equally strong for calcium and magnesium.

There is a limited amount of evidence to explain the possible mechanism whereby calcium and/or magnesium may play a role in protection against cardiovascular diseases. Experimentally, a moderate increase of calcium in the diet results in lower levels of circulating and organ cholesterol; this is speculated as a possible factor in the association noted between water hardness and cardiovascular diseases. Magnesium is theorized to protect against lipid deposits in arteries and also may have some anticoagulant properties that could protect against cardiovascular diseases by inhibiting blood clot formation. Also, there is evidence to indicate that there may be higher concentrations of calcium and magnesium in certain tissues among residents of hard water areas as compared to soft water areas.

PROTECTIVE ACTION OF TRACE ELEMENTS IN HARD WATER

There is a paucity of systematic data concerning the concentrations of trace elements as a correlate of hardness of water and cardiovascular disease rates. From a limited number of studies that have been carried out, if hard water contains protective beneficial elements (other than calcium and magnesium), vanadium, lithium, and possibly manganese and chromium emerge as candidates.

Lithium and vanadium have been reported to be negatively correlated with cardiovascular mortality. These negative correlations appear to persist and remain significant even after controlling for calcium and magnesium. The biological functions of these metals are obscure. It is speculated that lithium may have a specific influence on catecholamines and coronary-prone behavioral patterns. Vanadium is reported as an essential trace element in human nutrition and thought to inhibit hepatic cholesterol synthesis and reduce serum cholesterol. Increased intake of vanadium is believed therefore to reduce serum cholesterol. The mechanism is thought to be an inhibition of cholesterol synthesis, especially in young subjects.

A case is made that chromium, which is positively correlated with the hardness of tap water in North America (but not in the United Kingdom), may be causally involved. Experimentally, chromium deficiency produces elevated serum glucose and cholesterol levels and increased deposition of aortic plaques. Though quantitative estimates of daily chromium requirements cannot be given yet, it is thought that the chromium level in hard water may help protect against a deficiency. Similarly, it is speculated that hard water may protect against a deficiency of manganese which also experimentally is associated with decreased glucose tolerance.

HARMFUL ELEMENTS IN SOFT WATER

Soft water tends to be more corrosive than hard water. As a result certain trace metals are found in higher concentrations in soft than in hard water. Several such metals have been suggested as possible intermediaries in the increased cardiovascular disease rates associated with soft water. Based on very limited data, cadmium, lead, copper, and zinc have been suspected to be possibly involved in the induction of cardiovascular disease. These metals often occur in plumbing materials and have been found to leach into soft drinking water.

There is evidence that relatively low doses of cadmium can produce hypertension in rats. It is known that the metal can accumulate in human kidneys and produce renal damage and presumably could affect blood pressure. However, direct evidence linking cadmium in water to heart disease in humans is lacking.

Several studies have shown elevated levels of blood lead occurring among persons living in homes having lead plumbing and soft water, or both. But the relationship between these elevated blood lead levels and cardiovascular disease remains unclear.

There are limited data suggesting that the intake levels of copper and zinc from soft water may adversely affect cardiovascular disease rates. However, there are conflicting data from other studies. Still other studies suggest that the discrepancies may be due to the failure to examine critically the ionic form and the intake ratios of the suspect metals from all sources, particularly the Zn:Cu and the Cd:Zn ratios as well as various other metabolic variables.

OTHER FACTORS AND CONFOUNDING VARIABLES

From the above discussion, it is apparent that there is no shortage of hypotheses to explain how components of drinking water might affect cardiovascular function and disease. It is necessary to consider these hypotheses along with other factors and some confounding variables.

Several cations found predominantly in hard water are theorized to exert a beneficial effect on cardiovascular function, and other cations found in soft water, to exert a detrimental effect. The question often raised is whether drinking water can provide enough of these elements to have any significant impact on the pathogenesis of cardiovascular diseases when considered in the context of the total intake of these elements through other dietary and environmental pathways. Hard or mineralized water generally would supply less than 10–15% of the total dietary intake for calcium and magnesium.

Water provides even a smaller proportion of the total intake for the various suspect trace metals with the possible exception of lead. The largest proportion of trace metal intake from water compared to food is for zinc, but even for this water provides only about 4% of its total dietary intake. For all other suspect metals drinking water provides under 4% of total intake. The concentrations of lead in certain drinking waters may exceed 100 μg/liter as compared to an average adult daily dietary intake of about 300 μg.

Several investigators, however, point out that the amount of these elements provided through drinking water relative to other sources is less important than their chemical form. It is theorized that trace elements often occur in a chelated form in foods and may be less available metabolically than the ionized form that generally occurs in water. Also, the valence form of elements found in water may differ from that in foods and affect metabolic behavior.

Another possible variable is the different effect of hard and soft waters on the mineral composition of foods during cooking. It is theorized that soft water may remove a significantly higher proportion of various "protective" nutrients and elements from foods during cooking than do hard waters.

Most of the studies carried out to date correlate mortality rates with measurements made on raw rather than on finished water; the correlations were of lesser statistical significance when finished water was used.

There was considerable variation in the study design and methods among the numerous investigations reported. As previously noted, most of the studies report a statistically significant correlation between water hardness and one or more of several cardiovascular diseases. It is not possible, however, to quantitatively compare the data from many of these studies because of the different criteria and indices used in the specification of cause of death. The case for a causal association of water factors to any specific pathologic effects is thought to be further weakened by several reports of correlations of the water factor with other causes of death, such as bronchitis, infant mortality, malignancies, cirrhosis, and other noncardiovascular causes of death. Despite the consistent trend for most of the reported studies, a few studies have shown negative or conflicting results for different age and sex groups. For example, in Holland and Sweden, hard water was correlated with decreased cardiovascular mortality among women but not men, and an opposite finding emerged from a study in Newfoundland.

The strength and specificity of the correlative studies have varied depending on the sample sizes of the area and population. In general, the relationship appears stronger in larger and more populous areas.

To some extent these differences are probably due to a lack of sensitivity of correlation coefficients related statistically to the size of the sampling unit. Obviously, smaller geographical units with smaller populations would tend to have less stable death rates and consistency than larger ones, so that any variable will tend to correlate less well with smaller geographical and population bases. But it should be noted that the size of the metropolitan area and population density tend to correlate well with cardiovascular disease rates independently of water quality. This is attributed to various cultural and socioeconomic factors that appear to influence cardiovascular disease mortality rates. On the other hand, less urban areas are more likely to use relatively hard groundwater and, conversely, larger metropolitan areas are usually more dependent on softer surface waters. In a few studies where corrections for socioeconomic factors were attempted, the correlatons with hardness of water still exist but with a reduced statistical significance. It is possible that both urbanization and water mineralization have an effect on cardiovascular disease rates and could be interacting or acting separately.

Several studies have shown statistically significant correlations of death rates with various geographical and climatic variables, especially rainfall, independently of water-quality variables. Much more work must be done on the possible associations and interrelationships of variables such as rain, soil chemistry, and human nutrition with water-quality and cardiovascular disease rates.

From this review, it is clear that there is no shortage of hypotheses related to how the components of drinking water might affect cardiovascular function and disease. Despite the large body of evidence supporting the hypotheses, there are too many confounding variables and discrepancies in the data to permit any scientifically sound conclusions as to the specific role of water factors in the pathogenesis of cardiovascular diseases.

Summary—Water Hardness and Health

There is a large body of scientific information that indicates certain inorganic or mineral constituents of drinking water are correlated with increased morbidity and mortality rates. These constituents by usual definition are not considered to be "contaminants," as they often are associated with the level of "hardness" of drinking water and occur naturally or are picked up from water-treatment or distribution systems. Hardness is due primarily to the presence of ions of calcium and magnesium and is expressed as the equivalent quantity of calcium carbonate ($CaCO_3$). Water with less than 75 mg $CaCO_3$/liter is generally considered soft, and above 75 mg/liter as hard.

A voluminous body of literature suggests that in the United States and other developed nations, the incidence of many chronic diseases, but particularly cardiovascular diseases (heart disease, hypertension, and stroke), is associated with various water characteristics related to hardness. Most of these reports indicate an *inverse* correlation between the incidence of cardiovascular disease and the amount of hardness. A few reports also indicate a similar inverse correlation between the hardness of water and the risk from several noncardiovascular causes of death as well.

Several hypotheses are reported on how water factor(s) may effect health; these mostly involve either a protective action attributed to some elements found in hard water or harmful effects attributed to certain metals often found in soft water.

The theorized protective agents include calcium, magnesium, vanadium, lithium, chromium, and manganese. The suspect harmful agents include the metals cadmium, lead, copper, and zinc, all of which tend to be found in higher concentrations in soft water as a result of the relative corrosiveness of soft water.

It is evident from the review of the literature that there is considerable disagreement concerning the magnitude or even the existence of a "water factor" risk, the identity of the specific causal factor(s), the mode of action, and the specific pathologic effects.

Nevertheless, the preponderance of reported evidence reflects a consistent trend of statistically significant inverse correlations between the hardness of water and the incidence of cardiovascular diseases. As a result, there is a general impression that harmful elements in soft water and/or protective elements in hard water are causally implicated in the pathogenesis of cardiovascular and possibly other chronic diseases.

The wide spectrum of alleged associated effects, the lack of consistency in theorized or reported etiologic factors, the very small quantities of suspect elements in water relative to other sources, and the discrepancies between studies raise serious questions as to whether drinking water really serves as a vehicle of causal agents, is an indicator of something broader within the environment, or represents some unexplained spurious associations. Despite these uncertainties, the body of evidence is sufficiently compelling to treat the "water story" as plausible, particularly when the number of potentially preventable deaths from cardiovascular diseases is considered. In the United States, cardiovascular diseases account for more than one-half of the approximate 2 million deaths occurring each year. On the assumption that water factor(s) are causally implicated, it is estimated that optimal conditioning of drinking water could reduce this annual cardiovascular disease mortality rate by as much as 15% in the United States.

In view of this potential health significance, it is essential to ascertain whether water factors are causally linked to the induction of cardiovascular or other diseases and, if so, to identify the specific factors that are involved. Much more definitive information is needed in order to identify what remedial water treatment actions, if any, can be considered.

REFERENCES FOR TRACE METALS

Aberg, B., L. Ekman, R. Falk, U. Greitz, G. Persson, and J.O. Snihs. 1969. Metabolism of methyl mercury (^{203}Hg) compounds in man. Arch. Environ. Health 19:478-484.

Ackermann, W.C. 1971. Minor Elements in Illinois Surface Waters. Illinois State Water Survey Technical Letter 14.

Adamson, A.H., D.A. Valks, M.A. Appleton, and W.B. Shaw. 1969. Copper toxicity in housed lambs. Vet. Rec. 85:368-369.

Aikawa, J.K., E.L. Rhoades, and G.S. Gordon. 1952. Urinary and fecal excretion of orally administered Mg^{28}. Proc. Soc. Exp. Biol. Med. 98:39-31.

Albert, R.E., R.E. Shore, A.J. Sayers, C. Strehlow, T.J. Kneip, B.S. Pasternack, A.J. Friedhoff, F. Covan, and J.A. Cimino. 1974. Follow-up of children overexposed to lead. Environ. Health Perspect., Exp. Issue no. 7, pp. 33-39.

Alberts, J.J., J.E. Schindler, and R.W. Miller. 1974. Mercury determinations in natural waters by persulfate oxidation. Anal. Chem. 46:434-437.

Aldous, K.M., D.G. Mitchell, and K.W. Jackson. 1975. Simultaneous determination of seven trace metals in potable water using a Vidicon atomic absorption spectrometer. Anal. Chem. 47:1034-1037.

Alexander, F.W., H.T. Delves, and B. E. Clayton. 1973. The uptake and excretion by children of lead and other contaminants. *In* Environmental Health Aspects of Lead, Proc. Int. Symp., Amsterdam, Oct. 2-6, 1972. Luxembourg, Commission of the European Communities, pp. 319-331.

American Public Health Association. 1976. Standard Methods for the Examination of Water and Wastewater, 13th ed. Washington, D.C.

American Society for Testing and Materials. 1970. Annual Book of ASTM Standards, pt. 23, Water and atmospheric analysis. Philadelphia.

Andelman, J.B., and M.A. Shapiro. 1972. Changes in trace element concentrations in water treatment and distribution systems. *In* D.D. Hemphill, ed. Trace Substances in Environmental Health. University of Missouri, Columbia, pp. 87-91.

Andelman, J.B. 1974. The effect of water treatment and distribution on trace element concentrations. *In* A.J. Rubin, ed. Chemistry of Water Supply, Treatment, and Distribution, pp. 423-440. Ann Arbor Science Publishers, Inc. Ann Arbor, Michigan.

Anon. 1962. Molybdenum toxicity. Nutr. Rev. 20:152-154.

Asmangulyan, T.A. 1965. Determination of the maximum permissible concentration of molybdenum in open bodies of water. Hyg. and Sanit. (trans. of Gig. Sanit.) 30:5-11.

Bacon, A.P.C., K. Froome, A.E. Gent, T.K. Cooke, and P. Sowerby. 1967. Lead poisoning from drinking soft water. Lancet 1:264-266.

Baltisberger, R.J. and C.L. Knudson. 1974. The differentiation of submicrogram amounts of inorganic and organomercury in water by flameless atomic absorption spectrometry. Anal. Chem. Acta 73:265-272.

Barabannik, P.I., I.A. Mikhaliuk, R.P. Mnatsakanian, I.N. Tsvetkova, and G.S. Iatsula. 1961. Zinc, manganese, cobalt and iodine in potable artesian water in Kiev. Gig. Sanit. 26:95-97.

Barnard, W.M., and M.J. Fishman. 1973. Evaluation of the use of the heated graphite atomizer for the routine determination of trace metals in water. At. Absorpt. Newsl. 12:118-124.

Barnes, J.M., and H.B. Stoner. 1959. The toxicity of tin compounds. Pharmacol. Rev. 2:211-231, Part 1.

Barnett, P.R., M.W. Skougstad, and K.J. Miller. 1969. Chemical characterization of a public water supply. J. Am. Water Works Assoc. 61:61-67.

Barry, P.S.I. 1975. A comparison of concentrations of lead in human tissues. Br. J. Ind. Med. 32:119-139.

Bauer, G.C.H., A. Carlsson, and B. Lindquist. 1957. Metabolism of ^{140}Ba in man. Acta Orthop. Scand. 26:241-254.

Bauer, G.C.H., A. Carlsson, and B. Lindquist. 1956. A comparative study on the metabolism of ^{140}Ba and ^{45}Ca in rats. Biochem. J. 63:535-542.

Beattie, A.D., M.R. Moore, A. Goldberg, M.J.W. Finlayson, J.F. Graham, E.M. Mackie, J.C. Main, D.A. McLaren, R.M. Murdoch, and G.T. Stewart. 1975. Role of chronic low-level lead exposure in the aetiology of mental retardation. Lancet 1:589-592.

Beattie, A.D., M.R. Moore, W.T. Devenay, A.R. Miller and A. Goldberg. 1972. Environmental lead pollution in an urban soft-water area. Br. Med. J. 2:491-493.

Beeson, K.C., W.R. Griffitts, and D.B. Milne. 1977. Geochemistry and the Environment. Vol. II: Tin. National Academy of Sciences, Washington, D.C.

Berg, J.W., and F. Burbank. 1972. Correlations between carcinogenic trace metals in water supplies and cancer mortality. Ann. N.Y. Acad. Sci. 199:249-264.

Berglund, F. 1971. Reprt from an expert group. Methylmercury in fish, A toxicologic–epidemiologic evaluation of risks. Nord. Hyg. Tidskr. Supplement 4, Stockholm, Sweden.

Bisogni, J.J., Jr. and A.W. Lawrence. 1974. Determination of submicrogram quantities of monomethyl mercury in aquatic samples. Environ. Sci. Technol. 8:850-852.

Boettner, E.A., and F.I. Grunder. 1968. Water analysis by atomic absorption and flameless emission spectroscopy. *In* R.A. Baker, ed. Trace Inorganics in Water, pp. 236-246, Adv. Chem. Ser. no. 73. American Chemical Society, Washington D.C.

Bostrom, H., and P.O. Wester. 1967. Trace elements in drinking water and death rate in cardiovascular disease. Acta Med. Scand. 181:465-473.

Bowers, E. 1971. Ion-exchange softening. *In* Water Quality and Treatment, a Handbook of Public Water Supplies, 3d ed., pp. 341-377. Prepared by The American Water Works Association. McGraw-Hill Book Co., New York.

Brooks, P.P. Presley, and I.R. Kaplan. 1967. APDC-MIBK extraction system for the determination of trace elements in saline waters by atomic absorption spectrophotometry. Talanta 14:809-816.

Brown, D.R. 1975. Neonatal lead exposure in the rat: Decreased learning as a function of age and blood lead concentrations. Toxicol. Appl. Pharmacol. 32:628-637.

Brown, E., M.W. Skougstad, and M.J. Fishman. 1970. Methods for collection and analysis of water samples for dissolved minerals and gases. U.S. Geological Survey, Techniques of Water-Resources Invest. no. 5.

Browning, E. 1961. Toxicity of industrial metals. Butterworths, London, England.

Camp, T.R., and R.L. Meserve. 1974. Water and Its Impurities, 2nd ed., pp. 184-191. Dowden, Hutchinson and Ross Inc., Stroudsbrug, Pa.

Carson, T.L., G.A. VanGelder, G.C. Karas, and W.B. Buck. 1974. Slowed learning in lambs prenatally exposed to lead. Arch. Environ. Health. 29:154-156.

Chao, T.T., M.J. Fishman, and J.W. Ball. 1969. Determination of traces of silver in waters by anion exchange and atomic absorption spectrophotometry. Anal. Chem. Acta. 47:189-195.

Chapman, J.F., L.S. Dale, and J.W. Kelly. 1974. A carbon tube for the analysis of water by flameless atomic absorption spectrometry. Anal. Chem. Acta 69:207-210.

Chappell, W.R. 1973. Transport and biological effects of molybdenum in the environment. Progress Report, 1 Jan. 1973. University of Colorado and Colorado State University.

Chau, Y.K., and K. Lum-Shue-Chan. 1969. Atomic absorption determination of microgram quantities of molybdenum in lake waters. Anal Chem. Acta 48:205-212.

Chernoff, N. 1973. Teratogenic effects of cadmium in rats. Teratology 8(1):29-32.

Chuttani, H.K., P.S. Gupta, S. Gulati, and D.N. Gupta. 1965. Acute copper poisoning. Am. J. Med. 39:849-854.

Cohen, J.M., L.J. Kamphake, E.K. Harris, and R.L. Woodward. 1960. Taste threshold concentrations of metals in drinking water. J. Am. Water Works Assoc. 52:660-670.

Consolazio, C.F., L.O. Matoush, R.A. Nelson, R.S. Harding, and J.E. Canham. 1963. Excretion of sodium, potassium, magnesium, and iron in human sweat and the relation of each to balance and requirements. J. Nutr. 79:407-415.

Copenhaver, E.D., G.U. Ulrikson, L.T. Newman, and W. Fulkerson. 1973. Cadmium in the environment: An annotated bibliography. Oak Ridge National Laboratory. ORNL-EIS-73-17.

Cosgrove, J.F., and D.J. Bracco. 1973. Determination of minor metallic elements in the water environment. *In* L. Ciaccio, ed. Water and water pollution handbook, vol. 4, pp. 1315-1356. M. Dekker Co., New York.

Coussons, H. 1969. Magnesium metabolism in infants and children. Postgrad. Med. 46, 135-139.

Cralley, L.J. 1972. Uses and industrial exposures. *In* I.R. Tabershaw, ed. The Toxicology of Beryllium. U.S. Department of Health, Education, and Welfare, Public Health Service. Public Health Service Publication 2173, Washington, D.C.

Craun, G.F., and L.J. McCabe. 1975. Problems associated with metals in drinking water. J. Am. Water Works Assoc. 67:593-599.

Crump-Wiesner, H.J. and W.C. Purdy. 1969. Extraction of vanadium into isobutyl methyl ketone. Talanta 16:124-129.

Dangel, R.A. 1975. Study of corrosion products in the Seattle Water Department distribution system. Report, Environmental Protection Technology Series, EPA-670/2-75-036.

Davis, G.K. 1974. Copper and molybdenum. *In* Geochemistry and the Enviornment. Vol. I: The Relation of Selected Trace Elements to Health and Disease, pp. 68-79. National Academy of Sciences, Washington, D.C.

De Groot, A.P., V.J. Feron, and H.P. Til. 1973. Short-term toxicity studies of some salts and oxides of tin in rats. Food Cosmet. Toxicol. 11:19-30.

de No, L.R., and T.P. Feng. 1946. Analysis of the effect of barium upon nerve with particular reference to rhythmic activity. J. Cell. Comp. Physiol. 28:397-464.

Doherty, P.C., R.M. Barlow, and K.W. Angus. 1969. Spongy changes in the brains of sheep poisoned by excess dietary copper. Res. Vet. Sci. 10:303-304.

Dolinsek, F., and J. Stupar. 1973. Application of the carbon cup atomization technique in water analysis by atomic absorption spectroscopy. Analyst 98:841-850.

Durfor, C.N., and E. Becker. 1964. Public Water Supplies of the 100 Largest Cities in the United States, 1962. U.S. Geological Survey Water-Supply Paper 1812. U.S. Government Printing Office, Washington, D.C.

Durum, W.H. and J. Haffty. 1961. Occurrence of Minor Elements in Water. U.S. Geological Survey Circular 445, Washington, D.C.

Durum, W.H. 1974. Occurrence of some trace metals in surface and groundwaters. *In* Trace Metals in Water Supplies: Occurrence, Significance, and Control. Proceedings, 16th Water Quality Conference, University of Illinois, Urbana.

Durum, W.H., J.D. Hem, and S.G. Heidel. 1971. Reconnaissance of Selected Minor Elements in Surface Waters of the United States, October 1970. U.S. Geological Survey Circular 643, Washington, D.C.

Durum, W.H., S.G. Heidel, and L.J. Tison. 1960. World-wide runoff of dissolved solids. *In* International Association of Scientific Hydrology, General Assembly of Helsinki, 1960, pp. 618-628. Publication no. 51-55.

Dye, J.F., and J.L. Tuepker. 1971. Chemistry of the lime-soda process. *In* Water Quality and Treatment, a Handbook of Public Water Supplies, 3rd ed, pp. 313-340. Prepared by the American Water Works Associations. McGraw-Hill Book Co., New York.

Ediger, R.P. 1973. Review of water analysis by atomic absorption. At. Absorpt. Newsl. 12:151-157.

Ekman, L., U. Greitz, G. Persson, and B. Aberg. 1968. Omsattning av methylkvicksilver hos manniska. Nord. Med. 79:450-456.

Elwell, W.T., and J.A. Gidley. 1966. Atomic-absorption spectrophotometry, 2nd rev. ed. Pergamon Press, New York.

Everett, G.L., T.S. West, and R.W. Williams. 1974. The determination of tin by carbon filament atomic absorption spectrometry. Anal. Chem. Acta 70:291-198.

Everson, R.J., and H.E. Parker. 1974. Effect of hydrogen ion concentration on the determination of lead by solvent extraction and atomic absorption spectrophotometry. Anal. Chem. 46:1966-1970.

Falk, R., J.O. Snihs, L. Ekman, U. Greitz, and B. Aberg. 1971. Whole-body measurements on the distribution of mercury-203 in humans after oral intake of methylradiomercury nitrate. Acta. Radiol. 9:55-72.

Feldman, C. 1974. Perchloric acid procedure for wet-ashing organic for the determination of mercury (and other metals). Anal. Chem. 46:1606-1609.

Ferm, V.H. 1972. The teratogenic effects of metals on mammalian embryos. Adv. Teratol. 5:51-75.

Fernandez, F.J., and D.C. Manning. 1971. Atomic absorption analyses of metal pollutants in water using a heated graphite atomizer. At. Absorpt. Newsl. 10:65-69.

Fernandez, F.J. 1973. Atomic absorption determination of gaseous hydrides utilizing sodium borohydride reduction. At. Absorpt. Newsl. 12:93-97.

Friberg, L., M. Piscator, and G. Nordberg. 1971. Cadmium in the Environment. CRC Press, Cleveland.

Friberg, L., T. Kjellstrom, G. Nordberg, and M. Piscator. 1975. Cadmium in the Environment. III: A Toxicological and Epidemiological Appraisal. U.S. Environmental Protection Agency, Environmental Protection Series, EPA-650/2-75-049, Washington, D.C.

Friberg, M. Piscator, G.F. Nordberg and T. Kjellstrom. 1974. Cadmium in the Environment, 2nd Edition. CRC Press, Cleveland.

Furukawa, D.H. 1973. Removal of heavy metals from water using reverse osmosis. *In* Conference on Traces of Heavy Metals in Water Removal Processes and Monitoring, pp. 180-187. Princeton University, Princeton, N.J., Nov. 15-16, 1973. U.S. Environmental Protection Agency, EPA-902/9-74-001.

Gammill, J.C., B. Wheeler, E.L. Carothers, and P.F. Hahn. 1950. Distribution of radioactive silver solloids in tissues of rodents following injection by various routes. Proc. Soc. Exp. Biol. 74:691-695.

Gettler, A.C., C.P. Rhoads, and S. Weiss. 1927. A contribution to the pathology of generalized argyria with a discussion of the fate of silver in the human body. Am. J. Pathol. 3:631-651.

Goldwater, L.J., and T.W. Clarkson. 1972. Mercury. *In* D.H.K. Lee, ed. Metallic Contaminants and Human Health, pp. 17-55. Academic Press, New York.

Goldwater, L.J. 1971. Mercury in the environment. Sci. Am. 224:15-21

Goodman, L.S., and A. Gilman, eds. 1975. The Pharmacological Basis of Therapeutics. Macmillan Pub. Co., New York.

Gotsev, T. 1944. Blood pressure and heart activity. III. Action of barium on the circulation. Arch. Exp. Pathol. Pharmakol. 203:264-277.

Griffitts, W.R., W.H. Allaway, and D.H. Groth. 1977. Beryllium. *In* Geochemistry and the Enviornment. Vol. II: The Relation of Other Substances and Trace Elements to Health and Disease. National Academy of Sciences, Washington, D.C.

Gross, S.B., E.A. Pfitzer, D.W. Yeager, and R.A. Kehoe. 1975. Lead in human tissues. Toxicol. Appl. Pharmacol. 32:638-351.

Guy, R.D., and C.L. Chakrabarti. 1975a. Distribution of metal ions between soluble and particulate forms. International Conference on Heavy Metals in the Environment, Abstracts, Toronto, Ontario, Canada, Oct. 27-31.

Guy, R.D., and C.L. Chakrabarti. 1975. Analytical techniques for speciation of trace metals. International Conference on Heavy Metals in the Environment, Abstracts, Toronto, Ontario, Canada, Oct. 27-31. pp. 275-294.

Hadjimarkos, D.M. 1967. Effect of trace elements in drinking water on dental caries. J. Pediatr. 70:967-969.

Hambidge, K.M. 1971. Chromium nutrition in the mother and the growing child. *In* W. Mertz and W.E. Cornatzer, eds. Newer Trace Elements in Nutrition, pp. 169-194. Marcel Dekker, New York.

Hammerstrom, R.J., D.E. Hissong, F.C. Kopfler, J. Jayer, E.F. McFarron, and B.H. Pringle. 1972. Mercury in drinking water supplies. Am. Water Works Assoc. 64:60-61.

Harris, R.W., and W.R. Elsea. 1967. Ceramic glaze as a source of lead poisoning. J. Am. Med. Assoc. 202:544-546.

Hatch, W.R., and W.L. Ott. 1968. Determination of submicrogram quantities of mercury by atomic absorption spectrophotometry. Anal. Chem. 40:2085-2087.

Hem, J.D. 1970. Study and Interpretation of Chemical Characteristics of Natural Water, 2nd ed., p. 172. Geological Survey Water-Supply Paper 1473. U.S. Government Printing Office, Washington, D.C.

Hemphill, D.D., ed. 1972. Trace Substances in Enviornmental Health, vol. VI. University of Missouri.

Hill, W.R., and D.M. Pillsbury. 1939. Argyria: The Pharmacology of Silver. Williams & Wilkins Co., Baltimore.

Holtzman, N.A., and R.H.A. Haslam. 1968. Elevation of serum copper following copper sulfate as an emetic. Pediatrics 42:189-193.

Hopper, S.H., and H.S. Adams. 1958. Copper poisoning from vending machines. Public Health Rep. 73:910-914.

Hume, D.N. 1967. Analysis of water for trace metals. *In* Equilibrium Concepts in Natural Water Systems, pp. 30-44. Avd. Chem. Ser. no. 67, American Chemical Society, Washington, D.C.

Ichinose, N. 1974. Extraction and atomic absorption spectrometric determination of trace copper with zinc dibenzyldithiocarbamate. Anal. Chem. Acta 70:222-226.

International Agency for Research on Cancer. 1972. IARC Monographs on the Evaluation of the Carcinogenic Risk of Chemicals to Man, vol. I. World Health Organization, Geneva, Switzerland.

International Agency for Research on Cancer. 1973. IARC Monographs on the Evaluation of Carcinogenic Risk of Chemicals to Man. Vol. 2: Some Inorganic and Organometallic Compounds. World Health Organization, Geneva, Switzerland.

Issaq, H.J., and W.L. Zielinski, Jr. 1974. Hot atomic absorption spectrometry method for determination of mercury at the nanogram and subnanogram level. Anal. Chem. 46:1436-1438.

Jenne, E.A. Mercury in waters of the United States. 1970-1971. U.S. Department of the Interior, Geological Survey. Open-file report. Menlo Park, Calif. Apr. 1, 1972.

Jenne, E.A., and J.W. Ball. 1972. Time stability of aqueous ammonium pyrrolidine dithiocarbamate and its manganese and nickel complexes in methyl isobutyl ketone. At. Absorpt. Newsl. 11:60-61.

Jones, J.E., R. Manalo, and E.B. Flink. 1967. Magnesium requirements in adults. Am. J. Clin. Nutr. 10:632-635.

Joyner, T., M.L. Healy, D. Chakravarti, and T. Koyanagi. 1967. Preconcentration for trace analysis of sea water. Environ. Sci. Technol. 1:417-424.

Kaminski, E.E. 1974. Interference of aluminum in the atomic absorption determination of cadmium using sodium diethyldithiocarbamate as chelating agent. Anal. Chem. 46:1304-1305.

Karalekas, P.C., Jr., G.F. Craun, A.F. Hammonds, C.R. Ryan, and D.J. Worth. 1976. Lead and other trace metals in drinking water in the Boston metropolitan area. J. New Engl. Water Works Assoc. 90:150-172.

Karlsson, B., and L. Noren. 1965. Ipecacuanha and copper sulphate as emetics in intoxications in children. Acta Paediatr. Scand. 54:331-335.

Kehoe, R.A. 1953. Report on the physiological effects of some common inorganic salts in water on man and domestic animals. The Kettering Laboratory, University of Cincinnati.

Kehoe, R.A. 1961. The metabolism of lead in man in health and disease. The Harben Lectures, 1960. J. R. Inst. Public Health Hyg. 24:81-97, 129-143, 177-203.

Kehoe, R.A., J. Cholak, and E.J. Largent. 1944. The hygienic significance of the contamination of water with certain mineral constitutents. J. Am. Water Works Assoc. 36:645-657.

Kehoe, R.A., J. Cholak, and E.J. Largent. 1944. The concentrations of certain trace metals in drinking water. J. Am. Water Works Assoc. 36:637-644.

Kehoe, R.A., J. Cholak, and R.V. Story. 1940. Manganese, lead, tin, aluminum, copper and silver in normal biological material. J. Nutr. 20:85-98.

Kent, N.L., and R.A. McCance. 1941. The absorption and excretion of "minor" elements by man. II. Cobalt, nickel, tin, and manganese. Biochem. J. 35:877-883.

Kerber, J.D., and F.J. Fernandez, 1971. The determination of trace metals in aqueous solution with the Delves sampling cup technique. At. Absorpt. Newsl. 10:78-80.

King, B.G. 1971. Maximum daily intake of lead without excessive body lead-burden in children. Am. J. Dis. Child. 122:337-340.

Kinrade, J.D., and J.C. Van Loon. 1974. Solvent extraction for use with flame atomic absxrption spectrometry. Anal. Chem. 46:1894-1898.

Kirkbright, G.F. and M. Sargent. 1974. Atomic Absorption and Fluorescence Spectroscopy. Academic Press, New York.

Klein, M., R. Namer, E. Harpur, and R. Corbin. 1970. Earthenware containers as a source of fatal lead poisoning: Case study and public-health considerations. N. Engl. J. Med. 283:669-672.

Klimmer, O.R. 1968. Toxicologicl viewpoint on the application of organotin fungicides in agriculture. Pflanzenschutzberichte, 37:57-66.

Kolbye, A.C., Jr., K.R. Mahaffey, J.A. Fiorino, P.C. Corneliussen, and C.F. Jelinek. 1974. Food exposures to lead. Environ. Health Perspect. 7:65-74.

Konovalov, G.S., A.A. Ivanova, and T.K. Kolensnikova. 1966. Rare and dispersed elements (microelements) in the water and in the suspended substances in rivers of the European Territory of USSR. Gidrokhimi. Mater. (trans.) 42:94-111.

Kopp, J.F., and R.C. Kroner. 1967. Trace metals in waters of the United States. A five-year summary of trace metals in rivers and lakes of the United States (Oct. 1, 1962-Sept. 30, 1967). U.S. Department of the Interior, Federal Water Pollution Control Administration, Division of Pollution Surveillance, Cincinnati, Ohio.

Kopp, J.F. 1969. The occurrence of trace elements in water. *In* D.D. Hemphill, ed. Proceedings of the Third Annual Conference on Trace Substances in Environmental Health, 1969, pp. 59-73. University of Missouri, Columbia.

Korkisch, J., and A. Sorio. 1975. Determination of cadmium, copper and lead in natural waters after anion exchange separation. Anal. Chem. Acta 76:393-399.

Krasovskii, G.N., and S.A. Fridlyand. 1971. Experimental data for the validation of the maximum permissible concentration of cobalt in water bodies. Hyg. Sanit. (trans. of Gig. Sanit) 36:277-279.

Kubota, J., E.L. Mills, and R.T. Oglesby. 1974. Lead, Cd, Zn, Cu, and Co in streams and lake waters of Cayuga Lake basin, New York. Environ. Sci. Technol. 8:243-248.

L'vov, B.V. 1970. Atomic Absorption Spectrochemical Analysis. Adam Hilger, London.

Lancranjan, I., H.I. Popescu, O. Gavanescu, I. Klepsch, and M. Servanescu. 1975. Reproductive ability of workmen occupationally exposed to lead. Arch. Environ. Health 30:396-401.

Landrigan, P.J., S.H. Gehlbach, B.F. Rosenblum, J.M. Shoults, R.M. Candelaria, W.F. Barthel, J.A. Liddle, A.L. Smrek, N.W. Staehling, and J.F. Sanders. 1975. Epidemic lead absorption near an ore smelter. The role of particulate lead. N. Engl. J. Med. 292:123-129.

Lauwerys, R., J.P. Buchet, H. Roels, A. Berlin and J. Smeets. 1975. Intercomparison program of lead, mercury, and cadmium analysis in blood, urine, and aqueous solutions. Clin. Chem. 21:551-557.

Lieber, M. 1954. Contamination of ground water by cadmium. J. Am. Water Works Assoc. 46:541-547.

Linstedt, K.D., C.P. Houck, and J.T. O'Commor. 1971. Trace element removals in advanced waste water treatment processes. J. Water Pollut. Control Fed. 43:1507-1513.

Livingstone, D.A. 1963. Chemical composition of rivers and lakes. *In* M. Fleischer, ed. Data of geochemistry, 6th ed. Geological Survey Professional Paper 440-G. U.S. Government Printing Office, Washington, D.C.

Lockhart, E.E., C.L. Tucker, and M.C. Merrit. 1955. The effect of water impurities on the flavor of brewed coffee. Food Res. 10:598-605.

Logsdon, G.S., and J.M. Symons. 1973. Removal of trace inorganics in drinking water treatment unit processes. Am. Inst. Chem. Eng. Meet., Detroit, June 1973. Paper 482

Logsdon, G.S., and J.M. Symons. 1973. Removal of heavy metals by conventional treatment. Conference on Traces of Heavy Metals in Water Removal Processes and Monitoring, Princeton University, Princeton, N.J., Nov. 15-16, 1973, pp. 225-226. U.S. Environmental Protection Agency. EPA 902/9-74-001.

Logsdon, G.S., and J.M. Symons. 1973. Mercury removal by conventional water-treatment techniques. J. Am. Water Works Assoc. 5:554-562.

Lu, F.C., P.E. Berteau, and D.J. Clegg. 1972. The toxicity of mercury in man and animals. *In* Mercury Contamination in Man and His Environment, pp. 67-85. International Atomic Energy Agency, Vienna.

Lundgren, K.D., A. Swensson, and U. Ulfarvson. 1967. Studies in humans on the distribution of mercury in the blood and the excretion in urine after exposure to different mercury compounds. Scand. J. Clin. Lab. Invest. 20: 164-166.

Maines, I.S., K.M. Aldous, and D.G. Mitchell. 1975. Determination of lead in potable waters using Delves cup atomic-absorption spectrometer with signal integration. Environ. Sci. Technol. 9:549-551.

McCabe, L.J., and J.C. Vaughn. 1969. Trace metals content of drinking water from a large system. Presented at National Meeting, American Chemical Society, Minneapolis, Minn.

McCabe, L.J., J.M. Symons, R.D. Lee, and G.G. Robeck. 1970. Survey of community water supply systems. J. Am. Water Works Assoc. 62:670-687.

McKee, J.E., and H.W. Wolf (eds.). 1963. Water Quality Criteria, 2nd ed. The Resources Agency of California State Water Resources Control Board Publication no. 3-A (Reprint December, 1971). Sacramento.

McKee, J.E., and H.W. Wolf. 1976. Water Quality Criteria. California State Water Quality Control Board Publication no. 3-A, Sacramento.

Mertz, W. 1972. Human requirements: Basic and optimal. N.Y. Acad. Sci. Ann. 199:191-201.

Miller, R.F., N.O. Price, and R.W. Engel. 1959. The microelement (Zn, Mn, Cu, Mo, and Co) balance of 7-9 year old girls. Fed. Proc. 18:538.

Minear, R.A. 1975. Analytical techniques for measuring and monitoring trace metals. J. Am. Water Works Assoc. 67:9-14.

Monier-Williams, G.W. 1949. Trace Elements in Foods. Chapman-Hall, Ltd., London.

Monty, K.J. 1960. Effects of trace amounts of molybdenum. *In* Proceedings, Conference on Physiological Aspects of Water Quality, pp. 75-78. U.S.Public Health Service, Washington, D.C.

Moore, M.R., P.A. Meredith, A. Goldberg, K.E. Carr, P.G. Toner, and T.D.V. Lawrie. 1975. Cardiac effects of lead in drinking water of rats. Clin. Sci. Molecu. Med. 49:337-341.

Morik, J., and Z. Morlin. 1959. Pollution of the air of industrial regions by metals. Nepeqeszsegugy 40:288-293, reported in Chemical Abstracts, 57, 8850f (1962).

Mulford, C.E. 1966. Solvent extraction techniques for atomic absorption spectroscopy. At. Absorpt. Newsl. 5:88-90.

National Academy of Sciences-National Research Council. Environmental Studies Board. 1973. Water Quality Criteria 1972. EPA Report. EPA-R3-73-033. Washington, D.C.

National Academy of Sciences-National Research Council. Division of Medical Sciences. 1974. Medical and Biological Effects of Environmental Pollutants: Chromium. Washington, D.C.

National Academy of Sciences-National Research Council. Division of Medical Sciences. 1972. Lead: Airborne Lead in Perspective. Washington, D.C.

National Academy of Sciences-National Research Council. Assembly of Life Sciences. Committee on Toxicology. 1976. Recommendations for the Prevention of Lead Poisoning in Children. Washington, D.C.

National Academy of Sciences-National Research Council. Division of Medical Sciences. 1973. Medical and Biologic Effects of Environmental Pollutants: Manganese. Washington, D.C.

National Academy of Sciences-National Research Council. Division of Medical Sciences. 1975. Medical and Environmental Effects of Environmental Pollutants: Nickel. Washington, D.C.

National Academy of Sciences-National Research Council. Division of Medical Sciences. 1974. Medical and Environmental Effects of Environmental Pollutants: Vanadium. Washington, D.C.

National Academy of Sciences-National Research Council. Food and Nutrition Board. 1973. Toxicants Occurring Naturally in Foods, 2nd ed. Washington, D.C.

National Academy of Sciences-National Research Council. Food and Nutrition Board. 1974. Recommended Dietary Allowances, 8th ed. Washington, D.C.

National Technical Advisory Committee. 1969. Raw water quality criteria for public supplies. J. Am. Water Works Assoc. 61:133-138.

Naylor, L.M., and R.R. Dague. 1975. Simulation of lead removal by chemical treatment. J. Am. Water Works Assoc. 67:560-565.

Negus, S.S. 1938. The physiological aspects of mineral salts in public water supplies. J. Am. Water Works Assoc. 30:242-264.

Nicholas, P.O. 1968. Food-poisoning due to copper in the morning tea. Lancet 2:40-42.

Nilsson, R. 1971. Removal of metals by chemical treatment of municipal waste water. Water Res. 5:51-60.

Nix, J., and T. Goodwin. 1970. The simultaneous extraction of iron, manganese, copper, cobalt, nickel, chromium, lead and zinc from natural water for determination by atomic absorption spectrocopy. At. Absorpt. Newsl. 9:119-122.

Nordberg, G.F. (ed.) 1976. Effects and Dose-Response Relationships of Toxic Metals. Elsevier Scientific Publishing Co., Amsterdam.

Nordell, E. 1961. Water Treatment for Industrial and Other Uses, 2nd ed. Reinhold Publishing Co., New York.

Norgaard, O. 1954. Investigation with radioactive Ag into the resorption of silver through human skin. Acta Dermato-Venerol. 34:415-419.

Olcutt, C.T. 1950. Experimental argyrosis. V. Hypertrophy of the left ventricle of the heart in rats ingesting silver salts. Arch. Pathol. 49:138-149.

Oliver, S. 1974. Mood and trace metals in drinking water. Master of Science Thesis. The Johns Hopkins University, School of Hygiene and Public Health, Baltimore, Md.

Omang, S.H. 1971. Determination of mercury in natural waters and effluents by flameless atomic absorption spectrophotometry. Anal. Chem. Acta 53:415-419.

Paus, P.E. 1971. The application of atomic absorption spectroscopy to the analysis of natural waters. At. Absorpt. Newsl. 10:69-71.

Pickering, Q.H., and C. Henderson. 1966. The acute toxicity of some heavy metals to different species of warmwater fishes. Int. J. Air Water Pollut. 10:453-463.

Poller, R.C. 1970. The Chemistry of Organotin Compounds. Academic Press, New York.

Pomelee, C.S. 1953. Toxicity of beryllium. Sewage Ind. Wastes 25:1424-1428.

Price, W.J. 1972. Analytical Atomic Absorption Spectrometry. Heyden and Son, London.

Proctor and Gamble Co. 1974. Nitrilotriacetate Levels in Canadian Waters. Drinking Water Survey Progress Report no. 1.

Ramage, H. 1930. Mushrooms—Mineral content. Nature 126:279.

Ramamoorthy, S., and D.J. Kushner. 1975. Binding of heavy metal ions by river water. International Conference on Heavy Metals in the Environment, Abstracts, Toronto, Ontario, Canada, Oct. 27-31, pp. D-19-D-21.

Ramirez-Munoz, J. 1968. Atomic-Absorption Spectroscopy and Analyses by Atomic-Absorption Flame Photometry. Elsevier Publishing Co., New York.

Rattonetti, A. 1974. Determination of soluble cadmium, lead, silver, and indium in rainwater and stream water with the use of flameless atomic absorption. Anal. Chem. 46:739-742.

Renn, C.E., W.E. Chesney, and S.L. Chang. 1955. Effect of hyla 603K on cysts of E. histolytic and bactericidal efficiencies of hyla 603D filtrate. The Johns Hopkins University, Institute for Cooperative Research, Project Report PG 49.33.

Renshaw, G.D. 1973. The determination of barium by flameless atomic absorption spectrophotometry using a modified graphite tube atomizer. At. Absorpt. Newsl. 12:158-160.

Renshaw, G.D., C.A. Pounds, and E.F. Pearson. 1973. The quantitative estimation of lead, antimony and barium in gunshot residues by nonflame atomic absorption spectrophotometry. At. Absorpt. Newsl. 12:55-56.

Reynolds, R.J., and K. Aldous. 1970. Atomic Absorption Spectroscopy: A Practical Guide. Barnes and Noble, Scranton, Pa.

Robinson, J.W. 1975. Atomic Absorption Spectroscopy. Marcel Dekker Co., New York.

Roels, H.A. 1975. Response of some heme biosynthetic pathway parameters in men, women, and children moderately exposed to lead. *In* International Conference on Heavy Metals in the Environment, Abstracts, Toronto, Ontario, Canada, Oct. 27-31, pp. B-57-B-60.

Roshchin, I.V., A.V. Il'nitskaia, L.A. Lutsenko, and L.V. Zhidkova. 1965. Effect on organism of vanadium trioxide. Fed. Proc. 24:611-613.

Sachdev, S.L. and P.W. West. 1969. Concentration and determination of traces of metal ions. Anal. Chem. Acta 44:301-307.

Sachdev, S.L., and P.W. West. 1970. Concentration of trace metals by solvent extraction and their determination by atomic absorption spectrophotometry. Environ. Sci. Technol. 4:749-751.

Salvidio, E., I. Pannaccivlli, and A. Tizianello. 1963. Glucose-6-phosphate and 6-phosphogluconic dehydrogenase activities in the red blood cells of several animal species. Nature 200:372-373.

Sandstead, H.H. 1976. Interactions of cadmium and lead with essential minerals. *In* G.F. Nordberg. Effects and Dose-Response Relationships of Toxic Metals, pp. 511-526. Elsevier Scientific Publishing Co., Amsterdam.

Sandstead, H.H. 1974. Cadmium, zinc, and lead. *In* Geochemistry and the Environment. Vol. I: The Relation of Selected Trace Elements to Health and Disease, pp. 43-56. National Academy of Sciences, Washington, D.C.

Sayre, J.W., E. Charney, J. Vostal, and I.B. Pless. 1974. House and hand dust as a potential source of childhood lead exposure. Am. J. Dis. Child. 127:167-170.

Scanlon, J.W. 1975. Dangers to the human fetus from certain heavy metals in the environment. Rev. Environ. Health 2:39-64.

Scheinbert, I.H., and I. Sternlieb. 1965. Wilson's disease. Ann. Rev. Med. 16:119-134.

Schroeder, D.C., and G.F. Lee. 1975. Potential transformations of chromium in natural waters. Water Air Soil Pollut. 4:355-365.

Schroeder, H.A. 1970. Chromium American Petroleum Institute Air Quality Monograph No. 70-15. Washington, D.C.

Schroeder, H.A., and M. Mitchener. 1975. Life-term effects of mercury, methyl mercury, and nine other trace metals on mice. J. Nutr. 105:452-458.

Schroeder, H.A. 1974. The role of trace elements in cardiovascular disease. Med. Clin. N. Am. 58:381-396.

Schroeder, H.A., A.P. Nason, and I.H. Tipton. 1969. Essential metals in man: Magnesium. J. Chron. Dis. 21:815-841.

Schroeder, H.A., A.P. Nason, I.H. Tipton, and J.J. Balassa. 1966. Essential trace metals in man: Copper. J. Chron. Dis. 19:1007-1034.

Schroeder, H.A., J.J. Balassa, and I.H. Tipton. 1970. Essential trace elements in man: Molybdenum. J. Chron. Dis. 23:481-499.

Schroeder, H.A., J.J. Balassa, and I.H. Tipton. 1964. Abnormal trace elements in man: Tin. J. Chron. Dis. 17:483-502.

Schwarz, K., D.B. Milne, and E. Vinyard. 1970. Growth effects of tin compounds in rats maintained in a trace element-controlled environment. Biochem. Biophys. Res. Commun. 40:22-29.

Seaber, W.M. 1933. Barium as a normal constituent of Brazil nuts. Analyst 58:575-580.

Semmens, M.J. 1975. Unpublished data.

Semple, A.B., W.H. Parry, and D.E. Phillips. 1960. Acute copper poisoning; an outbreak traced to contaminated water from a corroded geyser. Lancet 2:700-701.

Shakman, R.A. 1974. Nutritional influence on the toxicity of environmental pollutants. A review. Arch. Environ. Health 28:105-113.

Shapiro, M.A., W.H. Hill, P.K. Chin, and Y. Kobayashi. 1962. Physiological Aspects of Water Quality. University of Pittsburgh, RG5309.

Shapiro, M.A., W.H. Hill, F.A. Rosenberg, and G.F. Lee. 1960. Report on research project at University of Pittsburgh. *In* Proceedings, Conference on Physiological Aspects of Water Quality, pp. 223-231. U.S. Public Health Service, Washington, D.C.

Shigematsu, T., M. Matsui, O. Fujino, and K. Kinoshita. 1975. Determination of manganese in natural waters by atomic absorption spectrometry with a carbon tube atomizer. Anal. Chiem. Acta 76:329-336.

Shouse, S.S., and G.H. Whipple. 1931. I. Effects of the intravenous injection of colloidal silver upon the hemopoietic system in dogs. J. Exp. Med. 53:413.

Sigworth, E.A., and S.B. Smith. 1972. Adsorption of inorganic compounds by activated carbon. J. Am. Water Works Assoc. 64:386.

Singer, P.C. 1974. Chemical processes for the removal of trace metals from drinking waters. *In* Trace Metals in Water Supplies: Occurrence, Significance, and Control. Proceedings, 16th Water Quality Conference, University of Illinois, Urbana, Feb. 1974.

Slavin, W. 1968. Atomic Absorption Spectroscopy. John Wiley-Interscience, New York.

Sollman, T. 1957. A Manual of Pharmacology, 8th ed. W.B. Saunders Co., Philadelphia.

Sterner, J.H., and M. Eisenbud. 1951. Epidemiology of beryllium intoxication. Arch. Ind. Hyg. Occup. Med. 4:123-151.

Stofen, D. 1973. The maximum permissible concentrations in the U.S.S.R. for harmful substances in drinking water. Toxicology 1:187-195.

Stokinger, H.E., and R.L. Woodward. 1958. Toxicologic methods for establishing drinking-water standards. J. Am. Water Works Assoc. 50(4):515-529.

Stokinger, H.E. 1972. *In* I.R. Tabershaw, ed. The Toxicology of Beryllium. Public Health Service Publication 2173. U.S. Department of Health, Education, and Welfare, Public Health Service, Washington, D.C.

Straub, C.P. 1964. Low Level Radioactive Wastes. U.S. Government Printing Office, Washington, D.C.

Streeten, D.H.P., M.M. Gerstein, B.M. Marmor, and R.J. Doisy. 1965. Reduced glucose tolerance in elderly human subjects. Diabetes 14:579-583.

Sunderman, F.W., Jr. 1971. Metal carcinogenesis in experimental animals. Food. Cosmet. Toxicol. 9:105-120.

Surles, T., J.R. Tuschall, Jr., and T.T. Collins. 1975. Comparative atomic absorption spectroscopic study of trace metals in lake water. Environ. Sci. Technol. 9:1073-1075.

Szostak, W. 1961. The role of magnesium in the body. Pol. Med. Wkly. 16(34):1421-1424.

Takeuchi, T. 1972. Biological reactions and pathological changes in human beings and animals caused by organic mercury contamination. *In* R. Hartung and B.D. Dinman, eds. Environmental Mercury Contamination, an International Conference, University of Michigan, Sept. 30-Oct. 2, 1970. Ann Arbor Science Publishers, Inc., Ann Arbor, Mich.

Tepper, L.B., and L.S. Levin. 1975. A survey of air and population lead levels in selected American communities. *In* F. Coulston and F. Korte, eds. Environmental Quality and Safety, Supplement vol. II, Lead, ed. by T.B. Griffin and J.H. Knelson, pp. 152-196. New York, Academic Press.

Ter Haar, G., and R. Aronow. 1975. Tracer studies of ingestion of dust by urban children. *In* F. Coulston and F. Korte, eds. Environmental Quality and Safety, Supplement vol. II, Lead, ed. by T.B. Griffin and J.H. Knelson, pp. 197-201. New York, Academic Press.

Tipton, I.H., P.L. Stewart, and P.G. Martin. 1966. Trace elements in diets and excreta. Health Phys. 12:1682-1689.

Todd, J.R. 1969. Chronic copper toxicity of ruminants. Proc. Nutr. Soc. 28:189-198.

Trace elements in clinical chemistry. 1975. Clin. Chem. 21:467-634. (Special Issue)

Traversy, W.J. 1971. Methods for Chemical Analysis of Waters and Wastewaters. Ottawa, Canada, Department of Fisheries and Forestry, Inland Waters Branch, Water Quality Division.

U.S. Environmental Protection Agency. 1975. Region V joint federal/state survey of organics and inorganics in selected drinking water supplies. Draft report. Chicago.

U.S. Environmental Protection Agency. 1973. Water programs. Guidelines establishing test procedures for analysis of pollutants. Fed. Reg. 38 (199): 28758-28760, Oct. 16.

U.S. Environmental Protection Agency. 1976. Methods for chemical analysis of waters and wastewater. Cincinnati, Ohio.

U.S. Environmental Protection Agency. 1975. Water programs. National interim primary drinking water regulations. Fed. Reg. 40(248), 59566-59588, Dec. 24.

U.S. Environmental Protection Agency. 1975. Scientific and technical assessment report on manganese. EPA 600/6-75-002. National Environmental Research Center, Research Triangle Park, N.C.

U.S. Environmental Protection Agency. 1975. Chemical analysis of interstate carrier water supply systems. EPA-430/9-75-005. Washington, D.C.

U.S. Environmental Protection Agency Order. 1976. Decision of the Administrator on the cancellation of pesticides containing mercury. FIFRA Dockets 246, Febuary 17.

U.S. Environmental Protection Agency. 1973. Water Quality Criteria, 1972. EPA.R.73.033, March.

U.S. Environmental Protection Agency. 1975. Preliminary Investigation of Effects on the Environment of Boron, Indium, Nickel, Selenium, Tin, Vanadium, and Their compounds. Vol. VI: Vanadium. EPA/560/2-75/005f. Washington, D.C.

U.S. Food and Drug Administration. 1975. Toxicity of the essential minerals—Information pertinent to establishing appropriate levels of single-mineral dietary supplements. Washington, D.C.

U.S. Geological Survey. 1959. Study and interpretation of the chemical characteristics of natural water. Water Supply Paper 1473. U.S. Geological Survey Sampling Data.

U.S. Geological Survey. 1970. Mercury in the Environment. A Compilation of Papers on the Abundance, Distribution, and Testing of Mercury in Rocks, Soils, Waters, Plants, and the Atmosphere. Professional Paper 713. Washington, D.C.

Underwood, E.J. 1971. Trace Elements in Human and Animal Nutrition, 3rd ed. Academic Press, New York.

Underwood, E.J. 1973. Trace elements. *In* Toxicants Occurring Naturally in Foods, 2nd ed., pp. 43-87. National Academy of Sciences, Washington, D.C.

Velhagin, K., Jr. 1953. Zur Hornhautargyrose. Klin. Mbl. Augenheilk. 122:36-42.

Von Nageli, C. 1893. Neu Deuschr. Allg. Schweig-Ges. Gesam. Naturu 33.

Walker-Smith, J., and J. Blomfield. 1973. Wilson's disease or chronic copper poisoning? Arch. Dis. Child. 48:476-479.

Wallace, R.A., W. Fulkerson, W.D. Shults, and W.S. Lyon. 1971. Mercury in the Environment: The Human Element. Oak Ridge National Laboratory. ORNL NSF-EP-1, Oak Ridge, Tenn.

West, F.K., P.W. West, and T.V. Ramakrishna. 1967. Stabilization and determination of traces of silver in waters. Environ. Sci. Technol. 1:717-720.

Wolf, H.W. Personal Communication (1975).

Wong, P.T.S., Y.K. Chau, and P.L. Luxon. 1975. Methylation of lead in the environment. Nature 253:263-264.

Wood, J.M. 1976. Metabolic cycles for toxic elements in the aqueous environment. *In* O. Bessey, Status of marine biomedical research. Environ. Health Perspect. 13:147-163.

World Health Organization. 1970. European Standards for Drinking Water, 2nd ed. Geneva, Switzerland.

World Health Organization. 1971. International Standards for Drinking Water, 3rd ed. Geneva, Switzerland.

World Health Organization. 1972. Evaluation of mercury, lead, cadmium and the food additives amaranth, diethylpyrocarbonate, and octyl gallate, p. 20. WHO Food Additives Series, no. 4. p. 20.

World Health Organization. 1973. Trace Elements in Human Nutrition, pp. 38-39. Technical Report Series no. 532. Geneva, Switzerland.

Wyllie, J. 1957. Copper poisoning at a cocktail party. Am. J. Public Health 47:617.

Yanagisawa, M., M. Suzuki, and T. Takeuchi. 1969. Extraction of manganese dithiocarbamate complexes for atomic absorption spectrophotometry. Anal. Chiem. Acta 43:500-502.

Zielhuis, R.L. 1975a. Dose-response relationships for inorganic lead. I. Biochemical and haematological responses. Int. Arch. Occup. Health 35:1-18.

Zielhuis, R.L. 1975b. Dose-response relationships for inorganic lead. II. Subjective and functional responses—chronic sequelae-no-response levels. Int. Arch. Occup. Health 35:19-35.

REFERENCES FOR ARSENIC AND SELENIUM

Abu-Erreish, G.M. 1967. On the nature of some selenium losses from soils and waters. M.S. Thesis. South Dakota State University, Brookings.

Albright, S.D. III, and J.M. Hitch. 1966. Rapid treatment of tinea versicolor with selenium sulfide. Arch. Dermatol. 93:460-462.

Aldrich, C.J. 1904. Leuconychia striata arsenicalis transversus. With report of three cases. Am. J. Med. Sci. 127:702-709.

Amor, A.J., and P. Pringle. 1945. A review of selenium as an industrial hazard. Bull. Hyg. 20:239-241.

Anderson, M.S., H.W. Lakin, K.C. Beeson, F.F. Smith, and E. Thacker. 1961. Selenium in Agriculture. U.S. Department of Agriculture Handbook 200. U.S. Government Printing Office, Washington, D.C.

Baird, R.B., S. Pourian, and S.M. Gabrielian. 1972. Determination of trace amounts of selenium in waste waters by carbon rod atomizaion. Anal. Chem. 44:1887-1889.

Baroni, C., G.J. Van Esch, and U. Saffiotti. 1963. Carcinogenesis tests of two inorganic arsenicals. Arch. Environ. Health 7:668-674.

Beath, O.A. 1962. Selenium poisoning in Indians. Sci. News Letter 81:254.

Beath, O.A. 1962a. The Story of Selenium in Wyoming. University of Wyoming, Laramie.

Beath, O.A., A.F. Hagner, and C.S. Gilbert. 1946. Some Rocks of High Selenium Content. Wyoming Geological Survey Bull. no. 36. The Geological Survey of Wyoming, University of Wyoming, Laramie.

Bergoglio, R.M. 1964. Mortalidad por cancer en zonas de aguas arsenicales de la Provincia de Cordoba, Republica Argentina. Prensa Med. Argent. 51:994-998.

Bertine, K.K., and E.D. Goldberg. 1971. Fossil fuel combustion and the major sedimentary cycle. Science 173:233-235.

Betteridge, D. 1965. Determination of selenium in hair by neutron-activation analysis. United Kingdom Atomic Energy Research Establishment Report no. AERER4881. London.

Bird, H.R., A.C. Groschke, and M. Rubin. 1949. Effect of arsenic acid derivatives in stiumlating growth in chickens. J. Nutr. 37:215-226.

Blau, M., and M.A. Bender. 1962. Se^{75}-selenomethionine for visualization of the pancreas by isotope scanning. Radiology 78:974.

Blau, M., and R.F. Manske. 1961. The pancreas specificity of Se^{75}-selenomethionine. J. Nucl. Med. 2:102-105.

Borgono. J.M., H. Venturino, and P. Vincent. 1976. Arsenic in the drinking water of the city of Antofogasta: Epidemiological and clinical study before and after the installation of a treatment plant. Presented at an International Conference on Environmental Arsenic. Co-sponsored by NIEHS and the Karolinska Institute. Fort Lauderdale, Fla.

Borgono, J.M., and R. Greiber. 1972. Epidemiological study of arsenicism in the city of Antofasgasta. *In* D.D. Hemphill, ed. Trace Substances in Environmental Health. Proceedings of the University of Missouri's 5th Annual Conference on Trace Substances in Environmental Health, June 29-July 1, 1971. University of Missouri, Columbia.

Boutwell, R.K. 1963. A carcinogenicity evaluation of potassium arsenite and arsanilic acid. J. Agric. Food Chem. 11:381-385.

Bowen, H.J.M., and P.A. Cawse. 1963. The determination of selenium in biological material by radioactivation. Analyst 88:721-726.

Braun, W. 1958. Carcinoma of the skin and the internal organs caused by arsenic: Delayed occupational lesions due to arsenic. Ger. Med. Mon. 3:321-324.

Brown, D.G., and R.F. Burk. 1973. Selenium retention in tissues and sperm of rats fed a Torula yeast diet. J. Nutr. 103:102-108.

Brown, D.G., R.F. Burk, R.J. Seely, and K.W. Kiker. 1972. Effect of dietary selenium on the gastrointestinal absorption of (^{75}SeO) in the rat. Int. J. Vit. Nutr. 42:588-591.

Broyer, T.C., D.C. Lee, and C.J. Asher. 1966. Selenium nutrition of green plants. Effect of selenite supply on growth and selenium content of alfalfa and subterranean clover. Plant Physiol. 41:1425-1428.

Buchan, R.F. 1947. Industrial selenosis. A review of the literature, report of five cases and a general bibliography. Occup. Med. 3:439-456.

Buck, W.B. 1969. Untoward reaction encountered with medicated feeds. *In* The Use of Drugs in Animal Feeds, Proceedings of a Symposium. Publ. no. 1679. National Academy of Sciences, Washington, D.C.

Buck, W.B., G.D. Osweiler, and G.A. Van Gelder. 1973. Clinical and Diagnostic Veterinary Toxicology. Kendall Hunt Publishing Co., Dubuque, Iowa.

Bull, R.C., and J.E. Oldfield. 1967. Selenium involvement in the oxidation by rat liver tissue of certain tricarboxylic acid cycle intermediates. J. Nutr. 91:237-246.

Burk, R.F., D.G. Brown, R.J. Seely, and C.C. Scaief III. 1972. Influence of dietary and injected selenium on whole-body retention, route of excretion, and tissue retention of $^{75}SeO^{2-}$ in the rat. J. Nutr. 102:1049-1055.

Burk, R.F., Jr., W.N. Pearson, R.P. Wood II, and F. Viteri. 1967. Blood-selenium levels and *in vitro* red blood cell uptake of ^{75}Se in kwashiorkor. Am. J. Clin. Nutr. 20:723-733.

Burk, R.F., R.J. Seely, and K.W. Kiker. 1973. Selenium: Dietary threshold for urinary excretion in the rat. Proc. Soc. Exp. Biol. Med. 142:214-216.

Buttner, W. 1963. Action of trace elements on the metabolism of fluoride. J. Dent. Res. 42:453-460.

Byers, H.G., T.J. Miller, K.T. Williams, and H.W. Lakin. 1938. Selenium occurrence in certain soils in the United States with a discussion of related topics. Third report, U.S. Department of Agriculture Technical Bulletin no. 601. U.S. Department of Agriculture, Washington, D.C.

Byron, W.R., G.W. Bierbower, J.B. Brouwer, and W.H. Hansen. 1967. Pathologic changes in rats and dogs from two-year feeding of sodium arsenite or sodium arsenate. Toxicol. Appl. Pharmacol. 10:132-147.

Campo, R.D., and R.J. Bieln. 1971. Acute toxic effects of sodium selenate on the epiphyseal plate of the rat. Calc. Tiss. Res. 7:318-330.

Cannon, H.L. 1974. Natural toxicants of geologic origin and their availability to man. *In* P.L. White and D. Robbins, eds. Symposium on Environmental Quality in Food Supply, pp. 143-164. Futura Publishers.

Caravaggi, C., F.L. Clark and A.R.B. Jackson. 1970. Acute selenium toxicity in lambs following intramuscular injection of sodium selenite. Res. Vet. Sci. 2:146-149.

Carey, W.F. 1968. Determination of arsenic in organic arsenates. J. Assoc. Off. Anal. Chem. 51:1300.

Carter, R.F. 1966. Acute selenium poisoning. Med. J. Aust. 1:525-528.

Cerwenka, E.A., Jr., and W.C. Cooper. 1961. Toxicology of selenium and tellurium and their compounds. Arch. Environ. Health 3:189-200.

Chau, Y.K., P.T.S. Wong, B.A. Silverberg, P.L. Luxon, and G.A. Bengert. 1976. Methylation of selenium in the aquatic environment. Science 192:1130-1131.

Clarke, E.G.C., and M.L. Clarke. 1967. Arsenic. *In* Garner's Veterinary Toxicology. 3rd ed. Williams & Wilkins Co., Baltimore.

Clayton, C.C., and C.A. Baumann. 1949. Diet and azo dye tumors: Effect of diet during a period when the dye is not fed. Cancer Res. 9:575-582.

Clinton, M., Jr. 1947. Selenium fume exposure. J. Ind. Hyg. Toxicol. 29:225-226.

Cohen, L.B. 1954. Use of "Selsun" in blepharitis marginalis. Am. J. Ophthal. 38: 560-562.

Cooper, W.C. 1967. Selenium toxicity in man. *In* O.H. Muth, ed. Symposium, Selenium in Biomedicine. AVI Publishing Co., Inc., Westport, Conn.

Cousins, F.B. 1960. A fluorimetric microdetermination of selenium in biological materials. Aust. J. Exp. Biol. Med. Sci. 38:11-16.

Crecelius, E.A., and R. Carpenter. 1974. Arsenic distribution in waters and sediments of the Puget Sound region. *In* Proceedings, First National Science Foundation Trace Contaminants Conference.

Cummings, J.G. 1966. Pesticides in the total diet. Res. Rev. 16:30.

Cummins, L.M., and J.L. Martin. 1967. Are selenocystine and selenomethionine synthesized *in vitro* from sodium selenite in mammals? Biochemistry 6:3162-3168.

Czapek, F., and J. Weil. 1893. Uber die wirkung des selens and Tellurs auf dem thierischen organismus. Naunyn-Schmiedeberg's Arch, Exp. Pathol. Pharmakol 32:438-455.

Davis, W.E. 1972. National inventory of sources emissions: Barium, boron, copper, selenium and zinc. Environmental Protection Agency. Air Programs. Leawood, Kansas. W.E. Davis and Associates, Contract no. 68-02-0100.

Diplock, A.T. 1976. Metabolic aspects of selenium action and toxicity. CRC Crit. Rev. Toxicol. 4:271-329.

Diplock, A.T., J. Green, J. Bunyan, D. Mchale, and I.R. Muthy. 1967. Vitamin E and stress. 3. The metabolism of D-α-tocopherol in the rat under dietary stress with silver. Br. J. Nutr. 21:115-125.

DiGuilio, W., and W. Beirwaltes. 1964. Parathyroid scanning with selenium^{75} labeled methionine. J. Nucl. Med. 5:417-427.

Douglas, C.P. 1969. Assessment of placental competance. Scot. Med. J. 14:162-170.

Ducoff, H.S., W.B. Neal, R.L. Straube, L.O. Jacobson, and A.M. Brues. 1948. Biological studies with arsenic^{76}. II. Excretion and tissue localization. Proc. Soc. Exp. Biol. Med. 69:548-554

Dudley, H.C., and J.W. Miller. 1937. Toxicology of selenium. IV. Effects of exposure to hydrogen selenide. U.S. Public Health Rep. 52:1217-1231.

Dudley, H.C., and J.W. Miller. 1941. Toxicology of selenium. VI. Effects of subacute exposure to hydrogen selenide. J. Ind. Hyg. Toxicol. 23:470-477.

Dudley, H.C. 1938. Selenium as a potential industrial hazard. U.S. Public Health Rep. 53:281-292.

Dudley, H.C. 1938. Toxicology of selenium. V. Toxic and vesicant properties of selenium oxychloride. U.S. Public Health Rep. 53:94-98.

Duggan, R.E., and G.Q. Lipscomb. 1969. Dietary intake of pesticide chemicals in the United States. June 1966-April 1968. Pesticide Monit. J. 2:153.

Durum, W.H. 1974. Occurrence of some trace metals in surface waters and ground waters. Proc. Water Qual. Conf. 16:17-25.

Durum, W.H., J.D. Hem, and S.G. Heidel. 1971. Reconnaissance of selected minor elements in surface waters of U.S. U.S. Geological Survey Circular 643.

Dutkiewicz, T., B. Dutkiewicz, and I. Balcerska. 1971. Dynamics of organ and tissue distriution of selenium after intragastric and dermal administration of sodium selenite. Bromatol. Chem. Toksykol. 4:475-481 (Chem. Abstr. 77:1476, 1972).

Eagle, H., and G.O. Doak. 1951. The biological activity of arsenobenzenes in relation to their structure. Pharmacol. Rev. 3:107-143.

Edmond, C.R. 1967. Dental caries etiology in New Guinea. Some contributions from analytical chemistry. Aust. Miner. Dev. Lab. Bull. 4:17-36.

Eisenberg, B.C. 1955. Contact dermatitis from selenium sulfide shampoo. Arch. Dermatol. Syphil. 72:71-72.

Feinglass, E.J. 1973. Arsenic intoxication from well water in the United States. N. Engl. J. Med. 288:828-830.

Ferm, V.H., and S.J. Carpenter. 1968. Malformation induced by sodium arsenate. J. Reprod. Fertil. 17:199-201.

Ferm, V.H., A. Saxon, and B.M. Smith. 1971. The teratogenic profile of sodium arsenate in the golden hamster. Arch. Environ. Health 22:557-560.

Fernandez, F.J., and D.C. Manning. 1971. The determination of arsenic at submicrogram levels by atomic absorption spectrophotometry. At. Absorpt. Newsl. 10:4.

Fernandez, F.J. 1973. Atomic absorption determination of gaseous hydrides utilizing sodium borohydride reduction. At. Absorpt. Newsl. 12:93-97.

Fitch, L.W.N., R.E.R. Grimmett, and E.M. Wall. 1939. Occurrence of arsenic in the soils and waters of the Waiotapu Valley and its relation to stock health. II. Feeding experiments at Wallaceville. N.Z.J. Sci. Tech. Sect. A21:146A-149A.

Fleischer, M. 1973. Natural sources of some trace elements in the environment. Proc. Environ. Resour. Conf. Nat. Environ. Res. Center, 3-10.

Flohe, L., W.A. Gunzler, and H.H. Schock. 1973. Glutathione peroxidase: a selenoenzyme. Fed. Eur. Biochem. Soc. Lett. 32:132-134.

Franke, K.W., and V.R. Potter. 1936. The effect of selenium containing foodstuffs on growth and reproduction of rats at various ages. J. Nutr. 12:205-214.

Franke, K.W., and A.L. Moxon. 1936. A comparison of the minimum fatal doses of selenium, tellurium, arsenic and vanadium. J. Pharmacol. Exp. Ther. 58:454-459.

Franke, K.W., and V.R. Potter. 1935. A new toxicant occurring naturally in certain samples of plant foodstuffs. IX. Toxic effects of orally ingested selenium. J. Nutr. 10:213-221.

Franke, K.W., and W.C. Tully. 1935. A new toxicant occurring naturally in certain samples of plant foodstuffs. V. Low hatchability due to deformities in chicks. Poult. Sci. 14:273-276.

Franke, K.W., A.L. Mxon, W.E. Poley, and W.C. Tully. 1936. A new toxicant occurring naturally in certain samples of plant foodstuffs. XII. Monstrosities produced by the injection of selenium salts into hens' eggs. Anat. Rec. 65:15-22.

Fritz, M.H. 1955. The treatment of dandruff and granulated eyelids with selenium sulfide (Selsun). Clin. Med. 2:695-696.

Frost, D.V. 1960. Arsenic and selenium in relation to the Food Additive Law of 1958. Nutr. Rev. 18:129-132.

Frost, D.V. 1972. The faces of selenium—Can selenophobia be cured? CRC Crit. Rev. Toxicol. 1:467-514.

Frost, D.V. 1967. Arsenicals in biology—Retrospect and prospect. Fed. Proc. 26:194-208.

Frost, D.V. 1967. Significance of the symposium. *In* O.H. Muth, ed. Symposium: Selenium in Biomedicine. AVI Publishing Co. Inc., Westport, Conn.

Frost, D.V., H.S. Perdue, B.T. Main, J.A. Kolar, I.D. Smith, R.J. Stein, and L.R. Overby. 1962. Further considerations on the safety of arsanilic acid for feed use. *In* Proceedings, 12th World's Poultry Congress, Sydney, Australia.

Frost, D.V. 1970. Tolerances for arsenic and selenium: A psycholdynamic problem. World Rev. Pest Control 9:6-28.

Gabbedy, B.J. and J. Dickson. 1969. Acute selenium poisoning in lambs. Aust. Vet. J. 45:470-472.

Gainer, J.H., and T.W. Pry. 1972. Effects of arsenicals on viral infections in mice. Am. J. Vet. Res. 33:2299-2307.

Gainer, J.H. 1972. Effects of arsenicals on interferon formation and action. Am. J. Vet. Res. 33:2579-2586.

Ganther, H.E., and C.A. Baumann. 1962. Selenium metabolism. I. Effects of diet, arsenic and cadmium. J. Nutr. 77:210-216.

Ganther, H.E. 1966. Enzymic synthesis of dimethyl selenide from sodium selenite in mouse liver extracts. Biochemistry 5:1089-1098.

Ganther, H.E. 1968. Selenotrisulfides. Foration by the reaction of thiols with selenious acid. Biochemistry 7:2898-2905.

Ganther, H.E. 1971. Reduction of the selenotrisulfide derivative of glutathione to a persulfide analog by glutathione reductase. Biochemistry 10:4089-4098.

Ganther, H.E. C. Goudie, M.L. Sunde, M.J. Kopecky, P. Wagner, S.H. Oh, and W.G. Hoekstra. 1972. Selenium: Relation to decreased toxicity of methylmercury added to diets containing tuna. Science 175:1122-1124.

Garrow, J.C., and C.P. Douglas. 1968. A rapid method for assessing intrauterine growth by radioactive selenomethionine uptake. J. Obstet. Gynecol. Br. Commonw. 75:1034-1039.

Geering, H.R., E.E. Cary, L.H.P. Jones, and W.H. Allaway. 1968. Solubility and redox criteria for the possible forms of selenium in soils. Soil. Sci. Soc. Am. Proc. 32:35-40.

Geyer, L. 1898. Ueber die chronischen Hautveranderungen beim Arsenicismus und Betrachtungen ueber die Massenerkrankungen in Reichenstein in Schlesien. Arch. Dermatol. Syphilol. 43:221-280.

Gilbert, L.M., W.G. Overend, and M. Webb. 1951. The inhibition of pancreas deoxyribonuclease. Exp. Cell Res. 2:349-365.

Ginsburg, J.M., and W.D. Lotspeich. 1963. Interrelations of arsenate and phosphate transport in the dog kidney. Am. J. Physiol. 205:707-714.

Ginsburg, J.M. 1965. Renal mechanism for excretion and transformation of arsenic in the dog. Am. J. Physiol. 208:832-840.

Giordano, W.G. 1963. One application treatment for tinea versicolor. J. Med. Soc. N.J. 60:186-187.

Glenn, M.W., R. Jensen, and L.A. Griner. 1964. Sodium selenate toxicosis: Pathology and pathogenesis of sodium selenate toxicosis in sheep. Am. J. Vet. Res. 25:1486-1494.

Glover, J.R. 1970. Selenium and its industrial toxicology. Ind. Med. 39:50-54.

Glover, J.R. 1954. Some medical problems concerning selenium in industry. Trans. Assoc. Ind. Med. Officers 4:94-96.

Glover, J.R. 1970. Selenium and its industrial toxicology. Ind. Med. 39:50-54.

Godwin, K.O., and C.N. Fuss. 1972. The entry of selenium into rabbit protein following the administration of $Na_2{}^{75}SeO_3$. Aust. J. Biol. Sci. 25:865-871.

Goldschmidt, V.M., and L.W. Strock. 1935. Zur Geochemi des Selen II Nachr. Ges. Wiss. Gottingen, Math-Physik. Klasse 1:123-142.

Goldsmith, J.R., M. Deane, J. Thom, and G. Gentry. 1972. Water Res. 6:1133-1136.

Graham, J.H., G.R. Mazzanti, and E.B. Helwig. 1961. Chemistry of Bowen's disease: Relationship to arsenic. J. Invest. Dermatol. 37:317-332.

Grant, C.A., B. Thafvelin, and R. Christell. 1961. Retention of selenium by pig tissues. Acta Pharmacol. Toxicol. 18:285-297.

Grasso, P., R. Abraham, R. Hendy, A.T. Diplock, L. Golberg, and J. Green. 1969. The role of dietary silver in the production of liver necrosis in vitamin E-deficient rats. Exp. Mol. Pathol. 11:186-199.

Grover, R.W. 1956. Diffuse hair loss associated with selenium (Selsun) sulfide shampoo. J. Am. Med. Assoc. 160:1397-1398.

Gunn, S.A., T.C. Gould, and W.A.D. Anderson. 1968. Specificity in protection against lethality and testicular toxicity from cadmium. Proc. Soc. Exp. Biol. Med. 128:591-595.

Hadjimarkos, D.M., and C.W. Bonhorst. 1958. The trace element selenium and its influence on dental caries susceptibility. J. Pediatr. 52:274-278.

Hadjimarkos, D.M., and C.W. Bonhorst. 1961. The selenium content of eggs, milk, and water in relation to dental caries in children. J. Pediatr. 59:256-259.

Hadjimarkos, D.M. 1970. Toxic effects of dietary selenium in hamsters. Nutr. Rep. Int. 1:175-179.

Halver, J.E. 1962. Progress in studies on contaminanted trout rations and trout hepatoma. NIH Report, April 11-12.

Halverson, A.W., D.T. Tsay, K.C. Triebwasser and E.I. Whitehead. 1970. Development of hemolytic anemia in rats red selenite. Toxicol. Appl. Pharmacol. 17:151-159.

Halverson, A.W., I.S. Palmer, and P.L. Guss. 1966. Toxicity of selenium to post-weanling rats. Toxicol. Appl. Pharmacol. 9:477-484.

Harr, J.R., and O.H. Muth. 1972. Selenium poisoning in domestic animals and its relationship to man. Clin. Toxicol. 5:175-186.

Harr, J.R., J.F. Bone, I.J. Tinsley, P.H. Weswig, and R.S. Yamamoto. 1967. Selenium toxicity in rats. II. Histopathology. *In* O.H. Muth, ed. Symposium: Selenium in Biomedicine, pp. 153-178. AVI Publishing Co., Inc., Westport, Conn.

Harvey, S.C. 1965. Arsenic. *In* L.S. Goodman and A Gilman, eds. The Pharmacological Bases of Therapeutics, 3rd ed. The Macmillan Co., New York.

Harvey, S.C. 1975. Heavy metals. *In* L.S. Goodman and A Gilman, eds. The Pharmacological Bases of Therapeutics, 5th ed. The Macmillan Co., New York.

Haynie, T.P., W.K. Otte, and J.C. Wright. 1964. Visualization of hyperfunctioning parathyroid adenoma using Se^{75}-selenomethionine and the photoscanner. J. Nucl. Med. 5:710-714.

Heinrich, M., Jr., and F.E. Kelsey. 1955. Studies on selenium metabolism: The distribution of selenium in the tissues of the mouse. J. Pharmacol. Exp. Ther. 114:28-32.

Heinrich, M.A., Jr., and D.M. MacCanon. 1960. Some effects of sodium selenite on the cardiovascular system. Toxicol. Appl. Pharmacol. 2:33-43.

Herigstad, R.R., C.K. Whitehair, and O.E. Olson. 1973. Inorganic and organic selenium toxicosis in young swine: Comparison of athologic changes with those in swine with vitamin E-selenium deficiency. Am. J. Vet. Res. 34:1227-1283.

Herrera, N.E., R. Gonzalez, R.D. Schwartz, A.M. Diggs, and J. Belsky. 1965. ^{75}Se-selenomethione as diagnostic agent in malignant lymphoma. J. Nucl. Med. 6:792-804.

Heuper, W.C., and W.W. Payne. 1962. Experimental studies in metal carcinogenesis. Chromium, nickel, iron, arsenic. Arch. Environ. Health 5:445-462.

Hidiroglou, M., K.J. Jenkins, and I. Hoffman. 1971. Teneurs en selenium dan les tissus des ruminants. Ann. Biol. Anim. Biochim. Biophys. 11:695-704.

Hill, A.B., and E.L. Faning. 1948. Studies in the incidence of cancer in a factory handling inorganic compounds of arsenic. I. Mortality experience in the factory. Br. J. Ind. Med. 5:1-6.

Holker, J.R., and J.B. Speakman. 1958. The action of selenium dioxide on wool. J. Appl. Chem. 8:1-3.

Holland, J.W. 1904. Arsenic. *In* F. Peterson and W.S. Haines, eds. A Textbook of Legal Medicine and Toxicology, vol. 2. W.B. Saunders & Company, Philadelphia.

Hollo, Z.M., and S. Zlatarov. 1960. The prevention of thallium death by selenate. Naturwissenschaften 47:87.

Holmberg, R.E., and V.H. Ferm. 1969. Interrelationships of selenium, cadmium, and arsenic in mammalian teratogenesis. Arch. Environ. Health 18:873-877.

Hood, R.D., and C.T. Pike. 1972. BAL alleviation of arsenate-induced teratogenesis in mice. Teratology 6:235-237.

Hood, R.D., and S.L. Bishop. 1972. Teratogenic effects of sodium arsenate in mice. Arch. Environ. Health 24:62-65.

Hopkins, L.L., Jr., A.L. Pope, and C.A. Baumann. 1966. Distribution of microgram quantities of selenium in the tissues of the rat and effects of previous selenium uptake. J. Nutr. 88:61-65.

Horwitz, W. 1970. Official Methods of Analysis of the Association of Official Analytical Chemists. 11th ed. Association of Official Analytical Chemists, Washington, D.C.

Hove, E., C.A. Elvehjem, and E.B. Hart. 1938. Arsenic in the nutrition of the rat. Am. J. Physiol. 124-205-212.

Hunter, F.T., A.F. Kip, and J.W. Irvine, Jr. 1942. Radioactive tracer studies on arsenic injected as potassium arsenite. J. Pharmacol. Exp. Ther. 76:207-220.

Hutchinson, J. 1888. On some examples of arsenic-keratoses of the skin and of arsenic-cancer. Trans. Pathol. Soc. (London) 39:352-363.

Hwang, S.W., and L.S. Schanker. 1973. Absorption of organic arsenical compounds from the rat small intestine. Xenobiotica 3:351-355.

International Agency for Research on Cancer. 1973. IARC Monographs on the Evaluation of the Carcinogenic Risk of Chemicals to Man. Vol. 2: Some Inorganic and Organometallic Compounds. World Health Organization, Lyon.

Ishibashi, M., T. Shigematsu, and Y. Nakagawa. 1953. Determination of selenium in sea water. Rec. Oceanogr. Work. Japan 1:44-48.

Jacobsson, S.O. 1966. Uptake of Se^{75} in tissues of sheep after administration of a single dose of Se^{75}-sodium selenite, Se^{75}-selenomethionine, or Se^{75}-selenocystine. Acta Vet. Scand. 7:303-320.

James, L.F., V.A. Lazar, and W. Binns. 1966. Effects of sublethal doses of certain minerals on pregnant ewes and fetal development. Am. J. Vet. Res. 27:132-135.

Jones, G.B., and K.O. Godwin. 1962. Distribution of radioactive selenium in mice. Nature 196:1294-1296.

Jones, G.B., and K.O. Godwin. 1963. Studies on the nutritional role of selenium. I. The distribution of radioactive selenium in mice. Aust. J. Agric. Res. 14:716-723.

Josephson, C.J., S.S. Pinto, and S.J. Petronella. 1951. Arsine: Electrocardiographic changes produced in acute human poisoning. Arch. Ind. Hyg. Occup. Med. 4:43-52.

Kanisawa, M., and H.A. Schroeder. 1967. Life term studies on the effects of arsenic, germanium, tin, and vanadium on spontaneous tumors in mice. Cancer Res. 27:1192-1195.

Kar, A.B., R.P. Das, and F.N.I. Mukergi. 1960. Prevention of cadmium-induced changes in the gonads of the rat by zinc and selenium: a study in antagonism between metals in the biological system. Proc. Nat. Inst. Sci. India. Part B, Suppl. 26:40-50.

Kar, A.B., R.P. Das, and J.N. Karkun. 1959. Ovarian changes in prepubertal rats after treatment with cadmium chloride. Acta Biol. Med. Ger. 3:372-399.

Kenzaburo, T. 1976. The various effects of arsenic in Japan according to type of exposure. International Conference on Environmental Arsenic. Fort Lauderdale, Fla.

Kharkar, D.P., K.K. Turekian, and K.K. Bertine. 1968. Stream supply of dissolved silver, molybdenum, antimony, selenium, chromium, cobalt, rubidium, and cesium to the ocean. Geochim. Cosmochim. Acta 32:285-298.

Klayman, D.L., and W.H.H. Gunther. 1973. Organic selenium compounds: Their chemistry and biology. Wiley-Interscience, New York.

Kraybill, H.F., and M.B. Shimkin. 1964. Carcinogenesis related to foods contaminated by processing and fungal metabolites. Adv. Cancer Res. 8:191-248.

Kroes, R., M.J. van Logten, J.M. Berkvens, T. de Vries, and G.J. van Esch. 1974. Study on the carcinogenicity of lead arsenate and sodium arsenate and on the possible synergistic effect of diethylnitrosamine. Food Cosmet. Toxicol. 12:671-679.

Ku, P.K., W.T. Ely, A.W. Groce, and D.E. Ullrey. 1972. Natural dietary selenium tocopherol and effect on tissue selenium. J. Anim. Sci. 34:208-211.

Kuttler, K.L., D.W. Marble, and C. Blincoe. 1961. Serum and tissue residues following selenium injections in sheep. Am. J. Vet. Res. 22:422-428.

Lakin, H.W., and H.G. Byers. 1941. Selenium in wheat and wheat products. Cereal Chem. 18:73-78.

Lakin, H.W., and D.F. Davidson. 1967. The relation of the geochemistry of selenium to its occurrence in soils. *In* O.H. Muth, ed. Symposium: Selenium in Biomedicine. First International Symposium, Oregon State University, 1966, AVI Publishing Co., Inc., Westport, Conn.

Lakin, H.W. 1972. Selenium accumulation in soils and its absorption by plants and animals. *In* H.L. Cannnon and H.C. Hopps, eds. Geochemical Environment in Relation to Health and Disease, pp. 45-54. Geological Society of America. Paper 140.

Lambert, J.L., P. Arthur, and T.E. Moore. 1951. Determination of trace amounts of selenium in water. Anal. Chem. 23:1101-1106.

Lambourne, D.A., and R.W. Mason. 1969. Mortality in lambs following overdosing with sodium selenite. Aust. Vet. J. 45:208.

Lanz, H. Jr., P.W. Wallace, and J.G. Hamilton. 1950. The metabolism of arsenic in laboratory animals using As^{74} as a tracer. Univ. Calif. Pub. Pharmacol. 2:263-282.

Ledet, A.E., J.R. Duncan, W.B. Buck, and F.K. Ramsey. 1973. Clinical, toxicological, and pathological aspects of arsanilic acid poisoning in swine. Clin. Toxicol. 6:439-457.

Lee, A.M., and J.F. Fraumeni, Jr. 1969. Arsenic and respiratory cancer in man: An occupational study. J. Nat. Cancer Inst. 42:1045-1052.

Lee, P., and J.S. Garrow. 1970. A clinical evaluation of the selenomethionine uptake test. J. Obstet. Gynacol. Br. Commonw. 77:983-986.

Lemley, R.E., and M.P. Merryman. 1941. Selenium poisoning in the human subject. Lancet 61:435-438.

Levan, A. 1945. Cytological reactions induced by inorganic salt solutions. Nature 156:751-752.

Levan, N.E. 1957. Selenium sulfide suspension in the treatment of tinea versicolor. Arch. Dermatol. 75:128-129.

Levander, O.A., and C.A. Baumann. 1966. Selenium metabolism. V. Studies on the distribution of selenium in rats given arsenic. Toxicol. Appl. Pharmacol. 9:98-105.

Levander, O.A., and C.A. Baumann. 1966. Selenium metabolism. VI. Effect of arsenic on the excretion of selenium in the bile. Toxicol. Appl. Pharmacol. 9:106-115.

Levander, O.A., and L.C. Argrett. 1969. Effects of arsenic, mercury, thallium and lead on selenium metabolism in rats. Toxicol. Appl. Pharmacol. 14:308-314.

Levander, O.A., and V.C. Morris. 1970. Interactions of methionine, vitamin E, and antioxidants in selenium toxicity in the rat. J. Nutr. 100:1111-1118.

Levander, O.A. 1972. Metabolic interrelationships and adaptations in selenium toxicity. Ann. N.Y. Acad. Sci. 192:181-192.

Levander, O.A., M.L. Young, and S.A. Meeks. 1970. Studies on the binding of selenium by liver homogenates from rats fed diets containing either casein or casein plus linseed oil meal. Toxicol. Appl. Pharmacol. 16:79-87.

Levander, O.A., V.C. Morris, and D.J. Higgs. 1973. Selenium as a catalyst for the reduction of cytochrome c by glutathione. Biochemistry 12:4591-4595.

Levander, O.S., and C.A. Baumann. 1966. Selenium metabolism. VI. Effect of arsenic on the excretion of selenium in the bile. Toxicol. Appl. Pharmacol. 9:106-115.

Lipmann, F. 1958. Biological sulfate activation and transfer. Science 128:575-580.

Lisella, F.S., K.R. Long, and H.G. Scott. 1972. Health aspects of arsenicals in the environment. J. Environ. Health 34:511-518.

Lopez, P.L., R.L. Preston and W.H. Pfander. 1968. *In vitro* uptake of selenium-75 by red blood cells from the immature ovine during varying selenium intakes. J. Nutr. 94:219-226.

Maag, D.D., J.S. Osborn, and J.R. Clopton. 1960. The effect of sodium selenite on cattle. Am. J. Vet. Res. 21:1049-1053.

Marshall, S.P., F.W. Hayward, and W.R. Meagher. 1963. Effects of feeding arsenic and lead upon their secretion in milk. J. Diary Sci. 46:580-581.

Mason, K.E., and J.O. Young. 1967. Effectiveness of selenium and zinc in protecting against cadmium-induced injury of the rat testis. *In* O.H. Muth, ed. Symposium: Selenium in Biomedicine, pp. 383-394. AVI Publishing Co. Inc., Westport, Conn.

Matson, E.J. 1956. Selenium sulfides as an antidandruff agent. J. Soc. Cosmet. Chem. 7:459-466.

Mautner, H.G., and J.J. Jaffe. 1958. The activity of 6-selenopurine and related compounds against some experimental mouse tumors. Cancer Res. 18:294-298.

Mautner, H.G., S.H. Chu, J.J. Jaffe, and A.C. Sartonelli. 1963. The synthesis and antineoplastic properties of selenoguanine selenocytosine and related compounds. J. Med. Chem. 6:36-39.

McConnell, K.P., and A.E. Kreamer. 1960. Incorporation of selenium-75 into dog hair. Proc. Soc. Exp. Biol. Med. 105:170-173.

McConnell, K.P., and D.M. Roth. 1962. ^{75}Se in rat intracellular liver fractions. Biochim. Biophys. Acta 62:503-508.

McConnell, K.P., and G.J. Cho. 1965. Transmucosal movement of selenium. Am. J. Physiol. 208:1191-1195.

McConnell, K.P., and O.W. Portman. 1952a. Toxicity of dimethyl selenide in the rat and mouse. Proc. Soc. Exp. Biol. Med. 79:230-231.

McConnell, K.P., and O.W. Portman. 1952b. Excretion of dimethyl selenide by the rat. J. Biol. Chem. 195:277-282.

McConnell, K.P. 1941. Distribution and excretion studies in the rat after a single subtoxic subcutaneous injection of sodium selenate containing radioselenium. J. Biol. Chem. 141:427-437.

McConnell, K.P., C.H. Wabnitz, and D.M. Roth. 1960. Time-distribution studies of selenium-75 in dog serum proteins. Tex. Rep. Biol. Med. 18:438-445.

Mealey, J., Jr., G.L. Brownell, and W.H. Sweet. 1959. Radioarsenic in plasma, urine, normal tissues, and intracranial neoplasms. Arch. Neurol. Psychiatry 81:310-320.

Middleton, J.M. 1947. Selenium burn of the eye. Report of a case, with a review of the literature. Arch. Ophthalmol. 38:806-811.

Miller, J.T., and H.G. Byers. 1935. A selenium spring. Ind. Eng. Chem. News Ed. 13:456.

Milner, J.E. 1969. The effect of ingested arsenic on methylcholanthrene-induced skin tumors in mice. Arch. Environ. Health 18:7-11.

Mizuta, N., M. Mizuta, F. Ito, T. Ito, H. Uchida, Y. Watanabe, H. Akama, T. Murakami, F. Hayashi, K. Nakamura, T. Yamaguchi, W. Mizuia, S. Oishi, and H. Matsumura. 1956. An outbreak of acute arsenic poisoning caused by arsenic contaminated soy-sauce (shoyu): A clinical report of 220 cases. Bull. Yamaguchi Med. Sch. 4(2,3):131-150.

Moeschlin, S. 1965. Poisoning: Diagnosis and Treatment, 1st Am. Ed. Grune and Stratton, New York.

Moody, J.P., and R.T. Williams. 1964a. The fate of arsanilic acid and acetylarsanilic acid in hens. Food Cosmet. Toxicol. 2:687-693.

Moody, J.P., and R.T. Williams. 1964b. The fate of 4-nitrophenylarsonic acid in hens. Food Cosmet. Toxicol. 2:695-706.

Morehouse, N.F. 1949. Accelerated growth in chickens and turkeys produced by 3-nitro-4-hydroxyphenylarsonic acid. Poult. Sci. 28:375-384.

Morette, A., and J.P. Diven. 1965. La determination du selenium dans l'eau ann. Pharm. Fr. 23:169-178.

Morris. V.C., and O.A. Levander. 1970. Selenium content of foods. J. Nutr. 100:1383-1388.

Morrow, D.A. 1968. Acute selenite toxicosis in lambs. J. Am. Vet. Med. Assoc. 152:1625-1629.

Morss, S.G., and H.S. Olcott. 1967. Absence of effect of tocopherol on acute oral toxicity of sodium selenite in the rat. Proc. Soc. Exp. Biol. Med. 124:483-485.

Motley, H.L., M.M. Ellis, and M.D. Ellis. 1937. Acute sore throats following exposure to selenium. J. Am. Med. Assoc. 109:1718-1719.

Moutschen, J., and N. Degraeve. 1965. Influence of thiol-inhibiting substances on the effects of ethyl methane sulphonate (EMS) on chromosomes. Experientia 21:200-202.

Moxon, A.L., and K.P. DuBois. 1939. The influence of arsenic and certain other elements on the toxicity of seleniferous grains. J. Nutr. 18:447-457.

Moxon, A.L. 1937. Alkali Disease or Selenium Poisoning. S. Dak. Agric. Exp. Stn. Bull. no. 311. Brookings, S. Dak.

Moxon, A.L. 1938. The effect of arsenic on the toxicity of seleniferous grains. Science 88:81.

Moxon, A.O., O.E. Olson, and W.V. Seawright. 1939. Selenium in Rocks, Soils and Plants. S. Dak. Agric. Exp. Stn. Tech. Bull. no. 2, Brookings, S. Dak.

Muth, O.H., and W. Binns. 1964. Selenium toxicity in domestic animals. Ann. N.Y. Acad. Sci. 111:583-590.

Muth, O.H., P.D. Whanger. P.H. Weswig, and J.E. Oldfield. 1971. Occurrence of myopathy in lambs of ewes fed added arsenic in a selenium-deficient ration. Am. J. Vet. Res. 32:1621-1623.

Nagai, H., R. Okuda, H. Nagaumi, A. Yagi, C. Mori, and H. Wada. 1956. Subacute and chronic arsenic poisoning in bottle-fed infants—Follow-up clinical observations. Ann. Paediatr. Jap. (Shonika Kiyo) 2(2):124-132. (In Japanese).

Nagai, I. 1959. An experimental study of selenium poisoning. Igaku Kenkyu (Acta Med.) 29:1505-1532.

National Academy of Sciences-National Research Council. 1976. Assembly of Life Sciences. Medical and Biologic Effects of Environmental Pollutants: Selenium. Washington, D.C.

National Institute for Occupational Safety and Health. 1974. NIOSH Manual of Analytical Methods. U.S. Department of Health, Education, and Welfare, Cincinnati, Ohio.

National Research Council. Agriculture Board, Committee on Animal Nutrition. Subcommittee on Selenium. 1971. Selenium in Nutrition. Washington, D.C.

Nelson, A.A., O.G. Fitzhugh, and H.O. Calvery. 1943. Liver tumors following cirrhosis caused by selenium in rats. Cancer Res. 3:230-236.

Nelson, W.C., M.H. Lykins, J. Mackey, V.A. Newill, J.F. Finklea, and D.I. Hammer. 1973. Mortality among orchard workers exposed to lead arsenate spray: A cohort study. J. Chron. Dis. 26:105-118.

Neubauer, O. 1947. Arsenical cancer: A review. Br. J. Cancer 1:192-251.

Nielsen, F.H., S.H. Givand and D.R. Myron. 1975. Evidence of a possible requirement for arsenic by the rat. Fed. Proc. 34:923. (Abstract)

Obermeyer, B.D., I.S. Palmer, O.E. Olson, and A.W. Halverson. 1971. Toxicity of trimethylselenonium chloride in the rat with and without arsenite. Toxicol. Appl. Pharmacol. 20:135-146.

Oelschager, W., and K.H. Menke. 1969. Uber Selengehalte pflanzlicher, tierischer and anderer stoffe. 2. Mitteilung Selen-und Schwfelgehalte in Nehrungsmitteln. Z. Ernaehrungswiss. 9:216-222.

Okamoto, Y., and W.H.H. Gunther. 1972. Organic selenium and tellurium chemistry. Ann. N.Y. Acad. Sci. 192:1-226.

Oliver, W.T., and C.K. Roe. 1957. Arsanilic acid poisoning in swine. J. Am. Vet. Med. Assoc. 130:177-178.

Olson, O.E., B.M. Schulte, E.I. Whitehead, and A.W. Halverson. 1963. Effect of arsenic on selenium metabolism in rats. J. Agric. Food Chem. 11:531-534.

Olson, O.E., E.I. Whitehead, and A.L. Moxon. 1942. Occurrence of soluble selenium in soils and its availability to plants. Soil Sci. 54: 47-53.

Olson, O.E., I.S. Palmer, and E.I. Whitehead. 1973. Determination of selenium in biological materials. *In* D. Glick, ed. Methods of Biochemical Analysis, vol. 21. John Wiley Sons, New York.

Osburn, H.S. 1957. Cancer of the lung in Gwanda. Cent. Af. J. Med. 3:215-223.

Osswald, H., and Kl. Goerttler. 1971. Leukosen bei der Maus nach diaplacentarer und postnataler Arsenik-Applikation. Dtsch. Gesamte Path. 55:289-293.

Ott, M.G., B.B. Holder, and H.L. Gordon. 1974. Respiratory cancer and occupational exposure to arsenicals. Arch. Environ. Health 29:250-255.

Overby, L.R., and L. Straube. 1965. Metabolism of arsanilic acid. I. Metabolic stability of double labeled arsanilic acid in chickens. Toxicol. Appl. Pharmacol. 7:850-854.

Overby, L.R., and R.L. Fredrickson. 1963. Metabolic stability of radioactive arsanilic acid in chickens. J. Agric. Food Chem. 11:378-381.

Overby, L.R., and R.L. Fredrickson. 1965. Metabolism of arsanilic acid. II. Localization and type of arsenic excreted and retained by chickens. Toxicol. Appl. Pharmacol. 7:855-867.

Painter, E.P. 1941. The chemistry and toxicity of selenium compounds, with special reference to the selenium problem. Chem. Rev. 28:179-213.

Palmer, I.S., and O.E. Olson. 1974. Relative toxicities of selenite and selenate in the drinking water of rats. J. Nutr. 104:306-314.

Palmer, I.S., D.D. Fischer, A.W. Halverson, and O.E. Olson. 1969. Identification of a major selenium excretory product in rat urine. Biochim. Biophys. Acta 177:336-342.

Parizek, J., and Z. Zahor. 1956. Effect of cadmium salts on testicular tissue. Nature 177:1036.

Parizek, J. 1964. Vascular changes at sites of estrogen biosynthesis produced by parenteral injection of cadmium salts. The destruction of the placenta by cadmium salts. J. Reprod. Ferti. 7:263-265.

Parizek, J. 1965. The peculiar toxicity of cadmium during pregnancy: "An experimental toxaemia of pregnancy" induced by cadmium salts. J. Reprod. Ferti. 9:111-112.

Parizek, J., I. Ostadalova, J. Kalouskova, A. Babicky, and J. Benes. 1971. The detoxifying effects of selenium interrelations between compounds of selenium and certain metals. *In*

W. Mertz and W.E. Cornatzer, eds. Newer Trace Elements in Nutrition, Marcel Dekker, Inc., New York.

Parizek, J., I. Ostadalova, J. Kalouskova, A. Babicky, L. Pavlik, and B. Bibr. 1971. Effect of mercuric compounds on the maternal tranmission of selenium in the pregnant and lactating rat. J. Reprod. Ferti. 25:157-170.

Parizek, J., I. Ostadolova, I. Benes, and A. Babecky. 1968. Pregnancy and trace elements: The protective effect of compounds of an essential trace element selenium-against the peculiar toxic effects of cadmium during pregnancy. J. Reprod. Ferti. 16:507-509.

Parizek, J., J. Kalouskova, A.A. Babicky, J. Benes, and L. Pavlik. 1974. Interaction of selenium with mercury, cadmium and other toxic metals. *In* W.G. Hoekstra, J.W. Suttie, H.E. Ganther and W. Mertz, eds. Trace Element Metabolism in Animals, 2nd ed. University Park Press, Baltimore.

Parker, C.A., and L.G. Harvey. 1961. Fluorometric determination of submicrogram amounts of selenium. Analyst 86:54-62.

Paton, G.R., and A.C. Allison. 1972. Chromosome damage in human cell cultures induced by metal salts. Mutation Res. 16:322-336.

Pedersen, N.D., P.D. Whanger, P.H. Weswig, and O.H. Muth. 1973. Selenium binding proteins in tissues of normal and selenium responsive myopathic lambs. Bioinorg. Chem. 2:33-45.

Penrose, W.R. 1974. Arsenic in the marine and aquatic environments: Analysis, occurrence, and significance. CRC Crit. Rev. Environ. Control 4(4):465-482.

Peoples, S.A. 1964. Arsenic toxicity in cattle. Ann. N.Y. Acad. Sci. 111:644-649.

Perry, K., R.G. Bowler, H.M. Buckell, H.A. Druett, and R.S. F. Shilling. 1948. Studies in the incidence of cancer in a factory handling inorganic compounds of arsenic. II. Clinical and environmental investigations. Br. J. Ind. Med. 5:6-15.

Pershagen, G., C.G. Elinder, and A.M. Balander. 1976. Mortality in an area surrounding an arsenic emitting plant. International Conference on Environmental Arsenic. Fort Lauderdale, Fla.

Peterson, P.J., and D.J. Spedding. 1963. The excretion by sheep of ^{75}selenium into red clover. The chemical nature of the excreted selenium and its uptake by three plant species. N.Z.J. Agric. Res. 6:13-23.

Petres, J., and A. Berger. 1972. Zum Einfluss anorganischen Arsens auf die DNS-Synthese menschlicher Lymphocyten in vitro. Arch. Dermatol. Forsch. 242:343-352.

Petres, J., and M. Hundeiker. 1968. "Chromosomenpulverisation" nach Arseneinwirkung auf Zellkulturen in vitro. Arch. Klin. Exp. Dermatol. 231:366-370.

Petres, J., D. Baron, and M. Hagedorn. 1976. Effects of arsenic on cell metabolism and cell proliferation. Cytogenic and biochemical studies. International Conference on Environmental Arsenic. Fort Lauderdale, Fla.

Petres, J., K. Schmid-Ullrich, and W. Wolf. 1970. Chromsomenaberrationen an menschlichen Lymphozyten bei chronischen Arsenchaden. Dtsch. Med. Wochenschr. 95:79-80.

Pinto, S.S., and B.M. Bennett. 1963. Effect of arsenic trioxide exposure on mortality. Arch. Environ. Health 7:583-591.

Potchen, E.J. 1963. Isotopic labeling of the rat parathyroid as demonstrated by autoradiography. J. Nucl. Med. 4:480-484.

Pringle, P. 1942. Occupational dermatitis following exposure to inorganic selenium compounds. Br. J. Dermatol. Syphilol. 54:54-58.

Radeleff, R.D. 1970. Veterinary Toxicology, 2nd ed. Lea and Febiger, Philadelphia.

Ransone, J.W., N.M. Scott, Jr., and E.C. Knoblock. 1961. Selenium sulfide intoxication. N. Engl. J. Med. 264:384-385.

Reynolds, E.S. 1901. An account of the epidemic outbreak of arsenical poisoning occurring in beer-drinkers in the north of England and Midland Countries in 1900. Lancet 1:166-170.

Rhian, M., and A.L. Moxon. 1943. Chronic selenium poisoning in dogs and its prevention by arsenic. J. Pharmacol. Exp. Ther. 78:249-264.

Ridgway, L.P., and D.A. Karnofsky. 1952. The effects of metals on the chick embryo: Toxicity and production of abnormalities in development. Ann. N.Y. Acad. Sci. 55:203-215.

Riley, J.F. 1968. Mast cells, co-carcinogens and anticarcinogenesis in the skin of mice. Expermentia 24:1237.

Robinson, H.M. Jr., and S.N. Yaffe. 1956. Selenium sulfide in the treatment of pityriasis versicolor. J. Am. Med. Assoc. 162:113-114.

Robinson, W.O. 1936. Selenium content of wheat from various parts of the world. Ind. Eng. Chem. Ed. 28:736-738.

Rosenfeld, I., and O.A. Beath. 1964. Selenium: Geobotany, Biochemistry, Toxicity and Nutrition. Academic Press, New York.

Rosenfeld, I. and O.A. Beath. 1947. The influence of various substances on chronic selenium poisoning. J. Pharmacol. Exp. Ther. 91:218-223.

Rossman, T.G., M.S. Meyn, and W. Troll. 1976. Effects of Arsenite on DNA Repair in Escherichia coli. International Conference on Environmental Arsenic. Fort Lauderdale, Fla.

Roth, F. 1957. The sequelae of chronic arsenic poisoning in Moselle vintners. Ger. Med. Month. 2:172-175.

Rotruck, J.T., A.L. Pope, H.E. Ganther, A.B. Swanson, D.G. Hafeman, and W.G. Hoesktra. 1973. Selenium: Biochemical role as a component of glutathione peroxidase. Science 179:588-590.

Rusiecki, W., and J. Brzezinski. 1966. Influence of sodium selenate on acute thallium poisonings. Acta Pol. Pharm. 23:69-74.

Schroeder, H.A., and J.J. Balassa. 1966. Abnormal trace elements in man: arsenic. J. Chron. Dis. 19:85-106.

Schroeder, H.A., and M. Mitchener. 1971a. Selenium and tellurium in rats: Effect on growth, survival and tumors. J. Nutr. 101:1531-1540.

Schroeder, H.A., and M. Mitchener. 1972. Selenium and tellurium in mice. Effects on growth, survival and tumors. Arch. Environ. Health. 24:66-71.

Schroeder, H.A., and M. Mitchener. 1971b. Toxic effects of trace elements on the reproduction of mice and rats. Arch. Environ. Health 23:102-106.

Schroeder, H.A., M. Kanisawa, D.V. Frost, and M. Mitchener. 1968. Germanium, tin, and arsenic in rats: Effects on growth, survival, pathological lesions and life span. J. Nutr. 96:37-45.

Schwarz, K. 1965. Role of vitamin E, selenium and related factors in experimental nutritional liver disease. Fed. Proc. 24:58-67.

Scott, M.L., and J.N. Thompson. 1971. Selenium content of foodstuffs and effects of dietary selenium levels upon tissue selenium in chicks and poults. Poult. Sci. 50:1742-1748.

Shamberger, R.J. 1970. Relationship of selenium to cancer. I. Inhibitory effect of selenium on carcinogenesis. J. Nat. Cancer Inst. 44:931-936.

Shapiro, J.R. 1972. Selenium and carcinogenesis. A review. Ann. N.Y. Acad. Sci. 192:215-219.

Shapiro, J.R. 1972. Selenium compounds in nature and medicine; selenium and human biology. *In* D.L. Klayman and W.H.H. Gunther, eds. Organic Selenium Compounds: Their Chemistry and Biology. John Wiley & Sons, New York.

Shortridge, E.H., P.J. O'Hara, and P.M. Marshall. 1971. Acute selenium poisoning in cattle. N. Z. Vet. J. 19:47-50.

Silver, A.S., and P.L. Wainman. 1952. Chronic arsenic poisoning following use of an asthma remedy. J. Am. Med. Assoc. 150:584-585.

Smith, M.I., and B.B. Westfall. 1937. Further field studies on the selenium problem in relation to public health. Public Health. Rep. 52:1375-1384.

Smith, M.I. 1941. Chronic endemic selenium poisoning. J. Am. Med. Assoc. 116:562-566.

Smith, M.I., E.F. Stohlman, and R.D. Lillie. 1937. The toxicity and pathology of selenium. J. Pharmacol. Exp. Ther. 60:449-470.

Snegireff, L.S., and O.L.M. Lombard. 1951. Arsenic and cancer. Observations in the metallurgical industry. Arch. Ind. Hyg. 4:199-205.

Sommers, S.C., and R.G. McManus. 1953. Multiple arsenical cancers of the skin and internal organs. Cancer 6:347-359.

Spencer, R.P., and M. Blau. 1962. International transport of selenium-75 selenomethionine. Science 136:155-156.

Stadtman, T.C. 1974. Selenium biochemistry. Science 183:915-922.

Strock, L.W. 1935. The distribution of selenium in nature. Am. J. Pharm. 107:144-157.

Tank, G., and C.A. Strovick. 1960. Effect of naturally occurring selenium and vanadium on dental caries. J. Dent. Res. 39:473-488.

Tarrant, R.F., and J. Allard. 1972. Arsenic levels in urine of forest workers applying silvicides. Arch. Environ. Health 24:277-280.

Taylor, F.B. 1963. Significance of trace elements in public, finished water supplies. J. Am. Water Works Assoc. 55:619-623.

Thapar, N.T., E. Guenthner, C.W. Carlson, and O.E. Olson. 1969. Dietary selenium and arsenic additions to diets for chickens over a life cycle. Poult. Sci. 48:1987-1993.

Thompson, J.N., and M.L. Scott. 1969. Role of selenium in the nutrition of the chick. J. Nutr. 97:335-342.

Tscherkes, L.A., M.N. Volgarev and S.G. Aptekar. 1963. Selenium-caused tumors. Acta Un. Int. Cancer 19:632-633.

Tseng, W.P., H.M. Chu, S.W. How, J. M. Fong, C.S. Lin, and S. Yeh. 1968. Prevalence of skin cancer in an endemic area of chronic arsenicism in Taiwan. J. Nat. Cancer Inst. 40:453-363.

Tseng, Wen-Ping. 1976. Effects and dose–response relationships of skin cancer and blackfoot disease with arsenic. International Conference on Arsenic. Fort Lauderdale, Fla.

Tsuchiya, K. 1976. Various effects of arsenic in Japan according to type of exposure. Presented at Int. Conf. Environ. Arsenic Res., Triangle Park, N.C., Oct. 5-8, 1976.

U.S. Department of Health, Education, and Welfare. 1975. National Institute for Occupational Safety and Health. Criteria for a Recommended Standard . . . Occupational Exposure to Inorganic Arsenic. New Criteria, 1975. Publ. no. (NIOSH)75-149. U.S. Government Printing Office, Washington, D.C.

U.S. Environmental Protection Agency, 1975. Chemical Analysis of Interstate Carrier Water Supply Systems. EPA-430/9/75-005. Washington, D.C.

U.S. Public Health Service. 1962. Drinking Water Standards. U.S. Department of Health, Education, and Welfare. Public Health Service Publ. no. 956. Washington, D.C.

Underwood, E.J. 1971. Trace Elements in Human and Animal Nutrition, 3rd ed. Academic Press, New York.

Voegtlin, C., and J.W. Thompson. 1923. Quantitative studies in chemotherapy. VI. Rate of excretion of arsenicals, a factor governing toxicity and parasiticidal action. J. Pharmacol. Exp. Ther. 20:85-105.

Volgarev, M.N., and L.A. Tscherkes. 1967. Further studies in tissue changes associated with sodium selenate. *In* O.H. Muth, ed. Symposium: Selenium in Biomedicine, pp. 179-184. First International Symposium, Oregon State University, 1966. AVI Publishing Co., Inc., Westport, Conn.

Vorhies, M.W., S.D. Sleight, and C.K. Whitehair. 1969. Toxicity of arsanilic acid in swine as influenced by water intake. Cornell Vet. 59:3-9.

Wadkins, C.L. 1960. Stimulation of adenosinetriphosphatase activity of mitochondria and submitochondrial particles by arsenate. J. Biol. Chem. 235:3300-3303.

Walker, G.W.R., and A.M. Bradley. 1969. Interacting effects of sodium monohydrogenarsenate and selenocystine on crossing over in Drosophila melanogaster. Can. J. Genet. Cytol. 11:677-688.

Watkinson, J.H. 1960. Fluorometric determination of traces of selenium. Anal. Chem. 32:981-983.

Watkinson, J.H. 1967. Analytical methods for selenium in biological material. *In* O.H. Muth, ed. Symposium: Selenium in Biomedicine. First International Symposium, Oregon State University. 1966. AVI Publishing Co., Inc., Westport, Conn.

Weiss, H.V., M. Koide, and E.D. Goldberg. 1971. Selenium and sulfur in a Greenland ice sheet; Relation of fossil fuel consumption. Science 172:261-263.

Weswig, P.H., S.A. Roffler, M.A. Arnold, O.H. Muth, and J.E. Oldfield. 1966. In vitro uptake of selenium-75 by blood from ewes and their lambs on different selenium regimens. Am. J. Vet. Res. 27:128-131.

Willcox, W.H. 1922. An address on acute arsenical poisoning. Br. Med. J. 2:118-124.

Williams, K.T., and H.G. Byers. 1935. Occurrence of selenium in the Colorado River and some of its tributaries. Ind. Eng. Chem. Anal. Ed. 7:431-432.

Wilson, L.G., and R.S. Bandurski. 1956. An enzymatic reaction involving adenosine triphosphate and selenate. Arch. Biochem. Biophys. 62:503-506.

Wright, P.L., and M.C. Bell. 1963. Selenium and vitamin E influence upon the *in vitro* uptake of Se^{75} by ovine blood cells. Proc. Soc. Exp. Biol. Med. 114:379-382.

Wright, P.L., and M.C. Bell. 1964. $Selenium^{75}$ metabolism in the gestating ewe and fetal lamb: effects of dietary α-tocopherol and selenium. J. Nutr. 84:49-57.

Wright, P.L., and M.C. Bell. 1966. Comparative metabolism of selenium and tellurium in sheep and swine. Am. J. Physiol. 211:6-10.

Wright, P.L. 1967. The absorption and tissue distribution of selenium in depleted animals. *In* O.H. Muth ed. Symposium: Selenium in Biomedicine. First International Symposium Oregon State University, 1966. AVI Publishing Co., Inc., Westport, Conn.

Zachariae, H., H. Sogaard, and A. Nyfors. 1974. Liver biopsy in psoriatics previously treated with potassium arsenite. Acta Derm. Venereol. 54:235-236.

Zaldivar, R. 1974. Arsenic contamination of drinking water and foodstuffs causing endemic chronic poisoning. Beitr. Pathol. Bd. 151:384-400.

REFERENCES FOR FLUORIDE, SODIUM, NITRATE, AND SULFATE

Abbie, A.A., and J. Schroder. 1960. Blood pressure in Arnhem Land aborigines. Med. J. Aust. 2:493-496.

Al-Alousi, W., D. Jackson, G. Crompton, and O.C. Jenkins. 1975. Enamel mottling in a fluoride and in a non-fluoride community; A study. Br. Dent. J. 138:9-15, 56-60.

American Academy of Pediatrics Committee on Nutrition. 1970. Infant methemoglobinemia: The role of dietary nitrate. Pediatrics 46:475-478.

American Academy of Pediatrics Committee on Nutrition. 1974. Salt intake and eating patterns of infants and children in relation to blood pressure. Pediatrics 53:115-121.

American Medical Association House of Delegates. 1957. Statement on fluoridation of public water supplies.

American Public Health Association. 1976. Standard Methods for the Examination of Water and Wastewater, 14th ed. Washington, D.C.

American Public Works Association. 1969. Water pollution aspects of urban runoff. Final report on the causes and remedies of water pollution from surface drainage of urban areas. Research project no. 120, conducted for the Federal Water Quality Administration, U.S. Department of the Interior.

An, A.S., V.A. Dudina, and N.I. Nedostupova. 1967. Outbreaks of intestinal disorders due to high sulfate concentration in drinking water. Hyg. Sanit. 32:264-266.

Ast, D.B., D.J. Smith, B. Wachs, and K.T. Cantwell. 1956. Newburgh-Kingston caries-fluorine study. XIV. Combined clinical and roentgenographic dental findings after ten years of fluoride experience. J. Am. Dent. Assoc. 52:314-325.

Bell, M.E., and T. G. Ludwig. 1970. The supply of fluoride to man. *In* Fluorides and Human Health, pp. 18-32. World Health Organization Monograph no. 59.

Berman, L.B., and D.R. Taves. 1973. Fluoride excretion in normal and uremic humans. Clin. Res. 21:100.

Bernstein, D.S., N. Sadowsky, D.M. Hegsted, C.D. Guri, and F.J. Stare. 1966. Prevalence of osteoporosis in high and low fluoride areas in North Dakota. J. Am. Med. Assoc. 198:499-504.

Berry, W.T. 1958. A study of the incidence of mongolism in relation to the fluoride content of water. Am. J. Ment. Defic. 62:634-636.

Bianchi, G., V. Fox, G. FiFrancesco, V. Bardi, and M. Radice. 1973. The hypertensive role of the kidney in spontaneously hypertensive rats. Eur. J. Clin. Invest. 3:313.

Binkerd, E.F., and O.E. Kolari. 1975. The history and use of nitrate and nitrite in the curing of meat. Food Cosmet. Toxicol. 13:655-661.

Bittner, J.J., and W.D. Armstrong. 1952. Lack of effect of fluoride ingestion on longevity of mice. J. Dent. Res. 31:495.

Blood, D.C., and J.A. Henderson. 1968. Veterinary Medicine, 3rd ed. Williams & Wilkins, Baltimore.

Boltz, D.F. March 1973. Recent development in methods for the determination of anions. Section V: Anions of nitrogen. Crit. Rev. Anal. Chem. 3:147-199.

Bosch, H.M., A.B. Rosenfield, R. Huston, H.R. Shipman, and F.L. Woodward. 1950. Methemoglobinemia and Minnesota well supplies. J. Am. Water Works Assoc. 42:161-170.

Bradley, W.B., A.O. Beath, and H.F. Eppson. 1939. Oat hay poisoning. Science 89:365.

Bradley, W.B., H.F. Eppson, and A.O. Beath. 1940. Livestock Poisoning by Oat-Hay and Other Plants Containing Nitrates, pp. 1-20. Wyo. Agric. Exp. Stn. Bull. no. 241.

Braun-Menendez, E., and M.R. Covian. 1948. Mecanismo de la hipertenion de las ratas totalmente nefrectomizadas. Rev. Soc. Argent. Biol. 24:130-141.

Brest, A.N. 1960. The therapeutic use of the thiazide derivatives in the treatment of hypertension. *In* J.H. Moyer and M. Fuchs, eds. Edema: Mechanisms and Management. W.B. Saunders Co., Philadelphia.

Brooks, J.B., W.B. Cherry, L. Thacker, and C.C. Alley. 1972. Analysis by gas chromatography of amines and nitrosamines produced *in vitro* and *in vitro* by Proteus mirabilis. J. Infect. Dis. 126:143-153.

Bryce, H.G. 1964. Industrial and utilitarian aspects of fluorine chemistry. *In* S.H. Simmons, ed. Fluorine Chemistry, vol. 1, pp. 295-498. Academic Press, New York.

Bubeck, R.C., W.H. Diment, B.L. Deck, A.L. Baldwin, and S.D. Lipton. 1971. Runoff of deicing salt: Effect on Irondequoit Bay, Rochester, New York. Science 172:1128-1131.

Buck, C.W. 1973. The persistence of elevated blood pressure first observed at age five. J. Chron. Dis. 26:101-104.

Burg, M.B. 1976. Renal handling of sodium chloride. *In* B.M. Brenner and F.C. Rector, eds. The Kidney, vol. 1. W.B. Saunders Co., Philadelphia.

Burgen, A.S.V., and N.G. Emmelin. 1961. Physiology of the salivary glands. Williams & Wilkins Co., Baltimore.

Burk, D., and J. Yiamouyiannis. 1975. Fluoridation and Cancer, July 21, Congressional Record.

Burns-Cox, C.J., and J.D. Maclean. 1970. Splenomegaly and blood pressure in an Orang-Asli community in West Malaysia. Am. Heart J. 80:718-719.

Burrell, R.J.W., W.A. Roach, and A. Shadwell. 1966. Esophageal cancer in the Bantu of the Transkei associated with mineral deficiency in garden plants. J. Nat. Cancer Inst. 36:201-214.

Caffey, F. 1955. On fibrous defects in cortical walls of growing tubular bones: Their radiologic appearance, structure, prevalence, natural course, and diagnostic significance. Adv. in Pediatr. 7:13-50.

Carlson, C.H., W.D. Armstrong, and L. Singer. 1960a. Distribution, migration and binding of whole blood fluoride evaluated with radiofluoride. Amer. J. Physiol. 199:187-189.

Carlson, C.H., W.D. Armstrong, and L. Singer. 1960b. Distribution and excretion of radiofluoride in the human. Proc. Soc. Exp. Biol. Med. 104:235-239.

Carslon, C.H., W.D. Armstrong, L. Singer, and L.B. Hinshaw. 1960c. Renal excretion of radiofluoride in the dog. Am. J. Physiol. 198:829-832.

Chen, P.S., Jr., F.A. Smith, D.E. Gardner, J.A. O'Brien, and H.C. Hodge. 1956. Renal clearance of fluoride. Proc. Soc. Exp. Biol. Med. 92:879-883.

Chiang, B.N., L.V. Perlman, M. Fulton, L.D. Ostrander, and F.H. Epstein. 1970. Predisposing factors in sudden cardiac death in Tecumseh, Michigan: A prospective study. Circulation 41:31-37.

Clifford, P. 1970. On the epidemiology of nasopharyngeal carcinoma. Int. J. Cancer 5:287-309.

Cohen, B., and N.B. Myant. 1959. Concentration of salivary iodide: A comparative study. J. Physiol. 145:595-610.

Coleman, T.G., R.D. Manning, R.A. Norman, and J. DeClue. 1975. The role of the kidney in spontaneous hypertension. Am. Heart J. 89:94-98.

Comly, H.H. 1945. Cyanosis in infants caused by nitrates in well water. J. Am. Med. Assoc. 129:112-116.

Conn, J.W. 1949. The mechanism of acclimatization to heat. Adv. Inter. Med. 3:373-393.

Conway, J., and P. Lauwers. 1960. Hemodynamic and hypotensive effects of long term therapy with chlorothiazide. Circulation 21:21-37.

Cook, H.A. 1970. Fluoride intake through tea by British children. Fluoride Q. Rep. 3:12-18.

Correa, P., W. Haenszel, C. Cuello, S. Tannenbaum, and M. Archer. 1975. A model for gastric cancer epidemiology. Lancet 2:58-59.

Crabtree, K.T. 1970. Nitrate variation in ground water. Technical Completion Report, OWRR B-044-Wis. Office of Water Resources Research.

Cruz-Coke, R., H. Donoso, and R. Barrera. 1973. Genetic ecology of hypertension. Clin. Sci. Mol. Med. 45(Suppl. 1):55-65.

Cruz-Coke, R., R. Etcheverry, and R. Nagel. 1964. Influence of migration on the blood pressure of Easter Islanders. Lancet 1:697-699.

Curtin, T.M., and W.T. London. 1966. Nitrate-nitrite intoxication in swine. Proceedings, United States Livestock Sanitary Association 60:339-348.

Dace, O., L. Kramer, D. Wiatrowski, H. Spencer. 1974. Dietary fluoride intake in man. J. Nutr. 104:1313-1318.

Dahl, L.K. 1958. Salt intake and salt need. N. Engl. J. Med. 258:1152-1157.

Dahl, L.K. 1960. Possible role of salt intake in the development of essential hypertension. *In* K.D. Bock and P.T.Cottier, eds. Essential Hypertension, An International Symposium, pp. 53-65. Springer-Verlag, Heidelberg.

Dahl, L.K. 1972. Salt and hypertension. Am. J. Clin. Nutr. 25:231-244.

Dahl, L.K., M. Heine, and K. Thompson. 1974. Genetic influence of the kidneys on blood pressure. Evidence from chronic renal homografts in rats with opposite predispositions to hypertension. Circ. Res. 40:94-101.

Dahl, L.K., M. Heine, and L. Tassinari. 1962. Effects of chronic excess salt ingestion. Evidence that genetic factors play an important role in susceptibility to experimental hypertension. J. Exp. Med. 115:1173-1190.

Dawber, T.R., W.B. Kannel, A. Kagan, R.K. Donabedian, P. McNamara, and G. Pearson. 1967. Environmental factors in hypertension. *In* J. Stamler, R. Stamler, and T. Pullman, eds. The Epidemioloty of Hypertension. Proceedings of an International Symposium, Chicago, pp. 255-288.1964, Grune and Stratton, Inc., New York.

DeWardener, H.E. 1973. The control of sodium excretion. *In* J. Orloff, and R.W. Ber.iner, eds. Handbook of Physiology, pp. 677-720. Section 8: Renal Physiology. American Physiological Society, Washington, D.C.

Dickey, E., W.D. Lembke, T.R. Peck, G. Stone, and W.H. Walker. 1972. Nitrate levels and possible sources in shallow wells. *In* Proceedings Second Allerton Conference on Environmental Quality and Agriculture, 1971, pp. 40-44. University of Illinois, Urbana. Special Publication No. 26.

Digesti, R.D., and H.J. Weeth. 1973. Effects of sulfate-water on cattle. Proc. West. Sect., Am. Soc. Anim. Sci. 24:259-263.

Dixon, W.J., and F.J. Massey. 1969. Introduction to Statistical Analysis, 3d ed. McGraw Hill, New York.

Dole, V.P., L.K. Dahl, G.C. Cotzais, H.A. Eder, and M.E. Krebs. 1950. Dietary treatment of hypertension. Clinical and metabolic studies of patients on the rice-fruit diet. J. Clin. Invest. 29:1189-1206.

Douglas, T.E. 1957. Fluoride dentrifice and stomatitis. Northwest Med. 56:1037-1039.

Druckrey, H., D. Steinhoff, H. Beuthner, H. Schneider, and P. Klarner. 1963. Prufung von Nitrit auf chronisch toxische Wirkung und Ratten. ArzneimiHelforschung 13:320-323.

Druckrey, H., R. Preussmann, S. Ivankovic, and D. Schmahl. 1967. Organotrope carcinogene Wirkungen bei 65 verschiedenen N-nitroso-verbindungen an BD ratten. Zeitschr. Krebsforsch. 69:103-201.

Earley, L.E. 1972. Sodium metabolism. *In* M.H. Maxwell and C.R. Kleeman, eds. Clinical Disorders of Fluid and Electrolyte Metabolism, 2nd ed., pp. 95-119. McGraw Hill, Inc. New York.

Epstein, F.H., and R.D. Eckoff. 1967. The epidemiology of high blood pressure-geographic distributions and etiologic factors. *In* J. Stamler, R. Stamler, and T.N. Pullman, eds. The Epidemiology of Hypertension. Proceedings of an International Symposium, Chicago, 1964, pp. 155-166. Grune and Stratton, Inc., New York.

Erickson, J.D., G.P. Oakley, Jr., J.W. Flynt, Jr., and S. Hays. 1976. Water fluoridation and congenital malformations: No association. J. Am. Dent. Assoc. 93:981-984.

Ericsson, Y., and U. Ribelius. 1971. Wide variations of fluoride supply to infants and their effect. Caries Res. 5:78-88.

Feltman, R. 1956. Prenatal and postnatal ingestion of fluorides: a progress report. Dent. Digest 62:353-357.

Feltman, R., and G. Kosel. 1961. Prenatal and postnatal ingestion of fluorides 14 years of investigation final report. J. Dent. Med. 16:190-198.

Ferrant, M. 1946. Methemoglobinemia: Two cases in newborn infants caused by nitrates in well water. J. Pediatr. 29:585-592.

Fisher, F., and M.J. Prival. 1973. Total Fluoride Intake. Center for Science in the Public Interest, Washington, D.C.

Fleming, H.S. 1953. Effect of fluorides on the tumor S37 after transplantation to selected locations in mice and guinea pigs. J. Dent. Res. 32:646.

Fodor, J.G., E.C. Abbott, and I.E. Rusted. 1973. An epidemiologic study of hypertension in Newfoundland. Can. Med. Assoc. J. 108:1365-1368.

Fong, Y.Y., and W.C. Chan. 1973. Bacterial production of dimethyl nitrosamine in salted fish. Nature 243:421-422.

Forbes. G., F.A. Smith, and M.F. Bryson. 1973. Effect of growth hormone on fluoride balance. Calc. Tiss. Res. 11:301-10.

Fry, B.W., D.R. Taves, and R.G. Merin. 1973. Fluorometabolites of methoxyflurane. Anethesiology 38:1-44.

Gavras, H., H.B. Brunner, E.D. Baughan, Jr., and J.H. Laragh. 1973. Angiotensin sodium interaction in blood pressure maintenance of renal hypertensive and normotensive rats. Science 180:1369-1372.

Gerdes, R.A., J.D. Smith, and H.G. Applegate. 1971. The effects of atmospheric hydrogen fluoride upon Drosophila melanogaster. I. Differential genotypic response. Atmos. Environ. 5:113-122.

Gibbons, R.J., and J. van Houte. 1975. Bacterial adherence in oral microbial ecology. Ann. Rev. Microbiol. 29:19-44.

Glanville, E.V., and R.A. Geerdink. 1972. Blood pressure of Amerindians from Surinum. Am. J. Phys. Anthropol. 37:251-254.

Goodman, L.S., and A. Gilman. 1975. The Pharmacologic Basis of Therapeutics, 5th ed. MacMillan Co., New York.

Greenberg, L.W., C.E. Nelsen, and N. Kramer. 1974. Nephrogenic diabetes insipidus with fluorosis. Pediatrics 54:320-322.

Greenblatt, M., S. Mirvish, and B.T. So. 1971. Nitrosamine studies: Induction of lung adenomas by concurrent administration of sodium nitrite and secondary amines in Swiss mice. J. Nat. Cancer. Inst. 46:1029-1034.

Greenblatt, M., V.R.C. Kommineni, and W. Lijinsky. 1973. Null effect of concurrent feeding of sodium nitrite and amino acids to MRC rats. J. Nat. Cancer. Inst. 50:799-802.

Greene, I., and E.P. Hiat. 1955. Renal excretion of nitrate and its effect on excretion of sodium and chloride. Am. J. Physiol. 180:149-182.

Greene, I., and E.P. Hiatt. 1954. Behavior of the nitrate ion in the dog. Am. J. Physiol. 176:463-367.

Gregor, O. 1974. Gastric cancer control. Neoplasmia 21:235-247.

Grimbergen, G.W. 1974. A double blind test for determination of intolerance to fluoridated water; Preliminary report. Fluoride 7:146-152.

Gross, E. 1964. Vergiftungen durch aufnakme von nitraten im trinlcwasser und in pflanzen bei kleinstkinderen und bei nutztieren. Arch. Hyg. Bakteriol. 148:28-39.

Gross, F. 1960. Adrenocortical function and renal pressor mechanisms. *In* K.D. Bock and P.T. Cottier, eds. Essential Hypertension, An International Symposium, pp. 92-111. Springer-Verlag, Berlin.

Gross, F. 1971. The renin-angiotensin system and hypertension. Ann. Int. Med. 75:777-787.

Gruener, N., H.I. Shuval, K. Behroozi, S. Cohen, and H. Shecter. 1973. Methemoglobinemia induced by transplacental passage of nitrites in rats. Bull. Environ. Contam. Toxicol. 9:44-48.

Guy, W.G., D.R. Taves, and W.S. Brey. 1976. Organic fluorocompounds in human plasma: Prevalence and characterization. *In* R. Filler, ed. Biochemistry Involving Carbon-Fluorine Bonds. ACS Symposium, Series 28.

Guyton, A.C., T.G. Colemen, A.W. Cowly, K.W. Scheel, R.D. Manning, Jr., and R.A. Norman, Jr. 1972. Arterial pressure regulation. Overriding dominance of the kidneys in long-term regulation and in hypertension. Am. J. Med. 52:584-594.

Hagan, T.L., M. Pasternack, and G.C. Scholz. 1954. Waterborne fluorides and mortality. Public Health Rep. 69:450-454.

Hamilton, M., G.W. Pickering, J.A.F. Roberts, and G.S.C. Sowry. 1954. The aetiology of essential hypertension. I. The arterial pressure in the general population. Clin. Sci. 13:11-35.

Hammerton, C. 1945. The corrosion of cement and concrete. Sewage Works J. 17:403-405.

Hanes, R.E., L.W. Zelazny, and R.E. Blaser. 1970. Effects of de-icing salts on water quality and biota; Literature review and recommended research. National Cooperative Highway Research Program Report 91, Highway Research Board, National Research Council, National Academy of Sciences-National Academy of Engineering, Washington, D.C.

Hanhijarvi, H., V.M. Anttonen, A. Pekkarinen, and I. Penttila. 1972. The effect of artificially fluoridated drinking water on the plasma ionized fluoride content in certain clinical diseases and in normal individuals. Acta Pharmacol. Toxicol. 31(I):104.

Harada, M, H. Ishiwata, Y. Nakamura, A. Tanimura, and M. Ishidate. 1975. Studies on *in vivo* formation of nitroso compounds. I. Changes of nitrite and nitrate concentrations in human saliva after ingestion of salted Chinese cabbage. J. Food Hyg. Soc. Jap. 16:11-18.

Harmeson, R.H., F.W. Sollo, Jr., and T.E. Larson. 1971. The nitrate situation in Illinois. J. Am. Water Works Assoc. 63:303-310.

Harmeson, R.H., T.E. Larson, L.M. Henley, R.A. Sinclair, and J.C. Neill. 1973. Quality of surface water in Illinois, 1966-71. Illinois State Water Survey Bulletin 56. Urbana.

Hatch, F.T., A.R. Wertheim, G.H. Eurman, D.M. Watkin, H.F. Froeb, and H.A. Epstein. 1954. Effects of diet in essential hypertension. III. Alterations in sodium chloride, protein and fat intake. Am. J. Med. 17:499-513.

Hawksworth, G., M.J. Hill, G. Gordillo, and C. Cuello. 1975. Possible relationship between nitrates, nitrosamines, and gastric cancer in S.W. Colombia. *In* P. Bogovski, ed. N-Nitroso Compounds in the Environment. International Agency for Research in Cancer. Scientific Publication no. 9. Lyon, in press.

Herskowitz, I.H., and I.L. Norton. 1963. Increased incidence of melanotic tumors in two strains of Drosophila melanogaster following treatment with sodium fluoride. Gen. 48:307-310.

Hill, M.J., G. Hawksworth, and G. Tattersall. 1973. Bacteria, nitrosamines and cancer of the stomach. Br. J. Cancer 28:562-567.

Hirayama, T. 1976. Changing patterns of cancer mortality in Japan with special reference to the decrease in stomach cancer mortality. Presented at a conference on Origins of Human Cancer, September 7-14, Cold Spring Harbor Laboratory.

Hodge, H.C. 1956. Fluoride metabolism: its significance in water fluoridation. J. Am. Dent. Assoc. 52:307-314.

Hodge, H.C., and F.A. Smith. 1965. Fluorine Chemistry, vol. IV, ed. by J.H. Simmons. Academic Press, New York.

Hodge, H.C., and F.A. Smith. 1970. Minerals: fluorine and dental caries. Advances in Chemistry Series no. 94:93-115.

Hodge, H.C., F.A. Smith, and I. Gedalia. 1970. Excretion of fluorider. *In* Fluorides and Human Health, pp. 141-161. World Health Organization Monograph Series no. 59. Geneva.

Hodge, H.D. 1961. Metabolism of fluorides. J. Am. Med. Assoc. 177:313-316.

Holl, K. 1937. The factors which play a role in the solution of lead by water. Ges. Ing. 58:323-328 (Abstr.: J. Am. Water Works Assoc. 29:293).

Hoobler, S.W., C. Tejada, M. Guzman, and A. Pardo. 1965. Influence of nutrition and acculturation on the blood pressure levels and changes with age in the highland Guatemala Indian Circ. 32(Suppl II):116.

Hoover, R.N. 1976. Fluoridated drinking water and the occurrence of cancer. J. Nat. Cancer Inst. In press.

Hutchinson, F.E. 1971. The effect of highway salt on water quality in selected Maine rivers. *In* Proceedings, Street Salting-Urban Water Quality Workshop, pp. 20-23. State University of New York College of Environmental Science and Forestry at Syracuse.

Ingleson, H., A.M. Sage, and R. Wilkinson. 1949. Effect of chlorination of drinking water on brass fittings. J. Inst. Water Eng. 3:81-91.

Jackson, D., P.M.C. James, and W.B. Wofe. 1975. Fluoridation in Anglesey. Br. Dent. J. 138:165-171.

Jaffe, E.R., and P. Heller. 1964. Methemoglobinemia in man. *In* C.V. Moore and E.B. Brown, eds. Progress in Hematology, vol. IV, pp. 48-71. Grune and Stratton, New York.

Jagiello, G., and L. Ja-Shein. 1974. Sodium fluoride as potential mutagen in mammalian eggs. Arch. Environ. Health 29:230-235.

Jowsey, J., R.K. Schenk, and F.W. Reutter. 1968. Some results of the effect of fluoride on bone tissue in osteoporosis. J. Clin. Endocrinol. Metab. 28:869-874.

Juncos, L.I., and J.V. Donadio, Jr. 1972. Renal failure and fluorosis. J. Am. Med. Assoc. 222:783-785.

Kahn, H.A., H.H. Medalie, H.N. Neufeld, E.G. Riss, and U. Goldbourt. 1972. The incidence of hypertension and associated factors. The Israel ischemic heart disease study. Am. Heart J. 84:171-172.

Kannel, W.B., W.P. Castelli, P.M. McNamara, and P. Sorlie. 1969a. Some factors affecting morbidity and mortality in hypertension: The Framingham Study. Milbank Mem. Fund Q. 47(3)Part 2:116-142.

Kannel, W.B., M.J. Schwartz, and P.M. McNamara. 1969. Blood pressure and risk of coronary heart disease: The Framingham Study. Dis. Chest 56:43-52.

Kellam, B. 1933. The action of water on concrete. Proc. Am. Soc. Testing Materials 33(Part I):389-296.

Kempner, W. 1948. Treatment of hypertensive vascular disease with rice diet. Am. J. Med. 4:545-577.

Kinlen, L. 1975. Cancer incidence in relation to fluoride level in water supplies. Br. Dent. J. 138:221-224.

Kirkendall, W.M., W.E. Connor, F. Abboud, S.P. Rastogi, T.A. Anderson, and M. Fry. 1972. The effect of dietary sodium on the blood pressure of normotensive man. *In* J. Geest and E. Koiw, eds. Hypertension '72, pp. 360-373. Springer-Verlag, New York.

Knotek, Z., and P. Schmidt. 1964. Pathogenesis, incidence, and possibilities of preventing alimentary nitrate methemoglobinemia in infants. Pediatrics 34:78-83.

Korotchenok, N.A. 1946. Limiting concentrations of some mineral consituents of drinking water in western Turkmenia. Chem. Abstr. 40:7459; Gig. Sanit. 10(6):13-15 (1945).

Kramer, L., D. Osis, E. Wiatrowski, and H. Spencer. 1974. Dietary fluoride in different areas in the United States. Am. J. Clin. Nutr. 27:590-594.

Langford, H.G., and R.L. Watson. 1971. A hypothesis about essential hypertension. Trans. Am. Clin. Climatol. Assoc. 83:125-132.

Langford, H.G., R.L. Watson, and B H. Douglas. 1968. Factors affecting blood pressure in population groups. Re. Assoc. Am. Phys. 81:135-145.

Langford, H.G., R.L. Watson, and J.G. Thomas. 1976. Salt intake and the treatment of hypertension. Am. Heart J., in press.

Langford, H.S., and R.L. Watson. 1975. Electrolytes and hypertension. *In* C. Paul, ed. Epidemiology and Control of Hypertension, pp. 119-128. Stratton Intercontinental Medical Book Corp., New York.

Larson, T.E., and L. Henley. 1966. Occurrence of nitrate in well waters. Final Report. Project 65-05G. University of Illinois Water Resources Center, Urbana.

Leone, N.C., M.B. Shimkin, F.A. Arnold, Jr., C.A. Stevenson, E.R. Zimmerman, P.B. Geiser, and J.E. Lieberman. 1954. Medical aspects of excessive fluoride in a water supply. Public Health Rep. 69:925-936.

Lockhart, E.E., C.L. Tucker, and M.C. Merritt. 1955. The effect of water impurities on the flavor of brewed coffee. Food Res. 10:598-605.

Lowenstein, F.W. 1961. Blood pressure in relation to age and sex in the tropics and subtropics. Lancet 1:389-392.

Macfayden, W.A. 1953. Sulfates in African inland waters. (Letter to the editor.) Nature 172:595.

Machle, W., and E.J. Largent. 1943. The absorption and excretion of fluoride: II. The metabolism at high levels of intake. J. Ind. Hyg. Toxicol. 25:112-123.

Machle, W., E.W. Scott, and E.J. Largent. 1942. The absorption and excretion of fluorides. Part I. The normal fluoride balance. Ind. Hyg. Toxicol. 24:199-204.

Maddock, I. 1967. Blood pressure in Melanesians. Med. J. Aust. 1:1123-1126.

Maddocks, I. 1961. Possible absence of essential hypertension in two complete Pacific island populations. Lancet 2:396-399.

Magee, P.N., and J.M. Barnes. 1967. Carcinogenic nitroso compounds. Adv. Can. Res. 10:163-246.

Maier, F.J. 1963. Manual of Water Fluoridation Practice. McGraw Hill, New York.

Mann, G.V., O.A. Roels, D.L. Price, and J.M. Merrill. 1962. Cardiovascular disease in African pygmies. A survey of the health status, serum lipids and diet of Pygmies in the Congo. J. Chron. Dis. 15:341-371.

Mann, G.V., R.D. Shaffer, R.S. Anderson, and H.H Sandstead. 1964. Carciovascular disease in the Masai. J. Atheroscler. Res. 4:289-312.

Manocha, S.L., H. Warner, and Z.L. Olkowski. 1975. Cytochemical response of kidney, liver and nervous system to fluoride ions in drinking water. Histochem. J. 7(11):343-355.

Marier, J.R., and D. Rose. 1966. The fluoride content of some foods and beverages. A brief survey using a modified Zr-spadns method. J. Food Sci. 31:941-946.

Meneely, G.R., and L.K. Dahl. 1961. Electrolytes in hypertension. The effects of sodium chloride. Med. Clin. N. Am. 45:271-283.

Miall, W.E., and S. Chinn. 1973. Blood pressure and aging. Results of a fifteen to seventeen year follow-up study in South Wales. Clin. Sci. Mol. Med. 45(Suppl. I):23-33.

Milham, P.J., A.S. Awad, R.E. Paull, and J.H. Bull. 1970. Analysis of plants, soils, and waters for nitrate by using an ion-selective electrode. Analyst 95:751-757.

Mirvish, S.S. 1972. Studies on N-nitrosation reactions. Kinetics of nitrosation, correlation with mouse feeding experiments, and natural occurrence of nitrosatable compounds (ureides and quanidines). *In* W. Nakahara, S. Takayama, T. Sugimura, and S. Odashima, eds. Topics in Chemical Carcinogenesis, pp. 279-295. University Park Press, Baltimore.

Mirvish, S.S. 1975a. Formation of N-nitroso compounds: Chemistry, kinetics, and *in vivo* occurrence. Toxicol. Appl. Pharmacol., in press.

Mirvish, S.S. 1975b. Blocking the formation of N-nitroso compounds with ascorbic acid in *vitro* and *in vivo*. *In* C.G. King and J.J. Burns, eds. Proc., Second Conference on Vitamin C. Ann. N.Y. Acad. Sce., in press.

Mohamed, A.H. 1968. Cytogenic effects of hydrogen fluoride treatment in tomato plants. J. Air Pollut. Cont. Assoc. 18:6, 395-398.

Mohamed, A.H. 1969. Cytogenetic effects of hydrogen fluoride in plants. Fluoride 2:76-84.

Mohamed, A.H. 1971. Induced recessive lethals in second chromosomes of Drosophia melanogaster by hydrogen fluoride. *In* H.M. Englung and W.T. Berry, eds. Proc. 2nd Internat. Clean Air Cong., pp. 158-161. Academic Press, New York.

Mohamed, A.H. 1970a. Chromosomal changes in maise induced by hydrogen fluoride gas. Can. J. Gen. Cyto. 12(3):614-620.

Mohamed, A.H., and P.A. Kemmer. 1970b. Genetic effects of hydrogen fluoride on Drosophila melanogaster. Fluoride 3(4):192-199.

Mohamed, A.H., H.G. Applegate, and J.D. Smith. 1966a. Cytological reactions induced by sodium fluoride in Allium Cepa root tip chromosomes. Can. J. Genet. Cytol. 8(2):241-244, 241-244.

Mohamed, A.H., J.D. Smith, and H.G. Applegate. 1966b. Cytological effects of hydrogen fluoride on tomato chromosomes. Can. J. Genet. Cytol. 8(3):575-583.

Mohamed, A.H., and M.E.W. Chandler. 1976. Cytological effects of sodium fluoride on mitotic and meiotic chromosomes of mice. Preprint.

Moore, E.W. 1952. Physiological effects of the consumption of saline drinking water. Bulletin of Subcommittee on Water Supply, National Research Council, Jan. 10, 1952. Appendix B, pp. 221-227.

Morie, G.P., C.J. Ledford, and C.A. Glover. 1972. Determination of nitrate and nitrite in mixtures with a nitrate ion electrode. Anal. Chim. Acta. 60:397-403.

Morse, W.R., and Y.T. Beh. 1937. Blood pressure amongst aboriginal ethnic groups of Szechwan Province, West China. Lancet 1:966-967.

Mucha, V., P. Kamensky, and J. Keleti. 1965. Genesis and prevention of alimentary nitrate methemoglobinemia in babies. Hyg. Sanit. 30:185-190.

Muhler, J.C. 1970. The Supply of Fluorides to Man. *In* Fluorides and Human Health, pp. 32-40. World Health Organization Monograph no. 59.

Mukherjee, R.N., and F.H. Sobels. 1968. The effects of sodium fluoride and iodoacetamide on mutation induction by x-irradiation in mature spermatozoa of Drosophila. Mutat. Res. 6:217-225.

Murrill, R.I. 1949. A blood pressure study of the natives of Ponape Island, Eastern Carolines. Human Biol. 21:47-59.

National Academy of Sciences. 1971. Biologic Effects of Atmospheric Pollutants—Fluorides. Washington, D.C.

National Academy of Sciences-National Research Council. 1971. Statement regarding the role of methoxyflurane in the production of renal dysfunction. Anesthesiology 34(6):505-509.

National Academy of Sciences-National Research Council. Environmental Studies Board. 1973. Water Quality criteria, 1972. EPA Report. EPA-R3-73-033. Washington, D.C.

Needleman, H.L., S.M. Pueschel, and K.J. Rothman. 1974. Fluoridation and the occurrence of Down's Syndrome. N. Engl. J. Med. 291:821-823.

Needleman, H.L., S.M. Pueschel, and K.J. Rothman. 1975. Fluoridation and Down's Syndrome. N. Engl. J. Med. 292(3):161-162.

Newberne, P.M., and R.C. Shank. 1973. Induction of liver and lung tumours in rats by the simultaneous administration of sodium nitrite and morpholine. Food Cosmet. Toxicol. 11:819-125.

O'Meara, W.F. 1968. Fluoride administration in single daily dose: A survey of its value in prevention of dental caries. Clin. Pediatr. 7:177-184.

Obe, G., and R. Slaci-Erben. 1973. Suppressive activity by fluoride on the induction of chromosome aberrations in human cells and alkylating agents *in vitro*. Mutat. Res. 19:369-371.

Okamoto, K., 1969. Spontaneous hypertension in rats. Int. Rev. Exp. Pathol. 7:227-270.

Okamura, T., and T. Matsuhisa. 1963. Fluorine and other related materials in rice. I. Fluorine content of lowland nonglutinous husked rice and its correlation with human mortality with cancer. Nippon Sakumotsu Gakkai Kiji 32:132-138.

Olson, J.R., F.W. Oehme, and D.L. Carnahan. 1972. Relationship of nitrate levels in water and livestock feeds to herd health problems on 25 Kansas farms. Vet. Med. Small Anim. Clin. 67:257-260.

Olson, O.E., and A.L. Moxon. 1942. Nitrate reduction in relation to oat-hay poisoning. J. Am. Vet. Med. Assc. 100:403-406.

Oreopoulos, D.G., D.R. Taves, S. Rabinovich, H.E. Meema, T. Murray, S.S. Fenton, and G.A. deVerber. 1974. Fluoride and dialysis osteodystrophy: Results of a double-blind study. Trans. Am. Soc. Art. Int. Organs 20:203-208.

Orgeron, J.D., J.D. Martin, and C.T. CAraway. 1957. Methemoglobinemia from eating meat with high nitrite content. Public Health Rep. 72:189-193.

Ostfeld, A.M., and O. Paul. 1963. The inheritance of hypertension. Lancet 3:575-579.

Page, L.B., and J.J. Sidd. 1973. Medical Management of Primary Hypertension. Little, Brown and Co., Boston.

Page, L.B. 1976. Epidemiologic evidence on the etiology of human hypertension and its possible prevention. Am. Heart J. 91:527-534.

Page, L.B., Damon, A., and R.C. Moellering. 1974. Antecedents of cardiovascular disease in six Solomon Islands societies. Circulation 49:1132-1146.

Palmer, A.W. 1903. Chemical survey of the water of Illinois. Report for the years 1897-1902. University of Illinois.

Parkins, F.M. 1974. Relationship of human plasma fluoride and bone fluoride to age. Calc. Tiss. Res. 16:335-338.

Perara, G.A., and D.W. Blood. 1947 The relationship of sodium chloride to hypertension. J. Clin. Invest. 26:1109-1118.

Peterson, N.L. 1951. Sulfates in drinking water. Official Bulletin. North Dakota Water and Sewage Works Conference, 18:6-11.

Petraborg, H.T. 1974. Chronic fluoride intoxication from drinking water: Preliminary report. Fluoride 7:47-52.

Pickering, G. 1965. Hyperpeisis: High blood pressure without evident cause. Essential Hypertension. Br. Med. J. 2:959-968.

Piskin, R. 1973. Evaluation of nitrate content of ground water in Hall County, Nebraska. Groundwater 11:4-13.

Prior, I.A., J.M. Stanhope, J. Grimley-Evans, and C.E. Salmond. 1974. The Tokelau Island migrant study. Int. J. Epidemiol. 3:225-232.

Prival, M.J., and F. Fisher. 1974. Adding fluorides to the diet. Environment 16(5):29-33.

Quissell, D.O., and J.W. Suttie. 1972. Development of fluoride-resistant strain of L cells: Membrane and metabolic characteristics. Am. J. Physiol. 223:596-603.

Rapaport, I. 1959. Nouvelles recherches sur le mongolisme. A propos du role pathogenique du fluor. Bull. Acad. Nat. Med. 143:367-379.

Rensburg, S.W.J., and W.H. Vos. 1966. The influence of excess fluorine intake in the drinking water on reproductive efficiency in bovines. Onderstepoort J. Vet. Res. 33(1):185-194.

Richards, F.M., and J.R. Knowles. 1968. Glutaraldehyde as a protein cross-linking reagent. J. Mol. Biol. 37:231-233.

Richards, L.F., W.W. Westmoreland, M. Tashiro, C.M. McKay, and J.T. Morrison. 1967. Determining optimum fluoride levels for community water supplies in relation to temperature. J. Am. Dent. Assoc. 74:389-397.

Ridder, W.E., and F.W. Oehme. 1974. Nitrates as an environmental, animal, and human hazard. Clin. Toxicol. 7:145-159.

Robertson, J.S. 1975. Water sodium: The problem of the bottle-fed neonate. WRC Drinking Water Quality and Public Health.

Roholm, K. 1937. Fluorine Intoxication. H.K. Lewis, London.

Royal College of Physicians. 1976. Fluoride, teeth, and health. Pitman Medical and Scientific Publishing Co., Ltd., London.

San Filippo, F.A., and G.C. Battistone. 1971. The fluoride content of a representative diet of the young adult male. Clin. Chim. Acta 31:453-457.

Sander, J., and F. Schweinsberg. 1972. Wechselbeziehungen zwischen nitrat, nitrit und kanzerogenen N-nitrosoverbindungen. Zbl. Bakt. Hyg. I. Abt. Orig. B. 156:299-340.

Sander, J., F. Schweinsberg, and H.P. Menz. 1968. Untersuchunge- ueber die entstehung cancerogener nitrosamine in magen. Hoppe-Seyler's Z. Physiol. Chem. 349:1691-1697.

Sattelmacher, P.G. 1962. Methemoglobinemia from nitrates in drinking water. Schriftenreiche des Vererins fur Wassar Boden und Lufthygiene, no 21.

Sauerbrunn, B.J.L., C.M. Ryan, and J.F. Shaw. 1965. Chronic fluoride intoxication with fluorotic radiculomyelopathy. Ann. Intern. Med. 63:1074-1078.

Schlesinger, E.R. 1956. Newburgh-Kingston Caries-fluorine study. XIII. Pediatric findings after ten years. J. Am. Dent. Assoc. 52:296-306.

Schneider, N.R., and R.A. Yeary. 1975. Nitrite and nitrate pharmacokinetics in the dog, sheep, and pony. Am. J. Vet. Res. 36:941-947.

Schuller, P.L., and E. Veen. 1967. Preservatives: A review of methods of analysis. J. Assoc. Off. Anal. Chem. 50:1127-1145.

Schuphan, W. 1965. The nitrate content of spinach (Spinacia oleracea) in relation to methemoglobinemia in infants. Z. Ernaehrungswiss. 5:207-209.

Scofield, C.S. 1936. The salinity of irrigation water. Smithsonian Institution Annual Report, 1935, pp. 275-287. Washington, D.C.

Scott, K.D., A.E. Kimberly, A.L. Van Horn, L.F. Ely, and F.H. Waring. 1937. Fluoride in Ohio water supplies. Its effect, occurrence and reduction. J. Am. Water Works Assoc. 29:9-25.

Selye, H., C.E. Hall, and E.M. Fowley. 1943. Malignant hypertension produced by treatment with desoxycorticosterone acetate and sodium chloride. Can. Med. Assoc. J. 49:88-92.

Shank, R.C. 1975. Toxicology of N-nitroso compounds. Toxicol. Appl. Pharmacol. 31:361-368.

Shaper, A.G., D.H. Wright, and J. Kyobe. 1969. Blood pressure and body build in three nomadic tribes of northern Kenya. East Afr. Med. J. 46:274.

Shea, J.J., S.M. Gillespie, and G.L. Waldbott. 1967. Allergy to fluoride. Ann. Allergy 25:388-391.

Shearer, L.A., J.R. Goldsmith, C. Young, O.A. Kearns, and B.R. Tamplin. 1972. Methemoglobin levels in infants in an area with high nitrate water supply. Am. J. Public Health 62:1174-1180.

Shuval, H.I., and N. Gruener. 1973. Health effects of nitrates in water. Final report. Office of Research and Development, U.S. Environmental Protection Agency, Washington, D.C. (Grant No. 06-012-3)

Shuval, H.I., and N. Gruener. 1972. Epidemiological and toxicological aspects of nitrates and nitrites in the environment. Am. J. Pub. Health 62:1045-1052.

Simon, C. 1966. Nitrite poisoning from spinach. Lancet 1:872.

Singer, L., and W.D. Armstrong. 1969a. Determination of fluoride procedure based upon diffusion of HF. Anal. Biochem. 10:495-500.

Singer, L., and W.D. Armstrong. 1969. Total fluoride content of human serum. Arch. Oral Biol. 14:1343-1347.

Singer, L., and W.D. Armstrong. 1973. Determination of fluoride in ultrafiltrates of sera. Biochem. Med. 8:415-422.

Singer, L., and W.D. Armstrong. 1960. Regulation of human plasma fluoride concentration. J. Appl. Physiol. 15:508-510.

Singer, R.H. 1968. Environmental nitrates and animal health. Southwest. Vet. 22:13-18.

Sinios, A., and W. Wodsak. 1965. Die spinatvergiftung des savglings. Dent. Med. Wochenschr. 90:1856-1863.

Slacik-Erben, R., and G. Obe. 1976. The effect of sodium fluoride on DNA synthesis, mitotic indices and chromosomal aberrations in human leukocytes treated with Trenimon *in vitro*. Mutat. Res. in press.

Smith, F.A. 1966. Handbook of Experimental Pharmacoloy, vol. XXII. Springer-Verlag, New York.

Smith, F.A., D.E. Gardner, and H.C. Hodge. 1950. Investigations on the metabolism of fluoride II Fluoride content of blood and urine as a function of the fluorine in drinking water. J. Dent. Res. 29:596-600.

Smith, G.E. 1970. Nitrate pollution of water supplies. Trace Subst. Environ. Health 3:273-287.

Smith, J.E., and E. Beutler. 1966. Methemoglobin formation and reduction in man and various animal species. Am. J. Physiol. 210:347-250.

Smith, S.O., and J.H. Baier. 1969. Report on nitrate pollution of ground water, Nassau County, Long Island. Bureau of Water Resources, Nassau County Department of Health, Mineola, New York.

Sollman, T. 1957. A Manual of Pharmacology, 8th ed. W.B. Saunders, Philadelphia.

Spencer, H., I. Lewin, E. Wistrowski, and J. Samachson. 1970. Fluoride metabolism in man. Am. J. Med. 49:807-813.

Spiegelhalder, B., G. Eisenbrand, and R. Preussman. 1976. The influence of dietary intake of nitrate on the nitrite content in human saliva: A factor of possible relevance for *in vivo* formation of N-nitroso compounds. Food Cosmet. Toxicol., in press.

Stamler, J., M. Kjelsberg, and Y. Hall. 1960. Epidemiologic studies on cardiovascular-renal disease. I. Analysis of mortality by age-race-sex-occupation. J. Chron. Dis. 12:440-455.

Stephany, R.W., and P.L. Schuller. 1974. De aanwezigheid van nitriet in menselijk speeksel en het N-nitrosamine probleem. In Berichten uit het Rijksin stituut voor de Volksgezondheid. waarin Liber Amicorum, pp. 184-190. Utrecht.

Strotz, C.R., and G.I. Shorr. 1973. Hypertension in the Papago Indians. Circulation 48:1299-1303.

Subbotin, F.N. 1961. Nitrates in the drinking water and their effect on the formation of methemoglobin. Gigi. Sanit. 2:13-17.

Tannenbaum, S.R., A.J. Sinskey, M. Weisman, and W. Bishop. 1974. Nitrite in human saliva. Its possible relationship to nitrosamine formation. J. Nat. Cancer Inst. 53:79-84.

Tannenbaum, S.R., M. Wiesman, and D. Fett. 1976a. The effect of nitrate intake on nitrite formation in human saliva. Food Cosmet. Toxicol. 14(6):549-552.

Tannenbaum, S.R., M.C. Archer, J.S. Wishnok, and W. Bishop. 1976a. Nitrosamine formation in saliva. Presented at the 4th Meeting on the Analysis and Formation of N-Nitroso Compounds, Tallinn, Estonia, Oct. 1-2, 1975. International Agency for Research on Cancer, World Health Organization, in press.

Tao, S., and J.W. Suttie. 1976. Evidence for a lack of an effect of dietary fluoride level on reproduction in mice. J. Nutr. 106(8):1115-1122.

Tarazi, R.C., H.P. Dustan, and E.D. Frohlich. 1970. Long-term thiazode therapy in essential hypertension. Evidence for persistent alteration in plasma volume and renin activity. Circulation 41:709-717.

Taves, D.R. 1976. Fluoride and Cancer Mortality, Cold Springs Harbor Symposium on Origins of Human Cancer, in press.

Taves, D.R. 1966. Normal human serum fluoride concentrations. Nature 211:192-193.

Taves, D.R. 1968a. Electrophoretic mobility of serum fluoride. Nature 220:582-583.

Taves, D.R. 1968b. Evidence that there are two forms of fluoride in human serum. Nature 217:1050-1051.

Taves, D.R. 1975. Safety of fluoridation. B.N.F. Bull. 15, 3:3, 193-198.

Taves, D.R. 1967. Use of urine to serum fluoride concentration ratios to confirm serum fluoride analyses. Nature 215:1380.

Taylor, A., and N.C. Taylor. 1964. The effect of sodium bromide on tumor growth. Cancer Res. 24:751-753.

Taylor, A., and N.C. Taylor. 1965. The effect of sodium fluoride on tumor growth. Proc. Soc. Exp. Biol. Med. 119:252-255.

Temple, P., and L. Weinstein. 1976. Personal communication.

Thomas, C.B. 1973. Genetic pattern of hypertension in man. *In* G. Onesti, K.E. Kim, and J.H. Moyer, eds. Hypertension: Mechanisms and Management, pp. 66-73. Grune and Stratton, Inc.

Thomas, W.A. 1927. Health of a carnivorous race. Study of the Eskimo. J. Am. Med. Assoc. 88:1559-1560.

Tobian, L. 1975. Current status of salt in hypertension. *In* O. Paul, ed. Epidemiology and Control of Hypertension, pp. 131-143. Stratton Intercontinental Medical Book Corp., New York.

Truswell, A.S., B.M. Kennelly, J.D.L. Hansen, and R.B. Lee. 1974. Blood pressure of Ikung bushmen in northern Botswana. Am. Heart J. 84:5-12.

U. S. Department of Health, Education, and Welfare. 1969. Natural Fluoride Content of Community Water Supplies.

U.S. Environmental Protection Agency. 1971. Environmental impact of highway de-icing. Storm and Combined Sewer Technology Branch, Edison Water Quality Research Laboratory. 11040 GKK 06/71.

U.S. Public Health Service. 1962. Drinking water standards. U.S. Department of Health, Education, and Welfare. Public Health Service Publication no. 956. Washington, D.C.

Ulvila, J.M., J.A. Kennedy, J.D. Lamberg, and B.H. Scribner. 1972. Blood pressure in chronic renal failure: Effect of sodium intake and furosemide. J. Am. Med. Assoc. 220:233-288.

United States National Center for Health Statistics. 1964. Vital and Health Statistics. Heart Disease in Adults, United States 1960-62. PHS Publication no. 1000, series 11, no. 6. U.S. Government Printing Office, Washington, D.C.

Usher, C.D., and G.M. Telling. Dec. 1975. The analysis of nitrate and nitrite in food stuffs. A critical review. Int. Agency Res. Cancer. Lyon, France.

van Logten, M.J., E.M. den Tonkelaar, R. Kroes, J.M. Berkvens, and G.J. van Esch. 1972. Long-term experiment with canned meat treated with sodium nitrite and glucono-δ-lactone in rats. Food Cosmet. Toxicol. 10:475-488.

Vertes, V., J.L. Cangiano, L.B. Berman, and A. Gould. 1969. Hypertension in end-stage renal disease. N. Engl. J. Med. 380:978-981.

Vogel, E. 1973. Strong antimutagenic effects of fluoride on mutation induction by Trenimon and I-phenyl-3,3-dimethyltriazenc in Drosophila melanogaster. Mutat. Res. 20:339-352.

Waldbott, G.L. 1962. Fluoride in clinical medicine. Int. Arch. Allergy 20(Suppl. 1):1-60.

Walser, M., and W.J. Rahill. 1965. Nitrate, thiocyanate and perchlorate clearance in relation to chloride clearance. Am. J. Physiol. 208:1158-1164.

Walton, G. 1951. Survey of literature relating to infant methemoglobinemia due to nitrate-contaminated water. Am. J. Public Health 41:986-996.

Weidmann, S.M., and J.A. Weatherell. 1970. Distribution in hard tissues. *In* Fluorides and Human Health, pp. 104-128. World Health Organization Monograph Series no. 59, Geneva.

Weinstein, L.H., D.C. McCune, J.F. Mancini, L.J. Colavito, D.H. Silberman, and P. vanLeuken. 1972. Studies on fluoro-organic compounds in plants. III. Comparison of the biosynthesis of fluoro-organic acids in Acacia georginae with other species. Environ. Res. 5:393-408.

Whipple, G.C. 1907. The value of pure water. J. Wiley & Sons, New York. 84 pp.

White, J.M., J.G. Wingo, L.M. Alligood, G.R. Cooper, J. Gutridge, W. Hydaker, R.T. Benack, J.W. Dening, and F.B. Taylor. 1967. Sodium ion in drinking water. I. Properties, analysis, and occurrence. J. Am. Diet. Assoc. 50:32-36.

White, J.W., Jr. 1975. Relative significance of dietary sources of nitrate and nitrite. J. Agric. Food Chem. 23:886-891.

Whitford, G.M., D.H. Pashley, and G.E. Stringer. 1976. Fluoride renal clearance: A pH-dependent event. Am. J. Physiol. 230:527-532.

Whitford, G.H., and D.R. Taves. 1973. Fluoride-induced diuresis: Renal tissue solute concentrations, functional, hemodynamic and histological correlates in the rat. Anesthesiology 39:416-427.

Whyte, H.M. 1958. Body fat and blood pressure of natives in New Guinea. Aust. Ann. Med. 7:36-46.

Widdowson, E.M., R.A. McCance, and C.M. Spray. 1951. Chemical composition of the human body. Clin. Sci. 10:113-125.

Winton, E.F., R.G. Tardiff, and L.J. McCabe. 1971. Nitrate in drinking water. J. Am. Water Works Assoc. 63:95-98.

Wold, H.L., and J.V. Denko. 1958. Osteosclerosis in chronic renal disease. Am. J. Med. Sci. 235:33-42.

World Health Organization. 1970. Fluorides and Buma Health. WHO Monograph Series no. 59, 364 pp.

Yiamouyiannis, J.A. 1975. A definite link between fluoridation and cancer death rate. National Health Federation, unpublished manuscript.

Zinner, S.H., P.S. LTvy, and E.H. Kass. 1971. Familial aggregation of blood pressure in childhood. N. Engl. J. Med. 284:401-404.

REFERENCES FOR WATER HARDNESS AND HEALTH

COMA Report. 1974. Diet and coronary heart disease. Report of the Advisory Panel of the Committee on Medical Aspects of Food Policy (Nitrution) on Diet in Relation to Cardiovascular and Cerebrovascular Disease. Department of Health and Social Security, London.

Craun, G.F., and L.J. McCabe. 1975. Problems associated with metals in drinking water. J. Am. Water Works Assoc. 67:593-599.

Heyden, S. 1976. The hard facts behind the hard-water theory and ischemic heart disease. J. Chron. Dis. 29:149-157.

International Atomic Energy Agency. 1973. Trace Elements in Relation to Cardiovascular Diseases. (WHO/IAEA joint research programme) Proc. research coordination meeting, Vienna, 1973. IAEA, Vienna, Technical Report IAEA-157.

Kobayashi, J. 1957. On the geographical relationship between the chemical nature of river water and death-rate from apoplexy. Ber. Ohara Inst. Landwirt. Biol. 11:11-21.

Medical Research Council. 1970. Report on Recommendations. Conference on Trace Elements and Disease in Man. London, July 6, 1970.

Neri, L.C., D. Hewitt, and G.B. Schreiber. 1974. Can epidemiology elucidate the water story. Am. J. Epidemiol. 99:75-88.

Sauer, H.I. 1974. Relationship between trace element content of drinking water and chronic diseases. *In* J.T. O'Conner, and A.R. Sapoznik, eds. Proceedings of the Sixteenth Water Quality Conference: Trace Metals in Water Supplies: Occurrence, Significance, and Control, Feb. 12-13, 1974, University of Illinois, Urbana-Champaign. Univ. Ill. Bull. 71:39-48, April 29, 1974.

Schroeder, H.A. 1960. Relation between mortality from cardiovascular disease and treated water supplies. J. Am. Med. Assoc. 172:98-104.

Schroeder, H.A., and L.A. Kraemer. 1974. Cardiovascular mortality, municipal water, and corrosion. Arch. Environ. Health 28:303-311.

Second meeting of investigators on trace elements in relation to cardiovascular diseases (Joint WHO/IAEA research programme) (unpublished WHO document CVD/73.4), 1973.

Sharrett, A.R., and M. Feinleib. 1975. Water constituents and trace elements in relation to cardiovascular disease. Prev. Med. 4:20-36.

Winton, E.F., and L.J. McCabe. 1970. Studies relating to water mineralization and health. J. Am. Water Works Assoc. 62:26-30.

VI

Organic Solutes

INTRODUCTION

Selection of Agents

In selecting agents to be included in the organic contaminants section of this report, a number of tabulations of organic contaminants detected in drinking water were examined. From these lists, agents were selected that have been reported to be present in one or more drinking-water supplies at relatively high concentrations and for which there were data to suggest toxicity in man or animals. Also included were several agents that exhibit a structural relationship to other compounds for which toxicity data were available and all of the agents listed in the current interim standards, as well as those specific compounds listed in the *Federal Register* of December 24, 1975. A total of 298 volatile organic compounds were considered and 74 of these were selected for evaluation.

Similar criteria were used to select the organic pesticides for inclusion in this report. Several additional agents were added after examination of the usage patterns for all major types of organic pesticides, as well as a number of agents that were considered to be potential contaminants of drinking-water supplies because of the large quantities produced. A total of 55 organic pesticides were selected for evaluation.

Evaluation of Toxicity

A critical review of the available literature on the toxicology of each agent (or group of related agents) was carried out as the first stage in the evaluation. Although the primary focus in these reviews was on carcinogenesis and other chronic toxic effects, test results and data on teratogenesis, mutagenesis, reproductive effects, metabolism, acute toxicity, and other types of studies were included when available. Information on the current production, manufacturing methods, and environmental distribution was included for some pesticides and other organic compounds.

In the second stage of the evaluation, both the quantity and quality of the information in each of the critical reviews was considered to determine whether the data would permit judgments to be made regarding carcinogenicity or estimation of a maximum no-observed-adverse-effect level.

The hazards of ingesting compounds that were assessed as confirmed or suspected carcinogens were evaluated in terms of dose-related risks, as described below and in Chapter II. It is recognized that extrapolation of high-dose animal bioassay data to low-dose human exposures is beset by limitations, and that it is difficult to reconcile the results of experiments on animals that may show different target-organ responses, and may metabolize carcinogens at different rates and by different pathways. Such risk assessment and extrapolation procedures are further compromised by the limited information that is available concerning the mechanisms by which these agents act (e.g., as initiators, promotors, modifiers) and the almost total lack of data regarding the potentially synergistic and antagonistic interactions of these agents with each other and with other environmental agents. Despite these and other uncertainties, the "risk estimate" approach has been adopted as the basis for analyzing the data on carcinogenicity rather than the "safety factor" approach.

After a substance had been identified as a carcinogen, the risk to man was expressed as the probability that cancer would be produced by continued daily ingestion over a 70 yr lifetime of 1 liter of water containing a standard quantity (1 μg/liter) of the substance in question. Estimates expressed in this form may then be used to calculate risk due to the concentrations actually found in drinking-water and the daily consumption.

To make such estimates from the results of animal feeding studies, two steps are necessary. The first involves conversion of the standard human dose to the physiologically equivalent dose in the animal. This was performed on the basis of relative surface area (details are given in Hoel *et al.*, 1975, Chapter II). The second step requires use of a risk model relating dose to effect. The model used for this purpose is

$$P(d) = 1 - e^{-(\lambda_0 + \lambda_1 d + \lambda_2 d^2 + \ldots \lambda_k d^k)}$$

where $P(d)$ is the lifetime probability that dose d (total daily intake) will produce cancer, K = the number of events in the carcinogenic process, and $\lambda_0, \lambda_1, \lambda_2$, etc. . . . are nonnegative parameters (see Chapter II). At low doses, the higher-order terms in d^2, d^3, etc., may be neglected and

$$P(d) \simeq 1 - e^{-(\lambda_0 + \lambda_1 d)} \simeq \lambda_0 + \lambda_1 d$$

λ_0 representing the background rate. When two or more sets of results of lifetime animal feeding studies were available, experimental values of $P(d)$, the fraction of test animals developing cancer, and d, the total daily dose, were fitted to the equation to determine how many of the terms $\lambda_0, \lambda_1 d, \lambda_2 d^2$, etc., were necessary to give the best fit. Corresponding values of λ_0, λ_1, or λ_0, λ_1 and λ_2, etc., were used to calculate $P(d)$ for the low-dose of interest, namely the animal dose that was physiologically equivalent to the standard dose for man. If the animal experiments involved only one dose level, the $\lambda_1 d$ term, alone, was used in the calculation. Upper confidence limits in the estimated low-dose risk were also calculated by use of maximum likelihood theory (Guess and Crump, 1976, Chapter II), and these values were tabulated. Since the animal data were obtained from lifetime feeding studies, the risk estimates calculated from them for the low-doses that were estimated to be physiologically equivalent to the human dose were taken to represent the lifetime risks for man. The background rate, obtained from the cancer incidence in the control groups of experimental animls and represented by the parameter λ_0, was excluded from the tabulated values of $P(d)$, which therefore represent the incremental risks due to ingestion of the compounds in water.

It was felt that predictions that are risk-related provide a more meaningful first approximation of hazard than safety-related predictions. The risk estimate approach may provide unique advantages for other areas of toxicological evaluations, such as mutagenesis, and it is recommended that the usefulness of this procedure be evaluated as a new predictive method in toxicology.

For agents that were not considered to be known or suspected carcinogens and for which there were adequate toxicity data from prolonged ingestion studies in man or animals, the more traditional approach was utilized of combining the maximum dose producing no-observed-adverse-effects with an uncertainty (risk) factor to calculate an

ADI (acceptable daily intake). Several alternative terms, other than ADI, were considered, but it was concluded that the introduction of new terms might well lead to confusion and that the use of a widely recognized and generally acceptable term would be preferable for this report. The ADI has been used previously as an internationally established standard for the toxicologic evaluation of food additives and contaminants and the concept is applicable to other ingestion exposure situations. The ADI represents an empirically derived value that reflects a particular combination of knowledge and uncertainty concerning the relative risk of a chemical. The uncertainty factors used to calculate ADI values in this report represent the level of confidence that was judged to be justified on the basis of the animal and human toxicity data. All calculations for an ADI were based on chronic feeding studies, but other considerations, e.g., mutagenicity, teratogenicity, and lack of sex and strain information, influenced the choice of the uncertainty factor. ADI values were not calculated for agents where the data were considered to be inadequate.

Since the calculation of the ADI values is based on the total amount of a chemical that is ingested, the ADI values calculated in this report do not represent a safe level for drinking water. However, a suggested no-anticipated-adverse-effect level has been calculated for these chemicals in drinking water using two hypothetical exposures (where water constitutes 1% and 20% of the total intake of the agent), and similar calculations can readily be made for other exposures.

Conclusions

The organic contaminants that have been identified in drinking water constitute a small percentage of the total organic matter present in water. Although approximately 90% of the volatile organic compounds in drinking water have been identified and quantified, these represent no more than 10% of the total organic material. Of the nonvolatile organic compounds comprising the remaining 90% of the total organic matter in water, only 5 to 10% have been identified. From the 74 nonpesticide organic compounds and 55 organic pesticides selected for study, 22 have been identified as known or suspected carcinogens, 46 as having sufficient toxicity data to permit the calculation of an ADI value or a suggested no-adverse-effect level for drinking water, 6 as mutagens and 7 as teratogens. There were 61 agents for which the toxicity data were judged to be inadequate for establishing any recommendations. (See Tables VI-63 and 64 in "Summary of Organic Solutes.")

It is evident that this effort constitutes only the beginning of a very large task. However, in preparing these reports and recommendations, an attempt has been made to use procedures that will enable efforts in the future to be focused on revisions and additions to the estimates, adding to and updating, rather than on redoing, the task. Also identified are certain priorities for the selection of agents to be studied and the research needs in toxicology and epidemiology to facilitate the evaluation of the potential health hazards associated with organic agents that are or may be present in our drinking-water supplies.

PESTICIDES: HERBICIDES

Chlorophenoxys

2,4-D

Introduction

2,4-D, or 2,4-dichlorophenoxyacetic acid, was introduced as a plant growth-regulator in 1942 (USEPA, 1974b). It is registered in the United States as an herbicide for control of broadleaf plants and as a plant growth-regulator. Domestic use of 2,4-D is estimated at 40-50 million pounds a year, approximately 84% of which is used agriculturally and about 16% nonagriculturally (mainly for forest brush control).

2,4-D is produced commercially by chlorination of phenol to form 2,4-dichlorophenol, which reacts with monochloroacetic acid to form 2,4-D (USEPA, 1974b). Commercial 2,4-D formulations are generally composed of the salts or esters (ethyl, isopropyl, butyl, amyl, heptyl, octyl, etc.) of the acid. Analysis of 28 samples of technical 2,4-D by gas chromatography showed that hexachlorodioxins were present in only one sample, at less than 10 ppm (Woolson *et al.*, 1972). The dioxin most likely to be formed, 2,7-dichlorodibenzo-*p*-dioxin, was not found. The major impurity in technical 2,4-D was identified as *bis*-(2,4-dichlorophenoxy)methane, at 30 ppm (Huston, 1972).

The solubility of 2,4-D in water is 540 ppm at 20°C; its major breakdown product, 2,4-dichlorophenol, is soluble at 4,500 ppm (USEPA, 1974b). The 2,4-D salts are in general highly soluble, but the esters are much less soluble.

2,4-D is chemically quite stable, but its esters are rapidly hydrolyzed to the free acid. Microbial degradation of 2,4-D contributes to its rapid breakdown (half-time, 1 week) in water (USEPA, 1974b). When exposed to sunlight or ultraviolet irradiation, aqueous 2,4-D solutions decompose to 2,4-dichlorophenol, 4-chlorocatechol, 2-hydroxy-4-chlorophenoxyacetic acid, 1,2,4-benzene triol, and polymeric humic acids. The overall breakdown rate of 2,4-D in aqueous solution is fairly high, and 2,4-dichlorophenol is even more photolabile. Most 2,4-D residues are retained in the soil, where breakdown usually occurs within 6 weeks.

Between 1964 and 1970, only 50 samples of food were found to be contaminated with 2,4-D; the concentrations detected were 0.021–0.16 ppm (USEPA, 1974b). Residues were found in 1% or less of dairy products, oils, fats and shortening, and fruit, in 1.9% of leafy vegetables, and in 22.1% of sugar and adjuncts.

2,4-D is found in water (Manigold and Schulze, 1969). Concentrations as high as 70 ppb have been detected in Oregon streams after aerial application to forestland (Hiatt, 1976). 2,4-D was detected in raw water at 0.05 μg/liter, in Lafayette, Indiana (USEPA, 1975j). The EPA has set an interim standard for 2,4-D in finished water of 0.1 mg/liter (USEPA, 1975i).

Metabolism

When 2,4-D with labeled carbon was administered orally to sheep, 96% of the dose was excreted unchanged in the urine in 72 h, slightly less than 1.4% in the feces (Clark *et al.*, 1964). When adult sheep and cattle were fed 2,4-D in the diet for 28 days at up to 2,000 ppm, the kidney contained the highest and the liver somewhat lower concentrations of 2,4-D and its breakdown product 2,4-dichlorophenol (Clark *et al.*, 1975). Withdrawal from treatment for 7 days resulted in almost complete elimination of 2,4-D and its major metabolite from the tissues.

In rats that received 1–10 mg of 2,4-D, there was almost complete excretion in the urine and feces in 48 h; at higher doses, some accumulation occurred in tissues (Khanna and Fang, 1966).

After subcutaneous injection of 2,4-D and its butyl and isooctyl esters into mice at 100 mg/kg, the esters were eliminated rapidly, and only 5-10% of the 2,4-D remained after 1 day (USEPA, 1974b). No 2,4-dichlorophenol was detected in extracts of the treated mice.

In feeding studies of 2,4-D with dairy cows and steers, unchanged 2,4-D was found only in the urine (Bache *et al.*, 1964a, b; Guteman *et al.*, 1963a, b; Lisk *et al.*, 1963). Other studies (Burchfield and Storrs, 1961; Klingman *et al.*, 1966) demonstrated that 2,4-D was eliminated in the milk of cows maintained in pastures treated with 2,4-D or its butyl or isooctyl ester.

The pharmacokinetic profile of 2,4-D has been determined in five male human volunteers (Sauerhoff *et al.*, 1976). After ingestion of a single 5-mg/kg oral dose, 2,4-D was eliminated from plasma in an apparent first-order process with an average half-life of 11.7 h. All subjects excreted 2,4-D in the urine with an average half-life of 17.7 h, mainly as free 2,4-D (82.3%), with a smaller amount excreted as a 2,4-D conjugate (12.8%).

Health Aspects

Observations in Man A 46-yr-old male farmer accidentally ingested a 2,4-D formulation; the dose was estimated to contain 2,4-D at 100 mg/kg, *S*-ethyldipropylthiocarbamate at 230 mg/kg, and epichlorohydrin at 2.3 mg/kg (Berwick, 1970). The clinical picture was indicative of 2,4-D poisoning with symptoms including fibrillary twitching and muscular paralysis. Serum glutamic oxalacetic transaminase, glutamic pyruvic transaminase, lactic dehydrogenase, aldolase, and creatine phosphate were increased, and both hemoglobinuria and myoglobinuria were observed. After recovery of the patient, there was also a 4-month loss of sexual potency.

In testing 2,4-D for possible use in disseminated coccidiomycosis, 18 intravenous doses were administered to a patient over a 33-day period, with no observed side effect (Seabury, 1963). The dosage was 15 mg/kg for the last 12 doses, except that the eighteenth was increased to 37 mg/kg. Following the nineteenth and final dose of 67 mg/kg, the patient exhibited fibrillary twitching and general hyporeflexia. The patient later died, apparently owing to the disease.

After a 23-yr-old man used 2,4-D in suicide, the lethal dose was estimated to be over 90 mg/kg (Nielsen *et al.*, 1965).

Assouly (1951) is reported to have taken 2,4-D daily at 8 mg/kg for 3 weeks without harmful effects. Data from Dow Chemical Co. (Johnson, 1971) on 220 workers exposed to 2,4-D at 0.43–0.57 mg/kg/day over a period of 0.5-22 yr showed no significant differences from data on an unexposed human population.

Observations in Other Species

Acute Effects The acute toxicity of 2,4-D is moderate in a number of animal species, with LD_{50} values of 100–541 mg/kg for rats, mice, guinea pigs, chicks, and dogs (Drill and Hiratzka, 1953; Rowe and Hymas, 1954). Salts and esters of 2,4-D show an even lower degree of acute toxicity.

The acute oral toxicity of the major 2,4-D breakdown product 2,4-dichlorophenol is 580 and 1,625 mg/kg for the rat and the mouse, respectively (Toxic Substances List, 1974).

Subchronic and Chronic Effects Young adult female rats were given oral doses of 2,4-D in olive oil at 0, 3, 10, 30, 100, and 300 mg/kg five times a week for 4 weeks (Rowe and Hymas, 1954). No adverse effects were noted at 30 mg/kg and below, but depressed growth rates, liver pathology, and gastrointestinal irritation occurred at 300 mg/kg. In another experiment (Rowe and Hymas, 1954), depressed growth, liver pathology, mortalities, and increased liver/body weight ratios were observed in rats fed 1,000 ppm 2,4-D for 113 days.

2,4-D was administered orally to dogs at dosage levels of 0, 2, 5, 10, and 20 mg/kg 5 days a week for 13 weeks (Drill and Hiratzka, 1953). Three of four animals receiving 20 mg/kg dose died within 49 days. These animals showed a definite decrease in the percentage of lympocytes in the peripheral blood. The surviving animals in all groups did not show any hematological abnormalities.

Dietary levels of 0, 5, 25, 125, 625, and 1,250 ppm technical grade 2,4-D were fed to female and male Osborne–Mendel rats for 2 yr (Hansen *et al.*, 1971). No significant effects were observed on growth, survival rate, organ weights, or hematologic parameters. There was also no elevated incidence of tumors over that seen in controls.

In a parallel study (Hansen *et al.*, 1971), groups of 6–8-month-old beagle dogs received 0, 10, 50, 100 and 500 ppm of technical 2,4-D for 2 years. No 2,4-D related effects were noted. None of the lesions observed in the 30 dogs were believed related to the treatment.

The no-adverse-effect level of 2,4-D in the dog has been established at 8 mg/kg/day (Lehman, 1965).

Mutagenicity 2,4-D was unable to induce point mutations in four microbial systems (Andersen *et al.*, 1971) and showed no activity in Drosophila (Vogel and Chandler, 1974). *Saccharomyces cerevisiae* strain D4 (5×10^6) was treated with 2 ml of an aqueous 2,4-D suspension (trade name, U46D-Fluid) (Siebert and Lemperle, 1974). The mitotic gene conversion frequency of the *ade 2* locus was increased fivefold above control values; that of the *trp 5* locus was increased sixfold above control values.

Carcinogenicity Studies on the in vitro and in vivo effect of 2,4-D on the growth of Ehrlich ascites tumor in BALB/c mice showed that the herbicide was inhibitory at 45 mg/kg or more (Walker *et al.*, 1972). There was no significant increase in the incidence of tumors in various mouse strains initially given 2,4-D or its esters at 46.4 mg/kg/day orally on days 7–28 followed by dietary feeding up to 323 ppm for 18 months (USEPA, 1974b). In another study, mice that received 2,4-D orally for their life span showed no increased incidence of tumor formation (Vettorazzi, 1975b).

A study (Arkhipor and Kozlova, 1974) reported that two rats developed fibroadenoma and one hemangioma 27–31 months after receiving one-tenth the LD_{50} of the amine salt of 2,4-D. Administration of 0.1 the LD_{50} dose of the amine salt orally or subcutaneously to mice produced no tumors after 33 months. The herbicide, however, had a cocarcinogenic effect in mice when it was applied to the skin with 3-methylcholanthrene. DNA synthesis was increased, and there was a loss of cell differentiation in cultured chicken muscle after treatment with high concentrations of 2,4-D (Haag *et al.*, 1975).

2,4-Dichlorophenol has not been tested for carcinogenicity alone (USEPA, 1974b), but it is an initiator for skin carcinogenesis (Boutwell and Bosch, 1959).

Reproduction In a three-generation, six-litter Osborne–Mendel rat reproduction study, no deleterious effects due to technical 2,4-D at dietary doses of 100 or 500 ppm were observed (Hansen *et al.*, 1971). At 1,500 ppm, however, 2,4-D, although affecting neither fertility of either sex nor litter size, sharply reduced the percentage of pups that survived to weaning and the weights of the weanlings.

Teratogenicity In studies of CD-1 mice, Courtney (cited in EPA, 1974b) found that 2,4-D at 221 mg/kg per day increased fetal mortality, but produced no cleft palates. Various 2,4-D esters (isopropyl ester at 147 mg/kg/day, *n*-butyl ester at 155 mg/kg/day, and isooctyl ester at 186 mg/kg/day) had no effect on the incidence of cleft palate or fetal mortality, but did affect fetal weight. A significant increase in cleft palate was found, however, after administration of the propylene glycol butyl ether ester at 195 mg/kg/day.

A statistically significant increase in the proportion of abnormal fetuses was reported in mice that received maximally tolerated subcutaneous doses of the isooctyl ester, and two isopropyl esters of 2,4-D (130, 100, and 94 μg/kg, respectively), in dimethyl sulfoxide (DMSO) solution (Mrak, 1969). DMSO itself, however, is a teratogen (Caujolle *et al.*, 1967).

Bage *et al.* (1973) observed teratogenic and embryotoxic effects in NMRI mice that received 50- or 110-mg/kg injections of 2,4-D on days 6–14 of gestation.

Pregnant rats were treated orally with 2,4-D at 12.5, 25, 50, 75, and 87.5 mg/kg/day (maximal tolerated dose) or equimolar doses of propylene glycol butyl ether ester of 2,4-D up to 142 mg/kg/day or isooctyl ester of 2,4-D up to 131 mg/kg/day on days 6–15 of gestation (Schwetz *et al.*,

TABLE VI-1 Toxicity of 2,4-D

Species	Duration of Study	Dosage Levels and No. of Animals Per Group	Highest No-Adverse-Effect Level or Lowest-Minimal-Effect Level	Effect Measured	Reference
Dog	13 weeks	0–14 mg/kg/day 4 animals/group	7.1 mg/kg/day	no toxic effect	Drill and Hiratzka, 1953
Dog			8.0 mg/kg/day	no toxic effect	Lehman, 1965
Dog	2 yr	0–500 ppm in diet 6 animals/group	500 ppm (12.5 mg/kg/day)[c,d]	no toxic effect	Hansen *et al.*, 1971
Rat	4 weeks	0–300 mg/kg/day 5–6 females/group	30 mg/kg/day	no toxic effect	Rowe and Hymas, 1954
Rat	days 6–15 of gestation	0–87.5 mg/kg/day 14–19 females/group	25 mg/kg/day	no fetotoxic effect	Schwetz *et al.*, 1971
Rat	2 yr	0–1,250 ppm in diet 50 animals/group	1,250 ppm (62.5 mg/kg/day)[d]	no toxic effect	Hansen *et al.*, 1971

Using an uncertainty factor of 1,000, the suggested no-adverse-effect level in drinking water is calculated as follows:

$$\frac{12.5}{1000} = 0.0125 \text{ mg/kg/day (ADI)},\ 0.0125 \times 70^{a} \times 0.1^{b} = 0.09 \text{ mg/liter}$$

[a]Assume average weight of human adult = 70 kg.
[b]Assume average daily intake of water for man = 2 liters, and that 20 percent of total intake is from water.
[c]Value from which the suggested no-adverse-effect level was calculated.
[d]Assume weight of rat = 0.4 kg and of dog = 10 kg; assume average daily food consumption of rat = 0.02 kg and of dog = 0.25 kg.

1971). Fetotoxic responses were seen at the high dosages, but teratogenic effects were not seen at any dosage. The authors suggested that the no-adverse effect dosage of 2,4-D (or the molar equivalent, in the case of the esters) was 25 mg/kg/day.

Prenatal studies on 2,4-D in Wistar rats showed that it induced fetotoxic effects and an increased incidence of skeletal anomalies after single oral doses of 100–150 mg/kg/day on days 6–15 of gestation (Khera and McKinley, 1972). At the highest dosage of 150 mg/kg/day, the isooctyl ester, and butyl ester, and butoxyethynol and dimethylamine salts of 2,4-D were all associated with significantly increased teratologic incidence. The butyl and isooctyl esters also tended to decrease fetal weight. At a lower dosage, 2,4-D and its salts and esters induced no apparent harmful effects.

Pregnant hamsters received technical 2,4-D (three samples) at 20, 40, 60, and 100 mg/kg/day orally on days 6–10 of gestation (Collins and Williams, 1971). Terata were produced occasionally with 2,4-D, and the fetal viability per litter decreased; but neither effect was clearly dose-related. The lowest dose causing fetal anomalies with the three technical 2,4-D samples was 60 mg/kg/day.

Conclusions and Recommendations

The acute toxicity of 2,4-D is moderate. No-adverse-effect doses for 2,4-D were up to 62.5 mg/kg/day and 10 mg/kg/day in rats and dogs, respectively. Based on these data, an ADI was calculated at 0.0125 mg/kg/day. The available data on subchronic and chronic toxicity and calculations of ADI are summarized in Table VI-1.

The acceptable daily intake of 2,4-D has been established at 0.3 mg/kg by FAO/WHO. On the basis of electron-capture gas chromatography, the detection limit for 2,4-D in water is 1 ppb.

There are substantial disagreements in the results of subchronic and chronic toxicity studies with 2,4-D, perhaps reflecting the use of different formulations or preparations. In view of these deficiencies and the variability of the results, additional, properly constituted toxicity studies should be undertaken.

2,4,5-T AND TCDD

Introduction

2,4,5-T, or 2,4,5-trichlorophenoxyacetic acid, was introduced in 1944 as a translocated, selective herbicide; it is applied after emergence and is effective on woody plants (Spencer, 1973; Thomson, 1975; Weed Society of America, 1974). 2,4,5-T and its salts and esters are registered in the United States for noncrop areas, especially on woody plants, pastures, and rangelands (Thomson, 1975). It is still used for weed control on rice and sugarcane. The 1971 U.S. production of 2,4,5-T and its derivatives is estimated at 6 million pounds (NAS, 1975).

2,4,5-T is produced by interaction of 2,4,5-trichlorophenol with the sodium salt of monochloroacetic acid (Spencer, 1973). Esters of 2,4,5-T are synthesized by esterification of the acid with the appropriate alkyl alcohol. The solubility of 2,4,5-T in water at 25°C is 278 ppm (Spencer, 1973); 2,4,5-T salts are water-soluble, but the esters are generally insoluble.

2,4,5-T is more stable than 2,4-D. The 2,4,5-T esters are rapidly hydrolyzed after spraying, and the 2,4,5-T is then further decomposed by bacterial action. The major product of 2,4,5-T photodecomposition is 2,4,5-trichlorophenol (Crosby and Wong, 1971). Other products identified including 4,6-dichlororesorcinol, 4-chlororesorcinol, 2,5-dichlorophenol, 2-hydroxy-4,5-dichlorophenoxyacetic acid, and 2,4,5-trichloroanisole.

2,4,5-T is rapidly adsorbed onto particulate matter or broken down in water. Nevertheless, in the period 1965–1968, 2,4,5-T was detected in surface water at concentrations of 0.01–0.07 ppb (Johnson, 1971).

Very little 2,4,5-T was found in food in analyses of raw agricultural products and in the Market Basket Survey samples (Advisory Committee on 2,4,5-T, 1971). Of about 10,000 food and feed samples examined from 1964 to 1969, only 25 contained trace amounts of 2,4,5-T (less than 0.1 ppm), and only two contained measurable amounts (0.19 and 0.29 ppm). The Advisory Committee on 2,4,5-T (1971) concluded that 2,4,5-T did not accumulate in the biosphere and that the risk of human exposure in food, air, or water was negligible.

Technical 2,4,5-T contains traces of the highly toxic compound 2,3,7,8-tetrachlorodibenzo-p-dioxin (TCDD) as an impurity (Advisory Committee on 2,4,5-T, 1971). In addition, about 0.0002% of 2,4,5-T is converted to TCDD when wood or brush containing 2,4,5-T is burned (Stehl and Lauparski, 1974). 2,4,5-T preparations formerly contained TCDD at 1–80 ppm, a concentration sufficiently high to cause chloracne in industrial workers and to impart specific toxic properties that were characteristic of TCDD to the 2,4,5-T. It has not been feasible to eliminate TCDD completely from technical 2,4,5-T, but it is now reported to be present in commercial 2,4,5-T at less than 0.1 ppm (Advisory Committee on 2,4,5-T, 1971).

Water transport of TCDD is limited, because it is soluble in water at only 0.2 ppb (Advisory Committee on 2,4,5-T, 1971). TCDD is decomposed photochemically (Crosby *et al.*, 1971, 1973). It is firmly bound to soil, where it tends to persist for more than a year.

The Advisory Committee on 2,4,5-T (1971) concluded that there was no indication that TCDD accumulates in air, water, or plants, although it might accumulate in soils after heavy applications of 2,4,5-T.

Metabolism

2,4,5-T is readily absorbed and rapidly excreted by animals, including man. Rats and pigs given single 100-mg/kg doses of the amine salt of 2,4,5-T showed plasma half-lives of 3 and 10 h, respectively (Erne, 1966a,b). There was little buildup in tissues, and the compound was excreted mainly in the urine.

During the first 24 h, 75% of the radioactivity was excreted in the urine and 8.2% in the feces of female Wistar rats that had been given 0.17, 4.3, and 41 mg/kg orally of ^{14}C-carbonyl labeled 2,4,5-T (Fang *et al.*, 1973). No ^{14}C was found in the expired air. Radioactivity was detected in all tissues, with the highest concentration appearing in the kidneys. Radioactivity was detected in the fetuses of pregnant rats, and the average half-life of 2,4,5-T radioactivity in the organs was 3.4 h for the adult rats and 97 h for the newborns.

The half-life values for the clearance of carbon-14 activity from the plasma of rats given single oral doses of ^{14}C-carboxyl-labeled 2,4,5-T at 4, 50, 100, and 200 mg/kg were 4.7, 4.2, 19.4, and 25.2 h, respectively (Piper *et al.*, 1973). Half-lives for elimination from the body were 13.6, 13.1, 19.3, and 28.9 h, respectively. Cumulative excretion over a 144 h period was 82.6, 92.9, 78.3, and 68.4% of the administered dose of 5, 50, 100, and 200 mg/kg, respectively. A small amount of an unidentified metabolite was detected in the urine at the two highest dosages.

In dogs given ^{14}C-carboxyl-labeled 2,4,5-T at 5 mg/kg, half-life values for clearance and from the body were 77.0 and 86.6 h, respectively (Piper *et al.*, 1973). This low rate of clearance may explain why 2,4,5-T is more toxic in dogs than in rats. Some 42% of the dose was elimated in the urine and 20% in the feces over a 9-day period. Three unidentified metabolites were found in the urine.

Five human male volunteers ingested a single 5-mg/kg dose of 2,4,5-T that contained TCDD at less than 0.05 ppm (Gehring *et al.*, 1973). Clearance of 2,4,5-T from the plasma and its excretion from the body occurred with a half-life of 23.1 h. Essentially all the 2,4,5-T was absorbed and excreted unchanged in the urine.

After oral administration of 2,4,5-T to rats and mice, the unchanged herbicide was the main excretion product in the urine (Grunow *et al.*, 1971; Grunow and Bohme, 1974). Other urinary metabolites were identified as the glycine and taurine conjugates of 2,4,5-T, as well as 2,4,5-trichlorophenol. In addition to 2,4,5-T, 2,4,5-trichlorophenol residues appeared in the tissues of sheep and cattle fed the herbicide (Clark *et al.*, 1975).

After a single oral 1-μg/kg dose of ^{14}C-labeled TCDD in rats, radioactivity was found only in the feces, and the half-life of radioactivity in the body was 30.4 days (Rose *et al.*, 1976). Liver and fat contained carbon-14 concentrations ten times greater than those in other tissues examined 22 days after ingestion. The carbon-14 activity in the liver was associated with TCDD. TCDD reaches essentially steady-state concentrations after 90 days of daily exposure, and that period is independent of the administered dose for the range of 0.01-1.0 μg/kg/day. TCDD is excreted primarily via the feces; only 4.5% of the radioactivity from an oral dose of labeled TCDD was eliminated in urine during 21 days (Allen *et al.*, 1975). A large percentage of the radioactivity remaining in the body at the end of this period was in the liver—over 90% within the microsomal fraction. TCDD apparently undergoes little if any metabolism (Fullerton *et al.*, 1974).

Health Aspects

Observations in Man Data compiled by Dow Chemical Company showed that 126 manufacturing personnel exposed to 2,4,5-T at an estimated 1.6–8.1 mg/day (0.02–0.12 mg/kg/day) for periods of up to 3 yr developed no herbicide-related illness (Advisory Committee on 2,4,5-T, 1971).

The results were entirely different in another plant, where the 2,4,5-T produced contained a high proportion of TCDD (Bleibey *et al.*, 1964; Poland *et al.*, 1971); 18% of the men suffered moderate to severe chloracne, and several cases of porphyria were found. Chromosomal analysis of 52 workers exposed for various periods up to 960 days to 2,4,5-T (containing TCDD at $<$1 ppm) at 1.6–8.1 mg/day failed to show any abnormalities (Johnson, 1971).

Observations in Other Species

Acute Effects Rowe and Hymas (1954) reviewed the early toxicologic information on 2,4,5-T and concluded that the oral LD_{50} for male rats, male mice, guinea pigs, and chicks were 500, 389, 381, and 310 mg/kg, respectively. They also concluded that the acute toxicity of the butyl, isopropyl, and amyl esters of 2,4,5-T in the rat, guinea pig, and chicken was all greater than that listed above. Johnson (1971) has reported acute oral toxicity studies with commercial 2,4,5-T in which the LD_{50} were 500 mg/kg in the rat and 380 mg/kg in the guinea pig. The oral LD_{50} of 2,4,5-T in the dog was greater than 100 mg/kg (Drill and Hiratzka, 1953). It is not clear, however, how much TCDD contamination was present in the 2,4,5-T used in these studies.

TCDD is extremely toxic, as shown by oral LD_{50} values ranging between 0.6 and 115 μg/kg for several animal species (Schwetz, 1973). In the rat, oral LD_{50}s were 22 and 45 μg/kg for males and females, respectively, with death occurring 9-47 days after administration. The guinea pig was much more sensitive, with LD_{50} values of 0.6 and 2.1 μg/kg for males and females, respectively. Limited data showed that dogs were less sensitive to TCDD than rabbits. The LD_{50} for TCDD was 114 μg/kg in 3-month-old male C57B1/6 mice (Vos *et al.*, 1974).

Rats that received a single 100 μg/kg dose of TCDD showed 43% mortality, severe liver damage, thymic atrophy, and icterus (Gupta *et al.*, 1973). Animals given 50 and 25 μg/kg showed severe and moderate thymic atrophy and liver damage. In guinea pigs given 3.0 μg/kg, there was a 90% mortality, the appearance of hemorrhage, atrophy of adrenal zona glomerulosa, and depletion of lymphoid organs.

Female rats given a single oral dose of TCDD of up to 300 μg/kg showed delayed mortality over a 90-day period (Greig *et al.*, 1973). It was not possible to estimate an LD_{50} value, because of the irregular distribution of deaths in the treatment groups. The mean time to death was 40.4 days for animals that received 200 μg/kg. The animals lost weight, and significant changes in liver constitution appeared after 3 days. The liver showed pathologic changes in later periods, particularly the formation of multinucleate parenchymal cells. Gastric hemorrhage and jaundice also were common. Pericardial edema and death in chickens followed a single oral dose of 25–50 μg/kg.

Subchronic and Chronic Effects In work by Dow Chemical Co. reported in 1961 (Advisory Committee on 2,4,5-T, 1971), the monopropylene, dipropylene, and tripropylene glycol butyl ether esters of 2,4,5-T were administered orally to rats over a 90-day period at up to 186 mg of 2,4,5-T/kg/day. At the highest dosage and at 62 mg/kg/day, toxicity was observed, but no deleterious effects were seen at dosages of 18.6 and 6.2 mg/kg/day.

Ninety-day feeding studies with 2,4,5-T containing TCDD at 0.5 ppm were reported in 1970 by McCollister and Kociba (Advisory Committee on 2,4,5-T, 1971). The herbicide was administered to rats at 3, 10, 30, and 100 mg/kg/day. No adverse effects were observed in animals that received 30 mg/kg/day or less, but growth was decreased and changes in serum enzyme concentrations were observed at 100 mg/kg/day.

Maternal mice given four to eight doses of a technical preparation containing 97.9% 2,4,5-T at 120 mg/kg/day often developed myocardial lesions, hypocellularity of the bone marrow, and depletion of lymphocytes in the thymus, spleen, or lymph nodes (Highman and Schumacher, 1974). To determine whether the previous effects were due to 2,4,5-T alone or to TCDD, further studies were conducted in which female mice received, on nine successive days, either technical 2,4,5-T or a purified preparation of 2,4,5-T orally at 60 and 120 mg/kg/day (Highman *et al.*, 1975). All mice given 60 mg/kg and some of which given 120 mg/kg appeared normal at sacrifice and showed little or no pathologic change. Mice susceptible to 120 mg/kg became ill or moribund after one to eight doses, and few survived 11 days; 34 of 66 moribund mice given the technical and 23 of 31 given the purified 2,4,5-T had myocardial lesions, and more showed lesions in other organs. These findings support the view that the lesions are due primarily to 2,4,5-T, rather than to dioxins in the technical preparation.

Drill and Hiratzka (1953) found no adverse effects in dogs that were fed 2,4,5-T five times a week for 90 days at 2.5 and 10 mg/kg. Four dogs treated at 20 mg/kg died during the experiment.

A study was conducted in which rats received TCDD at 0.001, 0.01, 0.1, or 1.0 μg/kg 5 days a week for 13 weeks (Kociba *et al.*, 1976). No discernible adverse effect occurred in rats that received 0.01 or 0.001 μg/kg TCDD, but 0.1 μg/kg caused degenerative changes in the liver and thymus, porphyria, altered serum enzyme concentrations, and loss in body weight.

Four-month-old male C57B1/6 mice received TCDD at 0.2, 1.0, 5.0, and 25 μg/kg orally once a week for 2 or 6 weeks (Vos *et al.*, 1974). Some deaths and growth retardation occurred in the 25-μg/kg group. Significantly increased liver and decreased thymus weights were found in the 1.0, 5.0, and 25-μg/kg groups. Total neutrophils were increased significantly, whereas hemoglobin values and mean corpuscular hemoglobin concentrations were decreased significantly after six doses of 25 μg/kg. Total serum proteins and globulins also were decreased. TCDD was porphyrogenic, probably as a result of liver damage. At the lowest dosage, 0.2 μg/kg, slight but consistent centrilobular fatty changes were observed in the liver.

Gross pathologic and histopathologic examinations were performed on rats, guinea pigs, and mice that received daily or weekly treatments with

TCDD for up to 8 weeks (Gupta *et al.*, 1973). In rats and guinea pigs, the dose ranged from a no-adverse-effect dose to one that produced death. Lymphoid organs, primarily the thymus, were consistently affected over a wide range of dosage in all species examined. Thymic atrophy is a very sensitive index of TCDD exposure. The severity of liver pathology was quite variable between species, the most severe effects being found in the rat and the degenerative and necrotic changes being markedly lower in the guinea pig and mouse.

Surprisingly, no adequate chronic toxicity tests have been conducted with 2,4,5-T. In a long-term exposure study, mice received 21.5 mg/kg daily from the first through the fourth week and thereafter received 60 ppm (equivalent to 9 mg/kg) in the diet until 18 months had elapsed (Innes *et al.*, 1969). It is presumed that all animals survived the test period, but this was not stated.

Dogs and rats are said to tolerate oral intake of 2,4,5-T at 10 mg/kg/day for long periods (Advisory Committee on 2,4,5-T, 1971).

Mutagenicity 2,4,5-T was unable to induce point mutations in four different microbial systems (Anderson *et al.*, 1972). Buselmaier *et al.* (1972) conducted host-mediated assays in NMRI mice with mutants of *Salmonella typhimurium* and *Serratia marcescens* and produced no mutagenic effect with 2,4,5-T at 500 mg/kg or the *n*-butyl ester of 2,4,5-T at 1,000 mg/kg. These investigators also reported on dominant lethal tests in NMRI mice; no adverse effect was noted with 2,4,5-T at 1,000 mg/kg. The herbicide had no mutagenic effect in *Drosophila melanogaster* (Vogel and Chandler, 1974). Inhibition of mitosis and the development of abnormalities in plants by 2,4,5-T formulations have been shown to be due to TCDD contamination (Jackson, 1972).

A great number of chromosomal abnormalities were induced in bone marrow cells of gerbils given 2,4,5-T at 150, 250, or 350 mg/kg (Majumdai and Hall, 1973).

Khera and Ruddick (1973) conducted dominant lethal tests in which male Wistar rats received TCDD orally at 4 or 8 μg/kg/day for 7 days. Later reproduction studies failed to show any dominant lethal mutations during 35 days after treatment. TCDD is apparently negative in a mutagenicity test with *Salmonella typhimurium* (Fullerton *et al.*, 1974). It also appears to have no potential for producing chromosomal aberrations in the bone marrow of male rats (Green and Moreland, 1975).

Although many reports indicate that TCDD is not mutagenic, Hussain *et al.* (1972) reported that TCDD is strongly mutagenic in various bacterial systems.

Carcinogenicity No significant increase in the incidence of tumors was seen in two strains of mice that received 2,4,5-T (containing TCDD at approximately 30 ppm) at 21.5 mg/kg/day from the end of the first week through the fourth week and at 60 ppm in the diet thereafter until the age of 18 months (Innes *et al.*, 1969).

In one experiment, intraperitoneal injections of TCDD at 1 and 10 mg/kg induced liver lesions that "appeared to be malignant" (Buu-Hoi *et al.*, 1972). The significance of this report is highly questionable, because the lowest TCDD dose was almost 50 times greater than the oral LD_{50} for female rats (Sparschu *et al.*, 1971).

Intraperitoneal 2,4,5-T at 50 mg/kg/day for 5 days inhibited *in vivo* development of Ehrlich ascites tumor in mice (Walker *et al.*, 1972).

Teratogenicity The results of a study by Bionetics Research Laboratories released in 1969 indicated that 2,4,5-T was teratogenic in two stocks of mice 113 mg/kg/day when given during organogenesis (Courtney *et al.*, 1970). Cleft palate, cystic kidneys, intestinal hemorrhage, and fetal mortality occurred in higher percentages of treated than of control mice, although a clear dose–response relation was not evident at low dosages. The 2,4,5-T sample used in this study contained TCDD at 27 ± 8 ppm, and TCDD itself is a teratogen.

To clarify these results, additional sudies were conducted on rats, mice, hamsters, rabbits, sheep, and rhesus monkeys with samples of 2,4,5-T containing varying concentrations of TCDD. No maternal effects, no increases in prenatal mortality, and no fetal malformations resulted when Sprague–Dawley rats were given daily oral doses of a 2,4,5-T preparation containing TCDD at 0.5 ppm on days 5–15 of gestation at up to 24 mg/kg (Emerson *et al.*, 1971). Slight impairment of fetal growth was observed at the highest dosage, i.e., 24 mg/kg/day. In another study by the same group (Johnson, 1971), female rats received were given a 2,4,5-T preparation containing TCDD at 0.5 ppm daily on days 6–15 of gestation at 50 and 100 mg/kg or on days 6–10 at 100 mg/kg. The only effects noted at the lower dosage were one case of intestinal hemorrhage and a slight increase in the frequency of delayed ossification of skull bones. Maternal deaths and reabsorptions occurred at 100 mg/kg/day.

2,4,5-T containing TCDD at 0.5 ppm TCDD was teratogenic in Charles River rats at 80 mg/kg/day, but no fetal or maternal effects were found when the animals received 50 mg/kg/day (Courtney and Moore, 1971). In Wistar rats, 2,4,5-T containing TCDD at less than 0.5 ppm induced fetopathy and increased incidence of skeletal anomalies after daily oral doses of 100–150 mg/kg on days 6–15 of gestation (Khera and McKinley, 1972).

Rats were given 50 mg/kg/day "pure" 2,4,5-T (probably containing TCDD at 0.05 ppm) to which TCDD was added at 0.01, 0.03, 0.06, 0.125, 0.5, or 1.0 μg/kg/day, on days 6-15 of gestation. Cleft palate occurred in some fetuses, mainly the ones that received the 2,4,5-T with TCDD added at 0.5 mg/kg/day (Advisory Committee on 2,4,5-T, 1971).

Teratogenic and embryotoxic effects were seen when NMRI mice were given 2,4,5-T at 50 and 110 mg/kg/day subcutaneously on days 6-14 of gestation (Bage et al., 1973).

Moore (cited by the Advisory Committee on 2,4,5-T, 1971) found no appreciable difference in teratogenic and embryolethal potency between 2,4,5-T as the free acid and its butyl, isooctyl, and butyl ether esters.

Konstantinova (1974) observed embryotoxic effects and maternal toxicity including CNS and hematologic effects after feeding 0.1, 0.42, and 4.2 mg/kg/day of 2,4,5-T butyl ester (0.082, 0.34, 3.4 mg 2,4,5-T equivalent/kg/day) to pregnant albino rats during their entire pregnancy. The no-adverse-effect level was reported to be 0.01 mg/kg/day (0.0082 mg 2,4,5-T equivalent/kg/day).

Studies in CD1, C57Bl/6J, and DBA/2J mice strains dosed with 50, 100, 113, 125, or 150 mg/ kg/day of 2,4,5-T containing <1, 0.5, or <0.05 ppm TCDD on days 6–15 of gestation showed some teratogenicity at dosages of 100 mg/kg/day in all three herbicide samples (Courtney and Moore, 1971). Maternal weight was depressed in the C57Bl strain at 100 mg/kg and increased fetal mortality was observed only in CD1 mice at 150 mg/kg.

In another study by the Bionetics Research Laboratories (Advisory Committee on 2,4,5-T, 1971), CD1 mice were given 2,4,5-T from two sources (both containing TCDD at <0.5 ppm) at 100 mg/kg/day subcutaneously on days 6–15 of gestation. Mean fetal weights were slightly reduced, and there was an increased incidence of cleft palate.

The teratogenic effect of technical 2,4,5-T was studied in large numbers of C57Bl/6, C3H-He, CALB/C, and A/JAX inbred strains and CL-1 stock micc (Gaines *et al.*, 1975). The animals were given daily oral doses of 2,4,5-T at 15-120 mg/kg on days 6–14 of gestation. A dosage of 15 mg/kg was teratogenic in A/JAX mice, whereas the other strains and the CD-1 mice showed teratogenicity at 30 mg/kg, the lowest dosage tested. Significant differences in types and frequencies of malformations were observed between the different mice strains.

With the dose–response relationship for the production of cleft palate in mouse fetuses, the ED_{50} single dose of 2,4,5-T (containing TCDD at <0.02 ppm) for NMRI mice was estimated to be 2,000 mg/kg/day (Neubert *et al.*, 1973).

Golden hamsters were treated orally on days 6-10 of gestation with

2,4,5-T at 20-110 mg/kg/day. The 2,4,5-T had seven sources that contained no detectable TCDD or TCDD at 34, 2.9, 0.5, and 0.1 ppm (Collins and Williams, 1971). 2,4,5-T was feticidal and teratogenic in the hamsters, with the incidence and severity of effects increasing with TCDD content. Significantly reduced fetal viability was observed with 2,4,5-T at 20 and 40 mg/kg/day and either no detectable TCDD or 0.5 ppm, whereas significantly increased fetal abnormalities were seen with the same 2,4,5-T samples at 80 and 100 mg/kg/day.

In studies with rabbits (Emerson *et al.*, 1971), no maternal or fetal effects were seen at 2,4,5-T dosages of 40 mg/kg/day.

In a study conducted in Sweden (Advisory Committee on 2,4,5-T, 1971), pregnant rhesus monkeys received 2,4,5-T (containing TCDD at 0.5 ppm) at levels of 5, 10, 20, and 40 mg/kg 3 times a week for 4 weeks between days 20 and 48 of gestation. There were no maternal effects, and all fetuses were apparently normal. Similar effects were seen in rhesus monkeys that received doses of 0.05, 1.0 and 10 mg/kg/day of 2,4,5-T (containing less than 0.05 ppm TCDD) on days 22 through 38 of gestation (Dougherty *et al.*, 1975).

TCDD proved to be a potent fetotoxic agent in various animal species. Fetal weights were slightly decreased and there was a slight increase in intestinal hemorrhage and edema in fetuses from Sprague–Dawley rats that had received TCDD at 0.125 μg/kg/day (Sparschu *et al.*, 1971). The number of fetuses was reduced and fetal death was increased at 0.5 μg/kg/day. No teratogenic effects were seen at 0.03 μg/kg/day.

Fetal kidney malformations were observed when Charles River rats received TCDD subcutaneously at 0.5 μg/kg/day on day 9, day 10, or days 13 and 14 of gestation (Courtney and Moore, 1971).

A low frequency of cleft palate and kidney abnormalities was observed in three mouse lines that received TCDD at 1.0 or 3.0 μg/kg/day (Courtney and Moore, 1971). With a dose–response relationship, Neubert *et al.* (1973) estimated that the ED_{50} causing cleft palate in fetuses was 40 μg/kg/day for NMRI mice. The "just nonteratogenic dose" for days 6–15 of gestation was estimated at 2 μg/kg/day for this mouse strain.

Gastrointestinal hemorrhage was noted in hamster fetuses after administration of TCDD at 0.5 μg/kg/day on days 6–10 of gestation (Advisory Committee on 2,4,5-T, 1971).

Conclusions and Recommendations

Although pure 2,4,5-T is moderately toxic, contamination of the herbicide with TCDD, which is very toxic, greatly increases the toxicity. No-adverse-effect doses were: for 2,4,5-T, 10 mg/kg/day in dogs and mice and up to 30 mg/kg/day in rats; and for TCDD, 0.01 μg/kg/day in rats. Based on these data ADI's were calculated at 0.1 mg/kg/day for 2,4,5-T and 10^{-4} μg/kg/day for TCDD. The available data on chronic 2,4,5-T and TCDD toxicity and calculations of ADI's are summarized in Tables VI-2 and VI-3.

There are substantial differences in the reported toxicity of 2,4,5-T, probably because of varying degrees of contamination with TCDD. A number of the subchronic, carcinogenicity, etc., studies should be repeated with 2,4,5-T of very high purity. Apparently, no adequate 2-yr chronic-toxicity studies have been conducted with 2,4,5-T, and 2-yr feeding studies are needed. The data available are largely from relatively short-term exposure experiments; these data, however, are fairly consistent. An exception is the Russian study in rats that reported toxic effects in mothers and their pups at extremely low maternal doses of 2,4,5-T butyl ester and a no-adverse-effect dosage only one-thousandth as high as that found by other investigators. The 2,4,5-T butyl ester used by Konstantinova may have been heavily contaminated with TCDD, but the reason for this large discrepancy is still unexplained and should be resolved.

2,4,5-TP AND MCPA

Introduction

2,4,5-TP, or 2,4,5-trichlorophenoxypropionic acid (Silvex), was introduced in 1952 as a selective herbicide for both before and after emergence (USEPA, 1975k; Spencer, 1973; Thomson, 1975; Weed Society of America, 1974). It is available as the amine as well as sodium salts and various esters. The U.S. production is estimated at 3 million pounds per year in 1971 (NAS, 1975) and 3.7–4.1 million pounds per year currently (USEPA, 1975k).

MCPA, or 2-methyl-4-chlorophenoxyacetic acid, was introduced in 1945 as a selective, translocated, postemergence herbicide (USEPA, 1975f; Spencer, 1973; Thomson, 1975; Weed Society of America, 1974). It is formulated as amine salts and low-volatility esters. Estimated domestic use of MCPA in 1973 was 3.5–4.5 million pounds (USEPA, 1975f).

2,4,5-TP is produced by reaction of 2,4,5-trichlorophenol with the sodium salt of α-chloropropionic acid (USEPA, 1975k). Commercial 2,4,5-TP contains TCDD at 0.1 ppm or less. It is soluble in water at 180 ppm at 25°C (Weed Science Society of America, 1974).

MCPA is manufactured by chlorination of o-cresol to form 2-methyl-4-

TABLE VI-2 Toxicity of 2,4,5-T and Esters

Species	Duration of Study	Dosage Levels and No. of Animals Per Group	Highest No-Adverse-Effect Level or Lowest-Minimal-Effect Level	Effect Measured	Reference
2,4,5-T					
Human	up to 3 yr	(126 manufacturing personnel)	0.02–0.12 mg/kg/day	no toxic effect	Advisory Committee on 2,4,5-T, 1971
Dog	90 days	0–20 mg/kg/day, 4 animals/group	10 mg/kg/day[c]	no toxic effect	Drill and Hiratzka, 1953
Dog			10 mg/kg/day[d]	tolerated	Advisory Committee on 2,4,5-T, 1971
Rat			10 mg/kg/day[d]	tolerated	Advisory Committee on 2,4,5-T, 1971
Mouse	days 6–14 of gestation	0–120 mg/kg/day 236–1,485 females/group[e]	15 mg/kg/day	teratogenicity	Gaines *et al.*, 1971
Hamster	days 6–10 of gestation	0–100 mg/kg/day 6 females/group[f]	20 mg/kg/day	reduced fetal viability	Collins and Williams, 1971

Rat	days 6–15 of gestation	0–24 mg/kg/day 25 females/ group[f]	24 mg/kg/day	depressed fetal growth	Emerson *et al.*, 1971
Rat	90 days	0–100 mg/kg/day 20 animals/ group[f]	30 mg/kg/day	no toxic effect	Johnson, 1971
2,4,5-T esters					
Rat	fed through entire pregnancy	0–3.4 mg/kg/day	0.01 mg/kg/day	no toxic effect	Konstantinova, 1974
Rat	90 days	0–186 mg/kg/day	18.6 mg/kg/day	no toxic effect	Advisory Committee on 2,4,5-T, 1971

Using an uncertainty factor of 100, the suggested no-adverse-effect level in drinking water is calculated as follows:

$$\frac{10}{100} = 0.1 \text{ mg/kg/day (ADI)}, \; 0.1 \times 70^{a} \times 0.1^{b} = 0.7 \text{ mg/liter}$$

[a]Assume average weight of human adult = 70 kg.
[b]Assume average daily intake of water for man = 2 liters, and that 20 percent of total intake is from water.
[c]Value from which the suggested no-adverse-effect level was calculated.
[d]Unknown TCDD content.
[e]TCDD content estimated at 0.1 ppm.
[f]TCDD content at 0.5 ppm.

TABLE VI-3 Toxicity of TCDD

Species	Duration of Study	Dosage Levels and No. of Animals Per Group	Highest No-Adverse-Effect Level or Lowest-Minimal-Effect Level	Effect Measured	Reference
Rat	13 weeks	0, 0.001, 0.01, 0.1, 1.0 μg/kg/day (12 males and 12 females)	0.01 μg/kg/day[c]	no toxic effect	Kociba *et al.*, 1976
Mouse	6 weeks	0, 0.2, 1.0, 0.14, 5.0, 0.71, 25 μg/kg/week (18–24 males)	0.2 μg/kg/week	liver pathology	Vos *et al.*, 1974
Rat	6–15 days	0, 0.03, 0.125, 0.5, 2.0, 8.0 μg/kg/day (10–31 females)	0.03 μg/kg/day	no toxic effect	Sparschu *et al.*, 1971

Using an uncertainty factor of 100, the suggested no-adverse-effect level in drinking water is calculated as follows:

$$\frac{0.01}{100} = 0.0001\ \mu g/kg/day\ (\text{ADI}),\ 0.0001 \times 70^{a} \times 0.1^{b} = 0.0007\ \mu g/liter$$

[a]Assume average weight of human adult = 70 kg.

[b]Assume average daily intake of water for man = 2 liters, and that 20 percent of total intake is from water.

[c]Value from which the suggested no-adverse-effect drinking-water level was calculated.

chlorophenol, and then coupling with monochloroacetic acid (USEPA, 1975f). Technical MCPA has a typical composition of: MCPA, 94–96%; 2-methyl-6-chlorophenoxyacetic acid, 1.5–3.0%; a mixture of 2-methyl-4,6-dichlorophenoxyacetic acid, 2-methylphenoxyacetic acid, 2-chlorophenoxyacetic acid, 4-chlorophenoxyacetic acid, and 2,6-dimethyl-4-chlorophenoxyacetic 0.5–1.5%; chloro-*o*-cresol, 0.5%; and water, 1.0%.

In the FDA Market Basket Survey during 1965-1968, 2,4,5-TP and MCPA were detected at maximal concentrations of less than 0.1 ppm and 0.4 ppm, respectively (Johnson, 1971). During the same period, 2,4,5-TP residues in surface waters from 15 western states ranged between 0.01 and 0.21 ppb. 2,4,5-TP was also detected in the finished water (USEPA, 1976d). The EPA has set an interim standard for 2,4,5-TP in finished water of 0.01 mg/liter (USEPA, 1975i).

Metabolism

The tissue distributions of 2,4,5-TP and its metabolite, 2,4,5-trichlorophenol, were determined in adult sheep and cattle fed for 28 days a diet containing 2,4,5-TP at 300, 1,000, and 2,000 ppm (Clark *et al.*, 1975). Significant residues of both were found only in the liver and kidneys of the treated animals.

The metabolism of MCPA has not been studied extensively, but a metabolite, 2-methyl-4-chlorophenol, was detected in milk of dairy cows and in kidneys of sheep and cattle (USEPA, 1975f). Some unaltered MCPA was detected in the milk, liver, and kidneys of dairy cows.

Health Aspects

Observations in Man No available data.

Observations in Other Species

Acute Effects The oral LD_{50} of 2,4,5-TP is reported to be 650 mg/kg and 500 mg/kg in rats (Toxic Substances List, 1974; Rowe and Hymas, 1954) and 850 mg/kg in guinea pigs. In rats and rabbits, the oral LD_{50} of the mixed butyl esters and propylene glycol esters ranged between 500 and 1,000 mg/kg (Rowe and Hymas, 1954).

The oral LD_{50} of MCPA is 700–1,410 mg/kg in rats, and 560 mg/kg in mice (Toxic Substances List, 1974; Vershuuren *et al.*, 1975), 550 mg/kg in female guinea pigs, 813 mg/kg in female rabbits, and 940 mg/kg in female chickens. LD_{50} values in the rat and mouse by intraperitoneal administration are 400 and 500 mg/kg, respectively.

Subchronic and Chronic Effects The propylene glycol butyl ether ester of Silvex (Kuron) was fed to male and female rats in the diet at 10, 30, 100, 300, and 600 mg/kg/day for 90 days (Mullison, 1966; USEPA, 1975k). Mortalities were observed at 600 mg/kg/day, growth decrease at 300 and 600 mg/kg/day, and increased liver weight at 30 mg/kg/day and above. No toxic effect was found in animals receiving 10 mg/kg/day.

In another 90-day study (Mullsion, 1966; USEPA, 1975k), male and female rats received the sodium salt of 2,4,5-TP in the diet at 100, 300, 1,000, 3,000, and 10,000 ppm. Growth was decreased at 300 ppm (277 ppm 2,4,5-TP equivalent) and above, and liver weight was increased at 100 ppm (2,4,5-TP equivalent, 92 ppm). Histopathologic examination showed liver and kidney damage at all dietary concentrations, except that the kidneys of females were not affected at 100 ppm.

Beagles were fed Kurosol SI (a formulation containing the potassium salt of 2,4,5-TP at 60%, or the equivalent of 2,4-TP at 53%) of 100, 300, and 1,000 ppm for 89 days (Mullison, 1966; USEPA, 1975k). No adverse effects were noted at 100 ppm or 300 ppm (2,4,5-TP equivalents 53 or 160 ppm), but growth decrease occurred at 1,000 ppm in females.

In a 90-day feeding study of MCPA in rats, growth retardation and increased kidney:body-weight ratios were observed at 400 ppm or more (Vershuuren *et al.*, 1975). The 50-ppm dietary content of MCPA was considered to be the no-adverse-effect content for rats by the authors. In another 90-day feeding study in Charles River rats (USEPA, 1975f), significant growth decrease was observed with technical MCPA at 100 ppm, and histopathologic alterations of liver and kidneys were seen in both sexes at 25 ppm or higher. In a later study with the same rat strain, no abnormalities were seen after 90 days in animals fed technical MCPA at 4, 8, and 16 mg/kg/day (note that 4 mg/kg/day is approximately equivalent to a dietary content of 25 ppm).

Some dogs that received daily oral doses of technical MCPA over a 13-week period died, and all showed severe weight loss at 50 mg/kg/day, whereas more moderate weight losses but no mortalities occurred at 25 mg/kg/day (USEPA, 1975f). In another 13-week study, decreased testicular weight and histopathologic changes of the testes and prostate were seen in dogs fed technical MCPA at 640 ppm.

Male and female rats were fed Kurosol SI at 10, 30, 100, and 300 ppm for 2 yr (Mullison, 1966; USEPA, 1975k). Increased kidney weight was seen in males that received 300 ppm, but there were no adverse effects at 10, 30, and 100 ppm. The no-adverse-effect concentration was considered to be 100 ppm (2,4,5-TP equivalent, 53 ppm) (Mullison, 1966). The same formulation was fed to beagles 56, 190, and 560 ppm for 2 yr (Mullison, 1966; USEPA, 1975k). Dogs fed 560 ppm showed severe liver pathology after 1 yr. At 190 ppm, liver pathology was seen in females sacrificed after 1 yr, but not in animals sacrificed at 2 yr; in males, no liver pathology was seen at 1 yr, but it was present at 2 yr. The no-adverse-effect content thus was 56 ppm (2,4,5-TP equivalent, 30 ppm) for males and 190 ppm (2,4,5-TP equivalent, 101 ppm) for females (Mullison, 1966). Another report cited 5 mg/kg/day as the no-adverse-effect dosage for 2,4,5-TP in rats and dogs in 2-yr feeding studies (Johnson, 1971).

When technical MCPA was fed to rats for 7 months, some deaths occurred at 2,500 ppm, and a significant reduction in weight occurred at 1,000 and 2,500 ppm (USEPA, 1975f). No apparent toxic effects were noted in animals that received 100 and 400 ppm (66.8 mg/kg/day).

Mutagenicity 2,4,5-TP did not cause point mutations in histidine-requiring mutants of *Salmonella typhimurium* or bacteriophage T (Anderson *et al.*, 1972).

MCPA has been found to be a weak mutagen in *Drosophila melanogaster* (Vogel and Chandler, 1974).

Carcinogenicity Young male and female mice of the (C57BL/6×C3H/Anf)F and the (C57BL/6×AKR)F strains received 2,4,5-TP orally at 46.4 mg/kg/day on days 7-28 and thereafter were placed on a diet containing 2,4,5-TP at 121 ppm for approximately 18 months (Innes *et al.*, 1969). There was no increase in the incidence of tumors above control values for either strain.

Teratogenicity Courtney (1975) examined the effect of 2,4,5-TP containing TCDD at less than 0.1 ppm on pregnant CD-1 strain mice and their offspring. Animals received daily 2,4,5-TP at 398 mg/kg/day orally or subcutaneously on days 12–15 of gestation. Controls had no cleft palates, whereas the herbicide produced 3% (oral) or 7% (subcutaneous) cleft palates in the fetuses. There was also a significant increase in maternal liver:body-weight ratios in the treated mice.

In a study conducted by Dow (USEPA, 1975k), Sprague–Dawley rats were given 2,4,5-TP at 25, 50, 75, 100, or 175 mg/kg/day on days 6–15 of gestation or 50, 75, or 100 mg/kg/day from day 6 of gestation through lactation. A few maternal deaths occurred at 100 mg/kg/day; the dosage of 75 mg/kg/day produced alopecia and vaginal bleeding. Minor alopecia was seen at 50 mg/kg/day. Terata were seen at 50 mg/kg/day, but were minor and related to incomplete ossification of the skull. Mean pup weights were significantly decreased at 50 mg/kg/day and above. The dosage with no-adverse-fetotoxic effects was considered to be 25 mg/kg/day.

The teratogenic potential of the propylene glycol butyl ether ester of 2,4,5-TP (containing TCDD at less than 0.05 ppm) was tested in rats (USEPA, 1975k). Significant increases in minor skeletal abnormalities were observed at 50 mg/kg/day; at 35 mg/kg/day of 2,4,5-TP. No overt teratogenicity was seen.

Female Wistar rats were fed MCPA (ethyl ester) at 1, 40, 500, 1,000, and 2,000 ppm in the diet on days 8–15 of gestation (USEPA, 1975f). Fetal mortalities occurred at 2,000 ppm, and a dose-dependent decrease in fetal weight and an increase in fetal abnormalities occurred at 1,000 ppm.

Female mice were fed technical MCPA at 5, 25, and 100 mg/kg/day on days 6–15 of gestation (USEPA, 1975f). Litter and mean pup weights were reduced at 100 mg/kg/day, but no major malformations were observed.

Pregnant Wistar rats were fed with MCPEE (the ethyl ester of MCPA) at 30, 500, 1,000, and 2,000 ppm (about 2.7, 30, 60, and 100 mg/kg/day) on days 8–15 of gestation (Yasuda and Maeda, 1972). No adverse effects were noted at 30 and 500 ppm, but 1,000 and 2,000 ppm caused a decrease in fetal weight and increased teratogenesis. The highest dosage also caused a reduction in maternal weight.

Conclusions and Recommendations

In 2-yr feeding studies the no-adverse-effect doses for 2,4,5-TP are at up to 5 mg/kg/day and 6.8 mg/kg/day in dogs and rats, respectively. In 90-day feeding studies no-adverse-effect doses were reported at up to 10 mg/kg/day for MCPA in rats, but histopathologic changes in livers and kidneys were reported once at 1.25 mg/kg/day. Based on these data ADI's were calculated at 0.00075 mg/kg/day for 2,4,5-TP and 0.00125 mg/kg/day for MCPA.

The available chronic toxicity data and calculations of ADI's on 2,4,5-TP and MCPA are summarized in Tables VI-4 and VI-5.

There is considerable variation in the no-adverse-effect and minimal-toxic-effect dosages found in the various subchronic-toxicity experiments with MCPA. The reasons for these differences are not apparent, and further work is needed to resolve them. There have been no 2-yr chronic-toxicity tests with MCPA, and such studies should be undertaken. Moreover, very little is known about the reproductive, mutagenic, and

TABLE VI-4 Toxicity of 2,4,5-TP (Silvex)

Species	Duration of Study	Dosage Levels and No. of Animals Per Group	Highest No-Adverse-Effect Level or Lowest-Minimal-Effect Level	Effect Measured	Reference
Dog	2 yr	0–300 ppm in diet	30 ppm (0.75 mg/kg/day)[c,d]	no toxic effect measured in males	Mullison, 1966; USEPA, 1975k
Rat	2 yr	0–160 ppm in diet 50 animals/group	53 ppm (2.6 mg/kg/day)[d]	no toxic effect	Mullison, 1966; USEPA, 1975k
Dog	89 days	0–534 ppm in diet	160 ppm (4.0 mg/kg/day)[d]	no toxic effect	Mullison, 1966; USEPA, 1975k
Rat	90 days	0–9,200 ppm in diet	92 ppm (4.6 mg/kg/day)[d]	increased liver weight, liver and kidney pathology	Mullison, 1966; USEPA, 1975k
Rat	90 days		5 mg/kg/day	no toxic effect	Johnson, 1971
Dog	2 yr		5 mg/kg/day	no toxic effect	Johnson, 1971
Rat	90 days	0–408 mg/kg/day	6.8 mg/kg/day	no toxic effect	Mullison, 1966; USEPA, 1975k

Using an uncertainty factor of 1,000, the suggested no-adverse-effect level in drinking water is calculated as follows:

$$\frac{0.75}{1{,}000} = 0.00075 \text{ mg/kg/day (ADI)},\ 0.00075 \times 70^{a} \times 0.1^{b} = 0.00525 \text{ mg/liter}$$

[a]Assume average weight of human adult = 70 kg.

[b]Assume average daily intake of water for man = 2 liters, and that 20 percent of total intake is from water.

[c]Value from which the suggested no-adverse-effect drinking-water level was calculated.

[d]Assume weight of rat = 0.4 kg and of dog = 10 kg; assume daily food consumption of rat = 0.02 kg and of dog = 0.25 kg.

TABLE VI-5 Toxicity of MCPA

Species	Duration of Study	Dosage Levels and No. of Animals Per Group	Highest No-Adverse-Effect Level or Lowest-Minimal-Effect Level	Effect Measured	Reference
Rat	90 days	0–100 ppm in diet	25 ppm (1.25 mg/kg/day)[c,d]	liver and kidney pathology	EPA, 1975f
Rat	90 days	0–200 ppm in diet	50 ppm (2.5 mg/kg/day)[d]	no toxic effect	Verschuuren, *et al.*, 1975
Dog	13 weeks	640 ppm	640 ppm (16 mg/kg/day)[d]	testicular damage	EPA, 1975f
Rat	90 days	0–16 mg/kg/day	16 mg/kg/day	no toxic effect	EPA, 1975f
Rat	7 months	0–2,500 ppm in diet	400 ppm (20 mg/kg/day)[d]	no toxic effect	EPA, 1975f
Dog	13 weeks	0–75 mg/kg/day orally, 6 animals/group	25 mg/kg/day	weight loss	EPA, 1975f

Using an uncertainty factor of 1,000, the suggested no-adverse-effect level in drinking water is calculated as follows:

$$\frac{1.25}{1{,}000} = 0.00125 \text{ mg/kg/day (ADI)}, \; 0.00125 \times 70^{a} \times 0.1^{b} = 0.009 \text{ mg/liter}$$

[a]Assume average weight of human adult = 70 kg.
[b]Assume average daily intake of water for man = 2 liters, and that 20 percent of total intake is from water.
[c]Value from which the suggested no-adverse-effect drinking-water level was calculated.
[d]Assume weight of rat = 0.4 kg and of dog = 10 kg; assume daily food consumption of rat = 0.02 kg and of dog = 0.25 kg.

carcinogenic properties of MCPA. Additional research is needed, particularly in view of the reported weak mutagenic activity of MCPA.

Further studies on 2,4,5-TP are also needed to determine whether the observed toxicity and teratogenicity are intrinsic in the herbicide or are due to contamination with TCDD.

There appears to be a complete lack of data on human toxicity related to either herbicide.

Benzoics

AMIBEN

Introduction

Amiben, or 3-amino-2,5-dichlorobenzoic acid (Chloramben) is used as a selective preemergence herbicide (Spencer, 1973; Thomson, 1975). It was introduced in 1958. Annual production of amiben in the United States is estimated at 20 million pounds (NAS, 1975). The herbicide is formulated as the ammonium salt and the methyl ester.

Amiben is synthesized by chlorination of benzoic acid, followed by interaction and reduction (Spencer, 1973). Water solubility of Amiben is 700 ppm at 25°C (Weed Science Society of America, 1974).

Metabolism

No available data.

Health Aspects

Observations in Man No available data.

Observations in Other Species

Acute Effects The oral LD_{50} of Amiben in rats is 3,500-5,620 mg/kg, and the dermal LD_{50} in rabbits is 3,136 mg/kg (Ben-Dyke *et al.*, 1970).

Chronic Effects Amiben was fed to Charles River rats over a period of 2 years at dietary concentrations of 100, 1,000, and 10,000 ppm (Hazelton *et al.*, 1964). No adverse effects were found on growth, food consumption, mortality, tumor incidence, hematologic characteristics, or tissue morphology.

TABLE VI-6 Toxicity of Amiben

Species	Duration of Study	Dosage Levels and No. of Animals Per Group	Highest No-Adverse-Effect Level or Lowest-Minimal-Effect Level	Effect Measured	Reference
Dog	presumably 2 yr	0–10,000 ppm, 8 animals/group	10,000 ppm (250 mg/kg/day)[c,d]	no toxic effect	Hazelton *et al.*, 1964
Rat	2 yr	0–10,000 ppm females, 70 animals/group	10,000 (500 mg/kg/day)[d]	no toxic effect	Hazelton *et al.*, 1964

Using an uncertainty factor of 1,000, the suggested no-adverse-effect level in drinking water is calculated as follows:

$$\frac{250}{1,000} = 0.25 \text{ mg/kg/day (ADI)}, \; 0.25 \times 70^{a} \times 0.1^{b} = 1.75 \text{ mg/liter}$$

[a]Assume average weight of human adult = 70 kg.
[b]Assume average daily intake of water for man = 2 liters, and that 20 percent of total intake is from water.
[c]Value from which the suggested no-adverse-effect drinking-water level was calculated.
[d]Assume weight of rat = 0.4 kg and of dog = 10 kg; assume daily food consumption of rat = 0.02 kg and of dog = 0.25 kg.

Male and female beagles were fed Amiben at concentrations of 100, 1,000, and 10,000 ppm for an unspecified period; there were no dose-related effects on mortality, growth, hematologic values, biochemical characteristics, or tissue histopathology (Hazelton *et al.*, 1964).

Mutagenicity No mutagenic activity for Amiben was noted in bacteria (Anderson *et al.*, 1972).

Carcinogenicity No available data other than the Hazelton study (Hazelton *et al.*, 1964).

Teratogenicity No available data.

Conclusions and Recommendations

The available data on Amiben are very sparse. Much additional information is needed regarding its chronic toxicity, teratogenicity, and carcinogenicity before limits can be confidently set. It is possible that many pertinent studies have been conducted by the manufacturer and could be made available for evaluation.

No-observed-adverse-effect doses for Amiben were at 250 mg/kg/day and 500 mg/kg/day in dogs and rats, respectively, in feeding studies. Based on these data an ADI was calculated at 0.25 mg/kg/day.

The limited data available and calculations of the ADI are summarized in Table VI-6.

DICAMBA

Introduction

Dicamba, or 2-methoxy-3,6-dichlorobenzoic acid, is used as a preemergence herbicide for control of annual broadleaf and grassy weeds (USEPA, 1975c). Annual production of Dicamba in the United States has been estimated at 6 million pounds (NAS, 1975), but total domestic use was believed to be 1.2 million pounds in 1974 (USEPA, 1975c).

Dicamba is synthesized from hexachlorobenzene via 1,2,4-trichlorobenzene to 2,5-dichlorophenol to 2-hydroxy-3,6-dichlorobenzoic acid (USEPA, 1975c). The composition of technical-grade Dicamba is 2-methoxy-3,6-dichlorobenzoic acid, 80–93%; 2-methoxy-3,5-dichlorobenzoic acid, 7–20%; and 3,6-dichlorosalicylic acid, 0.5–5%. Dicamba formulations usually involve the alkali metal or alkylamine salts, and it is often formulated in combination with other herbicides (MCPA, 2,4-D, etc.). Dicamba is soluble at 4,500 ppm in water. It is chemically resistant to breakdown, and it persists in soils for 7–10 months. It is not strongly adsorbed onto soils, and it is readily leached by runoff waters. Volatilization of Dicamba is low. It is resistant to oxidation and reasonably resistant to hydrolysis, but is degraded by ultraviolet light to 3,6-dichlorosalicylic acid and unidentified compounds.

In field tests, runoff-water residues of Dicamba from field plots were found to be 1.6–4.8 ppm after 24 h (Trichell *et al.*, 1968). Rapid loss occurs, however, in water.

No residues of Dicamba have been found in foods in the FDA "total diet" samples (Manske and Johnson, 1975).

Golavan (1970) reported that the smell and taste threshold for Dicamba in water was about 200 ppm. On the basis of various toxicity tests, the USSR recommended maximal permissible concentration of Dicamba in water is 15 ppm.

Metabolism

When ^{14}Carboxyl-labeled Dicamba was administered orally to male and female Charles River CD rats, 0.8–1.1% of the radioactive dose was recovered in the feces, 92.88–99.1% in the urine, 0.0–0.3% in the gastrointestinal tract, and 0.5-2.1% in the tissues after 72 h (Tye and Engel, 1967). In a second experiment, groups of Charles River CD rats were fed ^{14}C-labeled Dicamba in the diet at 10, 100, 1,000, 10,000, or 20,000 ppm over a 24-day period. Fecal excretion averaged 3.8–4.4%, whereas excretion in the urine was 97.4% of the administered radioactive dose. Approximately two-thirds of the urinary radioactivity was in unchanged Dicamba, and 12–20% was in the glucuronide conjugate of Dicamba. No evidence of the sulfate conjugate or of 3,6-dichlorosalicylic acid was found.

Urine contained 73% of the Dicamba fed to a Holstein cow after 7 days (St. John and Lisk, 1969). Unchanged Dicamba and 2,6-dichlorosalicylic acid have been identified in the urine of a heifer fed Dicamba (USEPA, 1975c).

In studies conducted in a model ecosystem (Yu *et al.*, 1975), Dicamba was shown to persist in water in conjugated and in anionic forms. It was slowly transformed to 5-hydroxydicamba in water (about 10% after 32 days) and was slowly decarboxylated. No evidence of food-chain magnification of Dicamba was obtained.

Health Aspects

Observations in Man No available data.

Observations in Other Species

Acute Effects Reported acute oral LD_{50} values for technical Dicamba in rats range between 757 and 2,900 mg/kg (Edson and Sanderson, 1965; USEPA, 1975c; Golavan, 1970). Salts of Dicamba showed similar acute toxicities to rats (oral LD_{50}, 1,000–2,000 mg/kg). The acute LD_{50} of technical Dicamba in male rats on intraperitoneal injection, however, was only 80 mg/kg. Male rats were more susceptible to orally administered technical dicamba (LD_{50}, 757 mg/kg) than were females (LD_{50}, 1,414 mg/kg). Inasmuch as pure Dicamba had an oral LD_{50} in female rats of more than 2,560 mg/kg, contaminants of the technical herbicide may be more toxic than the herbicide. The oral LD_{50} in rats of 3,6-dichlorosalicylic acid, the major Dicamba decomposition product, was 1,440 mg/kg.

The oral LD_{50} of technical Dicamba in mice was 1,189 mg/kg whereas oral LD_{50}'s for various Dicamba salts in mice, rabbits, guinea pigs, and chickens were over 4,640, 566, 566, and 673 mg/kg, respectively (Edson and Sanderson, 1965; USEPA, 1975c). Signs of acute Dicamba poisoning in animals include muscle spasms, bradycardia, and inhibited voluntary and involuntary reflexes. Death occurs within 3 days.

Subchronic and Chronic Effects Concentrations of Banvel D (Dicamba, 41.3%; dimethylamine, 14.6%; and water, 44.1%) ranging from 658 to 23,500 ppm were fed to weanling Charles River CD strain rats for 3 weeks, with no significant effect (USEPA, 1975c). In another study, male and female Sprague–Dawley rats were fed diets Banvel D at 100, 500, 800, and 1,000 ppm for 13 weeks. Hypersensitivity was noted in the rats fed 1,000 ppm (equivalent to Dicamba at 413 ppm). Moderate necrosis and vacuolization of the liver were seen in rats fed 1,000 ppm (equivalent to Dicamba at 413 ppm), slight liver pathology in rats fed 800 ppm (330 ppm Dicamba), and no adverse effect in rats fed 500 ppm (206 ppm Dicamba) (USEPA, 1975c). In a third study, Wistar rats were fed diets containing Dicamba at 31.6, 100, 316, 1,000, or 3,162 ppm for a 15-week period (Edson and Sanderson, 1965). Liver:body-weight ratios were increased in animals receiving Dicamba at 1,000 and 3,162 ppm, and the no-adverse-effect dosage was estimated to be 316 ppm (19.3 mg/kg/day).

Purebred beagles of both sexes were fed diets containing Dicamba at

100 or 250 ppm for 90 days (USEPA, 1975c). The only adverse finding was a slight yellowish cast to the liver in two of the four dogs on the 100-ppm diet and one of the four dogs on the 250-ppm diet.

Dicamba was administered orally to an unspecified strain of rat for 6 months at 0.075, 0.75, or 7.5 mg/kg/day (Kudzina and Golovan, 1972). Unspecified toxicity was seen at 7.5 mg/kg/day. In another study, Sprague–Dawley rats of both sexes were fed diets containing technical Dicamba (90% Dicamba) at 5, 50, 100, 250, or 500 ppm for 2 yr (USEPA, 1975c; Velsicol Chemical Corp., 1967). These diets did not produce differences in survival, body weight, food consumption, organ weights, hematologic values, or histopathologic findings.

Purebred beagles of both sexes were fed diets containing technical Dicamba (90% Dicamba) at 5, 25, or 50 ppm for 2 yr (USEPA, 1975c; Velsicol Chemical Corp., 1967). No major differences were seen between control and treated groups in mortality, growth, feed consumption, organ weights, hematologic values, or histopathology.

Mutagenicity No mutations were noted in the *Salmonella*/microsome test with Dicamba (USEPA, 1975c), and no mutagenic effects were noted in other systems (Anderson *et al*., 1972).

Carcinogenicity No evidence of tumor induction by Dicamba has been reported.

Reproduction In a three-generation Charles River CD rat reproduction study, no significant effects were observed in animals receiving diets containing Banvel D at up to 500 ppm (206 ppm Dicamba) (USEPA, 1975c; Velsicol Chemical Corp., 1967). A similar study in Sprague–Dawley rats showed no effect at a dietary Dicamba concentration of 500 ppm.

Teratogenicity A 20% reduction in hatchability was noted in chicken eggs into which Dicamba was injected at 200 ppm (USEPA, 1975c).

Conclusions and Recommendations

The acute toxicity of Dicamba is relatively low. Dicamba produced no adverse effect when fed to rats at up to 19.3 mg/kg/day and 25 mg/kg/day in subchronic and chronic studies. The no-adverse-effect dose in dogs was 1.25 mg/kg/day in a 2-yr feeding study. Based on these data an ADI was calculated at 0.00125 mg/kg/day. The available data on subchronic and chronic toxicity and calculations of ADI are summarized in Table VI-7.

A detection limit of 1 ppb for Dicamba by electron-capture gas chromatography has been reported (Norris and Montgomery, 1975).

Additional studies are needed to clarify the finding of toxicity in subchronic experiments on various strains of rats in the absence of adverse effects in rats fed higher Dicamba concentrations over a 2-yr period. Because toxicity was not observed in chronic toxicity studies in dogs, additional chronic studies should be conducted at higher dosages to establish a minimal-toxic-effect dosage.

Amides

ALACHLOR, BUTACHLOR, AND PROPACHLOR

Introduction

Among the several herbicidal compounds based on *N*-substituted acetanilide are the compounds Alachlor, or 2-chloro-2',6'-diethyl-*N*-(methoxymethyl)-acetanilide; Butachlor, or 2-chloro-2',6'-diethyl-*N*-(butoxymethyl)-acetanilide; and Propachlor, or 2-chloro-*N*-isopropyl-*N*-acetanilide. These are used as preemergence herbicides and, under the trade names of Lasso (Alachlor), Machete (Butachlor), and Ramrod (Propachlor), are achieving a strong position in that market. Alachlor and Propachlor have major use in corn and soybean producton, and Butachlor is used primarily in rice production. In the United States in 1971, farmers used 14.8 million pounds of Alachlor and 23.7 million pounds of Propachlor (NAS, 1975). It was estimated that 20 million pounds of Alachlor and 23 million pounds of Propachlor were produced in the United States in 1961 (NAS, 1975).

These compounds are slightly soluble in water: Alachlor at 242 ppm at 25°C, Butachlor at 23 ppm at 24°C, and Propachlor at 580 ppm at 20°C (Weed Science of America, 1974). They are rated as having good resistance to photodecomposition with no ultraviolet absorption above 280 nm, which lies below the minimal wavelength of solar radiation received at the earth's surface.

It has been reported that Alachlor and Propapachlor are labile in an aquatic environment, and there was no evidence to indicate that the metabolites or degradation products were accumulated in the biota (Yu, *et al.*, 1975).

Alachlor and Butachlor have been found in the finished water of New

TABLE VI-7 Toxicity of Dicamba

Species	Duration of Study	Dosage Levels and No. of Animals Per Group	Highest No-Adverse-Effect Level or Lowest-Minimal-Effect Level	Effect Measured	Reference
Rat	6 months	0–75 mg/kg/day	0.75 mg/kg/day	no toxic effect	Kudzina and Golovan, 1972
Dog	2 yr	0–50 ppm in diet, 6 animals/group	50 ppm (1.25 mg/kg/day)[c,d]	no toxic effect	EPA, 1975c
Rat	13 weeks	0–413 ppm in diet, 30 animals/group	206 ppm (10.3 mg/kg/day)[d]	no toxic effect	EPA, 1975c
Rat	15 weeks	0–3,162 ppm in diet, 20 males/group	316 ppm (19.6 mg/kg/day)[d]	no toxic effect	Edson and Sanderson, 1965

Using an uncertainty factor of 1,000, the suggested no-adverse-effect level in drinking water is calculated as follows:

$$\frac{1.25}{1000} = 0.00125 \text{ mg/kg/day (ADI)}, \; 0.00125 \times 70^{a} \times 0.1^{b} = 0.009 \text{ mg/liter}$$

[a]Assume average weight of human adult = 70 kg.

[b]Assume average daily intake of water for man = 2 liters, and that 20 percent of total intake is from water.

[c]Value from which the suggested no-adverse-effect drinking-water level was calculated.

[d]Assume weight of rat = 0.4 kg and of dog = 10 kg; assume daily food consumption of rat = 0.02 kg and of dog = 0.25 kg.

Orleans area at 2.9 μg/l for Alachlor and 1.21 μg/l for Butachlor (USEPA, 1975n).

Metabolism

Rapid excretion of ^{14}C(carbonyl)-Propachlor administered to rats was observed, with 54–64% of the carbon-14 appearing in the urine within 24 h (Lamboureux *et al.*, 1975). Three major urinary products were found, one of which was identified as the mercapturic acid resulting from glutathione conjugation with Propachlor. The mercapturic acid excreted within 24 h accounted for 20% of the dose. The other major metabolites were not identified, but were not related to glutathione conjugation.

Health Aspects

Observations in Man No available data.

Observations in Other Species

Acute Effects These products are generally well tolerated. Alachlor, as the emulsifiable concentrate, has a rat oral LD_{50} of 1,800 mg/kg; Butachlor, 3,300 mg/kg; and Propachlor, 710 mg/kg (Weed Science Society of America, 1974).

Subchronic and Chronic Effects Subchronic toxicities in rats are reported to be over 2,000 ppm in the diet, at least over 2,000 ppm, and over 133.3 mg/kg/day for Alachlor, Butachlor, and Propachlor, respectively. With Alachlor, the growth patterns of rats and dogs were normal at 20, 200, and 2,000 ppm for a 90-day period; some growth decrease was observed at a higher rate of feeding. Butachlor administration at those concentrations produced similar results, except for slight growth decrease at 2,000 ppm in rats. Increased liver weight was observed in female rats fed Butachlor at 200 and 2,000 ppm. Propachlor was tolerated, without adverse clinical effects or gross or microscopic pathology, by rats and dogs fed at 1.3–133.3 mg/kg/day for 90 days (Herbicide Handbook, 1974). However, Propachlor has been reported to cause dystrophic changes in the liver and kidneys of rats, mice, and rabbits when administered at 100–1,800 mg/kg. The effects depended on dosage and were accompanied by decreased activities of various enzyme markers of cellular organelles (Strateva *et al.*, 1974). No data on long-term toxicity are available.

Mutagenicity No available data.

Carcinogenicity No available data.

Teratogenicity No available data.

Conclusions and Recommendations

Although the toxicity data on this group of compounds are meager, they appear to be fairly well tolerated by mammals. Propachlor, the most toxic of the group, has received somewhat more attention.

Tolerances of 0.2–0.75 ppm for peanut, soybean, and other legume forages has been established for Alachlor; it is also tolerated at 0.05 ppm in fresh corn (kernels) and peanuts. A 0.02-ppm (negligible residue) tolerance for Alachlor applies to meat, eggs, and milk.

The maximal tolerated dosage of Propachlor without adverse effect is reported as 133.3 mg/kg/day in both rats and dogs. Other workers reported slight organ pathology in rats, mice, and rabbits at 100 mg/kg/day or higher; this agrees approximately with the former data. Both Alachlor and Butachlor are apparently tolerated by rats at up to 100 mg/kg/day in the diet, except for increased liver weight in female rats fed Butachlor.

The existing toxicity data for these compounds are largely those produced by the manufacturer for registration purposes. Based on the above available data, ADI's were calculated at 0.1, 0.1, and 0.01 mg/kg/day for Alachlor, Popachlor, and Butachlor, respectively. The available data on subchronic toxicity and calculation of ADI's are summarized in Table VI-8.

Apparently, no long-term toxicity studies have been completed that would contribute information on reproductive effects or carcinogenic potential of these acetanilides or their degradation products, which include aniline derivatives. These studies are needed.

PROPANIL

Introduction

Propanil, or 3',4'-dichloropropionanilide, is a preemergence herbicide registered for use in rice to control grasses, sedges, and some broadleaf weeds. Use in the United States has been primarily in the rice-growing regions of Texas, Arkansas, Louisiana, and Mississippi; little has been used in California. Domestic consumption was around 8–9 million pounds in 1973 (USEPA, 1975o). Propanil is produced by reaction of 3,4-dichloroaniline with propionic acid at high temperature (Melnikov, 1971). It is soluble in water at 500 ppm (Weed Science Society of America, 1974).

Metabolism

Propanil is hydrolyzed by the action of hepatic acylamidase, forming 3,4-dichloroaniline and propionic acid (Williams *et al.*, 1966). The enzyme has been shown to be present in the liver of rats, mice, rabbits, and dogs. Other conversions are brought about either on propanil itself or on dichloroaniline, giving rise to at least six metabolites in urine; these metabolites constitute about 95% of the urinary products (Yih *et al.*, 1970). Little radioactivity from labeled propanil appeared in tissues in short-duration experiments with rats, mice, and dogs; this indicates that the propensity for accumulation of propanil or its metabolites in tissues is slight (USEPA, 1975o).

Methemoglobin formation occurs in mice treated with propanil. After a large dose (400 mg/kg), cyanosis becomes apparent, although no other symptoms of toxicity occur (Chow *et al.*, 1975). The methemoglobin formation is due to the dichloroaniline liberated by acylamidase.

Health Aspects

Observations in Man No available data.

Observations in Other Species

Acute Effects Ambrose *et al.* found oral LD_{50} values of 1,384 mg/kg for rats and 1,217 mg/kg for dogs (Ambrose, 1972); these values were observed with technical propanil. Proprietary data summarized by Midwest Research Institute indicated that rats of both sexes tolerated repeated doses of up to 60 mg/kg for 30 days and dietary administration at up to 200 ppm for 90 days without any effects (USEPA, 1975o). Ambrose *et al.* (1972) fed technical propanil to Wistar rats for 90 days at 100, 333, 1,000, 3,300, 10,000, and 50,000 ppm in the diet. Mortality was 100% at 50,000 ppm; body weight was depressed at 3,300 and 10,000 ppm, and there was a significant increase in polychromatophilia and other evidence of hemolytic anemia. Dogs were unaffected by propanil fed at 2,000 ppm for 4 weeks, but 10,000 and 50,000 ppm caused decreased food consumption and weight loss (Ambrose *et al.*, 1972).

TABLE VI-8 Toxicity of Alachlor, Butachlor, and Propachlor

Species	Duration of Study	Dosage Levels and No. of Animals Per Group	Highest No-Adverse-Effect Level or Lowest-Minimal-Effect Level	Effect Measured	Reference
Propachlor					
Rat	90 days	1.3 to 133.3 mg/kg/day	133.3 mg/kg/day	no mortality, no organ path	Weed Science Society of America, 1974
Dog	90 days	1.3 to 133.3 mg/kg/day (number not available)	133.3 mg/kg/day	no mortality, no organ path	WSSA, 1974
Rat		100 to 1,800 mg/kg/day (number not available)	100 mg/kg/day[c,d]	distrophic liver and kidney	Strateva *et al.*, 1974
Alachlor					
Rat, Dog	90 days	20, 200, 2,000 ppm in diet (number not available)	2,000 ppm (100 mg/kg/day)[c,d]	no adverse effect	WSSA, 1974

Butachlor					
Rat, Dog	90 days	20, 200, 2,000 ppm in diet (number not available)	2,000 ppm (dog), 200 ppm (rat) (10 mg/kg/day)[c,d]	no adverse effect, increased liver weight	WSSA, 1974

Using an uncertainty factor of 1,000, the suggested no-adverse-effect levels in drinking water are calculated as follows:

Alachlor: $\frac{100}{1,000} = 0.1$ mg/kg/day (ADI), $0.1 \times 70^a \times 0.1^b = 0.7$ mg/liter

Butachlor: $\frac{10}{1,000} = 0.01$ mg/kg/day (ADI), $0.01 \times 70^a \times 0.1^b = 0.07$ mg/liter

Propachlor: $\frac{100}{1,000} = 0.1$ mg/kg/day (ADI), $0.1 \times 70^a \times 0.1^b = 0.7$ mg/liter

[a]Assume average weight of human adult = 70 kg.
[b]Assume average daily intake of water for man = 2 liters, and that 20 percent of total intake is from water.
[c]Value from which the suggested no-adverse-effect drinking-water level was calculated.
[d]Assume weight of rat = 0.4 kg and of dog = 10 kg; assume daily food consumption of rat = 0.02 kg and of dog = 0.25 kg.

Chronic Effects Two-year feeding trials with rats were conducted by Ambrose *et al.* (1972) with dietary concentrations of 100, 400, and 1,600 ppm. No effects were observed, except 1,600 ppm (of both sexes). Males experienced increased mortality at 20 months, females had significantly reduced hemoglobin concentrations, and both sexes experienced body-weight decrease and increased spleen:body-weight ratios. No histopathologic alternations were found.

Dog feeding studies with propanil at 100, 600, and 3,000 ppm (4,000 ppm after week 5) were carried out for 2 yr (Ambrose *et al.*, 1972). No mortalities occurred, nor were any clinical, gross pathologic or histopathologic changes found; the only effect observed was decreased feed efficiency at 4,000 ppm.

Mutagenicity Propanil and its degradation products, dichloroaniline and 3,3′,4,4′-tetrachloroazobenzene (TCAB), were tested for back mutations of *Aspergillus nidulans* (Prasad 1970). Propanil did not increase the frequency of reversion when added to fungal conidia in concentrations of 5–200 μg/ml of medium. However, 3,4-dichloroaniline and TCAB both caused severalfold increases in reversion rates. Propanil has also been found negative in tests of induction of point mutations in three microbial systems (Anderson *et al.*, 1972).

Carcinogenicity No available data.

Reproduction A three-generation reproduction study in Wistar rats was reported by Ambrose *et al.* (1972). Dietary concentrations of 100, 300, and 1,000 ppm were fed to groups of females for 11 weeks before they mated with males receiving similar diets. No changes in reproductive performance were found in any generation (to the F_3) at any dosage, nor were fetal abnormalities observed in fetuses born dead or alive or in rats necropsied with fetuses *in utero*.

Teratogenicity No available data.

Conclusions and Recommendations

Propanil is well tolerated by experimental animals on a chronic basis, and there is little or no indication of mutagenic or oncogenic properties of the compound. The highest no-adverse-effect concentration of propanil based on reproduction in the rat and acute, subchronic, and chronic studies in rats and dogs is 400 ppm in the diet. Based on these data an ADI was calculated at 0.02 mg/kg/day. The available data on chronic toxicity and calculations of ADI are summarized in Table VI-9.

Triazines

ATRAZINE, SIMAZINE, PROPAZINE, CYANAZINE

Introduction

These four herbicides are all derivatives of cyanuric chlorides and are closely related in environmental properties. Atrazine is 2-chloro-4-ethylamino-6-isopropylamino-*S*-triazine, Simazine is 2-chloro-4,6-diethylamino-*S*-triazine, Propazine is 2-chloro-4,6-diisopropylamino-*S*-triazine, and Cyanazine is 2-chloro-4-(1-cyano-1-methylethylamino)-6-ethylamino-*S*-triazine.

These herbicides are used largely in preemergence applications for corn, sorghum, and sugarcane, with minor use on pineapple, macadamia orchards, and turf grasses, especially Atrazine. Simazine is also used in citrus, deciduous fruits, pineapple, turf grasses, ornamentals, and nursery plantings (WSSA, 1974).

U.S. production is estimated as: Atrazine, 90 million pounds; Simazine, 5 million pounds; Propazine, 4 million pounds; and Cyanazine, 1 million pounds (NAS, 1975). Atrazine is the pesticide most heavily used in the United States.

The solubilities of the triazine herbicides in water at 25°C are: Atrazine, 70 ppm; Simazine, 5 ppm, Propazine, 8.6 ppm; and Cyanazine, 171 ppm (WSSA, 1974).

Atrazine was found in the New Orleans water supply at 4.7–5.1 ppb, and diethylatrazine at 0.27–0.51 ppb (USEPA, 1974a). Atrazine was monitored in down surface and ground water in Iowa by Richard *et al.* (1975). In the Skunk River residues declined from 12.0 ppb on June 9, 1974 to 0.250 ppb on September 12, and in Indian Creek from 42 ppb in June 9 to 0.300 ppb on August 25. The finished water supply of Cedar Rapids contained 0.483 ppb; Davenport, 0.405; Iowa City, 0.20; and Des Moines, 0.03 ppm. These seasonal changes in Atrazine content in water reflect agricultural runoff following spring preemergence application. All the water examined in Iowa contained atrazine.

Propazine, Simazine, and Cyanazine were also detected in finished water in the United States (USEPA, 1976d).

TABLE VI-9 Toxicity of Propanil

Species	Duration of Study	Dosage Levels and No. of Animals Per Group	Highest No-Adverse-Effect Level or Lowest-Minimal-Effect Level	Effect Measured	Reference
Rat	2 yr	100, 400, 1,600 ppm (50/group, equal F, M)	400 ppm (20 mg/kg/day)[c,d]	no adverse effect	Ambrose *et al.*, 1972
Dog	2 yr	100, 600, 4,000 ppm (4/group, equal F, M)	4,000 ppm (100 mg/kg/day)[d]	no adverse effect	Ambrose *et al.*, 1972
Rat	3-generation	100, 300, 1,000 ppm (20 F/group at start)	1,000 ppm (50 mg/kg/day)[d]	no reproductive effects	Ambrose *et al.*, 1972

Using an uncertainty factor of 1,000, the suggested no-adverse-effect level in drinking water is calculated as follows:

$$\frac{20}{100} = 0.02 \text{ mg/kg/day (ADI)},\ 0.02 \times 70^{a} \times 0.1^{b} = 0.14 \text{ mg/liter}$$

[a]Assume average weight of human adult = 70 kg.
[b]Assume average daily intake of water for man = 2 liters, and that 20 percent of total intake is from water.
[c]Value from which the suggested no-adverse-effect level was calculated.
[d]Assume weight of rat = 0.4 kg and of dog = 10 kg; assume average daily food consumption of rat = 0.02 kg and of dog = 0.25 kg.

Metabolism

In animals, the dominant metabolic reaction is *N*-dealkylation, and rats have produced 20 metabolites from Atrazine, including 4-amino-*N*-ethyl-,4-amino-*N*-isopropyl-, 4,6-diamino-, 4-amino-*N*-acetyl-, and 4-amino-*N*-isopropionyl-2-chloro-*S*-triazines. Rabbits also excreted *N*-(chloro-4-amino-*S*-triazinyl-6)-glucoside (Menzie 1969). No firm evidence of ring cleavage has been found in degradation studies with bacteria, plants, or animals.

Cyanazine degradation proceeds initially by hydrolysis of the nitrile group and slower hydrolysis of the 2-chloro group. 2-Hydroxycyanazine is the major metabolite found in rat feces. The rat also produces the 4-amino derivative and the *N*-acetylcysteinyl derivative and hydrolyzes; the cyano group to the corresponding amide and carboxy derivatives (Menzies, 1974).

In a laboratory model ecosystem study, with carbon-14 ring-labeled Atrazine, the environmental degradation products were 2-amino-4chloro-6-isopropylamino-*S*-triazine and 2-amino-4-chloro-6-ethylamino-*S*-triazine. There was only a slight degree of food-chain transfer of Atrazine (ecologic magnification 11 times in fish) or any of its degradation products (Metcalf and Sanborn, 1975).

Simazine residues from water treated at 2.5 ppm rose to a maximum of 2.2 ppm in bluegill after 28 days and declined to 0.76 ppm after 60 days; in bass, they rose to 1.50 ppm after 28 days and declined to 0.88 ppm after 60 days (USEPA, 1976c).

Health Aspects

Observations in Man No case of poisoning in man from Simazine, Atrazine, Propazine, or Cyanazine has been reported, although exposure to Simazine has caused acute and subacute dermatitis in the USSR, characterized by erythema, slight edema, moderate pruritus, and burning lasting 4–5 days (Elizarov, 1972).

Observations in Other Species

Acute Toxicity The acute oral toxicity of Simazine in rats, mice, rabbits, chickens, and pigeons was 5,000–>5,000 mg/kg. The acute dermal toxicity in rabbits was over 8.16 g/kg. For Atrazine, the oral LD_{50} is 3,080 mg/kg in rats and 1,750 mg/kg in mice. For Propazine, the oral LD_{50} is over 5,000 mg/kg in rats and mice. For Cyanazine the oral LD_{50}

is 334 mg/kg in rats, and the dermal LD_{50} is over 2,000 mg/kg in rabbits (WSSA, 1974).

Chronic Toxicity Simazine fed to rats for 2 yr at 1.0, 10, and 100 ppm produced no difference between treated and control animals in gross appearance or behavior. The rats fed 100 ppm had approximately twice as many thyroid and mammary tumors as the control animals, but it was stated that these were not attributable to Simazine (USEPA, 1976c).

Propazine at 250 mg/kg for 130 days produced no gross signs of toxicity or pathologic changes (WSSA, 1974).

Atrazine, in 2-yr chronic-feeding studies at 100 ppm in the diet of rats, produced no gross or microscopic signs of toxicity (WSSA, 1974).

Cyanazine in 2-yr feeding studies in rats and dogs showed no signs of toxic effects at levels up to 25 ppm (WSSA, 1974).

A 2-yr chronic-feeding study of Simazine in dogs with Simazine 80W fed at 15, 150, and 1,500 ppm showed only a slight thyroid hyperplasia at 1,500 ppm and slight increases in serum alkaline phosphatase and serum glutamic oxalacetic transaminase in several of the dogs fed 1,500 ppm (USEPA, 1976c).

Mutagenicity Simazine and Atrazine were inactive in a standard mutagenicity screen with microorganisms, e.g., Simazine was negative with four strains of *Salmonella typhimurium* (USEPA, 1976c). Plewa and Gentile (1975) demonstrated that extracts of maize seedlings grown on soil treated with Atrazine at recommended rates contain an agent that is highly mutagenic in *Saccharomyces cerevisiae* (D4). Further study (Gentile and Plewa, 1976) has shown that the kernels of maize grown on Atrazine-treated plots contain this mutagenic agent, which produces mutation rates up to 30 times that of untreated maize. These data strongly suggest that maize plants can metabolize Atrazine into a mutagenic agent and generate considerable concern about ubiquitous triazine residues in water supplies.

Carcinogenicity Atrazine, Propazine, and Simazine were fed to 2 strains of mice at 21.5, 46.4, and 215 mg/kg/day respectively for 80 weeks (Innes *et al.*, 1969). The incidences of hepatomas were: 4.24% in controls, 5.6% in Atrazine treated, 5.7% in Propazine treated, and 5.6% in Simazine treated.

Reproduction Simazine at 50 and 100 ppm in the diet had no adverse effects on reproduction of rats or offspring over three generations (USEPA, 1976c). Similar experiments with chickens and quail showed anomalies in the urogenital tracts of male chickens when eggs were sprayed with 0.5, 0.7, 1.0, and 1.5% aqueous solutions of Simazine (Didier and Lutz-Ostertag, 1972).

Teratogenicity No available data.

Conclusions and Recommendations

Atrazine, Propazine, and Simazine all appear to have low chronic toxicity. The only good carcinogenicity feeding study done on these compounds did not reveal a significant increase in cancer incidence over controls. On the basis of these chronic studies, an ADI was calculated for each of these compounds. The ADI for Atrazine is 0.0215 mg/kg/day, for Propazine 0.0464 mg/kg/day, and for Simazine 0.215 mg/kg/day. The available chronic toxicity data for Atrazine, Simazine, and Propazine are summarized in Table VI-10.

Uracil

BROMACIL

Introduction

Bromacil, or 5-bromo-3-*sec*-butyl-6-methluracil, is one of several substituted uracils that were introduced as broad-spectrum herbicides in 1972. Trade names include Hyvar, Krovar (Bromacil plus Diuron), and Isocil (Spencer, 1973). It is estimated that 3 million pounds of this agent was used in the United States in 1972 (von Rumker *et al.*, 1975) and 8 million pounds was produced in 1971 (NAS, 1975).

Bromacil is used primarily for the control of annual and perennial grasses and broadleaf weeds, both nonselectively on noncrop lands and selectively for weed control in a few crops (citrus and pineapple). It appears to act in plants by inhibiting photosynthesis and to be primarily abosrbed through the roots.

Bromacil is manufactured by the reaction of phosgene and ammonia with sec-butylamine to produce sec-butylurea, which reacts with ethylacetoacetate to produce 3-*sec*-butyl-6-methyluracil, which is then brominated to produce Bromacil (USEPA, 1975a).

Bromacil is soluble in water at 815 ppm at 25°C, and it is stable in water, aqueous bases, and common organic solvents. It decomposes slowly in strong acids (USEPA, 1975a).

Bromacil undergoes photochemical decomposition and is degraded in

TABLE VI-10 Toxicity of Simazine, Atrazine, and Propazine

Species	Duration of Study	Dosage Levels	Highest No-Adverse-Effect Level or Lowest-Minimal-Effect Level	Effect Measured	Reference
Simazine					
Rat	2 yr	0			Cited in EPA, 1976c
		1.0 ppm		tumors 13.5%	
		10 ppm			
		100 ppm		tumors 50%	
Rat	8 months	10 mg/kg/day		av. length life 200 days	Cited in EPA, 1976c
		50 mg/kg/day		av. length life 151 days	
		100 mg/kg/day		av. length life 126 days	
Dog	2 yr	0		thyroid/body ratio 0.006	Cited in EPA, 1976c
		12 ppm		thyroid/body ratio 0.009	
		120 ppm		thyroid/body ratio 0.009	
		1,200 ppm	<12 ppm	thyroid/body ratio	

Mouse	80 weeks	0		Hepatoma 4.2%	Innes *et al.*, 1969
		215 mg/kg/day	<215 mg/kg/day[a]	Hepatoma 5.6%	
Atrazine					
Mouse	80 weeks	0		Hepatoma 4.2%	Innes *et al.*, 1969
		21.5 mg/kg/day	21.5 mg/kg/day[b]	Hepatoma 5.6%	
Propazine					
Mouse	80 weeks	0		Hepatoma 4.2%	Innes *et al.*, 1969
		46.4 mg/kg/day	46.4 mg/kg/day[c]	Hepatoma 5.7%	

Using an uncertainty factor of 1,000, the suggested no-adverse-effect level for Simazine in drinking water is calculated as follows:

$$\frac{215}{1,000} = 0.215 \text{ mg/kg/day (ADI)},\ 0.215 \times 70^{d} \times 0.1^{e} = 1.505 \text{ mg/liter}$$

Using an uncertainty factor of 1,000, the suggested no-adverse-effect level for Atrazine in drinking water is calculated as follows:

$$\frac{21.5}{1,000} = 0.0215 \text{ mg/kg/day (ADI)},\ 0.0215 \times 70^{d} \times 0.1^{e} = 0.15 \text{ mg/liter}$$

Using an uncertainty factor of 1,000, the suggested no-adverse-effect level for Propazine in drinking water is calculated as follows:

$$\frac{46.4}{1,000} = 0.0464 \text{ mg/kg/day (ADI)},\ 0.0464 \times 70^{d} \times 0.1^{e} = 0.32 \text{ mg/liter}$$

[a,b,c]Values from which the suggested no-adverse-effect levels were calculated.
[d]Assume average weight of human = 70 kg.
[e]Assume average daily intake of water for man = 2 liters, and that 20 percent of total intake is from water.

soil. The degradation in soil appears to follow first-order kinetics and to be nonenzymatic. However, Bromacil is subject to microbial decomposition under moist soil conditions (USEPA, 1975a).

Metabolism

Bromacil is absorbed from the gastrointestinal tract and appears to be excreted primarily in the urine. The major metabolite in rodents and man is 5-bromo-3-*sec*-butyl-6-hydroxymethyluracil, which can be detected as a glucuronide conjugate. Other minor metabolites include 5-bromo-3-(2-hydroxy-1-methylpropyl)-6-methyluracil, 3-*sec*-butyl-6-hydroxymethyluracil, 5-bromo-3-(3-hydroxy-1-methylpropyl)-6-methyluracil, and an unidentified bromine-containing compound (Gardiner *et al.*, 1969). 5-Bromouracil was not found in hydrolyzed or nonhydrolyzed urine samples from humans exposed to Bromacil (USEPA, 1975a).

Health Aspects

Observations in Man No available data.

Observations in Other Species

Acute Effects The acute oral LD_{50} of Bromacil in rats is 5,200 mg/kg, and the acute inhalation toxicity is greater than 4.8 mg/liter per 4 h. The acute dermal toxicity of Bromacil was estimated to be at 5,000 mg/kg in rabbits. Application of Bromacil (80% wettable powder) to abraded guinea pig skin produced only mild irritation, without evidence of induced skin sensitization. Because Bromacil causes emesis in dogs, its acute oral toxicity has not been determined in this species, but oral doses of 250 mg/kg produce toxicity (weight loss or abnormal gait) in sheep, chickens, and cattle. Toxic symptoms in poisoned animals also include anorexia, depression, tympanites (in cattle and sheep), and increased respiratory rate (in dogs) (USEPA, 1975a).

Subchronic and Chronic Effects Male rats were given Bromacil (as a 15% aqueous solution of the 80% AI wettable powder) for 2 weeks (5 days/week) at 650, 1,035, and 1,500 mg/kg. There were six animals in each dose group; five rats died after 5 doses at the highest dosage level, and one died after 10 doses at the intermediate dosage. There were no deaths in the low-dosage group, but these animals exhibited focal cell hypertrophy and hyperplasia of the liver, which were also seen in the higher-dosage groups. In another subchronic study in which 10 male and 10 female rats were fed Bromacil at 50, 500, 2,500, 5,000, 6,000, and 7,500 ppm for 90 days, there were no signs of mortality or toxicity; but microscopic examination of the tissues from these animals revealed increased thyroid activity in rats fed 5,000 ppm higher (Zapp, 1965). Bromacil (83% AI wettable powder) was also fed to rats for 2 yr at 50, 250, and 1,250 ppm. Additional controls in this study were corn-oil-vehicle groups, and there were initially 36 male and 36 female rats per diet group. Rats from each diet group were sacrificed at the end of 3, 6, and 12 months of feeding; weight loss in the female rats fed 1,250 ppm was the only toxic effect observed. Histopathologic examination of the tissues from these rats revealed hyperplasia in the light and follicular cells of the thyroid, and there was a follicular cell adenoma in one of the females fed 1,250 ppm (Sherman *et al.*, 1963). A 2-yr feeding study in dogs has also been carried out with Bromacil in which three male and three female dogs were fed 0.005, 0.025, and 0.925% Bromacil. No toxic effects were observed, although one dog (0.005% diet) died from non-Bromacil effects (Hazelton Labs, 1966).

Mutagenicity The mutagenic potential of Bromacil has been investigated in several studies, because 5-bromouracil is mutagenic. However, 5-bromouracil is not a metabolite of Bromacil, and Bromacil was not found to be mutagenic in any of these tests (USEPA, 1975a).

Carcinogenicity No available data.

Reproduction No significant reproductive effects were observed in a two-generation rat study in which indexes of fertility, gestation, viability, and lactation were observed. The dosages for these studies were 50, 250, 1,250 ppm, and there were 12 male and 12 female rats in each group (USEPA, 1975a).

No gross manifestations of teratogenic effects were observed in the fetuses of rabbits fed Bromacil in the diet at 50, 250, 1,250 ppm (USEPA, 1975a).

Conclusions and Recommendations

Bromacil is low in both acute and chronic toxicity. It appears that 1,250 ppm is a no-adverse-effect dietary concentration of Bromacil in dogs. However, rats fed this concentration of Bromacil in the diet exhibited abnormal thyroid pathology. In a 2-yr feeding study the no-adverse-effect dose for rats was 12.5 mg/kg/day. Based on these data an ADI was

TABLE VI-11 Toxicity of Bromacil

Species	Duration of Study	Dosage Levels and No. of Animals Per Group	Highest No-Adverse-Effect Level or Lowest-Minimal-Effect Level	Effect Measured	Reference
Rat	14 days	0–1,500 mg/kg/day, 6 animals/group	650 mg/kg/day	liver hyperplasia	Zapp, 1965
Rat	90 days	0–7,000 ppm, 20 animals/group	2,500 ppm (125 mg/kg/day)[d]	no toxic effect	Zapp, 1965
Rat	2 yr	0–1,250 ppm, 72 animals/group	250 ppm[c,d] (12.5 mg/kg/day)	no toxic effect	Sherman, 1965
Dog	2 yr	0–0.125% of Bromacil, 6 animals/group	0.125% (63 mg/kg/day)[d]	no toxic effect	Hazelton Labs, 1966

Using an uncertainty factor of 1,000, the suggested no-adverse-effect level in drinking water is calculated as follows:

$$\frac{12.5}{1{,}000} = 0.0125 \text{ mg/kg/day (ADI)},\ 0.0125 \times 70^{a} \times 0.1^{b} = 0.086 \text{ mg/liter}$$

[a]Assume average weight of human adult = 70 kg.
[b]Assume average daily intake of water for man = 2 liters, and that 20 percent of total intake is from water.
[c]Value from which the suggested no-adverse-effect level was calculated.
[d]Assume weight of rat = 0.4 kg and of dog = 10 kg; assume average daily intake food consumption of rat = 0.02 kg and of dog = 0.25 kg.

calculated at 0.0125 mg/kg/day. The available data on chronic oral toxicity and calculations of ADI are summarized in Table VI-11.

Bipyridl

PARAQUAT

Introduction

Paraquat, or 1,1′-dimethyl-4,4′-dipyridylium, is a general weed-killer of the bipyridyl family of herbicides. It is available either as a dichloride or as a dimethysulfate salt. Both compounds are water-soluble. It is registered as a contact herbicide for noncrop use.

During recent years paraquat has been used extensively in California—374,009 lb in 1973, and 272,361 lb in 1974. In 1975, 248,070 lb were used during the first three quarters of the year (University of California Pesticide Data Bank, 1975). It is used primarily for general weed control and as a desiccant.

Paraquat kills plants by acting on the green parts, not on woody stems, and is rapidly inactivated by contact with clay in the soil. Apparently, the molecule itself can penetrate into the crystal lattice of clay minerals, where it is firmly bound by physical bonding (Hayes *et al.*, 1975). Under these circumstances, paraquat cannot be attacked by soil microorganisms, because they cannot penetrate the lattice. In the bound form, paraquat is biologically inert, and it has been demonstrated that it does not cause any harm to either plant or animal life. When paraquat is in an environment that does not have clay particles, it is readily degraded by microorganisms. Under these circumstances, it is generally accepted that paraquat is environmentally safe, because its associated toxicologic hazard presents no major problems.

Apparently, paraquat is not extensively metabolized in plants; it has been demonstrated that there is no metabolic breakdown of paraquat in tomato, broad bean, and maize (Weeds Science Society of America, 1974). The herbicidal activity and organic chemical reactions of paraquat formulations depend solely on the paraquat cation and are not influenced by the nature of the associated anion, because the salts are largely dissociated in aqueous solution.

Paraquat is readily decomposed by ultraviolet light. Two major decomposition products are 1-methyl-4-carboxypyridinium ion (Funderburk *et al.*, 1966) and methylamine hydrochloride. Experiments have demonstrated that paraquat solutions degrade rapidly in ultraviolet light, with very little remaining after 48 h of exposure.

Health Aspects

Observations in Man Paraquat is acutely toxic to man. As a result, many accidental and suicidal deaths have been reported (Kimbrough, 1974; Copland *et al.*, 1974; van Dijk *et al.*, 1975; Carson, 1972; Beebeejaum *et al.*, 1971). It has been estimated that a lethal dose in man is about 14 ml of a 40% solution of paraquat (Kimbrough, 1974). The symptoms of poisoning include burning of the mouth and throat, nausea and vomiting, respiratory distress, and transient effects on the kidneys, heart, and nervous system. Death is usually due to progressive fibrosis and epithelial proliferation in the lungs.

Dermal exposure to paraquat concentrates may result in severe skin irritation, while nosebleeds may result from exposure of the nasal mucosa, and several severe eye injuries have resulted from eye exposure. Absorption studies have shown that paraquat is readily absorbed through the skin of both humans and animals.

There is no effective antidote for paraquat poisoning in man, although a few patients have recovered after ingesting doses thought to be fatal (Jones and Owen-Lloyd, 1973; Galloway and Petrie, 1972).

Observations in Other Species

Acute Effects Paraquat is acutely toxic to both man and animals. The oral LD_{50} reported in rats is 110–173 mg/kg (Mehani, 1972; Murry and Gibson, 1972). In the mouse, the LD_{50} is 90–120 mg/kg. The LD_{50} in monkeys is 50 mg/kg, and in guinea pigs it is 22 mg/kg (Murry and Gibson, 1972).

Animals poisoned by inhalation do not show major damage to the lungs, as is usually found when paraquat is administered orally. Apparently, after ingestion it acts similarly to a powerful irritant, such as phosgene, and the changes in the lung are typical of such effects. Death at sufficiently high doses occurs within a short period, and animals that do not die within this period recover completely; delayed fibrosis does not occur (Conning, 1969).

Chronic Effects Two-year feeding studies with rats have shown that paraquat at up to 170 ppm in the diet does not produce significant abnormalities in any of the several characteristics investigated (Chevron

Chemical Co., 1975). Dogs fed paraquat at 7.2 and 34 ppm in the diet over a period of 27 months have not developed significant abnormalities. However, some changes were observed at 85 and 170 ppm.

Kimbrough and Gaines (1970) have conducted 90-day feeding studies in rats with dietary paraquat concentrations of 300, 400, 500, 600, and 700 ppm. Clinical signs of acute and chronic poisoning included diarrhea, wheezing, irregular and rapid breathing, and red stains around the snout. All animals that died showed morphologic changes in their lungs.

Mutagenicity No available data.

Carcinogenicity No available data.

Reproduction and Teratognicity Administration of paraquat to mice, at 1.67 and 3.35 mg/kg intraperitoneally or 20 mg/kg orally, daily on days 8–16 of gestation induced no significant teratogenic effects, although a slight increase in nonossification of sternebrae was observed (Bus *et al.*, 1975). The same investigators reported that, when paraquat was administered to rats on single days of gestation, an average of 7.6% of the fetuses were found dead or being resorbed. Radioactivity reaching the mouse embryo after intraperitoneal or oral administration of [^{14}C]Paraquat on the eleventh day of gestation was low.

Conclusions and Recommendations

Paraquat is a highly effective, general herbicide that is acutely toxic to man and animals in its concentrated form (20% liquid concentrate). Oral exposure to high doses of paraquat frequently results in death, which is usually due to progressive fibrosis and epithelial proliferation in the lungs. However, in 2-yr feeding studies in rats, paraquat did not produce any significant abnormalities.

Paraquat is rapidly inactivated by contact with clay particles in soil and is firmly bound physically. In this form, it is biologically inactive and apparently does not have any immediate or prolonged harmful effects. Thus, it is unlikely that paraquat would be found in large amounts in drinking water. Based on a 2-yr feeding study in rats, an ADI was calculated at 0.0085 mg/kg/day. The available toxicity data and calculations of ADI are summarized in Table VI-12.

TABLE VI-12 Toxicity of Paraquat

Species	Duration of Study	Dosage Levels and No. of Animals Per Group	Highest No-Adverse-Effect Level or Lowest-Minimal-Effect Level	Effect Measured	Reference
Rat	90 days	300–700 ppm, 10 females per group	300 ppm (15 mg/kg/day)[d]	diarrhea, irregular and rapid breathing	Kimbrough and Gaines, 1970
Rat	27–57 days	250 ppm		death in some cases	Clark *et al.*, 1966
Rat	2 yr	170 ppm	170 ppm (8.5 mg/kg/day)[c,d]	no adverse effect	Chevron Chemical Company, 1975

Using an uncertainty factor of 1,000, the suggested no-adverse-effect level in drinking water is calculated as follows:

$$\frac{8.5}{1,000} = 0.0085 \text{ mg/kg/day (ADI)}, \; 0.0085 \times 70^{a} \times 0.1^{b} = 0.06 \text{ mg/liter}$$

[a]Assume average weight of human adult = 70 kg.

[b]Assume average daily intake of water for man = 2 liters, and that 20 percent of total intake is from water.

[c]Value from which the suggested no-adverse-effect level was calculated.

[d]Assume weight of rat = 0.4 kg and average daily food consumption of rat = 0.02 kg.

Dinitroanile

TRIFLURALIN, NITRALIN, AND BENEFIN

Introduction

The dinitroaniline herbicides are an important group of compounds whose use is expanding. The most prominent member of the group is trifluralin, or α,α,α-trifluoro-2,6-dinitro-*N*-dipropyl-*p*-toluidine (Treflan), which was first marketed in 1963 for use on cotton. It is now registered on more than 50 crops. Other members of the group that have been used include nitralin, or 4-(methylsulfonyl)-2,6-dinitro-*N,N*-dipropylaniline (Planavin), and benefin, or *N*-butyl-*N*-ethyl-α,α,α-trifluoro-2,6-dinitro-*p*-toluidine (Balan). A summary of dinitroaniline compounds used or under development as herbicides is given by Helling (1976). These compounds are particularly effective against annual grasses and some broadleaf weeds.

It is estimated (NAS, 1975) that 11.4 million pounds of trifluralin and 2.7 million pounds of nitralin were used in the United States in 1971. Virtually all of this material was used in agriculture. Another estimate (Helling, 1976) indicates the consumption of about 17 million pounds of trifluralin in the United States in 1972. About 60% of the material is used on soybeans, 30% on cotton, and 10% on other crops. Most of the use is in the north-central and south-central states, especially Illinois, Iowa, and Mississippi, which consume about three-fourths of the total production. The dinitroaniline herbicides probably account for 8–10% by volume of domestic herbicide use. Because trifluralin is by far the most important member of this group, with respect to total volume of use, this report will concentrate on it, with some supporting information on several others.

Trifluralin is synthesized by the reaction of *p*-chlorobenzotrifluoride with fuming nitric acid to produce 3,5-dinitro-4-chlorobenzotrifluoride, which then reacts with di-*n*-propylamine to produce trifluralin. The technical material contains the desired product at more than 95%. It is soluble in water at 0.2–0.4 ppm at 25°C.

The dinitroanilines are strongly adsorbed by soil and moderately persistent in soil.

In the annual Market Basket Surveys conducted by the Food and Drug Administration, trifluralin residues have never been detected (Corneliussen, 1970, 1972; Manske and Corneliussen, 1974). Triflurain is tolerated at 0.05 ppm by most crops; exceptions are alfalfa hay (0.2 ppm), carrots (1 ppm), and mung beans (2 ppm). The FAO/WHO has not established an acceptable daily intake of trifluralin or any other dinitroaniline herbicide.

Trifluralin was detected in finished water in the United States (USEPA, 1976d).

Metabolism

Studies on the metabolism of trifluralin have been rather limited. Emmerson and Anderson (1966) studied the metabolism of trifluralin in rats and dogs. Approximately 80% of the ingested compound was excreted in the feces, the remainder in the urine. Analysis of the feces revealed the parent compound and one metabolite, the amino derivative resulting from reduction of one nitro group. Ten different materials in the urine were separated by thin-layer chromatography. Only three were identified; they were the products of nitro reduction or removal of one or both propyl groups.

Several investigators have reported on the behavior of trifluralin in dairy animals (Fisher *et al*., 1965; Golab *et al*., 1969; Williams and Feil, 1971). Trifluralin is dealkylated in the rumen, losing one or both propyl groups; the nitro groups are reduced to one or two amino groups. The two types of reactions occur simultaneously, leading to a trifluoromethyltriaminobenzene. Unidentified polar products were also produced in rumen fluid. The acute toxicity of some of these metabolites has been determined. Metabolites with free amino groups tend to be somewhat more acutely toxic in test species, although the maximal toxicity is still quite low, at 1,800 mg/kg for the diamino compound in the mouse.

Nelson *et al*. (1976) studied three structurally related dinitroaniline herbicides—trifluralin, profluralin, and fluchloralin—in rat hepatic microsomal systems. All three were extensively metabolized by both normal and phenobarbital-induced microsomal systems. Identification of the metabolites extractable with ethylacetate from the aqueous incubation mixtures indicated that aliphatic hydroxylation of the *N*-alkyl substituents, *N*-dealkylation, reduction of a nitro group, and cyclization to form benzimidazoles (and, in the case of fluchloralin, a quinoxaline) were the predominant metabolic routes for these herbicides *in vitro*. Of particular interest was the formation of the benzimidazole metabolites.

Health Aspects

Observations in Man No controlled studies have been conducted with dinitroaniline compounds in humans. Since 1969, 16 episodes of trifluralin poisoning have been reported. There have been no fatalities, and only one case required hospitalization. Ten of the 16 cases involved symptoms that appeared to be related to the solvent, rather than trifluralin itself. In general, adverse effects of dinitroaniline herbicides in humans have been few and minor (Verhulst, 1974).

Observations in Other Species

Acute Effects The dinitroaniline herbicides are very low in acute toxicity. The following oral LD_{50} values have been reported for various dinitroaniline compounds in rats: technical trifluralin, greater than 10,000 mg/kg; benefin, greater than 10,000 mg/kg; nitralin, greater than 6,000 mg/kg (Berg, 1976). The acute oral LD_{50} of the trifluralin emulsifiable concentrate formulation in rats is 3,700 mg/kg.

The acute oral toxicity of dinitroanilines in other animals is similarly low. The oral LD_{50} of trifluralin in mice is 5,000 mg/kg; of nitralin, greater than 2,000 mg/kg (Berg, 1976). The acute oral LD_{50} of trifluralin in dogs, chickens, and rabbits is greater than 2,000 mg/kg.

The dermal LD_{50}'s of trifluralin and nitralin in rabbits were greater than 2,000 mg/kg after 25 h of exposure (Worth, 1970). Rabbits exposed to 500 mg of technical trifluralin in a standard Draize skin irritation study had a score of zero, indicating no dermal irritation (Worth, 1970). Technical trifluralin also caused no damage when tested in rabbit eyes.

Subchronic and Chronic Effects Chickens, which are sensitive to the cataractogenic properties of compounds, were exposed to trifluralin. There was no effect in the trifluralin-treated chickens, whereas 14 of the 16 chickens in the positive control had obvious lens opacities by the third day of the study conducted by Worth (1970).

In a 10-day study of cattle, sheep, and chickens orally treated with trifluralin, benefin, and nitralin, the no-adverse-effect dosage was 100 mg/kg/day for trifluratin in cattle, sheep, and chickens. For benefin, poisoning and changes were observed at 25 mg/kg/day in cattle and 50 mg/kg/day in sheep and chickens. For nitralin, poisoning and death were observed at 250 mg/kg/day in cattle and 375 mg/kg/day in sheep; the no-adverse-effect dosage was 500 mg/kg/day in chickens (Palmer, 1972).

Harlan rats (six males and six females in each group) were fed technical trifluralin at 20, 200, 2,000, and 20,000 ppm in the diet for 2 yr. At the highest dosage level, rats showed significant growth retardation and bile duct proliferation and survived a maximum of 460 days. In all other groups, there were no significant differences between treated animals and controls in growth, mortality, food intake, efficiency of food utilization, gross pathologic effects, and microscopic examination of major organs and tissues. The no-adverse-effect dosage, therefore, was established as 2,000 ppm, which is equivalent to approximately 100 mg/kg/day, according to Elanco (1967). However, with the assumptions on food consumption and animal weight of this report, 2,000 ppm is equivalent to 333 mg/kg/day.

Another 2-yr study was conducted with 25 male and 25 female Cox rats fed trifluralin at 200, 1,000, and 2,000 ppm trifluralin. Several male rats at the two higher dosages exhibited enlargement of the thyroid. Two male rats at 1,000 ppm and one male at 2,000 ppm had pheochromocytomas. Neither of these responses was dosage-related. Hence, the no-adverse-effect dosage was reported to be 2,000 ppm (Elanco 1967).

Three studies on the chronic toxicity of trifluralin in dogs have been conducted. In one, eight mongrel dogs were given daily oral doses in capsules over a 2-yr period. One male and one female in each group were given 2.5 mg/kg, 5 mg/kg, and 25 mg/kg. Two females were given 10 mg/kg. There were no adverse effects at any dosage. In another study, beagles were treated at 1, 2.5, 5, and 10 mg/kg. With two animals per group (except for the lowest, which included four animals), no adverse effects were found at any dosage. In a 3-yr study, purebred beagles were given trifluralin orally at 10 and 25 mg/kg. Each treatment group included two animals of each sex, and a control group was established with three animals of each sex. At 25 mg/kg, an increased liver:body-weight ratio was observed. Therefore, the no-adverse-effect dosage was considered to be 10 mg/kg (Worth, 1970).

Two-year feeding studies of nitralin in rats and dogs have been conducted by the Stanford Research Institute (Burdett, 1968a,b). At dietary concentrations of 2.5, 10, 40, 160, and 2,000 ppm in both male and female rats, no adverse effects were found. Therefore, the no-adverse-effect dosage of nitralin is at least 2,000 ppm (333 mg/kg/day). Nitralin was also fed to 30 male and 30 female beagles in the diet at 2.5, 10, 40, 160, and 2,000 ppm for 2 yr. No adverse effects were seen at any dosage. Measured were weight gain, hematologic values, serum alkaline phosphatase levels, blood urea nitrogen, organ weight ratios between experimental animals and controls, and histopathology. Again, the no-adverse-effect dosage is at least as high as 2,000 ppm (40 mg/kg/day).

Mutagenicity In a large screening study of many herbicides, Anderson *et al.* (1972) noted that trifluralin did not induce point mutations in any of three microbial systems.

Carcinogenicity There are no reports of carcinogenic or tumorigenic effects of trifluralin or other dinitroaniline herbicides.

Reproduction Groups of 6 male and 12 female rats were fed trifluralin in the diet at 200 and 2,000 ppm in a four-generation reproduction study. There was a definite decrease in the fertility of the animals at 2,000 ppm in the third generation. There were also adverse effects on viability and lactation in the third generation. This was not the case at 200 ppm. The no-adverse-effect dosage, therefore, was 200 ppm in the diet, equivalent to 20 mg/kg/day (Elanco, 1967).

The dogs used in the chronic 3-yr study were interbred with animals in their same treatment group. Dosages were 10 and 25 mg/kg/day. A number of experimental difficulties in the study complicated interpretation of the results; however, the no-adverse-effect dosage was stated to be 10 mg/kg/day.

Teratogenicity Rats, dogs, and rabbits revealed no significant teratogenic effects in offspring (Elanco, 1967). In the dog study, one runt was produced at the highest dosage, but no other abnormalities or malformations were seen in any of the dogs at any dosage. In rabbits, at 1,000 mg/kg/day there was a significant reduction in weight during pregnancy of the does, which did not occur in the control group. At one of the intermediate dosages two of six fetuses had underdeveloped hind legs and hindquarters. This effect was not seen at higher dosages or in controls. Hence, it is not considered to be due to trifluralin.

Conclusions and Recommendations

The dinitroanilines are an increasingly important group of herbicides with an extremely low degree of toxicity in mammals. Trifluralin has been used in relatively large amounts in agriculture in the past, and its use is expected to increase. In addition, extensive development of other compounds in this group is under way. The group is likely to include a number of important herbicides in agricultural use for the foreseeable future.

The mode of action of the dinitroanilines has not been delineated at the cellular or molecular level in either plants or animals, although inhibition of mitosis has been observed in plants. No specific characteristic of dinitroaniline poisoning is observed in mammals. Hence, the toxicology of these compounds has been studied in laboratory animals with rather nonspecific indicators for the measurement of toxic end points.

Adequate studies of mammalian toxicity have been reported only for trifluralin, benefin, and nitralin. Fortunately, studies of the acute toxicity of other representatives of the group indicate that the toxicity of the

TABLE VI-13 Toxicity of Trifluralin

Species	Duration of Study	Dosage Levels and No. of Animals Per Group	Highest No-Adverse-Effect Level or Lowest-Minimal-Effect Level	Effect Measured	Reference
Rats	2 yr	20–20,000 ppm, orally, 12 animals/group	2,000 ppm	no adverse effect	Elanco, 1976
Rats	2 yr	200–2,000 ppm, orally, 50 animals/group	2,000 ppm	no adverse effect	Elanco, 1976
Dogs	2 yr	2.5–25 mg/kg/day, orally, 2 animals/group	25 mg/kg/day	no adverse effect	Elanco, 1976
Dogs	2 yr	1–10 mg/kg/day, 2 animals/group	10 mg/kg/day	no adverse effect	Elanco, 1976
Dogs	3 yr	10 and 25 mg/kg/day, orally, 4 animals/group	10 mg/kg/day[c] 25 mg/kg/day	no adverse liver-to-body-weight ratio	Worth, 1970
Rats	4 generations	0–2,000 ppm in diet, 18 animals/group	200 ppm 2,000 ppm	no adverse effect on fertility, viability of offspring, or lactation	Elanco, 1967

Using an uncertainty factor of 100, the suggested no-adverse-effect level in drinking water is calculated as follows:

$$\frac{10}{100} = 0.1 \text{ mg/kg/day (ADI)}, \; 0.1 \times 70^{a} \times 0.1^{b} = 0.7 \text{ mg/liter}$$

[a]Assume average weight of human adult = 70 kg.
[b]Assume average daily intake of water for man = 2 liters, and that 20 percent of total intake is from water.
[c]Value from which the suggested no-adverse-effect level was calculated.

various newer compounds is likely to be about the same. Conclusions on the safety of new compounds can probably be based on studies of trifluralin with some assurance of the reasonableness of extrapolation. The toxicology of the dinitroanilines appears to be straightforward; no reports indicate mutagenic or carcinogenic effects of these compounds. A single report on teratogenicity did not seem to show dose dependence and therefore could not place blame specifically on trifluralin. A no-adverse-effect dosage can thus be set for trifluralin that could be extended without difficulty to include all dinitroaniline herbicides that are structural analogues. The available data on chronic toxicity and a calculated ADI of 0.1 mg/kg/day are summarized in Table VI-13. This concentration can be easily detected in water by a number of analytic techniques.

In light of the recent report of benzimidazole metabolites from dinitroanilines and the vintage of *in vivo* metabolic studies, there is a need for additional studies on the metabolism of these compounds in mammalian systems. The toxicology of metabolites should be investigated. As new compounds are introduced for development, chronic toxicologic studies should be done, to be sure that no anomalous effect will be observed from them that could not have been predicted from previous work with trifluralin, benefin, and nitralin. Additional studies on the possibility of teratogenic effects of dinitroanilines need to be conducted.

Aldehyde

ACROLEIN

Introduction

Acrolein, or acrylaldehyde, is a colorless liquid, readily soluble in water. It is extremely volatile, and vapors of the compound are irritating and cause excessive lacrimation. Dilute solutions of Acrolein are effective in killing undesirable plant life in irrigation streams and ditches.

Acrolein is reportedly a common air pollutant arising from various manufacturing processes and is also a constituent of cigarette smoke (Sinkuvene, 1970).

Metabolism

No available data.

Health Aspects

Observations in Man No available data.

Observations in Other Species

Acute Effects The acute oral LD_{50} of aqueous Acrolein solutions is 42 mg/kg in rats and 28 mg/kg in mice (Newill, 1958). Water intake of male rats receiving Acrolein at 80 and 160 ppm and female rats receiving 160 ppm was markedly decreased. Dietary consumption of the male rats was decreased slightly at 160 ppm, whereas that of the females was unaffected.

Subchronic and Chronic Effects In a subchronic study conducted with male and female rats for 90 days, Acrolein was added to the drinking water at 5, 13, 32, 80, and 200 ppm. No hematologic, organ-weight, or pathologic changes could be attributed to the ingestion of Acrolein. However, water consumption was reduced by one-third at 200 ppm for the first 3 weeks. By the twelfth week, the animals had apparently adapted to the odor and taste of the Acrolein (Newell, 1958).

Three additional groups of male rats were given drinking water containing Acrolein at 600, 1,200, and 1,800 for 60 days. Only one of five animals died at 600 ppm, whereas all the animals died at 1,200 and 1,800 ppm (Newell, 1958). Death was apparently due to lack of water intake; they would not drink the unpalatable solutions. Tissues from the surviving animals 600 ppm did not show any gross or micropathologic abnormalities.

No chronic-toxicity studies are available.

Inhalation Toxicity A study by Watanabe and Aviado (1974) has indicated that mice that inhale Acrolein at 0.1 μg/ml daily for 5 weeks develop reductions in pulmonary compliance. Because mice that had been exposed to the vapor phase of cigarette smoke do not exhibit reduced pulmonary compliance, it was concluded that the amounts of Acrolein contained in cigarette smoke contribute little to compliance changes.

Inhalation studies with mongrel dogs have revealed that total-tract retention of Acrolein is about 8,170 when the animals were exposed to concentrations of 0.4–0.6 μg/ml (Egle, 1972). The daily average maximal permissible concentration of Acrolein in the atmosphere has been determined in rats (Gusev, 1966). For these studies, groups of rats were placed in inhalation chambers containing Acrolein at 0.01, 0.51, and 1.52

mg/m^3 for periods of a few days to several weeks. Various factors were measured, but there was considerable lung damage in the group exposed to 1.52 mg/m^3. It was concluded that 0.1 mg/m^3 should not be exceeded. In another study, the maximum one-time and daily average permissible concentrations of Acrolein in the atmosphere were recommended to be set at 0.03 mg/m^3 (Sinkuvene, 1970).

Other Toxicologic Effects Murphy (1965) demonstrated that Acrolein affects liver alkaline phosphatase and tyrosine-α-ketoglutarate transaminase activities in rats 5–12 h after injection (3 mg/kg 20 h before sacrifice) or inhalation of Acrolein. Murphy found that these effects could be prevented or substantially reduced by prior adrenalectomy or hypophysectomy or by pretreatment of the animals with chemicals that inhibit protein synthesis. According to Murphy, the data suggested that the irritant action of Acrolein stimulates the pituitary–adrenal system, leading to hypersecretion of glucocorticoids that act to induce or stimulate the synthesis of increased amounts of the enzyme proteins by the liver.

Studies have been conducted on the effect of Acrolein on DNA-dependent DNA polymerase of regenerating rat liver. Munsch *et al.* (1973) found that an Acrolein-enzyme interaction seems to be fully responsible for the impaired replication *in vitro*, whereas incubations of the substrates with Acrolein slightly but reproducibly increase the enzyme activity, and incubations of the template with Acrolein do not affect the duplication. When DNA polymerase was preincubated with increasing amounts of Acrolein, the template duplication was either activated at low molarities or inhibited above 8×10^{-5} *M*.

Acrolein appears to possess indirect sympathomimetic activity. It produced irreversible contractile responses in rat vas deferens that were not blocked by reserpine pretreatment (Beckner *et al.*, 1974). Acrolein also apparently interacts with tissue norepinephrine stores and affects nonspecific membrane calcium-binding sites.

Mutagenicity, Teratogenicity, and Carcinogenicity No available data.

Conclusions and Recommendations

Acrolein is an herbicide that is used primarily for the control of aquatic weeds. It is highly volatile and apparently does not persist for extended periods in an aqueous environment. Only limited acute- and subchronic-toxicity data are available. In view of the relative paucity of data on the mutagenicity, carcinogenicity, teratogenicity, and long-term oral toxicity of Acrolein, estimates of the effects of chronic oral exposure at low levels cannot be made with any confidence. It is recommended that studies to produce such information be conducted before limits in drinking water can be established.

PESTICIDES: INSECTICIDES

Clorinated Hydrocarbons

CYCLODIENES: ALDRIN, DIELDRIN, ENDRIN, CHLORDANE, HEPTACHLOR, AND HEPTACHLOR EPOXIDE

Introduction

The cyclodiene insecticides are all derivatives of hexachlorocyclopentadiene produced by the Diels-Alder, or diene, reaction. Their discovery and development date from the synthesis of chlordane by Julius Hyman in 1944 (U.S. Pats. 2,509,160 and 2,606,910). Perhaps 600 million pounds of these highly chlorinated, cyclic organic compounds have been dispersed into the soil, air, water, and food of the United States during the last 30 yr. Little is certain about the degradation and fate of these compounds; however, traces of them and their stable epoxide oxidation products are ubiquitous in the environment and are heavily bioconcentrated in the lipids of terrestrial and aquatic wildlife, humans, and foods, especially animal fats and milk.

The cyclodienes have been used principally as preemergence soil insecticides for the control of corn rootworms, wireworms, cutworms, etc.; as seed treatments; as soil poisons for control of termites and ants; and on cotton for the control of the boll weevil and bollworms.

Aldrin, or 1,2,3,4,10,10-hexachloro-1,4,4a,5,8,8a-hexahydro-*endo*-1,4-*exo*-5,8-dimethanonaphthalene, is soluble in water at 0.027 ppm at 25°C (Gunther *et al.*, 1968).

Dieldrin, or 6,7-epoxy aldrin, is soluble in water at 0.25 ppm at 25°C (Gunther *et al.*, 1968).

Endrin, or 1,2,3,4,10,10-hexachloro-6,7-epoxy-1,4,4a,5,6,7,8,8a-octahydro-*endo*-1,4-*endo*-5,8-dimethanonaphthalene, is soluble in water at 0.25 ppm at 25°C (Gunther *et al.*, 1968). Endrin is produced by condensing hexachlorocyclopentadiene with vinyl chloride to produce heptachlorbicyclo-(2.2.1)-2-heptene. This is condensed with cyclopentadiene to form isodrin and that is oxidized to the 6,7-epoxide with peracetic or perbenzoic acid (Brooks, 1973).

Chlordane, or 1,2,4,5,6,7,8,8-octachloro-2,3,3a,4,7,7a-hexahydro-4,7-methanoindene, is a viscous amber liquid soluble in water at about 0.009 ppm at 25°C. Chlordane is manufactured by condensing hexachlorocyclopendadiene with cyclopentadiene to form chlordene and chlorinating the latter to approximate $C_{10}H_6Cl_{18}$. The technical material contains about 60–75% of the *cis*- (m.p. 106.5-108°), and *trans*- (m.p. 104.5–106°) isomers together with unreacted chlordene and isomers of the $C_{10}H_5Cl_7$ product Heptachlor (Brooks, 1973).

Heptachlor, or 1,4,5,6,7,8,8-heptachloro-3a,4,7,7a-tetrahydro-4,7-methanondene, is soluble in water at about 0.056 ppm at 25°C (Park and Bruce, 1968). Heptachlor is produced from Chlordene by chlorination with sulfuryl chloride (Brooks, 1973).

Heptachlor epoxide, or 1,4,5,6,7,8,8-heptachloro-2,3-epoxy-3a,4,7,7a-tetrahydro-4,7-methanoindene, is soluble in water at 0.350 ppm (Park and Bruce, 1968).

Domestic production in 1971 estimates are (NAS, 1975): Chlordane, 25 million pounds; Aldrin, 10 million pounds; Heptachlor, 6 million pounds; Dieldrin, less than 1 million pounds; and Endrin, less than 1 million pounds. Because of their environmental persistence and carcinogenic behavior in laboratory animals, Aldrin and Dieldrin were banned by the EPA on October 1, 1974, and Chlordane and Heptachlor registrations for agricultural crops were suspended on April 1, 1976.

Because of their persistence the cyclodienes and their epoxides—*viz.*, Dieldrin, Heptachlor epoxide, and probably Oxychlordane—are found in surface waters virtually everywhere. In an extensive 1958–1965 survey of the rivers of the United States, Breidenbach *et al.* (1967) found the following average concentrations of the cyclodienes:

Aldrin, <0.001–0.006 ppb
Dieldrin, 0.08–0.122 ppb
Endrin, 0.008–0.214 ppb
Heptachlor, 0.0–0.0031 ppb
Heptachlor epoxide, <0.001–0.008 ppb
DDT, 0.008–0.144 ppb

The highest concentrations were generally found in the lower Mississippi basin. In 1964, 74% of the grab samples were positive for Dieldrin, 46% for Endrin, 10% for Aldrin, 17% for Heptachlor, and 25% for Heptachlor epoxide. In comparison, 44% were positive for DDT and 39% for DDE.

More than 500 grab samples of finished drinking water and related raw water from the Mississippi and Missouri rivers were analyzed by Schafer *et al.* (1969). More than 40% of the finished-water samples contained Dieldrin at up to 0.25 ppb, more than 30% contained Endrin, and 20% contained Chlordane at up to 0.5 ppb. Aldrin and Heptachlor were found occasionally.

An extensive investigation of surface, subsurface, and finished water in Iowa (Richard *et al.*, 1974) showed Dieldrin present at the following concentrations:

S. Skunk River	2–76 ppt
Indian Creek	4–30 ppt
Des Moines River	2–12 ppt
Raccoon River	1–12 ppt
Red Rock Reservoir	3–36 ppt
Rothbun Reservoir	2–22 ppt
Cedar Rapids (surface)	.042 ppt
Iowa River	22 ppt
Mississippi River	<0.5–7 ppt
Finished Waters	
Davenport	2 ppt
Iowa City	5 ppt
Des Moines	0.4–2 ppt

It was concluded that water-treatment plants were not removing substantial amounts of pesticides from raw water, even by filtration through activated-carbon beds.

The New Orleans water supply contained Dieldrin at 0.05–0.07 ppb (50–70 ppt) and Endrin at 0.004 ppb (USEPA, 1974a). The 10-city drinking-water survey (USEPA, 1975j) found Dieldrin at 1–2 ppt in

TABLE VI-14 Pesticides in Food

	Daily Dietary Intake, mg						
Pesticide	1965	1966	1967	1968	1969	1970	6-yr Average
Aldrin	0.001	0.002	0.001	T[a]	T	T	0.001
Dieldrin	0.005	0.007	0.001	0.004	0.005	0.005	0.005
Endrin	T	T	T	0.001	T	T	0.001
Heptachlor	T	—	T	T	T	T	T
Heptachlor epoxide	0.002	0.003	0.001	0.002	0.002	0.001	0.002

[a]T = trace.

drinking water of Miami, Seattle, Ottumwa (Iowa), and Cincinnati. Other cyclodienes identified in U.S. drinking water included Aldrin, Chlordane, Chlordene, Endrin (80 ppt), Heptachlor, and Heptachlor epoxide.

Standards have been proposed for the maximal permissible concentrations of the cyclodienes in finished water (Schafer *et al.*, 1969). Concentrations suggested in 1965–1966 and based on those of the Subcommittee on Toxicology in 1965 were: Aldrin, 32 ppb; Dieldrin, 18 ppb; Endrin, 1 ppb; Heptachlor, 78 ppb; Heptachlor epoxide, 18 ppb; and Chlordane, 52 ppb. The suggested DDT-T (DDT, DDE, and DDD combined) concentration was 42 ppb. These were drastically lowered in a 1967 recommendation (Ettinger and Mount, 1967) based on maximal reasonable stream allowances to: Aldrin, 0.25 ppb; Dieldrin, 0.25 ppb; Endrin, 0.1 ppb; Heptachlor, 1.0 ppb; Heptachlor epoxide, 1.0 ppb; and Chlordane, 0.15 ppb. The DDT-T allowance was 0.5 ppb.

The U.S. Public Health Service Advisory Committee recommended the following drinking-water standards in 1968 (Mrak, 1969): Aldrin, 17 ppb; Dieldrin, 17 ppb; Endrin, 1 ppb; Heptachlor, 18 ppb; and Heptachlor epoxide, 18 ppb.

The EPA has set an interim standard for Endrin in finished water of 0.0002 mg/liter (USEPA, 1975i).

Residues in Food The persistent organochlorine cyclodienes are present everywhere in the environment, are readily biomagnified through food chains, and are common trace contaminants of human food. Market Basket Surveys of the U.S. diet, collected in five major U.S. cities and designed to simulate the diet of a 16–19-yr-old male, have produced results summarized in Table VI-14 (NAS, 1975).

The combined residues for Aldrin and Dieldrin are very close to the FAO/WHO acceptable daily intake (ADI), which is 0.0001 mg/kg/day for Aldrin and Dieldrin vs. 0.00013 mg/kg/day in 1966. For Heptachlor and Heptachlor epoxide, the FAO/WHO ADI is 0.0005 mg/kg/day vs. 0.00005 mg/kg/day in 1966 (Mrak, 1969). It should be pointed out that recent studies showing increases in mouse hepatomas at the lowest dosages fed—i.e., 0.1 ppm—demonstrated that no-adverse-effect level for Aldrin and Dieldrin has never been determined and that the ADI is therefore too high.

Cyclodienes in Milk Residues of the cyclodienes in milk are particularly high because of the ingestion of these insecticides with forage. Dieldrin has the highest retention time of all pesticides in milk, approximately 100 days (Mrak, 1969). For example, analogues of 1971 milk samples from 12 grade B dairy farms in an intensive grain-producing

TABLE VI-15 Organochlorine Insecticides in Illinois from Cow's Milk, ppm

Insecticide	1971	1972	1973	Average
Chlordane	0.02	0.04	0.06	0.05
DDT	0.05	0.02	0.03	0.03
Dieldrin	0.08	0.04	0.08	0.07
Heptachlor	0.03	0.03	0.05	0.05
Lindane	T[a]	0.02	0.03	0.02

[a]T = trace.
NOTE: Of 200 samples analyzed, 87% were positive for Chlordane, 92% for DDT, 94% for Dieldrin, 93% for Heptachlor, and 81% for Lindane (Moore, 1975).

area of northwestern Illinois showed combined Aldrin and Dieldrin concentrations in butterfat of 0.1314–0.5560 ppm (average 0.2921). There was a definite correlation between the overall Dieldrin soil residue on each farm (0.0104–0.3859 ppm) and the concentration in the milk (Moore *et al.*, 1973). Consumption of this milk (composite Dieldrin concentration 0.22 ppm) by a 5-kg infant at 500 g/day would provide a daily Dieldrin intake of approximately 0.75 μg/kg, or 7.5 times the FAO/WHO ADI.

The general concentrations of organochlorine insecticides in Illinois milk in 1971–1973 are shown in Table VI-15 (Moore, 1975).

Of 200 samples analyzed, 87% were positive for Chlordane, 92% for DDT, 94% for Dieldrin, 93% for Heptachlor, and 81% for Lindane (Moore, 1975).

Food Chain Effects The cyclodiene insecticides—especially the epoxides Dieldrin, Heptachlor epoxide, and Oxychlordane—are very stable, both environmentally and biologically, and have high lipid-water partition coefficients. Thus, they pass through food chains and undergo biologic magnification (Lu *et al.*, 1975; Metcalf *et al.*, 1973).

These factors account for the bioaccumulation of these persistent products in human adipose tissue. The values shown in Table VI-16 indicate the average amounts found in fiscal year 1970–1974 in over 1,400 bioassays of U.S. human fatty tissues (NAS, 1975).

The presence of Oxychlordane was first discovered in 1972. The decreasing amounts of DDT-T clearly reflect the banning of this compound.

The human is at the top of the food pyramid; thus, persistent pesticide residues, such as those of the cyclodienes, are excreted in human milk; [see Table VI-17 (Curley and Kimbrough, 1969)]. Recent unpublished studies have also identified oxychlordane in human milk.

TABLE VI-16 Pesticides in Fatty Tissue

Insecticide	Concentration, ppm				
	1970	1971	1972	1973	1974
Dieldrin	0.27	0.29	0.24	0.24	0.20
Heptachlor epoxide	0.17	0.12	0.12	0.12	0.10
Oxychlordane	—	—	0.15	0.15	0.15
DDT-T	11.65	11.55	9.91	8.91	7.83

Dieldrin provides a graphic example of the propensity to persist in food chains and to accumulate in lipid tissues. Gannon *et al.* (1959) demonstrated that Dieldrin fed to chickens was stored in body fat to very much higher concentrations than when fed to steers, hogs, and lambs. For example, Dieldrin fed at 0.1 ppm was stored at 4.1 ppm, and that fed at 0.75 ppm was stored at 35.7 ppm. However, it was not until 1974 that it was demonstrated that as many as 20 million chickens in Mississippi fed on waste food stocks of soybean oil that had been processed on soybeans grown in Aldrin-treated soil containing illegal residues of Dieldrin (generally at 0.01–0.04 ppm) contained Dieldrin residues in their body fat greatly exceeding the FDA "safe limit" of 0.3 ppm and ranging up to 30 ppm (Moore, 1975). The chickens had to be destroyed as unfit for human consumption (Pesticide Chemical News, 1974).

Metabolism

The breakdown pathways of the cyclodienes are relatively complex (Brooks, 1973) and are still in the process of elucidation. Many of the degradation products are highly active neurotoxins—e.g., photodieldrin—and present a substantial degree of environmental hazard. The metabolic pathways can only be summarized here.

TABLE VI-17 Pesticides in Human Milk

Insecticide	Concentration, ppm	
	Mean	Range
Dieldrin	0.0073	0.0029–0.0146
Heptachlor epoxide	0.0027	<0.0001–0.0044
DDT-T	0.0027	0.0404–0.1563

Aldrin and Dieldrin The dominant reaction of Aldrin is epoxidation at the double bond to form the 6,7-epoxide dieldrin. This is a microsomal oxidation and occurs photochemically and biologically in soils, plant tissues, and in all animals studied (Gannon and Decker, 1958). Thus the very stable Dieldrin appears everywhere in the environment as the major contaminant following the use of Aldrin. Further biological or photochemical reaction of Dieldrin produces photodieldrin or 10-oxa-3,6-*exo*-4,5,13,13-hexachloro-$(6.3.1.1^{3,6}.1^{9,11}.0^{2,7}.0^{5,12})$- tridecane, a cagelike compound (Matsumura *et al.*, 1970). Photodieldrin is about 5 times more acutely toxic to laboratory animals then Dieldrin. Aldrin is also degraded in plants and animals to hexachloro-hexahydro-1,4-*endo*-methyl-enein-dene-5, 7-dicarboxylic acid (Klein *et al.*, 1973) and to aldrin-*trans*-diol. In animals 5-hydroxydieldrin, 9-keto-dieldrin, and keto-photodieldrin are also formed as excretory metabolites (Mathews *et al.*, 1971). The hydroxy degradation products are largely conjugated in animals before excretion.

Endrin This cyclodiene exists in the *endo–endo* configuration, which is inherently less stable than the *endo–exo* configuration of its stereoisomer dieldrin. Endrin isomerizes in light to form Δ-ketoendrin or 1,8-*exo*-9,10,11,11-hexachloropentacyclo$(6.2.1.1^{3,6}.0^{2,7}.0^{4,10}$-dodecan-5-one. In animals, Endrin is degraded, largely to 9-ketoendrin and 9-hydroxyendrin, but also to 5-hydroxyendrin (Baldwin *et al.*, 1970).

Heptachlor and Heptachlor Epoxide Heptachlor is rapidly oxidized to the 2,3-heptachlor epoxide (Davidow and Radomski, 1953). This is a microsomal oxidation and occurs both photochemically and biologically in soils, plant tissues, and all animals studied (Gannon and Decker, 1958). Thus, the stable heptachlor epoxide appears everywhere in the environment as the major contaminant after the use of Heptachlor. Heptachlor epoxide is more toxic to animals than heptachlor. Heptachlor differs from Aldrin, in that it is much more easily hydrolyzed, because of the allyclic C=C–CHCl structure, to form l-hydroxychlordene or 1-hydroxy-4,5,6,7,8,8-hexachloro-3a,4,7,7a-tetrahydro-4,7-methanoindene, which is converted to the 2,3-epoxide, an excretory metabolite in animals (Lu *et al.*, 1975). Heptachlor forms a photoproduct, photoheptachlor. Heptachlor epoxide forms photoheptachlor epoxide and slowly hydrolyzes to the diol (Menzie, 1974).

Chlordane Both the *cis*- and *trans*-Chlordanes form a single epoxide, Oxychlordane, or 1-*exo*-2-*endo*-4,5,6,7,8,8-octachloro-2,3-*exo*epoxy-2,3,-3a,4,7,7a-hexahydro-4,7-methanoindene (Schwemmer *et al.*, 1970). This has only recently been recognized as the major terminal residue in animal tissues and milk after ingestion of Chlordane (Barnett and Dorough, 1974). Oxychlordane is more toxic to animals than either of the Chlordane isomers. There is also evidence of the formation of hydrophilic degradation products, such as chlordanedihydrodiol and 1-hydroxy-2-chlorodihydrochlordene (Korte, 1967). Other degradation products identified include 1-hydroxychlordane and photochlordane, a cagelike compound (Menzie, 1974).

Health Aspects

The effects of the cyclodienes on animal and human health are very subtle and complex. These are the most hazardous of all pesticides, because of their persistence, fat storage, and central nervous system target site. Their effects can be reviewed only briefly here.

Observations in Man Human illness and death have been observed after poisoning during the manufacture, spraying, or accidental ingestion of the cyclodienes. Typical symptoms of poisoning result from stimulation of the central nervous system and include headache, blurred vision, dizziness, slight involuntary muscular movements, sweating, insomnia, bad dreams, nausea, and general malaise. More severe illness is characterized by jerking of muscles or groups of muscles and epileptiform convulsions, with loss of consciousness, involuntary incontinence of urine and feces, disorientation, personality changes, psychic disturbances, and loss of memory. Such seizures may recur for 2–4 months after cessation of exposure and are marked by abnormal encephalographic patterns. These symptoms of severe poisoning have developed in 10–20% of spraymen working in WHO house-spraying programs (Hayes, 1957, 1959), and such poisoning has not been eliminated in any spray program.

Epidemics of Endrin poisoning have occurred after the eating of bread made from flour accidentally contaminated with Endrin; there were 59 illnesses in one episode (Davies and Lewis, 1956) and 874, with 26 deaths, in Saudi Arabia (Weeks, 1967). At least 97 cases of fatal Endrin poisoning were recorded through 1965 (USEPA, 1973a). It appears that ingestion of Endrin at 0.2–0.25 mg/kg can produce convulsions in humans (Hayes, 1963).

Workers in a plant manufacturing and formulating Aldrin, Dieldrin, Isodrin, and Endrin had epileptiform convulsions (3.3%) and had encephalograms suggesting brain stem injury (20.5%). The encephalograms usually returned to normal within 3–6 months after exposure ceased (Hoogendem *et al.*, 1962).

TABLE VI-18 Acute Toxicity of Cyclodienes

	Oral LD_{50}, mg/kg		Dermal LD_{50}, mg/kg	
Substance	Male	Female	Male	Female
Aldrin	39	60	98	98
Dieldrin	46	46	90	64
Photodieldrin	9.6	—	—	—
Endrin	17.8	7.5	—	15
Chlordane	335	430	840	690
Heptachlor	100	162	195	250
Heptachlor epoxide	46.5	61.3	—	—
Endosulfan	43	18	130	74

Observations in Other Species

Acute Effects The acute dermal and oral LD_{50} values of the various cyclodienes and key degradation products in rats, as measured under uniform conditions, were given by Hayes (1963) and are summarized in Table VI-18.

Not only are such compounds as Endrin extraordinarily toxic (it is registered as a rodenticide), but the dermal toxicity is roughly equivalent to the oral toxicity.

Chronic Effects The results of chronic feeding of the cyclodienes to laboratory animals are extraordinarily severe, and true no-adverse-effect dosages have never been determined for some of the compounds, such as Dieldrin, Heptachlor, and Chlordane (Walker *et al.*, 1972). Toxicological evaluation is complicated by the *in vivo* conversion of the cyclodienes to epoxides by microsomal oxidation: Aldrin to Dieldrin, Heptachlor to Heptachlor epoxide (Davidow and Radowski, 1953), and Chlordane isomers to Oxychlordane (Schwemmer *et al.*, 1970). Dieldrin, Heptachlor epoxide, and Oxychlordane are very persistent and fat soluble and are the dominant metabolites stored in human and animal tissues and excreted in milk. The amounts of these cyclodienes found in human adipose tissues in 1970–1974 were: Dieldrin, 0.00–15.2 ppm (mean, 0.18 ppm); Heptachlor epoxide, 0.00–10.62 ppm (mean, 0.17 ppm); and Oxychlordane (mean, 0.15 ppm) (NAS, 1975).

Chlordane fed to rats at 2.5 ppm caused slight liver damage (Lehman, 1952). Heptachlor fed to rats at 0.3–1.0 ppm resulted in the accumulation of Heptachlor epoxide in the body fat. When it was fed to dogs at 1 mg/kg/day, three of four animals died in 265-424 days; at 5 mg/kg/day, death occurred in 21–22 days (Lehman, 1952). Aldrin fed to rats at 5 ppm produced no adverse effects; fed to dogs at 1 mg/kg/day, it caused death in 21–22 days (Lehman, 1952).

Dieldrin fed to rats at 5 ppm produced no adverse effect. When it was fed to dogs at 0.5 mg/kg/day, two of four animals died, in 14 and 201 days; at 1 mg/kg/day, both animals tested died, in 83 and 300 days; at 2 mg/kg/day, both animals died, in 22 and 35 days (Lehman, 1952). In recent studies, Dieldrin fed to mice at 2.5 and 5 ppm in the diet shortened the life span; at 0.1-1.0 ppm, it caused a progressive increase in malignant hepatomas (Walker *et al.*, 1972). Thus, the no-adverse-effect dosage has never been determined.

Endrin fed to rats at 1 and 5 ppm in the diet produced no obvious effects over the life span, except for liver enlargement at 5 ppm. When it was fed at 25 ppm, the life span was shortened, and diffuse degeneration was seen in brain, liver, kidneys, and adrenals. Mice fed Endrin at 0.1–4.0 ppm over their life span showed increased liver weights at 2 and 4 ppm and vascular damage of liver cells. Convulsions were observed in dogs fed 2 and 4 ppm, and autopsies revealed pathologic changes in the brain (USEPA, 1973a).

Aldrin, Dieldrin, and Endrin at very low dosages affect the central nervous system, producing encephalographic changes and altering behavior. Medved *et al.* (1964) found that cats fed Aldrin at 1 mg/kg/day or made to inhale 0.1 μg/liter of air had marked lowering of conditioned reflexes and of unconditioned food and orientation reflexes, which required up to 8 days to return to normal. Sheep fed Dieldrin at 0.5 and 2.5 mg/kg/day had abnormal encephalographic and behavioral responses (Sandler *et al.*, 1968, Van Gelder *et al.*, 1969).

Mutagenicity Dieldrin was not mutagenic in the *Salmonella*/microsome test (McCann, 1975). There is no available information on Aldrin, Endrin, Chlordane, Heptachlor, and Heptachlor epoxide.

Carcinogenicity The Mrak Commission (Mrak, 1969) judged Aldrin, Dieldrin, and Heptachlor as positive for tumor induction in one or more species of laboratory test animals. Dieldrin fed to mice (CF1) for 2 yr (Walker *et al.*, 1972) produced a dosage-dependent incidence of hepatomas. In males, the incidences were: controls, 7%; on 0.1-ppm Dieldrin, 21%; on 1-ppm Dieldrin, 28%; and on 10-ppm Dieldrin, 53%. In females, the incidences were: controls, 4%; on 0.1-ppm Dieldrin, 30%; on 1-ppm Dieldrin, 42%; and on 10-ppm Dieldrin, 62%. Although the malignant nature of these tumors was questioned by the experimenters, they were later declared as true metastatic malignancies by a panel of experts (USEPA, 1974d). Experiments with rats and dogs were less definitive (Walker et al., 1969). An additional 2-yr feeding study with Dieldrin and Photodieldrin has been reported by Walton *et al.* (1971).

Heptachlor epoxide fed to rats (CF11) over a 2-yr period at 0.5, 2.5, 5.0, 7.5, and 10 ppm in the diet produced increased numbers of tumors, mostly adrenal, in all groups, compared with controls. Even at 0.5 ppm, there was a 62.5% incidence of tumors in male rats, compared with 34.78% in controls, and 82.61% incidence in female rats, compared with 54.17% in controls. From these apparently unpublished results, Heptachlor epoxide was judged as a highly potent carcinogen (Kettering Laboratory, 1959).

Chlordane and Heptachlor were evaluated for carcinogenicity by the National Cancer Institute and were found to be carcinogenic in mice (B6C3E1), with a high incidence of hepatocellular carcinomas when fed over an 80-week period, and in rats, in which hepatic nodules and liver hyperplasia were produced. Chlordane fed at 56 ppm produced 88.9% hepatocellular carcinoma in male mice, compared with 10% in controls, and fed at 64 ppm produced 69.6% hepatocellular carcinoma in female mice, compared with 0% in controls. Heptachlor fed at 13.8 ppm produced 70.2% hepatocellular carcinoma in male mice, compared with 11.1% in controls, and fed at 18.0 ppm produced 69.0% hepatocellular carcinoma in female mice, compared with 10% in controls. It was judged that both Chlordane and Heptachlor are potent liver carcinogens in both sexes of mice (NCI, 1975).

Endrin was fed to rats at 2, 6, or 12 ppm in the diet for 2 yr without producing primary malignant hepatic tumors or increasing tumor incidence in any organs (Dieckmann *et al.*, 1970).

Davis and Fitzhugh (1962) fed Aldrin at 10 ppm in the diet to C_3HeB/Fe mice for 2 yr. There was a statistically significant increase in the number of benign liver tumors in the Aldrin-fed mice as compared to controls. This study is cited by the Mrak Commission (Mrak, 1969) to be positive evidence for tumor induction for this compound.

Aldrin fed to rats at 2.5, 12.5, and 25 ppm in the diet for 2 yr produced non-dosage-dependent tumors which were not significantly different from the tumor incidences in the controls (Cleveland, 1966).

Reproduction Endrin fed to mice at 5 ppm for 30 days produced significantly smaller litters than in controls. However, 7 ppm had no significant effect on mean litter size and litter production frequency when fed to Saskatchewan deer mice (*Peromyscus maniculatus*) over intermittent periods. Rats fed 2 ppm over three generations had no observable effect in fertility, gestation, viability, and lactation (cited in USEPA, 1973a).

When quail were fed 1 ppm, no eggs were produced during the reproductive period. Endrin fed at 10 ppm reduced egg production in pheasants and reduced survival of the chicks (cited in USEPA, 1973a).

Evidence presented at EPA hearings (1974d) indicated substantial effects of Dieldrin on animal reproduction. For example, raccoons fed Dieldrin at 2 and 6 ppm in the diet produced 20.0 and 20.2%, respectively, as many young as did untreated controls. Litter size was also reduced. In further study, raccoons fed Dieldrin at 2 ppm had abnormal estrous cycle, reduced ovulation rate, reduction of pregnancy to 25–30% of that in controls, increased resorption of embryos, and reduction in litter size. Dieldrin also influenced spermatogenesis, sperm quality, and fertility adversely in male raccoons.

Teratogenicity Aldrin, Dieldrin and Endrine were studied by Ottolenghi *et al.* (1974) in hamsters and mice. Single oral doses of approximately one-half the respective LD_{50} doses were given on days 7, 3, or 9 of gestation in the hamster and on day 9 of gestation in the mouse. A significant number of defects were produced in both species.

Chlordane was found not to be teratogenic in rats at 150 to 300 ppm in diet (Ingle, 1952).

Carcinogenic Risk Estimates

Dieldrin, Chlordane and Heptachlor have produced dose-related hepatomas when fed to mice (Walker *et al.*, 1972, and NCI, 1975). For each compound the available sets of dose–response data were individually considered as described in the risk section in the margin-of-safety chapter. Each set of dose–response data was used to statistically estimate both the lifetime risk and an upper 95% confidence bound on the lifetime risk at the low-dose level. These estimates are of lifetime human risks and have been corrected for species conversion on a dose-per-surface-area basis. The risk estimates are expressed as a probability of cancer after a lifetime consumption of 1 liter of water per day containing Q ppb of the compound of interest. For example a risk of $1\times10^{-6}\,Q$ implies a lifetime probability of 2×10^{-5} of cancer if 2 liters/day were consumed and the concentration of the carcinogen was 10 ppb (i.e., $Q=10$). This means that at a concentration of 10 ppb during a lifetime of exposure this compound would be expected to produce one excess case of cancer for every 50,000 persons exposed. If the population of the United States is taken to be 220 million people, this translates into 4,400 excess lifetime deaths from cancer or 62.8 per year. Since several data sets are typically available the range of the dose risk estimates are reported.

For Dieldrin at a concentration of 1 μg/liter ($Q=1$) the estimated risk for man would fall between 0.8-1.9$\times 10^{-4}$ Q. The upper 95% confidence estimate of risk at the same concentration would be between 1.9-2.4$\times 10^{-4}$ Q.

For Chlordane at a concentration of 1 μg/liter ($Q=1$) the upper 95% confidence estimated of risk for man would be between 0.96-1.8$\times 10^{-5}$ Q.

For Heptachlor at a concentration of 1 μg/liter ($Q=1$) the upper 95% confidence estimate of risk for man would be from 3.5 to 4.8$\times 10^{-5}$ Q.

Conclusions and Recommendations

The cyclodiene insecticides—particularly the persistent epoxides, Dieldrin, Endrin, Heptachlor epoxide, and Oxychlordane—present the greatest hazards of all residual pesticides in water. At low dosages, they are highly active hepatocarcinogens and have a dangerous effect on the central nervous system of man and higher animals, leading to apparently irreversible changes in encephalographic and behavioral patterns. They are highly persistent biologically and can accumulate in animal fats and milk.

In light of the above and taking into account the carcinogenic risk projections, it is suggested that very strict criteria be applied when limits for Dieldrin, Heptachlor, and Chlordane in drinking-water are established. Before limits for Aldrin, Endrin, and Heptachlor epoxide in drinking water can be established, more toxicological data must be gathered and evaluated. The available chronic-toxicity data are summarized in Tables VI-19, VI-20, VI-21, and VI-22.

DDT AND DDE

Introduction

DDT, or 2,2-*bis*-(*p*-chlorophenyl)-1,1,1-trichloroethane, was patented as an insecticide in 1939 by Swiss chemist Paul Muller. After a period of extensive use for the control of malaria, typhus, and other insect-transmitted diseases during World War II, it became the prototype of the synthetic insecticides. At the height of its use in the United States, in 1963, production was 176 million pounds, and DDT was registered for use on 334 agricultural commodities. DDT has been used very extensively all over the world, both in malaria control and in agriculture, and it is estimated that more than 4.4 billion pounds has been used for insect control since 1940, about 80% in agriculture. Because of the extensive environmental problems resulting from its stability and high lipid-water partitioning, DDT was banned for all but essential public-health use in the United States on January 1, 1973.

DDT is produced by condensing chlorobenzene with chloral. The technical product contains about 80–90% *p,p'*-isomer. DDT is soluble in water at 0.0012 ppm at 25°C.

The persistence of DDT, DDE [or 2,2-*bis*-(*p*-chlorophenyl)-1,1-dichloroethylene], and DDD [or 2,2-(*p*-chlorophenyl)-1,1-dichloroethane] has made them ubiquitous contaminants of water. The total residues are commonly referred to as "DDT-T." In an extensive 1958–1965 survey of the rivers of the United States, Breidenbach *et al.* (1967) found DDT in every river surveyed at 0.008–0.144 ppb, DDE at 0.002–0.011 ppb, and DDD at 0.004–0.080 ppb. The highest concentrations were generally found in the West and South, where 44% of the samples were positive for DDT and 38% for DDE. More than 500 grab samples of finished drinking water and related raw water from the Mississippi and Missouri rivers were analyzed by Schafer *et al*, (1969); more than 33% of the finished-water samples contained DDT-T.

An EPA study of over 700 water utilities serving airplane, train, and bus terminals showed DDT in six of 106 samples at 1–2 ppt and in 5 of 83 samples of finished water at 6-68 ppt (USEPA, 1975j).

In Iowa, Richard *et al.* (1975) assayed DDE in various surface, subsurface, and finished waters. Water from the South Skunk River near Ames contained DDE at 3–1,820 ppt, with the highest concentrations in June 1974. Similar results were found in Indian Creek (2–3,920 ppt), and in a drainage ditch near Fernald, Iowa (4–1,150 ppt). Surface water had DDE at 1–248 ppt (average, 68 ppt) in the Des Moines River, 2–250 ppt (average 59 ppt) in the Raccoon River, 8–350 ppt (average, 212 ppt) in the Red Rock Reservoir, and 5–1,121 ppt (average, 420 ppt) in the Rothbun Reservoir. Other surface-water values found were: Cedar River, 480 ppt; Iowa River, 350 ppt; Des Moines River, 74 ppt; and Mississippi River (near McGregor Iowa), 2 ppt. The Mississippi at New Orleans had DDE at 48 ppt. Finished water at Cedar Rapids contained DDE at 28 ppt, but other finished water had less than 0.5 ppt.

Lake Michigan contains DDT-T at an average of 6 ppt. Most fishes from Lake Michigan contain DDT residues in excess of the 7 ppm FDA "safe limit" and the overall biomagnification from water to fish may exceed a factor of 3×10^6.

Water standards have been proposed for DDT in finished water (Schafer *et al.*, 1969). The DDT-T concentration suggested in 1965–1966 and based on maximal acceptable concentrations of the Subcommittee

TABLE VI-19 Toxicity of Aldrin and Dieldrin

Species	Duration of Study	Dosage Levels and No. of Animals Per Group	Highest No-Adverse-Effect Level or Lowest-Minimal-Effect Level	Effect Measured	Reference
Dieldrin					
Mouse	132 weeks			liver tumors	Walker *et al.*, 1972
		0.0 ppm 288 M 297 F		M 6.9% F 9.5%	
		0.1 ppm 124 M 90 F	⩽0.1 ppm	M 21% F 30%	
		1.0 ppm 111 M 89 F		M 36% F 42.5%	
		10.0 ppm 176 M 148 F		M 53.4% F 62.3%	
Rat (CFE)	2 yr			renal and liver tumors	Walker *et al.*, 1969
		0.0 ppm 43 M 23 F		M 28% F 44%	
		0.1 ppm 23 M 23 F		M 26% F 65%	
		1.0 ppm 23 M 23 F	<0.1 ppm	M 22% F 61%	
		10.0 ppm 23 M 23 F		M 35% F 52%	

				increased liver/body weight ratio	Walker *et al.*, 1969
Dog (beagle)	2 yr	0.00 ppm 5 M 5 F		M 3.37% F 3.32%	
		0.005 mg/kg/day 5 M 5 F	<0.1 ppm	M 3.61% F 3.56%	
		0.5 mg/kg/day 5 M 5 F		M 4.28% F 4.51%	
[This compound is an animal carcinogen.]					
Aldrin					
				tumors	Cleveland, 1966
Rat	2 yr	0 38 M 53 F		M 7.89% F 11.32%	
		2.5 29 M 32 F		M 3.45% F 3.13%	
		12.5 30 M 36 F	<2.5 ppm	M 0 F 8.33%	
		25.0 26 M 33 F		M 3.85% F 3.03%	
Mice	2 yr	107 M 107 F 10 ppm	10 ppm	hepatic cell adenoma	Davis and Fitzhugh, 1962
[This compound is an animal carcinogen.]					

TABLE VI-20 Toxicity of Endrin

Species	Duration of Study	Dosage Levels	Highest No-Adverse-Effect Level or Lowest-Minimal-Effect Level	Effect Measured	Reference
Rat	2 yr	0			Deichman *et al.*, 1970
		2 ppm		"no primary malignant tumors"	
		6 ppm		"no primary malignant tumors"	
		12 ppm		"no primary malignant tumors"	
Dog (beagle)	19 months	0			
		1 ppm		increased liver/body ratio	Cited in EPA, 1973
		3 ppm		increased liver/body ratio	
Dog	2 yr (7 M and 7 F at each level)	0			Cited in EPA, 1973
		0.1 ppm			
		0.5 ppm	0.5 ppm		
		1.0 ppm			
		2.0 ppm		convulsions, increased liver/body ratio, cell depreciation	
		4.0 ppm		convulsions, increased liver/body ratio, cell depreciation	

[This compound is a suspected animal carcinogen.]

TABLE VI-21 Toxicity of Chlordane

Species	Duration of Study	Dosage Levels and No. of Animals Per Group	Highest No-Adverse-Effect Level or Lowest-Minimal-Effect Level	Effect Measured	Reference
				liver tumors (carcinoma)	National Cancer Inst., 1975
Mice (B6C3F$_1$)	90 weeks	0 ppm M 48 F 48	<30 ppm	M 20% F 0%	
		30 ppm		M 33% F 6.2%	
		56 ppm		F 88.9%	
		64 ppm		F 73.9%	
				liver[a] tumors (carcinoma)	National Cancer Inst., 1975
Rat (OM)	110 weeks	0 ppm M 7 F 10	<120 ppm	M 0% F 0%	
		121 ppm F 49		F 0%	
		203 ppm M 43		M 20%	
		241 ppm F 43		F 2.3%	
		407 ppm M 42		M 0%	

[This compound is an animal carcinogen.]

[a]Liver hyperplasia: M; 0% controls, low dose 3.8%, high dose 14.3%; F; controls 0, low dose 14.7%, high dose 40.9%.

TABLE VI-22 Toxicity of Heptachlor and Heptachlor Epoxide

Species	Duration of Study	Dosage Levels and No. of Animals Per Group	Highest No-Adverse-Effect Level or Lowest-Minimal-Effect Level	Effect Measured	Reference
Heptachlor					
				liver tumors (carcinoma)	National Cancer Inst., 1975
Mouse (B6C351)	90 weeks	0 ppm M 58 F 40	<6.1 ppm	M 11.1% F 10%	
		6.1 ppm M 49		M 28.6%	
		9.0 ppm F 46		F 10.4%	
		13.8 ppm M 47		M 80.8%	
		18.0 ppm F 42		F 69.0%	
Rat (OM)				liver tumors (carcinoma)	National Cancer Inst., 1975
	110 weeks	0 ppm M 10 F 10	<18.9 ppm	M 0 F 0	
		18.9 ppm F 48		F 12.5%	
		38.9 ppm M 43		M 2.3%	
		37.8 ppm F 47		F 8.5%	
		77.9 ppm M 45		M 11.1%	
[This compound is an animal carcinogen.]					
Heptachlor Epoxide				endocrine tumors	Kettering Laboratory, 1959
Rat (CFN)	2 yr	0 ppm M 23 F 24	<0.5 ppm	M 35% F 54%	
		0.5 ppm M 24 F 23		M 62.5% F 82.6%	
		2.5 ppm M 20 F 24		M 60% F 79.2%	
		5.0 ppm M 20 F 22		M 60% F 77%	
		7.5 ppm M 24 F 22		M 54% F 90.9%	
		10.0 ppm M 23 F 23		M 56% F 73.9%	
[This compound is a suspected animal carcinogen.]					

TABLE VI-23 Pesticides in Diet

Pesticide	Daily Dietary Intake, mg						
	1965	1966	1967	1968	1969	1970	6-yr Average
DDT	0.031	0.041	0.026	0.019	0.016	0.015	0.025
DDE	0.018	0.028	0.017	0.015	0.011	0.010	0.017
DDD	0.013	0.018	0.013	0.011	0.005	0.004	0.011
DDT-T	0.062	0.087	0.056	0.045	0.032	0.029	0.053

on Toxicology was 42 ppb. This was drastically lowered to 0.5 ppb, by Ettinger and Mount (1969), on the basis of a maximal reasonable stream allowance.

DDT and its breakdown products are ubiquitous and, because of biomagnification and persistence, are in virtually every food product. "Market-basket" surveys of the U.S. diet, collected in five major United States cities and designed to represent the diet of a 16- to 19-yr-old male, show the intakes in Table VI-23 (NAS, 1975).

Calculated as human intake in mg/kg/day, the combined DDT-T was about 0.2 that of the FAO/WHO Acceptable Daily Intake of 0.005 mg/kg/day. The dietary intake was 0.0089 mg/kg/day in 1965, 0.0010 in 1966, 0.0008 in 1967, and 0.0007 in 1968 (Mrak, 1969).

DDT in Milk DDT is present in milk, everywhere. Moore (1975) surveyed Illinois milk in 1971–1973 and found DDT at 0.05 ppm in 1971, 0.02 ppm in 1972, and 0.03 ppm in 1973. The human is at the top of the food pyramid, so human milk is especially contaminated. Curley and Kimbrough (1969) found DDT-T residues averaging 0.0784 ppm in U.S. samples (range, 0.0404–0.1563 ppm).

Metabolism and Degradation

Although DDT is highly stable and persistent, it does undergo a relatively complex series of degradative changes, both biologically and environmentally. The dominant reaction is dehydrochlorination to form DDE, which is much less toxic to insects and higher animals, but has about the same solubility in water (0.0013 ppm) and high lipid-water partitioning. DDE is almost nondegradable, both biologically and environmentally. Thus, DDE is the predominant residue stored in tissues, increasing in relative concentration for each trophic level (Woodwell *et al.*, 1967) and reaching about 70% of DDT-T in humans (Durham 1969). Nothing is certain about the degradation pathway of DDE.

DDT is also reductively dechlorinated in biologic systems to form DDD. DDD is less stable than DDT or DDE and is the first step on the degradation pathway in animals (Morgan and Roan, 1974) and in the environment (Metcalf, 1973). DDD is dehydrochlorinated to DDMU, or 2,2-*bis*-(*p*-chlorophenyl)-1-chloroethylene; reduced to DDMS, or 2,2-*bis*-(*p*-chlorophenyl)-l-chloroethane; dehydrochlorinated to DDNU, or 2,2-*bis*-(*p*-chlorophenyl)-ethylene; reduced to 1,l-*bis*-(*p*-chlorophenyl)-ethane; and eventually oxidized to DDA, or *bis*-(*p*-chlorophenyl)-acetic acid. This compound is much more soluble in water than DDT and is the ultimate excretory product of DDT ingestion and storage in higher animals and humans. Environmentally, DDT residues are converted to *p,p'*- dichlorobenzophenone.

DDT is also degraded to a slight extent by microsomal oxidase enzymes by attack at the α-H to form dicofol, or 1,l-*bis*-(*p*-chlorophenyl)-2,2,2-trichloroethanol. Very recently, a new anaerobic degradation pathway, found especially in sewage sludge, was discovered in the conversion by bacteria to form DDCN, or *bis*-(*p*-chlorophenyl)-acetonitrile (Metcalf, 1973).

The kinetics of storage and loss of DDT and DDE in humans has been investigated intensively (Durham, 1969; Morgan and Roan, 1974). In humans, DDT is stored in fat at about 10 times the concentration of intake. The average U.S. inhabitant in 1964 had DDT-T stored in his fat at 10 ppm; about 70% of this was DDE. Storage can reach very high values; e.g., a DDT formulator stored DDT-T at 1,131 ppm, 43% of it as DDE (Durham, 1969). Conversion of DDT to DDE in the human body is very slow, i.e., less than 20% over 3 yr. DDT is eliminated from the human body through first-order reduction to DDD and conversion to the more water-soluble DDA, with a biologic half-life of about 1 yr. DDE is eliminated much more slowly, with a biologic half-life of about 8 yr. Its pathway of elimination is unknown; it may be slowly excreted as DDE (Morgan and Roan, 1974).

Health Aspects

Observations in Man There are no definite examples of human fatality due to ingestion of DDT, but a dosage of 10 mg/kg has produced illness in some (but not all) subjects, without convulsions. Convulsions have frequently occurred at 16 mg/kg or higher. Human volunteers have consumed 35 mg/day (about 0.5 mg/kg/day) for as long as 25 months without ill effects (Hayes, 1963). These subjects stored 101–466 ppm in their body fat after 12 months and 105–659 ppm after 21 months.

DDT-T concentrations found in human fat over fiscal years 1970–1974, in over 1,400 bioassays of U.S. human tissues, were 11.65, 11.5, 9.91, 8.91, and 7.83 ppm in fiscal years 1970, 1971, 1972, 1973, and 1974, respectively (NAS, 1975).

The decline undoubtedly represents the effects of decreased use and the banning of DDT in 1973.

Observations in Other Species

Acute Effects The oral LD_{50} of DDT in rats is 113 mg/kg in males and 118 mg/kg in females. The dermal LD_{50} in female rats is 2,510 mg/kg (Hayes, 1963). DDE has an oral LD_{50} in rats of 880 mg/kg in males and 1,240 mg/kg in females. DDA has an oral LD_{50} in rats of 740 mg/kg in males and 600 mg/kg in females. The oral LD_{50} of DDT in dogs is 60-75 mg/kg, in rabbits is 250-400 mg/kg, and in mice is 200 mg/kg (Pimentel, 1971).

Chronic Effects When rats were fed DDT at 5–10 ppm over the lifetime, microscopic alterations were reported in liver cells, including centrilobular enlargement with increased oxyphilia and peripheral margination of the basophilic granules. These effects became moderate when DDT was fed at 50 ppm and were pronounced at 400 ppm; however, 50 ppm was tolerated without gross toxicity, and 100 ppm with only slight symptoms of poisoning (Lehman, 1952a). The high lipid-water partition results in pronounced fat storage; when DDT was fed at 1 ppm to rats for 15 weeks, it was stored in fat at 13 ppm in males and 18 ppm in females, and the corresponding values for 50 ppm were 284 and 588 ppm (Lang *et al.*, 1950). It has been estimated that fat storage occurs at about 20 times the dietary intake.

Mice fed DDT at 100 ppm in the diet had a considerably shortened life span, although this was not apparent at 50 ppm (Walker *et al.*, 1972).

Dogs tolerated daily DDT intakes of 10 mg/kg in corn oil for three years without gross effects, but died after a few months at 50 and 80 mg/kg (Lehman, 1952b).

Mutagenicity DDT was not mutagenic in the *Salmonella*/microsome test (McCann *et al.*, 1975).

Carcinogenicity The Mrak Commission (1969) judged DDT to be positive for tumor induction in one or more species of test animals. This, with its high persistence and rate of fat storage, has caused substantial environmental concern. Tarjan and Kemeny (1969) showed a generalized increase in frequency of tumors in five generations of mice after feeding DDT at 3 ppm, and Faur and Kemen (1969) found increased numbers of malignancies when DDT was fed to mice at 0.3–0.6 mg/kg of body weight. The WHO has repeated these studies and found that DDT fed to mice at 0.3 mg/kg/day over a lifetime produced a significant increase in liver tumors in males (WHO, 1973).

Teratogenicity Although the thickness of egg shells of birds was reduced by DDT (Hickey and Anderson, 1968), no teratogenic effects have been identified in chicks, mice (Ware and Good, 1967), or in rats (Ottoboni, 1969).

Carcinogenic Risk Estimates

Despite the positive results in mice, oral administration of DDT to rats has not provided convincing evidence of carcinogenicity. Feeding studies on dogs and monkeys have also not shown DDT to be carcenogenic, but these studies are of limited value due to small group size and short duration.

Studies on human workers occupationally exposed to DDT have not shown an increased incidence of cancer, but these studies are limited by time factors. Terminal cancer patients have been observed to have higher fat concentrations of DDT, but a causal relationship is difficult to prove (IARC, 1974).

Only the data from feeding studies in mice can be statistically treated to provide an estimate of risk for man. Several species of mice have developed hepatomas after oral exposure to DDT.

The available sets of dose response data were individually considered as described in the risk section in the margin-of-safety chapter. Each set of dose–response data was used to statistically estimate both the lifetime risk and an upper 95% confidence bound on the lifetime risk at the low-dose level. These estimates are of lifetime human risks and have been corrected for species conversion on a dose-per-surface-area basis. The risk estimates are expressed as a probability of cancer after a lifetime consumption of 1 liter of water/day containing Q ppb of the compound of interest. For example, a risk of $1 \times 10^{-6}\,Q$ implies a lifetime probability of 2×10^{-5} of cancer if 2 liters/day were consumed and the concentration of the carcinogen was 10 ppb (i.e., $Q = 10$). This means that at a concentration of 10 ppb during a lifetime of exposure this compound would be expected to produce one excess case of cancer for every 50,000 persons exposed. If the population of the U.S. is taken to be 220 million people this translates into 4,400 excess lifetime deaths from cancer or 62.8 per year. Since several data sets are typically available the range of the low-dose risk estimates are reported.

For DDT at a concentration of 1 μg/liter ($Q = 1$), there are several risk estimates depending on which feeding study is evaluated. Four studies (Innes *et al.*, 1969; Tomatis *et al.*, 1972; Walker *et al.*, 1972; and Thorpe and Walker, 1973) provide a risk to man of from $0.18\text{-}13.0 \times 10^{-6}\ Q$. The upper 95% confidence estimate of risk at the same concentration is from $0.65\text{-}20.0 \times 10^{-6}\ Q$.

Conclusions and Recommendations

DDT is of moderate acute toxicity to man and most other organisms. However, its extremely low solubility in water (0.0012 ppm) and high solubility in fat (100,000 ppm) result in great bioconcentration. Its principal breakdown product, DDE, has very similar properties. Both compounds are also highly persistent in living organisms, so the major concern about DDT toxicity is related to its chronic effects, which are summarized in Table VI-24.

In light of the above and taking into account the carcinogenic risk projections, it is suggested that very strict criteria be applied when limits for DDT and DDE in drinking-water are established.

METHOXYCHLOR

Introduction

Methoxychlor, or 2,2-*bis*-(*p*-methoxyphenyl)-1,1,1-trichloroethane, was introduced as an insecticide in 1945. It is a close relative of DDT and has been used as an insecticide of very low mammalian toxicity for home and garden, on domestic animals for fly control, for elm bark-beetle vectors of Dutch elm disease, and for blackfly larvae in streams. Methoxychlor is registered for about 87 crops—alfalfa; nearly all fruits and vegetables; corn, wheat, rice, and other grains; beef and dairy cattle; and swine, goats, and sheep—and for agricultural premises and outdoor fogging. Domestic use of methoxychlor as a substitute for DDT is increasing and is estimated at 10 million pounds a year (NAS, 1975).

Methoxychlor is produced by condensing anisole with chloral. About 88% of the technical product is the *p,p'*-isomer, and the principal impurity is the *p,p*-isomer. The *p,p'*-isomer is soluble in water at 0.26 ppm at 25°C (Kapoor *et al.*, 1970). Its major breakdown product, 2,2-*bis*-(*p*-hydroxy-

TABLE VI-24 Toxicity of DDT and DDE

Species	Duration of Study	Dosage Levels and No. of Animals Per Group	Highest No-Adverse-Effect Level or Lowest-Minimal-Effect Level	Effect Measured	Reference
Mouse	5 generation	0 (406 animals)		2.23% tumors 1.23% leukemia	Tarjan and Kemeny, 1969
		3 ppm (684 animals)	3 ppm	28.4% tumors 11.57% leukemia	
		0.3–0.6 mg/kg/day	<0.3 mg/kg/day	tumors	Faur and Kemeny, 1969
		0.3 mg/kg/day	<0.3 mg/kg/day	liver tumors	WHO, 1973
Rat	2 yr	5 ppm	<5 ppm	altered liver cells	Lehman, 1952a
		10 ppm		altered liver cells	
		50 ppm		moderate liver damage	
		100 ppm		slight chronic poisoning	
		400 ppm		pronounced liver damage, nervous tremors	
Dog	3 yr	10 mg/kg/day (in corn oil)	10 kg/day	no adverse effect	Lehman, 1952b
		50 mg/kg/day (in corn oil)		died	
		80 mg/kg/day (in corn oil)		died	
Man	21.5 months	0.5 mg/kg/day		fat storage to 105–659 ppm	Hayes, 1963

[This compound is an animal carcinogen.]

phenyl)-1,1,1-trichloroethane, is soluble in water at 76 ppm (Kapoor *et al.*, 1970).

The half-life of Methoxychlor in water is about 46 days. No residues of Methoxychlor were detected in 500 samples of finished drinking-water from the Mississippi and Missouri rivers (Schafer *et al.*, 1969) or in 101 samples from Hawaii. No Methoxychlor was found in the New Orleans drinking-water survey (USEPA, 1974a).

The average daily intake of Methoxychlor in the human diet over a 6-yr period (1965–1970) was less than 0.001 mg (NAS, 1975). The maximal U.S. residues found were: dairy products, 0.006 ppb; grain and cereal, 0.003 ppb; leaf vegetables, 0.033 ppb; and fruits, 0.023 ppb (USEPA, 1976e).

Tolerances of Methoxychlor on more than 80 raw agricultural commodities range from 1 to 100 ppm, with most at 14 ppm.

The EPA has set an interim standard for Methoxychlor in finished water of 0.1 mg/liter (USEPA, 1975i).

Metabolism

Unlike DDT, Methoxychlor is not highly bioconcentrated and stored in animal fatty tissue. For example, when Methoxychlor was fed to rats at 25 ppm, no fat storage was detected; at 100 ppm, only 1 ppm was stored; and at 500 ppm, storage in 4 weeks reached 36 ppm in males and 17 ppm in females, but rapidly declined, and no Methoxychlor could be detected in fat 2 weeks after Methoxychlor feeding was stopped (Kunze *et al.*, 1950). In contrast, DDT fed at 1 ppm under identical conditions was stored at 13 ppm in male and 18 ppm in female rats (Lang *et al.*, 1950). When green sunfish, *Lepomis cyanellus* and *Tilapia mossambica*, were exposed to Methoxychlor in water at 0.01 ppm for 31 days, the body residues were 2.7 and 2 ppm, compared with 40.2 and 106 ppm for DDT at the same concentration (Reinbold *et al.*, 1971).

Methoxychlor is rapidly excreted by animals as the *mono*-phenol and *bis*-phenol derivatives and their conjugates. When radiolabeled Methoxychlor was administered orally to mice, 98.3% was eliminated in 24 h (Kapoor *et al.*, 1970). *Tilapia mossambica* exposed to Methoxychlor at 0.003 ppm in water for 12 days contained 8 ppm; they were then transferred to clean water and contained only 0.0001 ppm after 15 more days (Reinbold *et al.*, 1971).

Methoxychlor is readily *O*-demethylated by microsomal oxidase enzymes in mouse liver (Kapoor *et al.*, 1970) to form principally 2-(*p*-hydroxyphenyl-2-(*p*-methoxyphenyl)-1,1,1-trichloroethane and 2,2-*bis*-(*p*-hydroxyphenyl)-1,1,1-trichloroethane (Kapoor *et al.*, 1970). These—with

2,2-*bis*-(*p*-hydroxyphenyl)-1,1-dichloroethane (produced by reductive dechlorination), 4,4′-dihydroxybenzophenone, and 4,4′-dihydroxydiphenylacetic acid—are the principal excretory products in mice (Kapoor *et al.*, 1970) and fish (Rienbold *et al.*, 1971). All these were found as degradation products in a laboratory model ecosystem, as well as traces of Methoxychlor ethylene (Kapoor *et al.*, 1970). In this system, Methoxychlor had an ecologic magnification of 1,545 compared with 84,500 for DDT and a biodegradability index of 0.94 compared with 0.015 for DDT (Kapoor *et al.*, 1973). Thus, Methoxychlor differs substantially from DDT in the presence of the methoxy degradophores that make it biologically much more degradable.

Health Aspects

Observations in Man There is no conclusive evidence of Methoxychlor intoxication in humans.

Observations in Other Species

Acute Effects Methoxychlor is one of the safest of all insecticides. The oral LD_{50} in rats is over 6,000 mg/kg; that in mice is 2,900 mg/kg; that in monkeys is over 2,500 mg/kg. The dermal LD_{50} in rabbits is over 2,800 mg/kg (USEPA, 1976e). The acute oral LD_{50} of 2,2-*bis*-(*p*-hydrophenyl)-1,1,1-trichloroethane, the principal metabolite, in mice is 600 mg/kg (Von Oettingen and Sharpless, 1946).

Chronic Effects Methoxychlor fed to rats at 10,000 ppm was toxic, but fed at 5,000 ppm for 52 weeks produced mortality comparable with that in untreated controls. There was some growth retardation at 2,500 ppm and above, but no gross pathologic changes were found. No tremors were observed at any time (Haag *et al.*, 1950). Methoxychlor fed to rats for 2 yr at 0.02% produced no abnormal gross pathology or histopathologic changes (Haag *et al.*, 1950). When fed to beagle dogs at 1, 2, and 4 g/kg/day over 6 months, Methoxychlor produced convulsions at the 2 and 4 g/kg and increased serum alkaline phosphatase and serum transaminase (Tegaris *et al.*, 1966). However, when fed at 300 mg/kg/day for 1 yr, in another study, it had no observed effects on body weight, hematology, or histopathology (USEPA, 1976e).

Mutagenicity In mutagenic evaluation with *Escherichia coli* WP 2TRY, Methoxychlor gave negative results (Ashwood-Smith *et al.*, 1972).

Carcinogenicity Methoxychlor fed in FDA studies for 2 yr to C3He/FeJ and BALB/cJ mice at 750 ppm in the diet showed no significant difference in incidence of hepatocellular hyperplasia and hepatoma between controls and treated in mice. Testicular tumors were found in BALB/cJ mice, and it was concluded from histologic examination that Methoxychlor caused a significant increase in the incidence of this tumor in BALB/cJ mice, but not in C3He/FeJ mice (USEPA, 1976e).

Reproduction Rats fed Methoxychlor at 1,000 ppm in the diet had normal reproduction. At 2,500 ppm, fewer rats mated, and many did not produce litters. At 5,000 ppm, none of the rats had litters or implantation (Harris *et al.*, 1974). Further studies with 200 ppm through three generations showed no gross or histopathologic changes in any tissues from rats of the F_3 generation.

Because of the possible resemblance of Methoxychlor detoxication phenols to diethylstilbestrol, additional studies were made to evaluate chronic feeding of Methoxychlor for estrogenic effects. The results showed both no adverse effect and uterine weight increase. The latter effect was found to be at least partially due to an unidentified contaminant in technical Methoxychlor (Tullner, 1961).

Teratogenicity No available information.

Conclusions and Recommendations

Methoxychlor, a close relative of DDT, has very low mammalian toxicity. In a 2-yr feeding study no adverse effect was observed at 200 ppm in rats. On the basis of these chronic data an ADI was calculated at 0.1 mg/kg/day. The available data on chronic toxicity and calculations of ADI are summarized in Table VI-25.

BENZENE HEXACHLORIDE (BHC) AND LINDANE

Introduction

"Benzene hexachloride" (BHC) is the common name used to designate the mixed isomers of 1,2,3,4,5,6-hexachlorocyclohexane. "Hexachlorocyclohexane" is the proper term for this compound; however, because it is more customary, the trivial name, "benzene hexachloride" (or BHC), will be used in this document.

BHC (technical grade) is a mixture of the eight possible isomers that constitute the different spatial arrangements of the six chlorine atoms on

TABLE VI-25 Toxicity of Methoxychlor

Species	Duration of Study	Dosage Levels and No. of Animals Per Group	Highest No-Adverse-Effect Level or Lowest-Minimal-Effect Level	Effect Measured	Reference
Mouse	2 yr	750 ppm		No carcinogenesis (C_3He/FcJ) increased testicular tumors (BALB/cJ)	USEPA, 1976e
Rat	2 yr	200 ppm	200 ppm (10 mg/kg/day)[c,d]	No adverse effect	Haag *et al.*, 1959
Rat	6 weeks	0.0 ppm (17 animals)			Harris *et al.*, 1974
		1,000 ppm (17 animals)		Normal reproduction	
		2,500 ppm (20 animals)		Retarded reproduction	
		5,000 ppm (25 animals)		Inhibited reproduction	
Dog (beagle)	6 months	0.0 ppm 1 g/kg/day (6 animals)		1/6 convulsions	Tegeris *et al.*, 1966
		2 g/kg/day (6 animals)		5/6 convulsions CNS effects, death	
		4 g/kg/day (6 animals)		6/6 convulsions, death	

Using an uncertainty factor of 100, the suggested no-adverse-effect level in drinking water is calculated as follows:

$$\frac{10}{100} = 0.1 \text{ mg/kg/day (ADI)},\ 0.1 \times 70^{a} \times 0.1^{b} = 0.7 \text{ mg/liter}$$

[a]Assume average weight of human adult = 70 kg.

[b]Assume average daily intake of water for man = 2 liters, and that 20 percent of total intake is from water.

[c]Value from which the suggested no-adverse-effect level was calculated.

[d]Assume weight of rat = 0.4 kg and average daily food consumption of rat = 0.02 kg.

the *trans*- (or chair) form of the ring. Its composition approximates 65% α isomer, 11% β, 13–14% γ, 8–9% δ, and 1% ϵ. The lowest-melting-point (112.8°C) isomer, which is also the most reactive known, is that designated as the γ isomer. The commercial insecticide Lindane is defined as a product containing at least 99% γ isomer (the remainder being other BHC isomers). Technical BHC is prepared by photochlorination of benzene. Production of the γ isomer for Lindane is achieved by selective crystallization (Melnikov, 1971).

The different isomers have different solubilities in water and different vapor pressures: α, 10 mg/liter and 0.06 torr; β, 5 mg/liter and 0.17 torr; and γ, 10 mg/liter and 0.14 torr (Melnikov, 1971; NAS, 1975). The relatively high water solubility and vapor pressure of Lindane cause it to have relatively low persistence in the environment. Lindane has been detected in the finished water of Streator, Illinois at 4 μg/liter (USEPA, 1975j).

The EPA has set an interim standard for Lindane in finished water of 0.004 mg/liter (USEPA, 1975i).

The insecticidal properties of BHC were discovered and developed for commercial use in pest control beginning in 1942. When it was found that virtually all the insecticidal activity of BHC resided in the γ-isomer, major development of the latter as an insecticide itself was rapid. Lindane has been marketed under a large number of trade names as an insecticide. It has had major use in insect control in domestic and commercial settings, in numerous agricultural and silvicultural applications, and in dips, sprays, and dusts for livestock and pets. Recent U.S. production has been under 1 million pounds a year (NAS, 1975).

Metabolism

Mammalian biotransformation of BHC isomers involves the formation of chlorophenols (trichlorophenol, tetrachlorophenol, and pentachlorophenol), which are excreted free and as conjugates of sulfuric and glucuronic acids (Grover and Sims, 1965; Freal and Chadwick, 1973). Freal and Chadwich (1973) hypothesized that Lindane is metabolized in the rat through a pentachlorocyclohexene to a series of trichlorobenzenes and tetrachlorobenzenes en route to the corresponding chlorophenols. In later work, however, Chadwick *et al.* (1975) established that Lindane is initially metabolized to a hexachlorocyclohexene intermediate, from which two tetrachlorophenols and three trichlorophenols are later derived. This mode of metabolism is apparently peculiar to the γ-isomer. Freal and Chadwich (1973) showed that pretreatment of rats with BHC isomers resulted in enhanced metabolism of Lindane to the chlorophenols; the effects decreased in the order $\alpha > \delta > \gamma >> \beta$.

Metabolism of isomers other than γ-BHC leads to trichlorophenols, not all identical with those formed from the γ-isomer; but apparently no tetrachlorophenol occurs. Mercapturic acid excretion has also been observed after administration of BHC isomers. This may be due in part to the glutathione-dependent dechlorination of chlorobenzenes otherwise formed during BHC degradation, which then gives rise to the chlorophenols (Freal and Chadwick, 1973). Portig *et al.* (1973) observed the direct glutathione-dependent conversion of α-BHC to a hydrophilic metabolite by a preparation of rat liver cytosol. This is similar to the known biodegradation of γ-BHC in insects, which is glutathione-dependent (Ishida and Dahm, 1965); the insect enzyme acts on α-BHC more readily than on γ-BHC, and the β-isomer is nonreactive. The mammalian enzyme activity is increased after pretreatment of the rat with α-BHC (Kraus *et al.*, 1973). Pentachlorobenzene and pentachlorophenol have so far been observed only as metabolites of Lindane in the rabbit (Karopolly *et al.*, 1973). The eliminated products, the free and conjugated chlorophenols, are much less toxic than the parent isomers, and some are being considered separately as contaminants in water.

Health Aspects

Observations in Man Surveys of human tissue for organochlorine insecticide residues frequently show the presence of the most persistent, the β-isomer of BHC. In a study on the concentration of organochlorine residues in fat and liver of terminal patients, the only BHC isomer noted was the beta. Its concentration in cancer patients did not differ significantly from that in people dying from infectious or other diseases (Radomski *et al.*, 1968). Chronic liver damage (cirrhosis and chronic hepatitis) has been found, in liver biopsy, in eight workers heavily exposed to BHC, DDT, or both for periods ranging from 5 to 13 yr. As far as was feasible, other conditions, such as alcoholism, were excluded as the cause of the cirrhosis (Schuttmann, 1968).

Over 30 cases of exposure to BHC or Lindane and 21 cases of exposure to BHC and DDT followed by the development of aplastic anemia have been reported in the literature (Loge, 1965; West, 1967; Woodliff *et al.*, 1966). No satisfactory animal model of that condition has been found and, despite efforts to study the question, a firm causal relationship between Lindane or technical BHC exposure and aplastic anemia cannot be stated. Development of leukemia after Lindane exposure was reported for two cases (Jedlicka, 1958). That causal relationship is also inconclusive in relation to insecticide exposure.

Observations in Other Species

Acute Effects Lindane is the most toxic of the isomers of BHC. It excites the central nervous system, producing hyperirritability, incoordination, convulsions, and death due to respiratory collapse. Its single-dose oral LD_{50} in rats is 88-300 mg/kg (Gaines, 1969; Riemschneider, 1949; Burkatskaya, 1959; Slade, 1945; Klosa, 1950; Woodward and Hogen, 1947; Copper *et al.*, 1951). The oral LD_{50} of technical BHC is 600-1,250 mg/kg; those of the other isomers are about 1,500 mg/kg (α), 2,000 mg/kg (β), and 100 mg/kg (δ) (Riemschneider, 1949; Burkatskaya, 1969; Slade, 1945; Klosa, 1950; Coper, 1951). The wide range in observed LD_{50} for Lindane presumably results from differences in rates of absorption of various preparations of the material and variations in rates of detoxification and excretion under different experimental conditions. Single oral doses of 10–25 mg/kg in corn oil were fatal to beagles (Cited in USEPA, 1973b), and domestic animals were poisoned by similar amounts (Wasserman *et al.*, 1960).

Subchronic and Chronic Effects Klimmer (1955) administered daily doses of Lindane, at 32 mg/kg of body weight, by stomach tube to male and female rats for 6 months. He observed nervous symptoms, fatty degeneration of the liver and renal tubular epithelium, vacuolization of the cerebral cells, and a marked increase in mortality. None of these effects was seen with a daily dose of 10 mg/kg during 17 months. Melis (1955) fed diets containing Lindane at 2, 3, 4, 5, or 10 ppm for 12 months to rats and found no abnormalities in general behavior, body weight, histology, or other characteristics.

Beagle dogs were not affected by Lindane in the diet at 7.5 mg/kg/day (Cited in USEPA, 1973b). Higher dosages produced central nervous system effects.

Under conditions of chronic administration, the γ-isomer is considerably less toxic than the other principal isomers or technical BHC. Fitzhugh *et al.* (1950) conducted 2-yr rat-feeding studies with the various isomers of BHC, using diets containing the α, β, and γ-isomers at 5–1,600 ppm. These experiments clearly showed that the γ-isomer was the least toxic, and the β-isomer, the most toxic. The organs injured were the liver and, to a lesser extent, the kidneys. In the case of Lindane, the lowest concentration causing significant liver changes was 100 ppm; no effect was noted below 50 ppm. Truhaut (1954) summarized data from 2-yr feeding studies in rats with Lindane in the diet at 25, 50, and 100 ppm. At 25 ppm, no evidence of histologic changes in the liver or kidney or any other toxic effects were seen. At the higher concentrations, hypertrophy of the liver was observed, and, at 100 ppm, a slight degree of fatty degeneration. These findings and dose relationships were confirmed by other workers (Ortega *et al.*, 1957). FAO/WHO (1967) accepted 25 ppm in the diet of rats as the maximal concentration causing no adverse effects.

The hypertrophic liver and fatty degenerative changes of liver at higher dosage are similar to those produced by other slowly metabolized organochlorine compounds. As might be expected, Lindane induces hepatic microsomal enzymes (Freal and Chadwick, 1973). That effect may preceed in time and dosage relationships the liver pathology already described (Hotterer and Schaffner, 1968).

Mutagenicity In a dominant lethal assay, Lindane was administered to male mice as a single intraperitoneal dose of 12.5, 25, or 50 μg/kg (corresponding to one-eighth, one-fourth, or one-half of the LD_{50}), and the mice later mated with successive series of females during a 7-day period. No mutations were observed, nor were any reproductive effects noted (Cited in USEPA, 1973b). Host-mediated testing produced mutagenic rates too low to be considered positive (Cited in USEPA, 1973b). However, it has been claimed that Lindane in cell-culture media at 0.1–10.0 μg/ml affected the mitotic activity and the karyotype of human lymphocytes cultivated *in vitro* (Tsoneva-Manua, *et al.*, 1971). In general, published reports indicate that Lindane does not have significant mutagenic potential.

Carcinogenicity An investigation in rats fed over a lifetime on diets containing technical BHC, α-BHC, β-BHC, or γ-BHC at 10–800 ppm did not show evidence of increased tumor incidence or carcinogenicity (Fitzhugh, *et al.*, 1950). In the same study, Lindane was also administered at 5–1,600 ppm as a solution in oil. The average life-span was significantly reduced when all compounds were given at 800 ppm and more, but the tumor incidence in animals receiving treatment was not greater than that in controls (Fitzhugh *et al.*, 1950). However, it should be noted that not all animals in the study underwent microscopic examination of organs. In a further experiment in which rats received diets containing γ-BHC at 25, 50, or 100 ppm for 2 yr, no significant increase in tumor incidence was observed (Truhant, 1954).

Prompted by epidemiologic evidence, however, and the very high use of BHC in Japanese agriculture, more recent investigations have been undertaken that have developed quite a different picture. Nagasaki *et al.* (1971, 1972a) showed hepatoma formation in all tested mice on diets containing technical BHC at 660 ppm; diets containing either 6.6 or 66 ppm did not produce tumors. No hepatic nodules or tumors occurred in 14 male controls; the spontaneous incidence of liver tumors in this strain of mice is reportedly very low.

In a later experiment, groups of male dd mice were fed the α, β, γ, or δ-isomer separately, each at 100, 250, or 500 ppm. The experiment was terminated at 24 weeks. Multiple liver tumors, up to 2.0 cm in diameter, were found in all animals given α-BHC at 500 ppm; whereas smaller nodules were found in 9 of 20 mice given 250 ppm and no lesions were found in mice given 100 ppm. No tumors were produced with any dosage of the other three isomers or in a similar group of 20 control mice (Nagasaki et al., 1972b).

Thorpe and Walker (1973) fed groups of male and female CF1 mice diets containing β-BHC at 200 ppm or γ-BHC at 400 ppm. The percentages of animals that had liver tumors were 24%, 73% and 93% in males and 23%, 43%, and 69% in females for the controls, 200-ppm β-BHC, and 400-ppm γ-BHC diets, respectively. Lung metastases were found in some males receiving β- and γ-BHC and in some females receiving γ-BHC. The incidence of other tumors was not increased by exposure to either isomer.

Coincidentally with the Thorpe and Walker study, another research group reported results of feeding groups of male CR/JO mice from 5 to 31 weeks old on diets containing technical BHC, pure α, pure β, pure γ, or a mixture of δ and ϵ at 600 ppm. Liver nodules were found in all groups except the β-group BHC (Goto, *et al.*, 1972). The tumors frequently appeared to be malignant in the case of animals administered diets containing α-BHC and the δ- and ϵ-BHC mixture. The findings were interpreted as indicating that α-BHC or its metabolites are most probably carcinogenic. In the same study, three Lindane metabolites, 1,2,4-trichlorobenzene, 2,3,5-trichlorophenol, and 2,4,5-trichlorophenol, were administered for 6 months in the diet at 600 ppm; these treatments produced no hepatic tumors.

Further study by the Japanese researchers confirmed the high carcinogenicity of α-BHC and showed that combination of it with either β-, γ- or δ-BHC had no synergistic or antagonistic effect on the induction of tumors by α-BHC. Related studies showed that technical polychlorinated biphenyl (Kanechlors) promoted the induction of hepatic tumors by α-BHC and β-BHC; mice fed γ-BHC with or without PCB's did not show neoplastic changes in the liver (Ito *et al.*, 1973).

The data on induction of liver tumors by γ-BHC in mice are seen to be somewhat contradictory. For example, Thorpe and Walker (1973) found γ-BHC to be somewhat tumorigenic in CFL mice, but the Japanese workers used other strains and found that they were not susceptible to tumorigenic action by γ-BHC (Nagasaki *et al.*, 1971, 1972a, 1972b). The acute toxicity of technical BHC and BHC isomers components also differs greatly among various mouse strains; the CFl strain is particularly susceptible to acute poisoning (Miura *et al.*, 1974). Such toxicity differences may be related to different rates of metabolism of BHC; if so, the tumorigenic effects may also be so related.

The first report of tumorigenic activity of γ-BHC in rats was made by Nagasaki *et al.* in 1972. Three groups of Wistar rats (seven per group) were fed diets containing each BHC isomer at 250, 500, and 1,000 ppm. In rats sacrificed at 24 weeks, the increased liver weight was recognized only in the 500 and 1,000 ppm groups with absence of hepatoma. At 48 weeks, one of seven rats in the 1,000 ppm γ-BHC group showed a hepatoma, which was 1.5 cm in diameter. Three other animals of the same group showed clear hypertrophic nodules without signs of malignant tumor, as did other dosage and isomers groups. On the basis of these findings, it was concluded that γ-BHC was carcinogenic in rats, but that rats were less sensitive than mice.

A study of hepatocellular carcinoma development in rats treated with various isomers of BHC was recently published (Ito *et al.*, 1975). Male Wistar-derived rats were administered BHC isomers in the diet for 72 weeks. Each treatment group included 18-24 animals. The dietary treatment levels were: α-BHC, 500, 1,000, and 1,500 ppm; β-BHC, 500 and 1,000 ppm; γ-BHC, 500 ppm; δ-BHC, 500 and 1,000 ppm. No neoplastic changes or other abnormal findings such as oval cell infiltration, fatty changes, fibrosis, or bile duct proliferation of the liver were observed in groups receiving 500 ppm of any isomer, but relative liver weight was increased in all groups receiving 500 ppm of any isomer, except those treated with 500 ppm δ-BHC. Tumors developed only in the livers of rats in groups given α-BHC. In a group treated with 1500 ppm α-BHC for 72 weeks, the liver increased in weight due to tumor growth; in 10 of 13 rats it had a slightly irregular surface with many nodules up to 2 cm in diameter. In groups, 12 out of 16 rats that received 1,000 ppm α-BHC for 72 weeks, and 5 out of 12 that received 1,000 ppm α-BHC for 48 weeks, developed liver tumors. No metastases were seen. No liver tumors developed in other dietary groups, and no tumors were seen in other organs of any experimental animals.

Reproduction Charles River C.D. rats receiving Lindane at 25, 50, and 100 ppm continuously in the diet during a three-generation study showed normal reproduction, with respect to litter size, breeding rate, and birth weight in all generations. No malformations were found. The only effect observed was the expected liver hypertrophy with hepatocyte enlargement (Cited in USEPA, 1973b).

Teratogenicity No available data.

Carcinogenic Risk Estimates

α-, β-, and γ-BHC have produced dose-related liver tumors when given orally to mice and rats (Ito *et al.*, 1973 and 1975, and Thorpe and Walker, 1973). For each compound the available sets of dose response data were individually considered as described in the risk section in the margin-of-safety chapter. Each set of dose–response data was used to statistically estimate both the lifetime risk and an upper 95% confidence bound on the lifetime risk and an upper 95% confidence bound on the lifetime risk at the low-dose level. These estimates are of lifetime human risks and have been corrected for species conversion on a dose-per-surface-area basis. The risk estimates are expressed as a probability of cancer after a lifetime consumption of 1 liter of water/day containing Q/ppb of the compound of interest. For example, a risk of $1 \times 10^{-6}\, Q$ implies a lifetime probability of 2×10^{-5} of cancer if 2 liters/day were consumed and the concentration of the carcinogen was 10 ppb (i.e., $Q=10$). This means that at a concentration of 10 ppb during a lifetime of exposure this compound would be expected to produce one excess case of cancer for every 50,000 persons exposed. If the population of the United States is taken to be 220 million people, this translates into 4,400 excess lifetime deaths from cancer or 62.8 per year. Since several data sets are typically available the range of the low-dose risk estimates are reported.

For α-BHC at a concentration of 1 μg/liter ($Q=1$) the upper 95% confidence estimate of risk for man would fall between 0.7 to $1.5 \times 10^{-6}\, Q$.

For β-BHC at a concentration of 1 μg/liter ($Q=1$) the estimated risk for man would be from 1.1 to $3.5 \times 10^{-6}\, Q$. The upper 95% confidence estimate of risk at the same concentration would be between 2.5-$5.8 \times 10^{-6}\, Q$.

For Lindane (γ-BHC) at a concentration of 1 μg/liter ($Q=1$) the estimated risk for man would be from 3.3 to $8.1 \times 10^{-6}\, Q$. The upper 95% confidence estimate of risk at the same concentration would be from 5.6-13×10^{-6}

Conclusions and Recommendations

The chronic toxicity of the BHC isomers is clearly related to the tumorigenic effects so far observed only in rodents. The α-isomer is the most strongly implicated; its activity is sufficient to account for the degree of hepatoma formation observed with technical BHC administration in mice. Lindane is a weaker tumorigen in mice, and is so far a questionable tumorigen in rats.

As of 1972, the FAO/WHO ADI for Lindane was set at 0.0125 mg/kg/day. Later, that value was reduced to 0.001 mg/kg/day and held under temporary status because of the newer data concerning carcinogenicity. A full-scale reevaluation of the chronic toxicity of Lindane is scheduled for 1977 by the FAO/WHO. The EPA has recently announced plans to issue a presumptive notice that Lindane is too hazardous for continued registered use, with the intention of reevaluating its administrative position on this insecticide.

In light of the above and taking into account the carcinogenic risk projections it is suggested that very strict criteria be applied when limits for BHC isomers are established. The available chronic toxicity data are summarized in Table VI-26.

KEPONE

Introduction

"Kepone" is the trade name of decachlorooctahydro-1,3,4-metheno-2H-cyclobuta(cd)pentalen-2-one; its common name is "chlordeone," as designated by the International Standards Organization. Kepone was introduced in 1958. More recently it has been produced solely by the Life Science Products Company for Allied Chemical in Hopewell, Virginia, with the total output purchased by Allied Chemical. The Hopewell plant was closed in July 1975, when a number of its workers were found to be seriously ill. In August 1975, the EPA ordered that sales and use of the compound be stopped and prohibited further manufacture.

Kepone was registered for the control of rootborers on bananas with a residue tolerance of 0.01 ppm. This constituted the only food or feed use of Kepone. Nonfood uses included wireworm control in tobacco fields and bait to control ants and other insects in indoor and outdoor areas.

The U.S. production of Kepone for 1974 and 1975 was approximately 850,000 lb/yr (Anonymous, 1976), and 99.2% of this was exported to Latin America, Europe, and Africa. The remaining 0.8% was used in the United States for ant and roach traps or baits.

Kepone was made by the dimerization of hexachlorocyclopentadiene in the presence of sulfur trioxide, followed by hydrolysis of the sulfonated intermediate to Kepone (Brooks, 1974). The technical product (over 90% pure) sublimes at 350°C (Spencer, 1973); it is relatively soluble in water (0.4% at 100°C), compared with most chlorinated hydrocarbon pesticides.

Residues of Kepone have not been investigated in Market Basket Studies by the FDA. Kepone was not found in adipose tissue of humans in the monitoring programs of the Technical Services Division, Office of Pesticide Programs, EPA.

Metabolism

Kepone is very stable in the environment. No degradation products have been reported, although ultraviolet irradiation produced dechlorinated products in a laboratory study (Alley *et al*., 1974). No metabolic products have been reported; cows fed 5.0 ppm in the diet for 60 days excreted 90 ppb of Kepone in milk 35 days after cessation of treated feeding (Smith and Arant, 1967).

Health Aspects

Observations in Man Kepone came to public attention after Life Science Products Company, which produced Kepone, was closed down when many employees became seriously ill with such afflictions as tremors, nausea, dizziness, impaired vision, and impotence. According to an internal report submitted to the Director of the Center for Disease Control by the Cancer and Birth Defects Division, Bureau of Epidemiology, Public Health Service, between March 1974 and July 1975, 62 (55%) of 113 workers at the plant had clinical findings that included nervousness, weight loss, pleuritic and joint pains, oligospermia, tremor, opsoclonia, and ataxia. Kepone was found in the blood of all 32 current employees, at 0.165–26 ppm. These were the first recorded cases of Kepone poisoning in humans. Illness incidence rates were highest for production workers and foremen and least for employees not working directly in production. The mean latency between start of employment and onset of symptoms was 6 weeks. Symptoms have persisted for as long as 6 months after employment was terminated (USPHS, 1976).

Companies using chlordecone have received Occupational Safety and Health Administration (OSHA) notices that this substance is hazardous and that its use should be strictly controlled. The OSHA suggested that

TABLE VI-26 Toxicity of BHC Isomers

Chemical Form and Animal Species	Duration of Study	Dosage Levels and No. of Animals Per Group	Highest No-Adverse-Effect Level or Lowest-Minimal-Effect Level	Effect Measured	Reference
Rat					
BHC (tech)	approx. 2 yr	10, 50, 100, 800 ppm (10 M, 10 F)	800 ppm	reduced lifespan, no increased tumor incidence	Fitzhugh *et al.*, 1950
α -BHC, -BHC	approx. 2 yr	10, 50, 100, 800 ppm (10 M, 10 F)	800 ppm		
γ -BHC	approx. 2 yr	5, 10, 50, 100, 400, 800, 1,600 ppm (10 M, 10 F)	800 ppm		
γ -BHC	2 yr	25, 50, 100 ppm	100 ppm	no increase in tumor incidence	Truhaut, 1954
α -BHC	78 weeks	500, 1,000, 1,500 ppm (18–24 M)	500 ppm	liver hypertrophy (nodular hyperplasia, carcinoma at 1,000 and 1,500 ppm)	Ito *et al.*, 1975
β-BHC	78 weeks	500, 1,000 ppm	500 ppm	liver hypertrophy	
γ -BHC	78 weeks	500 ppm	500 ppm	liver hypertrophy	
δ -BHC	78 weeks	500, 1,000 ppm	1,000 ppm	liver hypertrophy	
Mouse					
BHC (tech)	24 weeks	6.6, 66, 660 ppm (20 M, dd strain)	660 ppm	hepatoma (20/20)	Nagasaki *et al.*, 1971, 1972a
α -BHC	24 weeks	100, 250, 500 ppm (20 M, dd strain)	250 ppm	hepatic nodules (9/20), tumors at 500 (20/20)	Nagasaki *et al.*, 1972b
β-BHC	24 weeks	100, 250, 500 ppm (20 M, dd strain)	500 ppm	no adverse effect	
γ-BHC	24 weeks	100, 250, 500 ppm (20 M, dd strain)	500 ppm	no adverse effect	

				metastases	Walker, 1975
δ-BHC	110 weeks	400 ppm (29 M, 29 F; CF1 strain)	400 ppm	hepatic tumors, lung metastases	
BHC (tech)	26 weeks	600 ppm (20 M; ICR-JCL strain)	600 ppm	hepatic nodules, tumors	Goto *et al.*, 1972
α-BHC	26 weeks	600 ppm (20 M; ICR-JCL strain)	600 ppm	hepatic tumors, lung metastases	
β-BHC	26 weeks	600 ppm (20 M; ICR-JCL strain)	600 ppm	hepatic tumors, lung metastases	
δ -BHC	26 weeks	600 ppm (20 M; ICR-JCL strain)	600 ppm	hepatic tumors, lung metastases	
γ -BHC	26 weeks	300, 600 ppm	300 ppm	no adverse effect	
α -BHC	24 weeks	50, 100, 250 ppm (30 M, dd strain)	100 ppm	liver hypertrophy (hyperplasia, tumors at 250)	Ito *et al.*, 1975
β-BHC	24 weeks	50, 100, 250 ppm (30 M, dd strain)	250 ppm	liver hypertrophy	
γ -BHC	24 weeks	50, 100, 250 ppm (30 M, dd strain)	250 ppm	liver hypertrophy (slight)	
γ -BHC	80 weeks	12.5, 25, 50 ppm (NMRI strain)	50 ppm	no adverse effect	Herbst *et al.*, 1975

[These compounds are animal carcinogens.]

worker exposure to Kepone be kept below 100 $\mu g/m^3$ of air for up to 10 h/day or 40 h/week, over a working lifetime. There is no specific OSHA standard for this chemical.

According to a report in the March 1976 issue of the *Occupational Health Letter*, Kepone is the cause of sterility in exposed human males, in addition to harmful effects on the nervous system and liver. Philip S. Guzelin, spokesman for a team of researchers at the Medical College of Virginia, reported on studies of 23 former industrial workers heavily exposed to Kepone who exhibited overt signs and symptoms of toxicity. In their investigations, the concentration of Kepone in whole blood has been in parts per million, or thousands of times greater than the minimal detectable concentration, and concentrations measured in biopsies of liver, muscle, and adipose tissue have been several times those in whole blood. Effective therapy for Kepone-associated toxicity is unknown. In the absence of data on the pharmacokinetics of Kepone and the mechanisms of its toxicity, rational treatment of exposed or afflicted people is impossible.

Observations in other Species

Acute Effects The acute oral LD_{50}, in corn oil solution, is 114–140 mg/kg in rats and 65–77 mg/kg in rabbits. The acute oral LD_{50} of the formulated product is about 95 mg/kg in male albino rats. The acute dermal LD_{50} is 345–375 mg/kg in rabbits (Martin, 1972). The characteristic effect of this compound was the development of DDT-like tremors. Acute rat inhalation studies of 10% Kepone dust with exposures 2 and 10 times as severe as those likely under agricultural conditions produced no pathologic or other outward effects in rats (USEPA, 1976b).

Chronic Effects and Carcinogenicity Kepone has been reported to be oncogenic in rats (USEPA, 1961). Five groups of male and female albino rats were fed Kepone at 2, 5, 10, 25, 50, and 80 ppm for up to 2 yr. Oncogenic effects appeared only in rats receiving Kepone in their diets for 1–2 yr. None of 23 control rats examined developed hepatocellular carcinomas. Among the seven male rats fed at 25 ppm, liver lesions in one rat were diagnosed as hepatocellular carcinoma by pathologists and "evolving carcinoma" by one pathologist, who also found "evolving carcinoma" in a second male rat at this dosage. Among the 16 female rats that survived at 10 ppm, liver lesions in three were diagnosed as hepatocellular carcinoma by one pathologist. Among the nine female rats that survived at 25 ppm, liver lesions in one were diagnosed as "evolving carcinoma" by one pathologist (U.S. Department of Transportation, 1976). Tremors developed, ranging from slight at 25 ppm to severe at higher dosages.

The carcinogenesis bioassay data prepared by NCI (1976) show the oncogenic effects of chlordecone on both sexes of Osborne-Mendel rats and B6C3Fl mice. Chlordecone was administered orally at average dosages ranging from 8 to 26 ppm for rats and from 20 to 40 ppm for mice for 80 weeks. The mice were sacrificed after 90 weeks, and the rats after 112 weeks; moribund animals were sacrificed and necropsied. Clinical signs of toxicity were observed in both species, including generalized tremors and dermatologic changes. None of the 225 control rats developed hepatocellular carcinomas. Fourteen of the 68 male control mice developed hepatocellular carcinomas. Pathologic diagnosis revealed a statistically significant increase ($p < 0.05$) in the incidence of hepatocellular carcinomas in rats fed an average of 24 ppm (males) and 26 ppm (females) and in mice fed an average of 20 and 23 ppm (males) and 20 and 40 ppm (females). Extensive hyperplasia of the liver was also reported in both species (NCI, 1976).

Reproduction It has been reported in the literature that the administration of sublethal dosages of Kepone to male and female mice caused interference with the reproductive process. Hubert (1965) reported that the major physiologic effects of ingestion of sublethal dosages by laboratory mice, exclusive of the liver and tremor syndrome, involved the reproductive processes. The reproductive capacity of treated animals was inhibited or severely reduced. The females were largely responsible for the reduced reproduction. Data showed that the female hormonal system was disturbed. In a separate and independent mouse reproduction study (Good *et al.*, 1965), authors showed that the reproduction in mice was reduced at all dosages used (10.0–37.5 ppm); both the size and the number of litters were decreased. Increased dosage resulted in increased effects. The reproductive effects of Kepone in rats have apparently not been tested.

Mutagenicity and Teratogenicity There does not appear to be data on the mutagenic and teratogenic properties of Kepone.

Carcinogenic Risk Estimates

Kepone has produced dose-related hepatomas when fed to mice and rats (NCI, 1976). The available sets of dose response data were individually

TABLE VI-27 Toxicity of Kepone (Chlordecone)

Species	Duration of Study	Dosage Levels and No. of Animals Per group	Highest No-Adverse-Effect Level or Lowest-Minimal-Effect Level	Effect Measured	Reference
Rat	2 yr	0, 5, 10, 25, 50, 80 ppm in diet (40 males and 40 females)	5 ppm (0.25 mg/kg/day)	No hepatocellular carcinomas	EPA, 1961
Rat	112 weeks	8 ppm (50 males) 24 ppm (44 males) 18 ppm (49 females) 26 ppm (45 females)	8 ppm (0.4 mg/kg/day)	Hepatocellular carcinomas	NCI, 1976
Mice	90 weeks	20 ppm (48 males) 23 ppm (49 males) 20 ppm (50 females) 40 ppm (49 females)	20 ppm	Hepatocellular carcinomas	NCI, 1976

[This compound is an animal carcinogen.]

considered as described in the risk section in the margin-of-safety chapter. Each set of dose–response data was used to statistically estimate both the lifetime risk at the low dose level. These estimates are of lifetime human risks and have been corrected for species conversion on a dose-per-surface-area basis. The risk estimates are expressed as a probability of cancer after a lifetime consumption of 1 liter of water/day containing Q/ppb of the compound of interest. For example, a risk of $1 \times 10^{-6}\ Q$ implies a lifetime probability of 2×10^{-5} of cancer if 2 liters/day were consumed and the concentration of the carcinogen was 10 ppb (i.e., $Q = 10$). This means that at a concentration of 10 ppb during a lifetime of exposure this compound would be expected to produce one excess case of cancer for every 50,000 persons exposed. If the population of the United States is taken to be 220 million people, this translates into 4,400 excess lifetime deaths from cancer or 62.8 per year. Since several data sets are typically available the range of the low-dose risk estimates are reported.

For Kepone at a concentration of 1 μg/liter ($Q = 1$) the estimated risk for man would be between $2.2\text{-}6.0 \times 10^{-5}\ Q$. The upper 95% confidence estimate of risk at the same concentration would be from 1.4 to $8.0 \times 10^{-5}\ Q$.

Conclusions and Recommendations

Kepone is a very toxic compound and is persistent in the environment. Test results clearly suggest that liver lesions, including cancer, were induced in both sexes of rats and mice fed chlordecone. In addition, the time to detection of the first hepatocellular carcinoma observed at death was shorter for treated than for control mice and, in both sexes and both species, it appeared inversely related to the dose.

In light of the above and taking into account the carcinogenic risk projections it is suggested that very strict criteria be applied when limits for Kepone in drinking water are established. The available chronic oral toxicity data are summarized in Table VI-27.

Apparently, little is known about the pharmacokinetics of Kepone and its mechanisms of toxicity. There is a pressing need for systematic investigation of the absorption, distribution, biotransformation, and excretion of Kepone in humans and experimental animals, to gain an understanding of its toxicity and to provide a basis for rational therapy.

There is also very little information on the environmental transport mechanisms of Kepone and its degradation products, its persistence, and its degradation in soil. Kepone residues have been found in food crops grown in rotation with Kepone-treated tobacco.

TOXAPHENE

Introduction

Toxaphene, a complex mixture of largely uncharacterized chlorinated camphene derivatives, is the most heavily used and least understood organochlorine insecticide. The major reason that so little is known about either its structure or its metabolism is its complex nature: it is a mixture of at least 175 compounds, of which the structures of fewer than 10 are known (Casida *et al.*, 1974).

Toxaphene is widely used as a foliage insecticide on a variety of food, feed, and fiber crops (USEPA, 1974c). A tolerance of 7 ppm was established in 1950 for a variety of crops. More recently, tolerances of 5, 3, and 2 ppm have been established for small grains, for cotton seed, and for bananas and soy beans, respectively. In addition, there is a temporary tolerance of 7 ppm for residues in or on sugar beets and sunflower seeds. Similar foreign tolerances have also been established. A tolerance of 7 ppm for residues of Toxaphene in the fat of meat has also been established. Other regulations have established interim tolerances for Toxaphene residues in or on alfalfa at 1 ppm and in milk at 0.05 ppm.

Like many organochlorine insecticides, Toxaphene is known to be somewhat persistent in the environment, particularly in soil. The EPA has set an interim standard for Toxaphene in finished water for 0.005 mg/liter ($C_{10}H_{10}Cl_8$-Technical chlorinated camphene, 67–69% chlorine) (USEPA, 1975i).

Metabolism

Very little is known about the metabolism of Toxaphene in animals. In the rat, 52.6% of an oral dose of [^{36}Cl]Toxaphene was excreted within 9 days (Crowder and Dindal, 1974). Approximately 37% was found in the feces, and 15% in the urine. On extraction, most of the radioactivity occurred in the water fractions of urine and feces as ionic chloride. Animals given a second dose on the ninth day excreted Toxaphene in a similar manner, except that chlorine-36 excretion in feces was reduced. Less than 10% of the dose was found in selected tissues and organs 1 day after treatment.

Toxaphene has been found in milk of dairy cows given 20–140 ppm in the feed (Clayborn *et al.*, 1963). At lower concentrations, Zweig *et al.* (1963) reported that the amount of toxaphene in milk was less than 0.03 ppm. When the animals were removed from the toxaphene diets, the milk became uncontaminated within 2 weeks.

Health Aspects

Observations in Man Although some cases have been reported, acute Toxaphene poisoning in humans is rare. When Toxaphene was introduced, four cases of poisoning by ingestion in children under 4 yr old were reported (McGee *et al.*, 1952). The same study contained a description of severe toxaphene poisoning in adults after its misuse in agriculture. The authors estimated that three patients ingested toxaphene at 9.5–47 mg/kg.

Aside from accidental poisoning, human volunteers have participated in Toxaphene toxicity studies. In one study, 50 human volunteers inhaled mist containing Toxaphene at 0.0004 mg/liter for 10 min/day for 15 days; there were no subjective or objective results (USEPA, 1974c). In another study, a mist containing Toxaphene at 0.25 mg/liter of air was inhaled by 25 people for 30 min/day for 13 days; there was no evidence of local or systemic toxicity (USEPA, 1974c).

Observations in Other Species

Acute Effects Acute toxicity studies with Toxaphene have involved oral, dermal, intravenous, intraocular, and inhalation exposure. The toxicity of toxaphene is influenced by the solvent or vehicle used. When administered orally as a solution or emulsion, it is more toxic in a digestible vegetable oil than in an oil like kerosene. Toxicity of Toxaphene by skin absorption is much less from an inert dust than from an oily solution. The acute oral LD_{50} is 90 mg/kg in male rats and 80 mg/kg in female rats; the acute dermal LD_{50} is 1,075 mg/kg in male rats and 780 mg/kg in female rats (Gaines, 1960).

Administration of a 20% solution of Toxaphene in kerosene to the eyes of rabbits and guinea pigs for 14 consecutive days produced mild irritation of the eyelids with loss of hair around the eyelids. The eyes were not injured, and the irritation in the eyelid was abated within 10 days (USEPA, 1974c). In acute inhalation studies, 40% Toxaphene dust at 3.4 g/liter of air killed approximately half the exposed rats within 1 h.

Subchronic and Chronic Effects Ortega *et al.* (1951) have studied the subchronic toxicity of Toxaphene in small groups of rats fed 50 and 200 ppm in the diet for 9 months. No clinical signs of toxicity or inhibition of food consumption or growth rate were evident. However, only the liver, spleen, and kidneys were examined histologically. There was no apparent damage to the kidneys or spleen, but 3 of the 12 rats that received 50 ppm

TABLE VI-28 Toxicity of Toxaphene

Species	Duration of Study	Dosage Levels and No. of Animals Per Group	Highest No-Adverse-Effect Level or Lowest-Minimal-Effect Level	Effect Measured	Reference
Rat	9 months	50 ppm (12 animals)		Slight liver change in animals	Ortega *et al.*, 1951
Rat	9 months	200 ppm (12 animals)		Distinct liver change in 6 animals	Ortega *et al.*, 1951
Dog	44 days	160 ppm (2 animals)		Change in kidney tubules and liver parenchyma	Lackey, 1959
Dog	106 days	160 ppm (2 animals)			Lackey, 1949
Rat	2 yr	25 ppm, 100 ppm, and 400 ppm	25 ppm (1.25 mg/kg)[c,d]	No adverse effect liver change	Fitzhugh and Nelson, 1951

Using an uncertainty factor of 1,000, the suggested no-adverse-effect level in drinking water is calculated as follows:

$$\frac{1.25}{1000} = 0.00125 \text{ mg/kg/day (ADI)}, \; 0.00125 \times 70^{a} \times 0.1^{b} = 0.0086 \text{ mg/liter}$$

[a]Assume average weight of human adult = 70 kg.
[b]Assume average daily intake of water for man = 2 liters, and that 20 percent of total intake is from water.
[c]Value from which the suggested no-adverse-effect level was calculated.
[d]Assume weight of rat = 0.4 kg and average daily food consumption of rat = 0.02 kg.

showed slight liver changes, and 6 of the 12 rats fed 200 ppm showed distinct liver changes.

Degenerative changes in the kidney tubules and liver parenchyma have been reported in dogs fed Toxaphene at low dosages (Lacky, 1949); two dogs received 4 mg/kg/day (about 160 ppm) for 44 days, and two others received the same dosage for 106 days.

Chronic studies have been done in rats, guinea pigs, dogs, cattle, sheep, and rabbits. In rats fed at 25, 100, and 400 ppm in the diet for the conventional 2-yr period, only the liver showed significant changes, at 100 and 400 ppm (Fitzhugh and Nelson, 1951).

Toxaphene was administered daily to dogs in a dry diet for 2 yr. When it was fed at 40 ppm, there was slight degeneration of the liver; at 200 ppm, there was moderate degeneration of the liver (USEPA, 1974c).

Studies have also shown that, when Toxaphene is applied to the skin of many large animals (including cattle, sheep, goats, horses, and swine), adult animals can withstand higher dosages than immature animals. Also, applications of cotton patches treated with Toxaphene to the skin of 200 human subjects caused no primary irritation or sensitization.

Reproduction, Teratogenicity, Carcinogenicity, and Mutagenicity A three-generation reproductive study was conducted, according to currently accepted protocol for rats, with Toxaphene at 20 and 100 ppm (Kennedy *et al.*, 1973). No differences between control and Toxaphene-treated animals were reported, with respect to reproduction, performance, fertility, lactation, or viability, size, and anatomic structure of progeny. In mutagenicity studies, occurrence of mutagenic effects among the controls and the animals treated with Toxaphene were similar. No evidence of carcinogenic action was reported in any of the chronic-toxicity studies previously undertaken.

Conclusions and Recommendations

Toxaphene is a widely used organochlorine insecticide that apparently has not caused a great deal of environmental harm, although it has been used in agriculture for many years. Because it is a complex mixture of uncharacterized camphene derivatives, very little is known about its metabolism in plants or other higher organisms. Considerable information is available, however, on its toxicity in laboratory animals and various aquatic organisms. An ADI of 0.00125 mg/kg/day was calculated on the basis of the chronic toxicity data. The available toxicity data and calculations of ADI are summarized in Table VI-28.

A summary of the results of examination of over 100,000 samples of raw agricultural commodities by the FDA between 1963 and 1969 (Duggan *et al.*, 1971) shows that Toxaphene residues are seldom present. Thus, the possibility that large quantities of Toxaphene residues could be found in drinking water is not great.

Organophosphates

AZINPHOSMETHYL

Introduction

Azinphosmethyl, or *O,O*-dimethyl-*S*-4-oxo-1,2,3-benzotriazin-3(4H)-methylphosphorodithioate (Guthion), is a contact organophosphorus insecticide used on a variety of fruit, vegetable, nut, and forage crops. It was first registered for use in 1956, and there are no nonagricultural uses.

It is estimated that 2.7 million pounds of azinphosmethyl were used in the United States in 1971 (NAS, 1975), vitrually all applied to crops. This amounted to approximately 2% of the insecticides used in that year. The prime areas for the use of azinphosmethyl were the Northeast and Pacific states, followed by the Midwest.

Azinphosmethyl is produced by the reaction of *N*-bromethylazimidobenzoyl with sodium dimethyldithiophosphoric acid. It is soluble in water at 33 ppm at 25°C. The products of hydrolysis depend on the pH of the medium, but hydrolysis generally results in cleavage of the *S*-methylaryl bond. At a pH of 5, the half-life is 8.9 h at 70°C and 240 days at 20°C (Melnikov, 1971). In the only study found on the behavior of azinphosmethyl in water (Weiss and Gakstatter, 1965), its half-life in both laboratory and natural water systems was found to be 30–70 days at a pH of 5.1–8.4. The higher the pH, the less persistent the compound seemed to be.

The acceptable daily intake of azinphosmethyl has been established by the WHO/FAO at 0.0025 mg/kg. The tolerance established by the FDA in the United States is 2 ppm. The FDA's Market Basket Surveys for pesticide residues do not include azinphosmethyl, so its possible presence in food has not been studied.

Metabolism

There is apparently no information in the literature on the metabolism of azinphosmethyl in mammalian systems.

Health Aspects

Observations in Man The anticholinesterase effects of azinphosmethyl were studied in human subjects by administering it at 7, 8, and 9 mg/day for 4 weeks. There were five test subjects per dosage and two controls. Cholinesterase was measured twice a week before and during exposure. None of the dosages produced any significant decrease in red-cell or plasma cholinesterase (Rider *et al.*, 1970).

There are no reported cases of human poisoning by azinphosmethyl in the literature.

Observations in Other Species

Acute Effects Acute oral LD_{50}'s in rats of 7–13 mg/kg (Simson *et al.*, 1969), 10–18 mg/kg (Neumeyer *et al.*, 1969), and 12 mg/kg (Crawford *et al.*, 1970) have been reported. Oral LD_{50} values of 11 and 13 mg/kg were reported for female and male rats, respectively (Gaines, 1960). The oral LD_{50} is 20 mg/kg in mice (Crawford *et al.*, 1970) and 80 mg/kg in guinea pigs (DuBois *et al.*, 1957). The higher LD_{50} in guinea pigs might be the result of slower conversion of azinphosmethyl to its active oxygen analogue.

The toxicity by other routes is about the same as by the oral route. In rats, the subcutaneous LD_{50} is 9.25 mg/kg (Edery *et al.*, 1970), the intraperitoneal LD_{50} is 5.7 mg/kg in females and 11.6 mg/kg in males (DuBois *et al.*, 1957), and the dermal LD_{50} is 280 mg/kg (Simson *et al.*, 1969). The intraperitoneal and subcutaneous LD_{50}'s in mice are similar.

Subchronic and Chronic Effects Although there have been a number of studies of the effect of azinphosmethyl on *in vitro* and *in vivo* cholinesterase activity, none of these were designed to establish a no-adverse-effect or minimal-effect dosage. DuBois *et al.* (1957) did establish that azinphosmethyl was a relatively weak *in vitro* cholinesterase inhibitor, the I_{50} being $2 \times 10^{-4} M$, $7.7 \times 10^{-4} M$, and $7.7 \times 10^{-4} M$ for brain, submaxillary gland, and serum enzyme, respectively. The oxygen analogue of azinphosmethyl, however, would be expected to be far more active in such an *in vitro* assay.

Azinphosmethyl was fed to postweaning Wistar rats at 5, 20, and 50 ppm for 2 yr, with 40 of each sex in each dosage group. Twenty-three weeks after the beginning of the study, dosage of 2.5 ppm was added; after 47 weeks, the 50-ppm dosage was increased to 100 ppm. No adverse effects were observed in the 50-ppm group, but increasing the dosage to

100 ppm resulted in convulsive episodes in several animals and a consistent decrease in plasma and red-cell cholinesterase activity. The no-adverse-effect dosage was determined to be 50 ppm (Worden *et al.*, 1973).

The same authors (Worden *et al.*, 1973) conducted a 2-yr feeding study in dogs. Four cocker spaniels of each sex were fed 5, 20, and 50 ppm. Because no adverse effects were seen in the initial stages of the experiment, the dosage of 20 ppm was increased to 50 ppm, and the 50-ppm was increased to 100 ppm at 36 weeks. The 100-ppm dosage was increased to 150 ppm at 57 weeks and to 300 ppm at 83 weeks. The dosage of 150 ppm was "well tolerated," but 300 ppm had adverse effects. Slight effects were noted at dosages above 20 ppm, so the no-adverse-effect dosage, with cholinesterase decrease as the determining factor, was established as 20 ppm.

The WHO/FAO (1969) summarized proprietary data on rats and dogs in 2-yr feeding studies. For rats, probably on the basis of the same study as later published by Worden *et al.* (1973), the no-adverse-effect dosage was established as 2.5 ppm (0.125 mg/kg/day) with plasma cholinesterase as the factor measured. For dogs, 5 ppm (0.125 mg/kg/day) was the no-adverse-effect dosage when dogs were treated at 5, 10, 10, and 50 ppm in the diet. Serum cholinesterase and red-cell cholinesterase were the factors measured.

Mutagenicity No reports on mutagenicity testing of azinphosmethyl could be found.

Carcinogenicity Although not specifically designed to test carcinogenicity, the chronic toxicity studies of Worden *et al.* (1973) included observations on tumor incidence. There was no evidence that azinphosmethyl induced tumor formation, as the incidence of tumors was highest in the control group and lowest in the highest dosage azinphosmethyl group.

Reproduction There are no studies of the effect of azinphosmethyl on reproduction in the open literature.

Teratogenicity The chick embroyo test for teratogenic potential was negative for azinphosmethyl (Roger *et al.*, 1969). No terata were observed at dosages of 1 mg/egg or less.

There are no *in vivo* studies reported in the literature designed to test the teratogenic potential of the compound. However, in chronic-toxicity studies, there are no reports of abnormal offspring.

Conclusions and Recommendations

Azinphosmethyl is an organophosphorus insecticide whose principal application is in agriculture. Its mode of action is inhibition of the enzyme acetylcholinesterase. It has high acute toxicity, and its chronic toxicity is moderate. Based on 2-yr feeding studies in rats and dogs, an ADI at 0.0125 mg/kg/day was calculated. The available data and calculations of ADI are summarized in Table VI-29.

No specific methods for the analysis of azinphosmethyl in water have been reported. However, methods available for its determination in food materials and soils should be easily adaptable to water samples. Gas-chromatographic and other methods have been developed and are routinely applied for the analysis of azinphosmethyl. The sensitivity of these methods is well below that which would be required for the analysis of water samples with reasonable sample sizes.

There is a pressing need for studies on the metabolism of azinphosmethyl in mammalian systems. It is difficult to understand how a compound could have come to be so extensively used when so little is known of its fate in mammalian systems, as well as in soil and the environment.

Studies on the potential of azinphosmethyl for mutagenicity, teratogenicity, and carcinogenicity need to be conducted. There is almost nothing in the literature on the behavior of this compound in these respects.

Data on the behavior of azinphosmethyl in water and the likelihood of its appearing in drinking water are needed. Studies on its environmental transport would also be useful in this respect.

DIAZINON

Introduction

Diazinon, or *O,O*-diethyl *O*-(2-isopropyl-4-methyl-6-pyrimidinyl)-phosphorothioate, is a wide-spectrum organophosphorus insecticide and miticide extensively used in the United States on a wide variety of agricultural crops, ornamentals, domestic animals, lawns and gardens, and household pests.

In 1971, 3.2 million pounds of diazinon was used in the United States, accounting for about 2% of insecticide use (NAS, 1975). Most of this was on crops, with only small amounts used on livestock and for other purposes. The EPA estimates that diazinon use was 4.8–5.6 million pounds in 1974. According to the EPA, the peak of agricultural use of diazinon was in 1966, and it has been declining since. The two sources of

TABLE VI-29 Toxicity of Azinphosmethyl

Species	Duration of Study	Dosage Levels and No. of Animals Per Group	Highest No-Adverse-Effect Level or Lowest-Minimal-Effect Level	Effect Measured	Reference
Rats	2 yr	0–50 ppm orally, 80 animals/group	50 ppm	no adverse effect	Worden *et al.*, 1973
Dogs	2 yr	0–50 ppm orally, 8 animals/group	20 ppm	no adverse effect	Worden *et al.*, 1973
Rats	2 yr		2.5 ppm (0.125 mg/kg/day)[c,d]	no adverse effect	WHO/FAO, 1969
Dogs	2 yr	0–50 ppm	5 ppm (0.125 mg/kg/day)[c,d]	no adverse effect	WHO/FAO, 1969
Man	4 weeks	7, 8, 9 mg/day, 5 men/group	0.13 mg/kg/day[a]	no adverse effect	Rider *et al.*, 1970

Using an uncertainty factor of 10, the suggested no-adverse-effect level in drinking water is calculated as follows:

$$\frac{0.125}{10} = 0.0125 \text{ mg/kg/day (ADI)}, 0.0125 \times 70^{a} \times 0.1^{b} = 0.088 \text{ mg/liter}$$

[a]Assume average weight of human adult = 70 kg.
[b]Assume average daily intake of water for man = 2 liters, and that 20 percent of total intake is from water.
[c]Value from which the suggested no-adverse-effect level was calculated.
[d]Assume average weight of rat = 0.4 kg and of dog = 10 kg; assume average daily food consumption of rat = 0.02 kg and of dog = 0.25 kg.

data do not result in the same figures, but they do indicate the general range for the quantities of diazinon used. Major regions of agricultural use are the Pacific, Southeast, and Appalachian states. Large amounts of diazinon are also used in lawn and turf insect control in urban areas.

Diazinon is synthesized by a series of steps starting with isobutyronitrile, methanol, and methylacetoacetate. Technical diazinon is approximately 97–99% pure. Diazinon is soluble in water at 40 ppm at 20°C. Compared with other organophosphorus insecticides, diazinon is relatively stable to base and unstable to acid. The half-life at a pH of 3.14 is 0.5 day and at a pH of 10.9 is 6 days, compared with 185 days at a pH of 7.4 (Menzie, 1969).

A number of studies have indicated that diazinon is relatively nonpersistent in soil. Most diazinon applied is lost from the soil through chemical and biologic degradation within about 2 months of application (Getzin, 1966, 1968). There is little information available on the behavior of diazinon in an aquatic environment. Paris and Lewis (1973) reported that about 46% of the diazinon added to neutral aqueous solution remained after 2 weeks.

The acceptable daily intake of diazinon has been established by the WHO/FAO at 0.002 mg/kg. A large number of tolerances of diazinon in food have been established by the FDA. These generally range from as low as 0.75 ppm in vegetable crops to as high as 40 ppm in alfalfa as a forage crop. FDA Market Basket Surveys have found diazinon in about 2% of the food samples analyzed. In no case did the residue exceed the established tolerance limit (Duggan, 1968; Duggan *et al.*, 1971).

Metabolism

The metabolism of diazinon has been reviewed by Fukami and Shishido (1972). Its metabolism is due principally to four enzyme systems: mixed function oxidases, in which diazinon is converted to its oxygen analogue and the isopropyl moiety and the ring methyl group may be hydroxylated; hydrolases or phosphatases, which cleave the aryl phosphate bond from the aromatic ring, producing phosphoric acids and pyrimidinols; glutathione-dependent transferases, which cleave the aryl phosphate bond and conjugate the resulting pyrimidine moiety with glutathione; and nonspecific esterases, which, again, produce phosphoric acids.

Most *in vivo* animal studies have demonstrated the production of diazoxon, hydroxydiazinon (the isopropyl secondary carbon is hydroxylated), isohyroxydiazinon (the ring methyl group is hydroxylated), and a propylenediazinon metabolite. These metabolites must all be considered potentially toxic, because they are neutral phosphorus esters. However, the activity of all has been shown to be lower than that of the parent compound. These metabolites are minor components in the urine and feces of treated animals. Most of the diazinon administered is accounted for in the urine of animals by the various cleavage products, which are not considered to be toxicologically active. In none of the studies of diazinon metabolism has cleavage of the ring been reported.

Health Aspects

Observations in Man The WHO/FAO (1967) reported that diazinon causes no toxicologic effects in man at 0.02 mg/kg/day. This determination resulted from treatment of human subjects at 0.02, 0.025, and 0.05 mg/kg/day for 37 days. Plasma cholinesterase decrease was measured.

Observations in Other Species

Acute Effects The oral LD_{50} of diazinon in rats ranges from 56 to 800 mg/kg. This rather wide range may be accounted for by the use of various grades of purity of the material and different vehicles of administration. Bruce *et al.* (1955) reported an LD_{50} of 100–150 mg/kg for the 95% technical compound administered in corn oil. Schafer (1972) reported 150–220 mg/kg. Gaines (1969) reported 250 mg/kg in male and 285 mg/kg in female rats. The value of 800 mg/kg resulted from the use of "high purity" diazinon in a test with female rats (Sanderson and Edson, 1959). Several studies have demonstrated an effect of diet on the toxicity of diazinon (Boyd and Carsky, 1969; Boyd *et al.*, 1969). The LD_{50} ranged from 56 to 466 mg/kg, depending on the nutritional state of the animals used. Studies on the acute oral toxicity of diazinon to mice gave an LD_{50} of 82 mg/kg in females (Bruce *et al.*, 1955).

Intraperitoneal injection of diazinon in female rats gave an LD_{50} of 90 mg/kg (DuBois, 1961). Dermal toxicity in rats and rabbits was also determined. Gaines (1960) reported a dermal LD_{50} of 34 mg/kg in rats when the purified compound was administered in xylene, but 200 mg/kg in females and 180 mg/kg in males with the impure material (Gaines, 1969). The dermal LD_{50} of the 25W formulation was greater than 4,000 mg/kg, expressed as the active ingredient (Bruce *et al.*, 1955).

Subchronic and Chronic Effects Dogs were fed diazinon at 0.25, 0.75, and 75 ppm in the diet for 90 days. Each treatment group consisted of one male and one female; the control group had five dogs. Plasma cholinesterase and red-cell cholinesterase were measured. Red-cell cholinesterase was decreased only in the highest-dosage group, and plasma cholinesterase was decreased in the two higher groups. Thus, the no-adverse-effect dosage in this study was 0.25 ppm (Williams *et al.*, 1959).

Dogs were also used for an 8-month study in which diazinon was administered by gelatin capsule daily at 2.5, 5.0, 10.0, and 20.0 mg/kg. Three female and three male beagles were used for each group. Various hematologic factors and blood chemistry were measured monthly during the study and compared with preexposure data. Three of the dogs at the highest dosage died in the first month; one of the dogs at 10.0 mg/kg developed cholinergic symptoms, but recovered. There were no dose-dependent hematologic effects at any dosage. Unfortunately, cholinesterase decrease was apparently not measured in this study. For the factors measured, however, a no-adverse-effect dosage of 5.0 mg/kg could be concluded (Earl *et al.*, 1971).

Female Wistar rats were fed diets containing diazinon at 1, 5, 25, and 125 ppm for 15–16 weeks. There were 10 animals per group. Plasma cholinesterase and red-cell cholinesterase were measured throughout the test, and brain cholinesterase at termination. Red-cell cholinesterase was slightly decreased in the 5-ppm group, and no-adverse-effects were observed at any time in the 1-ppm group (Edson and Noakes, 1960).

Other subchronic-toxicity studies were conducted in dogs (Bruce *et al.*, 1955) and miniature swine (Earl *et al.*, 1971), but neither study lends itself to the calculation of a no-adverse-effect dosage.

The WHO/FAO summarized proprietary data in the development of an acceptable daily intake in diazinon for rats (WHO/FAO, 1971) and dogs (WHO/FAO, 1965). A 90-day feeding study with rats at 0.5, 1, 2, and 4 ppm in which plasma cholinesterase decrease was the effect measured gave a no-effect dosage of 2 ppm (0.1 mg/kg/day). For dogs treated with 0.02, 0.04, and 0.08 mg/kg/day for 31 days, the no-adverse-effect dosage was 0.02 mg/kg, when inhibition of plasma cholinesterase was used as the endpoint.

There are no chronic feeding studies with diazinon in the open literature. However, the WHO/FAO (1967) summarized a study in monkeys that resulted in the estimation of a no-adverse-effect dosage of 0.05 mg/kg/day. Monkeys were treated at 0.05, 0.5, and 5 mg/kg for up to 2 yr. Inhibition of red-cell and plasma cholinesterase was measured.

No delayed neurotoxicity resulted from treatment of chickens subcutaneously with diazinon in peanut oil at 5–80 mg/kg (Durham *et al.*, 1956).

Mutagenicity Diazinon has not been extensively tested for its mutagenic properties. One study (Tzoneba-Maneva *et al.*, 1969) on the effect of diazinon on mitosis in human lymphocytes reported chromosomal aberrations in 74% of the cells at 0.5 mg/ml. A dosage of 2.5 mg/ml produced a greater effect on mitosis than 0.5 and 5.0 mg/ml.

Carcinogenicity Data from chronic oral-toxicity studies have not shown any oncogenicity resulting from diazinon.

Reproduction No studies on the effect of diazinon on reproduction have been reported.

Teratogenicity The 4E formulation of diazinon was administered to pregnant rats by gavage on days 9, 10, 8–12, or 12–15 of gestation. One day before parturition, the pups were delivered by Cesarean section and examined for abnormalities. None were found to be dose-related (Dobbins, 1967). However, a higher incidence of urinary malformations, hydronephrosis and hydroureter were observed in the multiple-dose animals than in the controls.

When diazinon was administered intraperitoneally to rats on day 11 of gestation at dosages sufficient to produce toxicity, it was found to be "slightly teratogenic" (Kimbrough and Gaines, 1968).

Robens (1969) studied the teratogenic effects of diazinon in hamsters and rabbits. Hamsters were treated at 0.125 and 0.25 mg/kg on day 6, 7, or 8 of gestation, and rabbits received either 7 or 30 mg/kg/day on days 5–15 of gestation. No terata were produced in either case.

Studies by Earl *et al.* (1973) on the effect of diazinon at 1, 2, or 5 mg/kg/day on dogs and 5 and 10 mg/kg/day on miniature pigs revealed a variety of gross abnormalities in some that may have been caused by diazinon.

Conclusions and Recommendations

Diazinon is a widely used organophosphorus insecticide with applications in agriculture, homes and gardens, and structural pest control. It may well be used in situations that would lead to contamination of drinking-water. The mode of action of diazinon, as with other organophosphorus insecticides, is inhibition of the enzyme cholinesterase. Its acute toxicity, however, in comparison with other organophosphates, is only moderate. Its metabolism is straightforward and leads to metabolites that have little toxic potential. Subchronic- and chronic-feeding studies are sufficiently complete and indicate little problem with the use of diazinon. An ADI was calculated at 0.002 mg/kg/day based on these data. The available data and calculations of ADI are summarized in Table VI-30.

Gas-chromatographic and thin-layer chromatographic methods are available for the analysis of diazinon in water. These methods require extraction of the diazinon from the water before analysis. Sensitivity thus depends on the size of the sample used. The anytical sensitivity of the methods, however, is adequate to detect concentrations lower than the recommended no-adverse-effect concentration in samples of reasonable size.

The data needed for the toxicologic evaluation of diazinon are fairly complete, and there is no pressing need for research to evaluate its safety. There is little information available on the actual presence or absence of diazinon in drinking-water or in sources of drinking-water. Studies on the environmental transport and persistence of diazinon would be useful in this respect.

PHORATE AND DISULFOTON

Introduction

Phorate, or *O,O*-diethyl-*S*-[(ethylthio)methyl]phosphorodithioate phosphorodithioate (Thimet R), and disulfoton, or *O,O*-diethyl-*S*-[(2-ethylthio)ethyl]phosphorodithioate (Di-Syston R), are closely related, systemic organophosphorus insecticides. The compounds differ from each other structurally only in the number of carbon atoms in the aliphatic side chain of the molecules, disulfoton having one more than phorate. Their properties and uses are quite similar. The principal uses for both compounds are in soil applications for the control of sucking insects.

There is only one report of the finding of a food containing disulfoton in the FDA's Market Basket Survey of prepared food (Corneliussen, 1970)—in a leafy vegetable containing 0.002 ppm, well below the tolerance limit. Phorate has not been found in food.

From the standpoint of total volume of use, both phorate and disulfoton must be considered as major insecticides. In 1971, 4.2 million pounds of phorate and 4.1 million pounds of disulfoton were used in the United States (NAS, 1975). Each represented 2% of the total insecticide used that year. Virtually all the phorate and disulfoton is used on crops, with less than 100,000 pounds (primarily disulfoton) being used for home and garden applications. The use of these compounds is growing steadily, with indications that further increase will occur as a result of DDT cancellation. The use of these compounds is most extensive in the south-

TABLE VI-30 Toxicity of Diazinon

Species	Duration of Study	Dosage Levels and No. of Animals Per Group	Highest No-Adverse-Effect Level or Lowest-Minimal-Effect Level	Effect Measured	Reference
Dogs	90 days	0.25–75 ppm in diet, 2 animals/group	0.25 ppm	no adverse effect	Williams *et al.*, 1959
Dogs	8 months	0–20 mg/kg/day orally, 6 animals/group	5 mg/kg/day	no adverse effect	Earl *et al.*, 1971
Rats	15–16 weeks	0–125 ppm in diet, 10 animals/group	1 ppm (0.05 mg/kg/day)	no adverse effect	Edson and Noake, 1960
Rats	90 days	0–4 ppm in diet	2 ppm (0.1 mg/kg/day)	no adverse effect	WHO/FAO, 1971
Dogs	31 days	0–0.08 mg/kg/day in diet	0.02 mg/kg/day[c]	no adverse effect	WHO/FAO, 1965
Monkeys	2 yr	0–5 mg/kg/day	0.05 mg/kg/day	no adverse effect	WHO/FAO, 1967
Man	37 days	0–0.05 mg/kg/day	0.02 mg/kg/day[c]	no adverse effect	WHO/FAO, 1967

Using an uncertainty factor of 10, the suggested no-adverse-effect level in drinking water is calculated as follows:

$$\frac{0.02}{10} = 0.002 \text{ mg/kg/day (ADI)}, \; 0.002 \times 70^{a} \times 0.1^{b} \times 0.014 \text{ mg/liter}$$

[a]Assume average weight of human adult = 70 kg.
[b]Assume average daily intake of water for man = 2 liters, and that 20 percent of total intake is from water.
[c]Value from which the no-adverse-effect drinking-water level was calculated.

central states, followed by the western and north-central areas. Only small amounts are used in the Southeast and Northeast.

Both compounds are synthesized commercially by straightforward procedures that give high yields of relatively pure products. Phorate is prepared by the reaction of *O,O*-diethylphosphorodithioic acid with formaldehyde and methylmercaptan (Melnikov, 1971). It is soluble in water at 50 ppm. Disulfoton is prepared by the reaction of *O,O*-diethylphosphorodithioic acid with B-chloroethylethylsflfide (Melnikov, 1971). It is soluble in water at 25 ppm at 23°C. Both compounds are very susceptible to alkaline hydrolysis. Phorate has a half-life of 2 h in an aqueous solution at a pH of 8 and 70°C. It is much more stable in an acid medium (Sutherland *et al.*, 1964). Disulfoton is more resistant to hydrolysis, its half-life at a pH of 8 and at 70°C being 21.5 h; its half-life at a pH of 9 and at 70°C is 7.2 h (Muhlmann and Schrader, 1957).

The fate and significance of phorate and disulfoton in the environment have not been extensively studied. Both are highly toxic to the fish, crustaceans, and terrestrial wildlife that have been tested. However, there are no reported killings of wildlife, fish, or other aquatic organisms, probably because the use patterns of the compounds do not lead to contamination of the environments of such organisms. Information on the presence and persistence of phorate and disulfoton in water is unavailable.

Tolerances for phorate on many raw agricultural commodities have been established. These tolerances range from 0.1 to 3 ppm. Tolerances for disulfoton on 54 food and feed commodities have been established. These range from 0.1 to 12 ppm. The FAO/WHO has established a temporary acceptable daily intake for disulfoton—at 0.01 mg/kg—but not for phorate.

Metabolism

Because the oxidative metabolites of disulfoton and phorate resemble the parent compounds in toxicity, it is important to consider the extent of their metabolism in mammalian systems and in the environment that would lead to human exposure to them.

In studies of phorate in rats, Bowman and Casida (1958) showed that hydrolysis products were the principal urinary components, consisting of diethylphosphorodithioic acid, diethylphosphorothioic acid, and diethyl phosphoric acid. In general, oxidative metabolites are not found as components of excretory products of animals treated with phorate. However, DuBois *et al.* (1950) used rat liver slices to show that phorate is converted by mammalian systems to its oxidative products. The major metabolites of phorate in blood after oral administration to rats have been shown to be phorate sulfoxide and phoratoxon sulfone.

Disulfoton follows essentially the same metabolic routes as phorate. Initial rapid conversion to the sulfoxide is followed by oxidation to the sulfone and oxidative desulfuration to the disulfotoxon sulfoxide and sulfone. Hydrolysis competes with the oxidative process to form the various phosphoric acids (Bull, 1965). Metabolism of disulfoton in plants parallels that in mammals. The oxidative metabolites are formed first, followed by hydrolysis to phosphoric acids.

Health Aspects

Observations in Man

EPA accident files contain reports of 21 episodes of poisoning involving phorate for the period 1971–1973. Eleven were classified as agricultural, six as industrial, and four as having other causes. There have been no fatalities from phorate poisoning. There are no controlled studies of phorate in humans from which no-adverse-effect dosages could be derived.

Five human subjects were given disulfoton at 0.75 mg/kg for 30 days. Measurement of plasma and red-cell cholinesterase during the administration period and for 30 days thereafter showed no decrease in cholinesterase (Rider *et al.*, 1972).

Observations in Other Species

Acute Effects Both disulfoton and phorate have high acute toxicity in laboratory animals. The oral LD_{50} of phorate in rats is reported variously as 1.75 mg/kg (Hazleton, 1953); 2.71-4.11 mg/kg (Tusing, 1955); and 17.7 mg/kg (American Cyanamid, 1966; cited in USEPA, 1974e). The oral LD_{50} of disulfoton in male rats is reported variously as 12.5 mg/kg (Bombinski and DuBois, 1958; Wysocka-Paruszewska, 1970) and 6.8 mg/kg (Gaines, 1969) and in female rats as 2.6 mg/kg (Wysocka-Paruszewska, 1970; Bombinski and DuBois, 1958), 2.3 mg/kg (Gaines, 1969), and 2.8 mg/kg (McPhillips and Dar, 1967). Studies on the acute oral toxicity of phorate in other animals were not found. The acute oral LD_{50} of disulfoton in mice and guinea pigs are about the same as those in rats (Bombinski and DuBois, 1958; Stevens *et al.*, 1972).

Studies to determine the acute dermal LD_{50} of phorate gave values of 3 mg/kg in rats (Shaffer, 1958), 20 mg/kg in male guinea pigs (American Cyanamid, 1966; cited in USEPA, 1974e), and 71 mg/kg in rabbits

(American Cyanamid, 1966; cited in USEPA, 1974e). The acute dermal LD_{50} values of disulfoton are 6.0 mg/kg in females and 15.0 mg/kg in male rats (Gaines, 1969). The oxidative metabolites of phorate and disulfoton are at least as toxic as the parent compounds. Although specific information is not available in the open literature, the same toxicity relationships hold for disulfoton and its oxidative metabolites.

Subchonic and Chronic Effects Subchronic feeding studies have been carried out with phorate and its oxidative metabolites. Four groups of 10 male Carworth Farms rats were given 88% technical phorate in the diet at 1, 5, and 25 ppm for 28 days. Cholinesterase in the 1-ppm group was not decreased (Tusing, 1955). In a second rat study, the no-adverse-effect dosage was 0.66 ppm. Groups of 50 male and female rats each were fed 92% phorate for 13 weeks at 0.22, 0.66, 2.0, 6.0, 12.0, and 18.0 ppm (Tusing, 1956).

Groups of three dogs (two females and one male) received 92% phorate at 0.01, 0.05, 0.25, and 1.24 mg/kg 6 days/week for 13–15 weeks. The no-adverse-effect dosage was judged to be 0.01 mg/kg, although very slight decrease in plasma cholinesterase did result even then. Higher dosages caused significant depression of cholinesterase and mortality at the two highest dosages (Tusing, 1956).

Rat feeding studies showed higher subchronic toxicities on phorate oxidative metabolites (Rombinski *et al.*, 1958).

Studies of the subchronic toxicity of disulfoton have measured cholinesterase decrease in animals and the effect of repeated administration of the compound on their tolerance of it. However, none of these studies were designed to allow the extrapolation of a no-adverse-effect dosage of disulfoton based on cholinesterase decrease. There are no reports of long-term chronic feeding studies of either phorate or disulfoton.

Mutagenicity No available data.

Carcinogenicity No chronic feeding studies of phorate or disflfoton in which carcinogenicity could be evaluated have been reported.

Reproduction CFI mice from Carworth Farms were fed diets containing 98.7% phorate at 0.6, 1.5, and 3.0 ppm. Pups were weaned directly onto diets that were being fed to the parents for a three-generations reproduction study. Reproductive performance and lactation were evaluated. In addition, a rather complete series of pathology evaluations was done to establish that the no-adverse-effect level for reproductive

TABLE VI-31 Toxicity of Phorate

Species	Duration of Study	Dosage Levels and No. of Animals Per Group	Highest No-Adverse-Effect Level or Lowest-Minimal-Effect Level	Effect Measured	Reference
Rats	28 days	1–25 ppm in diet, 10 animals/group	1 ppm	no adverse effect	Tusing, 1955
Rats	13 weeks	0–18 ppm in diet, 100 animals/group	0.66 ppm	no adverse effect	Tusing, 1956
Dogs	13–15 weeks	0–1.24 mg/kg/day in diet, 3 animals/group	0.01 mg/kg/day[c]	slight cholinesterase depression	Tusing, 1956
Rats	13 weeks	0–2 ppm in diet, 100 animals/group	0.32 ppm	no adverse effect	American Cyanamid, 1968a,b

Using an uncertainty factor of 100, the suggested no-adverse-effect level in drinking water is calculated as follows:

$$\frac{0.01}{100} = 0.0001 \text{ mg/kg/day (ADI)}, \; 0.0001 = 70^{a} \times 0.1^{b} = 0.0007 \text{ mg/liter}$$

[a]Assume average weight of human adult = 70 kg.
[b]Assume average daily intake of water for man = 2 liters, and that 20 percent of total intake is from water.
[c]Value from which the suggested no-adverse-effect level was calculated.

performance was 1.5 ppm (American Cyanamid, 1965b; cited in USEPA, 1974e).

There are no published studies on the effects of disulfoton on reproduction.

Teratogenicity No teratogenicity studies of phorate have been reported. However, in the studies on reproductive performance reported above, no abnormalities, including skeletal changes, could be related to phorate administration. Phorate was also studied in the chick embryo test (Richert and Prahlad, 1972). Phorate in peanut oil was injected into eggs on the tenth day of incubation at 1.5 or 2.0 ppm. Controls received peanut oil only. Hatchability of the eggs was decreased in a dose-dependent manner. Malformations were produced, but these did not seem to be dose-related. The relevance of these studies to mammalian teratology is unclear.

There are no published reports of teratogenicity studies of disulfoton.

Conclusions and Recommendations

Phorate and disulfoton are widely used agricultural insecticides. They are organophosphorus compounds whose mode of action, inhibition of acetylcholinesterase, is well understood. Both have high acute toxicity in laboratory animals. Because of this and a known mode of action, studies on the possible chronic toxicity of these compounds have been neglected. There is very little toxicologic research on disulfoton reported in the open literature. There is a single subchronic-toxicity study, in which no adverse effects were observed after administration of 0.75 mg/kg/day for 30 days; this indicates that disulfoton would pose less hazard than phorate. Based on subchronic toxicity data, an ADI was calculated at 0.0001 mg/kg/day for both phorate and disulfoton. The available data and calculations of ADI are summarized in Table VI-31.

Phorate and disulfoton are converted in the environment and in mammalian systems to a series of highly toxic oxidative metabolites, which are known to be more potent cholinesterase inhibitors than the parent compounds (Curry *et al.*, 1961). These materials must be considered when evaluating the toxicity of phorate and disulfoton. Therefore, it is proposed that the derived no-adverse-effect dosages of these compounds be considered to include their oxidative metabolites as well.

Sensitive methods for analyzing residues of phorate and disulfoton are available. A gas-liquid chromatographic method is available that can detect 0.01 ppm in milk; and a cholinesterase-inhibition method can detect as little as 0.008 ppm in a 5-g crop sample. However, it is clear that the analytic methods available will be barely adequate for the analysis of these materials in drinking water. Particular care will have to be taken to ensure that sample sizes are great enough to allow detection of concentrations as low as 0.0007 ppm.

The most obvious research need for both these compounds is studies on chronic toxicity, including carcinogenicity and teratogenicity. Some of these studies may have been done by the manufacturers; if so, they should be made generally available to assist in the evaluation of toxicology by the scientific community.

There is also a need for corroboration of the no-adverse-effect cholinesterase-inhibition dosage in human subjects in a controlled study with at least two dosages. This would allow the extrapolation of a no-adverse-effect dosage with a higher degree of confidence and a lower uncertainty factor.

MALATHION

Introduction

Malathion, or *S*-1,2-*bis*(ethoxycarbonyl)ethyl-*O,O*-dimethylphosphorodithioate, is a wide spectrum, extensively used organophosphorus insecticide. Agricultural, home, and garden uses of malathion accounted for about two-thirds of the domestic use in 1972. The remaining one-third of malathion use was for industrial, commercial, and governmental purposes. Malathion was one of the earliest organophosphorus compounds to be developed as an insecticide and is registered for use on more than 130 crops against a wide spectrum of insects and mites.

Use of malathion in 1971 is estimated to have been approximately 3.6 million pounds (NAS, 1975). This amount represented approximately 2% of the total insecticide use in the United States that year. This was a smaller amount than reports indicated for 1964 and 1966, when the use was approximately 5 million pounds. It has been estimated that the use of malathion has increased since 1971 (USEPA, 1975e). The total quantity used in agriculture was distributed fairly evenly throughout all geographic regions of the United States, except for the northeastern states, where somewhat smaller amounts were used. The production of malathion involves a two-step process: first, *O,O*-dimethyldithiophosphoric acid is prepared by the reaction of methanol and phosphorus pentasulfide; the acid then reacts with diethylmaleate or diethylfumarate to produce malathion. The currently used process yields 94% malathion. Malathion is soluble in water at approximately 145 ppm at 25°C. The stability of malathion in solution is a function of pH (Spiller, 1961). Its half-life at a pH of 9 is 12, whereas it was hydrolyzed instantaneously at a pH of 12. No hydrolysis took place in 12 days in solutions at a pH of 5–7. Conrad *et al.* (1969) found no degradation in 7 days at a pH of 2, 4, or 6.

In studies of the persistence of malathion in water, it was determined that the half-life in raw river water was less than 1 week, whereas malathion remained stable in distilled water for 3 weeks (Eichelberger and Lichtenberg, 1971). This difference may result from biologic activity in the raw river water. These results are confirmed by studies conducted in Czechoslovakia in which malathion at a concentration of 10 ppm degraded almost completely within 10 days in "environmental water" (Jirk *et al.*, 1971). Lewis and Eddy (1959) applied malathion at 1, 3, and 6 pounds/acre to log ponds in Oregon for the control of mosquito larvae. Under these conditions, malathion was effective for 2.5–6 weeks. In studies in the Virgin Islands, where malathion is extensively used for insect control, only 2 of 49 water samples taken from cisterns contained malathion, and there the concentrations were extremely low. However, a malathion metabolite that was not identified was present in all samples (Lenon *et al.*, 1972). In general, malathion is degraded in water more rapidly than other organophosphorus insecticides under the same conditions. However, the question of the production of metabolites and their persistence in water is largely uninvestigated.

Malathion tolerances ranging from 0.1 to 8 ppm on food crops and as high as 135 ppm on forage crops have been established in the United States for 127 raw agricultural commodities. The tolerances of malathion on most food crops are 8 ppm. The WHO/FAO has established the acceptable daily intake of malathion at 0.02 mg/kg. Market Basket Surveys conducted by the FDA revealed that most of the organophosphorus-insecticide residues in food are malathion. The 4-yr average (1965–1969) malathion concentration was 0.00013 ppm, whereas the total organophosphate residues were 0.00017 ppm (Duggan *et al.*, 1971). The largest residues were present in grain and cereal products. None of the residue concentrations found in the Market Basket Surveys exceeded the acceptable daily intake of malathion.

Metabolism

After ingestion by mammals, malathion is rapidly absorbed from the digestive system. Distribution then is general, and very low concentrations of malathion are found in many tissues. The concentrations in liver and bone are generally somewhat higher than those in other tissues (March *et al.*, 1956).

Malathion is a phosphorodithioate insecticide and thus requires activation to the phosphate, if it is to become an active anticholinesterase agent (Metcalf and March, 1953). It has been shown that the conversion of malathion to malaoxon is a reaction carried out by the liver microsomal monooxygenase system (O'Brien, 1957). Competing with the activation of malathion are enzymes responsible for its degradation to nontoxic metabolites. These are generally characterized as phosphatases and carboxylesterases or aliesterases. Products of reactions catalyzed by these enzymes are malathion monoester, various phosphoric acids, and the demethylated product (Krueger and O'Brien, 1959; Cohen and Murphy, 1972; Cook and Yip, 1958). However, it has been shown that the degradation rate of malaoxon exceeds the activation rate of malathion, so there is generally little accumulation of the toxic activation product in mammalian systems (Dahm *et al.*, 1962).

The toxicity of malathion is potentiated by *O*-ethyl *O*-para-nitrophenyl phenylphosphorothioate, tri-*o*-tolylphosphate, and some other organophosphorus compounds. It is postulated that this potentiation results from the inhibition of carboxylesterase or aliesterase enzymes responsible for degradation of malathion in mammals. Presumably, this mechanism would lead to increased formation of malaoxon, the activation product, because the enzymes responsible for degradation of malaoxon would be inhibited (DuBois, 1972).

Health Aspects

Observations in Man Studies with human volunteers have resulted in the conclusion that up to 16 mg of malathion may be ingested daily for up to 47 days with no significant effect on plasma or red-cell cholinesterase activity. One group of five volunteers was fed 16 mg of malathion daily for 88 days (Rider *et al.*, 1959). During the last 41 days of the treatment, the subjects also received 3 mg of EPN. In a separate study (Moeller and Rider, 1962) 8, 16 and 24 mg/day per person for 47 days yielded the conclusion that the threshold of toxicity appeared to be 24 mg/day. Smaller amounts had no adverse effect in human subjects.

There are many recorded cases of malathion poisoning in humans, including many attempted suicides. These reports lead to the conclusion that relatively large quantities of malathion can be ingested by humans without mortality if proper therapy is applied after ingestion. Subjects who have ingested as much as 60 g have survived. However, as little as 5 g has resulted in mortality in some adults.

Observations in Other Species

Acute Effects The acute oral LD_{50} of malathion is 480–2,100 mg/kg in male and 739–1,000 mg/kg in female rats, depending on the vehicle of administration and the purity of the malathion (Hazleton and Holland, 1953; Frawley *et al.*, 1957; Kimmerle and Lorke, 1968; Gaines, 1969).

Mice appear to be less susceptible to malathion poisoning than rats, with males and females being about equally susceptible. LD_{50} values range between 720 mg/kg for 90% technical malathion and 3,330 mg/kg for 99% pure material (Hazleton and Holland, 1953; Golz and Shaffer, 1956). The acute oral LD_{50} is 570 mg/kg in guinea pigs (Hagan, 1953) and greater than 900 mg/kg in rabbits (Adkins *et al.*, 1955).

Acute toxicity by routes of administration other than oral is also relatively low. In rats, the intraperitoneal LD_{50} is 750 mg/kg (Kimmerle and Lorke, 1968; Brodeur and DuBois 1963), the subcutaneous LD_{50} is 1,000 mg/kg (Spiller, 1961), and the dermal LD_{50} is greater than 4,444 mg/kg (Gaines, 1969). The intraperitoneal LD_{50} of malathion in mice is reported to be 420-474 mg/kg (Hazleton and Holland, 1953) and 815 mg/kg (O'Brien *et al.*, 1958). The intraperitoneal LD_{50} in guinea pigs is 500 mg/kg (Spiller, 1961). The acute intraperitoneal LD_{50} of a 19% solution of malathion in dogs is reported to be 1.51 ml/kg (Guiti and Sadeghi, 1969).

Subchronic and Chronic Effects Subchronic oral toxicity studies of malathion in rats have been conducted for periods of 33 days (Golz and Shaffer, 1956), 8 weeks (Frawley *et al.*, 1957), 5 months (Kalow and Marton, 1961), and 6 months (Holland *et al.*, 1952). Malathion concentrations in these studies ranged from 100 to 5,000 ppm. At no dose in any study was there an evident effect on food intake, weight gain, or growth. At 100 ppm, no effects were observed, even on red-cell cholinesterase activity. In two studies, 500 ppm for 8 weeks also produced no adverse effect on whole-blood cholinesterase activity. At 1,000 ppm and higher, however, red-cell cholinesterase activity was significantly decreased.

Intraperitoneal injection of malathion in rats for 60 days resulted in a no-adverse-effect level of 100 mg/kg without mortality, but dosages of 200 and 300 mg/kg resulted in mortality rates of 60 and 100%, respectively (DuBois *et al.*, 1953).

Other studies on the subchronic toxicity of malathion with other experimental animals did not result in data that could be used to project a no-adverse-effect dosage of malathion or that would be useful in evaluating its toxicity and hazard in drinking-water.

Two studies on the chronic toxicity of malathion in rats have been reported. Hazleton and Holland (1953) fed malathion at 100, 1,000, and 5,000 ppm as the 65% technical material in 25% wettable powder. There was no mortality during the 2-yr test period, and no gross effects were observed at 100 and 1,000 ppm. At 5,000 ppm, food intake and weight gain were reduced. Significant decreases in plasma, red-cell, and brain cholinesterase were observed at 1,000 and 5,000 ppm, but not at 100 ppm. Hazleton and Holland also fed technical 90% malathion as a 25% wettable powder at the same dosages for 2 yr. Growth rate and food intake were not influenced, but a significant decrease in cholinesterase activity was observed at all dosages.

Golz and Shaffer (1956) administered 99% malathion as a 25% wettable powder in the diet of rats at 500, 1,000, 5,000, and 20,000 ppm for 2 yr. A significant decrease in red-cell cholinesterase activity was observed at all dosages. Reductions in growth and food intake were observed at 20,000 ppm. In view of the chronic feeding studies with rats, the WHO/FAO has established the no-effect concentration of malathion at 100 ppm (WHO/FAO, 1965).

Surprisingly, the only other chronic studies of malathion toxicity found in the literature involved chickens. Malathion at 250 and 2,500 ppm in the diet of male and female chickens for 2 yr produced no adverse effect on hatchability. At the higher dosage, plasma cholinesterase activity was decreased (WHO/FAO, 1965). Chickens fed for 15 weeks at 10,000 ppm all died (Frawley *et al.*, 1956).

Mutagenicity No information on the possible mutagenic effects of malathion was found in the literature.

Carcinogenicity No information on the possible oncogenic effects of malathion was found in the literature.

Reproduction In the studies of Kalow and Marton (1961), in which rats were fed malathion at 4,000 ppm in the diet, significant effects on reproduction were observed. The numbers of newborn rats that were alive at 7 days were 105 for controls and 56 for the treated animals. At weaning in 21 days, there were 75 live controls and 34 live treated animals. At 9 weeks after birth the average body weight of the treated group was significantly lower than that of the controls.

When malathion was injected into hen eggs at 25, 100, 200, 300, 400, and 500 ppm in acetone, the hatchability of the eggs was reduced to 85, 87, 62, 71, 42, and 6%, respectively. When malathion in corn oil was injected at 50, 100, and 200 ppm, hatchability was reduced to 84, 9, and

9% (Dunachie and Fletcher, 1969). Studies by other authors have confirmed the reduced hatchability of chicken eggs after malathion injection.

Teratogenicity No teratogenic effects were observed when rats were treated intraperitoneally with malathion at 900 mg/kg. This dosage was determined in preliminary studies to be the highest nonfatal dosage. On day 11 after insemination, pregnant rats were given a single intraperitoneal injection of malathion. No significant difference between treated females and controls relative to dead fetuses per litter, resorptions, average weight of fetuses, average weight of placenta, or fetal malformations were observed (Kimbrough and Gaines, 1968). The authors suggested that feeding studies would have been a more practical and significant approach to the study of teratogenic effects of malathion.

A variety of different studies have been conducted with malathion in the avian egg embryotoxicity assay. When malathion was injected on day 4 at 1 mg/egg, no teratogenic signs were detectable. The length of embryo parts indicated no difference between malathion eggs and controls. Embryonic cholinesterase was also not decreased (Upshall *et al.*, 1968). Roger *et al.* (1969) reported that malathion injected into the egg at 1 mg reduced hatchability to 70%, compared with control hatchability of 95%. Again, there was no indication of teratogenic effects.

Conclusions and Recommendations

Malathion is a widely used organophosphorus insecticide with a wide spectrum of activity and many diverse uses in agricultural, home, and garden applications. It is quite likely that malathion could appear as a contaminant of drinking water, although there are no reports of its having been found as yet. The mode of action of malathion is similar to that of other organophosphorus insecticides—inhibition of acetylcholinesterase. Its acute toxicity, however, is quite low, compared with that of other members of this class of insecticides, primarily because of its facile metabolism in mammalian systems, by carboxylesterase or aliesterase enzymes, to products of decreased or no toxicity. Its toxic potential, however, is illustrated by the possibility of potentiation when degradative enzymes are inhibited by other chemicals.

The chronic-toxicity information available in malathion is surprisingly sparse for a compound that has been so extensively used in the past. However, the two rat studies that have been reported, the subchronic administration of malathion to human volunteers, and the establishment of no-adverse-effect dosages in rats and humans on the basis of anticholinesterase activity allows the establishment of a no-adverse-effect concentration for drinking-water with a high degree of assurance of safety. An ADI was calculated at 0.02 mg/kg/day based on these data. The available toxicity data and calculations of ADI are summarized in Table VI-32.

Additional chronic toxicity data are needed for malathion, with particular concentration on long-term feeding studies in which teratogenicity, mutagenicity, and carcinogenicity are evaluated. Of particular importance would be a good study of the metabolism and persistence of malathion in water. In view of the extent of past use of malathion, continued monitoring for its presence in food materials and water is necessary.

PARATHION AND METHYL PARATHION

Introduction

Parathion, or *(O,O*-diethyl-*O-p*-nitrophenylphosphorothioate, and methyl parathion, or *O,O*-dimethyl-*O-p*-nitrophenylphosphorothioate, are closely related, highly toxic organophosphorus insecticides. Both have a wide spectrum of activity against insects and some mites, and both are registered for use on a large number of crops, including field, forage, and vegetable crops. Essentially all domestic use of both parathion and methyl parathion is in agriculture. Use of these compounds is concentrated in the south-central states, with smaller amounts used in the Southwest and Southeast, and much smaller amounts used in other regions of the country.

The EPA estimates that 51 million pounds of methyl parathion and 14 million pounds of parathion were produced in 1973 in the United States (USEPA, 1975g,h). Domestic use that year is estimated at 40 million pounds of methyl parathion and 10 million pounds of parathion. In 1971, parathion and methyl parathion together accounted for more than 22% of all insecticide used in the United States (NAS, 1975). The current figure is undoubtedly higher, because the prohibition of DDT has changed patterns of use of insecticides.

Parathion and methyl parathion are prepared by the reaction of diethyl or dimethyl phosphorothionochloridate with sodium *p*-nitrophenate. The chemical properties of the resulting insecticides are quite similar. Both are readily oxidized in air to the corresponding oxygen analogue (oxon), which is the toxic form of the material. Hydrolysis of the compounds virtually destroys insecticidal activity. Methyl parathion is hydrolyzed considerably faster than parathion in water (USEPA, 1975h). Parathion is soluble in water at 24 ppm at 25°C, and methyl parathion, at 55–60 ppm at 25°C (USEPA, 1975g,h).

Relatively little information is available on the persistence and fate of parathion and methyl parathion residues in water, especially under field conditions (Paris and Rewis, 1973). In general, parathion has been shown to be 2–3 times more persistent than methyl parathion in natural water systems. Although no specific data are available on the possible bioaccumulation or biomagnification of parathion and methyl parathion, their physical, chemical, and biological properties make it unlikely that these phenomena will occur in food chains or food webs.

The acceptable daily intake of parathion has been established at 0.0005 mg/kg (FAO/WHO, 1968), and of methyl parathion, 0.001 mg/kg (FAO/WHO, 1969). The residues of both compounds that have been found in the various Market Basket Surveys and similar studies have been well below the acceptable daily intakes established by the FAO/WHO. Neither substance has been identified in drinking water in the United States.

Metabolism

The metabolism of both parathion and methyl parathion has been extensively studied in a wide variety of organisms, including microorganisms, plants, insects, and mammals. Both compounds depend on oxidative activation by replacement of the thiono sulfur with oxygen for their toxicity. Competing with this intoxication reaction are hydrolysis reactions that result in detoxification. The ring nitro group can also be reduced, particularly in bovine rumen fluid, to an amino group; this results in amino parathion, whose toxicity is much lower.

These compounds are readily absorbed through the skin of animals exposed to their residues. They are rapidly transported throughout the system after absorption. Oxidative activation takes place primarily in the liver. A number of workers have shown that, in liver microsomal mixed-function oxidase systems, presence of reduced nicotinamide adenine dinucleotide phosphate and oxygen are responsible for this reaction. The conversion of parathion to paraoxon has been demonstrated both *in vivo* and *in vitro*.

Degradative reactions that result in detoxification of parathion and methyl parathion involve either demethylation or dearylation. The resulting desmethyl compounds and dimethyl phosphoric acids are essentially nontoxic. Urinary excretion of *p*-nitrophenol resulting from dearylation has been used as a test for parathion poisoning.

The only tissue accumulation of parathion or methyl parathion that

TABLE VI-32 Toxicity of Malathion

Species	Duration of Study	Dosage Levels and No. of Animals Per Group	Highest No-Adverse-Effect Level or Lowest-Minimal-Effect Level	Effect Measured	Reference
Rat	33 days	0, 100, 1,000, 5,000 ppm in diet	100 ppm (5 mg/kg/day)[d]	Depression of erythrocyte cholinesterase	Golz and Shaffer, 1956
Rat	8 weeks	0, 100, 500 ppm in diet	500 ppm (25 mg/kg/day)[d]	Depression of whole blood cholinesterase	Frawley *et al.*, 1957
Rat	5 months	0, 4,000 ppm in diet	—	Normal growth	Kalow and Marton, 1961
Rat	6 months	0, 1,000 ppm in diet	1,000 ppm (50 mg/kg/day)[d]	No adverse effects	Holland *et al.*, 1952
Rat	60 days	0, 100, 200, 300 mg/kg/day	100 mg/kg/day	No mortality	DuBois *et al.*,

		tech. 65% malathion		cholinesterase	Holland, 1953
Rat	2 yr	0, 100, 1,000, 5,000 ppm of tech. 90% malathion	none	Depression of cholinesterase	Hazleton and Holland, 1953
Rat	2 yr	0, 500, 1,000, 5,000, 20,000 ppm tech. 99% malathion	none	Depression of cholinesterase	Golz and Shaffer, 1956
Man	47 days	0, 8, 16, 24 mg/day	16 mg/day (0.23 mg/kg/day)[a,c]	Depression of cholinesterase	Moeller and Rider, 1962

Using an uncertainty factor of 10, the suggested no-adverse-effect level in drinking water is calculated as follows:

$$\frac{0.23}{10} = 0.023 \text{ mg/kg/day (ADI)}, \; 0.023 \times 70^{a} \times 0.1^{b} = 0.16 \text{ mg/liter}$$

[a]Assume average weight of human adult = 70 kg.
[b]Assume average daily intake of water for man = 2 liters, and that 20 percent of total intake is from water.
[c]Value from which the suggested no-adverse-effect level was calculated.
[d]Assume weight of rat = 0.4 kg and average daily food consumption of rat = 0.02 kg.

has been observed is the irreversible binding to esterase enzymes. The highest concentrations are in the liver and lung.

Health Aspects

Observations in Man The fatal dosage of parathion in man has been estimated at 1.43 mg/kg in one report (DuBois, 1958), and 2 mg/kg in another (Hayes, 1967). No information has been found on the lethal dosage of methyl parathion in man.

There are many literature citations of acute and subacute poisoning of humans by parathion, usually presented as individual case studies of accidental poisoning. Most of these reports do not lend themselves to calculations of LD_{50} or the establishment of no-adverse-effect dosages. There are, however, two studies that allow the establishment of a no-adverse-effect dosage of parathion in man. Edson *et al.* (1964) established that injection at 0.05 mg/kg/day in the diet for 42 days produced no decrease in red-cell cholinesterase; 0.1 mg/kg/day significantly reduced both plasma cholinesterase and red-cell cholinesterase. In another experiment (Rider *et al.*, 1969), prison volunteers were fed parathion at 3.0, 4.5, 6.0, and 7.5 mg/day. Assuming the average weight of a human adult to be 70 kg, these dosages would result in the ingestion of 0.043, 0.064, 0.086, and 0.11 mg/kg/day. At the highest dosage, plasma cholinesterase was decreased in one subject on day 4 and in all subjects by day 16; the decrease was to 28% of the control value. The three lower dosages resulted only in a slight decrease in plasma cholinesterase.

In the same series of studies, methyl parathion at dosages as high as 19 mg/day (0.27 mg/kg/day) for 4 weeks produced no significant change in plasma or red-cell cholinesterase.

Observations in Other Species

Acute Effects Both parathion and methyl parathion are among the most toxic of the organophosphorus insecticides. Acute oral LD_{50} values have been determined for a number of laboratory animals and other species. The oral LD_{50} of parathion ranges between 2 and 30 mg/kg in male and 1.75 to 6 mg/kg in female rats; the mean LD_{50} is 7.6 mg/kg in males and 3.5 mg/kg in females (USEPA, 1975h). Methyl parathion is somewhat less toxic. The oral LD_{50} is 5.8–16 mg/kg in male and 4.5–24 mg/kg in female rats; the means are 11.1 and 16.0 mg/kg (USEPA, 1975g).

The acute oral toxicity of parathion averages 23.0 mg/kg in male mice and 12.7 mg/kg in a mixed population (USEPA, 1975h). The acute oral toxicity of methyl parathion averages 18.5 mg/kg in mice (USEPA, 1975g). LD_{50} values of parathion in other animals are about the same as in rats and mice. LD_{50} values of 9.3–32.0 mg/kg in guinea pigs have been reported. In rabbits, 68 mg/kg has been reported. Toxicity of methyl parathion in guinea pigs and rabbits is lower than that in rats and mice. The LD_{50} is 417 mg/kg in guinea pigs and, according to two reports, 420 and 1,270 mg/kg in rabbits.

The high toxicity of parathion and methyl parathion is also reflected in the LD_{50} values determined by routes other than oral. The intraperitoneal LD_{50} of parathion ranges from 3.6–7 mg/kg in male rats and is 4 mg/kg in female rats. The dermal LD_{50} is about 21 mg/kg in male and 6.8–100 mg/kg in female rats. Inhalation toxicity is 0.0315 mg/liter for 4 h and 0.115 mg/liter for 1 h. The intraperitoneal LD_{50} of methyl parathion is 3.5 mg/kg, the dermal LD_{50} is 67 mg/kg, and inhalation toxicity is 0.2 mg/liter for 1 h in rats. The data reported for other animals for both parathion and methyl parathion are similar to those reported for rats.

Acute poisoning from parathion and methyl parathion is related to their inhibiting action on the enzyme acetylcholinesterase. Toxic manifestations generally occur only after more than 50% of the plasma cholinesterase is inhibited. If an animal survives acute poisoning, it takes about 4 weeks for plasma cholinesterase to return to normal.

Subchronic and Chronic Effects Edson and Noakes (1960) fed diets containing parathion to rats for 15 and 16 weeks, after which the survivors were sacrificed and examined. Feeding at 15.4 mg/kg/day (125 ppm in the diet) resulted in death of three of the 10 rats in the group. No mortality occurred at 2.4 mg/kg/day (25 ppm) or 0.52 mg/kg/day (5 ppm).

Edson *et al.* (1964) determined the no-adverse-effect dosage of parathion in rats to be 0.02 mg/kg/day when the compound was fed over an 84-day period. A minimal effect was found at 0.04 and 0.06 mg/kg/day. The criterion of effect was decreased in plasma cholinesterase activity.

The subchronic toxicity of parathion in dogs was studied by Frawley and Tuyat (1957). Parathion was incorporated into the diet of dogs at 1, 2, and 5 ppm, and animals were fed for 24 weeks. At 1 ppm (average, 0.021 mg/kg/day) a minimal but significant reduction in plasma cholinesterase occurred. At the higher dosages (2 ppm, or 0.047 mg/kg/day; 5 ppm, or 0.117 mg/kg/day), plasma cholinesterase was reduced by 60–70%. Hazleton and Holland (1950) gave 15% parathion wettable powder in gelatin capsules to dogs 6 days/week for 90 days. At 2 mg/kg/day, the dogs lived 3 weeks but exhibited toxic signs continuously. At 1 and 3 mg/kg/day, the animals survived the test period, but were nervous and irritable during the early stages of treatment; later, their behavior seemed normal. No gross pathology was evident, but histopathologic examination after termination of the experiment revealed degenerative changes in the liver.

Subchronic toxicity in other domestic animals has been reported. Oral doses as low as 8 mg/kg/day were lethal to a goat in 11 days. Other subchronic doses resulting in mortality ranged from 12 mg/kg for 5 days to 32 mg/kg for 10 days (Wilber *et al.*, 1955). In sheep, the maximal safe oral dose has been determined to be 10 mg/kg (Radeleff, 1958). In cattle, parathion given by capsule at 0.022 and 0.112 mg/kg/day for 81 days produced no noticeable adverse effects. In another study, 0.11 and 0.89 mg/kg/day had no adverse effects (Dahm *et al.*, 1950).

Subchronic-toxicity studies of methyl parathion are lacking for rats, mice, and guinea pigs. The only report of a subchronic-toxicity study of methyl parathion was reported by the FAO/WHO in 1969. A 12-week feeding study at 5, 20, and 50 ppm was conducted with dogs. Assuming that the dogs weighed 10 kg and consumed 200 g/day, the dosages were 0.1, 0.4, and 1.0 mg/kg/day. Significant decrease in plasma cholinesterase activity was observed at 50 ppm; no significant decrease was observed at 5 ppm; and decrease was questionable at 20 ppm.

Hazleton and Holland (1950) fed male rats for 104 weeks and female rats for 64 weeks parathion at 10, 25, 50, and 100 ppm in the diet. Mortality was 40% in male controls and 33% in female controls. Mortality in the test groups was not higher than that in the controls, even at the highest dosage. At 100 ppm, female rats did exhibit some evidence of toxicity. All females in the control and 10-ppm groups produced living litters. All but one female in the 50-ppm group bore living litters. No other chronic-toxicity studies of parathion or methyl parathion have been reported. A three-generation study of methyl parathion in rats (USEPA, 1975g) at 10 and 30 ppm showed no consistent effect in number of live or dead births, physical structure of newborn, litter size, weanling weights, or percentage survival to weaning. At the higher dosage, there was decreased reproductive performance in some instances. This was not apparent at 10 ppm, which approximates 0.5 mg/kg/day. A comparable study has not been reported for parathion.

A number of studies in avian species have indicated that effects of both parathion and methyl parathion are minimal. Shellenberger *et al.* (1968) reported that egg production in Japanese quail was inhibited and hatchability was reduced by methyl parathion at 60 ppm and parathion at

27 ppm. Mueller and Lochman (1972) fed subtoxic doses of parathion to yearling mallards to observe effects on egg production, fertility, hatchability, shell thickness, and progeny growth. The mallards were fed parathion at 10 ppm in the diet beginning 30 days before egg production and continuing for 90 days afterwards. Parathion had no adverse effect, except a reduction in mean shell thickness. Neill *et al.* (1971) reported a similar study with gray partridge that received parathion at 8 ppm. There was no adverse effect on egg production, fertility, and hatchability.

Mutagenicity The *in vivo* effects of parathion on guinea pig chromosomes have been studied (Dikshith, 1973). Male guinea pigs were given 0.05 mg intertesticularly. The animals were killed after 24 h and examined for chromosomal changes at metaphase. Abnormalities were induced by the treatment, which confirmed that cell division is inhibited by parathion at metaphase.

The effect of methyl parathion on chromosomes of cells *in vivo* was studied with ICR male mice that received intraperitoneal injections (Huang, 1973). Dosage ranged from 5 to 100 mg/kg. Direct toxicity resulted from the two higher dosages, 50 and 100 mg/kg. At the lower dosages, as seen in examination of bone marrow, methyl parathion caused no increase in the incidence of chromosomal aberrations.

Carcinogenicity There are no reports of oncogenic effects in experimental animals of either parathion or methyl parathion in long term feeding studies.

Teratogenicity Methyl parathion has been studied in both rats and mice to ascertain teratogenic effects (Tanimura *et al.*, 1967). Animals received intraperitoneal injections on day 12 (rats) and day 10 (mice) of gestation at dosages approaching the LD_{50}. All animals exhibited some symptoms of toxicity. No significant external or internal malfunctions were observed in rats. However, some embryotoxicity was observed in mice at the highest dosage, 60 mg/kg. Because of this, the FAO/WHO has determined that a higher safety factor is necessary for methyl parathion. Another study (Fish, 1966) gave essentially similar results for methyl parathion and parathion. Some embryotoxicity was observed, but no specific teratogenic effects were noted.

Conclusions and Recommendations

Parathion and methyl parathion are highly toxic organophosphorus insecticides that are widely used in commercial agriculture. Acute

TABLE VI-33 Toxicity of Parathion

Species	Duration of Study	Dosage Levels and No. of Animals Per Group	Highest No-Adverse-Effect Level or Lowest-Minimal-Effect Level	Effect Measured	Reference
Rat	16 weeks	5–125 ppm in diet	125 ppm	mortality	Edison and Noakes, 1960
Rat	84 days		0.02 mg/kg/day	no adverse effect	Edison *et al.*, 1964
Dog	24 weeks	1–5 ppm in diet	1 ppm	cholinesterase depression	Frawley and Fuyat, 1957
Dog	90 weeks	1–3 mg/kg/day, orally	1 mg/kg/day	behavioral effects	Hazleton and Holland, 1950
Man	30–42 days		0.05 mg/kg/day		Edison *et al.*, 1964
			0.043 mg/kg/day[c]	cholinesterase depression	Rider *et al.*, 1969

Using an uncertainty factor of 10, the suggested no-adverse-effect level in drinking water is calculated as follows:

$$\frac{0.043}{10} = 0.0043 \text{ mg/kg/day (ADI)},\ 0.0043 \times 70^{a} \times 0.1^{b} = 0.03 \text{ mg/liter}$$

[a]Assume average weight of human adult = 70 kg.
[b]Assume average daily intake of water for man = 2 liters, and that 20 percent of total intake is from water.
[c]Value from which the suggested no-adverse-effect level was calculated.

toxicity of both compounds is very high, but chronic toxicity does not appear to be a major consideration. The mode of action of these compounds is well known to be inhibition of acetylcholinesterase. Subchronic and chronic studies with the compounds have been primarily concerned, therefore, with measuring the decrease in cholinesterase enzymes as a result of oral treatment or incorporation in the diet of a variety of animals.

An ADI was calculated at 0.0043 mg/kg/day for both parathion and methyl parathion based on human data on parathion. The available toxicity data and calculation of the ADI are summarized in Tables VI-33 and VI-34.

The obvious scarcity of data on the toxicity of methyl parathion indicates a pressing need for research. It appears that the assumption has been made that methyl parathion is toxicologically the same as parathion and that extrapolations have been made from parathion toxicology to methyl parathion. The data on teratogenic effects of methyl parathion, however, indicate that this is not an acceptable procedure in this case. Furthermore, in the last several years, methyl parathion has greatly surpassed parathion in total volume of use, making the need for specific data on methyl parathion even more pressing. The first priority in developing new information must be on the possibility of teratological effects of methyl parathion.

Carbamates

ALDICARB AND METHOMYL

Introduction

Aldicarb [2-methyl-2-(methylthio)propionaldehyde *O*-(methyl carbamoyl)oxime] and methomyl [1-methylthioacetaldhyde *O*-(methyl-carbamoyl)oxime] are two representatives of a class of carbamate insecticides known as "oxime carbamates." These materials are systemic insecticides with high toxicity to mammals. There are only a few registered uses for aldicarb on food crops, including potatoes, peanuts, and sugar beets; most of the use of this compound is on cotton. Methomyl, on the other hand, is a broad spectrum insecticide registered on several agricultural crops and commercially grown ornamental plants, for use primarily against lepidopterous insects on cole crops, tobacco, lettuce, cotton, and tomatoes.

Methomyl accounted for about 1% of the insecticides used by farmers on crops, livestock, and for other purposes in 1971 (NAS, 1975); 1.1

TABLE VI-34 Toxicity of Methyl Parathion

Species	Duration of Study	Dosage Levels and No. of Animals Per Group	Highest No-Adverse-Effect Level or Lowest-Minimal-Effect Level	Effect Measured	Reference
Man	4 weeks		0.27 mg/kg/day	cholinesterase depression	Rider *et al.*, 1969
Dog	12 weeks		0.4 mg/kg/day	cholinesterase depression	FAO/WHO, 1969

[Data are considered inadequate for calculation of ADI.]

million pounds were used on crops. Although the amount of aldicarb used was less than 50,000 lbs in that year, the useage of this compound since then has probably increased. For methomyl, the principal use is in the Pacific states, which accound for over half of the total volume of application, followed by the Southeast, and then scattered use in other parts of the country. Aldicarb is not listed individually in the 1971 report and hence its use pattern is difficult to evaluate. However, it is estimated that most of its use is in the south-central states and the Southwest, where its use on cotton predominates. It is claimed that use of aldicarb has not reached a steady state and is expanding rapidly.

Both aldicarb and methomyl are synthesized by reacting the appropriate oxime with methyl isocyanate. Methomyl is produced by E. I. DuPont under the trademark Lannate and by Shell under the trademark Nudrin (Buchanan, 1971). The solubility of aldicarb in water is 0.6%, while methomyl dissolves to the extent of about 6%. Both compounds are very soluble in most organic solvents and both are quite stable in neutral or slightly acidic solutions. Generally, aldicarb persists in soil between 1 and 15 days. One does not expect to find residues of either aldicarb or methomyl in soil beyond the growing season during which it was applied.

Very little data on the behavior of aldicarb and methomyl in water are available. In a study of pond and lake water, half-lives of 5 days and 6 days were determined for aldicarb and methomyl (Moorefield, 1974).

Tolerances of aldicarb have been established on about 15 food and feed commodities. These tolerances range from 0.01 ppm in meat byproducts to 1 ppm in potatoes and sugar beet tops. Methomyl is registered on a wide variety of forage crops, fruits, vegetables, cotton, and tobacco. Tolerances generally range between 0.1 ppm to 10 ppm. Acceptable daily intake levels have not been established for either aldicarb or methomyl. None of the available data in Market Basket Surveys conducted by the Food and Drug Administration indicate any residues of either aldicarb or methomyl in food. Neither compound is routincly included in the Market Basket analyses, however.

Metabolism

As is the case with most carbamate insecticides, aldicarb is metabolized by both oxidative pathways and hydrolytic processes. Oxidation results in compounds which are also active cholinesterase inhibitors, while hydrolysis produces compounds of little or no insecticidal activity or toxicity to other organisms. Oxidation of aldicarb results in the sulfoxide and sulfone metabolites, both of which are active anticholinesterase agents (Bull *et al.*, 1967). Hydrolytic metabolites found include aldicarb oxime, the sulfoxide oxime, and sulfone oxime, indicating the importance of *N*-demethylation in the metabolism of the compound. Unidentified water-soluble metabolites have also been reported by a number of workers (Andrawes *et al.*, 1967).

Aldicarb is readily absorbed from the gastrointestinal tract of treated animals. Excretion of the radiolabeled compound administered to rats is primarily in the urine, as approximately 80% appears within 24 h, with an additional 1% in the feces. Only traces of the unchanged parent compound were found in the excreta. When aldicarb is labeled on the *N*-methyl carbon or the carbonyl carbon a large portion of the radioactivity is found in the expired air as $^{14}CO_2$ (Ryan, 1971). Very little aldicarb residues are found in the tissues or carcasses of treated animals.

In contrast to aldicarb, the metabolism of methomyl is primarily by the hydrolytic route. The principal metabolites found in the urine following treatment of rats with ^{14}C-labeled methomyl were the oxime-*O*-sulfate, the free oxime, the oxime glucuronide, and a trace of the parent compound. The absorption, excretion, and tissue distribution of methomyl follows a similar pattern to aldicarb. The expired air collected following the administration of methomyl to rats contained labeled CO_2 and acetonitrile (Knaak, 1971).

Health Aspects

Observations in Man In a single dose study three groups of 4 adult males each were given doses of aldicarb of 0.1, 0.05, and 0.025 mg/kg. At the high dose the subjects developed mild cholinergic symptoms. At the other doses there appeared to be a nonstatistically significant cholinesterase depression, although by 6 h after treatment cholinesterase levels in all subjects were normal. Inhibition of cholinesterase by aldicarb appears to be rapidly reversible (Union Carbide Corporation, no date; cited in USEPA, 1975m).

Although aldicarb is an extremely toxic chemical, there have been relatively few cited examples of accidental poisoning. Furthermore, in cases of poisoning, the symptoms appear to be readily reversible and subjects who are poisoned normally recover within a short time, sometimes even a few hours (Sexton, 1966).

Methomyl is a much newer insecticide and there are very few incidents of poisoning in man. There have been reports of occupational exposure poisonings resulting from methomyl when the compound was inhaled by workers in formulating plants. It is difficult, however, to evaluate such poisonings since workers who are occupationally exposed to methomyl are usually exposed to other organophosphorus insecticides as well. There have been no controlled studies of the occurrence of methomyl poisonings.

Observations in Other Species

Acute Effects The acute toxicity of aldicarb is probably the highest of any widely used insecticide. The acute rat oral LD_{50} of aldicarb is reported to be 0.8 mg/kg for males and 0.65 mg/kg for females in studies using the technical-grade compound suspended in peanut oil (Gaines, 1969). In corn oil the LD_{50} to rats was 0.9 mg/kg for males and 1.0 mg/kg for females (Weiden *et al.*, 1965). The dermal toxicity of aldicarb is also high, as values of 3 mg/kg for males and 2.5 mg/kg for females were reported in 24 h exposures of rats (Gaines, 1969).

The acute oral LD_{50} of aldicarb to the mouse was 0.3–0.5 mg/kg (Black *et al.*, 1973). The dermal LD_{50} to rabbits was 4.96 mg/kg in 24 h exposures (Weiden *et al.*, 1965).

The rat oral LD_{50} values for methomyl fall in the range between 15 and 27 mg/kg (Felton, 1968; Neumeyer *et al*, 1969; Ben-Dyke *et al.*, 1970). The LD_{50} values for oral administration of methomyl to mice were 28-49 mg/kg (Felton, 1968). These data were for technical methomyl in an unspecified solvent. The rat dermal LD_{50} of technical methomyl was greater than 1,000 mg/kg (Ben-Dyke *et al.*, 1970).

Subchronic and Chronic Effects Aldicarb was incorporated into the diet of CFE male and female rats in a 93 day study. Doses of 0.5, 0.1, 0.02, and 0 mg/kg/day were used. At the highest dose mortality was increased but not at the other levels. Survivors at all levels did not differ from controls with regard to pathology, organ weight, or plasma, erythrocyte, or brain cholinesterase levels. When aldicarb was fed at 3.2 mg/kg/day, the body weight of males and females was depressed. Both sexes experienced depression of plasma cholinesterase activity, whereas only the males experienced a depression of erythrocyte cholinesterase (Weil and Carpenter, 1969; cited in USEPA, 1975m).

In an effort to ascertain whether tolerance was developed to aldicarb by multiple dosing, cats were treated at 0.5, 1.0, and 1.5 mg/kg with a 7- to 8-day interval between doses. No evidence of tolerance was observed since the LD_{50} values were approximately the same after the third dose as after the first. Similarly, no sensitizing properties were observed for aldicarb when guinea pigs were treated (Carpenter and Smyth, 1965; Pozzani and Kinead, 1968).

No subchronic studies using methomyl were found in the literature. A

2 yr study of aldicarb in the diet of rats using dosage levels of 0, 0.1, 0.05, 0.025, and 0.005 mg/kg was conducted. Twenty males and 20 females were fed at each level. The following criteria of effect were measured: food consumption, mortality, life span, incidence of infection, liver and kidney weight as percentage of body weight, body weight gain, hematocrit, incidence of neoplasms, incidence of pathological lesions, and plasma, brain and erythrocyte cholinesterase levels. In no case did aldicarb-treated animals differ significantly from the controls for any of these parameters (Weil and Carpenter, 1965; cited in USEPA, 1975m).

Weil also reported a 2-yr feeding study in rats. Twenty animals of each sex were fed levels of 0.3 and 0.6 mg/kg/day of aldicarb sulfoxide, 0.6 and 2.4 mg/kg/day of aldicarb sulfone and mixtures of the two. No adverse effects were noted in the positive controls at 0.3 mg/kg/day of aldicarb, but the high dose of the sulfoxide/sulfone mixture caused increased mortality and plasma cholinesterase depression. Some increased mortality was observed in females at the high dose of the sulfoxide. No-adverse-effect levels in the 2-yr study were estimated to be 0.3 mg/kg/day of aldicarb, 0.3 mg/kg/day of aldicarb sulfoxide, 2.4 mg/kg/day of aldicarb sulfone, and 0.6 mg/kg/day of a 1-to-1 mixture of sulfoxide/sulfone (Weil; cited in USEPA, 1975m).

Long-term feeding studies of aldicarb in the diet of beagle dogs have been conducted. Four groups of 6 dogs each, 3 males and 3 females, were dosed at 0, 0.1, 0.05, and 0.025 mg/kg/day day for 2 yr. Criteria of effect included body weight changes, appetite, mortality, histopathology, hematology, biochemistry, and terminal liver and kidney weights. No statistically measurable deleterious effects were found even at the highest dosage rate. The no-adverse-effect level for dogs, therefore, was established as 0.1 mg/kg/day. This is the same as previously established for rats in 2-yr and 90-day studies (Weil and Carpenter, 1966; cited in USEPA, 1975m).

No chronic feeding studies using methomyl have been published.

Mutagenicity The only mention of mutagenicity studies of aldicarb was in connection with the reproduction study reported above in which a dominant lethal test in rats showed no-adverse effects at 0.7 mg/kg (Weil and Carpenter, 1974; cited in USEPA, 1975m). No studies of the mutagenicity of methomyl were found.

Reproduction A three-generation study has been conducted in which aldicarb was incorporated in the diet of a parent generation of rats 84 days before mating and into the diets of the subsequent generations at levels of 0.1 and 0.05 mg/kg/day. When the first generation offspring were 112 days old they were mated and their offspring collected and used as parents of F_3 generation pups. The presence of aldicarb at either dose did not appear to affect the acceptability of the food of any generation. Evaluation of the effect of aldicarb on reproductive performance was made by comparing indices for fertility, gestation, viability, lactation, mean weight of male pups and female pups, micropathology on weanlings of the F_3 generation and on 90-day adults of the F_3 generation. In none of these measures were any statistically significant differences found between treated and control animals at either dose (Weil and Carpenter, 1964; cited in USEPA, 1975m). A later report indicated aldicarb in the diet of rats at dosages up to 0.7 mg/kg/day had no effect on fertility, gestation, and survival (Weil and Carpenter, 1974; cited in USEPA, 1975m).

A three-generation reproduction study of methomyl was conducted in rats. Males and females were fed dietary levels of 50 and 100 ppm methomyl for three months after which the animals were mated. The F_1 generation was continued on the diets for three months after which time they were bred to produce a second generation. The procedure was repeated for a third generation. Each generation was subjected to a complete histopathological examination and various other measures of the possible effect of methomyl on reproductive capacity were evaluated. No adverse effects upon reproduction were found at either feeding level (Busey, 1968).

Teratogenicity In an evaluation of the teratogenic potential of aldicarb in the diet of the rat (Weil and Carpenter, 1966; cited in USEPA, 1975m), no effect was found at dosages of 0, 0.04, 0.02, and 1.0 mg/kg. The highest dose level was close to the oral LD_{50} value but no significant effects were found on fertility, gestation, viability of pups, or lactation. No congenital malformations were found.

In studies using New Zealand white rabbits fed 0, 50, and 100 ppm of methomyl in the diet, no teratogenic effects were found in fetuses and pups after complete evaluations, including skeletal clearing and alizarin staining (Union Carbide Corporation, 1968; cited in USEPA, in preparation).

Carcinogenicity Aldicarb was reported to be noncarcinogenic to mice (Weil and Carpenter, 1966; cited in USEPA, 1975m). C3H/HeJ male mice were painted with 0.125% aldicarb twice per week until the animals died. The incidence of tumors in this very susceptible strain was not significantly different from controls. No studies on the carcinogenicity of methomyl were found.

TABLE VI-35 Toxicity of Aldicarb

Species	Duration of Study	Dosage Levels and No. of Animals Per Group	Highest No-Adverse-Effect Level or Lowest-Minimal-Effect Level	Effect Measured	Reference
Rat	93 days	0–0.5 mg/kg/day	0.1 mg/kg/day	no adverse effects	Weil and Carpenter, 1969
Rat	2 yr	0–0.1 mg/kg/day, 40 animals/group	0.1 mg/kg/day[c]	no adverse effects	Weil and Carpenter, 1965
Dog	2 yr	0–0.1 mg/kg/day, 96 animals/group	0.1 mg/kg/day[c]	no adverse effects	Weil and Carpenter, 1966
Man	7 days	0.025–0.1 mg/kg/day, 4 animals/group	0.05 mg/kg/day	cholinesterase depression	Union Carbide Corp., no date

Using an uncertainty factor of 100, the suggested no-adverse-effect level in drinking water is calculated as follows:

$$\frac{1.1}{100} = 0.001 \text{ mg/kg/day (ADI)}, \quad 0.001 \times 70^{a} \times 0.1^{b} = 0.007 \text{ mg/liter}$$

[a]Assume average weight of human adult = 70 kg.
[b]Assume average daily intake of water for man = 2 liters, and that 20 percent of total intake is from water.
[c]Value from which the suggested no-adverse-effect level was calculated.

Conclusions and Recommendations

Aldicarb and methomyl are highly toxic, oxime-carbamate insecticides with increasing uses on food crops, cotton, and ornamentals. Both compounds act systemically and are readily metabolized and degraded in organisms and in the environment. It is not likely that either compound will appear as a major contaminant of drinking water. The mode of action of these materials is inhibition of acetylcholinesterase. Acute toxicity is quite high, but because of the rapid breakdown of the compounds in organisms and the environment, chronic toxicity is not a major problem.

The chronic toxicity data reported in the literature have not been sufficient as yet for WHO/FAO to establish an acceptable daily intake for either aldicarb or methomyl. An ADI at 0.001 mg/kg/day for aldicarb was calculated based on the available data. The available data on the chronic toxicity of aldicarb and calculations of ADI are summarized in Table VI-35.

In view of the relative paucity of data on the mutagenicity, carcinogenicity, and long-term oral toxicity of Methomyl, estimates of the effects of chronic oral exposure at low levels cannot be made with any confidence. It is recommended that studies to produce such information be conducted before limits in drinkng water can be established. The behavior of either compound in water and the possibility of their appearing in drinking-water is not understood and should be the subject of high-priority research. Effects in humans have not been well-documented and efforts should be made in this direction.

CARBARYL

Introduction

Carbaryl, or 1-naphthyl-*N*-methylcarbamate, is a wide-spectrum carbamate insecticide effective against a variety of insect pests. The first registration was issued in 1959, and more than 1,200 products containing Carbaryl are now registered with the EPA. It is used agriculturally, in homes and gardens, on animals, and in forests. In 1971, 17.8 million pounds of carbaryl were used in the United States (NAS, 1975). This represents 10% of all insecticide used during that year and two-thirds of the total use of carbamate insecticides. The present use of carbaryl is undoubtedly greater, because it is one of the more useful substitutes for DDT.

Carbaryl is prepared in the United States by a commercial process involving the conversion of naphthalene by tetralin oxidation to 1-naphthol. Phosgene is prepared from chlorine and carbon monoxide and reacts with 1-naphthol in toluene solution to produce naphthyl chloroformate, which reacts with methylamine to yield 1-naphthyl-*N*-methylcarbamate, which crystallizes and is separated by centrifugation. The principal contaminant of the commercial process is 2-naphthy-*N*-methylcarbamate. The FAO provisional limit established for this impurity is 0.05%. The tetralin oxidation process produces a material well within this tolerance. This impurity is of concern, because it adversely affects crop flavor and may be cataractogenic (Fitzhugh and Bushka, 1949). Carbaryl is soluble in water at 40 ppm at 30°C. Hydrolysis of carbaryl is slow in neutral solutions. Little is known about the fate of carbaryl in surface water. Laboratory studies with pond water have shown that carbaryl is chemically hydrolyzed very rapidly in pond water to 1-naphthol. Enrichment of the pond water with bacterial isolates enhanced the degradation of carbaryl and 1-naphthol (Hughes, 1971). As would be expected, the persistence of carbaryl in natural water is highly influenced by the pH and temperature of the aquatic environment (Aly and El-Dib, 1971). A study of the persistence of carbaryl in estuarine water and mud in laboratory aquaria revealed approximately 50% disappearance of carbaryl in 38 days at 8°C. Most of the decrease was accounted for by the production of 1-naphthol. At 20°C after 17 days, carbaryl had almost completely disappeared. Hydrolysis was accelerated by increasing temperature and by exposure to sunlight. It is evident from these studies that carbaryl is relatively nonpersistent in water.

Tolerances of carbaryl range from 5 ppm to 12 ppm on a wide variety of food crops and are generally 100 ppm on forage crops. The acceptable daily intake for carbaryl has been established by WHO/FAO at 0.01 mg/kg/day. Market Basket Surveys conducted by the Food and Drug Administration showed declining residues of carbaryl in composite samples from 1964–1970. The maximum level detected would result in a daily intake of 0.0021 mg/kg. Carbaryl was found in 7.4% of the samples in 1964, the year of its maximum detection.

Metabolism

The metabolism and degradation of carbaryl have been studied extensively in microorganisms, plants, insects, and mammalian systems, including cell cultures, *in vitro* preparations, and whole animals. The compound is readily metabolized in most systems. The predominant metabolites are 1-naphthol and its conjugates. Other hydroxylated metabolites are generally found in relatively minor quantities, depending on the plant or animal system investigated and the circumstances under which the tests are conducted. All the metabolites are less toxic to both insects and mammals than carbaryl. In general, metabolism of carbaryl and the appearance of its metabolites in water systems would create no significant hazard in addition to that of carbaryl itself.

Health Aspects

Observations in Man Male volunteers ingested carbaryl in daily doses of 0.06 and 0.13 mg/kg for a period of 6 weeks (Wills *et al.*, 1968). Blood chemistry, urinalysis, stool examination, and electroencephalographic studies showed no substantive changes that were attributed to carbaryl. A slight decrease in ability of the proximal convoluted tubules to reabsorb amino acids was noted in the higher-dose group, but the lower-dose group showed increased absorption, compared with controls. These slight deviations were reversed and absorption became normal after feeding ceased.

A number of studies of occupational exposure to carbaryl have been reported. None of these indicate a great hazard in spray applicators that use carbaryl (Hayes, 1971). Exposure of inhabitants of huts that had been treated with carbaryl resulted in measurable concentrations of 1-naphthol in urine (Vandekar, 1965). The maximal concentrations measured within 24 h after exposure were equivalent to 70% of that found to be the oral no-adverse-effect dosage in dogs. Blood cholinesterase in some of these subjects was decreased by 15% after a week of exposure.

In general, fatal human poisoning from exposure to carbaryl is extremely rare.

Observations in Other Species

Acute Effects The acute toxicity of carbaryl in laboratory animals is moderate. The acute oral LD_{50} of carbaryl suspended in 0.25% agar is 500 mg/kg in male and 610 mg/kg in female rats. The LD_{50} values were about the same when other media were used as a vehicle (Union Carbide Corp., 1957, 1958a; cited in USEPA, 1975l).

Acute toxicity in other animals is about the same as in rats. The acute oral LD_{50} in guinea pigs is 280 mg/kg when administered in 0.25% agar, and in rabbits under the same conditions, 710 mg/kg (Union Carbide Corp., 1957; cited in USEPA, 1975l).

The dermal toxicity of carbaryl is quite low. The dermal LD_{50} of the wettable powder formulation of carbaryl tested on rabbits was reported to be above 2,500 mg/kg (Union Carbide Corp., 1957; cited in USEPA, 1975l).

Intravenous injection of carbaryl in female rats (weight, 90–120 g) as a 5% solution in propylene glycol gave an LD_{50} of 17.8 mg/kg and in male rats, 23.5 mg/kg. Intraperitoneal injection in male rats gave an LD_{50} of 57–180 mg/kg. The intraperitoneal LD_{50} of carbaryl in male albino rabbits was 220 mg/kg (Union Carbide Corp., 1958a; cited in USEPA, 1975l).

Subchronic and Chronic Effects Feeding studies with carbaryl in rats gave a no-adverse-effect dosage of 66 mg/kg/day (Union Carbide Corp., 1956; cited in USEPA, 1975l); this dosage was fed over a 90-day period. In a later study, a dosage of 104 mg/kg/day gave no adverse effect in rats, whereas 167 mg/kg/day reduced growth, increased liver weight, and slightly decreased cholinesterase activity (Union Carbide Corp., 1958b; cited in USEPA, 1975l).

Carbaryl was fed in the diet of rats for 7 days at 50 and 250 mg/kg/day. There was no adverse effect at the lower dosage; the higher dosage reduced growth and decreased plasma, red-cell and brain cholinesterase. After 1 day on a diet free of carbaryl, cholinesterase rose to normal, indicating a high degree of reactivation of the carbamylated enzyme (Union Carbide Corp., 1968; cited in USEPA, 1975l).

In 2-yr feeding studies with rats, the no-adverse-effect dosage was 8.2 mg/kg/day; 18 mg/kg/day reduced growth and caused transient cloudy swelling of kidney tubules and cloudy swelling of central hepatic cords (Union Carbide Corp., 1958b; cited in USEPA, 1975l).

In dogs, no adverse effects were observed during 1 yr of oral administration by capsule 5 days/week at 7.2 mg/kg/day (Union Carbide Corp., 1958c; cited in USEPA, 1975l).

Mutagenicity No studies with mammals as test organisms have been reported to show mutagenicity due to treatment with carbaryl. In this dominant-lethal test, no evidence of mutagenicity was found (Weil *et al.*, 1973). A similar study with ICR-Ha Swiss mice gave similar results (Epstein *et al.*, 1972).

The bacterial systems *Bacillus subtilis* (Degiovanni-Donnelly *et al.*, 1968) and *Escherichia coli* (Ashwood Smith *et al.*, 1972) have been used to assess the mutagenic potential of carbaryl. Both yielded negative results. However, two studies with the fruit fly, *Drosophila melanogaster*, have indicated mutagenicity. A 1% suspension of carbaryl in sugar syrup produced a 0.25% mutation rate within 24 h (Brzheskii, 1972). Inclusion of 1, 5, and 10 ppm in diets gave black and white-eyed flies at all concentrations and more males than females at the medium dosage (Hogue, 1972). However, the relevance of these studies to mammalian mutagenesis is questionable.

Carcinogenicity Carbaryl has been extensively tested for carcinogenicity. All results obtained to date indicate that carbaryl is not a carcinogen.

Tests in A/Jax and C3H mice—strains that are especially susceptible to lung tumors and mammary tumors, respectively—that received subcutaneously injections of 10 mg of carbaryl in 0.25% agar showed no increased incidence of tumors, lung infection, or mortality (Union Carbide Corp., 1958a; cited in USEPA, 1975l). Several 2-yr studies have been conducted with rats and dogs, and an 80-week feeding study with CD-1 mice. In these studies, careful searches were made for tumors, and none attributable to carbaryl were found (Union Carbide Corp., 1958b, 1958c, 1963; cited in USEPA, 1975l).

Similar lifetime-exposure studies with carbaryl have been conducted in CF-E rats (Weil and Carpenter, 1965) and unspecified strains of rats and mice (Carpenter *et al.*, 1961; Weil and Carpenter, 1962; cited in USEPA, 1975l). All these studies culminated in the Bionetics study of 1969 (Innes *et al.*, 1969), in which over 100 pesticides were administered to mice at maximally tolerated dosages. Carbaryl was fed at a daily dose of 4.64 mg/kg for 18 months and was declared to be one of the compounds that did not increase the incidence of tumors. In addition, the Mrak Commission report listed carbaryl as one of only three pesticides that were judged as "not positive for carcinogenicity by appropriate tests in more than one species of test animal."

Reproduction The feeding of carbaryl to rats revealed no effects on reproduction or on growth rate and micropathology of pups. Dosages as high as 200 mg/kg/day were involved in these studies (Union Carbide Corp., 1965; cited in USEPA, 1975l). However, intubation with 100 mg/kg/day did show some decrease in the number of successful matings and the number of pups born alive (Union Carbide Corp., 1972; cited in USEPA, 1975l).

In the three-generation rat study the male rats that received dosages as high as 200 mg/kg/day by either oral intubation or incorporation into the

TABLE VI-36 Toxicity of Carbaryl

Species	Duration of Study	Dosage Levels and No. of Animals Per Group	Highest No-Adverse-Effect Level or Lowest-Minimal-Effect Level	Effect Measured	Reference
Rat	90 days		66 mg/kg/day	plasma cholinesterase depression; liver weight; growth	Union Carbide, 1956; cited in EPA, 1975
Rat	90 days	104, 167 mg/kg/day	104 mg/kg/day 167 mg/kg/day	no adverse effect plasma cholinesterase depression; liver weight; growth	Union Carbide, 1958b; cited in EPA, 1975
Rat	2 yr		8.2 mg/kg/day[c] 18 mg/kg/day	no adverse effect growth; swelling of kidney tubules and central hepatic cords	Union Carbide, 1958; cited in EPA, 1975
Dog	1 yr		7.2 mg/kg/day	no adverse effect	Union Carbide, 1958c; cited in EPA, 1975
Man	6 weeks	0.06, 0.13 mg/kg/day	0.13 mg/kg/day	blood chemistry; kidney function	Wills *et al.*, 1968

Using an uncertainty factor of 100, the suggested no-adverse-effect level in drinking water is calculated as follows:

$$\frac{8.2}{100} = 0.082 \text{ mg/kg/day (ADI)}.\ 0.082 \times 70^{a} \times 0.1^{b} = 0.574 \text{ mg/liter}$$

[a]Assume average weight of human adult = 70 kg.
[b]Assume average daily intake of water for man = 2 liters, and that 20 percent of total intake is from water.
[c]Value from which the suggested no-adverse-effect level was calculated.

diet mated with groups of virgin females. The females were killed midway through their gestation periods to observe the number of viable or dead fetuses and the number of early or late resorption sites (Weil and Carpenter 1965; cited in USEPA, 1975l).

Teratogenicity Teratogenic effects were not found in treated pregnant female rats in various schedules at 20, 100, and 500 mg/kg/day. The highest dosage was very close to the single-dose LD_{50} (Union Carbide Corp., 1965, 1966; cited in USEPA, 1975l).

Pregnant guinea pigs were treated by gastric intubation or by incorporation of carbaryl inthe diet in 64 dosage schedules at 50, 100, 200, and 300 mg/kg/day. No teratogenic effects were found (Union Carbide Corp., 1971; cited in USEPA, 1975l).

The observations of Dougherty *et al.* (1971) of possible reproductive effects of carbaryl in Rhesus monkeys were statistically analyzed (Weil *et al.*, 1972) and shown to be nonsignificant and not dose-related. No teratogenic effects were found at 20 mg/kg/day.

Conclusions and Recommendations

Carbaryl is a moderately toxic carbamate insecticide that is widely used in commercial agriculture and in homes and gardens. It was the first of this group of insecticides to be introduced and is still the most heavily used. The mode of action of carbaryl is inhibition of the acetylcholinesterase, although there is evidence that the inhibition is reversible under some conditions, in contrast with that caused by the organophosphorus insecticides. Hence, chronic studies have been concerned with measuring factors in addition to decrease in cholinesterase activity, to determine a no-adverse-effect dosage.

Long-term studies have been conducted in rats and dogs and have led to the establishment of no-adverse-effect concentrations for these species. In addition, corroborating studies have been done in rats and man for shorter periods. Carbaryl has a known mode of action, adequate chronic-toxicity studies have been done, and there is no evidence of teratogenicity, mutagenicity, or carcinogenicity. An ADI was calculated at 0.082 mg/kg/day based on these data. The available data and calculations of ADI are summarized in Table VI-36.

There are no pressing research needs with respect to carbaryl. Continued monitoring of the presence and amounts of carbaryl in food and water will be necessary.

PESTICIDES: FUNGICIDES

Dithiocarbamates

FERBAM, MANEB, ZINEB, NABAM, THIRAM, AND ZIRAM (AND ETU)

Introduction

Dithiocarbamate pesticides constitute a group of fungicides useful in seed dressing, as soil treatment, and to control numerous plant diseases. The total U.S. production of dithiocarbamate fungicides is around 40 million pounds a year, sufficient for them to rank as a major pesticide group (NAS, 1975). The compounds are salts and coordination complexes of *N*-methyl-, and ethylene-*bis*-dithiocarbamic acids (EBDC). The disulfide oxidation product (Thiram) of dimethyldithiocarbamic acid is a third important type. Dithiocarbamate fungicides are synthesized by reacting a suitable amine (dimethylamine or ethylenediamine) with carbon disulfide under alkaline conditions to yield the alkali salt of the alkyl dithiocarbamic acid. Reacting these water-soluble salts with aqueous solutions of salts of zinc, iron, or manganese results in the precipitation of the corresponding highly insoluble metallo-salts which are the major commercial products (Melnikov, 1971). Alternatively the metallo-salts are produced by reaction of metal oxides with the appropriate amine and carbon disulfide. In addition, certain coordination products are produced such as the ammoniate of zinc EBDC (with EBDC acid and cyclic anhydrosulfide) designated as Polyram and the zincate of manganese EBDC designated as Dithane M-45 (Melnikov, 1971). The EBDC salts and coordination products are relatively low in toxicity; however, the occurrence of ethylenethiourea (ETU) as a major decomposition product of EBDC presents a potential hazard since it is goitrogenic in laboratory animals and may produce thyroid carcinoma.

The zinc (Ziram) and iron (Ferbam) salts of dimethyldithiocarbamic acid are the major *N,N*-dimethyldithiocarbamate fungicides. Both have low solubility in water: Ziram, 65 ppm at 25°C; Ferbam, 120 ppm at 20°C. The compounds are widely used because of their relatively great fungicidal activity, simplicity of production, and low cost.

The zinc (Zineb), manganese (Maneb), and sodium (Nabam) salts of ethylene-*bis*-dithiocarbamic acid are the major ethlene-*bis*-dithiocarbamate (EBDC) fungicides. Amoben (the diammonium salt) and Nabam (the disodium salt) are sometimes used in preparation of Maneb and Zineb at the site of application, because they can be marketed as stable aqueous solutions. Mixing in the spray tank with zinc sulfate or manganese sulfate yields the precipitated Zineb and Maneb. Nabam is also used directly as a fungicide. Polyram (ammoniate of zinc EBDC) and Dithane M-45 (zincate of manganese EBDC) or Mancozeb (zinc complexes of Zineb and Maneb, respectively), and Dithane S-31 (nickel complex of Maneb) are other important market formulations. Except for the sodium and ammonium salts, all are extremely insoluble in water (Zineb, <1 ppm). These products are relatively low in toxicity; however, the occurrence of ethylene thiourea (ETU) as a major decomposition product of EBDC presents a potential hazard since it is goitrogenic in laboratory animals and may produce thyroid carcinoma.

Thiram, or tetramethylthiuramdisulfide, is an oxidation product of dimethyldithiocarbamic acid that has high fungicidal activity and is used particularly as a seed dressing. In addition to its agricultural use, it has important industrial uses, e.g., as a sensitizer in rubber synthesis. It is highly insoluble in water (Melnikov, 1971).

Metabolism

N,N-Dimethyldithiocarbamates The acute toxicity of *N,N*-dimethyldithiocarbamates is low. Oral LD_{50}'s in rats have been reported as: Ziram, 1,400 mg/kg; and Ferbam, $>4{,}000$ mg/kg (Hodge *et al.*, 1956).

When Ferbam labeled with radioactive carbon and sulfur was administered to Charles River male rats, uptake of 40–70% was observed during a 24-h period (Hodgeson *et al.*, 1975). In rats receiving [^{35}S]Ferbam, 22.7, 18.1, and 1.0% of the radioactivity was found in urine, expired air, and bile, respectively. Little sulfur-35 was found in tissues. With [^{14}C]Ferbam, 42.9 and 1.4% of the carbon-14 was found in the urine and the bile, respectively, and only 0.6% was recovered in expired air. The only expired metabolite was carbon disulfide. The metabolites in urine included inorganic sulfate, a dimethylamine salt, and a glucuronide of dimethyldithiocarbamate. With pregnant rats, [^{14}C]Ferbam radioactivity was shown to cross the placenta into the fetus in small but significant amounts. In lactating rats, [^{14}C]Ferbam treatment resulted in radioactivity in the milk, its absorption by the pups, and later excretion in the pups' urine. The authors reasoned that the significant metabolism occurs in the stomach, inasmuch as Ferbam is known to decompose to carbon disulfide and dimethylamine under acidic conditions. Ziram metabolism has apparently been studied only by Ismirova and Marinov (1975) in Bulgaria; although their work cannot be adequately interpreted, the appearance of a substantial part of the [^{35}S]Ziram metabolites as chloroform-soluble material indicates that a similar breakdown to carbon disulfide probably occurs.

Ethylene-bis-dithiocarbamates The acute toxicity of EBDC is low, except for the soluble salts. Nabam and Amoben have an oral LD_{50} of 400 mg/kg in rats (Merck Index, 1968; Melnikov, 1971). In contrast, the LD_{50} of Zineb, Maneb, Polyram, and Dithane M-45 is about 5 g/kg or greater (Melnikov, 1971). The toxic effects observed at very high dosages are probably the result of the metal component.

In animal metabolism studies with [^{14}C]Maneb, Siedler *et al.* (1970) showed that nearly 55% of the administered dose was excreted as the metabolites ethylenediamine, ethylene-*bis*-thiuram monosulfide [ETM], and ethylenethiourea (ETU); metabolite excretion was mainly in the feces. Radiocarbon was cleared rapidly and did not accumulate in tissues.

Health Aspects

Observations in Man No data available.

Observations in Other Species

Acute Effects

N,N-Dimethyldithiocarbamates The rat oral LD_{50} values are 0.1400 mg/kg for Ziram and >4,000 mg/kg for Ferbam (Hodge *et al.*, 1956).

Ethylene-bis-dithiocarbamates The acute toxicity of these fungicides are low except for the soluble salts. Nabam and Amoben have rat oral LD_{50} values of 400 mg/kg (Melnikov, 1971; Merck Index, 1968). In contrast, LD_{50} values for the Zineb, Maneb, Polyram, and Dithane M-45 are on the order of 5 g/kg or greater (Melnikov, 1971). The toxic effects observed at very high dose rates are likely the result of the metal component.

Thiram Thiram is considerably more toxic than most of the preceding dithiocarbamates, except Nabam and Amoben. Gaines (1969) reported oral LD_{50} values of 640 and 620 mg/kg in male and female rats, respectively. Other sources give the oral LD_{50} in rats as 780 mg/kg and in rabbits as 350 mg/kg (Melnikov, 1971; Merck Index, 1968).

Chronic Effects

N,N-Dimethyldithiocarbamates Long-term toxicity studies have indicated that Ziram and Ferbam are not tolerated as well as the acute-toxicity values would indicate.

Hodge *et al.* (1956) observed poor growth and development in rats fed Ferbam and Ziram at 0.25% of the diet. Both Ziram and Ferbam produced similar results, but Ziram was the more toxic when fed at 56 mg/kg to chickens (Rasul *et al.*, 1974).

Melnikov (1971) stated that dogs administered Ziram at 5 mg/kg in the diet for 12 months showed no harmful effects. But reproductive abnormalities have been produced in rats and chickens given approximately 50 mg/kg (Chepinoga *et al.*, 1970), and 10 mg/kg produced no adverse effects (Ryazonava, 1967). In another case, Ziram pretreatment of female rats at 50 mg/kg for 50 days resulted in marked reduction in fertility and litter size, but had no effect on male fertility in mice (Ghezzo *et al.*, 1972).

Ethylene-bis-dithiocarbamates The ethylene-*bis*-dithiocarbamates are generally well tolerated by laboratory animals during long-term administration, but it is difficult to define the threshold for toxic response, because the general presence of ethylenethiouea renders such decisions very difficult. ETU has been identified as a minor component of the commercial ethylene-*bis*-dithiocarbamate formulations (Johnson *et al.*, 1962; Bontoyan *et al.*, 1972) and is also formed metabolically (Seidler *et al.*, 1970) or developed under conditions of environmental degradation (Ludwig *et al.*, 1954; Vonk *et al.*, 1976). ETU is goitrogenic, like thiourea and thiouracil, which are prototypes of antithyroid drugs. ETU concentrates principally in the thyroid, which then undergoes hyperplasia in response to inhibition of thyroxin production and the later continual stimulation by TSH from the pituitary. When groups of male rats were fed ETU at 0.50, 100, 500, and 750 ppm for 1-4 months, effects were obtained at 100 ppm or greater. Body weight and food consumption decreased, the thyroid enlarged, and iodide uptake diminished in those animals. Histologic examinations of thyroid from the rats fed 500 and 750 ppm showed characteristic hyperplasia and adenomas, but sections of thyroid glands from rats fed 50 ppm were not different from the controls (Graham and Hansen, 1972). Weanling rats were fed Maneb or ETU over wide dosage ranges for 60 days, and similar effects were obtained (Sobotka, 1972). The highest dosage of Maneb used (1,500 ppm) contained ETU as a contaminant at a concentration approximating the lowest dietary dosage of ETU used in the study (5 ppm), indicating that the ETU contaminant concentration was insufficient to account for the effects of Maneb on the thyroid. However, the metabolic conversion of ethylene-*bis*-dithiocarbamate to ETU, and perhaps to other antithyroid metabolites, contributes greatly to the thyroid changes.

Mutagenicity No available data.

Carcinogenicity One report attributed carcinogenic action to Ziram after implanting 15 mg subcutaneously; malignant tumors occurred in seven of 20 rats so treated (Andrianova *et al.*, 1970). Because the dimethyldithiocarbamates are tertiary amines, they are candidates for possible nitrosation by reaction with nitrite at a low pH. Eisenbrand *et al.* (1974) demonstrated the formation of dimethylnitrosamine, a known carcinogen, after incubation of Ziram for 15 min in the rat stomach with an excess of nitrate. Ferbam was shown to behave similarly to Ziram during nitrosation. Ethylenethiourea does not arise from the dimethyldithiocarbamates, either as a metabolite or as a decomposition product, so it does not contribute to the toxicology of those fungicides. Hence, the goitrogenic and thyroid tumorigenic propensities of other dithiocarbamates are not associated with Ferbam or Ziram. Hodge *et al.* (1956), however, observed a small incidence of thyroid hyperplasia and tumors in rats given Ziram for 2 yr, but not in those given Ferbam. The authors were cautious in ascribing the hyperplasia to an effect of Ziram. Dogs treated for a year also showed no thyroid pathology (Hodge *et al.*, 1956).

TABLE VI-37 Summary of No-Adverse-Effect Levels Estimated in Rats for Ethylene-bis-dithiocarbamate Fungicides and ETU, with Respect to Thyroid Hyperplasia and Sequelae

Compound	Highest Levels with No Adverse Effect, ppm	Lowest Levels with Minimum Effect, ppm	Reference
Zineb	5,000	10,000	Smith, 1953
Maneb	100	1,000	Haskell Lab, 1957
Maneb	100	1,000	Larson, 1964
Maneb	100	500	Balin, 1969
Dithane M-45	1,000	2,510	Rohm and Haas, 1972
Dithane M-45	100	1,000	Larson, 1964
Dithane M-45	300	1,000	Larson, 1965
ETU	63.1	159	Rohm and Haas, 1972
ETU	50	100	Graham and Hansen, 1972

TABLE VI-38 Summary of Chronic Toxic Levels[a]

Compound	Animal	Highest Levels with No Adverse Effect, ppm	Lowest Level with Minimum Effect, ppm
Zineb	Mice	1,298	—
	Rats	—	500 (thyroid hyperplasia)
	Dogs	2,000	10,000 (thyroid hyperplasia)
Dithane M-45	Rats	100	1,000 (thyroid hyperplasia)
	Dogs	1,000	—
Polyram	Rats	100	—
	Dogs	300	—
Maneb	Mice	158	—
	Rats	25	250 (thyroid hyperplasia)
	Dogs	80	800 (clinical effects)
ETU	Mice	—	646 (hepatoma)
	Rats	—	175 (thyroid carcinoma)
	Rats	—	5 and 25 (increased vascularity of thyroid)
	Rats	—	125 (thyroid hyperplasia)
	Mice	—	215 (hepatoma)
Nabam	Mice	73	—

[a]Taken from USEPA, 1973. *The Toxicology and Environmental Hazards of the Ethylene Bisdithiocarbamate Fungicides and Ethylene Thiourea*, p. 261.

ETU was fed to 2 strains of mice at 215 mg/kg/day for 83 weeks (Innes *et al.*, 1969). Hepatomas developed in both sexes and strains. The production of thyroid carcinoma and hepatoma by ETU constitutes the ultimate effect of long-term ingestion of ethylene-*bis*-dithiocarbamates and ETU (Tables VI-37 and VI-38). Humans occupationally exposed to Thiram have experienced contact dermatitis (Vonk *et al.*, 1970) and ophthalmic disturbances (Sivitskaya, 1974).

Reproduction and Teratogenicity Both Maneb and Zineb were found to be slightly teratogenic in rats given large single doses (1–4 g/kg and 2–8 g/kg respectively; the maximal no-effect was Maneb at 0.5 mg/kg and Zineb at 1 g/kg (Petrova-Vergieva *et al.*, 1973)). Teratogenic effects have been demonstrated with ETU administered to rats and rabbits (K'ra, 1973). Daily doses of 5–80 mg/kg produced dosage-related abnormalities in rats when fed either from before conception to day 15 of pregnancy or from conception to day 15 of pregnancy. Rabbits were less sensitive.

ETU was also found to have a small mutagenic index value (Seiler, 1974).

Thiram is fairly well tolerated in long-term studies, but has been associated with teratogenic effects in mice (Roll, 1971; Matthiaschk, 1973); rats have not been shown to be affected (Khera, 1969). Reproduction abnormalities in rats have been observed, however, that involved disturbed estros cycle and reduced fertility (Davydova, 1973). Cytogenetic and mutagenic effects have been reported by Russian investigators (Kurinnyi *et al.*, 1972).

Immune System Effects Considerable interest has been shown in effects of dithiocarbamates on various aspects of the immune defense systems. Ziram administered in the diet of female rats at 2.5 mg/kg for 9 months resulted in decreased antibody formation, decreased phagocytic activity, and decreased complement activity. Lymphatic blastogenic centers in the spleen were also reduced (Shtenberg *et al.*, 1972).

Both Zineb and Maneb produce effects on the immune system similar to those of dimethyldithiocarbamates, but appear to be somewhat less active than Ziram. Zineb administered to rats and rabbits at 10 mg/kg/day produced no effects, but administration at 100 mg/kg led to reduction in antibody titers and phagocytic activity of leukocytes (Perelygin *et al.*, 1971). Maneb given 5 times a week for 4.5 months at 150 mg/kg resulted in reduced resistance to infection. Chlorine compounds, such as DDT and PCB, are far more active in this respect than Zineb or Maneb (Olefir, 1974).

Carcinogenic Risk Estimates for ETU

ETU has produced hepatomas when given orally to mice (Innes *et al.*, 1969). The available set of dose–response data was considered as described in the risk section in the margin of safety chapter. Each set of dose–response data was used to statistically estimate both the lifetime risk and an upper 95% confidence bound on the lifetime risk at the low dose level. These estimates are of lifetime human risks and have been corrected for species conversion on a dose per surface area basis. The risk estimates are expressed as a probability of cancer after a lifetime consumption of 1 liter of water/day containing Q/ppb of the compound of interest. For example, a risk of $1 \times 10^{-6}\,Q$ implies a lifetime probability of 2×10^{-5} of cancer if 2 liters/day were consumed and the concentration of the carcinogen was 10 ppb (i.e., $Q=10$). This means that at a concentration of 10 ppb during a lifetime of exposure to this compound would be expected to produce one excess case of cancer for every 50,000 persons exposed. If the population of the United States is taken to be 220 million people this translates into 4,400 excess lifetime deaths from cancer or 62.8 per year.

For ETU at a concentration of 1 μg/liter ($Q=1$) the estimated risk for man would be 1.6×10^{-6} Q. The upper 95% estimate of risk at the same concentration would be 2.2×10^{-6} Q.

Conclusions and Recommendations

The dithiocarbamate fungicides are low in acute toxicity and do not present alarming properties during long-term administration to experimental animals, except at very high dosages. An acceptable daily intake has been temporarily set by the FAO/WHO (in 1974) at 0.005 mg/kg for both the dimethyldithiocarbamates (including Thiram) and the ethylene-*bis*-dithiocarbamates (FAO/WHO, 1975). That value represents a fivefold lowering from the previous value used by FAO/WHO for all dithiocarbamate fungicides. That decision was based, for the dimethyldithiocarbamates, on the recent evidence of teratogenic and mutagenic effects, as well as the possibility of nitrosation to form carcinogenic nitrosamines. For the EBDC compounds, the ETU problem and its associated teratogenic, mutagenic, and carcinogenic effects prompted the lowered values.

It could be held that ETU in water should be considered independently as a contaminant separate from the parent compounds. In light of the above and taking into account the carcinogenic risk projections it is suggested that very strict criteria be applied when limits for ETU in drinking water are established.

Based on long-term feeding studies results, ADI's were calculated at 0.005 mg/kg/day for Maneb, Zineb and Dithane M-45; at 0.0125 mg/kg/day for Ziram; and at 0.005 mg/kg/day for Thiram. The toxicity data on these compounds and calculations of ADI's are summarized in Tables VI-37, VI-38, VI-39, and VI-40.

Phthalimides

CAPTAN AND FOLPET

Introduction

Captan, or *N*-trichloromethylthio-4-cyclohexene-1, 2-dicarboximide, and Folpet, or *N*-trichloromethylthiophthalimide, were introduced in 1949 and 1952, respectively, as contact fungicides. Trade names include, for

TABLE VI-39 Toxicity of Ethylenebisdithiocarbamates

Species	Duration of Study	Dosage Levels and No. of Animals Per Group	Highest No-Adverse-Effect Level or Lowest-Minimal-Effect Level	Effect Measured	Reference
Zineb					
Rat	30 days	500–10,000 ppm, 30 animals/group	10,000 ppm	thyroid hyperplasia	Smith *et al.*, 1953
Mouse	18 months	1,298 (464 mg/kg), 18 males, 18 females	1,298 ppm	no effect	Innes *et al.*, 1969
Maneb					
Rat	4 months	100 and 500 mg/kg, daily	500 mg/kg	thyroid hyperplasia, liver degeneration	Balin, 1973
Rat	14 weeks	0–10,000 ppm	1,000 ppm 100 ppm[c,d] (5 mg/kg/day)	thyroid hyperplasia, increased liver/body weight ratios	Haskell Laboratory for Toxicology and Industrial Medicine Report No. 16-57
Rat	90 days	0–10,000 ppm	1,000	thyroid hyperplasia	Larson, 1973

		18 males, 18 females			
Dithane—M-45					
Rat	8 weeks	0–2,510 ppm	2,510 ppm	thyroid weight increase	Rohm and Haas, 1972
			10 ppm	lowered thyroid iodide	Rohm and Haas, 1972
Rat	90 days	0–150 ppm	150 ppm	approx. threshold for thyroid pathology	Larson, 1964
Rat	90 days	0–10,000 ppm	1,000	thyroid hyperplasia	Larson, 1964

Using an uncertainty factor of 1,000, the suggested no-adverse-effect level in drinking water for Maneb and Zineb is calculated as follows:

$$\frac{5}{1000} = 0.005 \text{ mg/kg/day (ADI)},\ 0.005 \times 70^{a} \times 0.1^{b} = 0.035 \text{ mg/liter}$$

[a]Assume average weight of human adult = 70 kg.
[b]Assume average daily intake of water for man = 2 liters, and that 20 percent of total intake is from water.
[c]Value from which the suggested no-adverse-effect level was calculated.
[d]Assume weight of rat = 0.4 kg and average daily food consumption of rat = 0.02 kg.

TABLE VI-40 Toxicity of Ziram and Thiram

Compound and Species	Duration of Study	Highest No-Adverse-Effect Level or Lowest-Minimal-Effect Level	Effect Measured	Reference
Ziram				
Rat	6 months pre-treatment	50 mg/kg	infertility embryotoxicity	Chepinoga *et al.*, 1970
Rat		10 mg/kg	no adverse effect	Ryazanova, 1967
Rat	9 months	2.5 mg/kg	immune suppression	Shtenberg *et al.*, 1972
Rat	2 yr	0.25% 0.25% diet (12.5 mg/kg)[c] 0.025%	neurologic effect no adverse effect no adverse effect	Hodge *et al.*, 1956
Thiram				
Rat	3 generations	100 ppm (5 mg/kg/day)[c,d]	no adverse effect	Khera, 1969
Mouse	days 6–17 of gestation	250 mg/kg	teratologic threshold dosage	Roll, 1971

Using an uncertainty factor of 1000, suggested no-adverse-effect levels for Ziram and Thiram are calculated as follows:

Ziram: $\frac{12.5}{1000} = 0.0125$ mg/kg/day (ADI), $0.0125 \times 70^a \times 0.1^b = 0.088$ mg/liter

Thiram: $\frac{5}{1000} = 0.005$ mg/kg/day (ADI), $0.005 \times 70^a \times 0.1^b = 0.035$ mg/liter

[a]Assume average weight of human adult = 70 kg.
[b]Assume average daily intake of water for man = 2 liters, and that 20 percent of total intake is from water.
[c]Value from which the suggested no-adverse-effect level was calculated.
[d]Assume weight of rat = 0.4 kg and average daily food consumption of rat = 0.02 kg.

Captan: Merpan, Orthocide, Vancide 89, Vanguard K, Flit 406, and Amercide; and for Folpet: Phaltan and Folpan (Spencer, 1973). Domestic production of Captan was estimated at 17 million pounds in 1972 (NAC–NRC Pest Control, 1975); agricultural use of this agent was estimated at 6.5 million pounds in 1971 (vonRumker *et al.*, 1975). Folpet production was estimated to be about 1.4 million pounds in 1974 (USEPA, 1975d).

Captan and Folpet are both broad-spectrum contact fungicides that are effective against a fairly wide range of fungi that cause plant diseases. They act by inhibiting fungal mycelial growth, but do not eradicate established fungal infection (USEPA, 1975b).

Captan is manufactured in a two-step synthesis from tetrahydrophthalimide and perchloromethylmercaptan. The technical product contains about 92% Captan, with sodium chloride, water, and unreacted tetrahydrophthalimide constituting the remainder (USEPA, 1975b). Folpet is synthesized commercially by the reaction of perchloromethylmercaptan with sodium phthalimide in a cold aqueous system. The technical product is 90–95% pure, and the major impurities are unreacted phthalimide (4.5%), water and calcium carbonate (up to 2.5% each), and sulfur (USEPA, 1975d).

Technical Captan is soluble in water at less than 0.5 ppm and soluble in chlorinated solvents to the extent of 1–2%. Folpet is insoluble in water at room temperature and only slightly soluble in organic solvents (Spencer, 1973).

Captan is rapidly degraded in natural soil by chemical as well as biologic means (estimated half-life, days to weeks). It has not been reported to be present in water, air, or nontarget plants (USEPA, 1975b). Folpet is stable when dry, but hydrolyzes slowly in water at room temperature. It has been reported to undergo photodegradation on plant surfaces to phthalic acid, chloride, and inorganic sulfur compounds. In the presence of sulfhdryl compounds, Folpet degrades rapidly to sulfur, phthalimide, and hydrochloric acid (USEPA, 1975d).

Metabolism

Captan is rapidly absorbed from the gastrointestinal tract and rapidly destroyed in the blood. It does not accumulate in the tissues and reacts readily with thiol-containing compounds. The metabolites of Captan in mammalian systems have been indentified as tetrahydrophthalimide (which is further metabolized to 3-hydroxytetrahydrophthalamic acid, tetrahydrophthalimide epoxide, and 4,5-dihydroxytetrahydrophthalimide), chloride ions, thiophosgene, carbonyl sulfide, hydrogen sulfide, and a substituted thiazolidinethione (USEPA, 1975b). Folpet is rapidly absorbed in rats after oral administration. The breakdown products of Folpet are tetrahydrophthalimide and phthalimide (USEPA, 1975d).

Health Aspects

Observations in Man Captan was reported to be the thirty-ninth most frequently cited pesticide (11 cases in 1973) in the EPA Pesticide Accident Surveillance System (PASS), which lists accidents involving humans, animals, and plants (USEPA, 1975b). Folpet was involved in six cases of human poisoning between 1967 and 1975, according to the EPA Pesticide Episode Review System (USEPA, 1975d).

Observations in Other Species

Acute Effect The acute oral LD_{50} of Captan in rats is about 10 g/kg of body weight, and it appears that this agent is also relatively nontoxic after acute oral ingestion in other species, although the data in other species are limited (USEPA, 1975b). Sheep appear to be more susceptible to the acute toxic effects of Captan than rats (Palmer, 1963). There does not appear to be any sex difference in the susceptibility of rats to Captan, but protein-depleted animals are more susceptible to Captan, as well as to other pesticides (Boyd and Krijnen, 1971).

Folpet is also relatively nontoxic to rodents (oral LD_{50}, 10 g/kg), but an intraperitoneal LD_{50} of 40 mg/kg in rats has been reported (USEPA, 1975d). The dermal toxicity of Folpet is also low (greater than 22,600 mg/kg in rabbits), and an inhalation exposure of 14 mg/liter for 1 h killed one of 10 rats.

Subchronic and Chronic Effects Young male rats fed Captan in the diet at various dosages for 100 days exhibited an oral LD_{50} of 916 mg/kg/day, but some survivors had weight loss and inhibited spermatogenesis (Boyd and Carsky, 1971). Weight suppression was also noted in a 13-week study in which rats were fed Captan at a starting dietary dosage of 500 ppm. In this study, the dietary dosage was then increased weekly to reach 5,000 ppm at 4 weeks and 10,000 ppm at 7 weeks (Gray, 1954). The only toxic effect observed in a 2-yr rat study with Captan (Weir, 1956) was weight reduction in the female rats fed the highest dietary dosage (5,000 ppm). There was some weight loss also during the last 16 weeks of this 2-yr study in the female rats fed Captan at 1,000 ppm. Testicular atrophy was observed in 3 of 24 male rats fed Captan in the diet at 10,000 ppm for 54 weeks, and growth decrease in both male and female rats (Weir, 1956). In another 2-yr study, in which rats and mice were fed Captan in the diet at 1,000 and 2,000 ppm, no adverse effects on growth, mortality, or pathology were reported (Reyna *et al.*, 1973).

Weight loss was observed in one-fourth of dogs fed Captan (50 mg/kg/day) for 66 weeks. In this study, four groups of dogs (two males and two females each) were given Captan at 10, 25, and 50 mg/kg/day by capsule (6 days/week). After 10 weeks of exposure, the highest two dosages were increased to 50 and 100 mg/kg/day. At 18 weeks, these dosages were further increased to 100 and 300 mg/kg/day (Fogelman, 1955). Enlarged kidneys and livers were observed in dogs fed Captan at 4,000 ppm for 66 weeks in a study that also included dietary dosages of 400 and 12,000 ppm (Fitzhugh, 1963).

Dystrophic changes were seen in the kidneys, lungs, spleen, stomach, and intestinal tract of rabbits given Captan orally at 500 mg/kg/day for 14 days (Szuperski and Grabarska, 1973). Toxic effects were not seen in monkeys fed Captan at 25 mg/kg/day for 11 days or in pregnant monkeys fed Captan in the diet at 75 mg/kg/day for 14 days (FAO/WHO, 1975). However, fetal mortality was seen at 12.5 mg/kg/day in an 84-day study in which monkeys were fed Captan at 6.35, 12.5, and 25 mg/kg/day (Courtney, 1970). There were no gross lesions or toxic manifestations observed in swine fed Captan-treated corn for 3 months at concentrations equivalent to 540 ppm or in weanling pigs fed diets containing Captan at 420, 840, and 1,680 ppm for 119 days (USEPA, 1975b).

Folpet was fed to rats (10 animals at each dosage) in a 12-week subacute study at 1,000, 2,300 and 10,000 ppm, with no reported effects on behavior, mortality, or gross or microscopic pathology, although there was a significant decrease in weight gain in the animals fed the highest dietary dosage (Weir, 1957). Similar results were obtained in another study in which groups of 30 rats of each sex were fed the same dosages of Folpet in the diet for 17 months (Kay and Calandra, 1961). Male and female dogs were given Folpet daily (5 days/week) at 1, 250, 1,000, and 1,500 mg/kg/day for 17 months. No adverse effects were noted during this study or in dogs sacrificed at the end of 12 and 17 months of exposure (Kay and Calandra, 1961).

Mutagenicity Captan has been shown to be mutagenic in a number of microorganisms and in forward (but not in the reverse) mutation system with the *Neurospora crassa* test organism system (Malling and deSerres, 1970). Sex-linked recessive lethal mutations, translocations, and dominant lethal mutations were not seen in *Drosophila melanogaster*. Captan

TABLE VI-41 Toxicity of Captan

Species	Duration of Study	Dosage Levels and No. of Animals Per Group	Highest No-Adverse-Effect Level or Lowest-Minimal-Effect Level	Effect Measured	Reference
Rat	13 weeks	500–10,000 ppm	10,000 ppm (500 mg/kg/day)	Weight reduction	Gray, 1954
Rat	2 yr	0–2,000 ppm	2,000 ppm (100 mg/kg/day)	no adverse effect	Reyna *et al.*, 1973
Rat	2 yr	0–5,000 ppm	1,000 ppm (50 mg/kg/day)[c,d]	no adverse effect	Weir, 1956
Rat	66 weeks	10,000 ppm, 24 animals	10,000 ppm (500 mg/kg/day)	testicular atrophy	Weir, 1956
Dog	66 weeks	0–300 mg/kg/day, 4 animals/group	300 mg/kg/day	weight loss	Fogelman, 1955
Dog	66 weeks	0–12,000 ppm, 4 animals/group	4,000 ppm (100 mg/kg/day)	enlarged liver	Fitzhugh, 1963
Monkey	14 days	0–75 mg/kg/day	75 mg/kg/day	no toxic effect	FAO/WHO, 1970
Monkey	14 days	0–25 mg/kg/day	12.5 mg/kg/day	fetal mortality	Courtney, 1970
Pig	119 days	0–1,680 ppm	1,680 ppm (108 mg/kg/day)	no adverse effect	FAO/WHO, 1970

Using an uncertainty factor of 1,000, the suggested no-adverse-effect level in drinking water is calculated as follows:

$$\frac{50}{1000} = 0.05 \text{ mg/kg/day (ADI)}, \; 0.05 \times 70^a \times 0.1^b = 0.35 \text{ mg/liter}$$

[a]Assume average weight of human adult = 70 kg.
[b]Assume average daily intake of water for man = 2 liters, and that 20 percent of total intake is from water.
[c]Value from which the suggested no-adverse-effect level was calculated.
[d]Assume weight of rat = 0.4 kg, of dog = 10 kg, and of pig = 60 kg, average daily food consumption of rat = 0.02 kg, of dog = 0.25 kg, and of pig = 2.4 kg.

did not produce dominant lethal mutations when injected intraperitoneally into mice at 3.5 or 7 mg/kg (USEPA, 1975b). Both Captan and Folpet have been reported as positive mutagens in the *Salmonella* test by McCann *et al.* (1975).

Carcinogenicity There was no increase in the number of tumors in mice exposed to Captan or Folpet in a carcinogenesis test in which 18 female and 18 male mice (C57BL/6×AKR) were given the agents by gavage from day 7 to 28 (215 mg/kg) and fed Captan (560 ppm) or Folpet (603 ppm) for the rest of the 17-month exposure period (Innes *et al.*, 1969).

Reproduction Reproductive studies in rats with Captan at dietary dosages of up to 1,000 ppm revealed no damage and no adverse reproductive effects, except for a slightly lowered lactation index in the third generation of the animals fed the diet containing 1,000 ppm (USEPA, 1975b).

Teratogenicity Developmental anomalies were observed after single-dose administration of Captan (750 mg/kg) in pregnant hamsters on day 7 of gestation. No such effects were observed with a dosage of 500 mg/kg (USEPA, 1975b). In a three-generation rat study, the feeding of diets containing Captan at 1,000 ppm did not affect fertility, gestation, viability, or lactation index. Daily doses of Captan decreased sperm motility in rats (6–57 mg/kg/day) and in mice (20–25 mg/kg/day). The injection of Captan at 3–20 ppm into eggs resulted in an incidence of 7–8% malformations in the chick embryos, but later feeding studies in chickens did not reveal any terata (USEPA, 1975b).

Conclusions and Recommendations

Most of the chronic-oral-toxicity data on Captan and Folpet suggest that the no-adverse-effect or toxicologically safe dosage of these agents is about 1,000 ppm (50 mg/kg/day). However, on the basis of fetal mortality observed in monkeys exposed to Captan (12.5 mg/kg/day), the acceptable daily intake of Captan and Folpet has been established at 0.1 mg/kg of body weight by the FAO/WHO (cited in Vettorazzi, 1975).

Based on long-term feeding studies results in rats and dogs, ADI's were calculated at 0.05 mg/kg/day for Captan and 0.16 mg/kg/day for Folpet. The toxicity data calculations of ADI's are summarized in Table VI-41 for Captan and in Table VI-42 for Folpet.

TABLE VI-42 Toxicity of Folpet

Species	Duration of Study	Dosage Levels and No. of Animals Per Group	Highest No-Adverse-Effect Level or Lowest-Minimal-Effect Level	Effect Measured	Reference
Rat	12 weeks	0–10,000 ppm, 20 animals/group	10,000 ppm, (500 mg/kg/day)[d]	weight loss	Weir, 1957
Rat	17 months	0–10,000 ppm	3,200 ppm (160 mg/kg/day)[c,d]	no adverse effect	Weir, 1957
Dog	17 months	0–1,500 mg/kg/day	1,500 mg/kg/day	no adverse effect	Kay and Calandra, 1961
Mouse	17 months	215 mg/kg, 36 animals/group	215 mg/kg/day	no tumors	Innet *et al.*, 1969

Using an uncertainty factor of 1,000, the suggested no-adverse-effect in drinking water is calculated as follows:

$$\frac{160}{1{,}000} = 0.16 \text{ mg/kg/day (ADI)}, \; 0.16 \times 70^{a} \times 0.1^{b} = 1.1 \text{ mg/liter}$$

[a]Assume average weight of human adult = 70 kg.
[b]Assume average daily intake of water for man = 2 liters, and that 20 percent of total intake is from water.
[c]Value from which the suggested no-adverse-effect level was calculated.
[d]Assume weight of rat = 0.4 kg, and average daily food consumption of rat = 0.02 kg.

Other Fungicides

HEXACHLOROBENZENE

Introduction

Hexachlorobenzene (HCB, Anticarie, Perchlorobenzene) was introduced as a cereal and seed treatment in 1945 and is registered in the United States as a fungicide for various cereal, vegetable, and other crops (Thomson, 1975). U.S. production for pest control is estimated at only 700,000 pounds (NAS, 1975), but HCB is encountered in much larger quantities as an intermediate or waste by-product in various chemical syntheses, including that of pentachlorophenol, and as a contaminant of other pesticides, such as technical pentachloronitrobenzene (Borzelleca *et al.*, 1971) and DCPA (Kimbrough and Linder, 1974). HCB has also been identified as a prominent constituent of the air collected in the vicinity of a plant manufacturing perchloroethylene (Mann *et al.*, 1974).

HCB is produced commercially by exhaustive chlorination of benzene in the presence of a catalyst (Spencer, 1973). Analysis of three commercial HCB preparations showed that they contained pentachlorobenzene at 100-81,000 ppm (0.02-3.1%), octachlorodibenzo-*p*-dioxin at 0.05–212 ppm, and octachlorodibenzofuran (octa-CDF) at 0.35–58.3 ppm (Villanueva *et al.*, 1974). HCB has a very low solubility in water: only 6 ppb (Lu and Metcalf, 1975).

HCB is extremely lipophilic and resistant toward degradation. It has been identified in the tissues of marine birds (Gilbertson and Reynolds, 1972), predatory birds (Cromartie *et al.*, 1975; Vos *et al.*, 1968), and starlings (Nickerson and Barbehann, 1975); surface-water (Herzel, 1972), freshwater (Johnson *et al.*, 1974), and marine (Zitko, 1971) fish; and other aquatic organisms (Koeman *et al.*, 1969). HCB residues in edible freshwater fish reached 0.34 ppm, and in one case carp contained 62 ppm (Johnson *et al.*, 1974). Marine fish oils contained 0.06-0.38 ppm.

HCB residues have also been found in human adipose tissue and blood from different parts of the world (Abbott *et al.*, 1972; Acker and Schutle, 1970; Brady and Ciyali, 1972; Burns and Miller, 1975; Curley *et al.*, 1973; Siyali, 1972), in human milk (Graca *et al.*, 1974; Stacey and Thomas, 1975), and in food products (Manske and Corneliussen, 1974; Manske and Johnson, 1975; Smyth, 1972). The EPA established interim HCB tolerances of 0.5 ppm in the fat of cattle and other domestic animals and 0.3 ppm in fat or milk and other dairy products.

HCB has been detected at 0.010 ppb in raw and 0.006 ppb in finished U.S. drinking water (USEPA, 1975j).

Metabolism

In studies on the fate of [^{14}C]HCB in rats after intravenous administration, only 0.7 and 0.1% of the dose was recovered in feces and urine, respectively, over a 48-h period, and there was no conversion of the labeled HCB to [^{14}C]carbon monoxide or other volatile radioactive metabolites (Yang and Pittman, 1975). Fat contained the highest radioactivity.

Seven days after a single 5-mg/kg oral dose of [^{14}C]HCB in adult male rats, approximately 16% of the dose had been excreted in the feces and less than 1% in the urine (Mehendale *et al.*, 1975); 70% of the dose remained in the animal, with fat as the major depot. Metabolites in the urine included pentachlorobenzene, tetrachlorobenzene, pentachlorophenol, and four unknown compounds. The half-life of HCB in rats was found to be about 60 days (Morita and Ioshi, 1975). Storage of dieldrin in the adipose tissue of rats is markedly decreased by HCB in the diet (Avrahami and Gernert, 1972).

In studies with rhesus monkeys, 17.1 and 1.8% of an intravenous dose of [^{14}C]HCB was excreted in feces and urine, respectively, over a period of 100 days (Yang and Pittman, 1975). As in rats, fat retained the highest amount of radioactivity.

In another study (Villeneuve, 1975), adult male Sprague–Dawley rats received HCB at 1, 10, and 100 mg/kg for 14 days and the tissues were then analyzed for HCB. Two other groups, after 14 days of HCB feeding, were either fed an HCB-free diet *ad libitum* for 10 days or fed 25% of their normal food intake over the same period. HCB concentrations in tissues were fat $>$ liver $>$ lungs $>$ kidneys $>$ brain $>$ spleen $>$ heart $>$ muscle $>$ plasma. No appreciable losses of HCB occurred in the tissues over a 10-day period in the animals placed on a diet free of HCB. Animals fed restricted quantities of the HCB-free diet, however, showed a mobilization of HCB stored within fat depots, which resulted in transfer of the compound into plasma and other tissues. Death occurred in the animals when brain HCB concentration exceeded 300 ppm.

Koss *et al.* (1975, 1976) have recently studied the pharmacokinetics and metabolism of HCB in rats.

In vitro conversion of HCB to pentachlorophenol has been demonstrated in rat liver microsomal preparations (Lui and Sweeney, 1975), and a dechlorination system requiring reduced nicotinamide adenine dinucleotide phosphate in the liver and other tissues was found by Mehendale *et al.* (1975).

HCB crosses the placenta and accumulates in the fetus in a dose-dependent manner (Andrews and Courtney, 1976; Courtney *et al.*, 1976; Villeneuve *et al.*, 1974; Villeneuve and Hierlihy, 1975). In rats, the maternal liver had the highest HCB residue, followed by fetal liver, whole fetus, and fetal brain (Villeneuve and Hierlihy, 1975). This is in contrast with the results in rabbits, in which fetal liver contains HCB at concentrations 2–4 times higher than maternal liver.

Health Aspects

Observations in Man In the period 1955-1959, an outbreak of human poisoning occurred in Turkey as a result of the consumption of HCB-treated wheat (Cam and Nigogosyan, 1963; DeMatteis *et al.*, 1961; Schmid, 1960). Some deaths resulted, but the major syndrome was cutaneous porphyria, with skin lesions, porphyrinuria, and photosensitization. The estimated dosage was approximately 50–200 mg/day (0.71–2.9 mg/kg/day) for presumably long periods before toxic manifestations became apparent (Cam and Nigogosyan, 1963; Schmid, 1960).

Observations in Other Species

Acute Effects The acute toxicity of HCB is relatively low, as evidenced by oral LD_{50} values of 3,500 mg/kg in rats, 2,600 mg/kg in rabbits, and 1,700 mg/kg in cats (Christensen *et al.*, 1974). In another report (Spencer, 1973), the acute oral LD_{50} in rats was given as 10,000 mg/kg.

Subchronic and Chronic Effects HCB is considerably more toxic on prolonged exposure. Mortalities and severe weight loss occurred among Wistar rats and guinea pigs receiving daily 500 mg/kg oral doses of pure HCB over a period of 9–16 days (Villeneuve and Newsome, 1975). In a study by Hazelton Laboratories (USEPA, 1973c), rats were fed HCB at 5, 25, 125, and 625 ppm for 13 weeks. At 125 ppm, liver:body weight ratios were increased, and there were pathologic effects on the liver. No adverse effects were noted in animals fed 5 and 25 ppm.

In a study by Dow Chemical Company, gross and histopathologic alterations occurred in the livers of female weanling rats fed HCB at 30, 65, and 100 mg/kg/day for 30 days (USEPA, 1973c). No adverse changes were observed in rats fed 1, 3, or 10 mg/kg/day. In a second study by the same group, rats fed 20 mg/kg/day for 13 days developed neurotoxic symptoms and increased liver:body weight ratios; at 6 mg/kg/day, there was only slight skin twitching and nervousness, but a significant increase in liver:body weight ratio; no toxic effect was seen at 2 mg/kg/day.

Rats and rabbits fed HCB at 5,000 ppm in the diet died in 8–12 weeks, after showing severe neurologic symptoms (DeMatteis *et al.*, 1961). There was a substantial increase in urinary porphyrin excretion after about 6 weeks; at death, there was substantial tissue porphyrin deposition in the animals. Guinea pigs and mice were much more susceptible to HCB; animals fed 5,000 ppm died after 8–10 days with marked neurologic signs. Before death, the latter animals developed moderate to severe porphyria.

Male and female Charles River rats received diets containing HCB at 0.5, 2.0, 8.0, and 32.0 mg/kg/day over a period of 12 weeks (Kuiper-Goodman *et al.*, 1975a). Female rats were more sensitive than males to the toxic effects of HCB: 26% of the females and none of the males died at the highest dosage. Females also developed more severe porphyria, with high porphyrin concentrations in the liver. Males at the two highest dosages showed a siginificant increase in liver weight, and this was correlated with increased hepatic mixed-function oxidase activity and increases in the smooth endoplasmic reticulum. Additional information (Kuiper-Goodman *et al.*, 1975b), presumably on the same study, indicated that tissue HCB residues had reached a plateau before 104 days. Tissue HCB concentrations were highest in adipose tissue, after which the order was liver > brain > serum. At the two highest dosages—8 and 32 mg/kg/day—liver:body weight ratios were increased in both sexes. Pathologic examination showed increased hepatocyte size due to proliferation of smooth endoplasmic reticulum. This was correlated with increased activities of drug-metabolizing enzymes, which persisted long after animals were placed on an HCB-free diet. Females developed porphyria, which persisted after the rats were removed from the HCB diets.

Chronic ingestion of HCB at 2,000 ppm in the diet of adult male Sprague–Dawley rats resulted in hepatocellular degeneration and increases in the amounts of porphyrin and porphyrin precursors in the liver and excreta (Ocker and Schmid, 1961).

Male and female Sprague–Dawley rats were fed diets containing HCB at 10, 20, 40, 80, and 160 ppm for 9 or 10 months (Grant *et al.*, 1974). Porphyria developed in rats fed 40 ppm and above, and the prophyria was much more severe in females than in males. Weight gains were reduced in female rats fed 80 and 160 ppm. Rats of both sexes showed increased liver:body weight ratios after receiving 80 or 160 ppm. Hepatic mixed-function oxidase activity was increased in male rats fed 40 ppm or more, but was unaltered in females. The pharmacologic activities of pentobarbital and zoxazolamine, however, were shortened in rats of both sexes fed 20 ppm or above. HCB residues in liver were similar in males and females and were dose-dependent.

Groups of weanling Sherman rats were fed technical HCB at 100, 500, and 1,000 ppm for a 4-month period (Kimbrough and Linder, 1974). No rats died in the control and 100-ppm groups, 2 of 10 males and 14 of 20 females died at 500 ppm, and 3 of 10 males and 19 of 20 females died at 1,000 ppm. Increased ratios of liver, spleen, adrenal, lung, and kidney weights to body weights were found in weanling Sherman rats fed 500 and 1,000 ppm. Hyperplasia of the adrenal cortex and lung degeneration were observed in all HCB-fed groups, particularly in females. Pathologic effects on liver and heart were found in rats receiving 500 ppm and above, with females showing the most severe effects. Hemoglobin and hematocrit values were significantly decreased in females fed 100 ppm or more and in males fed 1,000 ppm.

Mixed-Function Oxidase Activity and Porphyria HCB has been shown to be associated with the production of porphyria in humans and experimental animals (Cam and Nigogosyan, 1963; DeMatteis *et al.*, 1961; Ocker and Schmid, 1961). In HCB-treated animals, there are substantial increases in liver weight, in smooth endoplasmic reticulum, in mixed-function oxidase activity, and in cytochrome P-450 content (Carlson and Tardiff, 1975; Grant *et al.*, 1974; Kuiper-Goodman *et al.*, 1975a,b; Turner and Green, 1974; Wade *et al.*, 1968). It is noteworthy that HCB apparently induces primarily the hepatic cytochrome P1-450 system, rather than the P-450 system (Turner and Green, 1974).

Porphyria resulting from ingestion of HCB is much more severe in female than in male animals (Grant *et al.*, 1974). HCB is known to induce increased activity of mitochondrial 5-aminolevulinic acid (ALA) synthetase (Myakoshi and Kikuchi, 1963). The HCB-induced porphyria, however, is not simply related to an increase in ALA synthetase activity, inasmuch as a twofold increase in the activity of that enzyme (the rate-limiting step in heme synthesis) cannot explain the observed massive increase in porphyrins in HCB-treated animals (Wada *et al.*, 1968). Moreover, although hemin normally exerts a feedback function to suppress ALA synthetase activity, HCB porphyria cannot be suppressed by hemin (Strik, 1973).

Recent evidence (Sweeney, 1976) suggests that a contaminant of technical HCB may be more active than HCB in producing porphyria in experimental animals. Porphyria develops in mice fed technical HCB at 1,000 ppm in about 6 weeks. To produce the same degree of porphyria in 6 weeks in mice with pure HCB, it was necessary to feed 2,500 ppm. Sweeney also presented preliminary evidence that HCB is actually converted by mixed-function oxidase systems in the liver to a reactive metabolite that then covalently binds to tissue macromolecules and that this produces the porphyria.

Mutagenicity For dominant-lethal tests, 4 groups of 15 male Wistar rats each were given HCB orally at 20, 40, or 60 mg/kg for 10 consecutive days (Khera, 1974). After mating trials, there were no significant differences between test and control groups.

Carcinogenicity HCB is currently being tested for carcinogenicity (IARC, 1974, 1975).

Reproduction HCB at dietary concentrations of 10, 20, 40, 80, 160, 320, and 640 ppm was fed to Sprague–Dawley rats, and four generations of rats were raised (Grant *et al.*, 1975). The two highest dietary concentrations were toxic to the F_0 generation, and 50 and 20%, respectively, of the females died. The viability index was zero in the F_1a and F_1b generations for rats fed 320 and 640 ppm and only 55% for the 160-ppm group. The lactation index decreased from 30% for the F_1a and F_1b generation pups to 0% for the F_2a and F_2b generation pups in the 160-ppm group, from 93% in the F_1a generation to 40% in the F_3b generation in the 80-ppm group.

Teratogenicity No gross abnormalities were present in rat pups, but weight gain was affected by HCB treatment.

Teratogenic studies were carried out in Wistar rats given HCB in single daily doses of 10, 20, 40, 60, 80, or 120 mg/kg on days 6–9, 10–13, 6–16, or 6–21 of gestation (Khera, 1974). The 80- and 120-mg/kg doses caused maternal neurotoxicity and a reduction in fetal weight. In the fetuses, the incidence of unilateral and bilateral fourteenth rib was significantly increased over control values when doses of 20 mg/kg/day or more were administered on days 10–13, 6–16, or 6–21 of gestation. Sternal defects in the fetus were observed after 20 mg/kg/day on days 6-21 of gestation. Because these effects were not reproduced in later trials at up to 80 mg/kg given during the period of organogenesis, however, the teratogenic potential of HCB in the rat is doubtful. Oral administration of pure HCB at 100 mg/kg to CD-1 mice on days 7–16 of gestation, however, produced cleft palates and some kidney malformations (Courtney *et al.*, 1976).

Conclusions and Recommendations

The acute toxicity of HCB is relatively low, but subchronic or chronic exposure of laboratory animals or humans to HCB results in the development of severe porphyria, especially in females. An ADI was calculated at 0.001 mg/kg/day based on a 10-month feeding study in rats. The toxicity data and calculations of ADI are summarized in Table VI-

43. A conditional acceptable daily intake of 0.0006 mg/kg/day was derived by the FAO/WHO as the upper limit for residues. The FAO/WHO suggested extreme caution with the compound and indicated that available information is insufficient to establish a firm acceptable intake for HCB.

HCB can be readily determined by electron capture gas chromatography at concentrations as low as 0.0001 ppb.

There are a number of puzzling differences in the highest no-effect and lowest minimal-toxic-effect dosages found for HCB in rats (Table VI-43). These differences may be the results of using different rat strains or different HCB formulations in the various studies. They may also result from the use of HCB of uncertain purity. The source of the observed variations should be established. No subchronic- or chronic-toxicity studies have been conducted with HCB in mammalian species other than rats. It is especially important to conduct 2-yr feeding experiments and carcinogenicity studies with HCB in two species, because HCB has been found to be extremely toxic on long-term exposure and is on the list of suspected carcinogens.

PENTACHLORONITROBENZENE

Introduction

Pentachloronitrobenzene (PCNB, quintozene, terrachlor) was introduced in the United States in 1955 and is currently registered in this country as a soil fungicide treatment (USEPA, 1976a). The 1971 production by the single U.S. manufacturer was estimated at 3 million pounds (USEPA, 1976a; Lawless *et al.*, 1972), 60–70% of which was consumed domestically. A 40–50% increase in production capacity has just been completed (USEPA, 1976a).

PCNB is produced commercially by exhaustive chlorination of nitrobenzene (USEPA, 1976a). Technical-grade PCNB contains an average of 97.8% PCNB, 1.8% hexachlorobenzene (HCB), 0.4% 2,3,4,5-tetrachloronitrobenzene (TCNB), and less than 0.1% pentachlorobenzene (Borzelleca *et al.*, 1971). PCNB is only slightly soluble in water (0.44 mg/liter at 20°C).

FDA residue studies from 1964–1969 found PCNB residues in 0.7% of the leaf and stem vegetables sampled (USEPA, 1976a). Residues ranged from less than 0.005–0.42 ppm, with an average of 0.01 ppm. A tolerance of 0.1 ppm has been established for a number of vegetable and other crops, except peanuts, for which it is 1.0 ppm.

TABLE VI-43 Toxicity of HCB

Species	Duration of Study	Dosage Levels and No. of Animals Per Group	Highest No-Adverse-Effect Level or Lowest-Minimal-Effect Level	Effect Measured	Reference
Quail	90 days	0–80 ppm in diet, 15 animals/group	1 ppm (0.14 mg/kg/day)[d]	no toxic effect	Vos *et al.*, 1971
Rat	9–10 months	0–160 ppm in diet, 12 animals/group	20 ppm (1 mg/kg/day)[c,d]	reduced sleeping time	Grant *et al.*, 1974
Rat	13 weeks	0–625 ppm in diet	25 ppm (1.25 mg/kg/day)[d]	no toxic effect	EPA, 1973c
Rat	13 weeks	0–200 mg/kg/day orally, 5 animals/group	2 mg/kg/day	no toxic effect	EPA, 1973c
Rat	12 weeks	0–32 mg/kg/day orally, 140 animals/group	2 mg/kg/day	no toxic effect	Kuiper-Goodman *et al.*, 1975a, 1975b
Rat	4 months	0–1,000 ppm in diet, 30 animals/group	100 ppm (5 mg/kg/day)[d]	adrenal hyperplasia and hematologic effects	Kimbrough and Linder, 1974
Rat	30 days	0–100 mg/kg/day	100 mg/kg/day	no toxic effect	EPA, 1973c

Using an uncertainty factor of 1,000, the suggested no-adverse-effect level in drinking water is calculated as follows:

$$\frac{1}{1{,}000} = 0.001 \text{ mg/kg/day (ADI)}, \; 0.001 \times 70^{a} \times 0.1^{b} = 0.007 \text{ mg/liter}$$

[a]Assume average weight of human adult = 70 kg.
[b]Assume average daily intake of water for man = 2 liters, and that 20 percent of total intake is from water.
[c]Value from which the suggested no-adverse-effect level was calculated.
[d]Assume weight of rat = 0.4 kg and average daily food consumption of rat = 0.02 kg.

Metabolism

After oral administration of PCNB to rabbits, 62% of the dose was found unchanged in the feces, 12% was excreted as pentachloroaniline (PCA), and 14% was excreted as *N*-acetyl-5-pentachlorophenylcystine (Betts *et al.*, 1955).

After feeding of technical PCNB for 33 weeks to rats (at up to 500 ppm) and for 2 yr to beagles (at up to 1,080 ppm), no PCNB was found in the tissues, but trace amounts of PCA and methylpentachlorophenylsulfide (MPCPS) were detected in various tissues and fat (Borzelleca *et al.*, 1971). In rats fed PCNB at 500 ppm, the impurity HCB was detected in the greatest quantities, with 29.7, 1.93, and 6.43 ppm in muscle, liver, and kidneys, respectively. HCB was also the major residue found in dogs, with 6.41, 9.48, 7.28, 7.57, 0.65, and 1.37 ppm in kidneys, brain, muscle, liver, fat, and blood of animals fed PCNB at 1,080 ppm. The impurity pentachlorobenzene also was detected, at lower concentrations, in the tissues of the PCNB-fed animals.

No PCNB was found in the body fat of rats fed diets containing PCNB at 50 or 500 ppm for 7 months (Kuchar *et al.*, 1969). Only trace amounts of pentachlorobenzene were found, but HCB appeared at 117 ppm in the fat of rats fed PCNB at 500 ppm. Small amounts of PCA and MPCPS were also detected in the body fat.

PCNB was not detected in maternal tissues or 22-day-old fetuses after daily oral administration of doses of 50, 100, and 200 mg/kg to rats on days 6–15 of gestation (Villeneuve and Khen, 1975). Similar doses of pentachlorobenzene, however, accumulated to an appreciable extent in both maternal and fetal tissues.

In mice, four daily oral doses of PCNB (500 mg/kg) led to the appearance of PCA and MPCPS metabolites in fatty tissue of pregnant mice and fetuses; this insicated transplacental passage of these metabolites (Courtney, 1973; Courtney *et al.*, 1976). PCNB was found mainly in the maternal tissues.

In dogs fed a diet containing PCNB at 5 or 1,080 ppm for 2 yr, no PCNB was detected in muscle, kidneys, fat, or liver, and only trace amounts in the urine at 1,080 ppm (Kucher *et al.*, 1969). PCNB was present in the feces at both dosages. Pentachlorobenzene and HCB were detected in all samples. The PCNB metabolites PCA and MPCPS were detected in various fractions at both dietary PCNB dosages.

The present evidence from metabolic studies indicates that PCNB is rapidly metabolized to 2 major metabolites (PCA and MPCPS) and 2 minor ones (TCNB and pentachlorothiophenol). Two impurities of technical PCNB, HCB and pentachlorobenzene, also are commonly found in tissue, urine, and feces. The major excretary route of PCNB and its metabolites is via the bile, and tissue retention is concentrated in body fat and to a lesser extent in muscle.

Health Aspects

Observations in Man No available data.

Observations in Other Species

Acute Effects PCNB is a relatively nontoxic pesticide. Oral LD_{50} values of 1,200 and 1,650 mg/kg were found in rats for unspecified PCNB dosages and formulations (Christensen *et al.*, 1974). Technical PCNB dissolved in corn oil yielded oral LD_{50} values of 1,710 and 1,650 mg/kg in male and female rats, respectively (FAO/WHO, 1970) and 1,743 mg/kg in male rats (Borzelleca *et al.*, 1971). The oral LD_{50} of PCNB in dogs is greater than 2,400 mg/kg (Finnegan *et al.*, 1958).

Subchronic and Chronic Effects Male and female weanling albino rats were fed diets containing PCNB for a period of 3 months (Finnegan *et al.*, 1958). The male rats showed significant loss of body weight at 2,400 ppm, and the females showed a slight weight loss at 5,000 ppm. There was a significant increase in the liver:body weight ratios at 63.5 ppm and above in the males, but only at 635 ppm and above in the females. The kidney:body weight ratios showed a significant increase in the male rats at 1,250 ppm, but no significant changes in the females.

In a chronic-toxicity study with rats, diets containing PCNB at 25, 100, 300, 1,000, or 2,500 ppm in a commercial powder (20% PCNB; 77% Pyrax ABB, a pyrophyllite carrier; and 3% Armour Sticker, an adherence aid) were fed over a 2-yr period (Finnegan *et al.*, 1958). Deaths during the 2-yr study, however, did not correlate with dietary concentrations of the fungicide. Female rats showed a slight growth suppression at 100 ppm PCNB and above, but no toxic effect at 25 ppm. The fungicide was a growth stimulant for males, especially at 300 ppm. No significant histopathologic or hematologic changes were observed at any dosage.

The same PCNB formulation was fed to mongrel dogs over a 1-yr period, but no significant effects were observed at dietary concentrations up to 1,000 ppm (Finnegan *et al.*, 1958). In another study (Borzelleca *et al.*, 1971), purebred beagles of both sexes were fed for 2 yr a diet containing technical PCNB at 5, 30, 180, and 1,080 ppm added in corn oil solution. No significant differences in body weight or food consumption were observed, although a few males, including controls, had lost weight by the end of the study. Hematocrit values were significantly decreased at 18 months for males fed 30 and 180 ppm, but there was no significant change in males fed 1,080 ppm. No changes were found in the females. Liver:body weight ratios were increased in dogs fed 1,080 ppm. Histologic examination after 1 yr showed no treatment-related lesions; after 2 yr, cholestatic hepatoses with secondary bile nephrosis were found in dogs fed 180 ppm and, to a greater extent, in those fed 1,080 ppm.

In a 2-yr feeding study (cited by FAO/WHO, 1970), groups of male and female dogs were fed diets containing PCNB (purity not specified) at 500, 1,000, or 5,000 ppm. Liver changes—including fibrosis, narrowing of hepatic cells, thick leukocyte infiltration, and increased size of the periportal region—occurred in all groups; the degree of damage was dose-related.

Because technical PCNB contains 1.8% HCB, it is important to consider the toxicity of this major contaminant. Chronic ingestion of 0.2% HCB in the diet of adult male Sprague–Dawley rats resulted in hepatocellular degeneration and profound increases in the amounts of porphyrin and porphyrin precursors in the liver and excreta (Ocner and Schmid, 1961). Increased ratios of liver, spleen, adrenal, lung, and kidney weights to body weight were found in weanling Sherman rats fed technical HCB at 500 and 1,000 ppm for a 4-month period (Kimbrough and Linder, 1974). Hyperplasia of the adrenal cortex, as well as lung pathology, was observed. Female rats developed much more severe porphyria than did males fed HCB at 40 ppm for 274 days (Grant *et al.*, 1974). Rats of both sexes showed increased liver:body weight ratios after the feeding of HCB at 80 and 160 ppm. Liver mixed-function oxidase activity, however, was increased only in males fed 40 ppm and above. Liver pathology and increased liver:body weight ratios were found in male and female Charles River rats fed HCB at 8 and 32 mg/kg/day over a 15-week period (Kuiper-Goodman *et al.*, 1975). Only females developed porphyria.

Mutagenicity PCNB produced a positive mutagenic response in host cell reactive deficient strain of *Escherichia coli* B/r ochre at 10–15 mg/kg (Clarke, 1971). PCNB had a negative mutagenic response, however, at a 2 mg/ml on *E. coli* Gal (a noninducible galactose-negative mutant of *E. coli* 343) (Mohn, 1971). *In vitro* mutagenic testing with mutant strains of *Salmonella typhimurium*, *Saccharomyces cerevisiae*, *E. coli*, and *Bacillus subtilus* in the presence of a liver microsomal preparation showed no effect from PCNB (Simmon *et al.*, 1976). Dominant-lethal tests with three concentrations of PCNB in the diets of mice failed to show any evidence of mutagenicity (Jorgenson *et al.*, 1976). PCNB was negative in the sex-linked lethal test in *Drosophila* (Vogel and Chandler, 1974).

Carcinogenicity PCNB is listed as a suspected carcinogen (IARC, 1973). Two mouse hybrid strains, (C57 B1/6×C3H/Anf) F_1 and (C47 B1/6×AKR) F_1, were given a maximal tolerated oral dose of PCNB (464 mg/kg in 0.5% gelatin) daily, from the age of 7 days to the age of 28 days (but the absolute dosage was not corrected for increasing body weight) (Innes *et al.*, 1969). The animals were then transferred to a diet containing PCNB at 1,206 ppm, which was fed for 17 months. A significantly increased incidence of hepatomas was observed in both strains; 2 of 18 male and 4 of 18 female (C57B1/6×C3H/Anf) F_1 mice developed hepatomas, compared with 8 of 79 and none of 87, respectively, in the controls. Of the (C57B1/6×AKR) F_1 mice, 10 of 17 males and 1 of 17 females developed hepatomas, compared with 5 of 90 and 1 of 82 in the controls. The incidence of other tumors was similar in the treated and control mice.

In another study, stock albino mice of each sex were painted twice a week with 0.2 ml of a 0.3% solution of PCNB in acetone for 12 weeks. This was followed by twice-weekly paintings with a 0.5% solution of croton oil in acetone for 20 weeks (Searle, 1966). A control group was treated with acetone alone and then croton oil. The total numbers of skin tumors at the end of the croton oil treatment were 12 in 9 surviving controls and 50 in 13 survivors of the PCNB group. One tumor in the PCNB group was a squamous-cell carcinoma, and one in the control group was also an infiltrating squamous-cell carcinoma.

Rats that received PCNB at 25–2,500 ppm as a commercial powder (containing 20% PCNB) in the diet for 25 months showed no malignant growths or histopathologic changes related to dietary dosages of the fungicide (Finnegan *et al.*, 1958). No tumors were reported in a 2-yr study in which rats received diets containing PCNB at 25–2,500 ppm.

No tumors were observed in mongrel dogs fed PCNB at 25–1,000 ppm for 1 yr (Finnegan *et al.*, 1958) or in purebred beagles fed PCNB at 5–1,080 ppm for 2 yr (Borzelleca *et al.*, 1971).

The PCNB metabolite TCNB produced a larger number of papillomas than PCNB when applied to the skin and then followed by croton oil treatment (Searle, 1966). Searle (1966) suggested that tumor production results from formation of a hydroxylamine derivative formed as an intermediate in the metabolic reduction of the nitro groups. The TCNB has a stable nitro group, whereas 36–37% of the absorbed dose of PCNB yields a mercapturic acid by displacement of the nitro group; this perhaps accounting for the higher incidence of tumors with TCNB.

Reproduction In a three-generation reproductive study in rats, no adverse effects on any factor appeared to result from dietary dosages of PCNB through 500 ppm (Borzelleca *et al.*, 1971).

Teratogenicity When technical PCNB was administered orally at 500 mg/kg to pregnant female C57B1/6 mice on days 7-11 of gestation, renal agenesis and cleft palate were produced with a high frequency in the offspring (Courtney, 1973; Courtney *et al.*, 1976). The major contaminant, HCB (11% of the technical PCNB preparation), produced cleft palates and some kidney abnormalities in mice and was probably the major active teratogenic constituent of commercial PCNB. Nevertheless, purified PCNB (HCB at <20 ppm) at 500 mg/kg also produced a significant, but much lower, incidence of cleft palate and an increased fetal mortality. Another impurity of technical PCNB, TCNB, and the PCNB metabolite PCA were not teratogenic in mice or rats.

When oral PCNB dosages of 100–1,563 ppm in corn oil were administered to Charles River albino rats on days 6–15 of gestation, no significant differences from controls were noted on examination of the fetuses on day 20 (Jordan and Borzelleca, 1973). Intubation of PCNB at 50, 100, and 200 mg/kg in rats on days 6–15 of gestation produced no significant effects in fetuses at day 20 (Khera and Villeneuve, 1975). No embryolethal or teratogenic effects were found in Charles River CD rats at dosages up to 125 mg/kg/day (Jordan *et al.*, 1975).

Carcinogenic Risk Estimates

PCNB has produced hepatomas when given orally to mice (Innes *et al.*, 1969). The available sets of dose–response data were individually considered as described in the risk section in the margin of safety chapter. Each set of dose–response data was used to statistically estimate both the lifetime risk and an upper 95% confidence bound on the lifetime risk at the low dose level. These estimates are of lifetime human risks and have been corrected for species conversion on a dose-per-surface-area basis. The risk estimates are expressed as a probability of cancer after a lifetime consumption of 1 liter of water/day containing Q/ppb of the compound of interest. For example a risk of $1 \times 10^{-6}\ Q$ implies a lifetime probability of 2×10^{-5} of cancer if 2 liters/day were consumed and the concentration of the carcinogen was 10 ppb (i.e., $Q = 10$). This means that at a concentration of 10 ppb during a lifetime of exposure this compound would be expected to produce one excess case of cancer for every 50,000 persons exposed. If the population of the United States is taken to be 220

TABLE VI-44 Summary of Chronic and Subchronic Toxicity Data for PCNB

Species	Duration of Study	Dosage Levels and No. of Animals Per Group	Highest No-Adverse-Effect Level or Lowest-Minimal-Effect Level	Effect Measured	Reference
Dog	2 yr	0–1,080 ppm in diet, 8 animals/group	5 ppm (0.125 mg/kg/day)[a]	no effect	Borzelleca *et al.*, 1971
Rat	2 yr	0–2,500 ppm in diet, 20 animals/group	25 ppm (1.25 mg/kg/day)[a]	no toxic effect in females	Finnegan *et al.*, 1958
Rat	3 months	0–5,000 ppm in diet, 14 animals/group	6.35 ppm (3.2 mg/kg/day)[a]	increased liver/body weight ratios in males	Finnegan *et al.*, 1958
Dog	2 yr	0–5,000 ppm in diet, 6 animals/group	500 ppm (12.5 mg/kg/day)[a]	liver pathology	FAO/WHO, 1970
Mouse C 57B1 C 47B1	17 months	0–1,206 ppm in diet, 8 animals/group	1,206 ppm	hepatomas (C57) 2/18 M; 4/18F; controls: 8/79M; 0/87F; (C47) 10/17M; 1/17F; controls: 5/90M; 1/82F	Innes *et al.*, 1969

[This compound is an animal carcinogen.]

[a]Assume weight of rat = 0.4 kg and of dog = 10 kg; assume average daily food consumption of rat = 0.02 kg and of dog = 0.25 kg.

million people this translates into 4,400 excess lifetime deaths from cancer or 62.8 per year.

For PCNB at a concentration of 1 μg/liter ($Q=1$) the estimated risk for man would be 9.1×10^{-8} Q. The upper 95% estimate of risk at the same concentration would be 1.4×10^{-7} Q.

Conclusions and Recommendations

PCNB has relatively low acute toxicity. Although without effect in the rat and dog, PCNB appears to be carcinogenic in two strains of mice. In light of the above and taking into account the carcinogenic risk projections, it is suggested that very strict criteria be applied when limits for PCNB in drinking water are established. The chronic-toxicity data are summarized in Table VI-44.

A lower limit of detection of PCNB by gas chromatography was 0.01 ppm. A temporary acceptable daily intake of PCNB has been established for humans by the WHO at 0.001 mg/kg.

Most of the subchronic- and chronic-toxicity studies on PCNB have used technical-grade material, which normally contains about 1.8% HCB, but in some cases as much as 11% HCB. It is therefore not clear whether HCB and other impurities significantly contribute to the observed toxicity of PCNB. Moreover, some of the studies have involved PCNB formulations containing relatively low concentrations of the fungicide. The subchronic and chronic studies, particularly the latter, should be repeated in two species with pure PCNB. Such studies are particularly warranted, because of the suspected carcinogenicity of PCNB. Additional long-term oncogenic studies should also be conducted in susceptible strains of mice and other experimental animals. In addition, the FAO/WHO has recommended (Vettorazzi, 1975b) further short-term studies to elucidate the difference in teratogenic activity between rats and mice; studies to explain the effects on the liver and bone marrow of dogs; and further studies on the toxicity of PCNB metabolites.

PESTICIDES: FUMIGANT

p-Dichlorobenzene

Introduction

p-Dichlorobenzene (PDB, Paracide) came into use as an insecticidal fumigant about 1915 (Spencer, 1973;Thomson, 1975). Because of its high vapor pressure, over 90% of PDB's use involves vapor production by sublimation (IARC, 1974); 50% of its use is as a space deodorant and sanitizer (in toilets and refuse containers), 40% in moth control, and 10% in other applications (Anon., 1973). Total U.S. use of PDB in 1972 was estimated at 68 million pounds (IARC, 1974); production was estimated at 60 million pounds (NAS, 1975) or as high as 100 million pounds (Von Rumker *et al.*, 1975). Uses include 25–30 million pounds per year for moth control (balls, crystals, powders), 25–30 million pounds per year for lavatory-space deodorant, and the remainder for other purposes. PDB is also used as an intermediate in the synthesis of dyes and other chemicals (IARC, 1974).

PDB is produced commercially by chlorination of benzene or chlorobenzene at high temperature in the presence of catalysts (IARC, 1974). The impurities in technical-grade PDB are *m* and *o* isomers. PDB is soluble in water at 80 ppm at 25°C (Spencer, 1973). *o*-, *m*-, and *p*-Dichlorobenzenes have been detected in U.S. drinking water at concentrations of 1–3 pbb.

Metabolism

After oral administration in rabbits, PDB is metabolized to 2,4-dichlorophenol and 2,5-dichlorocatechol conjugated with glucuronic or sulfuric acid (Azouz *et al.*, 1955). The same two metabolites of PDB have been identified in man (Hallowell, 1959; Pagnotto and Walkley, 1965), and the amount of 2,4-dichlorophenol in the urine can serve as an index of PDB exposure. The phenolic metabolites are excreted as glucuronide and sulfate conjugates (Hallowell, 1959).

o-Dichlorobenzene is metabolized in the rabbit to 3,4-dichlorophenol and smaller amounts of 2,3-dichlorophenol, 4,5-dichlorophenylmercapturic acid, 3,4-dichlorocatechol, and 3,4-dichlorocatechol (Azouz *et al.*, 1955).

Both *o*-dichlorobenzene and PDB bind to cellular constituents, apparently via initial formation of reactive arene oxide intermediates formed by action of liver mixed-function oxidase systems (Reid and Krishna, 1973). Although hepatic mixed-function oxidase activities are increased by treatment of rats with the *m* isomer, *o*-dichlorobenzene and PDB had no effect (Ariyoshi *et al.*, 1975).

Health Aspects

Observations in Man There is evidence that accidentally inhaled or ingested PDB is quite toxic to humans. One case of pulmonary granulomatosis (Weller and Crellin, 1953) and two cases of hemolytic anemia (Campbell and Davidson, 1970; Hallowell, 1959) have been reported after exposure to PDB. A case of allergic purpura after exposure to PDB has also been described (Nalbandian and Pearce, 1965).

Girad *et al.* (1969) reported five cases of blood disorders in subjects exposed to *o*-dichlorobenzene and/or PDB: two cases of chronic lymphoid leukemia, two cases of acute myeloblastic leukemia, and one case of myeloproliferative syndrome.

No evidence of toxicity or hematologic changes was found in workers after exposure to air containing *o*-dichlorobenzene at 1–44 ppm (average, 15 ppm) for many years (Hollingsworth *et al.*, 1958).

The U.S. Occupational Safety and Health Administration health standards for air contaminants require that no employee's exposure to PDB exceed an 8-h time-weighted average of 75 ppm in the workplace during any 8-h work shift (IARC, 1974).

Prolonged inhalation of PDB by two young women reportedly caused development of cataracts (Berliner, 1939). Attempts to produce cataracts in rats, guinea pigs, and rabbits (Berliner, 1939; Pike, 1944; Zupko and Edwards, 1949) by treatment with PDB, however, were unsuccessful.

Human adipose tissue in Japan contained PDB at an average of 2.3 ppm (Morita and Ohi, 1975). Ambient-air samples collected in Tokyo contained PDB at 2–4 $\mu g/m^3$, whereas closets and bedrooms where PDB moth preparations were used contained 105–1,700 $\mu g/m^3$.

Observations in Other Species

Acute Effects The LD_{50} of PDB in rats after intraperitoneal administration is 2,500 mg/kg (Hollingsworth *et al.*, 1956). The acute oral LD_{50} of PDB is 500–5,000 mg/kg in rats and 2,950 mg/kg in mice (Spencer, 1973). An oral LD_{50} of PDB of 500 mg/kg in rats and a minimal lethal subcutaneous dose of 142 mg/kg in mice have also been reported (Christensen *et al.*, 1974).

The oral LD_{50} of *o*-dichlorobenzene is 500 mg/kg in rats, whereas the minimal lethal dose after intravenous administration is 326 mg/kg in rats (Christensen *et al.*, 1974).

Subchronic and Chronic Effects Rabbits subjected to inhalation exposure to PDB at about 800 ppm for 8-h periods, 5 days/week for as long as 12 weeks, developed tremors, weakness, nystagmus, and reversible nonspecific eye changes (Pike, 1944). Pike (1944) indicated that this concentration of PDB is 5–10 times the concentration that humans would voluntarily tolerate. Rabbits fed PDB at 1,000 mg/kg for 5 days/week developed similar toxicity symptoms after several months (Pike, 1944).

Young adult female rats received oral doses of PDB suspension 5

TABLE VI-45 Toxicity of PDB and ODB

Species	Duration of Study	Dosage Levels and No. of Animals Per Group	Highest No-Adverse-Effect Level or Lowest-Minimal-Effect Level	Effect Measured	Reference
PDB					
Rat	27 weeks	0–376 mg/kg/day, orally, 10 females/group	13.4 mg/kg/day[c]	no toxic effect	Hollingsworth *et al.*, 1956
Rabbit	1 yr	0–1,000 mg/kg/day, orally, 5 animals/group	357 mg/kg/day	weight loss, tremors, liver pathology	Hollingsworth *et al.*, 1956
ODB					
Rat	7 months	0–0.1 mg/kg/day, orally, 7 animals/group	.01 mg/kg/day	hematologic, behavioral, enzyme changes	Varshavskaya, 1968
Rat	28 weeks	0–376 mg/kg/day, orally, 10 females/group	13.4 mg/kg/day[c]	no toxic effect	Hollingsworth *et al.*, 1968

Using an uncertainty factor of 1,000, the suggested no-adverse-effect level in drinking water for both PDB and ODB is calculated as follows:

$$\frac{13.4}{1{,}000} = 0.0134 \text{ mg/kg/day (ADI)}, \; 0.0134 \times 70^{a} \times 0.1^{b} = 0.094 \text{ mg/liter}$$

[a]Assume average weight of human adult = 70 kg.
[b]Assume average daily intake of water for man = 2 liters, and that 20 percent of total intake is from water.
[c]Value from which the suggested no-adverse-effect level was calculated.

days/week over a period of 27 weeks (Hollingsworth *et al.*, 1956). At 376 mg/kg, the liver showed slight cirrhosis and focal necrosis. At 188 mg/kg, slight increases in the average weights of liver and kidneys occurred.

Rabbits were given PDB orally at 1,000 mg/kg for 5 days/week for 31 weeks or 500 mg/kg for 5 days/week for 1 yr (Hollingsworth *et al.*, 1956). Mortalities occurred among animals given the higher dosage; weight loss, tremors, weakness, and liver pathology developed in rabbits at both dosages. No hematologic changes were observed.

Young adult female rats received *o*-dichlorobenzene orally at 18.8, 188, and 376 mg/kg for 5 days/week for 28 weeks (Hollingsworth *et al.*, 1958). At the highest dosage, liver and kidney weights increased, spleen weight decreased, and liver pathology developed. At 188 mg/kg, slight increases in liver and kidney weight occurred. No adverse effect was detected at the lowest dosage.

It is difficult to reconcile these results with those of Varshavskaya (1968), who treated male albino rats orally with *o*-dichlorobenzene in sunflower oil at 0.1, 0.01, and 0.001 mg/kg daily for a period of 7 months. Serum and tissue enzyme alterations, behavioral abnormalities, and a marked reduction in hemoglobin, red-cell, and leukocyte concentrations occurred in animals receiving 0.1 or 0.01 mg/kg/day. No toxic effect was seen in animals given 0.001 mg/kg/day.

Carcinogencity No adequate studies on which to evaluate carcinogenicity have been carried out, but an association in man between leukemia and exposure to PDB has been suggested (IARC, 1974, 1975). PDB and *o*-dichlorobenzene are listed as suspected carcinogens (IARC, 1974, 1975). PDB is reported (Parsons, 1942) to have induced a transplantable sarcoma after injection into an irradiated mouse.

Mutagenicity and Teratogenicity No available data.

Conclusions and Recommendations

PDB is used in such a manner that large amounts of it could enter surface water and humans could obtain substantial exposure by inhalation. In spite of its tremendous use in the United States (68 million pounds) and its suspected involvement in human blood dyscrasias, there is very little adequate information on its toxicity. An ADI was calculated at 0.0134 mg/kg/day based on the available data. The available toxicity data and calculations of ADI are summarized in Table VI-45.

Gas-chromatographic methods have been developed for PDB with a sensitivity of 380 pg/cm peak height, and PDB concentrations as low as 1.0 ppb in water have been analyzed.

Apparently, no chronic-toxicity studies have been performed with PDB. There is no information on the reproductive effects, teratogenicity, mutagenicity, or carcinogenicity of PDB. This lack of information is disturbing, in view of the suspected role of PDB in human leukemia and its apparent ability to undergo metabolic activation and covalent binding to tissue constituents. Particularly disturbing is the very high degree of toxicity in rats that received *o*-dichlorobenzene at 0.1 or 0.01 mg/kg/day. The no-adverse-effect dosage in that study (0.001 mg/kg/day) was 1/13,400 of that found in other similar rat studies. The reason for this marked difference should be established.

OTHER ORGANIC CONSTITUENTS

Acetaldehyde

Introduction

Acetaldehyde is used extensively in the manufacture of acetic acid, acetic anhydride, synthetic resins, and various dyes. It is soluble in water and biodegradable in water (Merck Index, 1968; EPA, 1975d). It has been found in 5 of the 10 water supplies surveyed by EPA with the highest concentrations in Philadelphia and Seattle at 0.1 μg/liter (EPA, 1975a).

Metabolism

Acetaldehyde is metabolized in the rat via aldehyde dehydrogenase to acetate, which ultimately breaks down to carbon dioxide (Forsyth *et al.*, 1973). It has been shown to interfere with mitochondrial oxygen consumption in rat liver and thus to interfere with energy production (Cederbaum *et al.*, 1974).

Health Aspects

Observations in Man In a study of the effects of acetaldehyde inhalation in dogs, Egle (1970) showed that exposure at 134 ppm for 30 min resulted in mild upper-respratory-tract irritation. Higher concentrations decreased the respiratory rate by inhibition of the central nervous system. Exposure at 50 ppm produced eye irritation; 200 ppm resulted in conjunctivitis (Silverman *et al.*, 1946). Although there have been no systematic studies bearing directly on the effect of acetaldehyde in man, the effects of ethyl alcohol are indicative of the effects of acetaldehyde, because it is the major metabolite of ethyl alcohol. Furthermore, there is extensive human experience with acetaldehyde, as it is the principal metabolic buildup product of disulfiram therapy.

Observations in Other Species

Acute Effects The oral LD_{50} is 1,900 mg/kg in rats (Smyth *et al.*, 1951) and 1,232 mg/kg in mice (Amirhanova and Latppova, 1967). Parenteral LD_{50}'s are 560 mg/kg in mice and 640 mg/kg in rats (Skog, 1950).

In studies of the effects of acetaldehyde inhalation in rats, 100% saturated air was shown to be fatal within 2 min of exposure. The lowest lethal concentration proved to be 16,000 ppm in 4 h; concentrations up to 4,000 ppm for 8 h produced no fatalities (Smyth *et al.*, 1951). The effects of chronic acetaldehyde inhalation have also been examined in hamsters (Kruysee *et al.*, 1975). Inhalation of acetaldehyde has been shown to affect both blood pressure and heart rate (McCloy *et al.*, 1974; Egle *et al.*, 1973; Egle, 1972). It has been suggested that these effects are mediated through the release of catecholamines.

Mutagenicity No available data.

Carcinogenicity Rats showed some focal spindle cell sarcomas when given acetaldehyde subcutaneously approximately 100 times, once or twice a week (Shubik and Hartwell, 1969).

Teratogenicity No available data.

Conclusions and Recommendations

Human exposure to acetaldehyde probably antedates recorded history, inasmuch as acetaldehyde is the major metabolite of ethyl alcohol. An additional source of widespread human exposure is tobacco smoke. The pharmacology and toxicology of acetaldehyde have been studied most extensively in its relationship to alcohol toxicity and human metabolism. Because of this background of human and laboratory experience, there appears to be no need to establish limits for acetaldehyde in drinking water.

Benzene

Introduction

Benzene is produced by petroleum refining, coal tar distillation, coal processing, and coal coking. The U.S. production of benzene in 1973 was over 10 billion pounds (USITC, 1975). It is used primarily as a chemical intermediate in the manufacture of styrene, cyclohexane, detergents, and pesticides.

It was reported that motor gasoline usually contains less than 5% benzene (Parkinson, 1971); the concentrations of benzene in the ambient air of gas stations were 0.001–0.008 mg/liter.

Benzene is slightly soluble in water (0.8 ppm by weight at 20°C). Four of the 10 water supplies surveyed by the EPA contained benzene (USEPA, 1975a,e) at levels between 0.1–0.3 μg/liter. The highest concentration of benzene reported in finished water was 10 μg/liter.

Metabolism

Benzene is excreted rapidly. The metabolic products in the rat of benzene are phenol, hydroquinone, catechol hydroxyhydroquinone, and phenylmercapturic acid. Conjugated phenols have been reported by Williams (1975). In human retention studies, Nomiyama and Nomiyama (1974) reported 30% retention in man when exposed to 52–62 ppm for 4 h in air; Hunter and Blair (1972) noted that humans retained 230 mg after exposure to 80–100 μg/liter for 6 h. Benzene metabolism has been shown to be inhibited by 3-amino-1,2,4-triazole.

Health Aspects

Observations in Man

Acute Effects Single exposures to benzene at 20,000 ppm have proved to be fatal in man. Industrial air concentrations of benzene have been reported to give rise to nausea, giddiness, headache, unconsciousness, convulsions, and paralysis (Browning, 1965; Eckardt, 1973).

Chronic Effects The chronic exposure of humans to benzene has been reported to produce thrombocytopenia, leukopenia, myelocytic anemia, and leukemia. Despite negative animal toxicity data, the evidence that benzene is a leukemogen for man is convincing. The pathogenesis of leukemia is usually preceded by many observed effects on the hematopoietic system (Snyder and Koosis, 1975; Mallory *et al.*, 1939; Browning, 1965; Gerarde, 1960). The NIOSH (1974) recommended the occupational exposure to benzene at not in excess of 10 ppm determined as a time-weighted average exposure for up to a 10-h workday. A recent review on the health effects of benzene (NAS, 1976) concludes that:

> Most cases of severe benzene intoxication have been reported in workers exposed to rather high concentrations of benzene under somewhat unhygienic working conditions. It is probable that all cases reported as "leukemia associated with benzene exposure" have resulted from exposure to rather high concentrations of benzene and other chemicals.
>
> It has been suggested in the literature that "benzene-induced leukemia" may occur only in individuals who are highly sensitive because of genetic constitution or because of synergistic action of other chemical or physical environmental agents. A co-leukemogenic role for benzene would explain the failure to induce leukemia in benzene-exposed animals.
>
> The state of the benzene literature makes it very difficult or impossible to reach a firm conclusion on the dose–response relationship in chronic exposure of humans to benzene. The details of the extent of exposures are either inadequate or absent. Even in cases where some concentrations of benzene are reported, the stated concentrations were based on occasional measurements of short durations. The role of benzene metabolism in its toxicity and the significance of benzene-induced chromosome aberrations are currently unclear. It appears that a metabolite of benzene may be responsible for its myelotoxic effects.
>
> Based on available literature, it can be concluded that benzene may be associated with leukemia; therefore, benzene must be considered as a suspect leukemogen. More definitive data are required for an accurate assessment of the myelotoxic, leukemogenic, and chromosome-damaging effects of benzene.

Observations in Other Species

Acute Effects In an acute study, it was shown that rabbits absorbed benzene through the skin and underwent anesthesia at 35,000–45,000 ppm. Benzene inhaled by mice at 60 mg/liter in air (18,750 ppm) caused lesions on lipoprotein membranes.

Chronic Effects In a series of chronic studies, bilateral cataracts were found in 50% of the rats exposed to benzene at 50 ppm for 600 h; at 60–883 ppm, rats became leukopenic. It has also been found that an inadequate dietary protein intake has some bearing on the development of benzene toxicity.

Mutagenicity Some preliminary work suggests that benzene may induce mutagenic chromosomal alterations. Forni *et al.* (1971) have reported an increased incidence of various kinds of chromosomal breaks or aberrations in workers occupationally exposed to benzene. These observations are complicated by the fact that there were simultaneous exposures to other compounds.

Carcinogenicity Although animal experiments have thus far proved negative, with respect to the carcinogenic properties of the compound (Ward *et al.*, 1975), there are some indications that benzene acts as a cocarcinogen (Dubroklotov, 1972; Smolik *et al.*, 1973).

Teratogenicity There is no reported evidence of benzene-induced teratogenicity.

Carcinogenic Risk Estimates

On review of the original data from the carcinogenicity study by Ward *et al.* (1975), it is concluded that the observed increased occurrence of granulocytic leukemia in benzene-treated animals is not statistically significant, even when time to response is incorporated into the analysis. Therefore, statistical extrapolation from these data would be unwarranted. An additional difficulty in extrapolation is posed by the fact that the experimental route of exposure was subcutaneous injection, whereas man's exposure would be through ingestion of drinking water.

Occupational studies on human exposure (Aksoy *et al.*, 1972; Ishimaru *et al.*, 1971; Aksoy *et al.*, 1974a,b; Thorpe, 1974) do not contain adequate information on degree of exposure or size of population at risk. In addition, because the workers in benzene-related occupations were probably exposed to other chemicals, extrapolation of benzene-induced cancer risk from such data as these would be tenuous.

Conclusions and Recommendations

The acute effects of benzene cover a wide range of signs and symptoms. The effects are transitory but may lead to more lasting chronic effects such as anemia; if exposure is continuous and great enough, leukemia is a strong possibility for susceptible members of the population. There are no dose–response data on animals and the data on humans are inadequate to calculate a risk estimate for benzene with mathematical models.

In summary, there is no adequate source of data (animal or human) on which to base a statistical extrapolation from high to low exposure. More data are needed on the mutagenicity and teratogenicity of benzene. The cocarcinogenic effect of benzene should be further explored. If data are available on industrial benzene exposure, then systematic monitoring should be started with a view to following the population groups at risk.

Before limits for benzene in drinking water can be established more extensive toxicological data must be gathered and evaluated.

Benzo(*a*)pyrene

Introduction

Benzo(*a*)pyrene is a ubiquitous polycyclic aromatic hydrocarbon that is produced largely, if not exclusively, in the pyrolysis of naturally occurring hydrocarbons. It was isolated early in pure form from coal tar, one of the so-called industrial carcinogens. Benzo(*a*)pyrene is found as a constituent in coal, petroleum, shale, and kerosene. It has been reported that it is present in the combustion products of fuels and cigarette smoke.

Benzo(*a*)pyrene is very persistent in water and is soluble at 0.004 mg/liter at 27°C (Davis, 1942). It has been detected in finished water (USEPA, 1976).

Metabolism

The primary routes of benzo(*a*)pyrene excretion in mice and rats are the hepatobiliary and gastrointestinal tracts. The dihydroxy-, 3-hydroxy-, and 6-hydroxy- derivatives have been found in the liver, bile, and bowel (Berenblum and Schoenthal, 1943; Falk *et al.*, 1962; Sims, 1967, 1970a,b).

Health Aspects

Observations in Man There is no firm evidence that benzo(*a*)pyrene alone produces toxicity, including teratogenicity, mutagenicity, or carcinogenicity in humans. On the other hand, mixtures of compounds which contain benzo(*a*)pyrene as a constituent have been associated with cancer in man. In such cases the exact role of benzo(*a*)pyrene is difficult to assess.

Observations in Other Species

Mutagenicity Although there is no substantive literature on the mutagenic effects of benzo(*a*)pyrene, there have been indications that its metabolites bind to DNA. Benzo(*a*)pyrene is a positive mutagen in the *Salmonella*/microsome test (McCann *et al.*, 1975).

Carcinogenicity The effects of benzo(*a*)pyrene have been examined for the most part in relation to carcinogenesis. In mice, a single oral 0.012-mg dose induced forestomach tumors (Pierce, 1961); in rats a single 100-mg dose (gavage) produced mammary tumors (Huggins and Yang, 1962). Single subcutaneous and intramuscular doses that induced tumor formation were 0.062 mg, 0.004 mg, and 0.0025 mg in C3II, C57, and CFW Swiss mice, respectively. In rats and hamsters, the parenteral carcinogenic doses were 0.05 mg and 0.01 mg, respectively.

In chronic oral studies, carcinogenic effects were observed in mice after the administration of benzo(*a*)pyrene at 40–45 ppm for 110 days (Rigdon and Neal, 1966, 1969). Donetenwill and Mohr (1962) reported stomach tumors in hamsters after biweekly oral administration of the compound for 1 month. In mice, chronic dermal administration of a 0.001% solution three times a week induced benign and malignant skin tumors (Wynder *et al.*, 1957). Rats and hamsters were also shown to be sensitive to the induction of skin tumors with benzo(*a*)pyrene (Nakano, 1937; Shubik *et al.*, 1960).

In a study of the transplacental carcinogenic effects of benzo(*a*)pyrene, 2–4 mg on days 11, 13, and 15 of pregnancy induced tumors in the offspring of treated mice (Bulay and Wattenberg, 1970; Bulay, 1970). No other abnormalities were observed.

Teratogenicity Rigdon and Rennels (1964) found one malformed fetus out of 7 litters of rats whose mothers had been exposed to benzo(*a*)pyrene at a level of 1 mg/g of diet during pregnancy. There were also many excess reabsorptions and dead fetuses.

Carcinogenic Risk Estimates

Numerous carcinogenesis studies have been conducted in rodents with oral administration of benzo(*a*)pyrene (IARC, 1973). Stomach tumors in mice have been observed in several studies, as well as leukemia and lung adenomas. In rats, mammary tumors and papillomas in the esophagus and forestomach have been found. In hamsters, tumors were found in the forestomach, esophagus, and intestine. No satisfactory human data are available.

In the above studies, the oral administration of benzo(*a*)pyrene showed evidence of dose–response relationships. However, it was generally fed for less than 6 months; this is not adequate for estimating lifetime effects. Thus, without specific biologic assumptions that relate short-term to lifetime effects, no reasonable risk estimates can be attempted.

Conclusions and Recommendations

The occurrence of upper-gastrointestinal-tract tumors in animals fed benzo(*a*)pyrene, skin tumors at sites painted with it, and subcutaneous sarcomas at sites where it was injected demonstrates that benzo(*a*)pyrene is a potent contact carcinogen. In light of the above it is suggested that strict criteria be applied when limits for benzo(*a*)pyrene in drinking-water are established. The available chronic toxicity data are summarized in Table VI-46.

Bromobenzene

Introduction

Bromobenzene (Monobromobenzene) is used as an intermediate in organic synthesis, and as additive in motor oil and fuels. During chlorination water treatment, bromobenzene can be formed in small quantities (USEPA, 1975d). It is insoluble in water (CRC Handbook of Chemistry and Physics, 1970–1971). Bromobenzene was found in finished water in the lower Mississippi River area (USEPA, 1972).

Metabolism

Bromobenzene appears to be metabolized in the rat to an intermediate that can produce tissue damage (Reid, 1973). This damage is blocked by prior administration of piperonyl butoxide; thus, the damage may be due to a toxic metabolite. The metabolite is apparently produced in the liver and transported to the kidneys by the circulation. Phenobarbital pretreatment increases the liver toxicity of bromobenzene, but has little or no effect on the kidneys (Reid *et al.*, 1971; Sipes *et al.*, 1974). Bromobenzene may be metabolized to an epoxide (which causes the liver damage), excreted in the bile, reabsorbed through the enterohepatic circulation, and metabolized in several steps to *S-P*-bromophenyl mercapturic acid, which is then excreted in the urine (Sipes *et al.*, 1947).

Health Aspects

Observations in Man Bromobenzene irritates the skin and is a central nervous system depressant in humans. Nothing is known about its chronic effects.

TABLE VI-46 Toxicity of Benzo(a)Pyrene

Species	Duration of Study	Dosage Levels and No. of Animals Per Group	Highest No-Adverse-Effect Level or Lowest-Minimal-Effect Level	Effect Measured	Reference
Mouse	110 days		40–45 ppm (oral)	stomach tumors	Rigdon and Neal, 1966, 1967, 1969
Hamster	1–5 months	biweekly administration	2–5 mg (oral)	stomach tumors	Donetenwill and Mohr, 1962
Mouse			0.001% solution (oral)	malignant skin tumors	Wynder *et al.*, 1957
Rat	150 days	weekly paintings, 15 animals	0.5–1% solution	skin tumors	Nakano, 1937
Hamster	40 weeks	biweekly paintings, 10 animals	0.01% solution	skin tumors	Shubik *et al.*, 1960

[This compound is a suspected human carcinogen.]

Observations in Other Species

Acute Effects In an inhalation study in rats, bromobenzene was administered daily for a 4-h period at 3 $\mu g/m^3$, without toxic effects; 20 $\mu g/m^3$ was a definite-effect dosage in similar tests (Shamilov, 1970).

Chronic Effects No available data.

Mutagenicity Bromobenzene was not mutagenic in the *Salmonella*/microsome test (McCann *et al.*, 1975).

Carcinogenicity There is no evidence that bromobenzene is carcinogenic in animals and man.

Teratogenicity No available data.

Conclusions and Recommendations

In view of the relative paucity of data on the carcinogenicity, teratogenicity, and long-term oral toxicity of bromobenzene, estimates of the effects of chronic oral exposure at low levels cannot be made with any confidence. It is recommended that studies to produce such information be conducted before limits in drinking water can be established. Since bromobenzene was negative on the *Salmonella*/microsome mutagenicity test, there should be less concern than with those substances that are positive.

Bromoform

Introduction

Bromoform (Tribromomethane) is used in pharmaceutical manufacturing, as an ingredient in fire-resistant chemicals and gauge fluid, and as a solvent for waxes, greases, and oils (USEPA, 1975d).

Bromoform is nonbiodegradable in water. It is soluble at 1 part per 800 parts of water (Merck Index, 1968). Bromoform results from chlorination of precursors in raw water. Of 80 water supplies surveyed, 26 were positive results for bromoform in finished water, with a concentration range of $<0.8–92$ µg/liter (USEPA, 1975a). Of the 83 Region V water supplies surveyed, 14% contained bromoform, at a mean concentration of less than 1 μg/liter; none of the raw water contained bromoform (USEPA, 1975b).

Metabolism

Lucas (1929) demonstrated in rabbits that bromoform administered rectally or by inhalation was biotransformed in the liver and that inorganic bromides were later found in tissues and urine. After rectal anesthesia with bromoform, 0.3–1.2% of the dose was recovered in the urine as sodium bromide.

Health Aspects

Observations in Man No data are available on the adverse health effects of bromoform in man. An air exposure limit based on animal studies is listed in the *Federal Register* (1972) as 0.5 ppm, or 5 mg/m^3.

Observations in Other Species

Acute Effects The subcutaneous LD_{50} in mice is 1,820 mg/kg (Kutob and Plaa, 1962). In an attempt to assess the liver toxicity of bromoform, Kutob and Plaa (1962) found that a subcutaneous dose of 278 mg/kg was negative in mice, whereas 1,113 mg/kg produced decreased liver function as well as hepatic histopathology. In rats, the maximal single oral dose survived was 6,578 mg/kg at 1 h, 2,099 mg/kg at 8 h, and 658 mg/kg at 24 h.

Dykan (1962) reported that injecting 100–200 mg/kg/day into guinea pigs for 10 days resulted in pathologic changes in kidney and liver.

Chronic Effects Inhalation by rats of 0.25 mg/liter of air for 4 h/day for 2 months produced disorders in prothrombin synthesis and glycogenesis in the liver and reduced renal filtration capacity; the threshold concentration was 0.05 mg/liter (Dykan, 1962).

Mutagenicity Weakly positive in *Salmonella* test (Simmon and Poole, 1976).

Carcinogenicity No available data.

Teratogenicity No available data.

Conclusions and Recommendations

In view of the relative paucity of data on the mutagenicity, carcinogenicity, teratogenicity and long term toxicity of bromoform, estimates of the effects of chronic oral exposure at low levels cannot be made with any confidence. It is recommended that studies to produce such information be conducted before limits in drinking water can be established.

tert-Butyl Alcohol

Introduction

tert-Butyl alcohol (1-butanol) is used as an alcohol denaturant, a solvent, a dehydration agent, and a chemical intermediate (The Condensed Chemical Dictionary, 1971). It is miscible in water (CRC Handbook of Chemistry and Physics, 1970–1971). In the 10–city survey, only the finished water of Cincinnati contained *tert*-butyl alcohol (USEPA, 1975a).

Metabolism

Gaillard and Derache (1964) found, after administering *tert*-butyl alcohol orally to rats at 2 g/kg, that there was rapid absorption into the blood; 0.98% was excreted in the urine. After intraperitoneal administration in rats at 0.84 g/kg (Rietbrock and Abshagen, 1971), exponential elimination from the blood occurred, but more slowly than that of other aliphatic alcohols; the blood half-life was 13 h. Transformation by glucuronidation (24%) is the only metabolic pathway known. The possible conjugation is between the hydroxyl group and glucuronic acid. There is potential for one of the methyl groups to be oxidized to B-hydroxyisobutyric acid (Williams, 1959). Oral administration of *tert*-butyl alcohol in rats elicited a threefold increase in liver microsomal enzyme activity 24 h later (Bechtel and Cornish, 1972).

Health Aspects

Observations in Man A slight erythema has been reported in man after exposure of skin to *tert*-butyl alcohol (Oettel, 1936), and it has been suggested that the compound is a skin irritant (Swartz and Tulipan, 1939). The U.S. occupational standard in air is listed in the *Federal Register* (United States Department of Labor, 1972) at 100 ppm. A threshold limit value (TLV) has been set at 100 ppm, or 300 mg/m^3 (ACGIH, 1971).

Observations in Other Species

Acute Effects The acute effects of *tert*-butyl alcohol have been examined in both mice and rats. The oral LD_{50} in rats is 3,500 mg/kg (Schaffarzick and Brown, 1957). In mice the subcutaneous LD_{50} is 5 ml/kg (Harada, 1937).

Chronic Effects No available data.

Mutagenicity No available data.

Carcinogenicity Hoshino *et al.* (1970) conducted a study to determine the carcinogenic activity of *t*-butyl alcohol. Mice treated with an initiating dose of 4-nitroquinoline-1-oxide were examined after 270 applications of *t*-butanol, and no increase in carcinogenic activity was found.

Teratogenicity No available data.

Conclusions and Recommendations

In view of the relative paucity of data on the mutagenicity, carcinogenicity, teratogenicity, and long term oral toxicity of *t*-butyl alcohol, estimates of the effects of chronic oral exposure at low levels cannot be made with any confidence. It is recommended that studies to produce such information be conducted before limits in drinking water are established.

e-Caprolactam

Introduction

e-Caprolactam (hexahydro-2H-azepin-2-one) is used in the manufacture of nylon, plastics, bristles, film, coatings, synthetic leather, plasticizers, and paint vehicles; as a cross-linking agent for curing polyurethanes; and in the synthesis of lysine (USEPA, 1975d). The United States production of *e*-caprolactam in 1973 was over 656 million pounds (USITC, 1975). This compound is soluble in water (CRC Handbook of Chemistry and Physics, 1970–1971) and has been found in finished water (USEPA, 1976).

Metabolism

e-Caprolactam is excreted by rats partly as lactam and partly as *e*-amino acid. Rabbits metabolize *e*-caprolactam completely (Goldblatt *et al.*, 1954).

Health Aspects

Observations in Man Skin contact with caprolactam can cause serious burns if contact is prolonged and confined. Exposure in airborne dust at 5 mg/m^3 causes skin irritation in some people but not at 1 mg/m^3. Sensitivity has not been related to race, skin pigmentation, or other common indices of sensitivity (Ferguson and Wheeler, 1973). The prevalence of dermatoses among workers in a caprolactam manufacturing plant showed that contact dermatitis and eczema of the hands were most prevalent. Dry erythematous squamous foci on smooth skin was a typical manifestation (Dovzhanskii *et al.*, 1972).

Light sensitivity of the eyes was produced by inhalation of caprolactam at 0.11 mg/m^3 and higher. The olfactory threshold was 0.30 mg/m^3 (Krichevskaya, 1968). An oral dose of 3–6 g was given daily for 3–5 yr for the treatment of obesity in 90 subjects. No toxic effects were observed. There was no effect on appetite, and only one person developed an allergy to caprolactam (Anonymous, 1964).

Observations in Other Species

Acute Effects The acute lethal dosages in laboratory species are 500–900 mg/kg parenterally and over 1,000 mg/kg orally.

In dogs an intravenous injection of 0.002 g/kg increased arterial pressure; 0.1 g/kg caused a brief cardiac arrest and a sharp decrease in arterial pressure, and then an increase to a pressure well above normal. Additional results indicated an effect on the peripheral, as well as the central, nervous system (Polushkin, 1964).

Chronic Effects In a behavioral study with rats, ill-defined changes in conditioned-reflex activities were seen at a daily oral dose of 15 mg/kg for 2 months. In another chronic study (Statsek *et al.*, 1974), guinea pigs were exposed to vapors of caprolactam (0.01-0.03 mg/liter) once every 2 days. On day 14 of the experiment, circulatory antibodies to caprolactam appeared. By day 30, serum antibodies were present in lung tissues; this suggested the development of a self-immunizing process.

Mutagenicity No available data.

Carcinogenicity No available data.

Teratogenicity No available data.

Reproduction Caprolactam at 120–150 mg/m^3 in air reduced rats' fecundity by causing heavy losses of embryos (Khadzhieva, 1969).

Conclusions and Recommendations

In view of the relative paucity of data on the mutagenicity, carcinogenicity, teratogenicity, and long-term oral toxicity of caprolactam, estimates of the effects of chronic oral exposure at low levels cannot be made with any confidence. It is recommended that studies to produce such information be conducted before limits in drinking water are established.

Carbon Disulfide

Introduction

Carbon disulfide is produced in petroleum and coal tar refining. Its principal uses are in the manufacture of rayon, rubber, chemicals, solvents, and pesticides (USEPA, 1975d). U.S. production in 1973 was over 77 million pounds (USITC, 1975). It is soluble in water (0.294% at 20°C) (Merck Index, 1968). Carbon disulfide was detected in 5 of the 10 water supplies surveyed by the EPA (1975a).

Metabolism

Absorption and elimination of carbon disulfide differs with species and route of administration. Most of the work on absorption and elimination has been related to inhalation toxicity. The little work with cutaneous exposure has shown a change in blood proteins and a change in zinc content (Brieger and Teisinger, 1967).

Carbon disulfide is 90% metabolized by the mixed-function oxidase enzyme system P-450 to inorganic sulfate (Dalvi *et al.*, 1975). A portion of the sulfur released by carbon disulfide is thought to react with sulfide groups of cysteine residues in the microsomal protein to form hydrosulfide (Catignani and Neal, 1975). Small amounts of the compound (0.5%) are excreted as thiourea, 5-mercaptothioazolidone, and inorganic constituents in the urine (Teisinger, 1974). Some portion of the compound (8–10%) is also excreted unchanged in the breath.

Inhalation-toxicity studies have shown that 18% of the carbon disulfide inhaled is exhaled unchanged. Of the remaining inhaled dose 70% is excreted as free or bound carbon disulfide and urinary sulfates, and 30% is stored in the body and slowly excreted as carbon disulfide and its metabolites.

Large concentrations of both free and bound carbon disulfide are found in the brain (guinea pig studies) and peripheral nerves (rat studies) of exposed animals. The ratio of bound to free carbon disulfide in the brain is 3:1. Blood and fatty tissues contain mainly bound carbon disulfide, while the liver contains mainly free. Carbon disulfide can also chelate trace metals, especially copper and zinc.

Health Aspects

Observations in Man The effects of carbon disulfide inhalation have been examined in the light of their central nervous system and vascular effects on man. The lowest lethal concentration has been reported as 4,000 ppm in 30 min; in the same study, a person subjected to a concentration of 50 mg/m^3 for 7 yr had central nervous system effects (Registry of Toxic Effects of Chemical Substances, 1975). Moderate chronic exposure at less than 65 mg/m^3 for several years has been reported by Cooper (1976) to cause polyneuropathy. In a study by Baranowska *et al.* (1966), humans have been shown to absorb 8.8–37.2 mg of carbon disulfide from an aqueous solution containing 0.33–1.67 g/liter. This was over a period of 1 h of hand-soaking.

The U.S. Occupational standards (TLV) recommend a maximum of 20 ppm. The standards allow a peak concentration of 100 ppm for 30 min in an 8-h period. The USSR has set a standard of 4 ppm as the safe maximum, and the Czechoslovakians maintain 10 ppm as the safe limit (Hamilton and Hardy, 1974).

Observations in Other Species

Acute Effects The effects of acute administration of carbon disulfide have been examined in a variety of animals with a variety of routes of administration. Intraperitoneal injection of 400 mg/kg proved to be the lowest lethal dose in guinea pigs (Davidson and Feinlab, 1972). An intravenous LD_{50} of 694 mg/kg in mice was reported by Hylin and Chin (1968).

In studies with subcutaneous injection, the LD_{50} was 300 mg/kg in rabbits (Merck Index, Christenson and Luginbyhl, 1975); toxic effects have been observed at 1.7 mg/kg in rabbits (Okamoto, 1959). An LD_{50} of 0.1 ml in mice was reported by Yudeles and Bessarabova (1955). Rats showed toxic subcutaneous effects at 1 mg/kg (Okamoto, 1959). Oral administration of carbon disulfide in rats produced toxic effects at 1 mg/kg (Freundt *et al.*, 1974a,b). Vinogradov (1966) showed that 1 ppm in the drinking water was nontoxic to rabbits; 70 ppm proved lethal.

Chronic Effects In a chronic study, Paterni *et al.* (1958) found that 6 mg/kg/day produced toxic effects in rabbits. The lowest lethal chronic dosage for rabbits was later shown to be 0.1 ml three times a week for 7 months (Michalova *et al.*, 1959). Both of these studies used intramuscular administration of carbon disulfide.

In another study, carbon disulfide applied topically produced a higher incidence of anemia in female than in male rats, and teratogenic effects were observed (Gut, 1969). When rats inhaled carbon disulfide at 10 mg/m^3, abnormalities of genitourinary and skeletal systems were found. Disturbances of ossification and blood formation and dystrophic changes in the liver and kidney were also noted (Bariliak *et al.*, 1975).

Mutagenicity No available data.

Carcinogenicity No available data.

Teratogenicity Bariliak *et al.* (1975) showed that the inhalation of 10 mg/m^3 was lethal to embryos before and after implanation. Carbon disulfide at 2.2 g/m^3 for 4 h/day proved embyrotoxic if given to female rats during gestation and had no effect on male rats (Sal'nikova and Chirkova, 1974). Inhalation of lower concentrations (0.34 mg/liter for 210 days caused disturbances of estrus (Rozewiski *et al.*, 1973). In a dominant-lethal test, inhalation of 10 mg/m^3 by male rats before copulation proved lethal to embryos (Bariliak *et al.*, 1975).

Conclusions and Recommendations

Carbon disulfide has been demonstrated to produce distrubances in reproduction as well as teratogenic effects in animals when inhaled. There is no data availale on teratogenicity following oral exposure.

In view of the relative paucity of data on the mutagenicity, carcinogenicity, and long-term oral toxicity of carbon disulfide, estimates of the effects of chronic oral exposure at low levels cannot be made with any confidence. It is recommended that studies to produce such information be conducted before limits in drinking water are established.

Carbon Tetrachloride

Introduction

Over 1 billion pounds of carbon tetrachloride (tetrachloromethane) was produced in the United States in 1973 (USITC, 1975). It is used mostly in the manufacture of chlorofluoromethanes, but also in grain fumigants, fire extinguishers, solvents, and cleaning agents.

Carbon tetrachloride is highly persistent and insoluble in water. Carbon tetrachloride was identified in District of Columbia drinking water at 5 μg/liter (Schneiman *et al.*, 1974). The EPA's 80-city survey showed that it was detected in 10 locations in trace amounts, at 3 μg/liter or less (USEPA, 1975a). The survey of 10 water utilities showed that it was present in eight supplies. The Region V survey of 83 water supplies indicated that carbon tetrachloride is not formed during chlorination water treatment (USEPA, 1975b).

Metabolism

Carbon tetrachloride in rats and humans is rapidly absorbed and distributed and is excreted primarily through the lungs. The excretion products are 85% parent compound, 10% carbon dioxide, and smaller quantities of other products, including chloroform. In animal studies, chloroform, hexachloroethane, and two unidentified metabolites were found in rabbits. The mechanism of metabolism is postulated to be a free-radical pathway (Paul and Rubinstein, 1963; Butler, 1961; Fowler, 1969; Hathway, 1974; Recknagel, 1967).

Health Aspects

Observations in Man Carbon tetrachloride is readily abosrbed from the gastrointestinal tract and by inhalation through the lungs. A fatal dose for children has been reported as low as 3 ml, but there is great variation in individual susceptibility. Intestinal absorption is enhanced by fats, oils, and alcohol (Masoud *et al.*, 1973).

Some persons exposed to carbon tetrachloride will develop severe liver damage with little or no evidence of renal involvement, while others will present with renal shutdown and no hepatic disease. The reasons for this are not known (Eckardt, 1965).

In eight instances of either acute or subacute carbon tetrachloride poisoning seven patients suffered renal insufficiency and six of these required dialysis. Two died from heart failure. None of the six survivors showed any evidence of liver damage (Dume *et al.*, 1969).

Following a large acute exposure the primary finding is of centrilobular necrosis. If exposure is not too massive repair may begin after 3 or 4 days and be complete in 3 weeks. Chronic exposure usually results chiefly in symptoms of gastrointestinal upset such as nausea and vomiting, and nervous system symptoms such as headache, drowsiness, and excessive fatigue. It is rare to find jaundice following either acute or chronic exposure (Browning, 1961).

Gastric symptoms have been reported following chronic inhalation of from 45 to 100 ppm carbon tetrachloride. When exposure is from 100 to 300 ppm the symptoms in addition to gastrointestinal upset include apathy or mental confusion and weight loss (Lewis, 1961).

Observations in Other Species

Acute Effects Oral LD_{50} values are 6.4 (5.4–7.6) ml/kg in young male Wistar rats (McLean and McLean, 1966), 4.73 (4.16–5.38) ml/kg in mature male Sprague–Dawley rats (Pound *et al.*, 1973) and 1.5 ml/kg in male and female mongrel dogs (Klaassen and Plaa, 1967). The intraperitoneal LD_{50} is 2.23 ml/kg in rats (Maling *et al.*, 1974). Toxicity indexes have been set up for both animals and man. Signs and symptoms of toxicity include dyspnea, cyanosis, proteinuria, hematuria, jaundice, hepatomegaly, optic neuritis, ventricular fibrillation, eye–nose–throat irritation, headache, dizziness, nausea, vomiting, abdominal cramps, and diarrhea.

Chronic Effects Biochemical and biologic lesions include hepatic cirrhosis and necrosis, renal damage, changes in blood enzymes (serum glutamic pyruvic transaminase and alkaline phosphatase), and increased serum bilirubin (Busuttil *et al.*, 1972; Litchfield and Gartland, 1974).

A variety of interactions have been described to relate carbon tetrachloride exposure to metabolic inhibitors and inducers and diet. Many studies have reported reduction or potentiation of toxicity indexes, including liver necrosis–cirrhosis and blood enzyme changes (McLean and McLean, 1966; Maling *et al.*, 1974; Barawill and Gornall, 1952; Cawthorne *et al.*, 1970; Traiger and Plaa, 1971; Litterst *et al.*, 1973).

Mutagenicity Carbon tetrachloride was negative in a host-mediated assay using NMRI mice and strains G46 and TA1950 of *Salmonella typhimurium his* (Braun and Schoneich, 1975). Carbon tetrachloride was also negative in an *in vitro Salmonella*/microsome mutagenicity assay (McCann *et al.*, 1975).

Carcinogenicity In a series of studies of the carcinogenic potential of carbon tetrachloride, hepatomas were found in mice, hamsters, and rats after administration by several routes, including oral. There was, however, no evidence of tumors in other organs within the time limits of the experiment (usually less than life span). The tumor response depended on both the dosage and the interval between doses. With intermittent exposure, it was found that total dose and duration were more important than the dosage (IARC, 1972; Murphy, 1975).

In a study with mice, oral administration of 0.1 ml twice a week for 20–26 weeks produced hepatomas that were interpreted by the investigators as indicative of focal nodular hyperplasia, not neoplasia (Confer and Stenger, 1965). Kawasaki (1965) reported that 0.2–0.3 ml/100 g injected subcutaneously every 2 weeks produced a low number of hepatomas in Wistar rats. A 1.3-ml/kg oral dose twice a week for 12 weeks in Buffalo rats was reported to cause cholangiofibrosis from proliferating bile ducts (Ruber and Glover, 1967). Oral administration to Syrian golden hamsters at 6.25–12.5 μl once a week for 30 weeks followed by 25 additional weeks of observation induced liver-cell carcinomas associated with postnecrotic cirrhosis and regenerative hyperplastic nodules (Della-Porta *et al.*, 1961).

Teratogenicity No teratogenic effects were seen when carbontetrachloride was administered to rats (Wilson, 1954).

Carcinogenic Risk Estimates

Carbon tetrachloride has been given orally in a number of studies with mice, rats, hamsters, and dogs (IARC, 1972). It has also been used as a positive control in cancer bioassays (NCI, 1976). In the trichloroethylene study, the carbon tetrachloride positive control produced much higher incidences of hepatocellular carcinomas than did trichloroethylene.

The available sets of dose–response data from the NCI trichloroethylene bioassay were individually considered as described in the risk section in the chapter on margin of safety. Each set of dose–response data was used to statistically estimate both the lifetime risk and an upper 95% confidence bound on the lifetime risk at the low dose level. These estimates are of lifetime human risks and have been corrected for species

TABLE VI-47 Toxicity of Carbon Tetrachloride

Species	Duration of Study	Dosage Levels and No. of Animals Per Group	Highest No-Adverse-Effect Level or Lowest-Minimal-Effect Level	Effect-Measured	Reference
Mouse	20–26 weeks		0.1 ml, twice a week (oral)	Nodular hyperplasia	Confer and Stenger, 1965
Rat	12 weeks		1.3 ml/kg twice a week (oral)	Cholangiofibrosis	Ruber and Glover, 1967
Rat (male)	78 weeks	0, 47, 94 mg/kg/day, 50 animals/group	47 mg/kg/day (oral)	Hepatomas	NCI, 1976
Rat (female)	78 weeks	0, 80, 150 mg/kg/day, 49 animals/group	80 mg/kg/day (oral)	Hepatomas	NCI, 1976
Hamster	30 weeks	6.25–12.5 μl/week, 20 animals	6.25 μl/week (oral)	Hepatomas	Della-Porta *et al.*, 1961

[This compound is an animal carcinogen.]

conversion on a dose-per-surface-area basis. The risk estimates are expressed as a probability of cancer after a lifetime consumption of 1 liter of water/day containing Q ppb of the compound of interest. For example, a risk of 1×10^{-6} Q implies a lifetime probability of 2×10^{-5} of cancer if 2 liters/day were consumed and the concentration of the carcinogen was 10 ppb (i.e., $Q=10$). This means that at a concentration of 10 ppb during a lifetime of exposure this compound would be expected to produce one excess case of cancer for every 50,000 persons exposed. If the population of the United States is taken to be 220 million people, this translates into 4,400 excess lifetime deaths from cancer or 62.8 per year. Since several data sets are typically available the range of the low dose risk estimates are reported. For carbon tetrachloride at a concentration of 1 μg/liter ($Q=1$) the projected risk for man would fall between 4.5-5.4×10^{-8} Q. The upper 95% confidence estimate of risk at the same concentration would be from 1.0–1.1×10^{-7} Q.

Conclusions and Recommendations

The acute-toxicity effects of carbon tetrachloride are best characterized as hepatic nodular hyperplasia and cirrhosis and renal dysfunction in both experimental animals and man. It had no mutagenic potential in *in vitro* and *in vivo* test systems. Its teratogenic potential has not been firmly established. Carcinogenic bioassays have produced hepatomas in mice, rats, and hamsters, associated in most cases with regenerative nodular hyperplasia or postnecrotic cirrhosis.

In light of the above and taking into account the risk projections it is suggested that very strict criteria be applied when limits for carbon tetrachloride in drinking water are established. The available chronic toxicity data are summarized in Table VI-47.

Chloral

Introduction

Chloral (trichloroacetaldehyde) is used in spraying and pouring of polyurethanes. Chloral is very soluble in water. It has been identified in six of the ten water supplies surveyed by EPA (1975a) at 5 μg/liter in the finished water of Philadelphia, 3.5 μg/liter in Seattle, and 2 μg/liter in Cincinnati (USEPA, 1975a).

Metabolism

Chloral is metabolized in man by alcohol dehydrogenase to trichloroethanol. This NADH-dependent reduction takes place in the liver and is accelerated by ethanol which regenerates NADH. Small amounts of chloral are metabolized to trichloroacetic acid. Trichloroethanol is excreted mainly in the urine as a conjugate of glucuronic acid (Goodman and Gilman, 1975).

Health Aspects

Observations in Man Chloral has been used extensively as a hypnotic in its hydrated form, chloral hydrate, which is more stable. It is quite irritating to skin and mucous membranes. A toxic oral dose for adults is approximately 10 g although death has been reported from 4 g. Therapeutic doses (0.5–1.0 g) produce hypnosis through its central depressant activity as well as such unpleasant effects as epigastric distress, nausea, vomiting, light-headedness, malaise, ataxia, and nightmares. An overdose of the compound can cause respiratory and cardiac effects. Chloral hydrate interacts with ethanol to increase skin temperature and heart rate and to inhibit motor reflexes (Goodman and Gilman, 1975).

Some European reports have set a maximal permissible concentration of 0.2 mg/liter (Stoefen, 1973).

Observations in Other Species

Acute Effects Acute oral LD_{50} values of chloral have been established as 285 mg/kg in rats, 1,100 mg/kg in mice, and 1,000 mg/kg in dogs. In an acute inhalation study, chloral hydrate at 0.06 mg/liter of air lowered growth rate in mice; some leukocytosis and decreased albuminobulin ratios were observed (Boitsov *et al.*, 1970). Chloral given to rats at 1 mg/kg altered concentrations of hemoblobin, serum cholesterol, and transaminases and decreased bromsulphalein retention (Kryatov, 1970).

Chloral has been reported to increase plasma prolactin content in rats. Its metabolite, chloral hydrate, inhibits protein synthesis *in vivo* and has been shown to block the metaphase in segmenting eggs, with some alteration in chromosomal structure.

Chronic Effects No available data.

Mutagenicity No available data.

Carcinogenicity No available data.

Teratogenicity No available data.

Conclusions and Recommendations

In view of the relative paucity of data on the mutagenicity, carcinogenicity, teratogenicity, and long-term oral toxicity of chloral, estimates of the effects of chronic oral exposure at low levels cannot be made with any confidence. It is recommended that studies to produce such information be conducted before limits in drinking water are established.

Chlorobenzene

Introduction

Chlorobenzene (Monochlorobenzene) is used in the manufacture of aniline, insecticides, phenol, and chloronitrobenzene and as an intermediate in the manufacture of dyestuffs (USEPA, 1975d). The U.S. production of chlorobenzene in 1973 was over 397 million pounds (USITC, 1975). During chlorination water treatment, chlorobenzene may be formed. It is insoluble in water (CRC Handbook of Chemistry and Physics, 1970–1971). Finished water in 9 of the 10 water supplies surveyed by the EPA (1975a) contained chlorobenzene, with 5.6 μg/liter in Terrebonne Parrish, Louisianna, and 4.7 μg/liter in New York City.

Metabolism

Although many foreign chemicals are metabolized to inactive substances, chlorobenzene appears to be converted to a metabolite that can produce tissue damage. This damage may be blocked by prior administration of piperonyl butoxide. The metabolite is apparently produced in the liver and transported to the kidneys by the circulation. Pretreatment of rats with phenobarbital increases the liver toxicity of chlorobenzene (Norton, 1975; Reid, 1973). Chlorobenzene may be metabolized to *S*-(*p*-chlorophenyl)mercapturic acid by several steps (Reid *et al.*, 1971). The hepatotoxic metabolite may be an epoxide (Sipes *et al.*, 1947) excreted in the bile, reabsorbed, and finally excreted by the kidneys.

Health Aspects

Observations in Man Chlorobenzene is irritating to the respiratory system and is a central nervous system depressant. The USSR has suggested 0.02 mg/liter as the maximal permissible concentration in drinking water (Stoefen, 1973). This was based on odor and taste.

Observations in Other Species

Acute Effects Chlorobenzene has an acute oral LD_{50} of 2,910 mg/kg in rats (Toxic Substances List, 1974).

Chronic Effects The no-effect dosage in rats after 7 months of administration was 0.001 mg/kg/day (Varsharskaya, 1968). Other studies have shown no-effect oral dosages of 54.5 mg/kg in dogs and 12.5 mg/kg in rats (Knapp *et al.*, 1971).

Mutagenicity No available data.

Carcinogenicity No available data.

Teratogenicity No available data.

Conclusions and Recommendations

In view of the relative paucity of data on the mutagenicity, carcinogenicity, teratogenicity, and long-term oral toxicity of chlorobenzene, estimates of the effects of chronic oral exposure at low levels cannot be made with any confidence. It is recommended that studies to produce such information be conducted before limits in drinking water are established.

***bis*(2-Chloroethyl)ether**

Introduction

bis(2-Chloroethyl)ether (dichloroethyl ether) is used as a soil fumigant; as an insecticide and acaricide; as a solvent for fats, waxes, greases, and cellulose esters; as a scouring agent for textiles; in paints, varnishes, and lacquers; as a paint remover; in dry cleaning; and in the manufacture of medicinals and pharmaceuticals (USEPA, 1975d).

bis(2-Chloroethyl)ether is moderately persistent and insoluble in water.

It can be formed during chlorination water treatment when ethyl ether is present. *bis*(2-Chloroethyl)ether has been identified in finished water at 0.5 μg/liter in Philadelphia and 0.44 μg/liter in New Orleans (USEPA, 1975a,c).

Metabolism

No data are available on the metabolism, absorption, or excretion of *bis*(2-chloroethyl)ether.

Health Aspects

Observations in Man Shrenk *et al.* (1933) exposed humans to *bis*(2-chloroethyl)ether and found that a concentration of 550 ppm was intolerable and caused irritation of the eyes and nasal passages. Concentrations of 100 ppm and 260 ppm were irritating, but tolerable; at 35 ppm, there was no irritation, but a nauseous odor persisted.

Observations in Other Species

Acute Effects The oral LD_{50} has been given as 75–150 mg/kg in rats (Smyth and Carpenter, 1948; Spector, 1956; Hake and Rowe, 1963) and 136 mg/kg and 126 mg/kg in mice and rabbits, respectively (Spector, 1956). The cutaneous LD_{50} was 410 mg/kg (Spector, 1956) and 90 mg/kg (Hake and Rowe, 1963) in rabbits and 0.3 ml/kg in guinea pigs (Smyth and Carpenter, 1948). Smyth and Carpenter (1948) reported that the material caused moderate to severe irritation to rabbits' eyes, but that apparent healing occurred within 24 h. They also exposed six rats to 1,000 ppm for 45 m. Three of the rats died within 14 days. In another inhalation study in rats (Carpenter *et al.*, 1949), exposure at 250 ppm for 4 h killed some exposed rats. In guinea pigs, 500–1,000 ppm produced immediate severe eye and nasal irritation, and exposure for 1.5-3.0 h caused respiratory disturbances and deaths with pulmonary lesions (Shrenk, 1933).

Chronic Effects In chronic studies, rats and guinea pigs were exposed to *bis*(2-chloroethyl)ether at an average of 414 mg/m³ for 2 h/day, 5 days/week, for 93 exposures during 130 days. No serious injury and only mild physiologic stress were noted (Hake and Rowe, 1963).

Mutagenicity No available data.

Carcinogenicity Berenblum (1935) painted a 1.0% solution in acetone on mice for 15 weeks and found no irritation. Van Duuren *et al.* (1972) applied *bis*(2-chloroethyl)ether in benzene once to mouse skin as an initiator and then applied phorbol myristate three times a week for 590 days. The compound did not show tumor-initiating activity. The same authors reported the development of sarcomas at two sites of injection out of 30 mice receiving one 1-mg subcutaneous injection of *bis*(2-chloroethyl)ether per week for their life spans. Seventy two mice were given oral *bis*(2-chloroethyl)ether at 100 mg/kg/day from week 7–28 of life. Afterwards, 300 ppm was fed in the diet until the age of 80 weeks. Male mice of two strains and the females of one strain had an increased incidence of hepatomas (Innes *et al.*, 1969). In another study rats were given 50 mg/kg and 25 mg/kg by intubation three times per week for 18 months and followed for 6 months. The compound was not carcinogenic (Ulland *et al.*, 1973).

Teratogenicity No available data.

Carcinogenic Risk Estimates

bis(2-Chloroethyl)ether has produced dose-related hepatomas when given orally to mice (Innes *et al.*, 1969). The female mice of one strain did not develop any hepatomas. The available sets of dose–response data were individually considered as described in the risk section in the chapter on margin of safety. Each set of dose–response data was used to statistically estimate both the lifetime risk and an upper 95% confidence bound on the lifetime risk at the low dose level. These estimates are of lifetime human risks and have been corrected for species conversion on a dose per surface area basis. The risk estimates are expressed as a probability of cancer after a lifetime consumption of 1 liter of water/day containing Q ppb of the compound of interest. For example a risk of $1\times10^{-6}\ Q$ implies a lifetime probability of 2×10^{-5} of cancer if 2 liters/day were consumed and the concentration of the carcinogen was 10 ppb (i.e., $Q=10$). This means that at a concentration of 10 ppb during a lifetime of exposure this compound would be expected to produce one excess case of cancer for every 50,000 persons exposed. If the population of the United States is taken to be 220 million people, this translates into 4,400 excess lifetime deaths from cancer or 62.8 per year. For *bis*(2-chloroethyl)ether at a concentration of 1 μg/liter ($Q=1$) the estimated risk for both sexes is $8.1\times10^{-7}\ Q$. The upper 95% confidence estimate is $1.2\times10^{-6}\ Q$.

Conclusions and Recommendations

Even though the acute and chronic effects of *bis*(2-chloroethyl)ether have not been fully established it has been shown to produce dose-related tumors when given orally to mice.

In view of this potential in humans and taking the risk estimates into account, it is suggested that very strict criteria be applied when limits for *bis*(2-chloroethyl)ether in drinking water are established.

The available chronic toxicity data are summarized in Table VI-48.

Chloroform

Introduction

The chief uses (96%) of chloroform, or trichloromethane (after conversion to chlorodifluoromethane), in the United States since 1970 have been as a refrigerant and aerosol propellant and in the synthesis of fluorinated resins. The remainder has been used as an industrial solvent, as a heat-transfer medium in fire extinguishers (with carbon tetrachloride), and as a pesticide (IARC, 1972) and was used directly in pharmaceuticals and toiletries. The FDA has issued final regulations to ban chloroform as an ingredient in any human drugs or cosmetic products effective July 29, 1976 (*Federal Register,* vol. 41, no. 126, June 1976). The U.S. production of chloroform in 1973 was over 250 million pounds (USITC, 1975).

Chloroform is not biodegradable in water. Its solubility is 1 ml/200 ml of water at 25°C (Merck Index, 1968). Chloroform is produced during chlorination water treatment. The recent EPA water-supply surveys of finished chlorinated drinking water indicated that 95–100% of the finished waters surveyed contained chloroform. The mean concentration was 20 μg/liter; the highest was 311 μg/liter, in Miami (USEPA, 1975a,b).

Metabolism

Chloroform is rapidly absorbed, distributed throughout body fat depots and tissues, and excreted rapidly in mice, rats, and humans. It is metabolized in part to carbon dioxide and methylene chloride. Free-radical formation is postulated from enzymatic degradation of the carbon-halogen bond, to account for hepatic damage. Inhibitors and activators of metabolizing enzymes have been found to alter tissue binding and subsequent renal and hepatic necrosis (Van Poznak, 1974; Cascorbi, 1973; Paul and Rubinstein, 1963; Fry *et al.*, 1972; Butler, 1961; Ilett *et al.*, 1973; Brown *et al.*, 1974).

TABLE VI-48 Toxicity of *Bis* (2-Chloroethyl) Ether

Species	Duration of Study	Dosage Levels and No. of Animals Per Group	Highest No-Adverse-Effect Level or Lowest-Minimal-Effect Level	Effect Measured	Reference
Rat	130 days		414 mg/m^3 (inhalation)	mild physiologic stress	Hake and Rowe, 1963
Mouse	80 weeks	0–100 mg/kg/day	100 mg/kg/day (oral)	hepatomas	Innes *et al.*, 1969

[This compound is a suspected animal carcinogen.]

Health Aspects

Observations in Man In a chronic clinical study, dentifrice containing 3.4% chloroform and mouthwash with 0.43% chloroform were given to subjects for 1–5 yr. The estimated daily ingestion was 0.3–0.96 mg/kg; no hepatotoxicity was observed (DeSalva *et al.*, 1975). In a 10-yr clinical study, daily ingestion of 1.6–2.6 g of chloroform in a cough suppressant, roughly equivalent to 23–37 mg/kg/day, resulted in some reversible hepatotoxicity (Wallace, 1959).

The NIOSH (1974) recommended the occupational exposure to chloroform at not in excess of 10 ppm determined as time-weighted average exposure for up to a 10-h workday.

Observations in Other Species

Acute Effects Oral LD_{50} values have been calculated for a variety of experimental animals: 0.8 (0.7–0.9), 0.9 (0.8–1.1), and 0.3 (0.2–0.5) ml/kg in Sprague–Dawley male rats weighing 300–470 g, males weighing 80–160 g, and males and females weighing 16–50 g, respectively (Kimura *et al.*, 1971); 0.33 (0.26–0.40), 0.20 (0.16–0.24), and 0.08 (0.07–0.10) ml/kg in male C5Bl/6, B6D2Fl/j, and DBA/2J mice, respectively (Hill *et al.*, 1975); and 1.0 ml/kg in male and female dogs. The intraperitoneal LD_{50} was 1.2 (1.0–1.3) ml/kg in male Swiss-Webster mice weighing 25–35 g (Klaassen and Ploa, 1966).

Mutagenicity No available data.

Carcinogenicity The carcinogenic effects of chloroform have been examined in mice and rats. A-strain mice were orally dosed with 0.1–1.6 ml/kg every 4 days for 30 doses. All experimental females survived, but hepatoma associated with liver necrosis was produced at 0.4 ml/kg. Of the five experimental males, three survived. Of the survivors, none had hepatoma or liver necrosis at 0.2 ml/kg, but 0.1 ml/kg induced kidney necrosis in males and not in females (Eschenbrenner, 1945).

In another study, $B6C3F_1$ strain male and female mice were given oral doses of chloroform at 138 or 277 mg/kg and 238 or 477 mg/kg, respectively, five times a week for 78 weeks. Animals were sacrificed at 92–93 weeks; hepatocellular carcinoma was observed in all groups. Nodular hyperplasia was found in low-dosage males without carcinomas. In male and female Osborne–Mendel rats, chloroform at 90 or 180 mg/kg in males and 100 or 200 mg/kg in females five times a week for 78 weeks produced kidney epithelial tumors; 24% occurred in high-dosage males and 8% in low-dosage males. Benign thyroid tumors were seen in the females (NCI, 1976).

Teratogenicity In a study to examine the teratogenicity of oral chloroform in rats and rabbits, subjects were given 20, 50, or 126 mg/kg on days 6–18 of gestation. Although there was no evidence of teratogenicity, offspring of both species had reduced weights (Thompson *et al.*, 1974).

Carcinogenic Risk Estimates

In a recent study conducted by the National Cancer Insitute (NCI) (1976), chloroform was administered to rats and mice orally in corn oil by gavage. Dose–response relationships were found for epithelial tumors of the kidneys and renal pelvis in the rats and hepatocellular carcinomas in the mice. The estimated risks for the mice and the rats were comparable within an order of magnitude.

A study by Roe (1976) also reported an increased incidence of hepatocellular carcinoma in female rats and in one strain of male mice when dosed orally with chloroform. When these results and those of the NCI are extrapolated, the risk extimates are remarkably consistent.

The available sets of dose–response data (Roe, 1976; NCI, 1976) were individually considered as described in the risk section in the chapter on margin of safety. Each set of dose–response data was used to statisically estimate both the life-time risk and an upper 95% confidence bound on the lifetime risk at the low-dose level. These estimates are of lifetime human risks and have been corrected for species conversion on a dose-per-surface-area basis. The risk estimates are expressed as a probability of cancer after a lifetime consumption of 1 liter of water/day containing Q/ppb of the compound of interest. For example a risk of $1\times10^{-6}\ Q$ implies a life-time probability of 2×10^{-5} of cancer if 2 liters/day were consumed and the concentration of the carcinogen was 10 ppb (i.e., $Q=10$). This means that at a concentration of 10 ppb during a lifetime of exposure this compound would be expected to produce one excess case of cancer for every 50,000 persons exposed. If the population of the United States is taken to be 220 million people, this translates into 4,400 excess lifetime deaths from cancer or 62.8 per year. Since several data sets are typically available the range of the low-dose risk estimates are reported. For chloroform at a concentration of 1 μg/liter ($Q=1$) the estimated risk for man would fall between 1.5-$17.0\times10^{-7}\ Q$. The upper 95% confidence estimate of risk at the same concentration would fall between 3.0-$22.0\times10^{-7}\ Q$.

Conclusions and Recommendations

Acute toxicity of chloroform to experimental animals and man is characterized by hepatic and renal lesions and damage, including necrosis and cirrhosis. This material, although highly embryotoxic, is apparently not highly teratogenic. Mutagenicity studies were not found in the literature. A carcinogenicity bioassay in mice demonstrated hepatomas in one study that were associated with liver necrosis; the number of animals used in each group was not adequate for statistical analysis. In a recent study with mice and rats, hepatocellular carcinomas and hepatic nodular hyperplasia were observed in both male and female mice, whereas kidney epithelial tumors were seen only in male rats. Data strongly support the contention that chloroform is carcinogenic in at least one strain of mouse and one strain of rat.

In light of the above and taking into account the risk projections, it is suggested that strict criteria be applied when limits for chloroform in drinking water are established.

The available chronic toxicity data are summarized in Table VI-49.

Cyanogen Chloride

Introduction

Cyanogen chloride (chlorine cyanide) is used in organic synthesis, tear gas, and fumigant gases. It is soluble in water (CRC Handbook of Chemistry and Physics, 1970–1971) and has been detected in the finished water of 8 of the 10 water supplies surveyed by the EPA (NORS, USEPA 1975a).

Metabolism

An *in vitro* study by Aldridge (1951) on cyanogen chloride metabolism in rat blood showed that hemoglobin and glutathione rapidly metabolize cyanogen chloride to cyanide. The glutathione is the key metabolizing agent. Hemoglobin transforms cyanogen chloride to a compound that is later metabolized by glutathione, to liberate cyanide (Aldridge, 1951). Although red cells convert cyanogen chloride to hydrogen cyanide, serum decomposes cyanogen chloride without producing hydrogen cyanide. The toxicity of cyanogen chloride is due to the formation of hydrogen cyanide (Aldridge and Evans, 1946).

TABLE VI-49 Toxicity of Chloroform

Species	Duration of Study	Dosage Levels and No. of Animals Per Group	Highest No-Adverse-Effect Level or Lowest-Minimal-Effect Level	Effect Measured	Reference
Mouse	96 weeks	0, 17, 60 mg/kg/day, 35–38 animals/group	60 mg/kg/day (oral)	Renal tumors	Roe, 1976
Mouse	96 weeks	0, 17, 60 mg/kg/day, 35–38 animals/group	17 mg/kg/day (oral)	Liver tumors	Roe, 1976
Rat	96 weeks	0.60 mg/kg/day, 49 animals/group	60 mg/kg/day (oral)	Total tumors	Roe, 1976
Rat	lifetime	0, 90, 180 mg/kg/day, 50 animals/group	90 mg/kg/day (oral)	Kidney tumors	NCI, 1976

[This compound is an animal carcinogen.]

Health Aspects

Observations in Man The effects of the inhalation of cyanogen chloride in man were examined in two studies by Flury (1931, 1941). It was found that the lowest lethal concentration (LC_{50}) was 48 ppm, and the lowest irritant concentration, 1 ppm.

Observations in Other Species

Acute Effects The effects of acute cyanogen chloride inhalation have been examined in a series of experimental animals. The LC_{50}'s have been reported as follows: in rats, 118 ppm in 30 min; in mice, 177 ppm in 30 min; in guinea pigs, 207 ppm in 30 min; in rabbits, 207 ppm in 30 min (Registry of Toxic Effects of Chemical Substances, 1975); in goats, 1.8 ppm in 2 min; in dogs, 48 ppm in 6 h; and in cats, 40 ppm in 18 min (Flury and Zernick 1931). The intravenous administration of cyanogen chloride in rats yielded an LD_{50} of 4 mg/kg (Leitch and Bauer, 1945). Subcutaneous administration of the compound in mice, dogs, and rabbits yielded LD_{50} values of 39, 5, and 20 mg/kg, respectively (Registry of Toxic Effects of Chemical Substances, 1975). The oral acute LD_{50} in rats was 6 mg/kg (Leitch and Bauer, 1945). Allen *et al.* (1948) studied the formation of cyanogen chloride by chlorination of sewage effluent; the threshold concentration for toxicity to fish at 17–22°C was 0.08 ppm.

The effects of subchronic, oral administration of cyanogen chloride in drinking water were examined in mice. Although 1 week of exposure produced no weight loss, one death was observed on the first day (National Defense Research Committee, 1943).

Chronic Effects No available data.

Mutagenicity No available data.

Carcinogenicity No available data.

Teratogenicity No available data.

Conclusions and Recommendations

The acute toxicity of cyanide is well known, but the chronic toxicity has been less studied.

In view of the relative paucity of data on the mutagenicity, carcinogenicity, teratogenicity, and long-term oral toxicity of cyanogen chloride, estimates of the effects of chronic oral exposure at low levels cannot be made with any confidence. It is recommended that studies to produce such information be conducted before limits in drinking water are established.

Di-*n*-Butylphthalate

Introduction

Di-*n*-butylphthalate (DBP) is used in the manufacture of plasticizers, plastics, and in cosmetics, explosives, solid rocket propellant, textile lubricating agents, safety glass, insecticides, printing inks, paper coatings, and adhesive (USEPA, 1975d). The U.S. production of di-*n*-butylphthalate in 1973 was about 38 million pounds (USITC, 1975).

This compound is insoluble in water (CRC Handbook of Chemistry and Physics, 1970–1971) and very persistent in the environment (USEPA, 1975d). Six of the 10 water supplies surveyed by the EPA (1975a) contained di-*n*-butylphthalate; the highest concentration was 5 μg/liter in Miami.

Metabolism

Williams (1959) suggested that di-*n*-butylphthalate is one of the phthalate esters likely to be hydrolyzed *in vivo*, yielding phthalic acid and an alcohol. No accumulation of dibutylphthalate or monobutylphthalate was found by Williams and Blanchfield (1975) in tissues of rats fed di-*n*-butylphthalate at 1 g/kg of feed for 12 weeks. These authors reported that 80-90% of a dose of [^{14}C]di-*n*-butylphthalate was metabolized and excreted in the urine in 48 h. Phthalic acid, monobutylphthalate, mono(3-hydroxybutyl)phthalic acid, and mono (4-hydroxybutyl)phthalate were found in the urine. Smith (1953) found that DBP was hydrolyzed *in vitro* by pancreatic lipases; this suggested that it is metabolized like fat that is normally in the diet.

Health Aspects

Observations in Man Fairhall (1957) reviewed a report of an accidental ingestion of 10 g of DBP. Hours after ingestion, the patient was nauseous and giddy. His eyes were inflamed and painful, with photophobia and lacrimation. Toxic nephritis occurred, and his urine contained red and white cells and albumin. The patient recovered fully.

Observations in Other Species

Acute Effects Di-*n*-butylphthalate has low acute and chronic toxicity. The single-dose oral LD_{50} in animals is reported to be 9 g/kg (Smith, 1953) and 12.5 g/kg (Nikonorow *et al.*, 1973). The intraperitoneal LD_{50} is reported to be 6.76–4.0 g/kg in mice (Hodge *et al.*, 1942; Karel *et al.*, 1947; Calley *et al.*, 1966).

Chronic Effects Smith (1953) fed rats a diet of 1.25% DBP for 1 yr. The dose was 1,600 mg/kg at the start and 525 mg/kg at termination. Half the rats died in the first week; those sacrificed at 1 yr had no specific gross or microscopic pathologic effects. Nikonorow *et al.* (1973) fed rats 0.125% of DPB in the diet for 1 yr and recorded six deaths in the 40 rats, compared with four in 40 untreated control rats. Daily intubation of 0.12 g/kg and 1.20 g/kg for 3 months produced only a single death at the high dosage in rats (Piekacz, 1971a). Both dosages were reported, however, to produce enlargement of the liver. Shibko and Blumenthal (1973) reported no effects in dogs given 18 mg/kg/day for 1 yr.

Mutagenicity No available data.

Carcinogenicity No chronic studies with animals have revealed signs of carcinogenesis at the time of death.

Teratogenicity Teratogenic effects of DBP were identified in a study by Singh *et al.* (1972a). Rats were given one-tenth, one-fifth, and one-third of the LD_{50} (3.2 g/kg) intraperitoneally on day 5, 10, or 15 of gestation. Partially dose-related resorption and a 20–30% incidence of skeletal abnormalities were found at the high dosage. Studies by Bower *et al.* (1970) in chicken eggs showed 79% mortality at 0.1 ml, 67% at 0.05 ml, compared with 47% for the oil controls.

Reproduction Reproduction studies reported by Piekacz (1971b) included treating female rats with DBP at 0.60 and 0.12 mg/kg for 3 months before mating. The low dosage produced two resorptions, the high dosage 22, and the controls four. Piekacz (1971b) also gave rats DBP orally daily at 1% or 5% of the LD_{50} for 12 weeks. The numbers of fetuses and resorption sites were statistically different in the 5% group as compared to the controls. Other groups of 10 rats were intubated daily with 1% and 5%

TABLE VI-50 Toxicity of di-*n*-Butyl-Phthalate

Species	Duration of Study	Dosage Levels and No. of Animals Per Group	Highest No-Adverse-Effect Level or Lowest-Minimal-Effect Level	Effect Measured	Reference
Rat	1 yr	0–525 mg/kg/day, 10 animals/group	110 mg/kg/day[c] (oral)	no adverse effect	Smith, 1953
Rat	1 yr	0, 0.125%, 40 animals/group	0.125% (oral)	no adverse effect	Nikonorow *et al.*, 1973

Using an uncertainty factor of 1,000, the suggested no-adverse-effect level in drinking water is calculated as follows:

$$\frac{110}{1{,}000} = 0.11 \text{ mg/kg/day (ADI)},\ 0.11 \times 70^{a} \times 0.1^{b} = 0.77 \text{ mg/liter}$$

[a]Assume average weight of human adult = 70 kg.

[b]Assume average daily intake of water for man = 2 liters, and that 20 percent of total intake is from water.

[c]Value from which the suggested no-adverse-effect level was calculated.

of the LD_{50} during pregnancy. The number of fetuses was reduced, and resorptions increased. DBP had a greater adverse effect than di(2-ethylhexyl)phthalate, with which it was compared.

Conclusions and Recommendations

The major effect of di-*n*-butylphthalate in animals involves disturbances in reproduction and teratogenicity. There is no data available on mutagenicity, and the chronic feeding studies did not show any evidence of carcinogenicity.

An ADI was calculated, on the basis of the chronic toxicity data, to be 0.11 mg/kg/day. The calculations and available chronic toxicity data are summarized in Table VI-50.

1,2-Dichloroethane

Introduction

1,2-Dichloroethane (ethylene dichloride) is used in the manufacture of vinyl chloride and tetraethyl lead; as an insecticidal fumigant; in tobacco flavoring; as a constituent of paint, varnish, and finish removers; as a metal degreaser; in soap and scouring compounds; in wetting and penetrating agents; and in chemical synthesis and ore flotation (USEPA, 1975d). The U.S. production was over 9 billion pounds in 1973 (USITC, 1975).

1,2-Dichloroethane is difficult to degrade biologically. One part is soluble in about 120 parts of water (Merck Index, 1968). The Region V survey of 83 water supplies concluded that it is not produced during chlorination of water. The survey also indicated that 13% of the finished water contained 1,2-dichloroethane, at a mean concentration of 1 μg/liter (USEPA, 1975b). Of the 80 water supplies surveyed in 1974, 26 contained 1,2-dichloroethane, at less than 0.2 to 6 μg/liter (USEPA, 1975a). A concentration of 8 μg/liter has been reported in New Orleans finished water (USEPA, 1974).

Metabolism

1,2-Dichloroethane is rapidly absorbed after oral or pulmonary exposure (Morgan *et al.*, 1970). It is metabolized in mice by enzymatic dehalogenation and oxidation through the 2-chloroethanol intermediate to the chloroacetic acid excretion product (Yllner, 1971). Both enzymatic dehalogenation and oxidation appear to take place in the liver (Morgan *et al.*, 1970). The principle target organs in the mouse are the liver, kidneys, and adrenals (Plaa and Larson, 1965).

Health Aspects

Observations in Man In man, exposure to high vapor concentrations of 1,2-dichloroethane results in irritation of the eyes, nose, and throat. Continued or repeated exposure to concentrations above the response threshold produce central nervous system depression and injury to the liver, kidneys, and adrenals (American National Standards Institute, 1970; AIHA, 1956, 1965). The accidental oral ingestion of a single dose of 0.5–1.0 g/kg has been reported to result in death; autopsy revealed liver necrosis and focal adrenal degeneration and necrosis (Wirtschafter and Schwartz, 1939; Yodaiken and Babcock, 1973).

Observations in Other Species

Acute Effects The acute oral LD_{50} of 1,2-dichloroethane has been established at 0.77 (0.67-0.89) ml/kg in rats (Smyth *et al.*, 1969). LC_{50} values for vapor inhalation are 12,000 ppm in 0.53 h, 3,000 ppm in 2.75 h, and 1,000 ppm in 7.20 h in rats (Spencer *et al.*, 1951). In one study with rabbits, the LD_{50} for skin penetration was determined to be 3.89 (3.40-54.46) ml/kg. The toxic effects of single acute exposures to 1,2-dichloroethane were central nervous system depression, lung irritation, and injury to the liver, kidneys, and adrenals (Gohlke and Schmidt, 1972).

Chronic Effects When animals were exposed to 1,2-dichloroethane vapor for 7 h/day, 5/days/week, for 6 months, the maximal concentrations that produced no adverse effect were 400 ppm in rabbits, 200 ppm in rats, and 100 ppm in monkeys and guinea pigs (Heppel *et al.*, 1946; Yllner, 1971). Significant chronic changes at higher concentrations included hepatic and renal damage. In other chronic studies, 500 ppm was not tolerated by rats, guinea pigs, or rabbits, and significant mortality occurred in the first 2 weeks; more than 90% of the animals were dead by the end of the fourth week. All the animals tolerated 100 ppm for a 17-week period (Yllner *et al.*, 1971; Hofman *et al.*, 1971).

Mutagenicity Brem *et al.*, (1974) have reported a mutagenic effect of 1,2-dichloroethane in *S. typhimurium* and DNA polymerase-deficient *E. coli*. It was the weakest, however, of the series of haloalkanes tested.

Carcinogenicity No available data.

Teratogenicity No available data.

Conclusions and Recommendations

1,2-Dichloroethane has been shown to be weakly mutagenic in two different mutagenicity screening tests. No data are available on its potential carcinogenicity.

In view of the relative paucity of data on teratogenicity, carcinogenicity, and long-term oral toxicity of 1,2-dichloroethane, estimates of the effects of chronic oral exposure at low levels cannot be made with any confidence. It is recommended that studies to produce such information be conducted before final limits in drinking water are established.

2,4-Dichlorophenol

Introduction

2,4-Dichlorophenol is used mainly in organic synthesis. In the aquatic environment 2,4-D (2,4-dichlorophenoxyacetic acid) is decomposed to 2,4-dichlorophenol by sunlight and then to simpler compounds. 2,4-Dichlorophenol is slightly soluble in water (CRC Handbook of Chemistry and Physics, 1970–1971) and the highest concentration detected in United States drinking water was 36 μg/liter (USEPA, 1975a).

Metabolism

2,4-Dichlorophenol is excreted as a conjugate of glucuronic acid. Up to 16% may be excreted as sulfate in the urine of rabbits.

Health Aspects

Observations in Man No studies have been conducted to determine the effects of 2,4-dichlorophenol in man.

Observations in Other Species

Acute Effects The effects of an acute oral dose of 2,4-dichlorophenol have been examined in a variety of experimental animals; the oral LD_{50} is 1.63 g/kg in mice and 4.5 g/kg in male rats (Kobayaski *et al.*, 1972). On acute, subcutaneous administration, the LD_{50} was 1.73 g/kg in rats (Deichman, 1943). The intraperitoneal LD_{50} was 420 mg/kg in rats (Farquharson, *et al.*, 1958).

Chronic Effects In a study of the chronic effects of 2,4-dichlorophenol, it was found that the maximum dose-producing no-observed-adverse-effect in mice was 100 mg/kg/day (Kobayaski *et al.*, 1972). Kongiel-Chablo (1968) found that the administration of 0.2–2,000 mg/liter in the drinking water produced no effects, either on cholinesterase or on serum glutamic oxaloacetic transaminase (SGOT) in rats.

Mutagenicity No available data.

Carcinogenicity Boutwell and Bosch (1959) found that the topical application of 0.3% dimethylbenzanthracene in benzene as an initiator and 20% (312 mg/kg) 2,4-dichlorophenol for 39 weeks promoted papillomas and carcinomas in mice.

Teratogenicity No available data.

Conclusions and Recommendations

There is one report suggesting that topical 1,2-dichlorophenol may act as a cocarcinogen in promoting papillomas and carcinomas in mouse skin.

In view of the relative paucity of data on the mutagenicity, carcinogenicity, teratogenicity, and long-term oral toxicity of 2,4-dichlorophenol, estimates of the effects of chronic oral exposure at low levels cannot be made with any confidence. It is recommended that studies to produce such information be conducted before limits in drinking water are established.

Di(2-ethylhexyl)phthalate

Introduction

Di(2-ethylhexyl)phthalate (DEHP) is commercially produced by the reaction of 2-ethylhexyl alcohol and phthalic anhydride. It is used in the manufacture of plasticizer, plastics, and organic pump fluid (USEPA, 1975d). The U.S. production of di(2-ethylhexyl)phthalate in 1973 was over 378 million pounds (USITC, 1975).

Di(2-ethylhexyl)phthalate is insoluble (CRC Handbook of Chemistry and Physics, 1970–1971) and biologically persistent in water (USEPA,

1975d). Four of the 10 finished waters analyzed by EPA contained this compound; the highest concentration was 30 μg/liter in Miami (USEPA, 1975a). The Region V survey indicated that di(2-ethylhexyl)phthalate was present in 20 of 53 finished-water supplies; the highest concentration was 17 μg/liter, in Cincinnati (USEPA, 1975b).

Metabolism

Shaffer *et al.* (1945) studied the metabolism of di(2-ethylhexyl)phthalate in rats, rabbits, dogs, and man, and it was shown to be hydrolyzed in all four. Oral doses were not completely absorbed. Dogs excreted 4–5% of an oral 2 g/kg dose as phthalate in 3 days, but rabbits excreted 26–65% phthalate in the same period. In man, 4–5% of a 10 g dose has been shown to be excreted as phthalate in the urine.

Williams and Blanchfield (1974) gave [^{14}C]DEHP as a single oral dose or in the diet to rats and found only limited retention and accumulation. Virtually all was excreted in urine or feces within 48 h. If the concentration was over 0.2% of the diet, the metabolic products were found in the feces. If only 10 ppm was fed, all excreted metabolic products were in the urine. Intravenous injected [^{14}C]DEHP in rats at 0.1 mg/kg was almost totally excreted as water-soluble metabolites in 24 h, according to Schulz and Rubin (1973).

Health Aspects

Observations in Man A dose of 10 g of DEHP in humans caused mild gastric disturbance and catharsis (Shaffer *et al.*, 1945).

Observations in Other Species

Acute Effects The single-dose oral LD_{50} of DEHP is variously reported to be from 26 to 34 g/kg in rats (Hodge, 1943; Shaffer *et al.*, 1945; Fassett, 1963; and Nikonorow *et al.*, 1973). Others have reported similarly high LD_{50}'s by other routes of administration and in other species (Calley *et al.*, 1966; Lawrence *et al.*, 1975).

Chronic Effects Nikonorow *et al.* (1973) fed DEHP at 0.35% to rats for 12 months and produced 30% mortality. Harris *et al.* (1956) fed various concentrations in the diet of rats and reported that those fed 0.5% for 2 yr had lower weight gain, and enlarged livers and kidneys, but no

TABLE VI-51 Toxicity of di(2-ethyl hexyl)phthalate

Species	Duration of Study	Dosage Levels and No. of Animals Per Group	Highest No-Adverse-Effect Level or Lowest-Minimal-Effect Level	Effect Measured	Reference
Rat	2 yr	0–0.2 g/kg/day, 64 animals/group	0.06 g/kg/day[c] (oral)	no adverse effect	Carpenter *et al.*, 1953
Guinea pig	1 yr	0–0.64 g/kg/day, 46 animals/group	0.019 g/kg/day (oral)	no adverse effect	Carpenter *et al.*, 1953
Rat	2 yr	0–0.4 g/kg/day, 86 animals/group	0.04–0.08 g/kg/day (oral)	no adverse effect	Harris *et al.*, 1956

Using an uncertainty factor of 100, the suggested no-adverse-effect level in drinking water is calculated as follows:

$$\frac{60}{100} = 0.6 \text{ mg/kg/day (ADI)},\ 0.6 \times 70^{a} \times 0.1^{b} = 4.2 \text{ mg/liter}$$

[a]Assume average weight of human adult = 70 kg.
[b]Assume average daily intake of water for man = 2 liters, and that 20 percent of total intake is from water.
[c]Value from which the suggested no-adverse-effect level was calculated.

micropathology. The 0.1% group was found to be comparable with the controls after 2 yr.

When DEHP was given to rats at 2,000 mg/kg/day for 21 days, partial hydrolysis to the monoester was associated with the development of hepatomegaly, dilation of the endoplasmic reticulum and mitochondria, and changes in the activity of several enzymes (Lake *et al.*, 1975). Carpenter *et al.* (1953) fed DEHP to rats for 2 yr and suggested that the no-adverse-effect dosage was 0.06–0.20 g/kg/day. In both guinea pigs and dogs fed for 1 yr, the same authors found the no-adverse-effect dosage to be 0.06 g/kg/day.

Mutagenicity No available data.

Carcinogenicity In subacute and chronic feeding studies with rats, guinea pigs, and dogs by Carpenter *et al.* (1953), Harris *et al.* (1956), and Nikonorow *et al.* (1973) there were no increased instances of tumor formation, compared with controls, in any of the test species.

Teratogenicity Nikonorow *et al.* (1973) studied the effect of DEHP (given before and during gestation) on reproduction in rats and found slightly lower fetal weights at 0.34 and 1.7 g/kg/day and slightly reduced placental weight at 1.7 g/kg/day. Peters and Cook (1973) found adverse effects on implantation under some conditions. Singh *et al.* (1972) studied the teratogenic potential of DEHP by intraperitoneal injections in rats on various days of gestation and found some gross fetal abnormalities and resorptions at 10 ml/kg. The chick embryo test reported by Bower *et al.* (1970) produced no abnormalities. Prehatching death was more common in controls than in test samples.

Massive single doses of DEHP (12.78, 19.17, and 25.56 ml/kg) in male mice produced changes in the percent of females impregnated, implants per pregnancy, fetal deaths per pregnancy, and litter size per pregnancy in inseminated females. Half the members of the 25.56 ml/kg group died (Singh *et al.*, 1974).

Conclusions and Recommendations

The available data on di(2-ethylhexyl)phthalate do not suggest that it might be a health hazard at the concentrations at which it has been found.

An ADI was calculated, on the basis of the chronic toxicity data, to be 0.6 μg/kg/day. The calculations and available chronic toxicity data are summarized in Table VI-51.

2,4-Dimethylphenol

Introduction

2,4-Dimethylphenol is one of the five isomers of xylenol (dimethylphenol). It is the cresylic acid or tar acid fraction of coal tar. It is used principally in the manufacture of phenolic antioxidants, pharmaceuticals, plastics, resins, solvents, disinfectants, insecticides, fungicides, rubber chemicals, wetting agents, and dyestuff (USEPA, 1975d). It is slightly soluble in water and has been found in finished water (USEPA, 1976).

Metabolism

The metabolism of 2,4-dimethylphenol in animals is very similar to that of the cresols. In rabbits the average percentages of metabolites isolated included: 2% as free nonacidic phenol; 13% as ethereal sulfate; 46% as ether glucuronide; and 64% as ether-soluble acid (Bray *et al.*, 1950).

Health Aspects

Observations in Man The adverse health effects of 2,4-dimethylphenol in man have not been examined.

Observation in Other Species

Acute Effects The effects of acute oral administration of 2,4-dimethylphenol have been examined in mice, rats, and rabbits. The oral LD_{50}'s are 809 mg/kg in mice (Uzhdovini *et al.*, 1974) and 3,200 mg/kg in rats (Registry of Toxic Effects of Chemical Substances, 1975; Uzhdovini *et al.*, 1974). No appreciable toxic effect has been seen at 273–425 mg/kg in rabbits (Uzhdovini *et al.*, 1974). Topical administration has been shown to be lethal to mice at 5,600 mg/kg; the topical LD_{50} in mice is 1,040 mg/kg (Registry of Toxic Effects of Chemical Substances, 1975; Uzhdovini *et al.*, 1974). The intraperitoneal LD_{50} is 150 mg/kg in mice.

Chronic Effects No available data.

Mutagenicity No available data.

Carcinogenicity In a study of the chronic effects of 2,4-dimethylphenol in mice, Boutwell and Bosch (1959) showed that topical application after the administration of 3% dimethylbenzanthracene (as an initiator) produced papillomas in 50% and carcinomas in 11% at 15 weeks; by 23 weeks, 18% developed carcinomas. When dimethylbenzanthracene was used as the initiator and 20% 2,4-dimethylphenol in benzene as the promoter, 24 weeks of intermittent topical application produced papillomas in 63% and carcinomas in 5% by 39 weeks, 42% developed carcinomas. When 10% 2,4-dimethylphenol was applied topically for 20 weeks in the absence of an initiator, 31% had papillomas, and no carcinomas were observed. By 24 weeks, 12% had carcinomas.

Teratogenicity No available data.

Conclusions and Recommendations

2,4-Dimethylphenol appears to be a topical cocarcinogen, but its role as a primary cancer-producing agent is uncertain. Its potential role in cancer production warrants consideration of further testing. An *in vitro* mutaginicity assay should be carried out to further evaluate its mutagenic potential.

In view of the relative paucity of data on the mutagenicity, carcinogenicity, teratogenicity and long-term oral toxicity of 2,4-dimethylphenol, estimates of the effects of chronic oral exposure at low levels cannot be made with any confidence. It is recommended that studies to produce such information be conducted before limits in drinking water are established.

Diphenylhydrazine

Introduction

Diphenylhydrazine is an intermediate in the production of benzidine. It is slightly soluble in water and the highest concentration detected in United States drinking water was 1 μg/liter (USEPA, 1975a).

Metabolism

No data are available on the metabolism of diphenylhydrazine in man or animals.

TABLE VI-52 Toxicity of Diphenylhydrazine

Species	Duration of Study	Dosage Levels and No. of Animals Per Group	Highest No-Adverse-Effect Level or Lowest-Minimal-Effect Level	Effect Measured	Reference
Rat	588 days		40 mg/kg/wk subcutaneously, 30 mg/kg/day orally	urinary, mammary, and liver tumors	Pliss, 1974
Rat	lifetime		2 mg/day (oral)	no increase in the incidence of tumors	Marhold *et al.*, 1968
Mouse	588 days		2 mg/kg/day (oral) 5 mg/kg/week (subcutaneous)	subcutaneous sarcomas and hepatomas	Pliss, 1974

[This compound is an animal carcinogen.]

Health Aspects

Observations in Man The adverse health effects of diphenylhydrazine in man have not been examined.

Observations in Other Species

Acute Effects The oral LD_{50} of diphenylhydrazine is 301 mg/kg in rats (Mason Research Institute Report, 1971).

Chronic Effects No available data.

Mutagenicity No available data.

Carcinogenicity In a study to examine the carcinogenic effects of this compound, 60 mg/kg administered subcutaneously produced a wide variety of benign and malignant tumors in Sherman rats (Spitz *et al.*, 1950). In a similar study, subcutaneous injection of 40–60 mg/kg/week or ingestion of 30 mg/kg/day for up to 588 days induced uterine, mammary, and liver tumors in rats (Pliss, 1974). An oral dose of 2 mg/day for the entire life span of Wistar rats produced no increase in the incidence of tumors (Marhold *et al.*, 1968). A subcutaneous dose of 5 mg/kg/week or 2 mg/kg/day for up to 588 days resulted in subcutaneous sarcomas and hepatomas in mice (Pliss, 1974).

Teratogenicity No available data.

Conclusions and Recommendations

Diphenylhydrazine is a suspected carcinogen in humans because of its structural relationship to benzidine, which is an established human bladder carcinogen. Recent studies in rats and mice have shown that diphenylhydrazine produces both benign and malignant tumors when administered subcutaneously. The results of oral ingestion studies are equivocal and not adequate to establish a cancer risk estimate.

In view of the relative paucity of data on the mutagenicity, teratogenicity and long-term oral toxicity of diphenylhydrazine, estimates of the effects of chronic oral exposure at low levels cannot be made with any confidence. It is recommended that studies to produce such information be conducted before limits in drinking water are established.

The available chronic toxicity data are summarized in Table VI-52.

Hexachloroethane

Introduction

Hexachloroethane (HCE) is used in organic synthesis, as a retarding agent in fermentation, as a substitute for camphor in nitrocellulose, in pyrotechnics and smoke devices, and in the manufacture of explosives, solvents, and medicines. It can be formed in small quantities by chlorination (USEPA, 1975). It is insoluble in water and very persistent. Of the 10 water supplies surveyed by the EPA (1975a), only Miami's finished water contained hexachloroethane, at 0.5 μg/liter.

Metabolism

Hexachloroethane was detected as a metabolite of carbon tetrachloride in rabbits following a 1 ml/kg dose in olive oil. Fat contained the highest concentration of HCE, muscle the lowest; tissue concentrations reached a peak at 24 h, but persisted for as long as 44 h (Fowler 1969).

Health Aspects

Observations in Man No studies have been conducted to examine the acute, subchronic, or chronic effects of hexachloroethane in man.

Observations in Other Species

Acute Effects The Toxic Substances List (1974) notes that the lowest reported acutely lethal dosages of HCE are 325 mg/kg administered intravenously in dogs and 4,000 mg/kg administered subcutaneously in rabbits.

In a study of the subacute effects of hexachlorethane by Tugarinova *et al.* (1963), 12 mice received 310 mg/kg orally once a day for 10 days. Macroscopic examination of the animals revealed no cumulative effects.

Chronic Effects Chronic experiments with 19 male rats (weighing 200–240 g) and 12 female and 8 male rabbits weighing (2,100–2,800 g) given hexachloroethane orally at 0.05 mg/kg/day for 5.5 months showed no signs of toxicity measured by body weight, motor reflexes, and blood chemistry. Histopathologic evaluation of brain, heart, liver, kidneys, spleen, stomach, and intestine were negative (Tugarinova *et al.*, 1963).

Mutagenicity No available data.

Carcinogenicity No available data.

Teratogenicity No available data.

Conclusions and Recommendations

In view of the relative paucity of data on the mutagenicity, carcinogenicity, teratogenicity, and long-term oral toxiciy of hexachloroethane, estimates of the effects of chronic oral exposure at low levels cannot be made with any confidence. It is recommended that studies to produce such information be conducted before limits in drinking water are established.

Hexachlorophene

Introduction

Hexachlorophene (HCP), or 2,2'-methylene-*bis*(3,4,6-trichlorophenol), has been used as an antibacterial agent in a wide variety of consumer products, including soaps and deodorants (Gump, 1969; Kimbrough, 1976.) It has also been used as an antifungal agent to treat various citrus fruits and vegetables.

HCP has been identified in surface water (Buhler *et al.*, 1973; Sims and Pfaender, 1975) at concentrations as high as 48 ppb. HCP in drinking-water at 0.01 ppb has also been reported (Buhler *et al.*, 1973; USEPA, 1975). HCP is practically insoluble in water (CRC Handbook of Chemistry and Physics, 1970–1971).

Metabolism

Studies in rabbits, rats, and cows (Wit and Van Genderen, 1962) with [^{14}C]HCP showed that it is absorbed orally, that most of what is absorbed is excreted via the feces within 5–7 days, and that in rabbits the half-life is 17.8 h. Gandolfi and Buhler (1974) demonstrated after intraperitoneal injection in rats that the major metabolite is a monoglucuronide and that there is extensive enterohepatic circulation. Absorption through the skin has resulted in mean blood concentrations of 0.2 μg/ml in adult humans (Feldman and Maibach, 1970; Butcher *et al.*, 1973) and 0.049 μg/ml in human infants (Plueckhahn, 1973).

Health Aspects

Observations in Man Wear *et al.* (1962) reported that an oral dose of 2–10 g (33-166 mg/kg) may be fatal in adults. Lustig (1963) cited the case of a 16-kg child that died after ingesting 200–300 mg (16 mg/kg), and Martinez *et al.* (1974) described the case of a 17-yr-old boy who ingested 1,350 mg and died 61 h later. In another case, an infant was accidentally given 37 mg/kg/day orally for 7 days; the child developed gastrointestinal irritation, dehydration, neuromuscular effects, and shock, but recovered completely (Pilapil, 1966). Shuman *et al.* (1974) reported that human neonates weighing less than 1,400 g at birth are very susceptible to central nervous system effects of the compound.

There are many reports in the literature concerning intoxication by HCP following accidental or suicidal ingestion or exposure to preparations containing this antibacterial agent (Kimbrough, 1976).

Children poisoned with HCP develop myelin edema; i.e., status spongiosus (Mullick, 1973; Shuman *et al.*, 1974). While humans undergoing treatment for *Clonorchis sinensis* tolerated a single 20 mg/kg oral dose of HCP, three successive 20 mg/kg/day doses of the antibacterial produced intoxication in treated patients (Chung *et al.*, 1963; Liu *et al.*, 1963).

Observations in Other Species

Acute Effects In acute studies, the oral LD_{50} in mice was reported to be 187 mg/kg (Gump, 1969), 80 mg/kg (Florostano, 1949), and 67 mg/kg (Chung *et al.*, 1963). Oral LD_{50} values for male and female Wistar rats were 58–87 and 63–87 mg/kg, respectively, (Nakaue *et al.*, 1973) while for Sherman strain rats they were 66 and 56 mg/kg, respectively (Gaines *et al.*, 1973). Juvenile rats are more resistant to HCP than adults and oral LD_{50}'s for 10-day, 32-day and adult rats were 9, 111, and 55 mg/kg, respectively (Nieminen *et al.*, 1973). Acute toxicity appears to be a function of age and extent of myelination of the central nervous system.

Dog pups given 15 mg/kg oral dose of HCP exhibited neurotoxicity and died, whereas an oral dose of 7.5 mg/kg HCP only produced excitability (Edds and Simpson, 1974). The oral LD_{50} for young dogs was estimated at 15–30 mg/kg.

The loss of pupillary response and blindness was found in sheep after receiving a single 20–80 mg/kg oral dose of HCP (Udall and Malone, 1970). Weanling rats given a single 100 mg/kg oral dose of HCP developed weakness of the hind legs and showed severe vacuolization in the myelinated areas of the brain (Kimbrough, 1973). Severe testicular degeneration and detectable liver changes, including increased mitotic activity, were found in rats given 75 mg/kg HCP (Thorpe, 1967).

Subchronic and Chronic Effects In a study of the subchronic effects of HCP, rats fed 0.02 and 0.04% HCP in the diet for 30 days showed mild toxicity with reduced growth at the lowest dose. At the higher dose, liver and kidney pathology developed (Gump, 1969). Rats fed 20, 65, and 200 ppm HCP for 90 days showed no evidence of toxicity (Vaterlaus and Hostynek, 1972). A similiar study was recently reported by Kennedy *et al.* (1976) in which male and female Charles River CD strain rats were fed dietary levels of 0, 20, 65, or 200 ppm commercial grade HCP (G-11) or received 6.5 mg/kg daily oral doses of HCP over a 90-day period. A moderate degree of vacuolization in the cerebellum was observed in 2 of 20 rats at the 200 ppm HCP level (20 mg/kg/day), but no signs of CNS disorders or other abnormalities were observed in the treated animals. In a second study with the same strain of rats (Kennedy *et al.*, 1976), daily 0, 20, and 40 mg/kg oral doses of HCP were administered for 6 weeks. Growth was depressed at 40 mg/kg/day HCP. Vacuolization of the brain was seen in animals given 40 mg/kg/day and, to a lesser extent, in those receiving 20 mg/kg/day. The histopathologic changes of the brain elicited by HCP were barely detectable after a recovery period of 84 days and hence are reversible.

In contrast to these results, considerably greater toxicity was found with HCP in other rat studies. Some Sherman rats fed 500 ppm HCP for 98 days died after developing severe hind limb paralysis with accompanying brain edema (Gaines *et al.*, 1973; Kimbrough and Gaines, 1971).

In a chronic study, no paralysis was seen in rats fed 20 and 100 ppm HCP for 258 days, but appreciable vacuolization of the brain occurred at the higher dose (Gaines *et al.*, 1973). With Wistar strain weanling rats fed for 112 days, 400 ppm (28.9 mg/kg/day) HCP produced paralysis and death (Nakaue *et al.*, 1973). Rats fed 200 ppm (14.9 mg/kg/day) developed an initial paralysis but recovered after about 2 weeks, while rats fed 100 ppm (7.7 mg/kg/day) appeared normal. Brain edema was seen, however, with decreasing severity in the groups fed 400, 200, and 100 ppm HCP. No adverse effects were observed at 50 ppm (3.7 mg/kg/day).

Mutagenicity The possible mutagenic effects of HCP were evaluated by a dominant lethal study in mice and a host-mediated assay in rats with *Salmonella typhimurium* (Arnold *et al.*, 1975). No evidence for mutagenicity was seen in mice given single doses of 2.5 or 5 mg/kg HCP (dominant

TABLE VI-53 Toxicity of Hexachlorophene

Species	Duration of Study	Dosage Levels and No. of Animals Per Group	Highest No-Adverse-Effect Level or Lowest-Minimal-Effect Level	Effect Measured	Reference
Rat	14 weeks	0–25 mg/kg/day, 10–12 animals/group	<5 mg/kg/day (oral)	toxicity and pathology	Kimbrough and Gaines, 1971
Rat	37 weeks	0–100 ppm in diet, 20 animals/group	20 ppm (1.16 mg/kg/day)[a,b]	no toxic effect	Gaines *et al.*, 1973
Rat	16 weeks	0–400 ppm in diet, 6 animals/group	50 ppm (3.7 mg/kg/day)[a]	no toxic effect	Nakaue *et al.*, 1973

Using an uncertainty factor of 1,000, the suggested no-adverse-effect level in drinking water is calculated as follows:

$$\frac{1.16}{1{,}000} = 0.00116 \text{ mg/kg/day (ADI)}, \; 0.00116 \times 70^{a} \; ^{3}\, 0.1^{b} = 0.008 \text{ mg/liter}$$

[a]Assume average weight of human adult = 70 kg.
[b]Assume average daily intake of water for man = 2 liters, and that 20 percent of total intake is from water.
[c]Value from which the suggested no-adverse-effect level was calculated.

lethal) or in rats fed 100 or 200 ppm HCP over a 90-day period (host-mediated).

Carcinogenicity Twice-weekly application of 1, 5, and 10 mg HCP on the skin of Swiss mice over their lifetime caused local and systematic toxicity, but no evidence of carcinogenicity was seen (Stenback, 1975).

Teratogenicity Kimmel *et al.* (1974) examined the teratogenic effects of vaginally administered HCP. Doses of 80 mg/kg (equivalent to about 1,000 ppm in the diet) and above were teratogenic in Charles River rats while a 20 mg/kg dose was without adverse effect. The defects produced at the highest dose (300 mg/kg) included hydrocephaly, microthalmia, wavy ribs, and urogenital defects. CD strain rats received oral doses of 1, 15, or 30 mg/kg/day HCP on days 6–15 of gestation while NZW rabbits were given 1, 3 or 6 mg/kg/day HCP on days 6–18 of gestation (Kennedy *et al.*, 1975b). Rat fetuses exposed to 30 mg/kg/day HCP had a low frequency of eye and skeletal defects (10/209 angulated ribs) while skeletal changes (3/175 had rib malformations) appeared in rabbit fetuses exposed to 6 mg/kg/day HCP. There was no increase in prenatal death at any dosage level.

Administration of HCP to three successive generations of albino rats at dietary levels of 12.5, 25, and 50 ppm failed to produce any changes with respect to mating, fertility, length of gestation, and number of deliveries (Kennedy *et al.*, 1975a). There was no detectable adverse effect on the mothers or on the progeny.

Conclusions and Recommendations

The principal effect of hexachlorophene is on the central nervous system, where reversible edematous vacuolation of the myelin sheaths of the white matter occurs if the plasma concentration is maintained over a long period at or above 1.2 μg/ml. Newborn humans and laboratory animals are more susceptible to this effect than adults.

An ADI was calculated on the basis of the available chronic toxicity data to be 0.0012 mg/kg/day.

The calculations and available chronic-toxicity data on animals are summarized in Table VI-53.

Hexachlorophene does not appear to be an active carcinogen or teratogen, although long-term chronic-toxicity studies integrating carcinogenicity and target organ toxicity are recommended, to assemble more data. Since there are no reported 2-yr chronic toxicity studies with HCP, it is suggested that such studies be undertaken before a final assessment of the long term hazards of HCP exposure are made.

o-Methoxyphenol

Introduction

o-Methoxyphenol (guaiacol) is produced in wood processing or by chemical synthesis. It is used in the manufacture of medicines, guaiacol compounds, and perfumes (Chemistry Dictionary, 1972). The solubility of *o*-methoxyphenol is 1 g in 60–70 ml of water (Merck Index, 1968). It has been detected in finished water in the lower Mississippi River area (USEPA, 1972).

Metabolism

Methoxyphenol is largely absorbed from the digestive tract and stored in the blood, kidneys, and respiratory organs (Jurgens, 1920). It is excreted by rabbits in combined form with sulfate (15%) and glucuronic acid (72%) (Stefano and Quirico, 1939).

Health Aspects

Observations in Man There have been no investigations of the adverse health effects of *o*-methoxyphenol in man.

Observations in Other Species

Acute Effects The LD_{50} was shown to be 3.74 mg/kg in rabbits (Stefano and Quirico, 1939). The minimal lethal injected dose in rats was shown to be 50 mg/kg by Tedschi and DeCicco (1954). They found that, when *o*-methoxyphenol was injected into pregnant rats, it was fatal to the fetus; when similar doses were injected into male animals, serious disorders of the testes and destruction of the germinal epithelium were observed. The oral LD_{50} in rats has been shown to be 725 mg/kg by Taylor *et al.* (1964).

The lethal oral dose of *o*-methoxyphenol in mice is 0.4 g/kg (Ono, 1920). Ono also found that a 0.15% solution caused paralysis of the heart muscle, and a 0.6% solution, paralysis of intestinal smooth muscle.

In toxicologic studies with *o*-methoxyphenol, it was found that the compound exerted a hemolytic action on cattle blood (Stefano and

Quirico, 1939) and interfered with RNA synthesis, protein synthesis, and, to a small degree, mitochondrial respiration in rats (Taylor *et al.*, 1964). Vanderhock and Lands (1973) reported the inhibition of fatty acid oxygenase in sheep vesicular gland tissue on exposure to *o*-methoxyphenol and Busacca (1919) found that the compound induced leukopenia that led to leukocytosis in rodents.

Chronic Effects No available data.

Mutagenicity No avialable data.

Carcinogenicity Methoxyphenol has been found to contribute to the carcinogenic effect of tobacco smoke in rats (Wynder and Hoffamn, 1963).

Teratogenicity No available data.

Conclusions and Recommendations

In view of the relative pauciy of data on the mutagenicity, carcinogenicity, teratogenicity, and long-term oral toxicity of *o*-methoxyphenol, estimates of the effects of chronic oral exposure at low levels cannot be made with any confidence. It is recommended that studies to produce such information be conducted before limits in drinking water are established.

Methyl Chloride

Introduction

Methyl chloride (chloromethane) is produced commercially by the chlorination of methane or the action of hydrochloric acid on methanol. It is used in the manufacture of silicones, synthetic rubber, tetraethyl lead, methyl cellulose, refrigerants, organic chemicals, and fumigants; as a low-temperature solvent, as a catalyst carrier in polymerization; as a methylating agent; as a propellant; and as an herbicide (USEPA, 1975d). The United States production of methyl chloride in 1973 was 544 million pounds (USITC, 1975).

Methyl chloride is slightly soluble in water (CRC Handbook of Chemistry and Physics, 1970–1971). Five of the 10 water supplies surveyed by the EPA (1975a) contained methyl chloride.

Metabolism

In breath-analysis studies of some aliphatic halogenated hydrocarbons, Morgan *et al.* (1972) demonstrated that methyl chloride did not have the rate of excretion that would be predicted on the basis of its partition coefficient compared with the other similar compounds studied. It was later postulated that this anomalous behavior of methyl chloride may be due to an enzyme-catalyzed methylation of red-cell sulfhydryl groups. This is in agreement with the findings of Redford-Ellis and Gowenlock (1971a), who showed that [^{14}C]*S*-methylglutathione (GSMe) and [^{14}C]*S*-methylcysteine (*S*-Me Cys) were formed from the interaction of radioactively labeled methyl chloride with human blood and liver, brain, and kidney homogenates.

Health Aspects

Observations in Man No documented information on the adverse health effects of methyl chloride in man is available.

Observations in Other Species

Acute Effects The effects of a single inhalation exposure to methyl chloride were examined as functions of time and dose in a variety of experimental animals. A concentration of 150,000–300,000 ppm proved lethal to most animals in a short period; 20,000–40,000 ppm proved dangerous in 30–60 m; 7,000 ppm produced no serious effects in up to 60 m of exposure; and 500–1,000 was ineffective for up to 8 h (Patty, vol. II, 1963).

Chronic Effects Smith and von Octtingen (1947a,b) exposed guinea pigs, mice, dogs, rabbits, and rats to methyl chloride at 1,000 ppm for 6 h/day, 6 days/week, for up to 175 days. This concentration was judged toxic on the basis of central nervous system (neuromuscular effects) and decreased survival. At 500 ppm, rats showed no effects; but the other animals, including two monkeys, showed some response. Effects were usually delayed with these lower concentrations and remained for months after exposure. Common signs among most species were loss of leg movement, muscle contractions, tremors, and hyperactive tendon reflexes. Three of 4 dogs died after four weeks or less of exposure, and the two monkeys died after 17 weeks of exposure. At 300 ppm, no effects were observed in any of the animals.

Evtushenko (1966) indicated that rats exposed to methyl chloride at 120 and 20 ppm showed formaldehyde in the blood and developed anemia and reticulocytosis. There were some undescribed pathologic central nervous system changes and some eye effects. On the basis of the above work a TLV of 2.5 ppm was suggested in the USSR.

Mutagenicity No available data.

Carcinogenicity No available data.

Teratogenicity No available data.

Conclusions and Recommendations

In view of the relative paucity of data on the mutagenicity, carcinogenicity, teratogenicity, and long-term oral toxicity of methyl chloride, estimates of the effects of chronic oral exposure at low levels cannot be made with any confidence. It is recommended that studies to produce such information be conducted before final limits in drinking water are established.

Methylene Chloride

Introduction

Methylene chloride (dichloromethane) is used in the manufacture of paint and varnish removers, insecticides and fumigants, solvents, cleaners, pressurized spray products, fire extinguishers, and Christmas tree bubble lights (Chemistry Dictionary, 1972). It is produced by chlorination of methane or methyl chloride. The United States production in 1973 was over a half-billion pounds (USITC, 1975).

Methylene chloride is soluble at about 1 part to 50 parts of water (Merck Index, 1968). It is formed during chlorination water treatment. The Region V survey showed that 8% of the finished-water supplies contained methylene chloride, but only 1% of the raw-water supplies. The mean concentration in finished water was <1 μg/liter (USEPA, 1975b). Nine of the 10 water supplies surveyed by the EPA (1975a) contained methylene chloride; Lawrence, Massachusetts had the highest concentration, 1.6 μg/liter.

Metabolism

DiVincenzo and Hamilton (1975) administered [^{14}C]methylene chloride to Sprague–Dawley rats at 412–930 mg/kg. Methylene chloride was largely eliminated unchanged in the expired air during the first 2 h. After 24 h, only 2% of the original dose remained in the body. This 2% was found mostly in the liver, kidneys, and adrenal glands.

It has been shown by DiVincenzo and Hamilton (1975) and Soucek (1961) that some methylene chloride is converted in the body to carbon monoxide; this results in an increase in carboxyhemoglobin concentration. Blood carbon monoxide content is not directly related to the exposure concentration of methylene chloride. A review of the literature shows that there is a wide variation in carboxyhemoglobin concentration in persons exposed to a given concentration of methylene chloride for a given period and a lack of consistent correlation in measurement or calculation of carboxyhemoglobin. Furthermore, the significance of increased blood carboxyhemoglobin has not been satisfactorily determined.

Health Aspects

Observations in Man Raleigh (1974) reported a study on 562 workers; 103 were reportedly in the highest-exposure group, being exposed to methylene chloride at 50–100 ppm. There was no increase in the incidence of cardiovascular, gastrointestinal (including liver), genitourinary, or central nervous system disease in the exposed groups, compared with a nonexposed worker population.

The NIOSH (1976) recommended that occupational exposure to methylene chloride not exceed 75 ppm determined as a time-weighted average exposure for up to a 10-h workday.

Observations in Other Species

Acute Effects The acute oral LD_{50} values are 1.6–2.3 ml/kg for rats (Kimura, *et al.*, 1971). The intraperitoneal LD_{50} values are 1.50 ml/kg for mice and 0.95 ml/kg for dogs (Klaassen and Plaa, 1967).

Chronic Effects In a chronic study, Bornmann and Loeser (1967) reported no adverse effects in rats maintained on drinking water containing methylene chloride at 2.25 g/18 liters for 91 days. In a study on the effects of methylene chloride inhalation, Heppel *et al.* (1944)

showed no adverse effects on dogs and rabbits in a 6-month exposure to 5,000 ppm; a slight weight reduction was observed, however, in guinea pigs. Some liver injury was found after 7.5 weeks at 10,000 ppm.

Mutagenicity Methylene chloride was negative in a *Drosophila* mutagenicity test (Filippova *et al.*, 1967).

Carcinogenicity No available data.

Teratogenicity Methylene chloride vapor was not teratogenic in rats and mice at 1,250 ppm (Schwetz *et al.*, 1975). Both species were exposed for 7 h daily on days 6 through 15 of gestation. No fetal toxicity or teratogenicity was found.

Conclusions and Recommendations

Methylene chloride was not teratogenic when inhaled in one species of rats and mice. In view of the relative paucity of data on the mutagenicity, carcinogenicity, and long-term oral toxicity of methylene chloride, estimates of the effects of chronic oral exposure at low levels cannot be made with any confidence. It is recommended that studies to produce such information be conducted before final limits in drinking water are established.

Methyl Methacrylate

Introduction

Methyl methacrylate is the monomer for polymethacrylate resins and used in impregnation of concrete. The U.S. production of it in 1973 was over 706 million pounds (USITC, 1975). This compound is slightly soluble in water (CRC Handbook of Chemistry and Physics, 1970–1971). The highest concentration of methymethacrylate detected in United States drinking water was less than 1 μg/liter (USEPA, 1975a).

Metabolism

Methyl methacrylate is metabolized in rat liver slices via the citric acid cycle. It undergoes hydroxylation to a primary alcohol followed by oxidation to an aldehyde; finally the compound is deformylated to pyruvic acid (Pantucek, 1969).

Health Aspects

Observations in Man In a study by Milkov *et al.* (1966), small amounts of methyl methacrylate vapor found in casting plants was found to induce functional abnormalities in the nervous system of plant workers. In another series of experiments, exposure to methacrylate glue in the placement of bone protheses was also found to induce severe hypotension and some cases cause death. The studies did not determine, however, whether the adverse reactions were the result of the methacrylate or bone marrow embolism (Newens and Voltz, 1972; Cooper, 1975; Breed, 1974).

Observations in Other Species

Acute Effects In acute studies, the oral LD_{50} of methyl methacrylate has been determined for a variety of experimental animals: guinea pig, 6.3 ml/kg; rat, 8.4–10 ml/kg; and dog, 5.0 ml/kg (Spealman *et al.*, 1945; Deichman, 1941). The intraperitoneal LD_{50} values have also been calculated: rats, 1.8 ml/kg; mouse 10 ml/kg; and guinea pig, 2.0 ml/kg. The LD_{50} values for the subcutaneous injection of methacrylate are: rat, 7.5 ml/kg; dog, 4.5 ml/kg; and guinea pig, 6.3 ml/kg (Spealman *et al.*, 1945).

Chronic Effects In chronic studies, rats and dogs were given drinking water containing 6, 60, and 2,000 ppm and 10, 100, and 1,000 ppm methyl methacrylate, respectively, for 2 yr. No clinical, laboratory or pathological evidence of toxicity was observed in either group of animals (Borzelleca *et al.*, 1964).

Mutagenicity No available data.

Carcinogenicity In a study by Lavorgna *et al.* (1972), subcutaneous implants of freshly polymerized methyl methacrylate for up to 39 months increased the incidence of local fibrosarcoma compared to a glass implant control in rats. In another study, Laskin *et al.* (1954) found that subcutaneous implants of polymerized methyl methacrylate induced local fibrosarcomas in mice.

Teratogenicity Doses of 0.13–0.44 ml/kg methyl methacrylate injected into pregnant rats on days 5, 10, and 15 of gestation were found to affect resorptions, fetal survival and fetal size at all doses. Hemangiomas were also observed in some fetuses from the highest dose group. No skeletal abnormalities were observed at any dose (Singh *et al.*, 1972a).

Conclusions and Recommendations

Chronic toxicity studies in rats and dogs indicate that ingested methyl methacrylate does not pose a serious threat to humans or animals. Teratogenicity studies with rats indicate that it can affect fetal growth and survival when injected during specific days of gestation. An ADI of 0.1 mg/kg/day was calculated on the basis of the available chronic toxicity data. The calculations and available chronic toxicity data are summarized in Table VI-54.

Nicotine

Introduction

Nicotine [1-methyl-2(3-pyridyl)pyrrolidine] is commercially produced by distilling tobacco. It is used in some drugs and insecticides, and in tanning. Nicotine is very soluble in water (Chemistry Dictionary, 1972). Of the 10 water utilities surveyed by the EPA (1975a), only the finished water of Miami contained nicotine at 3 μg/liter.

Metabolism

In a study of the metabolism of nicotine in rats, 8–12% of the compound was found to be excreted unchanged; 40% was excreted in 3 h, with complete excretion in 16 h. The major metabolite of nicotine is cotinine (Bowman *et al.*, 1959). In mice, dogs, and guinea pigs, exposure to nicotine smoke permits its detection in visceral storage compartments, including liver, kidneys, lungs, and brain (Bennett *et al.*, 1954).

Health Aspects

Observations in Man The symptoms of nicotine intoxication are nausea, vomiting, diarrhea, confusion, twitching, and convulsions. A dose of 40 mg of nicotine taken orally is fatal in man. Nicotine has also been shown to induce blood-sugar changes in 24 h; 0.3 mg/kg was the lowest no-effect dose (Wilson and DeEds, 1936a).

TABLE VI-54 Toxicity of Methyl Methacrylate

Species	Duration of Study	Dosage Levels and No. of Animals Per Group	Highest No-Adverse-Effect Level or Lowest-Minimal-Effect Level	Effect Measured	Reference
Rat	2 yr	0, 6, 60, 2,000 ppm in drinking water, 25 animals/group	2,000 ppm (100 mg/kg/day)[a,d]	no adverse effect	Borzelleca *et al.*, 1964
Dog	2 yr	0–1,000 ppm in drinking water, 2 animals/group	1,000 ppm	no adverse effect	Borzelleca *et al.*, 1964

Using an uncertainty factor of 1,000, the suggested no-adverse-effect level in drinking water is calculated as follows:

$$\frac{100}{1{,}000} = 0.1 \text{ mg/kg/day (ADI)},\ 0.1 \times 70^{b} \times 0.1^{c} = 0.7 \text{ mg/liter}$$

[a]Assume weight of rat = 0.4 kg and daily food consumption of rat = 0.02 kg.
[b]Assume average weight of human adult = 70 kg.
[c]Assume average daily intake of water for man = 2 liters, and that 20 percent of total intake is from water.
[d]Value from which the suggested no-adverse-effect level was calculated.

Observations in Other Species

Acute Effects The acute oral LD_{50} for mice in 230 mg/kg (Barlow and McLeod, 1969) and 10 mg/kg for rats (Kenaga, 1966). The acute symptoms include respiratory toxicity and transitory hyperglycemia in rats. A change in blood sugar has been observed after 2 h with doses of nicotine greater than 0.5 mg/kg.

Chronic Effects Nicotine has been shown to decrease the growth of rats after 100 days with doses of 12.5 mg/kg and in 200 days with doses of 10 mg/kg (Wilson and De Eds, 1936b).

Mutagenicity Nicotine was negative on a *Salmonella*/microsome mutagenicity assay (McCann *et al.*, 1975).

Carcinogenicity Nicotine has been found to act as a cocarcinogen when applied to mouse skin with benzo(a)pyrene and 12-0-tetradecanolylphorbol-13-acetate (Chemical Engineering News, 1976). Oxidized nicotine applied to the skin of mice resulted in lung adenomas. In another strain of mouse (CBA), commercial nicotine produced no lung tumors.

Teratogenicity Nicotine was teratogenic in mice when injected at 25 mg/kg on days 9-11 of gestation. Skeletal defects and occasional cleft palates were produced (Nishimura and Nakai, 1958). Nicotine was also teratogenic in swine at an oral dose of 1,058 ppm (Menges *et al.*, 1970).

Conclusions and Recommendations

At high doses, nicotine is quite toxic and lethal. Nicotine is metabolized readily, principally to cotinine. Nicotine is teratogenic in mice only at high doses. Evidence on carcinogenicity is equivocal, but it is a cocarcinogen.

In view of the relative paucity of data on the carcinogenicity and long-term oral toxicity of nicotine, estimates of the effects of chronic oral exposure at low levels cannot be made with any confidence. It is recommended that studies to produce such information be conducted before limits in drinking water are established.

Pentachlorophenol

Introduction

Pentachlorophenol (PCP) has been used since 1936 for wood preservation (Spencer, 1973). Domestic production of PCP is estimated at 46 million pounds a year (NAS, 1975).

PCP is produced commercially by the chlorination of phenol (Spencer, 1973). Commercial-grade PCP contains 88.4% PCP, 4.4% tetrachlorophenol, 6.2% higher-chlorinated phenoxyphenols, less than 0.1% trichlorophenol, and various dibenzo-*p*-dioxins and dibenzofurans (Johnson *et al.*, 1973; Schwetz *et al.*, 1974). The highly toxic tetrachlorodioxins are not found in technical PCP. PCP is soluble in water at 20 ppm at 30°C. It is not very volatile, as evidenced by a vapor pressure of 1.1×10^{-4} mm Hg at 20°C (Spencer, 1973). Concentrations of 0.70 and 0.06 μg/liter PCP have been observed in river and treated drinking water, respectively (Buhler *et al.*, 1973). The highest concentration of PCP reported in U.S. drinking water was 1.4 μg/liter (USEPA, 1975e).

Metabolism

A pharmacokinetic profile of pentachlorophenol in monkeys and an elimination study with [^{14}C]pentachlorophenol and its metabolites in rats have been conducted (submitted for publication in Toxicology and Applied Pharmocology). These studies showed that 90% of a 10 mg/kg dose of PCP in rats is eliminated rapidly with a half-life of from 13 to 17 h, depending on sex. PCP is excreted either as tetrachlorohydroquinone (16%) or as a PCP glucuronide conjugate in the urine (9%) or a free PCP (75%). The excretion pattern in monkeys was slower than in rats and almost all PCP was excreted unchanged in urine. It was suggested that the monkey may be a better animal model and more closely approximate human pharmacokinetics.

Health Aspects

Observations in Man Menon (1958) reported loss of appetite, respiratory difficulties, anesthesia, hyperpyrexia, sweating, dyspnea, and rapidly progressive coma in humans exposed to PCP.

A number of cases of human poisoning by PCP are reviewed by Armstrong *et al.* (1969). The minimum lethal dose for humans is estimated to be 29 mg/kg (The Toxic Substances List, 1974). Work done in the USSR has established a maximum permissible concentration of 40 ng/m^3 PCP in the air (Tabakova, 1969).

Observations in Other Species

Acute Effects The acute, oral LD_{50}'s for PCP are: 120–140 mg/kg for the mouse, 27–100 mg/kg for the rat, 100 mg/kg for the guinea pig, 100–130 mg/kg for the rabbit, and 150–200 mg/kg for the dog (Christensen *et al.*, 1974; Deichmann *et al.*, 1942; Knudsen *et al.*, 1974; McGavack *et al.*, 1941; Stohlman, 1951). The acute symptoms of intoxication are vomiting, hyperpyrexia, elevated blood pressure, increased respiration rate, and tachycardia. The LD_{50} after oral administration of PCP to male and female rats was 146 and 175 mg/kg and upon percutaneous exposure 320 and 330 mg/kg, respectively (Gaines, 1969).

Subchronic and Chronic Effects In a study to determine the subchronic toxicity of the compound, PCP was fed in the diet to groups of Wistar rats at concentrations of 0, 25, 50, and 200 ppm for a 90-day period (Knudsen *et al.*, 1974). Female rats receiving 200 ppm (10 mg/kg/day) PCP showed a reduced growth rate while liver weights were increased in male rats ingesting 200 and 50 ppm (2.5 mg/kg/day). After 6 weeks, rats fed 50 and 200 ppm PCP showed elevated hemoglobin and hematocrit values, whereas at 11 weeks hemoglobin and erythrocytes were significantly reduced in the same groups of animals. No PCP-related effects were seen in animals fed 25 ppm (1.25 mg/kg/day). In another experiment, male rats received 1,000 ppm (50 mg/kg/day) of technical or pure PCP for a 90-day period (Kimbrough and Linder, 1975). Both PCP samples caused an increase in liver weight. Much more severe histopathological changes occurred in the livers of rats given the technical PCP than in those given the pure PCP. In another 90 day study, Sprague–Dawley rats showed increased liver and kidney weights, elevated serum alkaline phosphatase, and depressed serum albumin levels in animals consuming 3 mg/kg/day of technical PCP (Johnson *et al.*, 1973). When a sample of improved PCP containing substantially reduced amounts of dioxins was fed to rats, no adverse effects were seen at 3 mg/kg/day. In animals receiving chemically pure PCP, kidney and liver weights were elevated at 30 and 10 mg/kg/day, respectively, but 3 mg/kg/day was without adverse toxicologic effect.

In a chronic study, liver weights were significantly increased in rats ingesting 500 ppm (25 mg/kg/day) technical PCP over an 8-month period (Kimbrough and Linder, 1975). No toxic effects were observed at 100 ppm (5.0 mg/kg/day) PCP.

TABLE VI-55 Toxicity of Pentachlorophenol

Species	Duration of Study	Dosage Levels and No. of Animals Per Group	Highest No-Adverse-Effect Level or Lowest-Minimal-Effect Level	Effect Measured	Reference
Rat	12 weeks	0–200 ppm in diet, 20 animals/group	25 ppm (1.25 mg/kg/day)	no toxic effect	Knudson *et al.*, 1974
Hamster	days 5–10 of gestation	1.25–20 mg/kg/day orally	2.5 mg/kg/day	no fetotoxic or embryotoxic effects	Hinkle, 1973
Rat	90 days	0–30 mg/kg/day in diet[a]	3 mg/kg/day[e]	no toxic effect	Johnson *et al.*, 1973
Rat	90 days	0–30 mg/kg/day in diet[b]	3 mg/kg/day	increased organ weights, serum enzyme changes	Johnson *et al.*, 1973
Rat	days 6–15 of gestation	0–50 mg/kg/day, orally, 20–20 animals/group[a]	5 mg/kg/day	teratogenic effects	Schwetz *et al.*, 1974
Rat	8 months	0–50 ppm in diet, 20 animals/group	100 ppm (5.0 mg/kg/day)	no toxic effect	Kimbrough and Linder, 1975
Rat	8 months	0–500 ppm in diet[a]	500 ppm (25 mg/kg/day)	no toxic effect	Goldstein *et al.*, 1976

Using an uncertainty factor of 1,000, the suggested no-adverse-effect in drinking water is calculated as follows:

$$\frac{3}{1{,}000} = 0.003 \text{ mg/kg/day (ADI)},\ 0.003 \times 70^{c} \times 0.1^{d} = 0.021 \text{ mg/liter}$$

[a]Pure PCP.
[b]Technical PCP.
[c]Assume average weight of human adult = 70 kg.
[d]Assume average daily intake of water for man = 2 liters, and that 20 percent of total intake is from water.
[e]Value from which the suggested no-adverse-effect level was calculated.

When female weanling rats were fed pure or technical PCP for 8 months, increased urinary porphyrin excretion and increased liver porphyrin levels were observed in animals fed 100 (5.0 mg/kg/day) or 500 ppm of the technical product (Goldstein *et al.*, 1976). None of the rats fed pure PCP became porphyric. Liver weights were increased in rats receiving 500 ppm (25 mg/kg/day) of technical PCP but were unchanged in animals fed 500 ppm of the pure phenol. Thus the porphyrin and other major liver changes induced by technical PCP are apparently due to contaminants, probably the chlorinated dibenzo-*p*-dioxins, rather than PCP.

Mutagenicity PCP proved negative in the sex-linked level test in *Drosophila* (Vogel and Chandler, 1974).

Carcinogenicity No available data.

Teratogenicity In a study to examine the potential teratogenicity of PCP, purified and commercial-grade PCP were administered to Sprague–Dawley rats on days 6–15, 3–11, and 12–15 of gestation (Schwetz *et al.*, 1974). PCP was embryotoxic and fetotoxic at doses of the commercial and pure phenol of 15 mg/kg and above. The no adverse effect dose level was 5 mg/kg for the commercial PCP, but at this same dose level, delayed ossification of the skull was observed after treatment with pure PCP.

Oral administration of 0, 1.25, 2.5, 5, 10, and 20 mg/kg PCP to hamsters on days 5–10 of gestation produced fetal death and/or resorptions at 5 mg/kg/day and above (Hinkle, 1973).

Conclusions and Recommendations

There are substantial disagreements in the results of several of the subacute and chronic toxicity experiments with PCP (Table VI-55), perhaps because of the use of inadequately characterized PCP preparations in these studies. In addition, 2-yr chronic toxicity experiments in one or more species have not yet been conducted with this extensively used chemical. High doses (>5 mg/kg/day) of PCP have been shown to be teratogenic in rats and hamsters administered during susceptible days of gestation. There is also a need for an adequate determination of the carcinogenic potential of this chemical.

On the basis of the available chronic toxicity data an ADI for pentachlorophenol has been calculated to be 0.003 mg/kg/day. The data and calculations are summarized in Table VI-55.

Phenylacetic Acid

Introduction

Phenylacetic acid is derived from benzyl cyanide. It is used in the manufacture of perfume, medicines, penicillin, fungicides, plant hormones, and flavorings (Chemistry Dictionary, 1972). Phenylacetic acid is slightly soluble in cold water. Of the 10 water supplies surveyed by the EPA (1975a), only the finished water of Seattle contained phenylacetic acid, at 4 μg/liter (NORS, USEPA, 1975a).

Metabolism

Phenylacetic acid and alkyl chloro derivatives are rapidly absorbed from human buccal tissues or membranes. Phenylacetic acid inhibits the activity of coenzyme A. At 0.5–1 mM/kg, it inhibits the acetylation of sulfanilamide (Lisunkin, 1965).

Health Aspects

Observations in Man The adverse health aspects of phenylacetic acid have not been examined in man.

Observations in Other Species

Acute Effects The oral LD_{50} of phenylacetic acid is 1,630 mg/kg in rats. In a study of the acute effects in mice, intraperitoneal injection of 300 mg/kg proved toxic; 11 of the 15 experimental animals died (Anderson *et al.*, 1936). The time to death varied from 10 minutes to 10 days.

Chronic Effects No available data.

Mutagenicity No available data.

Carcinogenicity Hoshino (1970) reported that phenylacetic acid did not promote tumor formation when the compound was given to rabbits intravenously and subcutaneously for 40 days.

Teratogenicity In a teratogenic study with rats, the administration of phenylacetic acid on the twelfth day of embryogenesis affected body weight, retarded skeletal ossification, and caused embryos to be resorbed at twice the rate of controls. The dosage was 0.2% of the LD_{50}, or 3.2 mg/kg (Anderson *et al.*, 1936).

Conclusions and Recommendations

In view of the relative paucity of data on the mutagenicity, carcinogenicity, teratogenicity, and long-term oral toxicity of phenylacetic acid, estimates of the effects of chronic oral exposure at low levels cannot be made with any confidence. It is recommended that studies to produce such information be conducted before limits in drinking water are established.

Phthalic Anhydride

Introduction

Phthalic anhydride is used in the manufacture of plasticizers, alkyl and polyester resins, synthetic fibers, dyes, pigments, pharmaceuticals, and insecticides (USEPA, 1975d). The U.S. production of this compound in 1973 was over 1 billion pounds (USITC, 1975). It is soluble at 1 part in 162 parts of water (Merck Index, 1968). It has been detected in finished water (USEPA, 1976).

Metabolism

Phthalic anhydride is apparently excreted largely unchanged by both animals and man. In man and dogs, the unchanged compound can be recovered in urine almost quantitatively (Williams, 1959). There is no firm evidence that phthalic anhydride is converted to phthalic acid in the body; if it is, it should occur as the acid in urine.

Health Aspects

Observations in Man In man, phthalic anhydride is an eye, skin, and mucous-membrane irritant (Friebel, 1956; Merlevede and Elskens, 1957; Baader, 1955; Menshick, 1955; Chezzi and Scotti, 1965).

Observations in Other Species

Acute Effects Fassett (1963a) recorded the acute oral LD_{50} as 800–1,600 mg/kg in rats and less than 100 mg/kg in guinea pigs. Vapor exposures, particularly to heated phthalic anhydride, produced congestion, irritation, and injury of lung cells (Friebel, 1956). Jacobs *et al.* (1940) reported that the compound sensitized the skin of guinea pigs. Freibel (1956) reported a study in which oral doses in rats (starting at 20 mg/kg/day) were doubled weekly; 0.89 g/kg was reached by the ninth week. Rats that died at the high dosage had severe nephrosis, with destruction of the tubular epithelium. Surviving animals had gastric ulceration.

Chronic Effects No available data.

Mutagenicity No available data.

Carcinogenicity No available data.

Teratogenicity No available data.

Conclusions and Recommendations

In view of the relative paucity of data on the mutagenicity, carcinogenicity, teratogenicity, and long-term oral toxicity of phthalic anhydride, estimates of the effects of chronic oral exposure at low levels cannot be made with any confidence. It is recommended that studies to produce such information be conducted before limits in drinking water are established.

Polychlorinated Biphenyls

Introduction

Polychlorinated biphenyls (PCB's) are mixtures of chlorinated biphenyls produced commercially by the chlorination of biphenyl. PCB's are used in the production of capacitors and transformers.

PCB's are highly persistent and can accumulate in the environment. They are soluble in water at 0.04–0.2 ppm. Trichlorinated, tetrachlorinated, and pentachlorinated biphenyls have been detected in a few water supplies: at 3.0 μg/liter in Winnebago, Illinois, and 0.1 μg/liter in Sellersberg, Indiana (USEPA, 1975b).

Metabolism

Oral feeding of a single dose of PCB's to rodents and rhesus monkeys has shown that intestinal absorption is rapid and 90% complete (Albro and Fishbein, 1972); Allen and Norback, 1976; Berlin *et al.*, 1973). The feces provide the major route of excretion; only traces of PCB's could be found in the urine of the animals. When the analysis of feces is limited to the determination of unchanged PCB's, the recovery of the administered dose is incomplete (Platonow *et al.*, 1972).

Berlin *et al.* (1975a,b) demonstrated in mice that, after a single oral dose of a [^{14}C]pentachlorbiphenyl, radioactivity rapidly entered the circulation and was distributed in the tissues, particularly in liver, kidneys, lungs, and adrenals; within 24 h, it had migrated to the fat, which remained the major reservoir of unchanged PCB's in the body, until only traces remained after 32 days.

The degradation and elimination of PCB congeners appear to take place via the hepatic microsomal enzyme system. Two possible mechanisms for biotransformation have been suggested by Ecobichon (1976). The first and most rapid mechanism involves the formation of an arene oxide intermediate and requires the presence of unsubstituted adjacent carbon atoms in the nucleus. The second and much slower uses a different hydroxylation system for isolated unsubstituted positions, as are found in highly chlorinated biphenyls. Two adjacent unsubstituted carbon atoms appear to be important in metabolism, in that their presence facilitates the formation of arene oxides by the hepatic mixed-function oxidases.

Polychlorinated biphenyls are known to be strong inducers of hepatic mixed-function oxidase enzymes. The potency increases with increasing chlorination of the biphenyl rings. The PCB's are somewhat unique in this regard in that they induce both Type I and Type II P-450, but this may be due in part to contaminants in the PCB's tested (USDHEW, 1976).

These effects raise a concern that such induction may increase metabolism of birth control hormones with possible harmful effects. Also to be considered is the possibility that environmental carcinogens may be activated at a faster rate (USDHEW, 1976).

Health Aspects

Observations in Man PCB's are liver toxins and cause chloracne and possibly peripheral neuropathy in man (Murai and Juroiwa, 1971).

There is no information on acute adverse effects on humans. Although Yusho disease (an acute outbreak of disease which occurred in Japan) has generally been ascribed to the ingestion of PCB's in rice oil (0.07 mg/kg/day for at least 50 days), recent evidence provided by Kuratsune *et al.* (1976) suggests that the rice oil was contaminated with polychlorinated dibenzofurans (PCDF's). These compounds may have played a significant role in the observed toxicity. Initial measurements of the concentrations of PCDF's in the PCB's suggested that these materials contributed at least as much to the toxicity as the PCB's themselves. Symptoms included excessive fatigue, headache, phymata in articular regions, fever, cough, digestive disturbances, numbness, and menstrual disorders. Physical signs consisted primarily of cutaneomucosal abnormalities, such as acneiform eruptions and black comedones on face, buttocks, and intertriginous sites; increased pigmentation of face, palpebral conjunctiva, gingiva, and nails; ocular signs consisting of swelling and hypersecretion of the meibomian gland and palpebral edema.

Recent surveys have indicated that PCB can be found in the milk of nursing mothers. The highest reported level was 10.6 ppm with a mean of 1.8 ppm for all samples (USDHEW, 1976).

This information is especially meaningful in light of Allen's recent work (1975). Female rhesus monkeys orally exposed to 2.5 and 5.0 ppm of PCB (Aroclor 1248) developed facial acne, erythema, subcutaneous edema conjunctivitis and loss of eyelashes. All infants born to PCB-exposed mothers had PCB's in their tissues at birth. These infants also developed skin lesions as a result of nursing PCB contaminanted milk. Fifty percent of the infants died within 4 months.

Observations in Other Species

Acute Effects Oral LD_{50}'s of Arachlor's (a trade name in which the last two digits indicate the percent chlorination) agents have been determined in rats: Arochlor 1240, 4.25 g/kg (Bruckner *et al.*, 1973); Arochlor 1254, 1.3–2.5 g/kg (Grant and Philips, 1974); Arochlor 1254, 4–10 g/kg in female Sherman rats (Kimbrough *et al.*, 1972); and Arochlor 1254 and 1260, 1,295 and 1,315 mg/kg, respectively, in weanling rats (Kimbrough, 1974).

Subchronic and Chronic Effects Tucker and Crabtree (1970) reported deaths in rats fed Arochlor at 1 g/kg for 28–53 days. Repeated daily oral administration of 300 mg of Aroclor 1221, 1242, or 1254 in rabbits for 14 weeks produced liver enlargement and damage and one death with

Aroclor 1254, but only minor changes with Aroclor 1221 (Koller and Zinkl, 1973). Allen *et al.* (1974) administered Aroclor 1248 at 25 mg/kg of diet to six female rhesus monkeys for 2 months, with production of facial edema, loss of hair, and acne a month after onset of feeding. Mink on diets containing PCB at 30 mg/kg (Aroclor 1242, 1248, and 1254 at 10 mg/kg each) demonstrated 100% mortality within 6 months (Aulerich *et al.*, 1973). Female mink fed a diet supplemented with Aroclor 1254 at 5 mg/kg for 9 months failed to produce offspring (Ringer *et al.*, 1972).

The oral administration of Aroclor 1242, 1254, and 1260 in rats for 18 months at 1, 10, and 100 mg/kg (Keplinger *et al.*, 1971) produced adverse effects only at 100 mg/kg. With Aroclor 1242 and 1254, there was an increase in liver weight and a reduction in litter survival at 100 mg/kg. Kimbrough *et al.* (1972) reported experiments in which male rats survived Aroclor 1260 at 1 g/kg for 8 months, but 8 of 10 females died at this dosage. With both Aroclor 1254 and 1260, there was a significant dose-dependent increase in liver weight in male rats down to 20 mg/kg in the diet; in female rats, liver enlargement occurred only at 500 mg/kg and higher.

The rhesus monkey is the only animal reported to show signs of poisoning similar to those seen in Yusho patients. Oral administration of Aroclor 1248 at 2.5 and 5.0 mg/kg produced periorbital edema, alopecia, erythema, and acneiform eruptions within 1–2 months. At 25 mg/kg, one of six died; at 100 and 300 mg/kg, the mortality approached 100% in 2–3 months. Survivors still showed signs of poisoning 8 months after exposure was discontinued (Allen and Norback, 1973; Allen *et al.*, 1974; Allen, 1975).

Mutagenicity Aroclor 1242 and Aroclor 1254 have not been found to have mutagenic potential when administered to rats as single or repeated large daily doses. Possible mutagenicity was assessed by cytogenetic analysis of bone marrow and spermatogonia (Green *et al.*, 1975).

Carcinogenicity There have been a number of carcinogenicity studies with mice and rats treated with combinations of PCB's. Only the study of Kimbrough *et al.* (1975) provided a true long-term chronic feeding study. They fed Sherman female rats Aroclor 1260 at 100 mg/kg in their diets for 21 months and sacrificed them at 23 months. At this dosage, 26 of 184 in the experimental group and one of 173 in the controls had hepatocellular carcinomas.

Teratogenicity One study (Kato *et al.*, 1972) demonstrated that PCB's could cross the placenta but produced no defects. Other studies (Funatsu *et al.*, 1972; Miller, 1971) have linked maternal ingestion of PCB with dark-brown staining of the skin of newborn babies.

Carcinogenic Risk Estimates

Only the study by Kimbrough *et al.* (1975) is of sufficient duration to permit a statistical extrapolation of risk to man. The available set of dose–response data was considered as described in the risk section in the chapter on margin of safety. The set of dose–response data was used to statistically estimate both the lifetime risk and an upper 95% confidence bound on the lifetime risk at the low-dose level. These estimates are of lifetime human risks and have been corrected for species conversion on a dose per surface area basis. The risk estimates are expressed as a probability of cancer after a lifetime consumption of 1 liter of water/day containing Q ppb of the compound of interest. For example, a risk of 1×10^{-6} Q implies a lifetime probability of 2×10^{-5} of cancer if 2 liters/day were consumed and the concentration of the carcinogen was 10 ppb (i.e, $Q=10$). This means that at a concentration of 10 ppb during a lifetime of exposure this compound would be expected to produce one excess case of cancer for every 50,000 persons exposed. If the population of the United States is taken to be 220 million people this translates into 4,400 excess lifetime deaths from cancer or 62.8/yr. For the PCB Arochlor 1260 at a concentration of 1 μg/liter ($Q=1$) the projected risk for man is 2.2×10^{-6} Q. The upper 95% confidence estimate of risk at the same concentration is 3.1×10^{-6} Q.

It should be noted that this extrapolation is based on a one-hit mathematical model which may be invalid for this chemical. In addition, the extrapolation pertains to Arochlor 1260 and not to any of the other polychlorinated biphenyls which make up this class of compounds. It would be impossible from this limited study to single out any one of the PCB's as the carcinogenic agent and it should be kept in mind that they may be acting synergistically.

Conclusions and Recommendations

Although there are considerable data on toxicity of mixtures of PCB's, there is a paucity of data on the pure congeners present in these mixtures. Whether chronic toxicity is related to the metabolism of the PCB's and their intermediates or to the highly chlorinated stored PCB's remains to be determined. Considerably more attention must be directed to the detection of impurities in PCB's at very low concentrations. Polyclorodibenzoforan may constitute only one of several significant contaminating compounds responsible for PCB toxicity. Populations at special risk—both the industrially exposed and those heavily exposed by the ingestion of contaminated foods—should be carefully evaluated.

Despite the current lack of evidence in the United States that dietary PCB's have any deleterious effects on health, there is a growing concern with long-range effects of the contamination of our ecosystem with these chemicals. There is an urgent need for epidemiologic studies of exposed populations, more precise identification of all sources of PCB contamination, and efforts directed at the control of disposal of PCB's. Because of the demonstrated carcinogenic potential, studies on individual congeners, both those metabolized and those stored by man, are urgent.

The available chronic toxicity data are summarized in Table VI-56.

Propylbenzene

Introduction

Propylbenzene (1-phenylpropane) is produced in petroleum refining and as a byproduct of cumene manufacture. It is used in the manufacture of methylstyrene and in textile dyeing (USEPA, 1975d). It is insoluble in water (CRC Handbook of Chemistry and Physics, 1970–1971). Two of the 10 water supplies surveyed by the EPA (1975a) contained propylbenzene in the finished water, at 0.05 μg/liter in Miami and 0.01 μg/liter in Cincinnati.

Metabolism

Propylbenzene is probably readily absorbed from the gastrointestinal tract and the lungs and excreted mainly in the urine of humans (Thienes and Haley, 1972). No information on tissue or organ storage was available. Metabolically, propylbenzene is characterized by high stability of the benzene nucleus (Smirnova and Stepanova, 1969). In rats, there appears to be a dual metabolic pathway: side-chain oxidation and ring hydroxylation, with the former preferred (Gerarde and Ahlstrom, 1966).

Health Aspects

Observations in Man Propylbenzene is irritating to the mucous membranes, eyes, nose, throat, and skin. Systemically, it causes depression of the central nervous system, headache, anorexia, muscular weakness, incoordination, nausea, vertigo, paresthesias, mental confusion, and

TABLE VI-56 Toxicity of PCB's

Species	Duration of Study	Dosage Levels and No. of Animals Per Group	Highest No-Adverse-Effect Level or Lowest-Minimal-Effect Level	Effect Measured	Reference
Mink	6 mo		30 mg/kg in diet	100% mortality	Aulerich *el al.*, 1973
Mink	9 mo.		5 mg/kg in diet	females failed to produce offspring	Ringer *et al.*, 1972
Rat	18 mo.	1, 10, 100 mg/kg	100 mg/kg in diet	adverse effects	Kiplinger *et al.*, 1971
Rat (female)	21 mo.	0, 100 mg/kg in diet, 173–184 animals/group (Aroclor 1260)	100 mg/kg	heptocellular carcinoma	Kimbrough *et al.*, 1975

[Aroclor 1260 is an animal carcinogen.]

unconsciousness. Possible effects on the liver, bone marrow, and heart are not known (Thienes and Haley, 1972).

Observations in Other Species

Acute Effects In one study, the LD_{50} was 7.5 g/kg in rats and 5.2 g/kg in mice (Smirnova and Stepanova, 1969). In another study, the LD_{50} in rats was shown to be 6.04 g/kg (Jenner *et al.*, 1964).

Chronic Effects In a 6-month subchronic oral study (Gerarde and Ahlstrom, 1966), groups of 15 rabbits were fed propylbenzene at 0.25 and 2.5 mg/kg/day. The test animals did not differ from the controls in general appearance, body weight, organ weights, and protein function of the liver. There was a 7% decrease in the red-cell count in the high-dosage group that was not significant. Hemosiderin was deposited in the spleens of the high-dosage animals, indicating red-cell destruction. There was a nonsignificant leukocyte increase in both dosage groups. Individual animals exhibited mild protein dystrophy of the liver and kidneys.

Mutagenicity No available data.

Carcinogenicity No available data.

Teratogenicity No available data.

Conclusions and Recommendations

In view of the relative paucity of data on the mutagenicity, carcinogenicity, teratogenicity, and long-term oral toxicity of propylbenzene, estimates of the effects of chronic oral exposure at low levels cannot be made with any confidence. It is recommended that studies to produce such information be conducted before limits in drinking water are established.

Styrene

Introduction

Styrene monomer is synthesized from ethylene and benzene. It is used in the manufacture of polystyrene plastics, resins, insulators, synthetic rubber, and protective coatings (Chemistry Dictionary, 1972). The United States production of styrene in 1973 was over 2.56 billion pounds (USITC, 1975). Styrene is insoluble in water. It has been detected in the finished water of three of the 10 water supplies surveyed by the EPA (1975a).

Metabolism

In a study conducted by El Masri *et al.* (1958), rabbits were given styrene orally, and the metabolites were determined. It was established that the main metabolite of styrene was hippuric acid, which accounted for 30–40% of the oral dose. Lesser metabolites were mandelic acid and phenylglycol, the latter being excreted as a monoglucuronide. Only about 2% of the styrene administered was eliminated unchanged in the expired air. Because phenylglycol itself yields hippuric acid, mandelic acid, and phenylglycol as metabolites, it is suggested that styrene may undergo perhydroxylation *in vivo* to its intermediate, phenylglycol. It was noted that the metabolites of styrene were almost completely excreted 1–2 days after administration of the single dose.

Health Aspects

Observations in Man Wolf *et al.* (1956), in the course of conducting inhalation studies on animals, exposed human subjects to various concentrations of styrene monomer. They reported very strong odor with eye and nasal irritation at 600 ppm, detectable odor with no irritation at 60 ppm, and no detectable odor at 10 ppm and less.

Stewart *et al.* (1968) exposed human volunteers to styrene vapors at approximately 50, 100, 200, and 375 ppm for periods of 1–7 h. Only at 375 ppm did the subjects experience subjective symptoms and objective signs of transient neurologic impairment. The vapors irritated the eyes and nose and in one subject produced a burning sensation of the facial skin. Neurologic effects were manifested by inability to perform a normal modified Romberg test, a decrease in the Crawford Manual Dexterity color and Pin Test score, and decreased performance on the Flannigan Coordination Test. Stewart *et al.* (1968) showed that the amount of styrene exhaled after an exposure indicated the extent of exposure. Urine hippuric acid content, however, was not a sensitive indicator.

Observations in Other Species

Acute Effects In an acute study, Spencer *et al.* (1942) exposed rats and guinea pigs to various vapor doses of the compound. At the lowest dose (650–1,300), the animals demonstrated eye and nose irritation. Styrene could be tolerated for only 8 h at 1,300–2,000 ppm. The maximum tolerated time without serious adverse effects was reduced to 1 h at 2,500 ppm; and 10,000 ppm proved lethal in 30–60 m.

Chronic Effects In a study of the chronic effects of styrene, Spencer *et al.* (1942) intubated rats 5 days/week for 28 days at 2.0, 1.0, 0.5, and 0.1 g/kg/day. Animals survived 0.5 g/kg, but lost weight, probably owing to gastrointestinal irritation. The no-adverse-effect dosage was 0.1 g/kg/day. Wolf *et al.* (1956) intubated rats daily, 5 days/week, for 185 days (132 doses), at doses of 66.7, 133, 400, and 667 mg/kg/day. The no-adverse-effect level was 133 mg/kg/day. The only dosage-related effects at higher dosages were increased liver and kidney weights. In the same study, rats, guinea pigs, rabbits, and monkeys were chronically exposed to styrene by inhalation. The no-observed-adverse-effect concentration was 650–1,300 ppm, with some species variability.

Mutagenicity No available data.

Carcinogenicity No available data.

Teratogenicity No available data.

Conclusions and Recommendations

Styrene at high concentrations is mainly an irritant whether ingested or inhaled. Humans have tolerated acute exposures of 200 ppm with no ill effects.

An ADI of 0.133 mg/kg/day was calculated on the basis of the available chronic toxicity data. The available chronic toxicity data and calculations are summarized in Table VI-57.

1,1,1,2-Tetrachloroethane

Introduction

1,1,1,2-Tetrachloroethane is used as a solvent and in the manufacture of insecticides, herbicides, soil fumigants, bleaches, paints, and varnishes (USEPA, 1975d). It is soluble in water at 1 g in 350 ml at 25°C. It is potentially formed during chlorination of water (USEPA, 1975d). It has been reported that the finished water of the District of Columbia contained tetrachloroethane at 1 μg/liter (Scheiman *et al.*, 1974) and that of New Orleans, 0.11 μg/liter (USEPA, 1974).

TABLE VI-57 Toxicity of Styrene

Species	Duration of Study	Dosage Levels and No. of Animals Per Group	Highest No-Adverse-Effect Level or Lowest-Minimal-Effect Level	Effect Measured	Reference
Rat	28 days	0–20 g/kg/day, intubated	0.1 g/kg/day	no adverse effect	Spencer *et al.*, 1942
Rat	185 days	0–667 mg/kg/day, intubated	133 mg/kg/day[c]	no adverse effect	Wolf *et al.*, 1956

Using an uncertainty factor of 1,000, the suggested no-adverse-effect level in drinking water is calculated as follows:

$$\frac{133}{1{,}000} = 0.133 \text{ mg/kg/day (ADI)},\ 0.133 \times 70^{a} \times 0.1^{b} = 0.9 \text{ mg/liter}$$

[a]Assume average weight of human adult = 70 kg.
[b]Assume average daily intake of water for man = 2 liters, and that 20 percent of total intake is from water.
[c]Value from which the suggested no-adverse-effect level was calculated.

Metabolism

Truhaut (1973) reported that 1,1,1,2-tetrachloroethane underwent hydrolytic dehalogenation in rats, guinea pigs, and rabbits; this resulted in the formation of trichloroethanol, which was eliminated primarily in the urine in the form of a conjugated glucuronic derivative (urochloralic acid). Oxidation into trichloroacetic acid was considerable only in rats. The only halogenated compound found in expired air was untransformed 1,1,1,2-tetrachloroethane.

In a study of the metabolism of 1,1,1,2-tetrachloroethane in mice, Yllner (1971a,b) administered the compound subcutaneously at 1.2–2.0 g/kg and followed the excretion in urine for 3 days. About half the dose (21–62%) was expired and unchanged. The part metabolized was excreted mainly as trichloroethanol (17–49% of the dose) and to a lesser extent as trichloroacetic acid (1–7%).

It is concluded that the metabolism of tetrachloroethane probably takes place mainly via a staged hydrolytic fission of carbon–chlorine bonds and oxidation to give first dichloroacetic acid and then glyoxylic acid. With part of the tetrachloroethane, a nonenzymic dehydrochlorination occurs, with the formation of trichloroethylene, which is also found in the breath. Trichloroethylene is probably the precursor of the trichloroethanol and trichloroacetic acid found in the urine.

Health Aspects

Observations in Man Minot and Smith (1921), cited by Parmenter, discovered the high percentage of large mononuclear cells found in the circulating blood of patients suffering from the early stages of tetrachloroethane poisoning. These findings were confirmed by Parmenter (1923), who observed that, during the appearance of early tolerance to tetrachloroethane fumes, its toxicity was measured best by the appearance of the differential count of the blood, which often went as high as about 30–40% in large mononuclear cells without clinical signs of disease. Parmenter listed the symptoms as occasional complaints of a tired feeling and, more often, gastric symptoms, such as lack of appetite and slight nausea, possibly a slight headache, and intercurrent remissions and exacerbations that caused absenteeism. He stated that a high mononuclear-cell count (20% or above) usually indicated poisoning, although this varied with individual tolerance. A large number of broken cells of this type indicated rapid progression of poisoning, in his opinion. McNally's

(1937) observations of industrial exposures agreed with the clinical observations of the foregoing authors.

In a study of 380 workers employed in the manufacture of bangles in small factories in India, Lobo-Mendonca (1963) tried to determine the degree of inhalation of tetrachloroethane that formed part of the environment of workers engaged in washing and handling bangles and production machinery around or in which tetrachloroethane was used as a cleaning agent. Interest centered on the high percentage of workers with nervous symptoms, such as headache, vertigo, nervousness, numbness, and tremors. Tetrachloroethane at 9–17 ppm induced tremors in 14% of the personnel; at 40–74 ppm, in 33%; at 50–61 ppm, in 41%; and at 65–98 ppm, in 50%.

Observations in Other Species

Acute Effects The oral LD_{50} of 1,1,1,2-tetrachloroethane was 800 mg/kg in rats and 1,500 mg/kg in mice (Truhaut *et al.*, 1974). Compared with 1,1,2,2-tetrachloroethane, 1,1,1,2-tetrachloroethane was one-half or one-third as toxic, but had hepatotoxic properties, which were dose-related, in different animal species. It induced microvacuoliation or central lobular necrosis or both in the liver. It also passed through the placental barrier and affected the fetus.

Chronic Effects In a study of the effects of chronic action of low concentrations of chlorinated hydrocarbons on the production of various classes of immunoblobulins, Shmuter (1972) used rabbits that inhaled chlorinated hydrocarbons at 2 mg/m^3 for 3 h/day for 8–10 months. Tetrachloroethane was found to be more harmful to total antibody formation than its pentachloro- or dichloro- analogues.

Mutagenicity No available data.

Carcinogenicity No available data.

Teratogenicity No available data.

Conclusions and Recommendations

In view of the relative paucity of data on the mutagenicity, carcinogenicity, teratogenicity, and long-term oral toxicity of 1,1,1,2-tetrachloroethane, estimates of the effects of chronic oral exposure at low levels cannot be made with any confidence. It is recommended that studies to produce such information be conducted before limits in drinking water are established.

Tetrachloroethylene

Introduction

Tetrachloroethylene (perchloroethylene) is used as solvent, heat-transfer medium, and in the manufacture of fluorocarbons (USEPA, 1975d). The U.S. production of this compound in 1973 was over 705 million pounds (USITC, 1975). It is insoluble in water (CRC Handbook of Chemistry and Physics, 1970–1971). During chlorination water treatment, it can be formed in small quantities (USEPA, 1975d). It has been found in the finished water of the New Orleans area at up to 5 μg/liter (USEPA, 1974). Eight of the 10 water utilities surveyed by the EPA (1975a) contained tetrachloroethylene, at 0.07–0.46 μg/liter.

Metabolism

There have been a number of studies pertaining to the metabolism of tetrachloroethylene in mice, rats, and humans (Yllner, 1961; Daniel, 1963; Ogata, 1971). The consensus appears to be that most of the material is expired unchanged and that very little (5%) is metabolized and later excreted in the urine or feces. However, experience with similar compounds indicates that the portion metabolized may be markedly greater at low doses than at high doses. Up to 10% remains in the body (very likely in the fat) after 4 days, but to judge by these reports there is little likelihood of cumulative toxicity.

Health Aspects

Observations in Man Rowe *et al.* (1952) showed central nervous system effects in man from single exposures at 200 ppm, but not at 100 ppm.

Observations in Other Species

Acute Effects In studies of the acute effects of tetrachloroethylene, the oral LD_{50} was shown to be 4,000 mg/kg in dogs and 5,000 mg/kg in rabbits (Registry of Toxic Effects of Chemical Substances, 1975).

Chronic Effects In a chronic study, Rowe *et al.* (1952) exposed groups of rats, rabbits, guinea pigs, and monkeys repeatedly to various concentrations of tetrachloroethylene (100–2,500 ppm) for various periods (13–179 exposures in 18–250 days). No adverse effects were observed at 100 ppm.

Mutagenicity No available data.

Carcinogenicity No available data.

Teratogenicity Schwetz *et al.* (1975) examined the teratogenic effects of tetrachloroethylene in rats and Swiss Webster mice. The animals were exposed at 300 ppm 7 h/day on days 6–15 of gestation. There was no significant maternal, embryonal, or fetal toxicity, nor was tetrachloroethylene teratogenic in either species.

Conclusions and Recommendations

Tetrachloroethylene is not teratogenic in one strain of rats and mice. In view of the relative paucity of data on the mutagenicity, carinogenicity, and long-term oral toxicity of tetrachloroethylene, estimates of the effects of chronic oral exposure at low levels cannot be made with any confidence. It is recommended that studies to produce such information be conducted before final limits in drinking water are established.

Toluene

Introduction

Toluene is formed in petroleum refining and coal tar distillation. It is used in the manufacture of benzene derivatives, caprolactam, saccharin, perfumes, dyes, medicines, solvents, TNT, and detergent and as a gasoline component (USEPA, 1975d). The U.S. production of toluene in 1973 was over 6.8 billion pounds (USITC, 1975). It is insoluble in water (CRC Handbook of Chemistry and Physics, 1970–1971). Six of the 10 water supplies surveyed by the EPA (1975a) contained toluene. It has been reported that the finished water of the New Orleans area contained toluene, at up to 11 μg/liter (USEPA 1975c).

Metabolism

In man and rabbits, Bakke and Scheline (1970) reported that approximately 80% of a dose of toluene was excreted in the urine as hippuric acid (benzoyl glycine), whereas most of the remainder was exhaled (Williams, 1959). These authors also reported that 0.4–1.1% was excreted as *o*- or *p*-cresol. In hydrolyzed urine, small amounts of benzyl alcohol were detected; this suggested that this may be an intermediate in the formation of benzoic acid.

Pretreatment of rats with phenobarbital increased the rate of disappearance of toluene from the blood (Ikeda and Ohtsuji, 1971) and shortened the sleeping time after injection of toluene; thus, induction of the hepatic microsomal enzyme system may stimulate toluene metabolism.

The reports of Ogata *et al.* (1970, 1971) tend to show that, at relatively low exposures to toluene, the excretion of hippuric acid is proportional to the exposure. They also demonstrated that, when human volunteers were exposed at up to 200 ppm, 68% of a calculated dose was excreted as hippuric acid.

Health Aspects

Observations in Man All the available information on acute human exposure to toluene suggests a narcotic effect. Benzoic acid and hippuric acid, the major metabolites of toluene, are relatively innocuous and have been used as a clinical measure of liver function. In these studies, subjects are given 6 g of sodium benzoate orally, and excretion of hippuric acid is measured over the next 4 h. Excretion over this period accounts for approximately 50% of the ingested dose. Thus, relatively large quantities of the known major metabolites produce no known toxic effects in man. In addition, benzoic acid is approved as an antimicrobial food additive at 1,000 ppm.

Many reports on long-term industrial exposure to toluene are available. Capellini and Allessio (1971) reported that 17 workers were exposed for several years to a mean atmospheric toluene concentration of 125 ppm, without any detectable change in blood characteristics or in liver function. Banfer (1961) reported on studies of 889 photogravure printers and helpers exposed for more than 3 yr to variable toluene concentrations (measured on only 1 day, maximal concentration was 400 ppm; generally, it was 200 ppm), with no hematologic abnormalities. Greenburg (1942) reported on 61 workers exposed to toluene at 100–1,100 ppm from 2 weeks to 5 yr. He reported no severe illness, but found some evidence of mild red-cell decrease, enlarged liver, and increased mean corpuscular hemoglobin concentration.

Forni *et al.* (1971) reported that people exposed to toluene (at approximately 200 ppm) for work periods of 3–15 yr showed a somewhat higher average rate of unstable chromosomal changes and calculated breaks, but the differences were not statistically significant.

The human exposure data suggest that some effects of narcosis are evident at around 200 ppm. This was the threshold limit value (TLV) suggested for control of industrial exposures from 1947 to 1971. The TLV was then lowered to 100 ppm, on the basis of irritation to eyes and upper respiratory tract. The NIOSH criteria document (1973) for a recommended standard for toluene indicated that a literature search failed to confirm any clinical or laboratory evidence of altered liver function in workers exposed to 80–300 ppm for many years.

Observations in Other Species

Acute Effects Svirbely *et al.* (1943) reported the minimal lethal acute inhalation concentration of toluene (containing 0.01% benzene) to be 20 mg/liter (5,300 ppm) in mice for a single 8-h exposure.

Chronic Effects Fabre *et al.* (1955) reported that two dogs chronically exposed for 8 h/day, 6 days/week, for 4 months to toluene (containing 0.1% benzene) at 2,000 ppm (7.5 mg/liter) and an additional 2 months at 2,660 ppm (10 mg/liter) showed signs of nervous system intoxication, incoordination, and paralysis of the hindlegs. Blood and bone marrow studies yielded normal results. Congestive changes were seen in lungs, heart, liver, kidneys, and spleen. Takeuchi (1969) exposed rats to toluene (99.9%) vapor at 200, 1,000, and 2,000 ppm for 8 h/day for 32 weeks. No significant changes in body weight or hematologic findings were reported.

Gerarde (1956) reported that rats given daily injections of toluene at 1 ml/kg in olive oil for 2 weeks showed no abnormalities with respect to peripheral blood, femoral bone marrow, or weight of thymus or spleen. In rabbits given toluene subcutaneously at 300 mg/kg/day for 6 weeks or 700 mg/kg/day for 9 weeks, no decrease in bone marrow function was found, as measured by uptake of tritium-labeled thymidine, nor was there any alteration in the formed elements of the peripheral blood.

Mutagenicity No available data.

Carcinogenicity No available data.

Teratogenicity No available data.

Conclusions and Recommendations

Other than central nervous system depression, the inhalation of toluene at less than 2,000 ppm has produced no adverse effects. In addition, the major metabolite of toluene, benzoic acid, is considered relatively nontoxic and is an approved food additive.

In view of the relative paucity of data on the mutagenicity, carcinogenicity, teratogenicity and long-term oral toxicity of toluene, estimates of the effects of chronic oral exposure at low levels cannot be made with any confidence. It is recommended that studies to produce such information be conducted before final limits in drinking water are established.

Trichlorobenzene

Introduction

Trichlorobenzene is produced by chlorination of monochlorobenzene. It is used as a solvent, dielectric fluid, lubricant, and heat-transfer medium; in polyester dyeing; and in termite preparations (USEPA, 1975d).

The U.S. production of 1,2,4-trichlorobenzene in 1973 was over 28 million pounds (USITC, 1975). It is insoluble in water (CRC Handbook of Chemistry and Physics, 1970–1971). Trichlorobenzene can be formed in small quantities during chlorination of drinking water (USEPA, 1975d). Of the 10 water supplies surveyed by the EPA (1975a), trichlorobenzene was only detected in the finished water of Lawrence, Massachusetts.

Metabolism

In metabolic studies with rabbits using each of the three isomeric trichlorobenzenes at 0.5 g/kg, 1,2,3-trichlorobenzene was the most rapidly metabolized, and 1,3,5-trichlorobenzene was least rapidly metabolized. In 5 days, 62% of the 1,2,3-trichloro isomer underwent glucuronic conjugation. The major metabolite was 2,3,4-trichlorophenol; small amounts of 3,4,5-trichlorophenol, 3,4,5-trichlorocatechol, and mercapturic acid were also detected. 1,3,5-Trichlorobenzene formed practically no ethereal sulfate or mercapturic acid, and the only phenol formed was 2,4,6-trichlorophenol (Jondorf *et al.*, 1955).

Along with tests on other halogenated benzenes, 1,3,5-trichlorobenzene was administered orally to rats at 2 mg/kg, and this chemical was found in the fat at greater concentrations than in liver, kidneys, heart, or blood. These studies were designed to show the possible effects of chlorinated substances from Rhine River water and how they might affect body burden in animal tissues and organs (Jacobs *et al.*, 1974).

Health Aspects

Observations in Man In one plant where benzene was chlorinated over a period of 4 yr, there was no apparent serious illness, liver function change, or alteration in blood components. One worker who inhaled a massive amount of trichlorobenzene experienced some hemorrhaging in the lungs (Erlicher, 1968).

Observation in Other Species

Acute Effects Acute-toxicity tests have been conducted in rats (CFE strain) and mice (CF No. 1 strain) by oral and percutaneous administration. The single-dose acute oral LD_{50} was 756 mg/kg in rats. The main signs of intoxication were decrease in activity at a low dose and convulsions at higher doses. Death occurred 5 days after exposure. The single-dose acute oral LD_{50} was 766 mg/kg in mice. Signs of intoxication were the same as in rats (Brown *et al.*, 1969).

Chronic Effects In chronic-skin-irritation studies with rabbits and guinea pigs, trichlorobenzene was not irritating, although some degreasing action took place after prolonged contact. After 3 weeks of exposure, there was some skin inflammation characterized by spongiosis and parakeratosis. Livers of guinea pigs were found to have necrotic foci (Brown *et al.*, 1969). Trichlorobenzene was also evaluated for its acnegenic potential in rabbits by applying 1,2,4-trichlorobenzene to the ears of rabbits for 13 weeks. There was no typical acneiform dermatitits, but there was some dermal irritation (Powers *et al.*, 1975).

Mutagenicity No available data.

Carcinogenicity No available data.

Teratogenicity No available data.

Conclusions and Recommendations

In view of the relative paucity of data on the mutagenicity, carcinogenicity, teratogenicity and long-term oral toxicity of trichlorobenzene, esimates of the effects of chonic oral exposure at low levels cannot be made with any confidence. It is recommended that studies to produce such information be conducted before limits in drinking water are established.

1,1,2-Trichloroethane

Introduction

1,1,2-Trichloroethane (vinyl trichloride) is used as solvent for fats, oils, waxes, and resins and in the synthesis of organic chemicals (USEPA, 1975d). It is insoluble in water (CRC Handbook of Chemistry and Physics, 1970–1971). During chlorination water treatment, 1,1,2-trichloroethane can be formed in small quantities (USEPA, 1975d). Of the 10 water supplies surveyed by the EPA (1975a), only the finished water of Miami contained 1,1,2-trichloroethane. It has also been found in the finished water of the New Orleans area, at less than 0.1 to 8.5 μg/liter (USEPA, 1975c).

Metabolism

Trichloroethane is excreted primarily by the lungs, with some elimination via the kidneys (Browning, 1965). The major metabolite in the mouse of this compound is chloroacetic acid; minor metabolites are 2,2-dichloroethanol, 2,2,2-trichloroethanol, oxalic acid, and trichoroacetic acid (Yllner, 1971a). In vitro, the compound is dechlorinated by a reconstituted rat liver microsomal mixed-function oxidase system (Gandolfi and Van Dyke, 1973).

Health Aspects

Observations in Man The adverse health aspects of this compound in man have not been examined. No toxic effects have been recorded in association with its applications in industrial solvents (Browning, 1965).

Observations in Other Species

Acute Effects LD_{50}'s of 1,1,2-trichloroethane were calculated to be: 0.58 (0.47–0.71) and 1.14 g/kg orally in rats (Smyth *et al.*, 1969; Union Carbide Corp., 1968); 0.35 (0.28–0.44) ml/kg and 3.7 (3.0–4.7) mM/kg intraperitoneally in male and female Swiss-Webster mice, respectively (Klaassen and Plaa, 1966; Gehring, 1968); and 3.73 (3.30–4.21) ml/kg dermally in rabbits (Smyth *et al.*, 1969; Toxicology Information Bulletin, 1968).

The hepatotoxicity of trichloroethane has been extensively examined in a variety of experimental animals. Cellular infiltration, vacuolation of hepatocytes, increased serum glutamic pruvic transaminase (SGPT) and prolonged retention of BSP (bromsulphalein) have been observed in studies with mice (Klaassen and Plaa, 1966). SGPT increases and the threshold doses have also been shown to be potentiated by isopropyl alcohol and acetone in mice treated with 1,1,2-trichloroethane at 0.05–0.14 ml/kg (Traiger and Plaa, 1974). In dogs, mild centrilobular necrosis, slight subcapsular necrosis, and vacuolation of the centrilobular hepatocytes have been observed, in combination with increased SGPT (Klaassen and Plaa, 1967).

In studies that sought to examine the nephrotoxicity of trichloroethane, the presence of hyaline droplets, nuclear pycnosis, hydropic degeneration, increased eosinophilia, tubular necrosis with karyolysis, and loss of epithelium of convoluted tubules in mice have been reported, in combination with a decrease in *p*-aminohippuric acid concentration and altered urinary PSP (phenolsulfonphthalein) excretion (Klaassen and Plaa, 1966). In dogs, tubular necrosis has been observed after exposure to trichloroethane, but it appeared to be less severe than that seen in mice; urinary PSP excretion was also modified in dogs (Klaassen and Plaa, 1967).

Chronic Effects No available data.

Mutagenicity No available data.

Carcinogenicity There are some indications that responses to trichloroethane are comparable both qualitatively and quantitatively with those to carbon tetrachloride (Browning, 1965).

Teratogenicity No available data.

Conclusions and Recommendations

In view of the relative paucity of data on the mutagenicity, carcinogenicity, teratogenicity, and long-term oral toxicity of 1,1,2-trichloroethane, estimates of the effects of chronic oral exposure at low levels cannot be made with any confidence. It is recommended that studies to produce such information be conducted before limits in drinking water are established.

Trichloroethylene

Introduction

Trichloroethylene (trichloroethene) is used primarily in metal degreasing. It is also used in dry-cleaning operations, as a solvent, in organic synthesis, and in refrigerants and fumigants (Frear, 1969). The U.S. production of this compound in 1973 was over 451 million pounds (USITC, 1975).

Trichloroethylene is slightly soluble in water (CRC Handbook of Chemistry and Physics, 1970–1971). It can be formed during chlorination of water (USEPA, 1975d). The 10-city survey indicated that finished water of five supplies contained trichloroethylene, at 0.1–0.5 μg/liter (USEPA, 1975a).

Metabolism

Butler (1949) indicated that trichloroacetic acid, trichloroethanol, and small amounts of chloroform and monochloroacetic acid were the metabolic products of trichloroethylene. Ikeda and Ohtsuji (1972) reported that rats excrete 5–7 times more trichloroethanol than trichloroacetic acid after exposure to trichloroethylene. The excretion of trichloroethylene and trichloroacetic acid in the urine has been used to some extent to measure trichloroethylene exposure.

Health Aspects

Observations in Man Exposure to trichloroethylene results in central nervous system depression, incoordination, and unconsciousness, as evidenced by its use as an anesthetic. Acute human exposures have occurred, but have not always been clear-cut cases of exposure to a single entity. The report of Feldman *et al.* (1970) concerned a person who was exposed to trichloroethylene vapors from an overheated degreasing unit. He experienced nausea, vomiting, blurred vision, and numbness of the face 10–12 h after exposure. The recovery of sensation in the face and motor function of facial muscles occurred slowly over an 18-month period. Sagawa *et al.* (1973) reported accidental exposure of a young woman to vapor and mist of trichloroethylene, which resulted in unconsciousness and a permanent residual disability with respect to mobility. In fatal cases of acute trichloroethylene exposure reported by Kleinfeld and Tabershaw (1954), there was no tissue abnormality at autopsy. Based on chronic exposure of human work populations there are no reported problems with respect to hepatotoxicity. Both Stewart *et al.* (1970) and Ikeda and Imamuru (1973) reported a rather prolonged (2–3 days) biologic half-life for trichloroethylene.

The NIOSH (1973) recommended the occupational exposure to trichloroethylene at not in excess of 100 ppm as a time-weighted average exposure for an 8-h work day.

Observations in Other Species

Acute Effects The acute oral LD_{50} of trichloroethylene in rats was 4,920 mg/kg (Registry of Toxic Effects of Chemical Substances, 1975). Comparative studies of acute toxicity of halogenated hydrocarbon solvents have also demonstrated that near-lethal doses of trichloroethylene are necessary to produce mild hepatic dysfunction (Klassen and Plaa, 1966). Baker (1958) reported severe changes in the cerebellum, particularly in the Purkinje cell layers in dogs exposed to 3,000 ppm of trichloroethylene vapor. The dogs were exposed from 2–8 h/day for up to 6 days.

Chronic Effects In a study of the chronic effects of trichloroethylene, a 6-month inhalation exposure to 3,000 ppm resulted in increased liver and kidney weights in mice and rats (Adams *et al.*, 1951).

Mutagenicity No available data.

Teratogenicity Schwetz *et al.* (1975) described the acute exposure of mice and rats to 300 ppm, 7 h/day, on days 6–15 of gestation. No embryonal or fetal toxicity was noted, nor were there any teratogenic effects.

Carcinogenicity Trichloroethylene was tested for carcinogenicity by NCI (1976) in a chronic feeding study. Both sexes of Osborne-Mendel rats and $B6C3F_1$ mice were used. Animals were exposed to two doses

(MTD and 1/2 MTD) by oral gavage 5 times/week for 78 weeks. All animals were then kept until terminal sacrifice at 90 or 110 weeks for mice and rats, respectively. The doses used were as follows: 1,097 and 549 mg/kg for both male and female rats and 2,339 and 1,169 mg/kg for male mice and 1,739 and 869 mg/kg for female mice. Significant dose-related hepatocellular carcinoma was seen in both male and female mice, but the rats were quite resistant to the carcinogenic effects of trichloroethylene.

Carcinogenic Risk Estimates

The statistical assessment of human cancer risk associated with trichloroethylene in drinking water is based on the results of a carcinogenesis bioassay experiment with animals (NCI, 1976). Trichloroethylene was dissolved in corn oil and administered by gavage to male and female $B6C3F_1$ mice 5 days/week for 78 weeks. The surviving mice were sacrificed at 90 weeks, and a complete necropsy and microscopic evaluation of all animals were conducted. Highly significant differences in the incidence of hepatocellular carcinomas were found between treated and control mice of both sexes.

The available sets of dose–response data were individually considered as described in the risk section in the chapter on margin of safety. Each set of dose–response data was used to statistically estimate both the lifetime risk and an upper 95% confidence bound on the lifetime risk at the low-dose level. These estimates are of lifetime human risks and have been corrected for species conversion on a dose/surface area basis. The risk estimates are expressed as a probability of cancer after a lifetime consumption of 1 liter of water/day containing Q ppb of the compound of interest. For example, a risk of $1 \times 10^{-6}\ Q$ implies a lifetime probability of 2×10^{-5} of cancer if 2 liters/day were consumed and the concentration of the carcinogen was 10 ppb (i.e., $Q = 10$). This means that at a concentration of 10 ppb during a lifetime of exposure this compound would be expected to produce one excess case of cancer for every 50,000 persons exposed. If the population of the United States is taken to be 220 million people this translates into 4,400 excess lifetime deaths from cancer or 62.8/yr. Since several data sets are typically available the range of the low-dose risk estimates are reported. For trichloroethylene at a concentration of 1 μg/liter ($Q = 1$) the estimated risk for man would be $0.36–1.1 \times 10^{-7}\ Q$. The upper 95% confidence estimate of risk at the same concentration is $0.55–1.6 \times 10^{-7}\ Q$.

It should be emphasized that these extrapolations are based on a number of unverifiable assumptions: extrapolation from high exposure to low exposure in mice, on the basis of a multistage mathematical model;

TABLE VI-58 Toxicity of Trichloroethylene

Species	Duration of Study	Dosage Levels and No. of Animals Per Group	Highest No-Adverse-Effect Level or Lowest-Minimal-Effect Level	Effect Measured	Reference
Mouse (male)	78 weeks	0, 1,169, and 2,339 mg/kg/day, gavage 20–50 animals/group	1,169 mg/kg/day	hepatomas	NCI, 1976
Mouse	78 weeks	0, 869, and 1,739 mg/kg/day, gavage 20–50 animals/group	869 mg/kg/day	hepatomas	NCI, 1976

[This compound is an animal carcinogen.]

extrapolation from mouse to man, on the basis of the surface-area rule; and extrapolation from gavage exposure to oral exposure assumed equal. These estimated human risks should be taken as crude estimates at best.

Conclusions and Recommendations

It is concluded that trichloroethylene has low toxicity, both acute and chronic. Only after high acute accidental exposures have effects been reported in humans. These have been related to the depressant effect on the central nervous system. No fetal toxicity or teratogenic effects have been reported. Carcinogenic bioassay demonstrated hepatocellular carcinoma in one strain of mice. The chronic toxicity data are summarized in Table VI-58.

Trichlorofluoromethane

Introduction

Trichlorofluoromethane (Freon ll) is used in the manufacture of aerosol sprays, refrigerants, blowing agents, and cleaning compounds and in fire extinguishers (USEPA, 1975d). The U.S. production of this compound in 1973 was over 333 million pounds (USITC, 1975). It has been reported that the finished water of Washington, D.C., contained less than 1 μg/liter of trichlorofluoromethane (Scheiman *et al.*, 1974).

Metabolism

When trichlorofluoromethane was inhaled by humans, recovery of the intact compound in exhaled air was 79–99% and in urine, 0.07–0.09%, and metabolites amounted to 0.2% or less (Mergner *et al.*, 1975). Terrill (1974) demonstrated that absoprtion of a fluorocarbon, F115, in dogs was 35–48 times greater by inhalation than by oral administration. Charlesworth (1975) indicated that the main factor affecting the fate of fluorocarbons is the body fat, where they are concentrated and slowly released into the blood at concentrations that should not cause any risk of cardiac sensitization. Blake and Mergner (1974) showed that inhalation of ^{14}C-labeled Freon 11 by dogs resulted in complete recovery in exhaled air (101.8%) in 1 h, recovery from urine of only 0.0095%, and no evidence of biotransformation. However, Niazi and Chiou (1975), who administered Freon 11 intravenously in dogs, demonstrated that, although the compound is rapidly eliminated from the bloodstream, it is then eliminated via three compartments with half-lives of 3.2, 16, and 93 min.

Health Aspects

Observations in Man By inhalation, large, acute doses have resulted in cardiac sensitization (arrhythmia) or bronchial constriction leading to death (Dollery *et al.*, 1970). The threshold limit value (ACGIH, 1967) is 1,000 ppm, or 5,600 mg/m^3.

Observations in Other Species

Acute Effects Slater (1965) gave a single oral dose of 2.5 g/kg to rats and reported no liver pathology. Lester and Greenberg (1950) reported that inhalation by rats of aerosol containing 6% Freon 11 resulted in loss of postural reflex, 8% resulted in loss of righting reflex, 9% resulted in unconsciousness, and 10% was lethal. Mice that inhaled 10% developed cardiac arrhythmia (Aviado and Belej, 1975); dogs that inhaled 2.5% had decreased myocardial function, including cardiac output (Aviado and Belej, 1975); and monkeys that inhaled 5% developed tachycardia and hypotension (Belej and Aviado, 1973).

Chronic Effects Kudo *et al.* (1971) reported that mice given oral doses of 15, 55, and 220 mg/kg/day for a month showed only slight effects on food utilization.

Mutagenicity No available data.

Carcinogenicity In a study by Epstein *et al.* (1967) mice given 0.1 ml of 10% solution solution at 1 and 7 days of age and 0.2 ml at 14 and 21 days of age were observed for 1 yr. No evidence of a carcinogenic effect of Freon 11 was found.

Teratogenicity Paulet *et al.* (1974) reported that inhalation at 200,000 ppm of a 9:1 mixture of Freon 12 and Freon 11 by rats on days 4–16 of gestation and rabbits on days 5–20 of gestation did not induce any embryotoxic or teratogenic effects.

Conclusions and Recommendations

In view of the relative paucity of data on the mutagenicity, carcinogenicity, and long-term oral toxicity of trichlorofluoromethane, estimates of the effects of chronic oral exposure at low levels cannot be made with any confidence. It is recommended that studies to produce such information be conducted before limits in drinking water are established.

Vinyl Chloride

Introduction

Vinyl chloride (chloroethene) monomer is not known to occur in nature. It is commercially synthesized by the halogenation of ethylene. In the United States, the vinyl chloride monomer is used primarily in the production of polyvinyl chloride resins for the building and construction industries. Because it has been confirmed that vinyl chloride monomer is a human and animal carcinogen, the sale of propellents and all aerosols containing it was banned in 1974 (USEPA, 1974; United States Consumer Product Safety Commission, 1974). The occupational standard for atmospheric vinyl chloride in the United States is 1 ppm (2.56 mg/m^3) or less for 8 h/day and 5 days/week. The U.S. production of vinyl chloride in 1973 was 5.35 billion pounds (USITC, 1975).

Vinyl chloride monomer is slightly soluble in water ($<0.11\%$ by weight at 25°C) (CRC Handbook of Chemistry and Physics, 1970–1971). Results of the 10-city survey (USEPA, 1975a) indicate that vinyl chloride was present in the finished water of Miami, at 5.6 μg/liter, and Philadelphia, at 0.27 μg/liter.

Metabolism

After inhalation of ^{14}C-vinyl chloride by rats, 2–12% of the 10- or 1,000-ppm dose was eliminated as vinyl chloride in the expired air within 72 h. The 10-ppm exposure produced the higher urinary excretion and lower expired amount. Pulmonary excretion was fast and followed first-order kinetics, but the slower urinary excretion of vinyl chloride metabolites followed a biphasic elimination pattern. Three urinary metabolites have been detected: *N*-acetyl-*S*-(2-hydroxyethyl)cysteine, thiodiglycolic acid, and an unidentified substance (McGowan *et al.*, 1975).

Oral doses of 0.05–1.0 mg/kg in rats yielded similar information. The pulmonary excretion was monophasic at these doses, and the urinary metabolites are the same. At an oral dose of 100 mg/kg, the pulmonary excretion is biphasic and a greater percentage of the administered dose is expired as vinyl chloride—67%, compared with 1 or 2% at the lower dose.

The above data all indicate a dose-dependent fate of vinyl chloride after inhalation or oral administration in rats. The primary mechanism of detoxification of vinyl chloride or its reactive metabolites involves conjugation with hepatic glutathione. The glutathione conjugates are then subject to hydrolysis, yielding the cysteine conjugates found in the urine. This is consistent with the observed decrease in hepatic nonprotein sulfhydryl groups in rats exposed to vinyl chloride (Hefner *et al.*, 1975).

Health Aspects

Observations in Man In studies of the acute effects of vinyl chloride in man, it has been shown to produce central nervous system dysfunction, sympathetic-sensory polyneuritis, and organic disorders of the brain (Smirnova and Granik, 1970). In a series of studies on workers in the polyvinyl chloride industry, scleromalike skin alterations, Raynaud's syndrome, and acroosteolysis were observed (Juehe and Lange, 1972; Juehe *et al.*, 1974; Berk *et al.*, 1975; Martsteller *et al.*, 1975).

To date, 48 cases of hepatic angiosarcoma have been diagnosed in industrial vinyl chloride workers around the world. All authenticated cases were found in workers engaged in closed-in plants handling very large quantities of liquefied vinyl chloride under pressure (Anon., 1974; Makk *et al.*, 1976). Exposure concentrations were high, probably ranging from 1,000 ppm to several thousands ppm.

Lesions of the skin, bones, liver, spleen, and lungs have also been reported after chronic exposure to the compound (Popper and Thomas, 1975; Gedigk *et al.*, 1975; Thomas and Popper, 1975).

Observations in Other Species

Acute Effects Because of the physical properties of vinyl chloride, the effects of oral exposure to it have not been examined. With respect to inhalation toxicity, vinyl chloride has been shown to produce lung congestion and some hemorrhaging, blood-clotting difficulties, and congestion of liver and kidneys in laboratory animals (Mastromatteo *et al.*, 1960). After 2 h at 5% vinyl chloride, rats showed moderate intoxication; 2 h at 15% provoked respiratory failure (Lester *et al.*, 1963).

Mutagenicity In a study by Malaveille *et al.* (1975), exposure of *Salmonella typhimurium* strains TA1530, TA1535, and G-46 to vinyl chloride increased the number of his+revertants/plate 16, 12 or 5 times over the spontaneous mutation rate. The mutagenic response for TA1530 strain was increased when S-9 liver fractions from humans, rats, or mice were added. Exposure of *S. typhimurium* to vinyl chloride gas produced no mutagenic effect without microsomal activation (Rannug *et al.*, 1974).

Carcinogenicity In a study to determine the carcinogenic effects of vinyl chloride inhalation, Viola (1970a,b) and Viola *et al.* (1971) reported that 30,000 ppm, 4 h/day, 5 days/week, for 12 months produced tumors of lungs, skin, and bones in Wistar rats. Along the same lines, 250–10,000 ppm, 4 h/day, 5 days/week, for 12 months was reported by Maltoni and Lefemine (1974a,b) to increase the incidence of cancer in rats. Zymbal gland carcinoma, angiosarcoma, and nephroblastoma were most prominent. Latency for the development of these cancers ranged from 59 to 83 weeks. In another study, in which lower concentrations (50 ppm) were used, a marked change in the latency for finding tumors indicated the possibility of a threshold for induction (Maltoni and Lefemine, 1975).

Teratogenicity Vinyl chloride was administered for 7 h/day on days 6–18 of gestation in mice, rats, and rabbits. It was concluded that, although maternal toxicity was observed, vinyl chloride alone did not cause significant embryonal or fetal toxicity and was not teratogenic in any of the species at the concentrations tested (John *et al.*, 1975).

Carcinogenic Risk Estimates

In a recent study by Maltoni *et al.* (1975), rats were given vinyl chloride in olive oil by gavage four or five times per week for 52 weeks and held for their life span. The available set of dose–response data was considered as described in the risk section in the chapter on margin of safety. Each set of dose–response data was used to statistically estimate both the lifetime risk and an upper 95% confidence bound on the lifetime risk at the low dose level. These estimates are of lifetime human risks and have been corrected for species conversion on a dose/surface area basis. The risk estimates are expressed as a probability of cancer after a lifetime consumption of 1 liter/day of water containing Q ppb of the compound of interest. For example a risk of $1 \times 10^{-6}\ Q$ implies a lifetime probability of 2×10^{-5} of cancer if 2 liters/day were consumed and the concentraton of the carcinogen was 10 ppb (i.e., $Q = 10$). This means that at a concentration of 10 ppb during a lifetime exposure this compound would be expected to produce one excess case of cancer for every 50,000 persons exposed. If the population of the United States is taken to be 220 million people this translates into 4,400 excess lifetime deaths from cancer or 62.8/yr. For vinyl chloride a concentration of 1 μg/liter ($Q = 1$) the estimated risk for man is $3.0 \times 10^{-7}\ Q$. The upper 95% confidence estimate at the same concentration is $4.7 \times 10^{-7}\ Q$.

TABLE VI-59 Toxicity of Vinyl Chloride

Species	Duration of Study	Dosage Levels and No. of Animals Per Group	Highest No-Adverse-Effect Level or Lowest-Minimal-Effect Level	Effect Measured	Reference
Rat	12 months		30,000 ppm, 4 h/day, 5 day/wk	tumors of skin and bones	Viola, 1970a, b; Viola *et al.*, 1971
Rat	12 months	0, 3.33, 16.65, and 50 mg/kg/day	16.65 mg/kg/day (gavage)	angiosarcomas	Maltoni *et al.*, 1975

[This compound is a human and animal carcinogen.]

Conclusions and Recommendations

Vinyl chloride has acute and chronic toxic effects in animals and man. In addition to its chronic toxicity, it has been clearly shown to be a carcinogen in animals and man, with dose- and time-related properties, and to be a mutagen in *in vitro* systems. Its carcinogenic property has been demonstrated by oral administration. This route is more effective (efficient) in producing the characteristic tumor, angiosarcoma, than is loading the atmosphere with similar amounts of vapor. In animal studies, vinyl chloride has induced a wide variety of tumors, in addition to the characteristic and otherwise rare angiosarcoma. The available chronic toxicity data are summarized in Table VI-59.

Xylenes

Introduction

Xylene (dimethylbenzene) is formed in petroleum, coal tar, and coal gas distillation. It is used in aviation gasolines, in rubber cements, in the manufacture of solvents and protective coatings, and in the synthesis of organic chemicals (USEPA, 1975d). The U.S. production of xylene in 1973 was over 5.94 billion pounds (USITC, 1975). Xylene is insoluble in water (CRC Handbook of Chemistry and Physics, 1970–1971). The finished water of the New Orleans area (USEPA, 1975c) contained xylene at 4.1 μg/liter.

Metabolism

Oxidation of xylene to phenolic metabolites has been reported by a number of investigators, including Bakke and Scheline (1970). A dosage of 100 mg/kg in rats gave the following results: *o*-xylene metabolized to 3,4-dimethylphenol (0.1% of dose) and 2,3 dimethylphenol (0.03% of dose); *m*-xylene metabolized to 2,4-methylphenol (0.9% of dose); *p*-xylene metabolized to 2,5-dimethylphenol (1.0% of dose). 2-Methylbenzyl alcohol was also reported as a metabolite of *o*-xylene. In man, Ogata *et al.* (1970) reported that 72% of absorbed *m*-xylene was excreted as *m*-methylhippuric acid within 18 h.

Health Aspects

Observations in Man Carpenter *et al.* (1975) exposed human volunteers to xylene at 460, 1,000, and 2,000 mg/m³ (approximately 100, 225, and 450 ppm) for 15 min. All volunteers detected the odor, and several reported olfactory fatigue and eye irritation at the higher concentrations. Morley *et al.* (1970) reported an exposure of three painters to xylene at an estimated 10,000 ppm. Two of the three were in this atmosphere for approximately 18 h. One died, with evidence of severe lung congestion and intra-alveolar hemorrhage; the two survivors experienced confusion for some time after recovery, had impairment of renal function with recovery at approximately 2 weeks, and may also have had minimal liver damage.

The NIOSH (1975) recommended a time-weighted average exposure not to exceed 100 ppm of xylene for a 10-h workday, 40-h workweek.

Observations in Other Species

Acute Effects The acute oral LD_{50} in rats, as reported by Wolf *et al.* (1956), was 4.3 g/kg. Inhalation studies reported by Lazarev (1929) indicated lethal effects in mice exposed to *o*-xylene at 30 mg/liter (6,900 ppm), *m*-xylene at 50 mg/liter (11,500 ppm, or *p*-xylene at 15–35 mg/liter (3,450–8,050 ppm). Cameron *et al.* (1938) reported some deaths in mice exposed to the various isomers at 2,000–4,000 ppm. Hine and Zuidema (1970) reported the xylenes to be moderately irritating to the skin of animals. Batchelor (1925) exposed rats to xylene vapor for 18–20 h/day. At 1,600 ppm, two of four rats died within 4 days. Initial signs were incoordination and irritation of the mucous membranes. The white-cell count was decreased after 4 days of exposure. Four rats exposed to 980 ppm for 7 days had hyperplastic bone marrow and spleen, with kidney congestion. One animal had a 32% reduction in white cells. One of eight rats exposed to 620 ppm for 7 days had a 30% reduction in white-cell count.

Subchronic and Chronic Effects Smyth and Smyth (1928) exposed guinea pigs to xylene at 300 ppm for 4 h/day, 6 days/week for 2 months. Slight liver and lung effects were reported at necropsy. Speck and Moeschlin (1968) found no adverse effects on the hematopoietic system after subcutaneous administration at 300 mg/kg/day for 6 weeks or 700 mg/kg/day for 9 weeks. The authors suggested that other reports of myelotoxicity of xylene are probably related to benzene contamination.

Fabre (1960) reported that rabbits exposed to benzene-free xylene (at 5 mg/liter, or 1,150 ppm) for 40–55 days had decreased red- and white-cell counts. Carpenter *et al.* (1975) exposed rats and dogs to *o*-xylene at 805, 460, or 175 ppm (3.5, 2.0, or 0.77 mg/liter) for 6 h/day, 5 days/week, for 13 weeks. No gross or microscopic lesions were reported, and all hematologic characteristics were comparable with those of control rats.

Mutagenicity No available data.

Carcinogenicity No available data.

Teratogenicity Xylene has been reported to produce developmental defects in chicken embryos (Kucera, 1968).

Conclusions and Recommendations

In view of the relative paucity of data on the mutagenicity, carcinogenicity, teratogenicity, and long-term oral toxicity of xylene, estimates of the effects of chronic oral exposure at low levels cannot be made with any confidence. It is recommended that studies to produce such information be conducted before final limits in drinking water are established.

SUMMARY—ORGANIC SOLUTES

The organic contaminants identified in drinking water make up a small fraction of the total organic matter present. Although approximately 90% of the volatile organics in drinking water have been identified and quantified, these represent no more than 10% of the total organic material. Only 5–10% of the nonvolatile organic compounds, which comprise the remaining 90% of the total organic material in water, have been identified.

Considered were 74 nonpesticide organic compounds of the approximately 309 volatile organic compounds so far identified in drinking water, and 55 pesticides. Some of the pesticides studied have not yet been detected in drinking water, but were included because they are or have been used in large quantities. A compound was selected for consideration if any of the following criteria applied:

1. Experimental evidence of toxicity in man or animals including carcinogenicity, mutagenicity, and teratogenicity.
2. Identified in drinking water at relatively high concentrations.

3. Molecular structure closely related to that of another compound of known toxicity.
4. Pesticide in heavy use that could result in contamination of drinking-water supplies.
5. Listed in the Safe Drinking Water Act or National Interim Primary Drinking Water Regulations.

Toxicological information about the compounds of interest was variable in quality and quantity and, in some instances, inadequate for a proper assessment of toxicity. Although the carcinogenic effect of these compounds was of primary concern, evidence for other toxic effects on target organ systems was also considered. Sufficient data were available for less than one-fourth of the nonpesticide organic compounds and three-fourths of the organic pesticides investigated to permit judgement as to either the carcinogenicity of the compound or the establishment of an Acceptable Daily Intake (ADI).*

The ADI represents an empirically derived value that reflects a particular combination of both knowledge and uncertainty concerning the relative safety of a chemical. When there is more confidence about data derived from animal experiments or observations on humans the uncertainty factor is smaller than when little is known about the potential toxicity of a chemical. These numbers are not meant to represent a guaranteed safety level, but rather to indicate a level at which exposure to the single chemical in question is not anticipated to produce an observable toxic response in man. The ADI values do not consider interactions (e.g. synergism, antagonism) among the many possible contaminants. Furthermore, the ADI numbers do not represent a safe level in drinking water, because they do not take into account what fraction of the potential contaminant intake may come from water.

Suggested no-adverse-health-effects concentrations in water have been calculated based on two sets of assumptions: (1) that 20% of total intake of a material is from water and 80% from other sources, and (2) that 1% of total intake is from water and 99% from other sources (See Table VI-61). Similar calculations can be made for other materials discussed in this report using such data as may be available with regard to concentration of the contaminant in food or other sources.

*The Committee considered several alternative terms, other than ADI, but concluded that the introduction of a substitute for ADI might well lead to confusion. The term "Acceptable Daily Intake" is used throughout the discussion because of its adoption by international organizations.

Because of the lack of consistency in the experimental data on the effects of many substances, "no-adverse-health-effect" levels cannot be firmly specified for all organic contaminants. Most of the materials considered have not been studied sufficiently to firmly establish their carcinogenic potential. Interactions such as additive toxicity, synergism, and antagonism have not been considered in development of risk assessments. What ultimately may be most important is the interaction of these compounds with each other and with other material in contributing to the total body burden resulting from multiple sources of contaminant exposure. For these reasons, the ADI is intended to be used only as a guide for assessment of toxicity from chronic exposure. Furthermore, an ADI is not meant to provide a basis for the continuing discharge of a compound into the environment.

In the present limited state of our knowledge concerning structure-activity relationships for carcinogenic and other toxic effects, one cannot consistently and accurately extrapolate these properties from one compound to another. Nevertheless, in certain specific instances (for example, the substitution of bromine for chlorine in a halogenated methane) it is presumed that the relationship is sufficiently strong to justify the suspicion that the related compounds may be similarly toxic.

The potential for existing concentrations of organic pesticides and other organic contaminants in drinking water to adversely affect health cannot be answered with certainty at this time. The key issue is whether or not certain organic chemicals found in very low concentrations can cause or increase the rate of cancer development in man. Even though several of these chemicals have demonstrated carcinogenicity in laboratory animals, the extrapolation of such results to man remains difficult for a number of reasons.

Because the bioassays that have been used to establish carcinogenicity of certain organic chemicals are conducted at doses that are hundreds to thousands of times greater than the levels at which these chemicals occur in water, the risks at these low levels must be obtained by extrapolation from higher doses. There is no hard evidence that low-level oral exposure to any of these chemicals produces cancer. An argument has been made that the dose levels used to establish carcinogenicity are so high that they overwhelm normal detoxification and/or repair mechanisms and produce cancer by some mechanism which does not occur under low-dose conditions. Experimental animals subjected to such high doses could be considered a population different from those exposed to lower doses that do not produce pathological alterations and changes in pharmacokinetic parameters, or biochemistry.

Extrapolating from laboratory animals to man would be more meaningful if comparative metabolic information between the different species were available. Some species do not metabolize a parent compound to its activated form, so that use of these species in toxicological bioassays is inappropriate if the compound undergoes activation in man. The converse is also true. Differences may also occur with respect to other parameters such as rates of biotransformation, absorption, excretion, and biological half-life.

Risk assessments based on extrapolations that fail to consider species differences with respect to sensitivity, tissue susceptibility, kinetics, pathology or biotransformation pathways may be inappropriate. This kind of information is not presently available.

In light of such uncertainties, a cautious approach must be adopted when dealing with potentially harmful chemicals. Even more uncertainty exists when one considers the possibility that some of these chemicals may also be mutagenic or teratogenic. The methodologies used to establish these effects are even less applicable to man than cancer bioassays.

For many of the organic compounds identified in drinking water, virtually no toxicity data are available. Ideally, all of these agents (as well as any new ones) should be subjected to an extensive battery of toxicity tests, including chronic bioassay. In practice, there is a need to determine those agents for which the generation of data is most pressing. The main factors identified in the assignment of priorities are:

1. The relative concentrations of the compounds and the number of people likely to be exposed as well as the identity of defined subpopulations exposed.
2. The number of water systems in which they occur.
3. Positive responses to *in vitro* mutagenic screening systems.
4. Positive responses to *in vitro* carcinogen prescreens (mammalian cell transformations).
5. Similarity of chemical structure of the test compound to those of other compounds having defined toxic properties (i.e. structure-activity relationships).
6. Relationship of dose from water to total body burden.

A number of assays using bacteria and yeast have shown promise in yielding high correlations between mutagenic activity and known carcinogenic activity for certain classes of materials. These may prove to be useful in establishing a first level screen for potential carcinogens.

CONCLUSIONS

Carcinogenicity

Table VI-60 lists those specific organic contaminants for which positive data on carcinogenesis exist. For these compounds, where adequate (lifetime) feeding studies were available, a statistical extrapolation of risk was performed.

The statistical methodology is described in detail in the chapter on Margin of Safety and Extrapolation. The numbers in Table VI-60 are upper 95% confidence estimates of cancer risk to man from a lifetime of exposure to a particular compound. These estimates have been corrected (animal dose to human dose) on a dose/surface area basis.

Bacterial Mutagenicity

In addition to examining data from animal feeding studies for the identification of suspect carcinogens, data for mutagenesis in bacteria, or other test systems were also examined. Available data are summarized as follows:

1. Benzo(*a*)pyrene, chlorodibromomethane, captan, and Folpet have been found to be mutagenic.
2. Bromoform and vinyl chloride, weakly mutagenic.
3. Carbon tetrachloride, bromobenzene, nicotine, DDE, dieldrin, carbaryl and trifluraline, nonmutagenic.

Teratogenicity

Data on teratogenic potential exist for 24 of the compounds under study. Hexachlorophene, nicotine, the phthalate esters, 2,4-D, 2,4,5-T, and folpet have been shown to be teratogens, while benzene, benzo(*a*)pyrene, carbon tetrachloride, PCB's, Captan, Carbaryl, Chlordan, DDT, Kepone, Malathion, Methylparathion, Mirex, Paraquat, and Parathion have been reported to be non-teratogenic. Nowhere is the paucity of toxicologic data more evident than in the data on teratogenesis.

Noncarcinogenic Toxicity

For 45 compounds there were sufficient data to calculate ADI's. These are summarized in Table VI-61. Occasionally an ADI was calculated

TABLE VI-60 Categories of Known or Suspected Organic Chemical Carcinogens Found in Drinking Water

Compound	Highest Observed Concentrations in Finished Water, μg/liter	Upper 95% Confidence Estimate of Lifetime Cancer Risk Per μg/liter[a]
Human carcinogen		
Vinyl chloride	10	4.7×10^{-7}
Suspected human carcinogens		
Benzene	10	I.D.
Benzo *(a)* pyrene	D.	I.D.
Animal carcinogens		
Dieldrin	8	2.6×10^{-4}
Kepone	N.D.	4.4×10^{-5}
Heptachlor	D.	4.2×10^{-5}
Chlordane	0.1	1.8×10^{-5}
DDT	D.	1.2×10^{-5}
Lindane (γ-BHC)	0.01	9.3×10^{-6}
β-BHC	D.	4.2×10^{-6}
PCB (Aroclor 1260)	3	3.1×10^{-6}
ETU	N.D	2.2×10^{-6}
Chloroform	366	1.7×10^{-6}
α-BHC	D.	1.5×10^{-6}
PCNB	N.D.	1.4×10^{-7}
Carbontetrachloride	5	1.1×10^{-7}
Trichloroethylene	0.5	1.1×10^{-7}
Diphenylhydrazine	1	I.D.
Aldrin	D	I.D.
Suspected animal carcinogens		
Bis (2-chloroethyl) ether	0.42	1.2×10^{-6}
Endrin	0.08	I.D.
Heptachlor epoxide	D.	I.D.

[a]See text for details (Introduction and Chapter II). I.D. = insufficient data to permit a statistical extrapolation of risk; N.D. = not detected; D = Detected but not quantified.

when less than lifetime exposure studies were available. The selection of responses by which toxicity was measured was variable.

For 29 organic contaminants and pesticides there were insufficient data to calculate ADI's. The available toxicological data are included in the text and the compounds are listed in Table VI-62. Even a superficial evaluation could not be done on 32 compounds due to inadequacy of toxicological data. These compounds are listed in Table VI-63, together with their reported occurences in drinking waters of the United States.

RESEARCH RECOMMENDATIONS

1. Because great uncertainty exists in connection with extrapolation of data from the present cancer bioassays, better premises and methodologies are needed to establish the extent to which humans are at risk from the low-level exposures to organic substances in water. There is a need to know the extent to which low-level exposure to a presumed carcinogen does in fact increase the probability of cancer during the lifetime of an individual.

It is recommended that work be done to better characterize current animal models and also develop new ones. Studies of the comparative metabolism of laboratory animals and man are urgently needed. It is necessary to know, for example, if a laboratory animal metabolizes a test compound in the same manner and rate as man. Better mutagenicity bioassays using mammalian cells should be developed. More work is needed in the area of interactions and synergism which these assay systems could more easily accommodate.

2. Organic material in water is thought by many to be responsible for contributing the initial reactants for many potentially harmful contaminants. To this end total organic carbon (TOC) in drinking water supplies must be better characterized and more extensively determined. Because many halogenated compounds are formed by chlorination of naturally occurring organic substances, research on methods for destruction or removal of organic precursors of halogenated compounds prior to chlorination would lead to reduction in chlorinated products and their accompanying health hazards.

3. Epidemiological studies to obtain quantitative measures of association between the frequency of malignant disease in humans and exposure to specific organic compounds found in drinking water are needed. In particular, ways are needed to obtain useful data from small populations of individuals occupationally exposed to drinking water contaminants. A major effort now needs to be directed at determining the health status of

TABLE VI-61 Organic Pesticides and Other Organic Contaminants in Drinking Water, Concentration, Toxicity, ADI, and Suggested No-Adverse-Effect Levels

Compound	Maximum Observed Concentrations in H_2O, μg/liter	Maximum Dose producing No Observed Adverse Effect, mg/kg/day	Uncertainty Factor[a]	ADI[b] mg/kg/day	Suggested No-Adverse-Effect Level from H_2O, μg/liter Assumption[c] 1	2
2,4-D	0.04	12.5	1,000	0.0125	87.5	4.4
2,4,5-T		10.0	100	0.1	700	35.0
TCDD		10^{-5}	100	10^{-7}	7×10^{-4}	3.5×10^{-5}
2,4,5-TP	detected[d]	0.75	1,000	0.00075	5.25	0.26
MCPA		1.25	1,000	0.00125	8.75	0.44
Amiben		250	1,000	0.25	1,750.0	87.5
Dicamba		1.25	1,000	0.00125	8.75	0.44
Alachlor	2.9	100	1,000	0.1	700.0	35.0
Butachlor	0.06	10	1,000	0.01	70.0	3.5
Propachlor		100	1,000	0.1	700.0	35.0
Propanil		20	1,000	0.02	140.0	7.0
Aldicarb		0.1	100	0.001	7	0.35
Bromacil		12.5	1,000	0.0125	87.5	4.4
Paraquat		8.5	1,000	0.0085	59.5	2.98
Trifluralin (also for Nitralin and Benefin)	detected	10	100	0.1	700.0	35.0
Methoxychlor		10	100	0.1	700.0	35.0
Toxaphene		1.25	1,000	0.00125	8.75	0.44
Azinphosmethyl		0.125	10	0.0125	87.5	4.4
Diazinon		0.02	10	0.002	14.0	0.7
Phorate (also for Disulfoton)		0.01	100	0.0001	0.7	0.035

Carbaryl		8.2	100	0.082	574	28.7
Ziram (and Ferbam)		12.5	1,000	0.0125	87.5	4.4
Captan		50	1,000	0.05	350	17.5
Folpet		160	1,000	0.16	1,120	56.0
HCB	6.0	1	1,000	0.001	7	0.35
PDB	1.0	13.4	1,000	0.0134	93.8	4.7
Parathion (and Methyl parathion)		0.043	10	0.0043	30	1.5
Malathion		0.2	10	0.02	140	7.0
Maneb (and Zineb)		5.0	1,000	0.005	35	1.75
Thiram		5.0	1,000	0.005	35	1.75
Atrazine	5.1	21.5	1,000	0.0215	150	7.5
Propazine	detected	46.4	1,000	0.0464	325	16.0
Simazine	detected	215.0	1,000	0.215	1,505	75.25
Di-n-butyl phthalate	5.0	110	1,000	0.11	770	38.5
Di (2-ethyl hexyl)	30.0	60	100	0.6	4,200	210.0
Hexachlorophene	0.01	1	1,000	0.001	7	0.35
Methyl methacrylate	1.0	100	1,000	0.1	800	35.0
Pentachlorophenol	1.4	3	1,000	0.003	21	1.05
Styrene	1.0	133	1,000	0.133	931	46.5

[a]Uncertainty factor—the factor of 10 was used where good chronic human exposure data was available and supported by chronic oral toxicity data in other species, the factor of 100 was used where good chronic oral toxicity data were available in some animal species, and the factor 1,000 was used with limited chronic toxicity data.

[b]Acceptable Daily Intake (ADI)—Maximum dose producing no observed adverse effect divided by the uncertainty factor.

[c]Assumptions: Average weight of human adult = 70 kg. Average daily intake of water for man = 2 liters.

1. 20% of total ADI assignment to water, 80% from other sources.
2. 1% of total ADI assigned to water; 99% from other sources.

[d]Detected but not quantified.

TABLE VI-62 Organic Pesticides and Other Organic Contaminants Found in Drinking Water, with Insufficient Data on Chronic Toxicity to Calculate an ADI

Compound	Highest Concentration in Finished Water, μg/liter
Acetaldehyde	0.1
Acrolein[a]	
Bromobenzene	detected[b]
Bromoform	detected
Carbon disulfide	detected
Chloral	5.0
Chlorobenzene	5.6
Cyanogen chloride	0.1
1,2-Dichloroethane	21.0
2,4-Dichlorophenol	36.0
2,4-Dimethylphenol	detected
e-Caprolactam	detected
Hexachloroethane	4.4
o-Methoxyphenol	detected
Methyl chloride	detected
Methylene chloride	7.0
Phenylacetic acid	4.0
Phthalic anhydride	detected
Propylbenzene	< 5.0
t-Butyl alcohol	0.01
Tetrachloroethane	4.0
Tetrachloroethylene	<5.0
Toluene	11.0
Trichlorobenzene	1.0
1,1,2-Trichloroethane	detected
Nicotine	3.0
Methomyl[a]	
Cyanazine	detected
Xylene	<5.0

[a]Not detected in finished water.
[b]Detected = detected but not quantified.

workers in industries where there is occupational exposure to compounds identified as animal carcinogens.

More accurate recordkeeping, a national death index, and more reliable analytical methods to monitor environmental exposure are needed.

4. There is a need for more and better toxicological data on compounds that could not be evaluated at this time, especially creosote, methyl parathion, and acrolein, all of which are used in large quantities. Data are needed in the area of low-level, chronic (lifetime) exposures.

Studies should include exposure to formulated products (i.e., mixtures) as well as pure compounds.

5. There should be a periodic reevaluation by newer, more sensitive and more predictive methodologies of those pesticides used in large volume.

TABLE VI-63 Organic Contaminants Found in Drinking Water with No Available Information on Chronic Toxicity

Compound	Highest Concentration in Finished Water, μg/liter	Highest Concentration in Raw Water, μg/liter
1,2-*Bis*(chloroethoxy) ethane	0.03	
Bis(2-chloroisopropyl) ether	1.58	
Bromochlorobenzenes	detected	
Bromodichloromethane	116	11
Butyl bromide	detected	
Chloroethyl methyl ether	detected	
Chlorodibromomethane	100	1.4
Chlorohydroxybenzophenone	detected	
Chloromethyl ethyl ether	detected	
Chloropropene	detected	
Crotonaldehyde	5.0	
Dibromobenzene	detected	
Dibromodichloroethane	0.63	
1,3-Dichlorobenzene	<3.0	
Dichlorodifluoroethane	detected	
Dichloroiodomethane	0.5	
1,1-Dichloro-2-hexano	1.0	
1,2-Dichloropropane	<1.0	
1,3-Dichloropropene	<1.0	
1,2-Dimethoxybenzene	detected	
4,6-Dinitro-2-aminophenol	detected	
Dioctyladipate	20.0	
Hexachloro-1,3-butadiene	0.07	
Isodecane	5.0	
Metachloronitrobenzene	detected	
Methylstearate	detected	
Nonane	4.0	
Octyl chloride	detected	
Pentachlorophenyl methyl ether	0.1	
1,1,3,3-Tetrachloroacetone	1.0	1.0
2,4,6-Trichlorophenol	detected	
Trimethylbenzene	6.1	

DEFINITIONS

The Safe Drinking Water Committee adopted the following working definitions prior to its review of the scientific literature of organic contaminants.

Carcinogen

The following definition is from "General Criteria for Assessing the Evidence for Carcinogenicity of Chemical Substances," report of the Subcommittee on Environmental Carcinogensis, NCI, 1976.

The term carcinogen is used in its broad sense, because in most of the current human epidemiologic approaches and certain animal bioassays it is not possible to differentiate clearly between initiating agents, promoting agents, and certain modifying factors. Any factor or combination of factors which increases the risk of cancer in humans is of concern regardless of its mechanism of action. The criteria listed here apply only to chemical agents.

A malignant neoplasm is composed of a population of cells displaying progressive growth and varying degrees of autonomy and cellular atypia. It displays, or it has the capacity for, invasion of normal tissues, metastases, and causing death to the host. Benign neoplasms are a less autonomous population of cells and exhibit little or no cellular atypia or invasion of normal tissues and do not metastasize. In particular cases, however, benign neoplasms may endanger the life of the host by a variety of mechanisms, including hemorrhage, encroachment on a vital organ, or unregulated hormone production. The cytologic and histologic criteria utilized in determining whether a lesion is benign or malignant differ depending upon the tissue in which the neoplasm arises. Evaluation of whether a specific lesion is benign or malignant should, therefore, follow standard criteria used by experimental oncologists and pathologists with the emphasis on correlation of the histopathologic pattern with the biologic behavior of the lesion or type of lesion. In equivocal cases, the diagnosis of a specific lesion may require a panel of experts, recognizing that they may not always agree.

Depending upon the particular case, benign neoplasms may represent a stage in the evolution of a malignant neoplasm and in other cases they may be "end points" that do not readily undergo transition to malignant neoplasms.

CRITERIA IN HUMAN STUDIES

An agent—which may comprise a combination of chemicals—is carcinogenic in man if it increases the incidence of malignant neoplasms (or a combinaton of benign and malignant neoplasms) in humans to levels that are significantly higher than those in a comparable group not exposed (or exposed at a lower dose) to the same agent. If all of the induced neoplasms are benign, rather than malignant, then, for the reasons given elsewhere in this document, the agent must be considered a possible carcinogen and it should, therefore, be very carefully evaluated as a health hazard.

Types of evidence suggesting that an agent is carcinogenic in humans include: neoplastic response directly related to exposure (both duration and dose); incidence and mortality differences related to occupational exposure; incidence and mortality differences between geographic regions related to different exposures rather than genetic differences and/or altered incidence in migrant populations; time trends in incidence or mortality related to either the introduction or removal of a specific agent from the environment; case control studies; and the results of retrospective-prospective and prospective studies of the consequences of human exposure. Clinical case reports may also provide early warning of a potential carcinogen. Negative epidemiologic data may not establish the safety of suspected materials. Negative data on a given agent obtained from extensive epidemiologic studies of sufficient duration are useful for indicating upper limits for the rate at which a specific type of exposure to that agent could affect the incidence and/or mortality of specific human cancers.

CRITERIA IN EXPERIMENTAL ANIMAL STUDIES

The carcinogenicity of a substance is established when the administration to groups of animals in adequately designed and conducted experiments results in increases in the incidence of one or more types of malignant neoplasms (or a combination of benign and malignant neoplasms) in the treated groups as compared to control groups maintained under identical conditions but not given the test compound. The increased incidence of neoplasms in one or more of the experimental groups should be evaluated statistically for significance, and the only major experimental variable between the control and the experimental group should be the absence or presence of the single test agent. Such increases may be regarded with greater confidence if positive results are observed in more than one group of animals or in different laboratories. The demonstration that the occurrence of neoplasms follows a dose-dependent relationship provides additional evidence of a positive result.

The occurrence of benign neoplasms raises the strong possibility that the agent in question is also carcinogenic since compounds that induce benign neoplasms frequently induce malignant neoplasms. In addition, benign neoplasms may be an early stage in a multistep carcinogenic process and they may progress to malignant neoplasms; also, benign neoplasms may themselves jeopardize the health and life of the host. For these reasons, if a substance is found to induce benign neoplasms in experimental animals it should be considered a potential human health hazard which requires further evaluation. In experiments where the increased incidence of malignant neoplasms in the treated group is of questionable significance, a parallel increase in incidence of benign tumors in the same tissue adds weight to the evidence for carcinogenicity of the test substance.

Mutagen

A chemical that is capable of producing a heritable change in genetic material. These changes may be either point mutations or chromosomal mutations and can occur in either somatic or germ cells.

Teratogen

An agent which acts during pregnancy to produce a physical or functional defect in the developing offspring.

Organoleptic Test

The use of odor and taste thresholds to establish permissible levels of exposure to chemicals.

Adverse Response

"With increasing dosage in the continuum of the dose–response relationship, the region is generally entered where the effects are clearly adverse. Thus, adverse effects may be defined as changes that:

1. Occur with intermittent or continued exposure and that result in impairment of functional capacity (as determined by anatomical, physiological, and biochemical, or behavioral parameters) or in a decrement of the ability to compensate for additional stress.

2. Are irreversible during exposure or following cessation of exposure if such changes cause detectable decrements in the ability organism to maintain homeostatis.

3. Enhance the susceptibility of the organisms to the deleterious effects of other environmental influences."

(Quoted from *Principles for Evaluating Chemicals in the Environment*, 1975, National Academy of Sciences, Washington, D.C.)

Toxicity

The intrinsic quality of a chemical to produce an adverse effect. The term includes capacity to induce teratogenic, mutagenic, and carcinogenic effects.

Safety

"Safety is the practical certainty that injury will not result from the substance when used in the quantity and in the manner proposed for its use."

(Quoted from *Evaluating the Safety of Food Chemicals*, 1970, National Academy of Sciences, Washington, D.C.).

Evaluation of Safety

"An estimation of the potential of the substance to cause injury and review and evaluation of sufficient data to warrant a conclusion that the conditions of proposed use will provide an intake so low in relation to the toxic dose that there is a practical certainty no harm can result."

(Quoted from FDA Papers, November 1971).

For the purpose of this study, the proposed use was limited only to exposure from drinking water.

Safety Factor or Uncertainty Factor

A number that reflects the degree or amount of uncertainty that must be considered when experimental data in animals are extrapolated to man. When the quality and quantity of data are high the uncertainty factor is low and when data are inadequate or equivocal, the uncertainty factor must be larger.

The following general guidelines have been adopted in establishing the uncertainty factors.

1. Valid experimental results from studies on prolonged ingestion by man, with no indication of carcinogenicity.

Uncertainty Factor = 10

2. Experimental results of studies of human ingestion not available or scanty (e.g., acute exposure only). Valid results of long-term feeding studies on experimental animals or in the absence of human studies, valid animal studies on one or more species. No indication of carcinogenicity.

Uncertainty Factor = 100

3. No long-term or acute human data. Scanty results on experimental animals. No indication of carcinogenicity.

Uncertainty Factor = 1,000

These uncertainty factors are used in every case as a divisor of the highest reported long-term dose which is observed not to produce any adverse effect.

REFERENCES—PESTICIDES

Abbott, D.C., G.B. Collins, and R. Goulding. 1972. Organochlorine pesticide residues in human fat in the United Kingdom 1969-1971. Br. Med. J. 2:553-556.

Acker, L., and E. Schulte. 1970. Appearance of chlorinated biphenyls and hexachlorobenzene along with insecticides in human milk and fat tissues. Naturwissenschaften 57:497.

Adkins, T.R., Jr., W.L. Sowell, and F.S. Arant. 1955. Systemic effect of selected chemicals on the bed bug and lone star tick when administered to rabbits. J. Econ. Entomol. 48:139-141.

Advisory Committee on 2,4,5-T. 1971. Report to the Administrator of the Environmental Protection Agency. 76 pp.

Allen, J.R., J.P. Van Miller, and D.H. Norback. 1975. Tissue distribution, excretion, and biological effects of [^{14}C]tetrachlorodibenzo-*p*-dioxin in rats. Food Cosmet. Toxicol. 13:501-505.

Alley, E.G., B.R. Layton, and J.P. Minyard, Jr. 1974. Identification of the photoproducts of the insecticides Mirex and Kepone. J. Agric. Food Chem. 22:442-445.

Allied Chemical Corp. General Chemical Division. 1961. Toxicological studies on decachlorooctahydro-1,3,4-methano-2H-cyclo-lenta[cd]pentalen-2-one (Compound No. 1189) (Kepone). U.S. Environmental Protection Agency Document no. 108253.

Aly, O.M. and M.A. El-Dib. 1971. Studies on the persistence of some carbamate insecticides in the aquatic environment. 1. Hydrolysis of Sevin, Baygon, Pyrolan, and Dimetilan in waters. Water Res. 5:1191-1205.

Ambrose, A.M., P.S. Larson, J.F. Borzelleca, and G.R. Hennigar, Jr. 1972. Toxicologic studies on 3′,4′-dichloropropionanilide. Toxicol. Appl. Pharmacol. 23:650-659.

American Cyanamid. 1965a. Thimet systemic insecticide: demyelination studies in white leghorn hens. Unpublished report. Cited in U.S. Environmental Protection Agency. 1974e. Initial Scientific and Minieconomic Review of Phorate (Thimet). Office of Pesticides Programs, Washington, D.C.

American Cyanamid. 1965b. Thimet systemic insecticide: successive generation studies with mice. Unpublished report. Cited in U.S. Environmental Protection Agency. 1974c. Initial Scientific and Minieconomic Review of Phorate (Thimet). Office of Pesticides Programs, Washington, D.C.

American Cyanamid. 1966. Toxicity data on 15 percent Thimet Granules. Unpublished report. Cited in U.S. Environmental Protection Agency. 1974e. Initial Scientific and Minieconomic Review of Phorate (Thimet). Office of Pesticides Programs, Washington, D.C.

Andersen, K.J., E.G. Leighty, and M.T. Takahashi. 1972. Evaluation of herbicides for possible mutagenic properties. J. Agric. Food Chem. 20:649-656.

Andrawes, N.R., H.W. Dorough, and D.A. Lindquist. 1967. Degradation and elimination of Temik in rats. J. Econ. Entomol. 60:979-987.

Andrews, J.E., and K.D. Courtney. 1976. Inter- and intralitter variation of hexachlorobenzene (HCB) deposition in fetuses. Toxicol. Appl. Pharmacol. 37:128, Abstr. no. 87.

Andrianova, M.M., and I.V. Alekseev. 1970. The carcinogenic properties of the pesticides Sevin, Maneb, Ziram and Zineb. Vopr. Pitan. 29 (6):71-74.

Anonymous. 1973. Chemical profile: 0-Dichlorobenzene. Aromatic organics. Chem. Mark. Rep. 204:9-11, Oct. 15.

Anonymous. 1976. Kepone—fish action level possible. Pestic. Chem. News 4(8):18-22.

Ariyoshi, T., K. Ideguchi, K. Iwasaki, and M. Arakaki. 1975. Relationship between chemical structure and activity. II. Influences of isomers in dichlorobenzene, trichlorobenzene, and tetrachlorobenzene on the activities of drug-metabolizing enzymes. Chem. Pharmacol. Bull. 23:824-830.

Arkhipov, G.N., and I.N. Kozlova. 1974. Cancerogenic properties of the herbicide ammonium 2,4-D amine salt. Vopr. Pitan. no. 5:83-84. (Chem. Abstr. 82:69002n 1975.)

Ashwood-Smith, M.J., J. Trevino, and R. Ring. 1972. Mutagenicity of Dichlorvos. Nature 240:418-420.

Assouly, M. 1951. Desherbants selectifs et substances de croissance. Apercu/technique. Effet pathologique sur l'homme au cours de la fabrication de l'ester de 2,4-d. Arch. Mal. Prof. 12:26-30. Cited in Food and Agricultural Organization of the United Nations/World Health Organization, 1971. 1970 evaluations of some pesticide residues in food FAO/AGP 1970/M/12/1; WHO/Food Add/71.42. p. 69.

Avrahami, M. and I.L. Gernert. 1972. Hexachlorobenzene antagonism to dieldrin storage in adipose tissue of female rats. N.Z. J. Agric. Res. 15:783 787.

Azouz, W.M., D.V. Parke, and R.T. Williams. 1955. Detoxication. LXII. The metabolism of halogenogenzeness. ortho- and para-dichlorobenzenes. Biochem. J. 59:410-415.

Bache, C.A., D.D. Hardee, R.F. Holland, and D.J. Lisk. 1964. Absence of phenoxy acid herbicide residues in the milk of dairy cows at high feeding levels. J. Dairy Sci. 47:298-299.

Bache, C.A., D.J. Lisk, D.G. Wagner, and R.G. Wagner. 1964. Elimination of 2-methyl-4-chlorophenoxyacetic acid and 4-(-2-methyl-4-chlorophenoxy) butyric acid in the urine from cows. J. Dairy Sci. 47:93-95.

Bage, G., E. Cekanova, and K.S. Larsson. 1973. Teratogenic and embryotoxic effects of herbicides di- and trichlorophenoxyacetic acids (2,4-D and 2,4,5-T). Acta Pharmacol. Toxicol. 32:408-416.

Baldwin, M.K., J. Robinson, and D.V. Parke. 1970. Metabolism of Endrin in the rat. J. Agric. Food Chem. 18:1117-1123.

Balin, P.N. 1969. Pathologicomorphological changes in the organism occurring under the chronic action of the pesticide Maneb. Vrach. Delo 10:95-99.

Barnett, J.R. and H.W. Dorough. 1974. Metabolism of Chlordane in rats. J. Agric. Food Chem. 22:612-619.

Beckner, J.S., P.M. Hudgins, and J.L. Egle, Jr. 1974. Effects of acetaldehyde, propionaldehyde, formaldehyde and Acrolein on contractility, ^{14}C-norepinephrine and ^{45}calcium binding in isolated smooth muscle. Res. Comman. Chem. Pathol. Pharmacol 9:471-488.

Beebeejaun, A.R., G. Beevers, and W.N. Rogers, 1971. Paraquat poisoning—prolonged excretion. Clin. Toxicol. 4:397-407.

Ben-Dyke, R., D.M. Sanderson, and D.N. Noakes. 1970. Acute toxicity data for pesticides. World Rev. Pest Control 9:119-127.

Berliner, M.L. 1939. Cataract following the inhalation of paradichlorobenzene vapor. Arch. Ophthalmol. 22: 1023-1034.

Berwick, P. 1970. 2,4-Dichlorophenoxyacetic acid poisoning in man. Some interesting clinical and laboratory findings. J. Am. Med. Assoc. 214:1114-1117.

Betts, J.J., S.P. James, and W.V. Thorpe. 1955. The metabolism of pentachloronitrobenzene and 2,3,4,6-tetrachloronitrobenzene and the formation of mercapturic acid in the rabbit. Biochem. J. 61:611-617.

Black, A.L., Y.C. Chiu, M.A.H. Fahmy, and T.R. Fukuto. 1973. Selective toxicity of *N*-sulfenylated derivatives of insecticidal methylcarbamate esters. J. Agric. Food Chem. 21:747-751.

Bleiberg, J., M. Wallen, R. Brodkin, and I.L. Applebaum. 1964. Industrially acquired porphyria. Arch. Dermatol. 89:793-797.

Bombinski, T.J., and K.P. DuBois. 1958. Toxicity and mechanism of action of Di-Syston. Arch. Ind. Health 17:192-199.

Bontoyan, W.R., J.B. Looker, T.E. Kaiser, P. Giang, and B.M. Olive. 1972. Survey of ethylenethiourea in commercial ethylenebisdithiocarbamate formulations. J. Assoc. Offic. Anal. Chem. 55:923-925.

Bontwell, R.K., and D.K. Bosch. 1959. The tumor-promoting action of phenol and related compounds for mouse skin. Cancer Res. 19:413-424.

Booth, N.H., and J.R. McDowell. 1975. Toxicity of Hexachlorobenzene and associated residues in edible animal tissues. J. Am. Vet. Med. Assoc. 166:591-595.

Borzelleca, J.F., P.S. Larson, E.M. Crawford, G.R. Hennigar, Jr., E.J. Kuchar, and H.H. Klein. 1971. Toxicologic and metabolic studies on pentachloronitrobenzene. Toxicol. Appl. Pharmacol. 18:522-534.

Bowman, J.S., and J.E. Casida. 1958. Further studies on the metabolism of Thimet by plants, insects, and mammals. J. Econ. Entomol. 51:838-843.

Boyd, E.M., and E. Carsky. 1969. Kwashiorkorigenic diet and diazinon toxicity. Acta Pharmacol. Toxicol. 27:284-294.

Boyd, E.M., and C. Krijnen. 1968. Toxicity of Captan and protein-deficient diet. J. Clin. Pharmacol. 8:225-234.

Boyd, E.M., and E. Carsky. 1971. The 100 day LD_{50} index of Captan. Acta Pharmacol. Toxicol. 29:226-240.

Boyd, E.M., E. Carsky, and C.J. Krijnen. 1969. The effects of diets containing from 0 to 81 per cent casein on the acute oral toxicity of Diazinon. Clin. Toxicol. 2:295-302.

Brady, M.N., and D.S. Siyali. 1972. Hexachlorobenzene in human body fat. Med. J. Aust. 1:158-161.

Breidenbach, A.W., C.G. Gunnerson, F.K. Kawahara, J.J. Lichtenberg, and R.S. Green. 1967. Chlorinated hydrocarbon pesticides in major river basins, 1957-65. Public Health Rep. 82:139-156.

Brodeur, J., and K.P. DuBois. 1963. Comparison of acute toxicity of anticholinesterase insecticides to weanling and adult male rats. Proc. Soc. Exp. Med. 114:509-511.

Brooks, G.T. 1974. Chlorinated Insecticides. CRC Press, Cleveland, Ohio.

Bruce, R.B., J.W. Howard, and J.R. Elsea. 1955. Toxicity of *0,0*-diethyl *0*-(2-isopropyl-6-methyl-4-pyrimidyl) phosphorothioate (Diazinon). J. Agric. Food Chem. 3:1017-1021.

Brzheskiy, V.V. 1972. Mutagenic properties of Sevin, a carbamate insecticide. Genetika 8:151-153.

Buchanan, J.B. 1971. Pesticidal substituted 0-carbamylhydroxymates. U.S. Patent no. 3,576,834 (to E.I. duPont de Nemours and Company).

Bull, D.L. 1965. Metabolism of Di-System by insects, isolated cotton leaves, and rats. J. Econ. Entomol. 58:249-254.

Bull, D.L., D.A. Lindquist, and J.R. Coppedge. 1967. Metabolism of 2-methyl-2-(methylthio) propionaldehyde *O*-(methylcarbamoyl) oxime (Temik, UC-21149) in insects. J. Agric. Food Chem. 15:610-616.

Burchfield, H.P., and E.E. Storrs. 1961. Residue analysis of 2,4-D and other chlorine containing herbidices in milk. Abstracts, American Chemical Society Meeting, Chicago, Ill. p. 19A.

Burdett, M. 1968a. A two-year toxicological investigation of Shell Compound SD 11831-Rat. Final Report, SRI Project BC 5451, Part I.

Burdett, M. 1968b. A two-year toxicological investigation of Shell Compound SD 11831-Dog. Final Report, SRI Project BC 5451, Part II.

Burkatskaia, E.N. 1959. On the toxicology of isomers of hexachlorocyclohexane. Farmakol. Toksikol. 22:272. (Chem. Abstr. 53:225ld., 1959.)

Burns, J.E., and F.M. Miller. 1975. Hexachlorobenzene contamination: Its effects in a Louisiana population. Arch. Environ. Health 30:44-48.

Bus, J.S., M.M. Preache, S.Z. Cagen, H.S. Posner, B.C. Eliason, C.W. Sharp, and J.E. Gibson. 1975. Fetal toxicity and distribution of Paraquat and Diquat in mice and rats. Toxicol. Appl. Pharmacol. 33:450-460.

Buselmaier, W., G. Roehrborn, and P. Propping. 1972. Mutagenitats-Untersuchungen mit Pestiziden im Host-Mediated Assay und mit dem Dominanten Letaltest an der Maus. Biol. Zentralbl. 91:311-325.

Busey, W.M. 1968. Three generation reproduction study of Lannate methomyl insecticide. Hazleton Laboratory Report. EPA Pesticide Petition no. 9F0184. Cited in Initial Scientific and Minieconomic Review of Methonyl, U.S. Environmental Protection Agency (In preparation).

Buu-Hoi, N.P., P.H. Chanh, G. Sesque, M.C. Azum-Gelade, and G. Saint-Ruf. 1972. Organs as targets of "dioxin" (2,3,7,8-tetrachlorodibenzo-*p*-dioxin) intoxication. Naturwissenschaften. 59:174-175.

Cam, C., and G. Nigogosyan. 1963. Acquired toxic porphyria cutanea tarda due to Hexachlorobenzene. Report of 348 cases caused by this fungicide. J. Am. Med. Assoc. 183:88-91.

Campbell, D.M., and R.J.L. Davidson. 1970. Toxic haemolytic anemia in pregnancy due to a pica for paradichlorobenzene. J. Obstet. Gynaecol. Br. Commonw. 77:657-659.

Carlson, G.P., and R.G. Tardiff. 1976. Effect of chlorinated benzenes on the metabolism of foreign organic compounds. Toxicol. Appl. Pharmacol. 36:383-394.

Carpenter, C.P., C.S. Weil, P.E. Palm, M.W. Woodside, J.H. Nair III, and H.F. Smyth, Jr. 1961. Mammalian toxicity of 1-naphthyl *N*-methylcarbamate (Sevin insecticide.) J. Agric. Food Chem. 9:30-39.

Carson, E.D. 1972. Fatal Paraquat poisoning in Northern Ireland. J. Forensic Sci. Soc. 12:437-443.

Carter, L.J. 1974. Cancer and the environment (I): A creaky system grinds on. Science 186:239-242.

Casida, J.E., R.L. Holmstead, S. Khalifa, J.R. Knox, T. Ohsawa, K. J. Palmer, and R. Y. Wong. 1974. Toxaphene insecticide: A complex biodegradable mixture. Science 183:520-521.

Caujolle, F.M.E., D.H. Caujolle, S.B. Cros, and M.M.J. Calvet. 1967. Limits of toxic and teratogenic tolerance of dimethyl sulfoxide. Ann. N.Y. Acad. Sci. 141:110-125.

Chadwick, R.W., L.T. Chuang, and K. Williams. 1975. Dehydrogenation: A previously unreported pathway of Lindane metabolism in mammals. Pestic. Biochem. Physiol. 5: 575-586.

Chepinoga, O.P., O.V. Chernov, L.V. Samosh, P.N. Balin, I.I. Khitsenko, M.A. Pilinskaya, L.V. Martson, N.A. Zadorozhnaya, N.P. Zastavnyuk, and A.I. Kurinnoi. 1970. Possible blastomogenic, mutagenic, and embryotropic effects of some carbamate pesticides. Vop. Gig. Toksikol. Pestits., Tr. Nauch. Sess. Akad. Med. Nauk USSR: 129-134 (Russ.).

Chevron Chemical Company. 1975. Paraquat poisoning; a physician's guide for emergency treatment and medical management. Chevron Environmental Health Center, San Francisco. 16 pp.

Chow, A.Y.K. and S.D. Murphy. 1975. Propanil (3,4-dichloropropionanilide)-induced methemoglobin formation in relation to its metabolism *in vitro*. Toxicol. Appl. Pharmacol. 33:14-20.

Claborn, H.V., H.D. Mann, M.C. Ivey, R.D. Radeleff, and G.T. Woodard. 1963. Excretion of Toxaphene and Strobane in the milk of dairy cows. J. Agric. Food Chem. 11:286-289.

Clark, D.E., J.E. Young, R.L. Younger, L.M. Hunt, and J.K. McLaran. 1964. The fate of 2,4-dichlorophenoxyacetic acid in sheep. J. Agric. Food Chem. 12:43-45.

Clark, D.E., J.S. Palmer, R.D. Radeleff, H.R. Crookshank, and F.M. Farr. 1975. Residues of chlorophenoxy acid herbicides and their phenolic metabolites in tissues of sheep and cattle. J. Agric. Food Chem. 23:573-578.

Clarke, C.H. 1971. The mutagenic specificities of Pentachloronitrobenzene and Captan, two environmental mutagens. Mutat. Res. 11:247-248.

Cleveland, F.P. 1966. A summary of work on Aldrin and Dieldrin toxicity at the Kettering laboratory. Arch. Environ. Health 13:195-198.

Cohen, S.D., and S.D. Murphy. 1972. Inactivation of malaoxon by mouse liver. Proc. Soc. Exp. Biol. Med. 139:1385-1389.

Collins, T.F.X., and C.H. Williams. 1971. Teratogenic studies with 2,4,5-T and 2,4-D in the hamster. Bull. Environ. Contam. Toxicol. 6:559-567.

Conning, D.M., K. Fletcher, and A.A.B. Swan. 1969. Paraquat and related bipyridyls. Br. Med. Bull. 25:245-249.

Cook, J.W. and G. Yip. 1958. Malathionase, II. Identity of a Malathion metabolite. J. Assoc. Offic. Agric. Chem. 41:407-411.

Coper, H., H. Herken, and J. Klempau. 1951. Pharmacology and toxicology of chlorinated cyclohexanes. Arch. Exp. Pathol. Pharmakol. 212:463-471.

Copland, G.M., A. Kolin, and H.S. Shulman. 1974. Fatal pulmonary intra-alveolar fibrosis after Paraquat ingestion. N. Engl. J. Med. 291:290-292.

Corneliussen, P.E. 1970. Pesticide residues in total diet samples. V. Pestic. Monit. J. 4:89-105.

Corneliussen, P.E. 1972. Pesticide residues in total diet samples. VI. Pestic. Monit. J. 5:313-330.

Courtney, K.D. 1973. The effect of Pentachloronitrobenzene on fetal kidneys. Toxicol. Appl. Pharmacol. 25:455.

Courtney, K.D. 1975. Prenatal Development Index: a means of evaluation. Presented at the 15th Annual Meeting of the Teratology Society, May 11-14, Pocono Manor, Pennsylvania. Teratology 11:15A.

Courtney, K.D., and J.A. Moore. 1971. Teratology studies with 2,4,5-trichlorophenoxyacetic acid and 2,3,7,8-tetrachlorodibenzo-*p*-dioxin. Toxicol. Appl. Pharmacol. 20:396-403.

Courtney, K.D., D.W. Gaylor, M.D. Hogan, H.L. Falk, R.R. Bates, and I. Mitchell. 1970. Teratogenic evaluation of 2,4,5-T. Science 168:864-866.

Courtney, K.D., M.F. Copeland, and A. Robbins. 1976. The effects of Pentachloronitrobenzene, Hexachlorobenzene, and related compounds on fetal development. Toxicol. Appl. Pharmacol. 35:239-256.

Crawford, C.R., and J. Doull. 1970. Antagonism of the lethal effects of dipterex and Guthion with atropine and related drugs. Fed. Proc. 29:349. Abstr. no. 589.

Cromartie, E., W.L. Reichel, L.N. Locke, A.A. Belisle, T.E. Kaiser, T.G. Lamont, B.M. Mulhern, R.M. Prouty, and D.M. Swineford. 1975. Residues of organochlorine pesticides and polychlorinated biphenyls and autopsy data for bald eagles, 1971-72. Pestic. Monit. J. 9:11-14.

Crosby, D.G., and A.S. Wong. 1970. The effects of light on phenoxyherbicides. Abstracts, 160th American Chemical Society Meeting, Chicago, Ill. Pest-022.

Crosby, D.G., A.S. Wong, J.R. Plimmer, and E.A. Woolson. 1971. Photodecomposition of chlorinated dibenzo-*p*-dioxins. Science 173:748-749.

Crosby, D.G., K.W. Moilanen, and A.S. Wong. 1973. Environmental generation and degradation of dibenzodioxins and dibenzofurans. Environ. Health Perspect. 5:259-266.

Crowder, L.A., and E.F. Dindal. 1974. Fate of ^{36}Cl-Toxaphene in rats. Bull. Environ. Contam. Toxicol. 12:320-327.

Curley, A., and R. Kimbrough. 1969. Chlorinated hydrocarbon insecticides in plasma and milk of pregnant and lactating women. Arch. Environ. Health 18:156-164.

Curley, A., V.W. Burse, R.W. Jennings, E.C. Villanueva, L. Tomatis, and K. Akazaki. 1973. Chlorinated hydrocarbon pesticides and related compounds in adipose tissue from people of Japan. Nature 242:338-340.

Curry, A.N., L. M. Kress, and R.A.L. Paylor. 1961. Determination of residues of phorate and its insecticidally active metabolites by cholinesterase inhibition. J. Agric. Food Chem. 9:469-477.

Dahm, P.A., B.E. Kopecky, and C.B. Walker. 1962. Activation of organophosphorus insecticides by rat liver microsomes. Toxicol. Appl. Pharmacol. 4:683-696.

Dahm, P.A., F.C. Fountaine, J.C. Pankaskie, R.C. Smith, and F.W. Atkeson. 1950. The effects of feeding Parathion to dairy cows. J. Dairy Sci. 33:747-757.

Davidow, B., and J.L. Radomski. 1953. Isolation of an epoxide metabolite from fat tissues of dogs fed Heptachlor. J. Pharmacol. Expt. Ther. 107:259-265.

Davies, G. M., and I. Lewis. 1956. Outbreak of food-poisoning from bread made of chemically contaminated flour. Br. Med. J. 2:393-398.

Davis, K.J., and O.G. Fitzhugh. 1962. Tumorigenic potential of aldrin and dieldrin for mice. Toxicol. Appl. Pharmacol. 4:187-189.

Davydova, T.B. 1973. The effect of tetramethyl thiuram disulfide (Thiram) inhaled on the estrous cycle and the reproductive function of mammals. Gig. Sanit. 39:108-110.

De Matteis, F., B.E. Prior, and C. Rimington. 1961. Nervous and biochemical disturbances following hexachlorobenzene intoxication. Nature 191:363-366.

Deichmann, W.B., W.E. MacDonald, J. Radomski, E.B. Blum, M. Bevilacqua, and M. Keplinger. 1970. The tumorigenicity of aldrin, dieldrin, and endrin in the albino rat. Ind. Med. Surg. 39:314.

Devine, J.M., and G. Zweig. 1969. Note on the determination of some chlorophenoxy herbicides and their esters in water. J. Assoc. Offic. Anal. Chem. 52:187-189.

DeGiovanni-Donnelly, R., S.M. Kolbye, and P.O. Greeves. 1968. The effects of IPC, CIPC, Sevin and Zectran on Bacillus subtilis. Experientia 24:80-81.

Didier, R., and Y. Lutz-Ostertag. 1972. Action de la simazine sur le tractus genital de l'embryon de poulet et de caille *in vivo* et *in vitro*. C.R. Soc. Biol. 166:1691-1693.

Dikshith, T.S.S. 1973. *In vivo* effects of Parathion on guinea pig chromosomes. Environ. Physiol. Biochem. 3:161-168.

Dobbins, P.K. 1967. Organic phosphate insecticides as teratogens in the rat. J. Fla. Med. Assoc. 54:452-456.

Dougherty, W.J., L. Golberg, and F. Coulston. 1971. The effect of Carbaryl on reproduction in the monkey *(Mucacca mulatta)*. Toxicol. Appl. Pharmacol. 19:365. Abstr. no. 11.

Dougherty, W.J., M. Herbst, and F. Coulston. 1975. The non-teratogenicity of 2,4,5-trichlorophenoxyacetic acid in the Rhesus monkey *(Macacca mulatta)*. Bull. Environ. Contam. Toxicol. 13:477-482.

Drill, V.A., and T. Hiratzka. 1953. Toxicity of 2,4-dichlorophenoxyacetic acid and 2,4, 5-trichlorophenoxyacetic acid. A report on their acute and chronic toxicity in dogs. Arch. Ind. Hyg. Occup. Med. 7:61-67.

Duggan, R.E. 1968. Pesticide residue levels in foods in the United States from July 1, 1963, to June 30, 1967. Pestic. Monit. J. 2:2-46.

Duggan, R.E., G.Q. Lipscomb, E.L. Cox, R.E. Heatwole, and R.C. Kling. 1971. Pesticide residue levels in foods in the United States from July 1, 1963, to June 30, 1969. Pestic. Monit. J. 5:73-212.

Dunachie, J.F., and W.W. Fletcher. 1969. An investigation of the toxicity of insecticides to birds' eggs using the egg-injection technique. Ann. Appl. Biol. 64:409-423.

Durham, W.F. 1969. Body burden of pesticides in man. Ann. N.Y. Acad. Sci. 160:183-195.

Durham, W.F., T.B. Gaines, and W.J. Hayes, Jr. 1956. Paralytic and related effects of certain organic phosphorus compounds. Am. Med. Assoc. Arch. Ind. Health 13:326-330.

DuBois, K.P. 1972. The interaction of environmental chemicals with drugs. Drug Inf. J. 6:53-58.

DuBois, K.P. 1958. Insecticides, rodenticides, herbicides, household hazards. Postgrad. Med. J. 24:278-288.

DuBois, K.P. 1961. Potentiation of the toxicity of organophosphorus compounds. Adv. Pest Control Res. 4:117-151.

DuBois, K.P., D.R. Thursh, and S.D. Murphy. 1957. Studies on the toxicity and pharmacologic actions of the dimethoxy ester of benzotriazine dithiophosphoric acid (DBD, Guthion). J. Pharmacol. Exp. Ther. 119:208-218.

DuBois, K.P., J. Doull, and J.M. Coon. 1950. Studies on the toxicity and pharmacological action of octamethyl pyrophosphoramide (OMPA: Pestox III). J. Pharmacol. Exp. Ther. 99:376-393.

DuBois, K.P., J. Doull, J. Deroin, and O. K. Cummings. 1953. Studies on the toxicity and mechanism of action of some new insecticidal thionophosphates. Arch. Ind. Hyg. Occup. Med. 8:350-358.

Earl, F.L., B.E., Melveger, J.E. Reinwall, G.W. Bierbower, and J.M. Curtis. 1971. Diazinon toxicity-comparative studies in dogs and miniature swine. Toxicol. Appl. Pharmacol. 18:285-295.

Earl, F.L., E. Miller, and E.J. VanLoon. 1973. Reproductive, teratogenic, and neonatal effects of some pesticides and related compounds in beagle dogs and miniature swine. *In* W. B. Deichmann, ed. Pesticides and the Environment: A Continuing Controversy, pp. 253-266. Intercontinental Medical Book Corp., New York.

Edery, H., D. Soroker, and W. Kuhnberg. 1970. Antidotal action of new oximes in experimental organophosphate intoxication. Israel J. Med. Sci. 6:209-218.

Edson, E.F., and D.N. Noakes. 1960. The comparative toxicity of six organophosphorus insecticides in the rat. Toxicol. Appl. Pharmacol. 2:523-539.

Edson, E.F. 1964. No-effect levels of three organophosphates in the rat, pig, and man. Food Cosmet. Toxicol. 2:311-316.

Edson, E.F., and D.M. Sanderson. 1965. Toxicity of the herbicides, 2-methoxy-3,6-dichlorobenzoic acid (Dicamba) and 2-methoxy-3,5,6-trichlorobenzoic acid (Tricamba). Food Cosmet. Toxicol. 3:299-304.

Edwards, C.A. 1964. Factors affecting the persistence of insecticides in soil. Soils Fertil. 27:451-454.

Egle, J.L., Jr. 1972. Retention of inhaled formaldehyde, propionaldehyde, and acrolein in the dog. Arch. Environ. Health 25:119-124.

Eichelberger, J.W., and J.J. Lichtenberg. 1971. Persistence of pesticides in river water. Environ. Sci. Technol. 5:541-544.

Eisenbrand, G., O. Ungerer, and R. Preussman. 1974. Rapid formation of carcinogenic *N*-Nitrosamines by interaction of nitrite with fungicides derived from dithiocarbamic acid *in vitro* under simulated gastric conditions and *in vivo* in the rat stomach. Food Cosmet. Toxicol. 12:229-232.

Elanco Products Co. 1967. Report on Trifluralin. FDA Pesticide Petition no. 7F0555, Section C. Cited in Initial Scientific and Minieconomic Review of Trifluralin, U.S. Environmental Protection Agency (In preparation).

Elizarov, G.P. Vestn. 1972. Professional'nye zabole vaniia kozhi, vyzvannye simazinom i protazinom. Dermatol. Venerol. 46:27-9.

Emerson, J.L., D.J. Thompson, R.J. Strebing, C.G. Gerbig, and V.B. Robinson. 1971. Teratogenic studies on 2,4,5-trichlorophenoxyacetic acid in the rat and rabbit. Food Cosmet. Toxicol. 9:395-404.

Emmerson, J.L., and R.C. Anderson. 1966. Metabolism of Trifluralin in the rat and dog. Toxicol. Appl. Pharmacol. 9:84-97.

Engst, R., W. Schnaak, and H.J. Lewerenz. 1971. Studies on the metabolism of the fungicidal ethylene-*bis*-dithiocarbamates Maneb, Zineb and Nabam. Part V. Toxicology of the degradation products. Z. Lebnsm. Unters. Forsch. 146(2):91-97.

Epstein, S.S., E.Arnold, J. Andrea, W. Bass, and Y. Bishop. 1972. Detection of chemical mutagens by the dominant lethal assay in the mouse. Toxicol. Appl. Pharmacol. 23:288-325.

Erne, K. 1966a. Distribution and elimination of chlorinated phenoxyacetic acids in animals. Acta Vet. Scand. 7:240-256.

Erne, K. 1966b. Animal metabolism of phenoxyacetic herbicides. Acta Vet. Scand. 7:264-271.

Ettinger, M.B. and D.I. Mount. 1967. A wild fish should be safe to eat. Environ. Sci. Technol. 1:203-205.

Fang, S.C., E. Fallin, M.L. Montgomery, and V.H. Freed. 1973. The metabolism and distribution of 2,4,5-trichlorophenoxyacetic acid in female rats. Toxicol. Appl. Pharmacol. 24:555-563.

Farm Chemicals Handbook. 1976. Meister Publishing Co., Willoughby, Ohio.

Faur, N., and T. Kemeny. 1968. Effects of long-term ingestion of small amounts of DDT on blood picture of mice (BALB/c). Hyg. Sanit. 33(1-3):248-250. (Translation of Gig. Sanit.)

Felton, J.C. 1968. Insecticidal activity of some oxime carbamates. J. Sci. Food Agric. Suppl. 32-38.

Finnegan, J.K., P.S. Larson, R.B. Smith, Jr., H.B. Haag, and G.R. Hennigar. 1958. Acute and chronic toxicity studies on pentachloronitrobenzene. Arch. Int. Pharmacodyn. 114:38-52.

Fish, S.A. 1966. Organophosphorus cholinesterase inhibitors and fetal development. Am. J. Obstet. Gynecol. 96:1148-1154.

Fishbein, L. 1976. Environmental health aspects of fungicides. I. Dithiocarbamates. J. Toxicol. Environ. Health. 1:713-735.

Fisher, D.E., L.E. St. John, Jr., W.H. Gutenmann, D.G. Wagner, and D.J. Lisk. 1965. Fate of Banvel T, Ioxynil, Tordon, and Trifluralin in the dairy cow. J. Dairy Sci. 48:1711-1715.

Fitzhugh, O.G., and W. Buschke. 1949. Production of cataract in rats by β-tetralol and other derivatives of naphthalene. Arch. Ophthalmol. 41:572-582.

Fitzhugh, O.G., and A.A. Nelson. 1951. Comparison of chronic effects produced in rats by several chlorinated hydrocarbon insecticides. Fed. Proc. 10:295.

Fitzhugh, O.G., A.A. Nelson, and J.P. Frawley. 1950. The chronic toxicities of technical Benzenehexachloride and its alpha, beta, and gamma isomers. J. Pharmacol. Exp. Ther. 100:59-66.

Fogelman, R. 1954. Report of Hazelton Laboratories on Captan, EPA Pesticide Petition no. 15. Cited in U.S. Environmental Protection Agency. 1975. Initial Scientific and Minieconomic Review of Captan, p. 46. EPA-540/1-75-012.

Food and Agriculture Organization of the United Nations. 1970. 1969 Evaluations of some pesticides in food. The Monographs. FAO/PL:1969/M/17/1. WHO/Food Add./70.38. 243 pp.

Food and Agriculture Organization of the United Nations Working Party of Experts on Pesticide Residues. 1968. 1967 Evaluations of some Pesticide Residues in Food, the Monographs, issued jointly by FAO and WHO. FAO/PL:1967/M/11/1. WHO/Food Add./68.30.

Food and Agriculture Organization of the United Nations. 1975. Pesticide Residues in Food. Report of the 1974 Joint FAO/WHO meeting. Technical Report Series 574. FAO Agricultural Studies no. 97. World Health Organization, Geneva.

Food and Agriculture Organization of the United Nations. 1967. Evaluation of some pesticide residues in food. FAO. PL:CP/15, WHO/Food Add/67.32. Geneva.

Food and Agriculture Organization of the United Nations. Working Party of Experts on Pesticide Residues. 1973. 1972 Evaluations of some pesticide residues in food. The Monographs. World Health Organization, Geneva.

Food and Agriculture Organization of the United Nations. 1965. Evaluation of the toxicity of pesticide residues in food. FAO Meeting Report, no. PL: 1965/10/1; WHO/Food Add./27.65. Rome. 194 pp.

Food and Agriculture Organization of the United Nations. Working Party of Experts on Pesticide Residues. 1969. 1968 Evaluations of some Pesticide Residues in Food, the Monographs, issued jointly by FAO and WHO, FAO/PL:1968/m/9/1. WHO/Food Add./69.35.

Food and Agriculture Organization of the United Nations/World Health Organization. 1971. 1970 evaluations of some pesticide residues in food. FAO/AGP. 1970/M/12/1; WHO/Food Add./71.42.

Frawley, J.P., and H.N. Fuyat. 1957. Effect of low dietary levels of parathion and systox on blood cholinesterase of dogs. J. Agric. Food Chem. 5:346-348.

Frawley, J.P., H.N. Fuyat, E.C. Hagan, J.R. Blake, and O. G. Fitzhugh. 1957. Marked potentiation in mammalian toxicity from simultaneous administration of two anti cholinesterase compounds. J. Pharmacol. Exp. Ther. 121:96-106.

Frawley, J.P., R.E. Zwickey, and H.N. Fuyat. 1956. Myelin degeneration in chickens with subacute administration of organic phosphorus insecticides. Fed. Proc. 15:424. Abstr. no. 1380.

Freal, J.J., and R.W. Chadwick. 1973. Metabolism of hexachlorocyclohexane to chlorophenols and effect of isomer pretreatment on lindane metabolism in rat. J. Agric. Food Chem. 21: 424-427.

Fukami, J., and T. Shishido. 1972. Selective toxicity of Diazinon and other non-systemic insecticides. *In* A.S. Tahori, ed. Insectidides: Proceedings of the Second International IUPAC Congress of Pesticide Chemistry, Tel-Aviv, 1971, vol. 1. Gordon and Breach Publishers, New York.

Fullerton, R.W., M.B. Carlson, and A.R. Nolting. 1974. Final report on the 2,4,5-T Scientific Workshop, Washington, D.C. March 8-9, 1974. U.S. Department of Agriculture, Office of the General Counsel, Washington, D.C. 45 pp.

Funderburk, H.H. Jr., N.S. Megi, and J.M. Lawrence. 1966. Photochemical decomposition of Diquat and Paraquat. Weeds 14(3):240-243.

Gaines, T.B. 1960. The acute toxicity of pesticides to rats. Toxicol. Appl. Pharmacol. 2:88-99.

Gaines, T.B. 1969. Acute toxicity of pesticides. Toxicol. Appl. Pharmacol. 14:515-534.

Gaines, T.B., J.F. Holson, Jr., C.J. Nelson, and H.J. Schumacher. 1975. Analysis of strain differences in sensitivity and reproducibility of results in assessing 2,4,5-Teratogenicity in mice. Toxicol. Appl. Pharmacol. 33:174. Abstr. no. 130.

Galloway, D.B., and J.C. Petrie. 1972. Recovery from severe Paraquat poisoning. Postgrad. Med. J. 48:684-686.

Gannon, N., and G.C. Decker. 1958. The conversion of Aldrin to Dieldrin on plants. J. Econ. Entomol. 51:8-11.

Gannon, N., R.P. Link, and G.C. Decker. 1959. Storage of Dieldrin in tissues of steers, hogs, lambs, and poultry fed Dieldrin in their diets. J. Agric. Food Chem. 7:826-828.

Gannon, N.H., and J.H. Bigger. 1958. Conversion of Aldrin and Heptachlor to their epoxides in soil. J. Econ. Entomol. 51:1-2.

Gardiner, J.A., R.W. Reiser, and H. Sherman 1969. Identification of the metabolites of Bromacil in rat urine. J. Agric. Food Chem. 17:967-973.

Gehring, P.J., C.G. Kramer, B.A. Schwetz, J.Q. Rose, and V.K. Rowe. 1973. The fate of 2,4,5-trichlorophenoxyacetic acid (2,4,5-T) following oral administration to man. Toxicol. Appl. Pharmacol. 26:352-361.

Gentile, J., and M. Plewa. 1976. Mutat. Res. (In Press).

Gentile, J.M., and J. Plewa. 1975. A bio-assay for screening host-mediated proximal mutagens in agriculture. Mutat. Res. 31:317. Abstr. no. 21.

Getzin, L.W., and I. Rosefield. 1966. Persistence of Diazinon and Zinophos in soils. J. Econ. Entomol. 59:512-516.

Getzin, L.W., and R.K. Chapman. 1960. The fate of Phorate in soils. J. Econ. Entomol. 53:47-51.

Getzin, L.W. 1968. Persistence of Diazinon and Zinophos in soil: effects of autoclaving, temperature, moisture, and acidity. J. Econ. Entomol. 61:1560-1565.

Ghezzo, F.; L. Corradini, C. Guglielmini and V. Ninfo. 1972. Toxic effects of dithiocarbamates on enzymic systems. Quad. Sclavo Diagn. Clin. Lab. 8(1):485-494.

Gilbertson, M., and L.M. Reynolds. 1972. Hexachlorobenzene (HCB) in the eggs of common terns in Hamilton Harbour, Ontario. Bull. Environ. Contam. Toxicol. 7:371-373.

Girard, R., F. Tolot, P. Martin, and J. Bourret. 1969. Hemopathies graves et exposition a des derives chlores du benzene (a propos de 7 cas). J. Med. Lyon 50:771-773.

Golab, T., R. I. Herberg, E.W. Day, A.P. Raun, F.J. Holzer, and G.W. Probst. 1969. Fate of carbon-14 Trifluralin in artificial rumen fluid and in ruminant animals. J. Agric. Food Chem. 17:576-580.

Golovan, D.J. 1970. Experimental validation of permissible concentration of dianate (Dicamba) and 2,3,6-trichlorobenzoic acid in water bodies. Hyg. Sanit. 35(10-12):14-18.

Golz, H.H., and C.B. Shaffer. 1956. Malathion: Summary of Pharmacology and Toxicology. American Cyanamid Co., New York, 2-14. Cited in U.S. Environmental Protection Agency. Initial Scientific and Minieconomic Review of Malathion, p. 66. EPA-540/1-75-005.

Good, E.E., G.W. Ware, and D.F. Miller. 1965. Effects of insecticides on reproduction in the laboratory mouse. I. Kepone. J. Econ. Entomol. 58:754-757.

Goto, M., M. Hattori, and T. Miyagawa. 1972. Ecological Chemistry. Toxizitat von a-BHC in mausen. Chemosphere 1(4):153-154.

Graca, I., A.M.S. Silva Fernandes, and H.C. Mourao. 1974. Organochlorine insecticide residues in human milk in Portugal. Pestic. Monit. J. 8:148-156.

Graham, S.L., and W.H. Hansen. 1972. Effects of short-term administration of ethylenethiourea upon thyroid function of the rat. Bull. Environ. Contam. Toxicol. 7:19-25.

Grant D.L., G.V. Hatina, and W.E.J. Phillips. 1975. Effect of Hexachlorobenzene on rat reproduction. Toxicol. Appl. Pharmacol. 33:167, Abstr. no. 113.

Grant, D.L., F. Iverson, G.V. Hatina, and D.C. Villeneuve. 1974. Effects of Hexachlorobenzene on liver porphyrin levels and microsomal enzymes in the rat. Environ. Physiol. Biochem. 4:159-165.

Grant, D.L., F. Iverson, G.V. Hatina, and D.C. Villeneuve. 1974. Effects of Hexachlorobenzene on liver porphyrin levels and microsomal enzymes in the rat. Toxicol. Appl. Pharmacol. 29:101. Abstr. no. 66.

Gray, E. 1954. Report of Hazelton Labs on Captan, EPA Pesticide Petition no. 15. Cited in the U.S. Environmental Protection Agency. 1975b. Initial Scientific and Minieconomic Review of Captan, p. 45. EPA-540/1-75-012.

Green, S., and F.S. Moreland. 1975. Cytogenetic evaluation of several dioxins in the rat. Toxicol. Appl. Pharmacol. 33:161. Abstr. no. 99.

Greig, J.B., G. Jones, W.H. Butler, and J.M. Barnes. 1973. Toxic effects of 2,3,7,8-tetrachlorodibenzo-*p*-dioxin. Food Cosmet. Toxicol. 11:585-595.

Grover, P.L., and P. Sims. 1965. The metabolism of -2,3,4,5,6-pentachlorocyclohex-1-ene and hexachlorocyclohexane in rats. Biochem. J. 96:521-525.

Grunow, W., and C. Bohme. 1974. Uber den Stoffwechsel von 2.4.5-T und 2.4-D bei Ratten und Mausen. Arch. Toxicol. 32:217-225.

Grunow, W., C. Bohme, and B. Budczies. 1971. Renale Ausscheidung von 2,4,5-T bei Ratten. Food Cosmet. Toxicol. 9:667-670.

Guiti, N., and D. Sadeghi, 1969. Acute toxicity of Malathion in the mongrel dog. Toxicol. Appl. Pharmacol. 15:244-245.

Gunther, F.A., W.E. Westlake, and P.S. Jaglan. 1968. Reported solubilities of 738 pesticide chemicals in water. Residue Rev. 20:1-148.

Gupta, B.N., J.G. Vos, J.A. Moore, J.G. Zinkl, and B.C. Bullock. 1973. Pathologic effects of 2,3,7,8-tetrachlorodibenzo-*p*-dioxin in laboratory animals. Environ. Health Perspect. 5:125-140.

Gusev, M.I., A.I. Svechnikova, I.S. Dronov, M.D. Grebenskova, and A.I. Golovina. 1966. Determination of the daily average maximum permissible concentration of Acrolein in the atmosphere. Hyg. Sanit. 31(1-3):8-13.

Gutenmann, W.H., D.D. Hardee, R.F. Holland, and D.J. Lisk. 1963. Disappearance of 4-(2,4-dichlorophenoxy) butyric acid herbicide in the dairy cow. J. Dairy Sci. 46:991-992.

Gutenmann, W.H., D.D. Hardee, R.F. Holland, and D.J. Lisk. 1963. Residue studies with 2,4-dichlorophenoxyacetic acid herbicide in the dairy cow and in a natural and artificial rumen. J. Dairy Sci. 46:1287-1288.

Haag, D., K. Goerttler, and D. Preiss. 1975. The influence of non-cytotoxic concentrations of the herbicide 2,4-dichlorophenoxyacetic acid on the DNA synthesis in cultured vertebrate cells. Arch. Toxicol. 33:91-102.

Haag, H.B., J.K. Finnegan, P.S. Larson, W. Riese, and M.L. Dreyfuss. 1950. Comparative chronic toxicity for warm-blooded animals of 2,2-*bis*-9p-chlorophenyl)-1,1,1-trichloroethane (DDT) and 2,2-*bis*-(p-methoxyphenyl)-1,1,1-trichloroethane (DMDT), methoxychlor. Arch. Int. Pharmacodyn. 83:491-504.

Hagan, E.C. 1953. Acute toxicity of *O,O*-dimethyl dithiophosphate of diethyl mercaptosuccinate (4049). Fed. Proc. 12:327. Abstr. no. 1079.

Hallowell, M. 1959. Acute haemolytic anaemia following the ingestion of para-dichlorobenzene. Arch. Dis. Child. 34:74-75.

Hansen, W.H., M.L. Quaife, R.T. Habermann, and O.G. Fitzhugh. 1971. Chronic toxicity of 2,4-dichlorophenoxyacetic acid in rats and dogs. Toxicol. Appl. Pharmacol. 20:122-129.

Harris, C.I. 1967. Movement of herbicides in soil. Weeds 15:214-216.

Harris, S.J., H.C. Cecil, and J. Bitman. 1974. Effect of several dietary levels of technical Methoxychlor on reproduction in rats. J. Agric. Food Chem. 22:969-973.

Haskell Laboratory for Toxicology and Industrial Medicine Report no. 16-57. 1957. The toxicity of manganese ethylenebisdithiocarbamate (Maneb). Private communication to E.I. DuPont deNemours. Quoted from U.S. Environmental Protection agency. Toxicology and environmental hazards of the ethylenebisdithiocarbamate fungicides and ethylene thiourea. 1973.

Hayes, M.H.B., M.E. Pick, and B.A. Toms. 1975. Interactions between clay minerals and bipyridylium herbicides. Residue Rev. 57:1-25.

Hayes, W.J. Jr. 1963. Clinical Handbook of Economic Poisons. U.S. Department of Health, Education, and Welfare, Public Health Service Communicable Disease Center, Atlanta, Ga. Public Health Service Publication no. 476.

Hayes, W.J., Jr. 1957. Dieldrin poisoning in man. Public Health Rep. 72:1087-1091.

Hayes, W.J., Jr. 1959. The toxicity of Dieldrin to man. Report on a survey. Bull. WHO 20:891-912.

Hayes, W.J., Jr. 1967. Toxicity of pesticides to man: risks from present levels. Proc. R. Soc. Lond. Ser. B. 167(1007):101-127.

Hayes, W.J., Jr. 1971. Studies on exposure during the use of anticholinesterase pesticides. Bull. WHO 44:277-288.

Hazelton, L.W., O.E. Paynter, and R.J. Weir. 1964. Safety evaluation studies on 2,5-dichloro-3-aminobenzoic acid (Amiben). Toxicol. Appl. Pharmacol. 6:349, Abstr. no. 26.

Hazleton, L.W., and E.G. Holland. 1953. Toxicity of Malathon: summary of mammalian investigations. Arch. Ind. Hyg. Occup. Med. 8:399-405.

Hazleton, L.W., and E.G. Holland. 1950. Pharmacology, and toxicology of Parathion. Adv. Chem. Series 1(31):31-38.

Hazleton, L.W. 1953. Acute oral toxicity of experimental insecticide 3911. Unpublished report of the American Cyanamid Co. Cited in U.S. Environmental Protection Agency.

1974e. Initial Scientific and Minieconomic Review of Phorate (Thimet). Office of Pesticides Programs, Washington, D.C.

Helling, C.S. 1976. Dinitroaniline herbicides in soils. J. Environ. Qual. 5:1-15.

Herbst, M., I. Weisse, and H. Koellmer. 1975. A contribution to the question of the possible hepatocarcinogenic effects of Lindane. Toxicology 4:91-96 Pestic. Abstr. no. 75-1442.

Herzel, F. 1972. Organochlorine insecticides in surface waters in Germany—1970 and 1971. Pestic. Monit. J. 6:179-187.

Hiatt, V. 1976. Personal communication.

Hickey, J.J., and D.W. Anderson. 1968. Chlorinated hydrocarbons and eggshell changes in raptorial and fish-eating birds. Science 162:271-273.

Highman, B., and H.J. Schumacher. 1974. Pathologic effects of a preparation of 2,4,5-trichlorophenoxyacetic acid on maternal mice. Toxicol. Appl. Pharmacol. 29:134, Abstr. no. 152.

Highman, B., T.B. Gaines, and H.J. Schumacher. 1975. Sequential histopathologic changes induced in mice by a technical and a purified preparation of 2,4,5-trichlorophenoxyacetic acid. Toxicol. Appl. Pharmacol. 33:161. Abstr. no. 98.

Hodge, H.C., E.A. Maynard, W.L. Downs, R.D. Coye, Jr., and L.T. Steadman. 1956. Chronic oral toxicity of ferric dimethyldithiocarbamate (Ferbam) and zinc dimethyldithiocarbamate (Ziram). J. Pharmacol. Exp. Ther. 118:174-181.

Hodgson, J.R., J.C. Hoch, T.R. Castles, D.O. Helton, and C.C. Lee. 1975. Metabolism and disposition of Ferbam in the rat. Toxicol. Appl. Pharmacol. 33:505-513.

Holland, E.G., L.W. Hazleton, and D.L. Hanzal. 1952. Toxicity of Malathon (*0,0*-dimethyl dithiophosphate of diethyl mercaptosuccinate). Fed. Proc. 11:357.

Hollingsworth, R.L., V.K. Rowe, F. Oyen, H.R. Hoyle, and H.C. Spencer. 1956. Toxicity of paradichlorobenzene. Arch. Ind. Health 14:138-147.

Hollingsworth, R.L., V.K. Rowe, F. Oyen, T.R. Torkelson, and E.M. Adams. 1958. Toxicity of *o*-dichlorobenzene. Arch. Ind. Health 17:180-187.

Hoogendam, I.J., P.J. Versteeg, and M. DeVlieger. 1962. Electroencephalograms in insecticide toxicity. Arch. Environ. Health 4:86-94.

Hoque, M.Z. 1972. Carbaryl, a new chemical mutagen. Curr. Sci. 41:855-856.

Huang, C.C. 1973. Effect on growth but not on chromosomes of the mammalian cells after treatment with three organophosphorus insecticides. Proc. Soc. Exp. Biol. Med. 142:36-40.

Huber, J.J. 1965. Some physiological effects of the insecticide Kepone in the laboratory mouse. Toxicol. Appl. Pharmacol. 7:516-524.

Hughes, L.B. 1971. A study of the fate of Carbaryl insecticide in surface waters. Diss. Abstr. Int. 32(6):3108B.

Hussain, S., L. Ehrenberg, G. Lofroth, and T. Gejvall. 1972. Mutagenic effects of TCDD [2,3,7,8-tetrachlorodibenzo-*p*-dioxin] on bacterial systems. Ambio 1:32-33.

Huston, B.L. 1972. Identification of three neutral contaminants in production grade 2,4-D. J. Agric. Food Chem. 20:724-727.

Hutterer, F., F. Schaffner., F.M. Klion, and H. Popper. 1968. Hypertrophic hypoactive smooth endoplasmic reticulum: A sensitive indicator of hepatotoxicity exemplified by Dieldrin. Science 161:1017-1019.

Ingle, L. 1952. Chronic oral toxicity of Chlordan to rats. Arch. Ind. Hyg. Occup. Med. 6:357-367.

Innes, J.R.M., B.M. Ulland, M.G. Valerio, L. Petrucelli, L. Fishbein, E.R. Hart, A.J. Pallotta, R.R. Bates, H.L. Falk, J.J. Gart, M. Klein, I. Mitchell, and J. Peters. 1969. Bioassay of pesticides and industrial chemicals for tumorigenicity in mice. A preliminary note. J. Nat. Cancer Inst. 42:1101-1114.

International Agency for Research on Cancer. 1974. IARC Monographs on the Evaluation of Carcinogenic Risk of Chemicals to Man. Vol. 5: Some Organochlorine pesticides. Lyon, France.

International Agency for Research on Cancer. 1975. Report on an assessment of the carcinogenic potential of contaminants detected in drinking water in the U.S., including recommendations for further study. Lyon, France.

International Agency for Research on Cancer. 1974. IARC Monographs on the Evaluation of Carcinogenic Risk of Chemicals to Man. Vol. 7: pp. 231-244. Lyon, France.

Ishida, M. and P. Dahm. 1965. Metabolism of benzene hexachloride isomers and related compounds *in vitro*. I. Properties and distribution of the enzyme. J. Econ. Entomol. 58: 383-392.

Ismirova, N., and V. Marinov. 1972. Distribution, and release of ^{35}S-Ziram 24 hrs. after its oral administration in female rats. Eksper. Med. Morf. 11(3):152-156.

Ito, N., H. Nagasaki. M. Arai, A. Masayuki, S. Makiura, S. Sugihara, and K. Hirao. 1973. Histopathologic studies on liver tumorigenesis induced in mice by technical polychlorinated biphenyls and its promoting effect on liver tumors induced by benzene hexachloride. J. Nat. Cancer Inst. 51:1637-1646.

Ito, N., H. Nagasaki, H. Aoe, S. Sugihara, Y. Miyata, M. Arai, and T. Shirai. 1975. Development of hepatocellular carcinomas in rats treated with benzene-hexachloride. J. Nat. Cancer Inst. 54:801-805.

Ito, N., H. Nagasaki, M. Arai, S. Sugihara, and S. Makiura. 1973. Histologic and ultrastructural studies on the hepatocarcinogenicity of benzene hexachloride in mice. J. Nat. Cancer Inst. 51:817-826.

Jackson, W.T. 1972. Regulation of mitosis. III. Cytological effects of 2,4,5-trichlorophenoxyacetic acid and of dioxin contaminants in 2,4,5-T formulations. J. Cell. Sci. 10:15-25.

Jedlica, V.L., Z. Hermankaska, I. Smida, and A. Kouba. 1958. Paramyeloblastic leukaemia appearing simultaneously in two blood cousins after simultaneous contact with gammexane (hexachlorocyclohexane). Acta. Med. Scand. 161:447-451.

Jirik, V., J. Pokorny, and H. Culikova. 1971. Investigation of the degradation of organosphosphate insecticide Fosfotion in surface water. Cesk. Hyg. 16,177-182.

Johnson, E.I., and J.F.C. Tyler. 1962. Occurrence of ethylenethiourea in thiocarbamate fungicides and its detection in fruit juice. Chem. Ind. (Lond.), pp. 305-306.

Johnson, J.E. 1971. The public health implications of widespread use of the phenoxy herbicides and picloram. BioScience 21:899-905.

Johnson, J.L., D.L. Stalling, and J.W. Hogan. 1974. 1974. Hexachlorobenzene (HCB) residues in fish. Bull. Environ. Contam. Toxicol. 11:393-398.

Jones, G.R., and P. Owen-Lloyd. 1973. Recovery from poisoning by 20% Paraquat. Br. J. Clin. Pract. 27:69-70.

Jordan, R.L., and J.F. Borzelleca. 1973. Teratogenic studies with Pentachloronitrobenzene in rats. Toxicol. Appl. Pharmacol. 25:454-455. Abstr. no. 40.

Jordan, R.L., F. Sperling, H.H. Klein, and J.F. Borzelleca. 1975. A study of the potential teratogenic effects of Pentachloronitrobenzene in rats. Toxicol. Appl. Pharmacol. 33:222-230.

Jorgenson, T.A., C.J. Rushbrook, and G.W. Newell. 1976. *In vivo* mutagenesis investigations of ten commercial pesticides. Abstr. no. 41.

Kalow, W., and A. Marton. 1961. Second-generation toxicity of Malathion in rats. Nature 192:464-465.

Kapoor, I.P., R.L. Metcalf, A.S. Hirwe, J.R. Coats, and M.S. Khalsa. 1973. Structure activity correlations of biodegradability of DDT analogs. J. Agric. Food Chem. 21:310-315.

Kapoor, I.P., R.L. Metcalf, R.F. Nystrom, and G.K. Sangha. 1970. Comparative metabolism of Methoxchlor, Methiochlor, and DDT in mouse, insects, and in a model ecosystem. J. Agric. Food Chem 18:1145-1152.

Kaufman, D.D., and P.C. Kearney. 1970. Microbial degradation of 5-triazine herbicides. Pestic. Rev. 32:235-265.

Kay, J.H., and J.C. Calandra. 1961. Chronic oral toxicity of Phaltan in albino rats and dogs. Industrial Bio-test Laboratores, Northbrook, Ill. Pesticide Petition no. 283c. Cited in U.S. Environmental Protection Agency. Initial Scientific and Minieconomic Review of Folpet. In preparation.

Kenaga, E.E. 1966. Pesticide reference standards of the Entomological Society of America. Entomol. Soc. Bull. 12(2):117-127.

Kennedy, G.L., Jr., J.P. Frawley, and J.C. Calandra. 1973. Multigeneration reproductive effects of three pesticides in rats. Toxicol. Appl. Pharmacol. 25:589-596.

Kettering Laboratory. 1959. The physiological effects of the introduction of heptachlor epoxide in varying levels of concentration into the diet of CFN rats. University of Cincinnati, Department of Preventive Medicine and Industrial Health, Cincinnati, Ohio.

Khanna, S., and S.C. Fang. 1966. Metabolism of C^{14}-labeled 2,4 -dichlorophenoxyacetic acid in rats. J. Agric. Food Chem. 14:500-503.

Khera, K.D., and W.P. McKinley. 1972. Pre- and postnatal studies on 2,4,5-trichlorophenoxyacetic acid, 2,4-dichlorophenoxyacetic acid, and their derivatives in rats. Toxicol. Appl. Pharmacol. 22:14-28.

Khera, K.S., and D.C. Villeneuve. 1975. Teratagenicity studies on halogenated benzenes (pentachloro-, pentachloronitro-, and hexabromo-) in rats. Toxicology 5:117-122.

Khera, K.S. 1969. Perinatal toxicity of pesticides. Can. Med. Assoc. J. 100:167-172.

Khera, K.S. 1973. Ethylenethiourea: Teratogenicity study in rats and rabbits. Teratology 7:243-252.

Khera, K.S. 1974. Teratogenicity and dominant lethal studies on hexachlorobenzene in rats. Food Cosmet. Toxicol. 12:471-477.

Khera, K.S., and J.A. Ruddick. 1973. Polychlorodibenzo-*p*-dioxins: Perinatal effects and the dominant lethal test in Wistar rats. *In* E.H. Blair, ed. Chlorodioxins—Origin and Fate, pp. 70-84. Advances in Chemistry Series 120, American Chemical Society, Washington, D.C.

Kimbrough, R.D., and R.E. Linder. 1974. The toxicity of technical hexachlorobenzene in the Sherman strain rat. A preliminary study. Res. Commun. Chem. Pathol. Pharmacol. 8:653-664.

Kimbrough, R.D., and T. B. Gaines. 1970. Toxicity of Paraquat and its effects on rat lungs. Toxicol. Appl. Pharmacol. 17:679-690.

Kimbrough, R.D., and T.B. Gaines. 1968. Effect of organic phosphorus compounds and alkylating agents on the rat fetus. Arch. Environ. Health 16:805-808.

Kimbrough, R.D. 1974. Toxic effects of the herbicide Paraquat. Chest, 65, 65s-67s (April 1974 Suppl.).

Kimmerle, G., and D. Lorke. 1968. Toxicology of insecticidal organophosphates. Pflanz-Nachr. Bayer 21:111-142.

Klimmer, O.R. 1955. Experimentelle Untersuchungen Uber die toxikologie insecticider chlorieter kohlenwasserstoffe. (Experimental studies on the toxicology of insecticidal chlorinated hydrocarbon). I. Arch. Exp. Pathol. Pharmakol. 227:183-195.

Klingman, D.L., C.H. Gordon, G. Yip, and H.P. Burchfield. 1966. Residues in the forage and in milk from cows grazing forage treated with esters of 2,4-D. Weeds 14:164-167.

Klosa, J. 1950. Diskussions: zur toxikologie der hexachlorocyclohexane. Pharmazie 5:615-616.

Knaak, J.B. 1971. Biological and nonbiological modifications of carbamates. Bull. WHO 44:121-131.

Kociba, R.J., P.A. Keeler, C.N. Park, and P.J. Gehring. 1976. 2,3,7,8-Tetrachlorodibenzo-*p*-dioxin (TCDD): Results of a 13-week oral toxicity study in rats. Toxicol. Appl. Pharmacol. 35:553-574.

Koeman, J.H., M.C. ten Noever de Brauw, and R.H. deVos. 1969. Chlorinated biphenyls in fish, mussels and birds from the river Rhine and the Netherlands coastal area. Nature 221:1126-1128.

Konrad, J.G., G. Chesters, and D.E. Armstrong. 1969. Soil degradation of malathion, a phosphorodithioate insecticide. Soil. Sci. Soc. Am. Proc. 33:259-262.

Konstantinova, T.K. 1974. Experiments on the effects of 2,4,5-T butyl ester on pregnant animals and on the development of their offspring. Gig. Sanit. 39(8):101-102. (Pestic. Abstr. 8:37, no. 75-0149, 1975.)

Korte, F. 1967. Metabolism of ^{14}C-labelled insecticides in microorganisms, insects and mammals. Botyu-Kagaku 32:46-59.

Koss, G., and W. Koransky. 1975. Studies on the toxicology of hexachlorobenzene. I. Pharmacokinetics Arch. Toxicol. 34:203-212.

Koss, G., W. Koransky, and K. Steinbach. 1976. Studies on the toxicology of hexachlorobenzene. II. Identification and determination of metabolites. Arch. Toxicol. 35:107-114.

Kraus, P., G. Noack, and J. Protig. 1973. Biodegradation of alpha-hexachloro-cyclohexane. II. Glutathione-mediated conversion to hydrophilic substance by particulate fractions of rat liver and by homogenates of various organs. Naunyn-Schmied's Arch. Pharmacol. 279:199-202.

Krueger, H.R., and R.D. O'Brien. 1959. Relationship between metabolism and differential toxicity of Malathion in insects and mice. J. Econ. Entomol. 52:1063-1067.

Kuchar, E.J., F.O. Geenty, W.P. Griffith, and R.J. Thomas. 1969. Analytical studies of metabolism of Terraclor in beagle dogs, rats, and plants. J. Agric. Food Chem. 17:1237-1240.

Kudzina, G.D., and D.I. Golovan. 1972. Comparative sanitary-toxicological and cell culture evaluation of the chlorobenzoic acid herbicide group. Vrach. Delo 1:125-128. (Health Aspects Pestic. 5:454, no. 72-1954, 1972.)

Kuiper-Goodman, T., D. Grant, G. Korsrud, C.A. Moodie, and I.C. Munro. 1974. Toxic effects of hexachlorobenzene in the rat: Correlations of electron microscopy with other toxic parameters. Toxicol. Appl. Pharmacol. 29:101, Abstr. no. 67.

Kunze, F.M., E.P. Laug, and C.S. Prickett. 1950. The storage of Methoxychlor in the fat of the rat. Proc. Soc. Exp. Biol. Med. 75:415-416.

Kurinnyi, A.I., and T.I. Kondratenko. 1972. Effect of fungicides (dithiocarbamic acid derivatives) on chromosomes of bone marrow cells in mice. Tsitol. Genet. 6:225-228.

Lackey, R.W. 1949. Observations on the acute and chronic toxicity of Toxaphene in the dog. J. Ind. Hyg. Toxicol. 31:117-120.

Lamoureux, G.L., and K.L. Davison. 1975. Mercapturic acid formation in the metabolism of Propachlor, CDAA, and Fluordifen in the rat. Pestic. Biochem. Physiol. 5: 497-506.

Larson, P.S. 1964. Unpublished data. Toxicologic study on the effect of adding dithane M-22 and M-45 to the diet of rats for a period of three months. Private communication to Rohm and Haas. Quoted from U.S. Environmental Protection Agency. Toxicology and environmental hazards of the ethylenebisdithiocarbamate fungicides and ethylene thiourea. 1973.

Larson, P.S., A.M. Ambrose, and J.F. Borzelleca. 1965. Unpublished data. Toxicologic study on the effect of adding dithane M-45 to the diet of rats for a period of 90 weeks.

Private communication to Rohm and Haas. Quoted from U.S. Environmental Agency. Toxicology and environmental hazards of the ethylenebisdithiocarbamate fungicides and ethylene thiourea.

Laug, E.P. A.A. Nelson, O.G. Fitzhugh, and F.M. Kunze. 1950. Liver cell alteration and DDT storage in the fat of the rat induced by dietary levels of 1 to 50 ppm DDT. J. Pharmacol. Exp. Ther. 98:268-273.

Lawless, E.W., R. von Rumker, and T.L. Ferguson. 1972. Pollution potential in pesticide manufacturing. Final Report to the Midwest Research Institute on Contract no. 68-01-0142 for the Environmental Protection Agency, Office of Water Programs. June 1972 (NTIS Nos. PB-213, 782/3). Technical Studies Report:TS-00-72-04.

Lehman, A. 1952. Chemicals in foods: A report to the Association of Food and Drug officials on current developments. Part II, Pesticides. Section V: Pathology. U.S. Assoc. Food Drug Offic. Q. Bull. 16:126-132.

Lehman, A. 1952. Chemicals in foods: A report to the Association of Food and Drug officials on current developments. Part II. Pesticides. Section III. Subacute and chronic toxicity. U.S. Assoc. Food Drug Offic. Q. Bull. 16:47-53.

Lehman, A.J. 1965. Summaries of Pesticide Toxicity, pp. 13-14. Association of Food and Drug Officials of the U.S., Topeka, Kan.

Lenon, H., L. Curry, A. Miller, and O. Patulski. 1972. Insecticide residues in water and sediment from cisterns on the U.S. and British Virgin Islands. Pestic. Monit. J. 6:188-193.

Lewis, L.F., and G.W. Eddy. 1959. Control of mosquito larvae in log ponds in Oregon. J. Econ. Entomol. 52:259-260.

Lisk, D.J., W.H. Gutenmann, C.A. Bache, R.G. Warner, and D.G. Wagner. 1963. Elimination of 2,4-D in the urine of steers fed 4-(-2,4-DB) or 2,4-D. J. Dairy Sci. 46:1435-1436.

Loge, J.P. 1965. Aplastic anemia following exposure to benzene hexachloride (Lindane). J. Am. Med. Assoc. 193:110-114.

Lu, P.-Y., and R.L. Metcalf. 1975. Environmental fate and biodegradability of benzene derivatives as studied in a model aquatic ecosystem. Environ. Health Perspect. 10:269-284.

Lu, P.-Y., R.L. Metcalf, A.S. Hirwe, and J.W. Williams. 1975. Evaluaton of environmental distribution and fate of hexachlorocyclopentadiene, Chlordene, Heptachlor, and Heptachlor epoxide in a laboratory model ecosystem. J. Agric. Food Chem. 23:967-973.

Luczak, J.E., Brudny, Z. Chmielewska, J. Traczynk, J. Jurkiewicz, I. Krzeczkowska, F. Suidak, and M. Lewtah. 1973. Persistent pesticides in waters used for community purposes in the cities of Kralcow and Warsaw and in the provinces of Gdansk, Olsztyn, and Lodz. Rocz. Panstw. Zakl. Hig. 24:101-107. (Polish)

Ludwig, R.A., G.D. Thorn, and D.M. Miller. 1954. The mechanism of fungicidal action of disodium ethylenebisdithiocarbamate (Nabam). Can. J. Bot. 32:48-54.

Lui, H., and G.D. Sweeney. 1975. Hepatic metabolism of hexachlorobenzene in rats. FEBS Lett. 51:225-226.

Majumdar, S.K., and R.C. Hall. 1973. Cytogenetic effects of 2,4,5-T on in vivo bone marrow cells of Mongolian gerbils. J. Hered. 64:213-216.

Malling, H.V., and F.J. deSerres. 1970. Captan—a potent fungicide with mutagenic activity. Environ. Mutagen Soc. Newsl. 3:37. Abstr. no. 15, 1st Annual Meeting, Environmental Mutagen Society.

Manigold, D.B., and J.A. Schulze. 1969. Pesticides in selected western streams—A progress report. Pestic. Monit. J. 3:124-135.

Mann, J.B., H.F. Enos, J. Gonzalez, and J.F. Thompson. 1974. Development of sampling and analytical procedure for determining hexachlorobenzene and hexachloro-1,3-butadiene in air. Environ. Sci. Technol. 8:584-585.

Manske, D.D., and P.E. Corneliussen. 1974. Pesticide residues in total diet samples (VII). Pestic. Monit. J. 8:110-124.

Manske, D.D., and R.D. Johnson. 1975. Pesticide residues in total diet samples (VIII). Pestic. Monit. J. 9:94-105.

March, R.B., T.R. Fukuto, R.L. Metcalf, and M.G. Maxon. 1956. Fate of phosphorous-32-labeled Malathion in the laying hen, white mouse, and American cockroach. J. Econ. Entomol. 49:185-195.

Martin, H. 1972. Pesticide Manual. 3rd ed. British Crop Protecton Council, London, England.

Matthiaschk, G. 1973. Uber den Einfluss von L-Cystein auf die Teratogenese durch Thiram (TMTD), bei NMRI-Mausen. Arch. Toxikol. 30:251-262.

McCann, J., E. Choi, E. Yamasaki, and B.N. Ames. 1975. Detection of carcinogens as mutagens in the *Salmonella*/microsome test: Assay of 300 chemicals. Proc. Nat. Acad. Sci. 72(12):5135-5139.

McGee, L.C., H.L. Reed, and J.P. Fleming. 1952. Accidental poisoning by Toxaphene. J. Am. Med. Assoc. 149:1124-1126.

McPhillips, J.J., and M.S. Dar. 1967. Resistance to the effect of carbachol on the cardiovascular system and on the isolated ileum of rats after subacute administration of an organophosphorus cholinesterase inhibitor. J. Pharmacol. Exp. Ther. 156:507-513.

Medved', L.I., E.I. Spynu, and I.S. Kagan. 1964. The method of conditioned reflexes in toxicology and its application for determinng the toxicity of small quantities of pesticides. Residue Rev. 6:42-74.

Mehani, S. 1972. The toxic effects of Paraquat in rabbits and rats. Ain Shams Med. J. 23 (6):599-601.

Mehendale, H.M., M. Fields, and H.B. Matthews. 1975. Metabolism and effects of hexachlorobenzene on hepatic microsomal enzymes in the rat. J. Agric. Food Chem. 23:261-265.

Melis, R. 1955. Tolerance of small doses of lindane by warm-blooded animals. I. Effect of Lindane administered in the diet of albino rats in proportions of 2 to 10 ppm. Nuovi. Ann. Ig. Microbiol. 6(2):90-104.

Melnikov, N.N. 1971. Halogen derivatives of alicyclic hydrocarbons. Residue Rev. 36:42-66.

Melnikov, N.N. 1971. Chemistry of pesticides. Translated as Residue Reviews vol. 36. Springer-Verlag. pp. 371-372.

Menzie, C.M. 1969. Metabolism of Pesticides. U.S. Department of the Interior, U.S. Bureau of Sport Fisheries and Wildlife. Special Scientific Report: Wildlife no. 127. Washington, D.C.

Menzie, C.M. 1972. Fate of pesticides in the environment. Ann. Rev. Entomol. 17:199-222.

Menzie, C.M. 1974. Metabolism of pesticides, an update. U.S. Department of the Interior, Fish and Wildlife Service. Special Scientific Report-Wildlife no. 184. Washington, D.C.

Merck Index, 8th ed. 1968. Merck & Co., Rahway, N.J.

Metcalf, R.L. and J.R. Sanborn. 1975. Pesticides and Environmental Quality in Illinois. Ill. Nat. Hist. Sur. Bull. 31(9):381-436.

Metcalf, R.L., and R.B. March. 1953. Further studies on the mode of action of organic thionophosphate insecticides. Ann. Entomol. Soc. Am. 46:63-74.

Metcalf, R.L. 1973. A century of DDT. J. Agric. Food Chem. 21:511-519.

Metcalf, R.L., I.P. Kapoor, P.Y. Lu, C.K. Schuth, and P. Sherman. 1973. Model ecosystem studies of the environmental fate of six organochlorine pesticides. Environ. Health Perspect. Exp. Issue no. 4:35-44.

Miura, K., T. Ino, and S. Iizuka. 1974. Comparison of susceptibilities to the acute toxicity of BHC in strains of experimental mice. Jikken Dobutsu 2(3):198. (Pestic. Abstr. 8:255, 75-0921, Apr. 1975.)

Miyakoshi, T., and G. Kikuchi. 1963. Studies on experimental porphyria. I. Increased synthesis of δ-aminolevulinic acid in allyl-isopropylacetamide-induced rat. Tohuku J. Exp. Med. 79:199-208.

Moeller, H.C., and J.A. Rider. 1962. Plasma and red blood cell cholinesterase activity as indications of the threshold of incipient toxicity of ethyl-*p*-nitrophenyl thionobenzene-phosphonate (EPN) and Malathion in human beings. Toxicol. Appl. Pharmacol. 4:123-130.

Mohn, G. 1971. Microorganisms as test systems for mutagenicity. Arch. Toxicol. 28:93-104.

Moore, S., III. 1975. Proc. 27th Illinois Custom Spray Operators Training School, p. 217, Urbana, Ill. Jan. 8-9.

Moore, S., III, W.N. Bruce, D.E. Kuhlman, and R. Randell. 1973. A study of the sources of insecticide residues in milk on dairy farms in Illinois—1971. Pestic. Monit. J. 6:233-237.

Moorefield, H.H. 1974. Data on Temik aldicarb pesticide environmental impact. Cited in U.S. Environmental Protection Agency. 1975m. Initial Scientific and Minieconomic Review of Aldicarb. EPA-540/1-75-013.

Morgan, D.P., and C.C. Roan. 1974. The metabolism of DDT in man. Essays Toxicol. 5:39-97.

Morita, M., and G. Ohi. 1975. Para-dichlorobenzene in human tissue and atmosphere in Tokyo metropolitan area. Environ. Pollut. 8:269-274.

Morita, M., and S. Oishi. 1975. Clearance and tissue distribution of hexachlorobenzene in rats. Bull. Environ. Contam. Toxicol. 14:313-318.

Mrak, E.M. Chairman. 1969. Report of the Secretary's Commission on Pesticides and Their Relationship to Environmental Health. U.S. Department of Health, Education, and Welfare. Washington, D.C.

Muhlmann, R., and G. Schrader. 1957. Hydrolyse der insektiziden phosphorsaureester. Z. Naturforsch. Teil B 12:196-208.

Muller, H.D., and D.C. Lockman. 1972. Fecundity, and progeny growth following subacute insecticide ingestion by the mallard. Poult. Sci. 51:239-241.

Mullison, W. R. 1966. Some toxicological aspects of Silvex. Southern Weed Conference, Proceedings, 19th Annual Meeting. Jacksonville, Florida, pp. 420-435.

Munsch, N., A. deRecondo, and C. Frayssinet. 1973. Effects of Acrolein on DNA synthesis in vitro. FEBS Lett. 30:286-290.

Murphy, S.D. 1965. Mechanism of the effect of Acrolein on rat liver enzymes. Toxicol. Appl. Pharmacol. 7:833-843.

Murphy, S.D., Chairman. 1975. Report: Assessment of health risk from organics in drinking water, Environmental Protection Agency. Science Advisory Board. April 30, 1975.

Murray, R.E. and J.E. Gibson. 1972. A comparative study of Paraquat intoxication in rats, guinea pigs and monkeys. Exp. Mol. Pathol. 17:317-325.

Nagasaki, H., S. Tomii, T. Mega, M. Murugami, and N. Ito. 1971. Development of hepatomas in mice treated with benzene hexochloride. Gann 62:431.

Nagasaki, H., S. Tomii, T. Mega, M. Murugami, and N. Ito. 1972a. Carcinogenicity of benzene hexachloride (BHC). *In* W. Nakahara, S. Takayama, T. Sugimura, and S. Odashima, eds. Topics in Chemical Carcinogenesis, pp. 343-553. Univ. Tokyo Press, Tokyo.

Nagasaki, H., S. Tomii, T. Mega, M. Murugami and N. Ito. 1972b. Hepatocarcinogenic effect of α-, β-, γ-, and δ isomers of benzene hexachloride in mice. Gann 63:393.

Nagasaki, H., S. Tomii, T. Tsumashika, M. Marukami, M. Arai, and N. Ito. 1972. On the experimental tumorigenesis of the liver of mice and rats by the induction of BHC isomers, α-, β-, γ-, and δ. Nippon Gangakkai Kiji (Poc. Jap. Cancer Assoc.) 31:33; Health Aspects Pestic. 6:388 (73-1720).

Naishtein, S.Y., V.A. Zhulinskaya, and E.M. Yurovskaya. 1973. The stability of certain organophosphorus pesticides in the soil. Gig. Sanit. 1973(7):42-45.

Nalbandian, R.M., and J.R. Pearce. 1965. Allergic purpura induced by exposure to p-dichlorobenzene. Confirmation by indirect basophil degranulation test. J. Am. Med. Assoc. 194:828-829.

National Academy of Sciences-National Research Council. Committee on Toxicology. 1976. Health Effects of Benzene: A Review. Washington, D.C. 23 pp.

National Academy of Sciences-National Research Council. Environmental Studies Board. 1975. Pest control: An Assessment of Present and Alternative Technologies. Vol I: Contemporary Pest Control Practices and Prospects: The Report of the Executive Committee. Washington, D.C. 506 pp.

National Cancer Institute. 1975. Preliminary report on the carcinogenesis bioassay of chlordane and heptachlor. Draft document. Carcinogenesis Program, Division of Cancer Cause and Prevention, National Institutes of Health, Bethesda, Md.

National Cancer Institute. 1976. Report on carcinogenesis bioassay of technical grade chlordecone. (Kepone) Carcinogenesis Program, Division of Cancer Cause and Prevention, National Institute of Health, Bethesda, Md.

National Institute for Occupational Safety and Health. 1973. Criteria for a recommended standard . . . occupational exposure to trichloroethylene, HSM 73-11025. U.S. Government Printing Office, Washington, D.C.

National Institute for Occupaional Safety and Health. 1974. Criteria for a recommended standard . . . occupational exposure to benzene, HEW Publication no. (NIOSH) 74-137. U.S. Government Printing Office, Washington, D.C.

National Institute for Occupational Safety and Health. 1974. Criteria for a recommended standard . . . occupational exposure to chloroform, HEW Publication no. (NIOSH) 75-114. U.S. Government Printing Office, Washington, D.C.

National Institute for Occupational Safety and Health, 1975. Criteria for a recommended standard . . . occupational exposure to xylene. HEW Publication no. (NIOSH) 75-168. U.S. Government Printing Office, Washington, D.C.

Neill, D.D., H.D. Muller, and J.V. Shutze. 1971. Pesticide effects on the fecundity of the gray partridge. Bull. Environ. Contam. Toxicol. 6:546-551.

Nelson, J.O., P.C. Kearney, J.R. Plimmer, and R.E. Menzer. 1976. Metabolism of Trifluralin, Profluralin, and Fluchloralin by rat liver microsomes. Pestic. Biochem. Physiol., in press.

Neubert, D., P. Zens, A. Rothenwallner, and H.J. Merker. 1973. A survey of the embryotoxic effects of TCDD in mammalian species. Environ. Health Perspect. 5:67-79.

Neumeyer, J., D. Gibbons, and H. Trask. 1969. Pesticides. Chem. Week 104:37-68. Part I, April 12; Part II, April 26, p. 37-68.

Newell, G.W. 1958. Report: Acute and subacute toxicity study of Acrolein. Stanford Research Institute. SRI Project no. S-868-2.

Nickerson, P.R., and K.R. Barbehenn. 1975. Organochlorine residues in starlings, 1972. Pestic. Monit. J. 8:247-254.

Nielsen, K., B. Kaempe, and J. Jensen-Holm. 1965. Fatal poisoning in man by 2,4-dichlorophenoxyacetic acid (2,4-D); Determination of the agent in forensic materials. Acta Pharmacol. Toxicol. 22;224-234.

Norris, L.A., and M.L. Montgomery. 1975. Dicamba residues in streams after forest spraying. Bull. Environ. Contam. Toxicol. 13:1-8.

O'Brien, R.D. 1957. Properties and metabolism in the cockroach and Malathion and Malaoxon. J. Econ. Entomol. 50:159-164.

O'Brien, R.D., G.D. Thorn, and R.W. Fisher. 1958. New organophosphate insecticides developed on rational principles. J. Econ. Entomol. 51:714-71z.

Ockner, R.K., and R. Schmid. 1961. Acquired porphyria in man and rat due to hexachlorobenzene intoxication. Nature 189:499.

Olefir, A.I. 1973. Effect of chronic carbamate pesticide poisoning on immunologic reactivity and infection resistance. Vrach. Delo. 8:137-140; Pestic. Abstr. 7:95, Abstr. no. 74-0429.

Ortega, P., W.J. Hayes, Jr., and W.F. Durham. 1957. Pathologic changes in the liver of rats after feeding low levels of various insecticides. Arch. Pathol. 64:614-622.

Ottoboni, A. 1969. Effect of DDT on reproduction in the rat. Toxicol. Appl. Pharmacol. 14:74-81.

Ottolenghi, A.D., J.K. Haseman, and F. Suggs. 1974. Teratogenic effects of Aldrin, Dieldrin and Endrin in hamsters and mice. Teratology 9:11-16.

Pagnotto, L.D. and J.E. Walkley. 1965. Urinary dichlorophenol as an index of para-dichlorobenzene exposure. Am. Ind. Hyg. Assoc. J. 26:137-142.

Palmer, J.S. 1963. Tolerance of sheep to Captan. J. Am. Vet. Assoc. 143:513-514.

Palmer, J.S. 1972. Toxicity of 45 organic herbicides to cattle, sheep, and chickens. U.S. Department of Agriculture Production Research Report 137, 41 pp.

Paris, D.F., and D.L. Lewis. 1973. Chemical and microbial degradation of ten selected pesticides in aquatic systems. Residue Rev. 45:95-124.

Park, K.S., and W.N. Bruce. 1968. The determination of water solubility of Aldrin, Dieldrin, Heptachlor, and Heptachlor epoxide. J. Econ. Entomol. 61:770-774.

Parsons, L.D. 1942. On early tumour formation in pure-line mice treated with carcinogenic compounds and the associated blood and tissue changes. J. Pathol. Bacterial. 54:321-330.

Payne, L.K., and M.H.J. Weiden. 1965. Mellon Institute Report no. 31-143. EPA Pesticide Petition no. 9F0798.

Perelygin, V.M., M.B. Shpirt, O.A. Aripov, and V.I. Ershova. 1971. Effects of some pesticides on immunological reactivity. Gig. Sanit. 36(12):29-33.

Pesticide Chemical News. 1974. Senate may act next week on indemnity bill for Dieldrin-contaminated chickens. 2:17, April 3.

Petrova-Vergieva, T., and L. Ivanova-Tchemishanska. 1973. Assessment of the teratogenic activity of dithiocarbamate fungicides. Food Cosmet. Toxicol. 11:239-244.

Pike, M.H. 1944. Ocular pathology due to organic compounds. J. Mich. State Med. Soc. 43:581-584.

Piper, W.N., J.Q. Rose, M.L. Leng, and P.J. Gehring. 1973. The fate of 2,4,5-trichlorophenoxyacetic acid (2,4,5-T) following oral administration to rats and dogs. Toxicol. Appl. Pharmacol. 26:339-351.

Plewa, M.J., and J.M. Gentile. 1976. Mutagenicity of atrazine: A maize-microbe bioassay. Mutat. Res. 38:287-292.

Poland, A.P., D. Smith, G. Metter, and P. Possick. 1971. A health survey of workers in a 2,4-D and 2,4,5-T plant. Arch. Environ. Health 22:316-327.

Pope, J.D., Jr., W.S. Cox III, and A.R. Grzenda. 1966. Determination of Silvex and its low volatile esters in water and muds. *In* Advances in Chemistry Series no. 60, pp. 200-206. Americn Chemical Society, Washington, D.C.

Portig, J., P. Kraus, S. Sodomann, and G. Noack. 1973. Biodegradation of alpha-hexachlorocyclohexane. I. Glutathione-dependent conversion to a hydrophilic metabolite by rat liver cytosol. Naunyn-Schmied's Arch. Pharmacol. 279:185-198.

Pozzani, U.C., and E.R. Kinead. Mellon Inst. Report no. 31-143. EPA pesticide petition no. 9F0798. Cited in U.S. Environmental Protection Agency. May 1975. p. 29. Initial Scientific and Minieconomic Review of Aldicarb. EPA 540/1-75-013.

Prasad, I. 1970. Mutagenic effects of the herbicide 3',4'-dichloropropionanilide and its degradation products. Can. J. Microbiol. 16:369-372.

Radeleff, R.D. 1958. The toxicity of insecticides and herbicides to livestock. Adv. Vet. Sci. 4:265-276.

Radomski, J.L., W.B. Deichmann, and E.E. Clizer. 1968. Pesticide concentrations in the liver, brain, and adipose tissue of terminal hospital patients. Food Cosmet. Toxicol. 6:209-220.

Rasul, A.R., and J. McC. Howell. 1974. The toxicity of some dithiocarbamate compounds in young and adult domestic fowl. Toxicol. Appl. Pharmacol. 30:63-78.

Reinbold, K.A., I.P. Kapoor, W.F. Childers, W.N. Bruce, and R.L. Metcalf. 1971. Comparative uptake and biodegradability of DDT and Methoxychlor by aquatic rganisms. Ill. Nat. Hist.Surv. Bull. 30(6):405-417.

Reyna, M., G. Kennedy, and M. Keplinger. 1973. Eighteen-month carcinogenic study with Captan technical in Swiss white mice. Unpublished report, Industrial Bio-Test Labs., Inc., Northbrook, Ill. Cited in U.S. Environmental Protection Agency. Initial Scientific and Minieconomic Review of Captan, p. 78. EPA 540-1/1-75-012.

Richard, J.J., G.A. Junk, M.J. Avery, N.L. Nehring, J.S. Fritz, and H. Svec. 1975. Analysis of various Iowa waters for selected pesticides: Atrazine, DDE, and Dieldrin—1974. Pestic. Monit. J. 9:117-123.

Richert, E.P., and K.V. Prahlad. 1972. The effect of the organophosphate *O,O*-diethyl *S*-[(ethylthio) methyl] phosphorodithioate on the chick. Poult. Sci. 51:613-619.

Rider, J.A., H.C. Moeller, E.J. Puletti, and J.I. Swader. 1969. Toxicity of Parathion, Systox, Octamethyl pyrophosphoramide, and Methyl parathion in man. Toxicol. Appl. Pharmacol. 14:603-611.

Rider, J.A., H.C. Moeller, J. Swader, and R.G. Devereaux. 1959. A study of the anticholinesterase properties of EPN and Malathion in human volunteers. Clin. Res. 7:81-82.

Rider, J.A., J.I. Swader, and E.J. Puletti. 1970. Methyl parathion and Guthion anticholinesterase effects in human subjects. Fed. Proc. 29:349.

Rider, J.A., J.I. Swader, and E.J. Puletti. 1972. Anti-cholinesterase toxicity studies with Guthion, Phosdrin, Di-syston, and Trihion in human subjects. Fed. Proc. 31:520. Abstr. no. 1730.

Ried, W.D., and G. Krishna. 1973. Centrolobular hepatic necrosis related to covalent binding of metabolites of halogenated aromatic hydrocarbons. Exp. Mol. Pathol. 18:80-99.

Riemschneider, R. 1949. Ein beitrag zur toxicologie kontakt—insektizider substanzen. Anz. Schaedlingskd. 22:1-3.

Robens, J. F. 1969. Teratologic studies of Carbaryl, Diazinon, Norea, Disulfiram and Thiram in small laboratory animals. Toxicol. Appl. Pharmacol. 15:152-163.

Roger, J.C., D.G. Upshall, and J.E. Casida. 1969. Structure-activity and metabolism studies on organophosphate teratogens and their alleviating agents in developing hen eggs with special emphasis on Bidrin. Biochem. Pharmacol. 18:373-392.

Rohm and Haas. 1973. Unpublished data, progress report. Dose–response relationships—dithane, M-45, and ethylenethiourea. Quoted from U.S. Environmental Protection

Agency. Toxicology and environmental hazards of the ethylenebisdithiocarbamate fungicides and ethylene thiourea.

Rohm and Haas. 1973. Unpublished data. Mutagenic Study, 1972. Quoted from U.S. Environmental Protection Agency. 1973. Toxicology and environmental hazards of the ethylenebisdithiocarbamate fungicides and ethylene thiourea.

Roll, R. 1971. Teratologische Untersuchnugen mit Thiram (TMTD) an zwei Mausestammen. Arch. Toxikol. 27:173-186.

Rose, J.Q., J.C. Ramsey, T.H. Wentzler, R.A. Hummel, and P.J. Gehring. 1976. The fate of 2,3,7,8-tetrachloro-*p*-dioxin following single and repeated oral doses to the rat. Toxicol. Appl. Pharmacol. 36:209-226.

Rowe, V.K., and T.A. Hymas. 1954. Summary of toxicological information on 2,4-D and 2,4,5-T type herbicides and an evaluation of the hazards to livestock associated with their use. Am. J. Vet. Res. 15:622-629.

Ryan, A.J. 1971. The metabolism of pesticidal carbamates. CRC Crit. Rev. Toxicol. 1:33-54.

Ryazonova, R.A. 1967. The effect of the toxic chemicals Ziram and Zineb on reproductive function in experimental animals. Hyg. Sanit. 23(1-3):187-192.

Sanborn, J.R., B.M. Francis, and R.L. Metcalf. 1976. The degradation of selected pesticides in soil: A review of the published literature. U.S. Environmental Protection Agency, Office of Research and Development Cincinnati, Ohio.

Sanderson, D.M., and E.F. Edson. 1959. Oxime therapy in poisoning by six organophosphorus insecticides in the rat. J. Pharmacol. (London) 11:721-728.

Sandler, B.E., G.A. Van Gelder, W.B. Buck, and G.G. Karas. 1968. Psych. Rep. 23:451-455.

Sauerhoff, M.W., W.H. Braun, G.E. Blau, and J.E. LeBeau. 1976. The fate of 2,4-dichlorophenoxyacetic acid (2,4-D) following oral administration to man. Toxicol. Appl. Pharmacol. 37:136. Abstr. no. 106.

Schafer, E.W. 1972. The acute oral toxicity of 369 pesticidal, pharmaceutical, and other chemicals to wild birds. Toxicol. Appl. Pharmacol. 21:315-330.

Schafer, M.L., J.T. Peeler, W.S. Gardner, and J.E. Campbell. 1969. Pesticides in drinking water. Waters from the Mississippi and Missouri rivers. Environ. Sci. Technol. 3:1261-1269.

Scheiman, M.A., R.A. Saunders, and F.E. Saallfeld. 1974. Organic contaminants in the District of Columbia water supply. J. Biomed. Mass. Spectrom. 1:209-211.

Schmid, R. 1960. Cutaneous porphyria in Turkey. New Engl. J. Med. 263:397-398.

Schuttmann, W. 1968. Chronische Leberer-krankungen nach beruflicher Einwirkung von Dichlorodiphenyltrichlorothan (DDT) und Hexachlorocyclohexan (HCH). Int. Arch. Gewerbepathol. Gewerbehyg. 24:193-210.

Schwemmer, B., W.P. Cochrane, and P.B. Polen. 1970. Oxychlordane, animal metabolite of Chlordane: Isolation and synthesis. Science 169:1087.

Schwetz, B.A., G.L. Sparschu, and P.J. Gehring. 1971. The effect of 2,4-dichlorophenoxyacetic acid (2,4-D) and esters of 2,4-D on rat embryonal, foetal and neonatal growth and development. Food Cosmet. Toxicol. 9:801-817.

Schwetz, B.A., J.M. Norris, G.L. Sparschu, V.K. Rowe, P.J. Gehring, J.L. Emerson, and C.G. Gerbig. 1973. Toxicology of chlorinated dibenzo-*p*-dioxins. Environ. Health Perspect. 5:87-99.

Scott, H.D., and R.E. Phillips. 1972. Diffusion of selected herbicides in soil. Soil Sci. Soc. Am. Proc. 36:714-719.

Seabury, J.H. 1963. Toxicity of 2,4-dichlorophenoxyacetic acid for man and dog. Arch. Environ. Health 7:202-209.

Searle, C.E. 1966. Tumor initiatory activity of some chloromononitrobenzenes and other compounds. Cancer Res. 26:12-17.

Seidler, H., M. Haertig, W. Schnaak, and R. Engst. 1970. Studies on the metabolism of some insecticides and fungicides in the rat. Part II: Distribution and decomposition of C^{14}-labelled Maneb. Nahrung 14(5):363-373.

Seiler, J.P. 1974. Ethylenethiourea (ETU), a carcinogenic and mutagenic metabolite of ethylene-*bis*-dithiocarbamate. Mutat. Res. 26:189-191.

Sexton, W.F. 1966. Report on Aldicarb. EPA Pesticide Petition no. 9F0798, Section C. Cited in U.S. Environmental Protection Agency. 1975. Initial Scientific and Minieconomic Review of Aldicarb. EPA 540/1-75-013.

Shaffer, C.B. 1958. Thimet and formulations, toxicity by skin absorption. Unpublished report of the American Cyanamid Co. Cited in U.S. Environmental Protection Agency. 1974. Initial Scientific and Minieconomic Review of Phorate (Thimet). Office of Pesticides Programs, Washington, D.C.

Shellenberger, T.E., B.J. Gough, and L.A. Escuriex. 1968. Comparative toxicity evaluations of organophosphate pesticides with wildlife. Ind. Med. Surg. 37:537.

Sherman, H. *et al.* 1963. Report 12-66, EPA Pesticide Petition no. 6F-499, 1975. Cited in EPA 540.

Shmuter, L.M. 1972. The effect of the chronic action of low concentrations of chlorinated hydrocarbons on the production of various classes of immunoglobulins. Gig. Sanit. 37(2):36-40 (Trans.).

Shtenberg, A.I., Y.I. Ashmenskas, and I.A. Kusevitskiy. 1972. Immunobiological body reactivity changes under the effect of some pesticides belonging to the group of carbamine and dihiocarbamine compounds. Vop. Pitan. 30(1):55-57.

Siebert, D., and E. Lemperle. 1974. Genetic effects of herbicides: Induction of mitotic gene conversion in Saccharomyces cerevisiae. Mutat. Res. 22:111-120.

Simmon, V.F., D.C. Poole, and G.W. Newell. 1976. *In vitro* mutagenic studies of twenty pesticides. Toxicol. Appl. Pharmacol. 37:109. Abstr. no. 42.

Simson, R.E., G. R. Simpson, and D.J. Penney. 1969. Poisoning with monocrotophos, an organophosphorus pesticide. Med. J. Aust. 2:1013-1016.

Sinkuvene, D.S. 1970. Hygienic evaluation of Acrolein as an air pollutant. Hyg. Sanit. 35(1-3):325-329.

Sivitskaia, I.I. 1974. State of the organ of vision in persons working in contact with TMTD. Oftalmol. Zh. 28:286.

Siyali, D.S. 1972. Hexachlorobenzene and other organochlorine pesticides in human blood. Med. J. Aust. 2:1063-1066.

Slade, R.E. 1945. Specific poisons. Endeavor 4:148-153.

Smith, J.C., and F.S. Arant. 1967. Residues of Kepone in milk from cows receiving treated feed. J. Econ. Entomol. 60:925-927.

Smith, R.B., Jr., J.K. Finnegan, P.S. Larson, P.F. Sahyoun, M.L. Dreyfuss, and H.B. Hagg. 1953. Toxicologic studies on zinc and disodium ethylene bisdithiocarbamates. J. Pharmacol. Exp. Ther. 109:159-166.

Smyth, R.J. 1972. Detection of Hexachlorobenzene residues in dairy products, meat fat, and eggs. J. Assoc. Offic. Anal. Chem. 55:806-808.

Sobotka, T. 1971. Comparative effects of 60-day feeding of Maneb and of ethylenethiourea on thyroid electrophoretic patterns of rats. Food Cosmet. Toxicol. 9:537-540.

Sobotka, T.J., R.E. Brodie, and M.P. Cook. 1972. Behavioral and neuroendocrine effects in rats of postnatal exposure to low dietary levels of Maneb. Dev. Phychobiol. 5:137-148.

Sparschu, G.L., F.L. Dunn, and V.K. Rowe. 1971. Studies of the teratogenicity of 2,3,7,8-tetrachlorodibenzo-*p*-dioxin in the rat. Food Cosmet. Toxicol. 9:405-412.

Spencer, E. Y. 1973. Guide to the Chemicals Used in Crop Protection. Publication no. 1093. Research Branch, Agriculture Canada, Ottawa, Canada. 542 pp.

Spiller, D. 1961. A digest of available information on the insecticide Malathion. Adv. Pest Control Res. 4:249-335.

St. John, L.E., Jr., and D.J. Lisk. 1969. Metabolism of Banvel-D herbicide in a dairy cow. J. Dairy Sci. 52:392-393.

Stacey, C.I., and B.W. Thomas. 1975. Organochlorine pesticide residues in human milk, Western Australia—1970-71. Pestic. Monit. J. 9:64-66.

Stehl, R.H., and L.L. Lamparski. 1974. Analysis of combustion product of 2,4,5-T for 2,3,7,8-tetrachlorodibenzo-*p*-dioxin. Dow Chemical Company, Midland, Mich. To be published.

Stevens, J.T., R.E. Stitzel, and J.J. McPhillips. 1972. The effects of subacute administration anticholinesterase insecticides on hepatic microsomal metabolism. Life Sci. 11:423-431.

Strateva, A., A. Velizarov, and A. Georgiev. 1974. Morphological and enzymohistological studies on some internal organs of experimental animals during the influence of RAMROD under acute experimental conditions. Khig. Zdraveopaz. 17:283-287. (CA 82: 93927p).

Strik, J.J.T.W.A. 1973. Chemical porphyria in Japanese quail (*Coturnix c. japonica*). Hoppe-Seyler's Z. Physiol. Chem. 850.

Sutherland, G.L., P.A. Giang, and T.E. Archer. 1964. Thimet. *In* G. Zweig, ed. Analytical Methods for Pesticides, Plant Growth Regulators and Food Additives, vol. 2. Academic Press, New York.

Szuperski, T., and A. Grabarska. 1972. Changes in internal organs of rabbits after experimental oral administration of Captan fungicide. Zesz. Nauk. Szk. Roln. Olsztynie., 28:279-284, Cited in U.S. Environmental Protection Agency. 1975. Initial Scientific and Minieconomic Review of Captan, p. 87. EPA-540/1-75-012.

Tanimura, T., T. Katsuya, and H. Nishimura. 1967. Embryotoxicity of acute exposure to Methyl parathion in rats and mice. Arch. Environ. Health 15:609-613.

Tarjan, R., and T. Kemeny. 1969. Multigeneration studies on DDT in mice. Food Cosmet. Toxicol. 7:215-222.

Tegeris, A.S., F.L. Earl, H.E. Smalley, Jr., and J.M. Curtis. 1966. Methoxychlor toxicity. Arch. Environ. Health 13:776-787.

Thomson, W.T. 1974. Agricultural Chemicals. Book III. Fumigants, Growth Regulators, Repellants, and Rodenticides. Thomson Publications, Indianapolis, Ind. 164 pp.

Thomson, W.T. 1975. Agricultural Chemicals. Book II. Herbicides. Thomson Publishers, Fresno, Calif. 256 pp.

Thomson, W.T. 1976. Agricultural Chemicals. Book IV. Fungicides. Thomson Publications, Fresno, Calif. 164 pp.

Thorpe, E., and A.I.T. Walker. 1973. The toxicology of Dieldrin (HEOD). II. Comparative long-term oral toxicity studies in mice with dieldrin, DDT, Phenobarbitone, β-BHC and γ-BHC. Food Cosmet. Toxicol. 11:433-442.

Tomatis, L., V. Turusov, N. Day, and R.T. Charles. 1972. Effect of long-term exposure to DDT on CF-1 mice. Int. J. Cancer 10:489-506.

Totaro, S. 1961. Le transaminasi e l'aldolasi sieriche nella intossicazione sperimentale subacuta da paradichlorobenzene. Folia Med. (Napoli) 44:586-594.

Toxic Substances List. 1974. Christensen, H.E., T.T. Luginbyhl, and B.S. Carroll, eds. National Institute for Occupational Safety and Health. HEW Publication no. (NIOSH)74-134. Government Printing Office, Washington, D.C. 904 pp.

Trichell, D.W., H.L. Morton, and M.G. Merkle. 1968. Loss of herbicides in runoff water. Weed Sci. 16:447-449.

Truhaut, R. 1954. Communication au symposium international de la prevention du cancer, Sao Paulo. Cited by FAO/WHO Expert Committee on Pesticide Residues. Evaluation of some pesticide residues in food; p. 130. WHO/Food Add. 67:32, FAO, PL:CP/15. Geneva, 1967.

Tullner, W.W., and J.H. Edgcomb. 1962. Cystic tubular nephropathy and decrease in testicular weight in rats following oral Methoxychlor treatment. J. Pharmacol. Exp. Ther. 138:126-30.

Turner, J.C., and R.S. Green. 1974. Effect of Hexachlorobenzene on microsomal enzyme systems. Biochem. Pharmacol. 23:2387-2390.

Tusing, T.W. 1955. Toxicological studies of experimental insecticide 3911. Unpublished report of the American Cyanamid Co. Cited in U.S. Environmental Protection Agency. 1974. Initial Scientific and Minieconomic Review of Phorate (Thimet). Office of Pesticides Programs, Washington, D.C.

Tusing, T.W. 1956. 13-Week subacute Thimet feeding study in male and female rats. Unpublished report of the American Cyanamid Co. Cited in U.S. Environmental Protection Agency. 1974. Initial scientific and Minieconomic Review of Phorate (Thimet). Office of Pesticide Programs, Washington, D.C.

Tye, R., and D. Engel. 1967. Distribution and excretion of Dicamba by rats as determined by radiotracer technique. J. Agric. Food Chem. 15:837-840.

Tsoneva-Maneva, M. T., F. Kaloyanova, and V. Georgieva. 1969. Mutagenic effect of Diazinon on human peripheral blood lymphocytes in vitro. Eksp. Med. Morfol. 8(3):132-136. (CA 72:89210a, 1970)

Tzoneva-Maneva, M.T., E. Kaloyanova, and V. Georgieva. 1971. Influence of Diazinon and Lindane on the mitotic activity and the caryotype of human lymphocytes cultivated *in vitro*. Bibl. Haematol. 38:344-347. (CA 77:15302).

U.S. Department of Transportation. Coast Guard. 1976. Pollution by oil and hazardous substances. Fed. Reg., vol. 41, no. 59, pp. 12628-12634, March 25, 1976.

U.S. Department of Health, Education, and Welfare. Survey of compounds which have been tested for carcinogenic activity; 1970-1971 volume. DHEW Publication no. (NIH) 73-453. Public Health Service Publication no. 149. U.S. Government Printing Office, Washington, D.C.

U.S. Environmental Protection Agency. Final Report in preparation. Initial Scientific and Minieconomic Review of Methomyl. Office of Pesticide Programs.

U.S. Environmental Protection Agency. 1961. Kepone. EPA Document no. 108253.

U.S. Environmental Protection Agency. 1972a. An evaluation of DDT and Dieldrin in Lake Michigan. Ecological Research Series EPA-R3-72-003 Aug.

U.S. Environmental Protection Agency. 1972b. Region VI. Surveillance and Analysis Division. Industrial Pollution of the Lower Mississippi River in Louisiana.

U.S. Environmental Protection Agency. 1973a. Aspects of pesticidal use of Endrin on man and the environment. Office of Toxic Substances, Washington, D.C.

U.S. Environmental Protection Agency. 1973b. Unpublished Report. BHC-Lindane. Criteria and Evaluation Division, Office of Pesticide Programs, Washington, D.C. 280 pp.

U.S. Environmental Protection Agency. 1973c. Environmental contamination from Hexachlorobenzene. Office of Pesticide Programs, Washington, D.C. 27 pp.

U.S. Environmental Protection Agency. 1973d. The toxicology and environmental hazards of ethylenebisdithiocarbamate fungicides and ethylenethiourea, Report of the Special Pesticide Review Group. (Privileged Document.)

U.S. Environmental Protection Agency. 1974a. Draft Analytical Report New Orleans Area Water Supply Study. Prepared and submitted by Lower Mississippi River Facility, Slidell, La. Surveillance and Analysis Division, Region VI, Dallas, Tex. EPA-906/10-74-002.

U.S. Environmental Protection Agency. 1974b. The herbicide 2,4-D. Office of Pesticides Programs, Washington, D.C. 207 pp.

U.S. Environmental Protection Agency. 1974c. Report: Aspects of pesticidal use of toxaphene and strobane on man and the environment. In press.

U.S. Environmental Protection Agency. 1974d. Respondent's First Proposed Findings of Fact on Environmental Effects of Aldrin and Dieldrin. Office of Pesticide Programs, Washington, D.C. 134 pp.

U.S. Environmental Protection Agency. 1974e. Initial Scientific and Minieconomic Review of Phorate (Thimet). Office of Pesticides Programs, Washington, D.C.

U.S. Environmental Protection Agency. 1975a. Initial Scientific and Minieconomic Review of Bromacil. EPA-540/1-75-006. Office of Pesticide Programs, Washington, D.C.

U.S. Environmental Protection Agency. 1975b. Initial Scientific and Minieconomic Review of Captan. Office of Pesticide Programs. EPA-540/1-75-012. Washington, D.C.

U.S. Environmental Protection Agency. 1975c. Initial Scientific and Minieconomic Review of Diacamba. Office of Pesticide Programs, Washington, D.C.

U.S. Environmental Protection Agency. 1975d. Draft Report. Initial Scientific and Minieconomic Review of Folpet. Office of Pesticide Programs, Washington, D.C.

U.S. Environmental Protection Agency. 1975e. Initial Scientific and Minieconomic Review of Malathion. EPA-540/1-75-005. Office of Pesticide Programs, Washington, D.C.

U.S. Environmental Protection Agency. 1975f. Initial Scientific and Minieconomic Review. No. 21, MCPA. Office of Pesticide Programs, Washington, D.C.

U.S. Environmental Protection Agency. 1975g. Initial Scientific and Minieconomic Review of Methyl Parathion. EPA-540/1-75-004. Office of Pesticide Programs, Washington, D.C.

U.S. Environmental Protection Agency. 1975h. Initial Scientific and Minieconomic Review of Parathion. EPA-540/1-75-001. Office of Pesticide Programs, Washington, D.C.

U.S. Environmental Protection Agency. 1975i. National interim primary drinking water regulations. Fed. Reg. vol. 40, no. 248, pp. 59566-59588, Dec. 24, 1975.

U.S. Environmental Protection Agency. 1975j. Preliminary assessment of suspected carcinogens in drinking water. Report to Congress. Office of Toxic Substances, Washington, D.C. EPA-560/4-75-005. PB-25096/.

U.S. Environmental Protection Agency. 1975k. 2-(2,4,5-Trichlorophenoxy) propionic acid. Silvex. Suspect chemical review. Office of Pesticide Programs, Washington, D.C.

U.S. Environmental Protection Agency. 1975l. Draft Report. Aspects of pesticidal uses of Carbaryl (Sevin) on man and the environment. Office of Pesticide Programs, Washington, D.C.

U.S. Environmental Protection Agency. 1975m. Initial Scientific and Minieconomic Review of Aldicarb. EPA-540/1-775-013. Office of Pesticide Programs, Washington, D.C.

U.S. Environmental Protection Agency. 1975n. New Orleans Area Water Supply Study. Analysis of Carbon and Resin Extracts. Prepared and submitted to the Lower Mississippi River Branch, Surveillance and Analysis Division, Region VI, by the Analytical Branch, Southeast Environmental Research Laboratory, Athens, Ga.

U.S. Environmental Protection Agency. 1975o. Initial Scientific and Minieconomic Review no. 19. Propanil. Office of Pesticide Programs, Washington, D.C.

U.S. Environmental Protection Agency. 1976a. Initial Scientific Review of PCNB. EPA-540/1-75-016. Office of Pesticide Programs, Washington, D.C. 65 pp.

U.S. Environmental Protection Agency. 1976b. Kepone. A summary prepared by the Criteria and Evaluation Division, Office of Pesticide Programs, Washington, D.C.

U.S. Environmental Protection Agency. 1976c. Draft Report. Initial Scientific and Minieconomic Review, Simazine. Office of Pesticide Programs. EPA Contract 68-01-1904

U.S. Environmental Protection Agency. 1976d. Organic Compounds Identified in Drinking Water in the U.S. Health Effects Research Laboratory, Cincinnati, Ohio.

U.S. Environmental Protection Agency. 1976e. Initial Scientific and Minieconomic Review. No. 24. Methoxychlor. Office of Pesticide Programs, Washington, D.C. J. Agric. Food Chem. 11:70-72.

U.S. International Trade Commission. 1975. Syntheic Organic Chemicals U.S. Production and Sales, 1973. ITC Publication 728. U.S. Government Printing Office, Washington, D.C.

U.S. Public Health Service. 1976. Kepone poisoning—Virginia. An internal report. Atlanta, Ga. Communicable Disease Center. (Unpublished, for administrative use only.)

Union Carbide Corporation. Aldicarb report. EPA Pesticide Petition no. 1F1008, Section C. Cited in U.S. Environmental Protection Agency. 1975m. Initial Scientific and Minieconomic Review of Aldicarb. EPA 540/1-75-013. p.36.

Union Carbide Corporation. 1956. Subacute oral toxicity studies on compound 7744. Internal report no. 19-106. Cited in Aspects of pesticidal uses of Carbaryl (Sevin) on man and the environment. U.S. Environmental Protection Agency. 1975. Office of Pesticide Programs. Draft report.

Union Carbide Corporation. 1957. The toxicity of the insecticide Sevin (compound 7744: *N*-methyl 1-naphthyl carbamate). Internal report no. 20-89. Cited in Aspects of pesticidal uses of Carbaryl (Sevin) on man and the environment. U.S. Environmental Protection Agency. 1975. Office of Pesticide Programs. Draft report.

Union Carbide Corporation. 1958a. Miscellaneous toxic effects and mechanism of action of insecticide Sevin. Internal Report no. 21-90. Cited in Aspects of pesticidal uses of Carbaryl (Sevin) on man and the environment. U.S. Environmental Protection Agency. 1975. Office of Pesticide Programs. Draft report.

Union Carbide Corporation. 1958b. Chronic oral feeding of Sevin to rats. Internal Report no. 21-88. Cited in Aspects of pesticidal uses of Carbaryl (Sevin) on man and the environment. U.S. Environmental Protection Agency. 1975. Office of Pesticide Programs. Draft report.

Union Carbide Corporation. 1958c. Chronic toxicity of Sevin for dogs. Internal report no. 21-89. Cited in Aspects of pesticidal uses of Carbaryl (Sevin) on man and the Environment. U.S. Environmental Protection Agency. 1975. Office of Pesticide Programs. Draft report.

Union Carbide Corporation. 1963. Results of eighty weeks of inclusion of Sevin in the diet of mice. Internal report no. 26-53. Cited in Aspects of pesticidal uses of Carbaryl (Sevin) on man and the environment. U.S. Environmental Protection Agency. 1975. Office of Pesticide Programs. Draft report.

Union Carbide Corporation. 1965. Results of a three generation reproduction study on rats fed Sevin in their diets. Internal report no. 28-53. Cited in Aspects of pesticidal uses of Carbaryl (Sevin) on man and the environment. U.S. Environmental Protection Agency. 1975. Office of Pesticide Programs. Draft report.

Union Carbide Corporation. 1966. Evaluation of the teratogenic potential of the insecticide Sevin in rats. Internal report no. 29-49. Cited in Aspects of pesticidal uses of Carbaryl (Sevin) on man and the environment. U.S. Environmental Protection Agency. 1975. Office of Pesticide Programs. Draft report.

Union Carbide Corporation. 1968. EPA Pesticide Petition no. 9F0814. Cited in Initial Scientific and Minieconomic Review of Methomyl. Union Carbide Corporation. 1968. Sevin: results of feeding in the diet of rats for one week, and for one week plus one day on control diets. Internal Report no. 31-160. Cited in U.S. Environmental Protection

Agency. 1975l. Aspects of pesticidal uses of Carbaryl (Sevin) on man and the environment. Office of Pesticide Programs. Draft Report.

Union Carbide Corporation. 1971. Study of guinea pig teratology of Sevin fed in the diet versus stomach intubation. Internal report no. 34-81. Cited in U.S. Environmental Protection Agency. 1975l. Aspects of pesticidal uses of Carbaryl (Sevin) on man and the environment. Office of Pesticide Programs. Draft report.

Union Carbide Corporation. 1972. Sevin: Comparative study of dietary inclusion versus stomach intubation on three generations of reproduction, on teratology, and on mutagenesis. Internal report no. 35-65. Cited in U.S. Environmental Protection Agency. 1975. Aspects of pesticidal uses of Carbaryl (Sevin) on man and the environment. Office of Pesticide Programs. Draft report.

University of California, Davis. 1975. Pesticide Data Bank, Food Protection and Toxicology Center. Department of Environmental Toxicology. Pesticides use report.

Upshall, D.G., J.C. Roger, and J.E. Casida. 1968. Biochemical studies on the teratogenic action of Bidrin and other neuroactive agents in developing hen eggs. Biochem. Pharmacol. 17:1529-1542.

Usher, C.D., and G.M. Telling. 1975. Analysis of nitrate and nitrite in foodstuffs: A critical review. J. Sci. Food Agric. 26:1793-1805.

van Dijk, A., R.A.A. Maes, R.H. Drost, J.M.C. Douze, and A.N.P. van Heyst. 1975. Paraquat poisoning in man. Arch. Toxicol. 34:129-136.

Van Gelder, G.A., B.E. Sandler, B. Buck, J.B. Maland, and G.G. Karas. 1969. Behavioral and electrophysiological effects of Dieldrin in sheep. Ind. Med. Surg. 38:111-114.

Vandekar, M. 1965. Observations on the toxicity of Carbaryl, Folithion, and 3-isopropylphenyl *N*-methylcarbamate in a village-scale trial in southern Nigeria. Bull. WHO 33:107-115.

Varshavskaya, S.P. 1968. Comparative toxicologic characteristics of chlorobenzene and dichlorobenzene (ortho- and para-isomers) in relation to the sanitary protection of water bodies. Hyg. Sanit. 33:17-23.

Verhulst, H. 1974. Personal communication to Eli Lilly and Co. Cited in Initial Scientific and Minieconomic Review of Trifluralin. U.S. Environmental Protection Agency. In preparation.

Verschuuren, H. G., R. Kroes, and E. M. den Tonkelaar. 1975. Short-term oral and dermal toxicity of MCPA and MCPP. Toxicology 3:349-359.

Vettorazzi, G. 1975. Toxicological decisions and recommendations resulting from the safety assessment of pesticide residues in food. CRC Crit. Rev. Toxicol. 4:125-183.

Vettorazzi, G. 1975b. State of the art of the toxicological evaluation carried out by the Joint FAO/WHO Expert Committee on Pesticide Residues. I. Organohalogenated pesticides used in public health and agriculture. Residue Rev. 56:107-134.

Villanueva, E.C., R.W. Jennings, V.W. Burse, and R.D. Kimbrough. 1974. Evidence of chlorodibenzo-*p*-dioxin and chlorodibenzofuran in hexachlorobenzene. J. Agric. Food Chem. 22:916-917.

Villeneuve, D.C., and K.S. Khera. 1975. Placental transfer of halogenated benzenes (pentachloro-, pentachloronitro-, and hexabromo-) in rats. Toxicol. Appl. Pharmacol. 33:146-147.

Villeneuve, D.C., and S.L. Hierlihy. 1975. Placental transfer of Hexachlorobenzene in the rat. Bull. Environ. Contam. Toxicol. 13:489-491.

Villeneuve, D.C. and W.H. Newsome. 1975. Toxicity and tissue levels in the rat and guinea pig following acute Hexachlorobenzene administration. Bull. Environ. Contam. Toxicol. 14:297-300.

Villeneuve, D.C. 1975. The effect of food restriction on the redistribution of Hexachlorobenzene in the rat. Toxicol. Appl. Pharmacol. 31:313-319.

Villeneuve, D.C., L.G. Panopio, and D.L. Grant. 1974. Placental transfer of Hexachlorobenzene in the rabbit. Environ. Physiol. Biochem. 4:112-115.

Vogel, E. and J.L.R. Chandler. 1974. Mutagenicity testing of cyclamate and some pesticides in *Drosophila melanogaster*. Experientia 30:621-623.

Von Oettingen, W.F., and N.E. Sharpless. 1946. The toxicity and toxic manifestations of 2,2-*bis*-(*p*-chlorophenyl)-1,1,1-trichloroethane (DDT) as influenced by chemical changes in the molecule. A contribution to the relation betwen chemical constitution and toxicoloical action. J. Pharmacol. Exp. Ther. 88:400-413.

Von Rumker, R., E.W. Lawless, and A.F. Meiners. 1975. Production, distribution, use and environmental impact potential of selected pesticides. EPA-540/1-74-001. Environmental Protection Agency, Washington, D.C. 439 pp.

Vonk, J.W., and A. Kaars Sijpesteijn. 1970. Fate in plants of ethylenebisdithiocarbamate fungicides and their decomposition products. Ann. Appl. Biol. 65:489-496.

Vonk, J.W., and A. Kaars Sijpesteijn. 1976. Formation of ethylenethiourea from 5,6-dihydro-3*H*-imidazo[2,1-c]1,2,4-dithiaazole-3-thione by microorganisms and reducing agents. J. Environ. Sci. Health Pestic. Food Contam. Agric. Wastes B11(1):33-47.

Vos, J.G., H.A. Breeman, and H. Benschop. 1968. The occurrence of the fungicide hexachlorobenzene in wild birds and its toxicological importance: A preliminary communication. Meded. Rijksfac. Landbouwwet. Gent 33:1263-1269.

Vos, J.G., J.A. Moore, and J.G. Zinkl. 1974. Toxicity of 2,3,7,8-tetrachlorodibenzo-*p*-dioxin (TCDD) in C57B1/6 mice. Toxicol. Appl. Pharmacol. 29:229-241.

Vos, J.G., P.F. Botterweg, J.J.T.W.A. Strik, and J.H. Koeman. 1972. Experimental studies with HCB in birds. TNO-Nieuws 27:599-603.

Wada, O., Y. Yano, G. Urata, and K. Nakao. 1968. Behavior of hepatic microsomal cytochromes after treatment of mice with drugs known to disturb porphyrin metabolism in liver. Biochem. Pharmacol. 17:595-603.

Walker, A.I.T., D.E. Stevenson, J. Robinson, E. Thorpe, and M. Roberts. 1969. The toxicology and pharmacodynamics of Dieldrin (HEOD): Two-year oral exposures of rats and dogs. Toxicol. Appl. Pharmacol. 15:345-373.

Walker, A.I.T., E. Thorpe, and D.E. Stevenson. 1973. The toxicology of Dieldrin (HEOD). I. Long-term oral toxiciy studies in mice. Food Cosmet. Toxicol. 11:415-432.

Walker, E.M., Jr., R.H. Gadsden, L.M. Atkins, and G.R. Gale. 1972. Some effects of 2,4-D and 2,4,5-T on Ehrlich ascites tumor cells *in vivo* and *in vitro*. Ind. Ed. Surg. 41:22-27.

Walton, M.S., V.B. Bastone, and R.L. Baron. 1971. Subchronic toxicity of Photodieldrin, a photodecomposition product of Dieldrin. Toxicol. Appl. Pharmacol. 20:82-88.

Ware, G.W., and E.E. Good. 1967. Effects of insecticides on reproduction in the laboratory mouse II. Mirex, Telodrin and DDT. Toxicol. Appl. Pharmacol. 10:54-61.

Wassermann, M., G. Sandulescu, S. Iliescu, and G. Mandric. 1960. Investigation of the medium conditions and the working pathology of fly insecticides. Chronic poisoning by hexachlorocyclohexane I. Sanitary hygienic conditions in working with fly insecticides. Arch. Mal. Prof. Med. Trav. Secur. Soc. 21:195-200.

Watanabe, T., and D.M. Aviado. 1974. Functional and biochemical effects on the lung following inhalation of cagarette smoke and constituents. II. Skatole, Acrolein, and acetaldehyde. Toxicol. Appl. Pharmacol. 30:201-209.

Weed Science Society of America. 1974. Herbicide Handbook. Weed Science Society of America, Champaign, Ill. 430 pp.

Weeks, D.E. 1967. Endrin food-poisoning: A report on four outbreaks caused by two separate shipments of endrin-contaminated flour. Bull. WHO 37:499-512.

Weiden, M.H.J., H.H. Moorefield, and L.K. Payne. 1965. *O*-(Methylcarbamoyl)oximes: A new class of carbamate insecticides-acaracides. J. Econ. Entomol. 58:154-155.

Weidner, C.W. 1974. Degradation in groundwater and mobility of herbicides. Nat. Tech. Inf. Serv. PB-239 242. 69 p. (M.S. Thesis, University of Nebraska, Lincoln).

Weil, C. Mellon Institute Report no. 35-72, Section C, EPA Pesticide Petition no. 3F1414. Cited in U.S. Environmental Protection Agency. 1975m. Initial Scientific and Minieconomic Review of Aldicarb. EPA-540/1-75-013. Office of Pesticide Programs, Washington, D.C.

Weil, C., and C. Carpenter. 1964. Mellon Institute Report no. 27-158, EPA Pesticide Petition no. OF1008. Cited in U.S. Environmental Protection Agency. 1975m. Initial Scientific and Minieconomic Review of Aldicarb. EPA 540/1-75-013.

Weil, C. and C. Carpenter. 1965. Mellon Institute Report 28-123, EPA Pesticide Petition no. 9FO798. Cited in U.S. Environmental Protection Agency. 1975m. Initial Scientific and Minieconomic Review of Aldicarb. EPA 540/1-75-013.

Weil, C., and C. Carpenter. 1966. Mellon Institute Report no. 29-5. EPA Pesticide Petition no. 9F0798. Cited in U.S. Environmental Protection Agency. 1975m. Initial Scientific and Minieconomic Review of Aldicarb. EPA 540/1-75-013.

Weil, C., and C. Carpenter. 1969. Mellon Institute Report 26-47, Section C, EPA Pesticide Petition no. 9FO798. Cited in U.S. Environmental Protection Agency. 1975m. Initial Scientific and Minieconomic Review of Aldicarb. EPA 540/1-75-013.

Weil, C., and C. Carpenter. 1974. Three generation reproductive and dominant lethal study in rats. Mellon Institute Rerport no. 37-90. Cited in U.S. Environmental Protection Agency. 1975m. Initial Scientific and Minieconomic Review of Aldicarb. EPA 540/1-75-013.

Weil, C.S, and C.P. Carpenter. 1965. Draft report. Results of a three-generation reproduction study on rats fed Sevin in their diets. Mellon Institute Report no. 38-53. 18 pp. Cited in U.S. Environmental Protection Agency. 1975l. Aspects of pesticidal uses of Carbaryl (Sevin) on man and the environment. Office of Pesticide Programs.

Weil, C.S., and C.P. Carpenter. 1962. Draft report. Studies on carcinogenesis completed in 1962. Mellon Institute Report no. 25-122. 6 pp. Cited in U.S. Environmental Protection Agency. 1975l. Aspects of pesticidal uses of Carbaryl (Sevin) on man and the environment. Office of Pesticide Programs.

Weil, C.S., M.D. Woodside, C.P. Carpenter, and H.F. Smythe, Jr. 1972. Current status of tests for Carbaryl for reproductive and teratogenic effect. Toxicol. Appl. Pharmacol. 21:390-404.

Weil, C.S., M.D. Woodside, J.B. Bernard, N.L. Condra, J.M. King, and C.P. Carpenter. 1973. Comparative effect of Carbaryl on rat reproduction and guinea pig teratology when fed either in the diet or by stomach intubation. Toxicol. Appl. Pharmacol. 26:621-638.

Weir, R. 1956. Report of Hazelton Laboratories on Captan. EPA Pesticide Petition no. 15. Cited in U.S. Environmental Protection Agency. 1975. Initial Scientific and Minieconomic Review of Captan. EPA-540/1-75-012. p. 46.

Weir, R. 1957. Subacute feeding of phthalimide analog of Captan. Hazelton Laboratory EPA Folder File no. TF 464. Cited in EPA C-77353.

Weiss, C.M., and J.H. Gakstatter. 1965. The decay of anti-cholinesterase activity of organic phosphorus insecticides on storage in water of different pH. Proc. 2nd-Int. Water Pollut. Res. Conf., Tokyo (1964). Adv. Water Pollut. Res. 1:83-95. Pergamon Press.

Weller, R.W., and A.J. Crellin. 1953. Pulmonary granulomatosis following extensive use of paradichlorobenzene. Arch. Int. Med. 91:408-413.

West, I. 1967. Lindane and hematologic reactions. Arch. Environ. Health. 15:97-101.

Wiersma, G.B., H. Tai, and P.F. Sand. 1972. Pesticide residue levels in soils, FY 1969—National Soils Monitoring Program. Pestic. Monit. J. 6:194-228.

Wilber, C.G., and R.A. Morrison. 1955. The physiological action of Parathion in goats. Am. J. Vet. Res. 16:308-313.

Williams, C.H., and K.H. Jacobson. 1966. An acylamidase in mammalian liver hydrolyzing the herbicide 3,4-dichloropropionanilide. Toxicol. Appl. Pharmacol. 9:495-500.

Williams, M.W., H.N. Fuyat, and O.G. Fitzhugh. 1959. The subacute toxicity of four organic phosphates to dogs. Toxicol. Appl. Pharmacol. 1:1-7.

Williams, P.P., and V.J. Feil. 1971. Identification of Trifluralin metabolites from rumen microbial cultures: Effect of Trifluralin on bacteria and protozoa. J. Agric. Food Chem. 19:1198-1204.

Wills, J.H., E. Jameson, and F. Coulston. 1968. Effects of oral doses of Carbaryl on man. Clin. Toxicol. 1:265-271.

Woodard, G., and E.L. Hagen. 1947. Toxicological studies on the isomers and mixtures of isomers of benzene hexachloride. Fed. Proc. 6:386.

Woodliff, H.J., P.M. Connor, and J. Scopa. 1966. Aplastic anemia associated with insecticides. Med. J. Aust. 1:628-629.

Woodwell, G.M., C.F. Wurster, Jr., and P.A. Isaacson. 1967. DDT residues in an east coast estuary: A case of biological concentration of a persistent insecticide. Science 156:821-824.

Woolson, E.A., R.F. Thomas, and P.D.J. Ensor. 1972. Survey of polychlorodibenzo-*p*-dioxin content in selected pesticides. J. Agric. Food Chem. 20:351-354.

Worden, A.N., G. H. Wheldon, P.R.B. Noel, and L.E. Mawdesley-Thomas. 1973. Toxicity of Gusathion for the rat and the dog. Toxicol. Appl. Pharmacol. 24:405-412.

World Health Organization. 1973. Safe Use of Pesticides. Tech. Rep. Ser. no. 513. Geneva.

Worth, H.M. 1970. The toxicological evaluation of Benefin and Trifluralin. Pesticides Symposia 6th Conference, August, 1968, Halos and Assoc., Miami, pp. 263-267.

Wysocka-Paruszewska, B. 1970. The urine level of 4-hydroxy-3-methoxymandelic acid in the urine of rats poisoned with phosphorus organic insecticides. Diss. Pharmacol. Pharmacol. 22:485-489.

Yang, R.S.H., and K.A. Pittman. 1975. Fate of [^{14}C]hexachlorobenzene in the rhesus monkey and the rat. Toxicol. Appl. Pharmacol. 33:147. Abstr. no. 63.

Yasuda, M., and H. Maeda. 1972. Teratogenic effects of 4-chloro-2-methylphenoxyacetic acid ethylester (MCPEE) in rats. Toxicol. Appl. Pharmacol. 23: 326-333.

Yih, R.Y., and D.H. McRae. 1970. Studies on metabolism of 3',4'-dichloropropionoanilide in rats. Unpublished proprietary information reviewed by Midwest Research Institute. Initial scientific and minieconomic review, no. 19. 1975.

Yu, C.-C., G.M. Booth, D.J. Hansen, and J.R. Larsen. 1975. Fate of Alachlor and Propachlor in a model ecosystem. J. Agric. Food Chem. 23:877-879.

Yu, C-C., D.J. Hansen, and G.M. Booth. 1975. Fate of Dicamba in a model ecosystem. Bull. Environ. Contam. Toxicol. 13:280-283.

Zapp, J.A. 1965. Report on Bromacil. EPA Pesticide Petition no. 6F0499, 1975. Cited in EPA 540.

Zitko, V. 1971. Polychlorinated biphenyls and organochlorine pesticides in some freshwater and marine fishes. Bull. Environ. Contam. Toxicol. 6:464-470.

Zupko, A.G., and L.D. Edwards. 1949. A toxicological study of *p*-dichlorobenzene. J. Am. Pharm. Assoc. 38:124-131.

Zweig, G., E.L. Pye, R, Sitlani, and S.A. Peoples. 1963. Residues in milk from dairy cows fed low levels of Toxaphene in their daily ration. J. Agric. Food Chem. 11:70-72.

REFERENCES—OTHER ORGANIC CONSTITUENTS

Adams, E.M., H.C. Spencer, V.K. Rowe, D.D. McCollister, and D.D. Irish. 1951. Vapor toxicity of trichloroethylene determined by experiments on laboratory animals. Arch. Ind. Hyg. Occup. Med. 4:469-481.

Aksoy, M., K. Dincol, S. Erdem, and G. Dincol. 1972. Acute leukemia due to chronic exposure to benzene. Am. J. Med. 52:160-166.

Aksoy, M., S. Erdem and G. Dincol. 1974a. Leukemia in shoe-workers exposed chronically to benzene. Blood 44:837-841.

Aksoy, M., S. Erdem, K. Dincol, T. Hepyuksel, and G. Dincol. 1974b. Chronic exposure to benzene as a possible contributory etiologic factor in Hodgkin's disease. Blut 28:293-298.

Aksoy, M., S. Erdem, G. Erdogan, and G. Dincol. 1974c. Acute leukemia in two generations following chronic exposure to benzene. Hum. Hered. 24:70-74.

Albro, P.W., and L. Fishbein. 1972. Intestinal absorption of polychlorinated biphenyls in rats. Bull. Environ. Contam. Toxicol. 8:26-31.

Aldridge, W.N., and C.L. Evans. 1946. The physiological effects and fate of cyanogen chloride. Q. J. Exp. Physiol. 33:241-266.

Aldridge, W.N. 1951. The conversion of cyanogen chloride to cyanide in the presence of blood proteins and sulphydryl compounds. Biochem. J. 48:271-276.

Allen, J.R. 1975. Response of the nonhuman primate to polychlorinated biphenyl exposure. Fed. Proc. 34:1675-1679.

Allen, J.R., and D.H. Norback. 1973. Polychlorinated biphenyl- and triphenyl- induced gastric mucosal hyperplasia in primates. Science 179:498-499.

Allen, J.R., and D.H. Norback. 1976. Pathobiological response of primates to polychlorinated biphenyl exposure. *In* Conference Proceedings. National Conference on Polychlorinated Biphenyls (November 1975, Chicago, Illinois), pp. 43-49. Environmental Protection Agency, Office of Toxic Substances, Washington, D.C.

Allen, J.R., L.A. Carstens, and D.A. Barsotti. 1974. Residual effects of short-term, low-level exposure of nonhuman primates to polychlorinated biphenyls. Toxicol. Appl. Pharmacol. 30:440-451.

Allen, L.A., N. Blizard, and A.B. Wheatland. 1948. Formation of cyanogen chloride during chlorination of certain liquids. Toxicity of such liquids to fish. J. Hyg. 46:184-193.

American Conference of Governmental Industrial Hygienists. 1971. Documentation of the Threshold Limit Values for Substances in Workroom Air, 3rd ed. Cincinnati, Ohio.

American Industrial Hygiene Association. 1956. 1,2-Dichloroethane (Ethylene dichloride), Hygenic Guide Series. Am. Ind. Hyg. Assoc. J. 17:447-448.

American Industrial Hygiene Association. 1965. 1,2-Dichloroethane (Ethylene chloride ethylene dichloride, glycol dichloride). Hygienic Guide Series. Am. Ind. Hyg. Assoc. J. 26:435-438.

American National Standards Institute. 1970. American national standard: Acceptable concentrations of ethylene dichloride: Approved September 5, 1969 (ANSI Z37.21-1969).

Amirkhanova, G.F., and Z.V. Latypova. 1967. Toxicity of acetaldehyde during its oral administration to animals. Nauch. Tr. Kazan. Med. Inst. 24:26-27. (CA 71:111003 p. 1969.)

Anonymous. 1974. How hazardous to health is vinyl chloride? J. Am. Med. Assoc. 228:1355.

Anonymous. 1964. How toxic is caprolactam? Food Cosmet. Toxicol. 2:222-223, 1363-1364.

Armstrong, R.W., E.R. Eichner, D.E. Klein, W.F. Barthel, J.V. Bennet, V. Jonsson, H. Bruce, and L.E. Loveless. 1969. Pentachlorophenol poisoning in a nursery for newborn infants. II. Epidemiologic and toxicologic studies. J. Pediatr. 75:317-325.

Arnold, D.W., G.L. Kennedy, Jr., and M.L. Keplinger. 1975. Mutagenic evaluation of hexachlorophene. Toxicol. Appl. Pharmacol. 33:185.

Aulerich, R.J., R.K. Ringer, and S. Iwamoto. 1973. Reproductive failure and mortality in mink fed on Great Lakes fish. J. Reprod. Fertil. Suppl. 19:365-376.

Aviado, D.M., and M.A. Belej. 1975. Toxicity of aerosol propellants in the respiratory and circulatory systems. V. Ventricular function in the dog. Toxicology 3: 79-86.

Baader, E.W. 1955. Illnesses caused by Phthalic Acid and its Compounds. Arch. Gewerbepath. Gewerbehyg. 13:419-453. Abstr. in Arch. Ind. Health. 13:401-402; 1956.

Baker, A. 1958. The nervous system in trichloroethylene intoxication: An experimental study. J. Neuropathol. Exp. Neurol. 17:649-655.

Bakke O.M., and R.R. Scheline. 1970. Hydroxylation of aromatic hydrocarbons in the rat. Toxicol. Appl. Pharmacol. 16:691-700.

Banfer, W. 1961. Studies on the effect of pure toluene on the blood picture of photogravure printers and helper workers. Zentralbl Arbeitsmed. 11:35-40, (in German).

Baranowska and Dutkiewicz. 1966. Influence of concentration and temperature of carbon disulfide solutions on its absorption through human skin. Ann. Acad. Med. Lodz. 8:169-74 (in Polish). Chem. Abs. 70:31443w, Feb. 24, 1969)

Bardawill, C.J., and A.G. Gornall. 1952. The influence of dietary protein on liver injury due to carbon tetrachloride in dogs. Can J. Med. Sci. 30:272-283.

Bariliak, I.R., I.A. Vasil'eva, and L.P. Kalinovskaia. 1975. Effect of small concentrations of carbon disulfide and hydrogen disulfide on intrauterine developments in rats. Arkh. Anat. Gistol. Embriol. 68(5):77-81 (in Russian).

Barlow, R.G., and L.J. McLeod. 1969. Some studies on cytisine and its methylated derivatives. Br. J. Pharmacol. 35:161-174.

Barrett, H.M., J.G. Cunningham, and J.H. Johnston. 1939. A study of the fate in the organism of some chlorinated hydrocarbons. J. Ind. Hyg. Toxicol. 21:479-490.

Batchelor, J.J. 1927. The relative toxicity of benzol and its higher homologues. Am. J. Hyg. 7:276-298.

Bechtel, D.H. and H.H. Cornish. 1972. Effect of the butyl alcohols on liver microsomal enzymes. Toxicol. Appl. Pharmacol. 22:298-299.

Belej, M.A., and D.M. Aviado. 1973. Acute fluorocarbon toxicity in rhesus monkey. Fed. Proc. 32:814. Abstr. no. 3359.

Bennett, D.R., Larson, P.L., and Tedeschi, R.C. 1954. Studies on the fate of nicotine in the body. VII. Observations on the excretion of nicotine and its metabolites by the dog. Arch. Int. Pharmacodyn. 98:221-227.

Berenblum, I. 1935. Experimental inhibition of tumour induction by mustard gas and other compounds. J. Pathol. Bacterial. 40:549-558.

Berenblum, I., and R. Schoental. 1943. The metabolism of 3,4-benzpyrene in mice and rats. 1. The isolation of a hydroxy and a quinone derivative, and a consideration of their biological significance. Cancer Res. 3:145-150.

Berlin M., J.C. Gage, and S. Holm. 1975a. Distribution and metabolism of polychlorobiphenyls. Proc. Int. Symp. Recent Adv. Environ. Pollut. Paris, June 24-28, 1974, vol. II.

Berlin, M., J. Gage, and S. Holm. 1975b. Distribution and metabolism of 2,4,5,2′,5′-pentachlorobiphenyl. Arch. Environ. Health 30:141-147.

Berlin, M., J.C. Gage, and S. Holm. 1973. The metabolism and distribution of -2,4,5,2,5-pentachlorobiphenyl in the mouse. *In* PCB Conference, 2d Wenner-Glenn Center, 1972, National Swedish Environment Protection Board/Publications, 1973-1974E, pp. 101-108.

Blake, D.A., and G.W. Mergner. 1974. Inhalation studies on the biotransformation and elimination of [^{14}C] trichlorofluromethane and [^{14}C] dichlorodifluoromethane in beagles. Toxicol. Appl. Pharmacol. 30:396-407.

Boitsov, A.N., Y.S. Rotenberg, and V.G. Mulenkova. 1970. Toxicological evaluation of chloral in the process of its liberation during spraying and pouring of polyurethane foams. Gig. Tr. Prof. Zabol. 14(6):26-29 (in Russian).

Bornmann, G., and A. Loeser. 1967. Chronic toxic effect of dichloromethane. Z. Lebensm.-Unters. Forsch. 136:14-18.

Borzelleca, J.F., P.S. Larson, G.R. Hennigar, Jr., E.G. Huf, E.M. Crawford, and R.B. Smith, Jr. 1964. Studies on the chronic oral toxicity of monomeric ethyl acrylate and methyl methacrylate. Toxicol. Appl. Pharmacol. 6:29-36.

Boutwell, R.K. and D.K. Bosch. 1959. The tumor-promoting action of phenol and related compounds for mouse skin. Cancer Res. 19:413-424.

Bower, R.K., S. Haberman, and P.D. Minton. 1970. Teratogenic effects in the chick embryo caused by esters of phthalic acid. J. Pharmacol. Exp. Ther. 171:314-324.

Bowman, E.R., L.B. Turnbull, and H. McKennis, Jr. 1959. Metabolism of nicotine in the human and excretion of pyridine compounds by smokers. J. Pharmacol. Expt. Ther. 127:92-95.

Braun, R., and J. Schoneich. 1975. The influence of ethanol and carbon tetrachloride on the mutagenic effectivity of cyclophosphamide in the host-mediated assay with *Salmonella typhimurium*. Mutat. Res. 31:191-194.

Bray, H.G., Brenda G. Humphris, and W.V. Thorpe. 1950. Metabolism of derivatives of toluene. V. Fate of the xylenols in the rabbit, with further observations on the metabolism of the xylenes. Biochem. J. 47:395-399.

Breed, A.L. 1974. Experimental production of vascular hypotension, and bone marrow and fat embolism with methylmethacrylate cement. Clin. Orthop. Relat. Res. 102:227-244.

Brem, H., A.B. Stein, and H.S. Rosenkranz. 1974. The mutagenicity and DNA-modifying effect of haloalkanes. Cancer Res. 34:2576-2579.

Brieger, H., and J. Teisinger, eds. 1967. Toxicology of Carbon Disulphide. Proceedings of the lst International Symposium. Excerpta Medica Foundation, Amsterdam. pp. 271

Brown, B.R., Jr., I.G. Sipes, and A.M. Sagalyn. 1974. Mechanisms of acute hepatic toxicity: Chloroform, halothane, and glutathione. Anesthesiology 41:554-561.

Brown, V.K.H., C. Muir, and E. Thorpe. 1969. The acute toxicity and skin irritant properties of 1,2-4trichlorobenzene. Ann. Occup. Hyg. 12:209-212.

Browning, E. 1965. Toxicity and metabolism of industrial solvents. Elsevier Publishing Company, Amsterdam.

Browning, E. 1961. Toxicology of organic compounds of industrial importance. Annu. Rev. Pharmacol. 1:397-430.

Bruckner, J.V., K.L. Khanna, and H.H. Cornish. 1973. Biological responses of the rat to polychlorinated biphenyls. Toxicol. Appl. Pharmacol. 24:434-448.

Bryan, W.R., and M.B. Shimkin. 1943. Quantitative analysis of dose–response data obtained with three carcinogenic hydrocarbons in strain C3H male mice. J. Nat. Cancer Inst. 3:503-531.

Buhler, D.R., M.E. Rasmusson, and H.S. Nakaue. 1973. Occurrence of hexachlorophene and pentachlorophenol in sewage and water. Environ. Sci. Tech. 7:929-934.

Bulay, O.M. 1970. The study of development of lung and skin tumours in mice exposed *in utero* to polycyclic hydrocarbons. Acta Med. Turc. 7:3-38.

Bulay, O.M., and L.W. Wattenberg. 1970. Carcinogenic effects of subcutaneous administration of benzo(*a*)pyrene during pregnancy on the progeny. Proc. Soc. Exp. Biol. Med. 135:84-86.

Busacca. 1919. Action of phenol and guaiacol on leucocytes. Arch Farm Sper. 28: 139-51.

Busuttil, A., W.C. Alston, C.H.W. Horne, and R.N.M. MacSween. 1972. Effect of experimental cirrhosis in rats on serum aminotransferase levels. Rev. Eur. Etude Clin. Biol. 17:979-982.

Butcher, H.R., W.F. Ballinger, D.L. Gravens, N.E. Dewar, E.F. Ledlie, and W.F. Barthel. 1973. Hexachlorophene concentrations in the blood of operating room personnel. Arch. Surg. 107:70-74.

Butler, T. 1949. Metabolic transformations of trichloroethylene. J. Pharmacol. Exp. Ther. 97:84-92.

Butler, T.C. 1961. Reduction of carbon tetrachloride *in vivo* and reduction of carbon tetrachloride and chloroform *in vitro* by tissue and tissue constituents. J. Pharmacol. Expt. Ther. 134:311-319.

Calley, D., J. Autian, and W.L. Guess. 1966. Toxicology of a series of phthalate esters. J. Pharmacol. Sci. 55:158-162.

Cameron, G.R., J.L.H. Paterson, G.S.W. de Saram, and J.C. Thomas. 1938. The toxicity of some methyl derivatives of benzene with special reference to pseudocumene and heavy coal tar naphtha. J. Pathol. Bacteriol. 46:95-107.

Capellini, A., and L. Alessio. 1971. The urinary excretion of hippuric acid in workers exposed to toluene. Med. Lavoro 62:196-201, (in Italian).

Carpenter, C.P., C.S. Weil, and H.F. Smyth, Jr. 1953. Chronic oral toxicity of Di(2-Ethylhexyl)Phthalate for rats, guinea pigs and dogs. Arch. Ind. Hyg. Occup. Med. 8:219-226.

Carpenter, C.P., E.R. Kinkead, D.L. Geary, Jr., L.J. Sullivan, and J.M. King. 1975. Petroleum hydrocarbon toxicity studies. V. Animal and human/response to vapors of mixed xylenes. Toxicol. Appl. Pharmacol. 33:543-558.

Carpenter, C.P., H.F. Smyth, Jr., and U.C. Pozzani. 1949. The assay of acute vapor toxicity, and the grading and interpretation of results on 96 chemical compounds. J. Ind. Hyg. Toxicol. 31:343-346.

Cascorbi, H.F. 1973. Biotransformation of drugs used in anesthesia. Anesthesiology 39:115-125.

Catignani, L., A. Neal. 1975. Evidence for the formation of a protein bound hydrodisulfide resulting from the microsomal mixed function oxidase catalyzed desulfuration of carbon disulfide. Biochem. Biophys. Res. Commun. 65(2):629-636.

Cawthorne, M.A., J. Bunyan, M.V. Sennitt, J. Green, and P. Grasso. 1970. Vitamin E and hepatotoxic agents. 3. Vitamin E, synthetic antioxidants and carbon tetrachloride toxicity in the rat. Br. J. Nutr. 24:357-384.

Cederbaum, A.I., C.S. Lieber, and E. Rubin. 1974. The effect of acetaldehyde on mitochondrial function. Arch. Biochem. Biophys. 161:26-39.

Charlesworth, F.A. 1975. The fate of fluorocarbons inhaled or ingested. Food Cosmet. Toxicol. 13:572-574.

Chung, H.L., W.C. Ts'ao, H.C. Hsu, C.H. Kuo, H.Y. K'o, P.S. Mo, H.Y. Chang, H.T. Chuo, and W.H. Chou. 1963. Hexachlorophene (G-11) as a new specific drug against Clonorchiasis sinensis. Chinese Med. J. 82:691-701.

Confer, D.B. and R.J. Stenger. 1965. Tumors of the liver in C3H mice after long-term carbon tetrachloride administration. A light and electron microscopic study. Am. J. Pathol. 46:19a. Abstr. no. 7.

Cooper, P. 1975. Acrylic cement reactions. Food Cosmet. Toxicol. 13:390-393.

Cooper, P. 1976. Carbon disulphide toxicology: the present picture. Food Cosmet. Toxicol. 14:57-59.

CRC Handbook of Chemistry and Physics, 1970-1971, 51st ed. Chemical Rubber Co., Cleveland, Ohio.

Dalvi, R., L. Hunter, and A. Neal. 1975. Toxicological implications of the mixed-funct oxidase catalyzed metabolism of carbon dislfide. Chem. Biol. Interact. 10(5):347-

Daniel, J.W. 1963. The metabolism of ^{36}Cl-labelled trichloroethylene and tetrachloroet lene in the rat. Biochem. Pharmacol. 12:795-802.

Davidson, M., and M. Feinleib. 1972. Carbon disulfide poisoning: A review. Am. Hear 83(1):100-14.

Deichmann, W. 1941. Toxicity of methyl, ethyl, and *n*-butyl methacrylate. J. Ind. Hy Toxicol. 23:343-351.

Deichmann, W., W. Machle, K.V. Kitzmiller, and G. Thomas. 1942. Acute and chron effects of pentachlorophenol and sodium pentachlorophenate upon experiment animals. J. Pharmacol. Exp. Ther. 76:104-117.

Deichmann, W. 1943. The toxicity of chlorophenols for rats. Fed. Proc. 2:76-77.

Della-Porta, G., B. Terracini, and P. Shubik. 1961. Induction with carbon tetrachloride liver-cell carcinomas in hamsters. J. Nat. Cancer Inst. 26:855-863.

DeSalva, S., A. Volpe, G. Leigh, and T. Regan. 1975. Long-term safety studies of chloroform-containing dentrifice and mouth rinse in man. Food Cosmet. Toxico 13:529-532.

DiVincenzo, G.D., and W.J. Krasavage. 1974. Serum ornithine carbamyl transferase as liver response test for exposure to organic solvents. Am. Ind. Hyg. Assoc. J. 35:21-29

DiVincenzo, G.D. and M.L. Hamilton. 1975. Fate and disposition of [^{14}C]-methylen chloride in the rat. Toxicol. Appl. Pharmacol. 32:385-393.

Dollery, C.T., G.H. Draffan, D.S. Davies, F.M. Williams, and M.E. Connelly. 1970. Bloo concentrations in man of fluorinated hydrocarbons after inhalation of pressurize aerosols. Lancet 1164-1166.

Dontenwill, W., and U. Mohr. 1962. Experimental studies on the problem of the origin o cancer of the respiratory tract I. Th different effects of benzpyrene on the epithelium o the skin, mouth and trachea in the hamster. Z. Krebsforch. 65:56-61.

Dovzhanskii, S.I., A.P. Suvorov, N.N. Ardentov, M.I. Granovskii, L.T. Dolzhikov, and M.B. Khonin. 1972. Dermatoses and their prevention at a chemical fibers combine. Gig Tr. Prof. Zabol. 16:47-49.

Dubrokhotov, V. B. 1972. The mutagenic influence of benzene and toluene unde experimental conditions. Gig. Sanit. 37(10):36-39.

Dume, T., W. Herms, E. Schroeder, and E. Wetzels. 1969. Clinical aspects and therapy o carbon tetrachloride poisoning. Dtsch. Med. Wochenschr. 94(33):1646-1651.

Dykan, V.A. 1962. Changes in liver and kidney functions due to methylene bromide and bromoform. Nauchn. Tr. Ukr. Nauchn.-Issled. Inst. Gig. Tr. Profzabol. 29:82-90.

Dykan, V.A. 1964. Problems on toxicology, clinical practice, and work hygiene in the production of bromine-organic compounds. Gigiena (Kiev:Zdorov'e) Sb., pp. 100-103

Eckardt, R.E. 1965. Toxic effects of carbon tetrachloride. J. Am. Med. Assoc. 194:1337-1338.

Eckhardt, R.E. 1973. Recent developments in industrial carcinogens. J. Occup. Med. 15:904-907.

Ecobichon, D.J. 1976. Enzymatic and other biochemical responses to selected PCP's. *In* Conference Proceedings, National Conference on Polychlorinated Biphenyls (Novembe 1975, Chicago, Illinois). Environmental Protection Agency, Office of Toxic Substances Washington, D.C. pp. 57-66.

Edds, G.T., and C.F. Simpson. 1974. Hexachlorophene-pHisohex toxicity in pups. Am. J Vet. Res. 35:1005-1007.

Egle, J.L., Jr. 1970. Retention of inhaled acetaldehyde in man. J. Pharmacol. Exp. The 174:14-19.

Egle, J.L., Jr. 1972. Effects of inhaled acetaldehyde and propionaldehyde on blood pressure and heart rate. Toxicol. Appl. Pharmacol. 23:131-135.

Egle, J.L., Jr., P.M. Hudgins, and F.M. Lai. 1973. Cardiovascular effects of intravenous acetaldehyde and propionaldehyde in the anesthetized rat. Toxicol. Appl. Pharmacol. 24:636-644.

El Masri, A.M., J.N. Smith, and R.T. Williams. 1958. Biochem. J. 68:199-204.

Epstein, S.S., S. Joshi, J. Andrea, P. Clapp, H. Falk, and N. Mantel. 1967. Synergistic toxicity and carcinogenicity of "Freons" and piperonyl butoxide. Nature 214:526-528.

Erlicher, H. 1968. Beobachtungen und erfahrungen in der industrie betreffend die giftigkeit (physiopathologische wirkung) der dampfe gechlorter benzole (mono-*bis*-hexachlorbenzol) Zentralbl. Arbeitsmed. Arbeitsschultz 18:204-205.

Eschenbrenner, A. 1945. Induction of hepatomas in mice by repeated oral administration of chloroform, with observations on sex differences. J. Nat. Cancer Inst. 5:251-255.

Evtushenko, G. Yu. 1966. Problems of methyl chloride toxicology. Gig. Tr. Prof. Zabol. 10(10):20-25.

Fabre, R., R. Truhaut, and S. Laham. 1960. Toxicological research on replacement solvents for benzene. IV. Study of xylenes. Arch. Mal. Prof. 21:301-313.

Fabre, R., R. Truhaut, S. Laham, and M. Peron. 1955. Toxicological research on substitute solvents for benzene II. A study of toluene. Arch Mal. Prof. 16:197-215 (in French).

Fairhall, L.T. 1957. Industrial Toxicology, 2nd ed. Williams & Wilkins, Baltimore.

Falk, H.L., P. Kotin, S.S. Lee, and A. Nathan. 1962. Intermediary metabolism of benzo(*a*)pyrene in the rat. J. Nat. Cancer. Inst. 28:699-724.

Farquharson, M.E., J.C. Gage, and J. Northover. 1958. The biological action of chlorophenols. Br. J. Pharmacol. 13:20-24.

Fassett, D.W. 1963. Aldehydes and acetals. *In* F.A. Patty, ed. Industrial Hygiene and Toxicology, vol. II, pp. 1959-1989. Interscience Publ. New York.

Federal Register, vol. 41, no. 126, part V, June 29, 1976. DHEW, FDA, Human drug and cosmetic products; Chloroform as an ingredient. pp. 26842-26846.

Feldman, R.G., R.M. Mayer, and A. Taub. 1970. Evidence for peripheral neurotoxic effect of trichloroethylene. Neurology 20:599-606.

Feldman, R.J., and H.I. Maibach. 1970. Absorption of some organic compounds through the skin in man. J. Invest. Dermatol. 54:399-404.

Ferguson, W.S., and D.D. Wheeler. 1973. Caprolactam vapor exposures. Am. Ind. Hyg. Assoc. J. 34:384-389.

Filippova, L.M., O.A. Pan'shin, and R.G. Kostyanovskii. 1967. Chemical Mutagens. IV. Genetic activity of geminal systems. Genetika (8):134-148.

Florestano, H.J. 1949. Tuberculocidal activity and toxicity of some diphenylmethane derivatives. J. Pharmacol. Exp. Ther. 96:238-249.

Flury, F. 1928. Modern occupational intoxications from the aspect of pharmacology and toxicology. Arch. Exp. Pathol. Pharmakol. 138:65-82.

Forni, A., A. Cappellini, E. Pacifico, and E.C. Vigliani. 1971. Chromosome changes and their evolution in subjects with past exposure to benzene. Arch. Environ. Health 23:385-391.

Forni, A., E. Pacifico, and A. Limonta. 1971. Chromosome studies in workers exposed to benzene or toluene or both. Arch Environ. Health 22:373-378.

Forsyth, G.W., H.T. Nagasawa, and C.S. Alexander. 1973. Acetaldehyde metabolism by the rat heart. Proc. Soc. Exp. Biol. Med. 144:498-500.

Fowler, J.S.L. 1969. Carbon tetrachloride metabolism in the rabbit. Br. J. Pharmacol. 37:733-737.

Freundt, K.J., G.P. Liebaldt, and K.H.M. Sieber. 1974a. Effect of barbiturates on the liver of rats exposed to carbon disulfide vapour. Int. Arch. Arbeitsmed. 32:297-303.

Freundt, K.J., K.J. Schauenburg, and P. Eichhorn. 1974b. Effect of acute exposure to carbon disulfide vapour upon some components of the hepatic microsomal enzyme system in rats. Arch. Toxicol. 32:233-240.

Friebel, H., E. Gross, L. Immisch-Seehausen, K.H. Linke, and S. Sommer. 1956. Toxicity of pure and crude phthalic acid anhydride in the industrial production of phthalic acid. Arch. Gewerbepath. Gewerbehyg. 14:465-482. Abstr. Bull. Hyg. 31:1124.

Fry, B.J., T. Taylor, and D.E. Hathway. 1972. Pulmonary elimination of chloroform and its metabolite in man. Arch. Int. Pharmacodyn. 196:98-111.

Funatsu, I., F. Yamashita, Y. Ito, S. Tsugawa, T. Funatsu, T. Yoshikane, M. Hayashi, T. Kato, M. Yakushiji, G. Okamoto, S. Yamasaki, T. Arima, T. Kuno, H. Ioe, and I. Ide. 1972. Polychlorbiphenyls (PCB) induced fetopathy. I. Clinical observation. Kurume Med. J. 19:43-51.

Gaillard, D., and R. Derache. 1964. Rates of metabolism of various alcohols in the rat. C.R. Soc. Biol. 158:1605-1608.

Gaines, T.B. 1969. Acute toxicity of pesticides. Toxicol. Appl. Pharmacol. 14:515-534.

Gaines, T.B., R.D. Kimbrough, and R.E. Linder. 1973. The oral and dermal toxicity of hexachlorophene in rats. Toxicol. Appl. Pharmacol. 25:332-343.

Gandolfi, A.J., and D.R. Buhler. 1974. Biliary metabolites and enterohepatic circulation of hexachlorophene in the rat. Xenobiotica 4(ll):693-704.

Gandolfi, A.J., and R.A. Van Dyke. 1973. Dechlorination of chloroethane with a reconstituted liver microsomal enzyme system. Biochem. Biophys. Res. Commum. 53:687-692.

Gandolfi, A.J., and D.R. Buhler. 1977. Metabolism of hexachlorophene in the rabbit. J. Ag. Food Chem. 25:21-25.

Gehring, P.J. 1968. Hepatotoxic potency of various chlorinated hydrocarbon vapours relative to their narcotic and lethal potencies in mice. Toxicol. Appl. Pharmacol. 13:287-298.

Gerarde H.W. 1956. Toxicological studies on hydrocarbons. II. A comparative study of the effect of benzene and certain mono-*n*-alkylbenzenes on hemopoiesis and bone marrow metabolism in rats. Arch. Ind. Health 13:468-474.

Gerarde, H.W. 1960. Toxicology and Biochemistry of Aromatic Hydrocarbons. pp. 97-108. Elsevier Publishing Company, New York.

Gohlke, R., and P. Schmidt. 1972. Zur subakuten wirkung geringer konzentrationen chlorierter athane ohne und mit zusatzlicher athanolbelastung auf ratten. II. Histologische, histochemische und morphometrische untersuchungen. Int. Arch. Arbeitsmed. 30:299-312.

Goldblatt, M.W., M.E. Farquharson, G. Bennett, and B.M. Askew. 1954. *e*-Caprolactam. Br. J. Ind. Med. ll:l-l0.

Goldstein, J.A., R.E. Linder, P. Hickman, and H. Bergman. 1976. Effects of pentachlorophenol on hepatic drug metabolism and porphyria related to contamination with chlorinated dibenzo-*p*-dioxins. Toxicol. Appl. Pharmacol. 37:145-146.

Grant, D.L., and W.E.J. Phillips. 1974. The effect of age and sex on the toxicity of Aroclor 1254, a polychlorinated biphenyl, in the rat. Bull. Environ. Contam. Toxicol. 12:145-152.

Green, S.G., J.V. Carr, K.A. Palmer, and E.J. Oswald. 1975. Lack of cytogenetic effects in bone marrow and spermatagonial cells in rats treated with polychlorinated biphenyls (Aroclors 1242 and 1254). Bull. Environ. Contam. Toxicol. 13:14-22.

Greenburg, L., M.R. Mayers, H. Heimann, and S. Moskowitz. 1942. The effects of exposure to toluene in industry. J. Am. Med. Assoc. 118:573-578.

Gump, W.S. 1969. Toxicological properties of hexachlorophene. J. Soc. Cosmet. Chem. 20:173-184.

Gut, R. 1969. Sex differences in sensitivity to some chemicals. Prac. Lek. 21(10): 453-458.

Hake, C.L., and V.K. Rowe. 1963. Ethers. *In* F.A. Patty, ed. Industrial Hygiene and Toxicology, vol. II., 2nd ed., pp. 1655-1718. Interscience, New York.

Hamilton, A., and L. Hardy. 1974. Industrial Toxicology, 3rd ed. Publishing Sciences Group, Acton, Mass.

Harada, M. 1937. Pharmacological and histological studies on amblyopia. Jap. J. Med. Sci. IV Pharmacol. 10:85-89.

Harris, R.S., H.C. Hodge, E.A. Maynard, and H.J. Blanchet, Jr. 1956. Chronic oral toxicity of 2-ethylhexyl phthalate in rats and dogs. Arch. Ind. Health 13:259-264.

Hathway, D.E. 1964. Chemical, biochemical and toxicological differences between carbon tetrachloride and chloroform. A critical review of recent investigations of these compounds in mammals. Arzneim-Forsch. 24:173-176.

Hefner, R.E., Jr., P.G. Watanabe, and P.J. Gehring. 1975. Preliminary studies of the fate of inhaled vinyl chloride monomer in rats. Ann. N.Y. Acad. Sci. 246:135-148.

Heppel, L.A., P.A. Neal, T.L. Perrin, K.M. Endicott, and V.T. Porterfield. 1946. The toxicology of 1,2-dichloroethane (ethylene dichloride) V. The effects of daily inhalations. J. Ind. Hyg. Toxicol. 28:113-120.

Heppel, L.A., P.A. Neal, T.L. Perrin, M.L. Orr, and V.T. Porterfield. 1944. Toxicology of dichloromethane (methylene chloride). I. Studies on effects of daily inhalation. J. Ind. Hyg. Tox. 26(1):8-16.

Hill, R.N., T.L. Clemens, D.K. Liu, E.S. Vesell, and W.D. Johnson. 1975. Genetic control of chloroform toxicity in mice. Science 190:159-161.

Hine, C.H., and H.H. Zuidema. 1970. The toxicological properties of hydrocarbon solvents. Ind. Med. Surg. 39:215-220.

Hinkle, D.K. 1973. Fetotoxic effects of pentachlorophenol in the golden Syrian hamster. Toxicol. Appl. Pharmacol. 25:455.

Hodge, H.C. 1943. Acute toxicity for rats and mice of 2-ethyl hexanol and 2-ethyl hexyl phthalate. Proc. Soc. Exp. Biol. Med. 53:20-23.

Hodge, H.C., M.R. Goldstein, and M. Wrightington. 1942. Acute toxicity for mice of phthalic acid and certain derivatives. Proc. Soc. Exp. Biol. Med. 49:471-473.

Hofmann, H. Th., H. Birnstiel, and P. Jobst. 1971. Zur inhalationstoxicitat von 1,1-und 1,2-dichlorathan. Arch. Toxikol. 27:248-265.

Hoshino, H., G. Chihara, and F. Fukuoka. 1970. Detection of potential weak carcinogens and procarcinogens. II. Carcinogenicity of tertiary butyl hydroperoxide. Gann 61:121-124.

Horvath, M., and E. Frantik. 1971. Assessment of the relative noxious potency of industrial chemicals. A procedure for the quantitative comparison of their effects in animal experiments. Neurotoxicity threshold limit value. *In* Helen Peskova, ed. Proceedings of the Scientific Meeting, Medical Faculty of Hy 5th, Prague, 1969, pp. 23-28.

Huggins, C., and N.C. Yang. 1962. Induction and extinction of mammary cancer. A striking effect of hydrocarbons permits analysis of mechanisms of causes and cure of breast cancer. Science 137:257-262.

Hunter, C.G., and D. Blair. 1972. Benzene: Pharmacokinetic studies in man. Ann. Occup. Hyg. 15:193-199.

Hylin, W., and B.H. Chin. 1968. Volatile metabolites from dimethyldithio carbamate fungicide residues. Bull. Environ. Contam. Toxicol. 3(6):322-332.

Ideda, M., and H. Ohtsuji. 1972. A comparative study of the excretion of Fujiwara reaction-positive substances in urine of humans and rodents given trichloro- or tetrachloro-derivatives of ethane and ethylene. Br. J. Ind. Med. 29:99-104.

Ikeda, M., and T. Imamura. 1973. Biological half-life of trichloroethylene and tetrachloroethylene in human subjects. Int. Arch. Arbeitsmed. 31:209-224.

Ikeda, M., and H. Ohtsuji. 1971. Phenobarbital-induced protection against toxicity of toluene and benzene in the rat. Toxicol. Appl. Pharmacol. 20:30-43.

Ilett, K.F., W.D. Reid, I.G. Sipes, and G. Krishna. 1973. Chloroform toxicity in mice: Correlation of renal and hepatic necrosis with covalent binding of metabolites to tissue macromolecules. Exp. Mol. Pathol. 19:215-229.

Innes, J.R.M., B.M. Ulland, M.G. Valerio, L. Petrucelli, L. Fishbein, E. R. Hart, A.J. Pallotta, R.R. Bates, H.L. Falk, J.J. Gart, M. Klein, I. Mitchell, and J. Peters. 1969. Bioassay of pesticides and industrial chemicals for tumorigenicity in mice: A preliminary note. J. Nat. Cancer Inst. 42:1101-1114.

Ishimaru, T., H. Okada, T. Tomiyasu, T. Tsuchimoto, T. Hoshino, and M. Ichimaru. 1971. Occupational factors in the epidemiology of leukemia in Hiroshima and Nagasaki. Am. J. Epidemiol. 93:157-165.

Jacobs, A., M. Blangetti, and E. Hellmund. 1974. Accumulation of noxious chlorinated substances from Rhine River water in the fatty tissue of rats. Vom Wasser 43:259-274.

Jacobs, J.L., T.S. Golden, and J.J. Kelley. 1940. Immediate reactions to anhydrides of wheal-and-erythema type. Proc. Soc. Exp. Biol Med. 43:74-77.

John, J.A., B.A. Schwetz, B.K.J. Leong, F.A. Smith, K.D. Nitschke, H.D. Haberstroh, F.J. Murray, M.F. Balmer, and P.J. Gehring. 1975. The effects of maternally inhaled vinyl chloride on embryonal and fetal development in mice, rats and rabbits. Report, Dow Chemical Company.

Johnson, R.L., P.J. Gehring, P.J. Kociba, and B.A. Schwetz. 1973. Chlorinated dibenzodioxins and pentachlorophenol. Environ. Health Perspect. 5:171-175.

Jondorf, W.R., D.V. Parke, and R.T. Williams. 1955. Studies in detoxication 66: The metabolism of halogenobenzenes. 1:2:3-1:2:4 and 1:3:5-trichlorobenzenes. Biochem. J. 61:512-521.

Juehe, S., and C.E. Lange. 1972. Schleroderma-like skin alterations, Raynaud's syndrome, and acroosteolysis in workers in the polyvinyl chloride industry. Dtsch. Med. Wochenschr. 97:1922-1923.

Juehe, S., C.E. Lange, G. Stein, and G. Veltman. 1974. On the so-called vinyl chloride disease. A new occupational illness. Berufs-Dermatosen, 22, 4-22.

Jurgens, G. 1920. Tissue storage of guaiacol and pyrocatecholacetic acid. Z. Exp. Pathol. Ther. 21:213-215.

Karel, L., B.H. Landing, and T. S. Harvey. 1947. The intraperitoneal toxicity of some glycols, glycol esters, glycol esters and phthalates in mice. Fed. Proc. 6:342.

Kato, T., M. Yakushiji, H. Tuda, A. Arima, K. Takahashi, M. Shimomura, M. Miyahara, M. Adachi, Y. Tashiro, M. Matsumoto, I. Funatsu, F. Yamashita, Y. Ito, M. Tsugawa, T. Funatsu, T. Yoshikane, and M. Hayashi. 1972. Polychlorobiphenyls (PCB) induced fetopathy. II. Experimental studies: Possible placental transfer of polychlorobiphenyls in rats. Kurume Med. J. 19:53-59.

Kawasaki, H. 1965. Development of tumor in the course of spontaneous restoration of carbon tetrachloride induced cirrhosis of the liver in rats. Kurume Med. J. 12:37-42.

Kenaga, E.E. 1966. Entomol. Soc. Am. Bull. 12(2):117-127.

Kennedy, G.L., Jr., I.A. Dressler, W.R. Richter, M.L. Keplinger, and J.C. Calandra. 1976. Effects of hexachlorophene in the rat and their reversibility. Toxicol. Appl. Pharmacol. 35:137-145.

Kennedy, G.L., Jr., S.H. Smith, M.L. Keplinger, and J.C. Calandra. 1975a. Effect of hexachlorophene on reproduction in rats. J. Agric.. Food Chem. 23:866-868.

Kennedy, G.L., Jr., S.H. Smith, M.L. Keplinger, and J.C. Calandra. 1975b. Evaluation of the teratological potential of hexachlorophene in rabbits and rats. Teratology 12:83-88.

Keplinger, M.L., O.E. Fancher, and J.C. Calandra. 1971. Toxiologic studies with polychlorinated biphenyls. Toxicol. Appl. Pharmacol. 19:402-403.

Khadzhieva, E.D. 1969. Effect of caprolactam on the reproductive functions of albino rats. Hyg. Sanit. 34(7-9):28-32.

Kimbrough, R.D. 1974. The toxicity of polychlorinated polycyclic compounds and related chemicals. Crit. Rev. Toxicol. 2:445-498.

Kimbrough, R.D. 1973. Review of the toxicity of hexachlorophene, including its neurotoxicity. J. Clin. Pharmacol. 13:439-444.

Kimbrough, R.D. 1976. Hexachlorophene: Toxicity and use as an antibacterial agent. *In* W.J. Hayes, Jr., ed. Essays in toxicology, vol. 7, pp. 99-120. Academic Press, New York.

Kimbrough, R.D., and T.B. Gaines. 1971. Hexachlorophene effects on the rat brain. Study of high doses by light and electron microscopy. Arch. Environ. Health 23:114-118.

Kimbrough, R.D., and R.E. Linder. 1975. The effect of technical and 99% pure pentachlorophenol on the rat liver. Light microscopy and ultrastructure. Toxicol. Appl. Pharmacol. 33:131-132.

Kimbrough, R.D., R.E. Linder, and T.B. Gaines. 1972. Morphological changes in livers of rats fed polychlorinated biphenyls: Light microscopy and ultrastructure. Arch. Environ. Health 25:354-364.

Kimbrough, R.D., R.A. Squire, R.E. Linder, J.D. Strandberg, R.J. Montali, and V.W. Burse. 1975. Induction of liver tumors in Sherman strain female rats by polychlorinated biphenyl Aroclor 1260. J. Nat. Canc. Inst. 55:1453-1459.

Kimmel, C.A., W. Moore, Jr., D.K. Hysell, and J.F. Stara. 1974. Teratogenicity of hexachlorophene in rats. Comparison of uptake following various routes of administration. Arch. Environ. Health 28:43-48.

Kimura, E.T., D.M. Ebert, and P.W. Dodge. 1971. Acute toxicity and limits of solvent residue for sixteen organic solvents. Toxicol. Appl. Pharmacol. 19:699-704.

Klaasen, C.D., and G.L. Plaa. 1966. Relative effects of chlorinated hydrocarbons on liver and kidney function in mice. Toxicol. Appl. Pharmacol. 9:139-151.

Klaasen, C.D., and G.L. Plaa. 1967. Relative effects of various chlorinated hydrocarbons on liver and kidney function in dogs. Toxicol. Appl. Pharmacol. 10:119-131.

Klaassen, C.D., and G.L. Plaa. 1969. Comparison of the biochemical alterations elicited in livers from rats treated with carbon tetrachloride, chloroform, 1,1,2-trichloroethane, and 1,1,1-trichloroethane. Biochem. Pharmacol. 18:2019-2027.

Kleinfeld, M., and Tabershaw, I. 1954. Trichloroethylene toxicity. Arch. Ind. Hyg. Occup. Med. 10:134-41.

Knapp, W.K., Jr., W.M. Busey, and W. Kundzins. 1971. Subacute oral toxicity of monochlorobenzene in dogs and rats. Toxicol. Appl. Pharmacol. 19. Abstr. no. 81.

Knudsen, I., H.G. Verschuuren, E.M. Den Tonkelaar, R. Kroes, and P.F.W. Helleman. 1974. Short-term toxicity of pentachlorophenol in rats. Toxicology 2:141-152.

Kobayashi, S., S. Toida, H. Kawamura, H. S. Chang, T. Fukuda, and K. Kawaguchi. 1972. Chronic toxicity of 2,4-dichlorophenol in mice. A simple design for the toxicity of residual metabolites of pesticides. Toho Igakkai Zasshi 19(3/4):356-362 (in Japanese).

Koller, L.D., and J.G. Zinkl. 1973. Pathology of polychlorinated biphenyls in rabbits. Am. J. Pathol. 70:363-373.

Kongiel-Chablo, I. 1968. Effect of chlorophenols in water on some enzymes in animals. Rocz Panstw. Zakl. Hig. 19(5):531-540 (in Polish).

Krichevskaya, I.M. 1968. Biological effect of caprolactam and its sanitary-hygienic assessment as an atmospheric pollutant. Hyg. Sanit. 33(1-3):24-30,

Kruysse, A., V.J. Feron, and H.P. Til. 1975. Repeated exposure to acetaldehyde vapor. Studies in Syrian golden hamsters. Arch. Environ. Health 30:449-452.

Kryatov, I.A. 1970. Hygienic evaluation of sodium *p*-chlorobenzene sulfonate and chloral as water pollutant. Hyg. Sanit. (USS 35:333-338.

Kucera, J. 1968. Exposure to fat solvents: A possible cause of sacral agenesis in man. J. Pediatr. 72:857-859.

Kudo, K. S., Toida, S. Matsuura, T. Sasaki, and H. Kawamura. 1971. Comparison of Freon-11S and Freon-11. Acute, subacute toxicity and irritation of mucous membrane. Toho Igakkai Zasshi 18(2):363-367.

Kuratsune, M., Y. Masuda, and J. Nagayama. 1976. Some of the recent findings concerning Yusho. *In* Conference Proceedings. National Conference on Polychlorinated Biphenyls (November 1975, Chicago, Illinois), pp. 14-29.

Kutob, S.D., and G.L. Plaa. 1962. A procedure for estimating the hepatotoxic potential of certain industrial solvents. Toxicol. Appl. Pharmocol. 4:354-361.

Lake, B.G., S.D. Gangolli, P. Grasso, and A.G. Lloyd. 1975. Studies on the hepatic effects of orally administered di-(2-ethylhexyl) phthalate in the rat. Toxicol. Appl. Pharmacol. 32:355-367.

Laskin, D.M., I.B. Robinson, and J.P. Weinmann. 1954. Experimental production of sarcomas by methyl methacrylate implants. Proc. Soc. Exp. Bi. Med. 87:329-332.

Lavorgna, J.J., N.A. Burstein, A.L. Schiller, and W.H. Harris. 1972. The carcinogenesis of plastics used in orthopedic surgery. An assessment of the incidence in rats and the possible relevance to man. Clin. Orthop. Relat. Res. 88:223-227.

Lawrence, W.H., M. Malik, J.E. Turner, A.R. Singh, and J. Autian. 1975. A toxicological investigation of some acute, short-term, and chronic effects of administering di-2-ethylhexyl phthalate (DEHP) and other phthalate esters. Environ. Res. 9:1-11.

Lazarev, N.Y. 1929. Toxicity of various hydrocarbon vapors. Arch. Exp. Pathol. Pharmakol. 143:223-233.

Leitch, J.L., and V.E. Bauer. 1945. 19. Oral toxicity of cyanogen chloride in water to rats. U.S. Chemical Warfare Service, Edgewood Arsenal, Md. Medical Division Report no. 19.

Lester, D., and L. Greenberg. 1950. Acute and chronic toxicity of some halogenated derivatives of methane and ethane. Arch. Ind. Hyg. Occup. Med. 2:335-344.

Lester, D., L.A. Greenberg, and W.R. Adams. 1963. Effects of single and repeated exposures of humans and rats to vinyl chloride. Am. Ind. Hyg. Assoc. J. 24:265-275.

Lewis, C.E. 1961. The toxicology of carbon tetrachloride. J. Occup. Med. 3:82-86.

Litchfield, M.H. and C. J. Gartland. 1974. Plasma enzyme activity and hepatocellular changes in the beagle dog after single or repeated administration of carbon tetrachloride. Toxicol. Appl. Pharmacol. 30:117-28.

Litterst, C.L., T.M. Farber, and E.J. VanLoon. 1973. Potentiation of CCl_4-induced hepatotoxicity in the dog by chronic exposure to phenobarbital. Toxicol. Appl. Pharmacol. 25:354-362.

Liu, J., C-N. Wang, J-H. Yu, M-N. Wang, C-F. Cang, and S. Cheng. 1963. Hexachlorophene in the treatment of Clonorchiasis sinensis. Chinese Med. J. 82:702-711.

Lobo-Mendonca, R. 1963. Tetrachloroethane—A survey. Br. J. Ind. Med. 20:50-56.

Lucas, G.H.W. 1929. A study of the fate and toxicity of bromine and chlorine containing anesthetics. J. Pharmacol. Exp. Ther. 34:223-237.

Lustig, F.W. 1963. A fatal case of hexachlorophene ("Phisohex") poisoning. Med. J. Australia 50:737.

Makk, L., F. Delmore, J.L. Creech, Jr., L.L. Ogden II, E.H. Fadell, C.L. Songster, J. Clanton, M.N. Johnson, and W.M. Christopherson. 1976. Clinical and morphologic features of hepatic angiosarcoma in vinyl chloride workers. Cancer 37(1):149-163.

Malaveille, C., H. Bartsch, A. Barbin, A.M. Camus, R. Montesano, A. Croisy, and P. Jacquignon. 1975. Mutagenicity of vinyl chloride, chloroethyleneoxide, chloroacetaldehyde and chloroethanol. Biochem. Biophys. Res. Commun. 63(2):363-370.

Maling, H.M., B. Highman, M.A. Williams, W. Saul, W.M. Butler, Jr., and B.B. Brodie. 1974. Reduction by pretreatment with dibenamine of hepatotoxicity induced by carbon tetrachloride, thioacetamide, or dimethylnitrosamine. Toxicol. Appl. Pharmacol. 27:380-394.

Mallory, T.B., E.A. Gall, and W.J. Brickley. 1939. Chronic exposure to benzene (benzol). III. The pathologic results. J. Ind. Hyg. Toxicol. 21:355-393.

Maltoni, C., A. Ciliberti, L. Gianni, and P. Chieco. 1975. The oncogenic effects of vinyl chloride administered by oral route in the rat. Gli Ospedali della Vita 2(6):65-66.

Maltoni, C., and G. Lefemine. 1974a. Carcinogenicity bioassays of vinyl chloride. I. Research plan and early results. Environ. Res. 7(3):387-405.

Maltoni, C., and G. Lefemine. 1974b. The potential of the planned experiment in the prediction of the risk of ambient carcinogens. An example: Vinyl chloride. Atti Accad. Naz. Lincei Cl. Scil, Fis., Mat., Nat., Rend. 56:(Series 8, fasc. 3)1-11.

Maltoni, C. and G. Lefemine. 1975. Carcinogenicity bioassays of vinyl chloride: Current results. Ann. N.Y. Acad. Sci. 246:195-218.

Marhold, J., M. Matrka, M. Hub, and F. Ruffer. 1968. The possible complicity of diphenyline in the origine of tumours in the manufacture of benzidene. Neoplasma 15:3-10.

Martinez, A.J., R. Boehm, and M.G. Hadfield. 1974. Acute hexachlorophene encephalopathy: clinico-neuropathological correlation. Acta Neuropathol. (Berl.) 28:93-103.

Mason Research Institute. 1971. Progress report, Contract NIH-71-2144.

Masoud, A.N., and J.T. Elder, A.L. Czerwinski. 1973. Chemistry and pharmacology of common acute poisoning in children. Paediatrician 2:2-37.

Mastromatteo, E., A.M. Fisher, H. Christie, and H. Danziger. 1960. Acute inhalation toxicity of vinyl chloride to laboratory animals. Am. Ind. Hyg. Assoc. J. 21:394-398.

McCann, J., E. Choi, E. Yamasaki, and B.N. Ames. 1975. Detection of carcinogens as mutagens in the Salmonella/Microsome Test: Assay of 300 chemicals. Proc. Nat. Acad. Sci. USA 72:5135-5139.

McCloy, R.B., Jr., A.V. Prancan, and J. Nakano. 1974. Effects of acetaldehyde on the systematic, pulmonary, and regional circulations. Cardiovasc. Res. 8:216-226.

McCollister, D.D., W.H. Beamer, G.J. Atchison, and H.C. Spencer. 1951. The absorption, distribution and elimination of radioactive carbon tetrachloride by monkeys upon exposure to low vapor concentrations. J. Pharmacol. Exp. Ther. 102:112-124.

McGavack, T.H., L.J. Boyd, F.V. Piccione, and R. Terranova. 1941. Acute and chronic intoxications with sodium pentachlorophenate in rabbits. J. Ind. Hyg. Toxicol. 23:239-251.

McGowan, G.R., P.G. Watanabe, and P.J. Gehring. 1975. Vinyl chloride urinary metabolites. Isolation and identification. In manuscript.

McLean, A.E.M., and E.K. McLean. 1966. The effect of diet and 1,1,1-trichloro-2,2-*bis*-(*p*-chlorophenyl)ethane (DDT) on microsomal hydroxylating enzymes and on sensitivity of rats to carbon tetrachloride poisoning. Biochem J. 100:564-571.

McNally, W.D. 1937. Industrial exposures and the worker as affected thereby. Ind. Med. 6:270-283.

Menges, R.W., L.A. Selby, C.J. Marienfeld, W.A. Aue, and D.L. Greer. 1970. A tobacco-related epidemic of congenital limb deformities in swine. Environ. Res. 3:285-302.

Menon, J.S. 1958. Tropical hazards associated with the use of pentachlorophenol. Br. Med. J. 2:1156-1158.

Menschick, H. 1955. Dangers to health in the production of phthalic anhydride. Arch. Gewerbepathol. U. Gewerbehyg. 13:454-475. Abstr. in Arch. Ind. Health. 13:402-404.

Merck Index. 1968. 8th ed. Merck & Co., Inc., Rahway, N.J.

Mergner, G.W., D.A. Blake, and M. Helrick. 1975. Biotransformation and elimination of ^{14}C-trichlorofluromethane (FC-11) and ^{14}C-dichlorofluoromethane (FC-12) in man. Anesthesiology 42:345-351.

Merlevede, E., and J. Elskens. 1957. The Toxicity of phthalic anhydride, maleic anhydride and the phthalates. Arch. Belges Med. Sociale. Hyg. Med. Travail Med. Legale 15:445-457. Abstr. in Bull. Hyg. 33:115.

Michalova, C., V. Bartonicek, and V. Zastava. 1959. Organotoxic effect of carbon disulfide after parenteral poisoning of rabbits. Arch. Gewerbepathol. Gerwerbehyg. 16:653-65.

Milkov, L., T.B. Popova, N.I. Ponomareva, E.N. L'vovksaya, K.A. Lopukhova, and A.M. Dzhezhev. 1966. Some data on the health status of workers engaged in the processing of plastics by die casting. Labor Hyg. Occup. Dis. 10:22-27. (Translated).

Miller, R.W. 1971. Cola-colored babies. Chlorobiphenyl poisoning in Japan. Teratology 4:211-212.

Minot, G.R., and L.W. Smith. 1921. The blood in tetrachloroethane poisoning. Arch. Intern. Med. 28:687-902.

Morgan, A., A. Black, and D.R. Belcher. 1970. The excretion in breath of some aliphatic halogenated hydrocarbons following administration by inhalation. Ann. Occup. Hyg. 13:219-233.

Morgan, A., A. Black, and D.R. Belcher. 1972. Studies on the absorption of halogenated hydrocarbons and their excretion in breath using ^{38}Cl tracer techniques. Ann. Occup. Hyg. 15:273-283.

Morley, R., D.W. Eccleston, C.P. Douglas, W.E.J. Greville, D.J. Scott, and J. Anderson. 1970. Xylene poisoning—A report of one fatal case and two cases of recovery after prolonged unconsciousness. Br. Med. J. 3:442-443.

Mullick, F.G. 1973. Hexachlorophene toxicity—Human experience at the Armed Forces Institute of Pathology. Pediatrics 51:395-399.

Murai, Y., and Y. Kuroiwa. 1971. Peripheral neuropathy in chlorobiphenyl poisoning. Neurology 21:1173-1176.

Nakano, K. 1937. Experimental production of malignant tumors by 3,4-benzopyrene and 1,2,5,6-dibenzanthracene. Osaka Igakki Zasshi. 36:483.

Nakaue, H.S., F.N. Dost, and D.R. Buhler. 1973. Studies on the toxicity of hexachlorophene in the rat. Toxicol. Appl. Pharmacol. 24:239-249.

National Academy of Sciences-National Research Council. Commission on Natural Resources. Environmental Studies Board. Pest Control: An Assessment of Present and Alternate Technologies. Vol. I: Contemporary Pest Control Practices and Prospects: The Report of the Executive Committee. National Academy of Sciences, Washington, D.C. 506 pp.

National Cancer Institute. 1976. Carcinogenesis Bioassay of Trichloroethylene. CAS/No.79-01-6 NCI-CG-TR-2, Washington, D.C. XIX. 197pp.

National Cancer Institute. 1976. Report on carcinogenesis bioassay of chloroform.

National Defense Research Committee of the Office of Scientific Research and Development, Division 9. 1943. Informal Monthly Progress Report on Toxicity of Chemical

Warfare Agents. Informal Monthly Report No. 9-4-1-6, p. 42. (Available from Library of Congress, Photoduplication Service. Reel 460 of OSRD, Div. 9.)

National Institute for Occupational Safety and Health. 1975. Suspected Carcinogens: A subfile of the NIOSH Toxic Substances List. Washington, D.C.

National Institute for Occupational Safety and Health 1973. Criteria for a Recommended Standard . . . Occupational Exposure to Trichloroethylene. HSM 73-11025. U.S. Government Printing Office. Washington, D.C.

National Institute for Occupational Safety and Health. 1974. Criteria for a Recommended Standard . . . Occupational Exposure to Chloroform, HEW Publication no. (NIOSH) 75-114. U.S. Government Printing Office. Washington, D.C.

National Institute for Occupational Safety and Health. 1974. Criteria for a Recommended Standard . . . Occupational Exposure to Benzene. HEW Publication no. (NIOSH) 74-137. U.S. Government Printing Office. Washington, D.C.

National Institute for Occupational Safety and Health. 1975. Criteria for a Recommended Standard . . . Occupational Exposure to Xylene. HEW Publication no. (NIOSH) 75-168. U.S. Government Printing Office. Washington, D.C.

Newens, A.F., and R.G. Volz. 1972. Severe hypotension during prosthetic hip surgery with acrylic bone cement. Anesthesiology 36:298-300.

Niazi, S., and W.L. Chiou. 1975. Fluorocarbon aerosol propellants. IV. Pharmacokinetics of trichloromonofluoromethane following single and multiple dosing in dogs. J. Pharm. Sci. 64:763-769.

Nieminen, L., K. Bjondahl, and M. Mottonen. 1973. Effect of hexachlorophene on the rat brain during ontogenesis. Food Cosmet. Toxicol. ll(4):635-639.

Nikonorow, M., H. Mazur, and H. Piekacz. 1973. Effect of orally administered plasticizers and polyvinyl chloride stabilizers in the rat. Toxicol. Appl. Pharmacol. 26:253-259.

Nishimura, H., and K. Nakai. 1958. Developmental anomalies in offspring of pregnant mice treated with nicotine. Science 127:877-878.

Nomiyama, D., and H. Nomiyama. 1974. Respiratory retention, uptake and excretion of organic solvents in man. Benzene, toluene, *n*-hexane, trichloroethylene, acetone, ethyl acetate and ethyl alcohol. Int. Arch. Arbeitsmed. 32:75-83.

Norton, T.R. 1975. Metabolism of toxic substances. *In* L.J. Casarett and J. Doull, eds. Toxicology: The Basic Science of Poisons, pp. 45-132. Macmillan, New York.

Oettel, H. 1936. Einwirkung organischer Flussigkeiten auf die Haut. Arch. Exp. Pathol. Pharmakol. 183:641-696.

Ogata, M., Y. Takatsuka, and K. Tomokuni. 1971. Excretion of hippuric acid and *m*- or *p*-methylhippuric acid in the urine of persons exposed to vapours of toluene and *m*- or *p*-xylene in an exposure chamber and in workshops, with specific reference to repeated exposures. Br. J. Ind. Med. 28:382-385.

Ogata, M., Y. Takatsuka, and K. Tomokuni. 1971. Excretion of organic chlorine compounds in the urine of persons exposed to vapours of trichloroethylene and tetrachloroethylene. Br. J. Ind. Med. 28:386-391.

Ogata, M., K. Tomokuni, and Y. Takatsuka. 1970. Urinary excretion of hippuric acid and *m*- and *p*- methylhippuric acid in the urine of persons exposed to vapours of toluene and *m*- or *p*-xylene as a test of exposure. Br. J. Ind. Med. 27:43-50.

Okamoto, S. 1959. Metabolism of acetylcholine in the central nervous system in carbon disulfide poisoning. Tokyo Jikeikai Ika Daigaku Zasshi 74:1184-1191.

Ono, J. 1920. The effects of the entrance of the sulfonic group on pharmacological action. Kyoto Igaku Zassi 17:317-319.

Pantucek, M. 1969. On the metabolic pathway of methyl methacrylate. Febs Lett. 2:206 Abstr. 1873, cited in Food Cosmet. Toxicol. 8:105, 1970.

Parmenter, D.C. 1923. Further observations on the control and prevention of tetrachlorethane poisoning. J. Ind. Hyg. Toxicol. 5:159-161.

Paterni, L., G. Pusic, and S. Teodori. 1958. Slow carbon disulfide poisoning and high cholesterol diet in the rabbit. Folia Med. 41:705-22.

Patty, F.A. 1963. Industrial Hygiene and Toxicology, 2nd ed. Interscience, New York.

Paul, B.B., and D. Rubinstein. 1963. Metabolism of carbon tetrachloride and chloroform by the rat. J. Pharmacol. Ex. Ther. 141:141-148.

Paulet, G., S. Desbrusses, and E. Vidal. 1974. Absence d'effet teratogene des fluorocarbones chez le rat et le lapin. Arch. Mal. Prof. 35:658-662.

Peirce, W.E. 1961. Tumour promotion by lime oil in the mouse forestomach. Nature 189:497-498.

Peters, J.W., and R.M. Cook. 1973. Effect of phthalate esters on reproduction in rats. Environ. Health Perspect. 3:91-94.

Piekacz, H. 1971a. The effect of dioctyl and dibutyl phthalates on rats during oral administration in prolonged experiments. Part II. Investigation of subacute and chronic toxicity. Rocz. Panstw. Zakl. Hig. 22:292-307.

Piekacz, H. 1971b. The effect of dibutyl and dicotyl phthalates on rats during oral administration in prolonged experiments. Part III. Influence on reproduction and development of the fetus. Roczn. Panstw. Zakl. Hig. 22:519-526.

Pilapil, V.R. 1966. Hexachlorophene toxicity in an infant. Am. J. Dis. Child. 111:333-336.

Plaa, G.L., and R.E. Larson. 1965. Relative nephrotoxic properties of chlorinated methane, ethane, and ethylene derivatives in mice. Toxicol. Appl. Pharmacol. 7:37-44.

Plaa, G.L., E. A. Evans, and C.H. Hine. 1958. Relative hepatotoxicity of seven halogenated hydrocarbons. J. Pharmacol. Exp. Ther. 123:224-229.

Platonow, N.S., R.M. Liptrap, and H.D. Geissinger. 1972. The distribution and excretion of polychlorinated biphenyls (Aroclor 1254) and their effect on urinary gonadal steroid levels in the boar. Bull. Environ. Contan. Toxicol. 7:358-365.

Pliss, G.B. 1974. Carcinogenic properties of hydrazobenzene. Vop. Onkol. 20:53-57. (CA 81:46159t).

Plueckhahn, V.D. 1973. Infant antiseptic skin care and hexachlorophene. Med. J. Aust. 1:93-100.

Polushkin, B.V. 1964. K toksikologii i farmakologii kaprolaktama. Farmakol. Toksikol. Moskva 2:234. Abstr. in Food Cosmet. Toxicol. 2:754.

Pound, A.W., L. Horn, and T. A. Lawson. 1973. Decreased toxicity of dimethylnitrosamine in rats after treatment with carbon tetrachloride. Pathology 5:233-242.

Powers, M., W.B. Coate, and T.R. Lewis. 1975. Repeated topical applications of 1,2,4-trichlorobenzene: Effects on rabbit ears. Arch. Environ. Health 30:165-167.

Raleigh, R.L. 1974. Conversation and memorandum to Dr. Stanley C. Mazaleski.

Rannug, U., A. Johansson, C. Ramel, and C.A. Wachtmeister. 1974. The mutagenicity of vinyl chloride after metabolic activation. Ambio 3(5):194-97.

Recknagel, R.O. 1967. Carbon tetrachloride hepatotoxicity. Pharmacol. Rev. 19:145-208.

Redford-Ellis, M., and A.H. Gowenlock. 1971a. Studies on the reaction of chloromethane with human blood. Acta. Pharmacol. Toxicol. 30:36-48.

Redford-Ellis, M., and A.H. Gowenlock. 1971b. Studies on the reaction of chloromethane with preparations of liver, brain and kidney. Acta. Pharmacol. Toxicol. 30:49-58.

Reid, W.D., B. Christie, G. Krishna, J.R. Mitchell, J. Moskowitz, and B.B. Brodie. 1971. Bromobenzene metabolism and hepatic necrosis. Pharmacology 6:41-55.

Reid, W.D. 1973. Mechanism of renal necrosis induced by bromobenzene or chlorobenzene. Exp. Mol. Pathol. 19:197-214.

Reuber, M.D., and E.L. Glover. 1967. Cholangiofibrosis in the liver of Buffalo strain rats injected with carbon tetrachtrachloride. Br. J. Exp. Pathol. 48:319-322.

Reynolds, E.S., and A.G. Yee. 1968. Liver parenchymal cell injury. VI. Significance of early glucose 6-phosphatase suppression and transient calcium influx following poisoning. Lab. Invest. 19:273-281.

Rietbrock, N., and U. Abshagen. 1971. Pharmakokinetik und stoffwechsel aliphatischer alkohole. Arzneim.-Forsch. 21(9):1309-1319.

Rigdon, R.H., and E.G. Rennels. 1964. Effect of feeding Benz[*a*]pyrene on reproduction in the rat. Experientia 20:224-226.

Rigdon, R.H., and J. Neal. 1966. Gastric carcinomas, and pulmonary adenomas in mice fed benzo(*a*)pyrene. Tex. Rep. Biol. Med. 24:195-207.

Rigdon, R.H., and J. Neal. 1969. Relationship of leukemia to lung and stomach tumors in mice fed benzo(*a*)pyrene. Proc. Soc. Exp. Bio. Med. 130:146-148.

Ringer, R.K., R.J. Aulerich, and M. Zabik. 1972. Effect of dietary polychlorinated biphenyls on growth and reproduction of mink. *In* Proceedings American Chemical Society Meeting (164th A.C.S. Meeting, New York), vol. 12, pp. 149-154.

Roe, F.J.C. 1976. Unpublished report. Preliminary report of long-term tests of chloroform in rats, mice and dogs.

Rowe, V.K., D.D. McCollister, H.C. Spencer, E.M. Adams, and D.D. Irish. 1952. Vapor toxicity of tetrachloroethylene for laboratory animals and human subjects. Arch. Ind. Hyg. Occup. Med. 5:566-579.

Rozewicki, S., S. Stanosz, and L. Samochowiec. 1973. Effect of chronic poisoning with carbon disulfide on the hormonal activity in rat ovaries. Med. Pr. 24(2):133-139 (in Polish).

Sagawa, K., H. Nishitani, H. Kawai, Y. Kuge, and M. Ikeda. 1973. Transverse lesion of spinal cord after accidental exposure to trichloroethylene. Int. Arch. Arbeitsmed. 31: 257-264.

Salnikova, L.S., and E.M. Chirkova. 1974. Gonadotropic and embryotropic effect of carbon disulphide. Gig. Tr. Prof. Zabol. (12):34-37 (in Russian).

Schaffarzick, R.W., and B.J. Brown. 1952. Anticonvulsant activity and toxicity of methylparafynol (Dormison) and some other alcohols. Science 116:663-665.

Scheiman, M.A., R.A. Saunders, and F.E. Saafeld. 1974. Organic contaminants in the District of Columbia water supply. J. Biomed. Mass. Spectrom. 1:209-211.

Schrenk, H.H., F.A. Patty, and W.P. Yant. 1933. Acute response of guinea pigs to vapors of some new commercial organic compounds. VII. Dichloroethylether. Public Health Rep. 48:1389-1398.

Schulz, C.O., and R.J. Rubin. 1973. Distribution, metabolism and excretion of di-2-ethylhexylphthalate in the rat. Environ. Health Perspect. 3:123-129.

Schwetz, B.A., P.A. Keeler, and P.J. Gehring. 1974. The effect of purified and commercial grade pentachlorophenol on rat embryonal and fetal development. Toxicol. Appl. Pharmacol. 28:151-161.

Schwetz, B.A., B.K.J. Leong, and P.J. Gehring. 1975. The effect of maternally inhaled trichloroethylene, perchloroethylene, methyl chloroform, and methylene chloride on embryonal and fetal development in mice and rats. Toxicol. Appl. Pharmacol. 32: 84-96.

Shaffer, C.B., C.P. Carpenter, and H.F. Smyth, Jr. 1945. Acute and subacute toxicity of di(2-ethylhexyl)phthalate with note upon its metabolism. J. Ind. Hyg. Toxicol. 27:130-135.

Shamilov, T.A. 1970. Toxicity characteristics and hazards of bromobenzene. Gig. Tr. Prof. Zabol. 13(9):56-8 (abstract only). (CA 72: #35489e, 1970)

Shibko, S,I., and H. Blumenthal. 1973. Toxicology of phthalic acid esters used in food-packaging materials. Environ. Health Perspectives 3:131-137.

Shubik, P., and J.L. Hartwell. 1969. Survey of compounds which have been tested for carcinogenic activity. Suppl. no. 2, HEW, Public Health Service. PHS Publ. no. 149.

Shubik, P., G. Pietra, and G. Della Porta. 1960. Studies of skin carcinogenesis in the Syrian golden hamster. Cancer Res. 20:100-105.

Shuman, R.M., R.W. Leech, and E.C. Alvord, Jr. 1974. Neurotoxicity of hexachlorophene in the human. I. A clinicopathologic study of 248 children. Pediatrics 54:689-695.

Silverman, L., H.F. Schulte, and M.W. First. 1946. Further studies on sensory response to certain industrial solvent vapors. J. Ind. Hyg. Toxicol. 28:262-266.

Simmon, V.F. and D.C. Poole. 1976. *In vitro* microbiological mutagenicity studies of eight compounds. Interim Report, April 1.

Sims, P. 1967. The metabolism of benzo(*a*)pyrene by rat-liver homogenates. Biochem. Pharmacol. 16:613-618.

Sims, P. 1970a. Qualitative and quantitative studies on the metabolism of a series of aromatic hydrocarbons by rat liver preparations. Biochem. Pharmacol. 19:795-818.

Sims, P. 1970b. The metabolism of some aromatic hydrocarbons by mouse embryo cell cultures. Biochem. Pharmacol. 19:285-297.

Singh, A.R., W.H. Lawrence, and J. Autian. 1972. Embryonic-fetal toxicity and teratogenic effects of a group of methacrylate esters in rats. J. Dent. Res. 51:1632-1638.

Singh, A.R., W.H. Lawrence, and J. Autian 1972a. Teratogenicity of phthalate esters in rats. J. Pharm. Sci. 61:51-55.

Singh, A.R., W.H. Lawrence, and J. Autian. 1974. Mutagenic and antifertility sensitivities of mice to di-2-ethylhexyl phthalate (DEHP) and dimethoxyethyl phthalate (DMEP). Toxicol. Appl. Pharmacol. 29:35-46.

Sipes, I.G., P.L. Gigon, and G. Krishna. 1974. Biliary excretion of metabolites of bromobenzene. Biochem. Pharmacol. 23(2):451-455.

Skog, Erik. 1950. A toxicological investigation of lower aliphatic aldehydes. I. Toxicity of formaldehyde, acetaldehyde, propionaldehyde and butyraldehyde as well as of acrolein and crotonaldehyde. Acta Pharmacol. Toxicol. 6:299-318.

Slater, T.F. 1965. A note on the relative toxic activities of tetrachloromethane and trichloro-fluoro-methane on the rat. Biochem. Pharmacol. 14:178-180.

Smirnova, R.D., and I.M. Stepanova. 1969. Experimental determinations of the maximum permissible concentration of propylbenzene in water bodies. USSR Literature on Water Supply and Pollution Control—A Survey, by B. S. Levine. Clearinghouse for Federal Scientific and Technical Information. U.S. Department of Commerce 10:122-128.

Smirnova, N.A., and N.P. Granik. 1970. Long-term side effects of acute occupational poisoning by certain hydrocarbons and their derivatives. Gig. Tr. Prof. Zabol. 14(5):50-51.

Smith, C.C. 1953. Toxicity of butyl stearate, dibutyl sebacate, butyl phthalate and methoxyethyl oleate. Arch. Ind. Hyg. Occup. Med. 7:310-318.

Smith, W.W., and W.F. von Oettingen. 1947b. The acute and chronic toxicity of methyl chloride. II. Symptomatology of animals poisoned by methyl chloride. J. Ind. Hyg. Toxicol. 29:123-128.

Smith, W.W., and W.F. von Oettingen. 1947a. The acute and chronic toxicity of methyl chloride. I. Mortality resulting resulting from exposures to methyl chloride in concentrations of 4,000 to 300 parts per million. J. Ind. Hyg. Toxicol. 29:47-52.

Smolik, R., G.K. Grzbek-Hryncewicz, A. Lange, and W. Zatonski. 1973. Serum complement level in workers exposed to benzene, toluene and xylene. Int. Arch. Arbeitsmed. 31:243-247.

Smyth, H.F., and H.F. Smyth, Jr. 1928. Inhalation experiments with certain lacquer solvents. J. Ind. Hyg. 10:261-71.

Smyth, H.F., Jr., and C.P. Carpenter. 1948. Further experience with the range finding test in the industrial toxicology laboratory. J. Ind. Hyg. Toxicol. 30:63-68.

Smyth, H.F., Jr., C.P. Carpenter, and C.S. Weil. 1951. Range finding toxicity data. List IV. Arch. Ind. Hyg. Occup. Med. 4:119-122.

Smyth, H.F., Jr., C.P. Carpenter, C.S. Weil, U.C. Pozzani, J.A. Striegel, and J.C. Nycum. 1969. Range-finding toxicity data: VII. Am. Ind. Hyg. Assoc. J. 30:470-476.

Snyder, R., and J.J. Kocsis. 1975. Current concepts of chronic benzene toxicity. CRC Crit. Rev. Toxicol. 3:265-288.

Soucek, B. 1961. Retention and excretion of methyl chloride and other chlorides of methane in mice. Folia Med. 44:219-226.

Spealman, R.J., R.J. Main, H.B. Haag, and P.S. Larson. 1945. Monomeric methyl methacrylate: Studies on toxicity. Ind. Med. 14:292-298.

Speck, B., and S. Moeschlin. 1968. The Effect of toluene, xylene, chloramphenicol and thiouracil on bone marrow — Experimental autoradiographic studies with 3H-thymidine. Schweiz Med. Wochenschr. 98:1684-1686.

Spector, W.S., ed. 1956. Handbook of Toxicology. Vol. I: Acute Toxicities of Solids, Liquids, and Gases to Laboratory Animals. Saunders, Philadelphia.

Spencer, H.C., D.D. Irish, E.M. Adams, and V.K. Rowe. 1942. The response of laboratory animals to monomeric styrene. J. Ind. Hyg. Toxicol. 24:295-301.

Spencer, H.C., V.K. Rowe, E.M. Adams, D.D. McCollister, and D.D. Irish. 1951. Vapor toxicity of ethylene dichloride determined by experiments on laboratory animals. Arch. Ind. Hyg. Occup. Med. 4:482-493.

Statsek, N.K., S.E. Yalkut, E.F. Gor-achevskaya, and D.V. Zinchenko. 1974. Experimental study of the allergic effect of caprolactam. Gig. Tr. Prof. Zabol. 18:54-55.

Stefano, B., and P. Quirico. 1939. The pharmacological action of guaiacol. Arch Farmacol. Sper. 67:190-206.

Stenback, F. 1975. Hexachlorophene in mice: Effects after long-term percutaneous applications. Arch. Environ. Health 30:32-35.

Stewart, R.D., H.C. Dodd, E.D. Baretta, and A.W. Schaffer. 1968. Human exposure to styrene vapor. Arch. Environ. Health 16:656-662.

Stewart, R.D., E.A. Boettner, R.R. Southworth, and J.C. Cerny. 1963. Acute carbon tetrachloride intoxication. J. Am. Med. Assoc. 183:994-997.

Stofen, D. 1973. The maximum permissible concentrations in the U.S.S.R. for harmful substances in drinking water. Toxicology 1:187-195.

Stohlman, E.F. 1951. The toxicity of some related halogenated derivatives of phenol. Public Health Rep. 66:1303-1312.

Stokinger, H.E., and R.L. Woodward. 1958. Toxicologic methods for establishing drinking-water standards. J. Am. Water Works Assoc. 50:515-529.

Svirbely, J.L., R.C. Dunn, and W.F. vonOettingen. 1943. The acute toxicity of vapors of certain solvents containing appreciable amounts of benzene and toluene. J. Ind. Hyg. Toxicol. 25:366-373.

Swartz, L., and L. Tulipan. 1939. A Textbook of Occupational Diseases of the Skin. Lea and Febiger, Philadelphia.

Tabakova, S.A. 1969. Experimental data for hygienic standards for dipterex. Hyg. Sanit. 34(10-12):187-193.

Takeuchi, Y. 1969. Experimental studies on the toluene poisoning—chiefly on the findings of peripheral blood and adrenal gland. Ind. Health 7:31-45.

Taylor, J.M., P.M. Jenner, and W.I. Jones. 1964. A comparison of the toxicity of some allyl, propenyl, and propyl compounds in the rat. Toxicol. Appl. Pharmacol. 6:378-387.

Tedeschi, E.G., and A. DeCicco. 1954. The antivitamin E action of thymol, curvacrol, and guaiacol. Boll. Soc. Ital. Biol. Sper. 30:727-729.

Teisinger, J. 1974. New advances in the toxicology of carbon disulfide. Am. Ind. Hyg. Assoc. J. 35(2):55-6l.

Thiemes, C. H., and T. J. Haley. 1972. Clinical Toxicology. Lea and Febiger, Philadelphia. p. 126.

Thompson, D.J., S.D. Warner, and V.B. Robinson. 1974. Teratology studies on orally administered chloroform in the rat and rabbit. Toxicol. Appl. Pharmacol. 29:348-357.

Thorpe, E. 1967. Some pathological effects of hexachlorophene in the rat. J. Comp. Pathol. 77:137-142.

Thorpe, J.J. 1974. Epidemiologic survey of leukemia in persons potentially exposed to benzene. J. Occup. Med. 16:375-382.

Toxic Substances List. 1974. Christensen, H.E., T.T. Luginbyhl, and B.S. Carroll, eds. National Institute for Occupational Safety and Health. HEW Publication no. (NIOSH)74-134. U.S. Government Printing Office, Washington, D.C.

Traiger, G.J., and G.L. Plaa. 1974. Chlorinated hydrocarbon toxicity: potentiation by isopropyl alcohol and acetone. Arch. Environ. Health 28:276-278.

Traiger, G.J., and G.L. Plaa. 1971. Differences in the potentiation of carbon tetrachloride in rats by ethanol and isopropanol pretreatment. Toxicol. Appl. Pharmacol. 20:105-12.

Trout, M.E. 1973. Hexachlorophene in perspective. J. Clin. Pharmacol. 13:451-457.

Truhaut, R. 1973. Metabolic transformations of l,l,l,2-tetrachloroethane in the rat, guinea pig and rabbit. J. Eur. Toxicol. 6:2ll-217.

Truhaut, R., N.P. Lich, H. Duterte-Catella, G. Molas, and V.N. Yuen. 1974. Contribution to the toxicological study of tetrachloro-1,1,1,2-ethane. Arch. Mal. Prof. 35:593-608.

Tucker, R.K., and D.G. Crabtree. 1970. Handbook of Toxicity of Pesticides to Wildlife. U.S. Department of the Interior, Bureau of Sport Fisheries and Wildlife. Resource Pub. 84, Washington, D.C.

Tugarinova, V.I., V.E. Miklashevskii, N.P. Alekseeva, and G.P. Yakovleva. (n.d.). Experimental determination of limits of allowable tetrachlorethane (TCLE) and hexachlorethane (HCLE) concentrations in water. USSR Lit. on Water Supply Pollut. Control. 5:145-154.

U.S. Department of Labor. 1972. Occupational Safety and Health Administration. Occupational safety and health standards. Fed. Reg. 37:22101-22356.

U.S. International Trade Commission. 1975. Synthetic Organic Chemicals. U.S. Production and Sales.

Udall, V., and J.C. Malone. 1970. Optic nerve atrophy after drug treatment. Proc. Eur. Soc. Study Drug Toxicity XI, pp. 244-248.

Ulland, B., E.K. Weisburger, and J.H. Weisburger. 1973. Chronic toxicity and carcinogenicity of industrial chemicals and pesticides. Abstract of Paper Presented at Twelfth Annual Meeting of the Society of Toxicology. Toxicol. Appl. Pharmacol. 25:446.

Uzhdovini, E.R., I.K. Astaf'eva, and A.A. Mamaeva. 1974. Acute toxicity of lower phenols. Gig. Tr. Prof. Zabol. (2):58-59 (in Russian CA 81:418q)

USEPA. 1972. Region VI Surveillance and Analysis Division, "Industrial Pollution of the Lower Miss. River in Louisiana."

USEPA. 1974. Draft Analytical Report New Orleans Area Water Supply Study. Surveillance and Analysis Division, Region VI, Dallas, Tex. EPA-906/10-74-002.

USEPA Advisory Committee. 1975. Report: Assessment of health risk from organics in drinking water.

USEPA. 1975a. Preliminary assessment of suspected carcinogens in drinking water. Report to Congress, Washington, D.C. EPA-56014-75-005 PB. 260961.

USEPA. 1975b. Region V Joint Federal/State Survey of Organics and Inorganics in Selected Drinking Water Supplies.

USEPA. 1975c. Analysis of carbon and resin extracts. New Orleans Area Water Supply Study. Analysis of Carbon and Resin Extracts.

USEPA. 1975d. Identification of Organic Compounds in Effluents from Industrial Sources.

USEPA. 1976. Organic Compounds Identified in Drinking Water in the U.S. Health Effects Research Laboratory, Cincinnati, Ohio.

USHEW. 1973. PHS. National Institute for Occupational Safety and Health Criteria for Recommended Standard, Occupational Exposure to Toluene, V. 99 pp. ITS Publ. HSM 73-11023.

Van Poznak, A. 1974. Biotransformation of diethyl ether ad chloroform. Int. Anesthesiol. Clin. 12:35-40.

Vanderhoek, J.Y., and W.E.M. Lands. 1973. The inhibition of the fatty acid oxygenase of sheep vesicular gland by antioxidants. Biochim. Biophys Acta. 296(2):382-385.

VanDuuren, B.L., C. Katz, B.M. Goldschmidt, K. Frenkel, and A. Sivak. 1972. Carcinogenicity of halo-ethers. II. Structure-activity relationships of analogs of bis(chloromethyl)ether. J. Nat. Cancer Inst. 48:1431-1439.

Varshavskaya, S.P. 1968. Comparative toxicological characteristics of chlorobenzene and dichlorobenzene (ortho-and para-isomers) in relation to the sanitary protection of water bodies. Hyg. Sanit. 33 (10-12): 17-23.

Vaterlaus, B.P., and J.J. Hostynek. 1972. The tolerance of hexachlorophene. Givaudan-Eskolko A.G. Comp., Zurich, Switzerland, p. 17.

Vinogradov, P.B. 1966. Experimental determination of the maximum permissible concentration of carbon disulfide in reservoirs. Gig. Sanit. 31(1):13-8.

Viola, P.A. 1970a. Pathology of vinyl chloride. Med. Lavoro 61:174-180.

Viola, P.L. 1970b. Cancerogenic effect of vinyl chloride. Abstr. Tenth Int. Cancer Conf., Houston, Tex. 56:742 Abstr. no. 29.

Viola, P.L., A. Bigotti, and A. Caputo. 1971. Oncogenic response of rat skin, lungs, and bones to vinyl chloride. Cancer Res. 31:516-522.

Vogel, E., and J.L.R. Chandler. 1974. Mutagenicity testing of cyclamate and some pesticides in *Drosphila melanogaster.* Experientia 30:621-623.

Wallace, C.J. 1959. Hepatitis and nephrosis due to cough syrup containing chloroform. Calif. Med. 73:442.

Wallgren, H. 1960. Relative intoxicating effects on rats of ethyl, propyl, and butyl alcohols. Acta Pharmacol. Toxicol. 16:217-22.

Ward, J.M., J.H. Weisburger, R.S. Yamamoto, T. Benjamin, C.A. Brown, and E.K. Weisburger. 1975. Long term effect of benzene in C57BL/6N mice. Arch. Environ. Health 30:22-25.

Watanabe, P.G., G.R. McGowan, P.J. Gehring. 1976. Fate of [^{14}C]-vinyl chloride after single oral administration in rats. Toxicol. Appl. Pharmacol. 36:339-352.

Watanabe, P.G., G.R. McGowan, E.O. Madrid, and P.J. Gehring. 1976. Fate of [^{14}]-vinyl chloride following inhalation exposure in rats. Toxicol. Appl. Pharmacol. 37:49-59.

Watrous, W.M., and G.L. Plaa. 1972. The nephrotoxicity of single and multiple doses of aliphatic chlorinated hydrocarbon solvents in male mice. Toxicol. Appl. Pharmacol. 23:640-649.

Wear, J.B. Jr., R. Shanahan, and R.K. Ratliff. 1962. Toxicity of ingested hexachlorophene. J. Am. Med. Assoc. 181:587-89.

Williams, D.T., and B.J. Blanchfield. 1975. The retention, distribution, excretion and metabolism of dibutyl phthalate-7-^{14}C in the rat. J. Agric. Food Chem. 23:854-858.

Williams, D.T., and B.J. Blanchfield. 1974. Retention, excretion and metabolism of di(2-ethylhexyl)phthalate administered orally to the rat. Bull. Environ. Contam. Toxicol. 11:371-378.

Williams, R.T. 1959. Detoxication Mechanisms. John Wiley & Sons, Inc. New York.

Wilson, R.H., and F. DeEds. 1936a. Chronic nicotine toxicity. I. Feeding of nicotine sulfate, tannate and bentonite. J. Ind. Hyg. Toxicol. 18:553-564.

Wilson, R.H., and F. DeEds. 1936b. II. Effect of nicotine-containing diets on the blood sugar concentration of the albino rat. J. Ind. Hyg. Toxicol. 18:565-570.

Wirtschafter, Z.T., and E.D. Schwartz. 1939. Acute ethylene dichloride poisoning. J. Ind. Hyg. Toxicol. 21:126-131.

Wit, J.G., and H. van Genderen. 1962. Some aspects of the fate of hexachlorophene (2,2'methylene bis (3,4,6-trichlorophenol) in rabbits, rats and dairy cattle. Acta Physiol. Pharmacol. Neer. 11:123-132.

Wolf, M.A., V.K. Rowe, D.D. McCollister, R.L. Hollingsworth, and F. Oyen. 1956. Toxicological studies of certain alkylated benzenes and benzene: experiments on laboratory animals. Arch. Ind. Health 14:387-398.

World Health Organization. 1973. International Agency for Research on Cancer. IARC Monographs on the Evaluation of Carcinogenic Risk of Chemicals to Man, vol. 3. International Agency for Research on Cancer, Lyon.

World Health Organization. 1972. IARC Monograph on the Evaluation of Carcinogenic Risks of Chemicals to Man, vol. I, pp. 53-65.

Wynder, E.L., L. Fritz, and N. Furth. 1957. Effect of concentration of benzopyrene in skin carcinogenesis. J. Nat. Cancer Inst. 19:361-370.

Yant, W.P., H.W. Shoaf, and J. Chronyak. 1930. Observations on possibility of methyl chloride poisoning by ingestion with food and water. Public Health Rep. 45: 1057-1065.

Yllner, S. 1971a. Metabolism of 1,1,1,2-tetrachloroethane in the mouse. Acta. Pharmacol. Toxicol. 29:471-480.

Yllner, S. 1971b. Metabolism of 1,1,3,2-tetrachloroethane-^{14}C in the mouse. Acta. Pharmacol. Toxicol. 29:499-512.

Yllner, S. 1971c. Metabolism of 1,1,2-trichloroethane-1,2-^{14}C in the mouse. Acta. Pharmacol. Toxicol. 30:248-256.

Yllner, S. 1971d. Metabolism of 1,2-dichloroethane-^{14}C in the mouse. Acta. Pharmacol. Toxicol. 30:257-265.

Yllner, S. 1961. Urinary metabolites of ^{14}C-tetrachloroethylene in mice. Nature 191:820.

Yodaiken, R.E., and J.R. Babcock. 1973. 1,2-Dichloroethane poisoning. Arch. Environ. Health 26:281-284.

Yudeles, A.L., and R.V. Bessarabova. 1955. Antidote effects against experimental carbon disulfide poisoning. Farmikol. Toksikol. 18(3):50-52.

VII

Radioactivity In Drinking Water

Since it was discovered that ionizing radiation produces detrimental biological effects, many national and international groups have studied the sources and levels of radiation to which the human population is exposed, and have estimated the corresponding biological effects. Some of these groups have also been responsible for establishing permissible levels of exposure. Consequently, there is a large body of information on the biological effects of ionizing radiation. The Subcommittee on Radioactivity in Drinking Water has relied heavily on the reports of those other groups and has abstracted and summarized pertinent sections. In some cases it was possible to take new published and unpublished information into account in this assessment of the probable effects of the radioactivity in drinking water on the population of the United States.

Among the groups whose reports were used were: the National Academy of Sciences Advisory Committee on the Biological Effects of Ionizing Radiation (BEIR), the United Nations Scientific Committee on the Effects of Atomic Radiation (UNSCEAR), the International Commission on Radiological Protection (ICRP), and the National Council on Radiation Protection and Measurements (NCRP).

BACKGROUND RADIATION

The natural ionizing radiation, to which all people are exposed, includes cosmic rays and products of the decay of radioactive elements in the

TABLE VII-1 Estimated Total Annual Whole-Body Doses from Natural Radiation in the United States (from BEIR Committee, 1972)

Source	Annual Doses, mrem
Cosmic rays	44
Terrestrial radiation	
External	40
Internal	18
Total	102

earth's crust and atmosphere. Part of the terrestrial radiation dose is from sources external to the body, and part is due to the inhalation and ingestion of radioactive elements in air, food, and water. In the United States, this unavoidable background radiation gives, on the average, an annual dose of about 100 mrem to the population (Table VII-1). There is, however, great variability in the amount of background radiation, which depends on regional geological characteristics and altitude. It has been found, for example, that the annual background dose in Colorado is 100 mrem (or more) higher than that in Louisiana (BEIR Committee, 1972). Mankind has always lived with such radiation, to which, however, the radionuclides in drinking water contribute but a small share.

ABUNDANCE OF RADIONUCLIDES IN WATER

Minute traces of radioactivity are normally found in all drinking water. The concentration and composition of these radioactive constituents vary from place to place, depending principally on the radiochemical composition of the soil and rock strata through which the raw water may have passed.

Many natural and artificial radionuclides have been found in water, but most of the radioactivity is due to a relatively small number of nuclides and their decay products. Among these are the following emitters of radiation of low linear energy transfer (LET): potassium-40 (^{40}K), tritium (^{3}H), carbon-14 (^{14}C), and rubidium-87 (^{87}Rb). In addition, high-LET, alpha-emitting radionuclides, such as radium-226 (^{226}Ra), the daughters of radium-228 (^{228}Ra), polonium-210 (^{210}Po), uranium (U), thorium (Th), radon-220 (^{220}Rn), and radon-222 (^{222}Rn), may also be present in varying amounts.

Natural Radionuclides

SOURCES OF LOW-LET RADIATION

Some of the radionuclides that are responsible for the natural radioactivity in drinking water come from radioactive elements, and their decay products, that were incorporated in the earth at its formation, and others are produced continuously by cosmic ray bombardment. Tritium is produced by cosmic ray interactions with atmospheric oxygen and nitrogen. It is then oxidized to tritiated water, which mixes into the hydrosphere. Tritium concentrations in water supplies vary from about 10 to 25 pCi/liter (Jacobs, 1968).

In similar fashion, carbon-14, produced by cosmic ray [$^{14}N(n,p)^{14}C$] interactions with atmospheric nitrogen (UNSCEAR, 1972, p. 29), is oxidized to $^{14}CO_2$, which is generally found at a concentration corresponding to about 6 pCi ^{14}C per gram of carbon. In water containing about 1 mg of carbon per liter, a concentration of 0.006 pCi/liter might be expected. In ocean water, the concentration might be about 0.1 pCi/liter (NCRP, 1975, p. 35).

Of all the natural radionuclides that occur in water and emit low-LET radiation, potassium-40 is likely to be the most significant. This primordial radionuclide occurs as a constant percentage (0.0118%) of total potassium. Adults in the United States ingest about 2,300 pCi of potassium-40 per day, but almost all of it is derived from foodstuffs. Since potassium concentrations in man seem to be under homeostatic control, wide fluctuations in drinking-water potassium would have negligible effects on internal concentrations. Assuming that there is 0.2% potassium in soft tissue, a dose rate of 19 mrad per year has been estimated; of this, 17 mrad are due to beta radiation (UNSCEAR, 1972, p. 30). In 1970, some California drinking water, for example, contained up to 4 pCi/liter of potassium-40. Consumption of 2 liters per day of such water might contribute as much as 8 pCi per day, but this is a negligible fraction of the total daily intake of 2,300 pCi of a nuclide that is the largest natural contributor to total body somatic and genetic dose.

SOURCES OF HIGH-LET RADIATION

Radionuclides that are produced by the decay of uranium-238 and thorium-232 are widely distributed throughout the earth's crust. The majority of them are alpha-emitters and include isotopes of polonium, radon, and radium (UNSCEAR, 1972, p. 31). Concentrations of uranium in drinking water are extremely variable, apparently ranging from 0.02 to

200 μg/liter in fresh waters. The thorium content of drinking water has not been extensively measured, but its concentration in the human skeleton is about 1 fCi/g of ash; the corresponding abundance of uranium in the skeleton is about 10 times greater.

The natural alpha-emitters that occur in drinking water appear to be bone seekers. Of these, radium-226 and its daughters and the daughters of radium-228 probably have the greatest potential for producing radiation doses of some consequence to man. The radium-226 content of fresh surface water is variable, ranging from 0.01 to about 0.1 pCi/liter. Some groundwater may contain up to 100 pCi/liter. Drinking water obtained from surface supplies generally does not contain significant amounts of radium, and treatment processes, such as flocculation and water-softening, can remove the bulk of radium from water.

In the Midwest of the United States there is an area where groundwaters contain significant levels of radium-226 and radium-228. This area—primarily in Iowa, Illinois, Wisconsin, and Missouri—includes an estimated population (1960 census) of approximately 1 million persons. The weighted mean concentration of radium-226 has been estimated to be approximately 5 pCi/liter (Peterson *et al.*, 1966). Rowland, Lucas, and Stehney (1975) have reported that approximately 500,000 people in Illinois and Iowa have drinking water supplies whose radium-226 content is 3–6 pCi/liter; about 300,000 people, 6–9 pCi/liter; and about 120,000 people live in areas where well water contains 9–80 pCi/liter of radium-226. A personal communication (Rowland, Lucas, and Stehney, 1976) from the same investigators stated that, of the last group, 113,000 people drink water that contains less than 20 pCi/liter, and 5,700, 20-25 pCi/liter. The one community (1,200 persons) that had a well in which 80 pCi/liter of radium-226 was found, now uses water from a well containing only 3 pCi/liter.

In addition, a survey in 1966 that was designed to locate water supplies with high concentrations of radium found water supplies with more than 3 pCi of radium-226 per liter in areas other than those of the northern Midwest described above (Hickey and Campbell, 1968). These supplies served approximately 145,000 people. Thus, it appears that in the entire United States approximately 1.1 million people consume water that contains more than 3 pCi/liter of radium-226.

The major additional contribution to the alpha-emissions in drinking water is due to the decay of radium-228; although other alpha-emitting natural radionuclides have been found in drinking water, they occur in exceedingly small concentrations. For example, one analysis of water containing 5 pCi of radium-228 per liter was found to contain less than

0.02 pCi/liter of thorium isotopes and only 0.03 pCi/liter of uranium (Stehney, 1960).

Two other radium isotopes may be present in drinking water, but although both radium-223 and radium-224 may contribute to the gross alpha activity of water measured soon after drawing from the tap, their contributions to the long-term dose deposited in the skeleton are negligible because they have short half-lives. However, radium-228, which decays by beta emission, and therefore does not contribute to gross alpha activity in drinking water, will, as a result of its subsequent decay scheme, give rise to a series of alpha-emitting daughter products. It is these radium-228 daughter products, and radium-226 and its daughters, that produce, in our opinion, the major alpha-particle dose to the tissues of the body, particularly to the skeleton. Thus, when discussing radium in drinking water, it is essential to distinguish between the isotopic mixture measured in freshly drawn drinking water and the long-term alpha dose that might be accumulated in tissue.

Because of the different decay schemes for radium-226 and radium-228, different alpha doses are received under equilibrium conditions from each of these two radium isotopes. In waters of low alpha-particle radioactivity, the activity concentration of radium-228 is generally equal to that of radium-226, whereas at high radioactivity concentrations it is only half that of radium-226 (Lucas and Krause, 1960).

The abundance of the radioactive gas radon-222, which is formed by the decay of radium-226, is not highly correlated with the radium concentration in fresh water. Radon concentration is generally 1 pCi/liter in surface water, but activity concentrations in groundwater are typically a few thousand times greater. Some mineral or spa waters, however, may contain 500,000 pCi/liter.

Consumption of water containing 1 μCi of radon-222 will result in a stomach dose of about 20 mrads, but the doses to other organs will be lower by at least a factor of 10 (UNSCEAR 1975, p. 35). Furthermore, consumption of 2 liters per day of water containing 1 nCi/liter of radon-222 would deliver an annual stomach dose of about 12 mrad.

In three large American cities, the total daily intake of uranium, radium-226, radium-228, and lead-210 in water have all been quoted to range approximately between 0.01 and 0.05 pCi/day (NCRP, 1975, p. 92). When compared with other components of the diet, drinking water usually contributes less than about 2% of these alpha-emitting radionuclides to the daily dietary intake (NAS-NRC, 1973). The greatest dose potential from alpha-radiation from naturally occurring radionuclides in drinking water will be related to the ingestion of radium-226 in areas where its concentration is high.

Artificial Radionuclides

To some extent, all drinking water obtained from surface sources will reflect contamination from atmospheric testing of nuclear weapons. Extensive measurements have been made of the contribution of airborne fission products to drinking water contamination and in particular to the levels that were produced by testing weapons before the Nuclear Test Ban Treaty of 1963. The sharp decrease in radioactive fallout since that date has been followed by a corresponding decrease in the radioactivity of surface water. Although the analyses are not very extensive, the temporal characteristics provide some information that is useful in predicting the transport and fate of radionuclides in water. Some of the longer-lived radionuclides still persist from early tests, together with smaller quantities of fission products injected irregularly into the atmosphere from the testing of weapons by nontreaty nations.

Many of the states conduct periodic surveys of the radioactivity of drinking water. Unfortunately, these consist, for the most part, in counting only the gross beta and gross alpha activity in the water. In addition, there is a considerable body of data on the temporal patterns and regional concentrations of the fission products strontium-90 and cesium-137, the physical half-lives of which are about 30 yr.

There appears to be a fairly good correlation between the measurement of solids in finished water and radioactivity content measured as beta activity (Figure VII-1). It is likely that potassium-40 in soil suspensions might account for such an observation. Because they account for a major part of the potential dose from nuclear fission and activation products, and because of their biological significance, considerable attention has been devoted to strontium-90, cesium-137, iodine-131, tritium, and carbon-14 as potential water contaminants. These, however, are not necessarily correlated with the solids content of drinking water.

Sources of man-made radionuclides, in addition to atmospheric weapons tests, include local discharge of radiopharmaceuticals and the possible entry of radioactivity into watersheds from the use and processing of nuclear fuel to produce electric power.

RADIOPHARMACEUTICALS

The release of radioactive materials in the exhaust air and liquid wastes from medical institutions has been studied many times in different locales. No evidence yet suggests a drinking-water hazard from medical effluents. This conclusion is based on data collected in many surveys

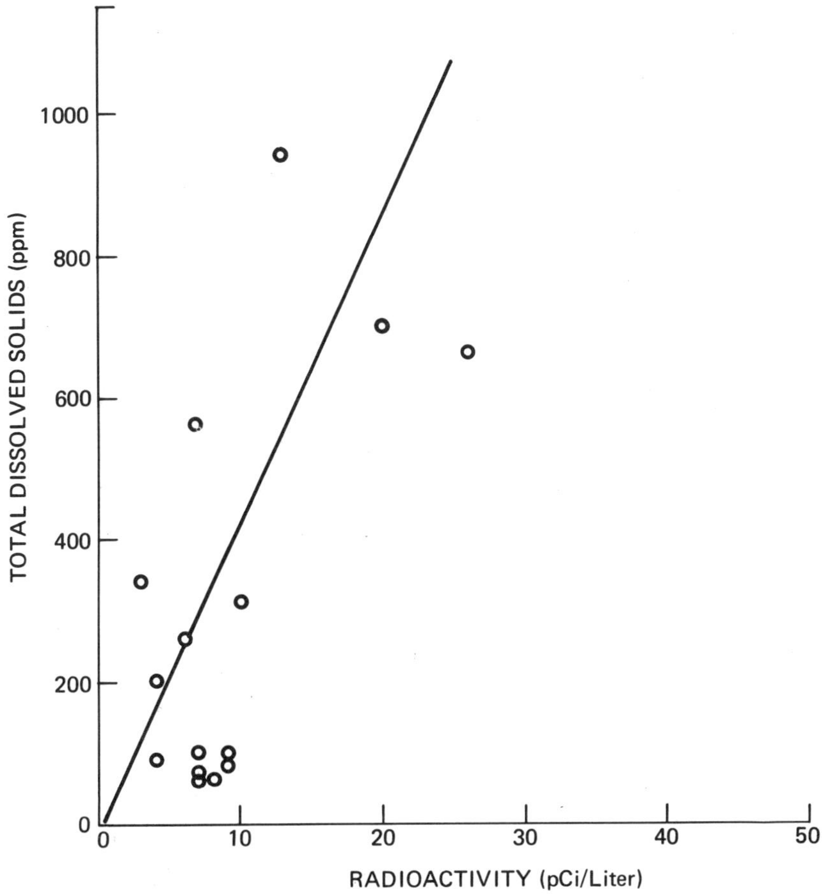

FIGURE VII-1 Relationship between total dissolved solids and radioactivity of California domestic water. Goldberg (1976).

(Sodd *et al.*, 1975; Gesell *et al.*, 1975; Klement *et al.*, 1972; Kaul and Loose, 1975). The agents to which particular attention was given in these surveys were radioactive iodine and technetium-99m. Both are widely used in medical practice, and there is special concern over the iodine isotopes, because of their potential effects on the thyroid gland.

Since 1950, eight groups have reported on the extent of release of radioisotopes in areas of the United States where there were active clinical nuclear medicine programs. Because of recent rapid increases in the numbers and kinds of procedures being conducted, Sodd *et al.* (1975) studied the use and discharge of iodine-125, iodine-131, and technetium-99m in the Cincinnati area. They measured the radioactivity from these nuclides in the influent, effluent, and sludge at the sewage-treatment plant, as well as the activity in the Ohio River 10 miles above and 5 miles below the plant. Gesell *et al.* (1975) conducted a similar survey of medical usage and concentrations in sewage of iodine-131 and technetium-99m in the Houston area. The general conclusions reached by both groups indicated that the effect on levels of radioactivity in drinking water of the medical usage of radioisotopes that they studied appears to be of negligible importance.

The Cincinnati study was centered about the largest sewage treatment plant serving that city. This plant receives the effluent from 10 hospitals that use radionuclides in clinical nuclear medicine. Approximately 60% of the patients were outpatients, so control of biological wastes was not attempted. Radioactivity in the sludge accumulated at the plant exceeded that in the water. Sludge concentrations of iodine-131 and technetium-99m were measurable, but that of iodine-125 was below the limit of detectability (10 pCi/liter).

It was estimated that between 10% and 30% of the total amount of technetium-99m given to patients in Cincinnati hospitals was discharged in sewage effluent into the Ohio River. Typically, about 300 mCi/week of this nuclide were estimated to reach the river, where dilution with river water was calculated to give concentrations downstream of about 1 pCi/liter. In fact, analysis of river water showed identical values upstream and downstream of 3-4 ± 3 pCi/liter. These are lower, by a factor of about a million, than the current maximum permissible concentration (6 μCi/liter; NRC, 1976) of technetium-99m in water for the general population. Comparable results were obtained for iodine-131. Smaller amounts were used, and the concentrations in sludge and water were lower than those of technetium. No differences between upstream and downstream levels were detected. Under the assumption that the same dilution had occurred, the medical uses of iodine-131 in the area were calculated to produce a maximal increase in concentration in the river of about 0.3 pCi/liter. This value is about one thousandth of the current maximum permissible concentration of iodine-131 in water (300 pCi/liter; NRC, 1976) for the general population.

Thus, at present, given current rates of use, patterns of disposal, and radiation protection guidelines, many orders of magnitude separate the concentrations of radioactivity in drinking water due to medical uses of radioisotopes from conceivably hazardous levels. Projections of the rate of increase in use of radiopharmaceuticals have been made by the Environmental Protection Agency (Klement *et al.*, 1972). They estimate that there may be a 12-fold increase in the medical use of these agents by the year 2000, on the basis of the annual increments in whole-body radiation dose from the use of these agents in medicine. This represents a very small incursion, and probably will not be measurable.

NUCLEAR FUEL CYCLE ACTIVITIES

Among the major effluents from the use and processing of nuclear fuel are tritium, plutonium, and krypton. Of these, only tritium, which is released as a gas, and plutonium can possibly enter water supplies. The predominant form of plutonium release from nuclear power and processing plants is as an aerosol that will have little or no impact on drinking water. Although a single incident has occurred in which as much as 18,750 Ci of plutonium were released from liquid storage on a local basis, none apparently reached off-site water supplies (AEC, 1974, pp. 49-50). The usual rate of release from liquid storage at controlled sites is about 1 mCi/yr. Continuing improvement in methods of storage should further reduce this rate. Nevertheless, the adequacy of monitoring water supplies in the vicinity of nuclear facilities should be reviewed periodically.

Because of its exceedingly long half-life (1.7×10^7 yr), the possible consequences of the release of iodine-129 during nuclear fuel reprocessing were considered. This radionuclide has a specific activity of about 173 μCi/g. In a recent review, Soldat (1976) calculated that the maximal isotope ratios of $^{129}I:^{127}I$ would be about 10^{-6} in water near nuclear facilities. His calculations indicate that consumption of 2 liters/day of water containing iodine-129 at 1 pCi/liter deliver an annual thyroid dose of about 5 mrem to an adult and about 10 mrem to an infant. Peak activities in water have been reported to be about 0.01 pCi/liter, which would correspond to an annual thyroid dose of about 0.05 mrem to an adult.

RADIATION DOSE CALCULATIONS

Estimates of the radiation doses expected to be produced by radionuclides ingested in water were calculated by means of the methods and parameters given in NCRP Report 22 (NBS Handbook 69, 1963 revision) and ICRP Publication 2 (ICRP, 1959). To approximate the equilibrium levels that take into account build-up, retention, decay, and elimination of various radionuclides, annual doses were computed for the fiftieth year of constant intake of 1 pCi/year, and 2 liters per day of water containing 1 pCi/liter. These doses are presented in Table VII-2. At earlier times, the annual doses may be lower than those shown, and for a few long-lived radionuclides (e.g. ^{90}Sr, ^{226}Ra), they may never reach equilibrium, but the values in Table VII-2 are within 20% of the theoretical equilibrium levels. These values were obtained by using the NCRP and ICRP metabolic and dosimetric models for all radionuclides, except for the isotopes of the alkaline earth elements radium and strontium, which are discussed below.

ISOTOPES OF ALKALINE EARTH ELEMENTS

For the alkaline earth elements, the recent metabolic model of ICRP Publication 20 (1973) was used.

In its 1959 report on permissible doses (ICRP, 1959*), Committee II of the ICRP used an exponential model of retention for all radionuclides to calculate maximum permissible concentrations in water. The committee pointed out, however, that there was good evidence that retention of radium-226 and other bone-seeking radionuclides is best represented by a power function model (Norris *et al.*, 1958). In the case of radium-226, the calculated body burden from intake at constant daily rate for 50 yr is about a factor of 10 smaller by the power function model than by the ICRP exponential model. This may be shown by use of the equations and the values for metabolic parameters that are given in the ICRP report. Ingestion of 1 pCi of radium-226 per day in water is assumed in the sample calculations given below.

According to the ICRP exponential model, the amount of a radionuclide, qf_2, that accumulates in an organ from constant ingestion rate, a, is given by:

$$qf_2 = af_w \frac{\tau}{0.693}\left(1-e^{-0.693\,T/\tau}\right)$$

where $q=$ total amount in the body, f_2 = fraction of q in the organ of reference (0.99 for bone), f_w = fraction of radionuclide ingested in water

*The maximum permissible concentrations of radionuclides in ICRP 1959 and NCRP 1963 are identical.

TABLE VII-2 Adult Equilibrium Annual Dose Factors for Some Radionuclides in Water[a]

	Millirem per Year in Year 50 of Constant Intake at				
	1 pCi per year			1 pCi/liter; 2 liter/day	
Nuclide	Total Body	Organ Specific	Organ	Total Body	Organ Specific
^{3}H	1.1×10^{-7}	—		8.2×10^{-5}	—
^{14}C	5.7×10^{-7}	—		4.2×10^{-4}	—
^{40}K	2.4×10^{-5}	—		2.0×10^{-2}	—
^{54}Mn	8.7×10^{-7}	1.4×10^{-5}	GI (LLI)	6.4×10^{-4}	1.0×10^{-2}
^{87}Rb	4.3×10^{-6}	—		3.1×10^{-3}	—
^{89}Sr	5.6×10^{-7}[b]	7.1×10^{-5}	Bone	4.1×10^{-4}[b]	5.2×10^{-2}
$^{90}Sr+D$	3.2×10^{-6}[b]	6.3×10^{-3}	Bone	2.3×10^{-3}[b]	4.6×10^{0}
$^{95}Zr+D$	6.6×10^{-9}	3.0×10^{-5}	GI (LLI)	4.8×10^{-6}	2.0×10^{-2}
^{99}mTc	8.9×10^{-9}	4.1×10^{-7}	GI (LLI)	6.5×10^{-6}	3.0×10^{-4}
^{129}I	9.2×10^{-6}	7.2×10^{-3}	Thyroid	6.7×10^{-3}	5.3×10^{0}
$^{131}I+D$	3.4×10^{-6}	1.9×10^{-3}	Thyroid	2.5×10^{-3}	1.4×10^{0}
^{134}Cs	1.2×10^{-4}	—		8.9×10^{-2}	—
$^{137}Cs+D$	7.1×10^{-5}	—		5.2×10^{-2}	—
$^{144}Ce+D$	2.6×10^{-8}	1.7×10^{-4}	GI (LLI)	1.9×10^{-5}	1.2×10^{-1}
$^{210}Pb+D$	5.4×10^{-4}	1.2×10^{-2}	Kidney	3.9×10^{-1}	9.0×10^{0}
^{210}Po	8.6×10^{-5}	2.5×10^{-3}	Kidney	6.3×10^{-2}	1.8×10^{0}
$^{226}Ra+D$	8.7×10^{-4}[b]	2.2×10^{-2}	Bone	2.7×10^{-1}[b]	1.6×10^{1}
$^{228}Ra+D$	8.1×10^{-4}[b]	2.2×10^{-2}	Bone	5.9×10^{-1}[b]	1.6×10^{1}
$^{232}Th+D$	4.9×10^{-5}	1.8×10^{-3}	Bone	3.6×10^{-2}	1.3×10^{0}
$^{238}U+D$	4.5×10^{-5}	7.7×10^{-4}	Bone	3.2×10^{-2}	5.6×10^{-1}
^{239}Pu	1.9×10^{-5}	7.9×10^{-4}	Bone	1.0×10^{-2}	5.8×10^{-1}

[a]Based on NCRP Report no. 22 (1963 rev.); Soldat *et al.*, 1975; and alkaline earth values as described in text.
[b]Values are soft tissue doses, not total body doses.
Factors in left-hand columns also give total dose accumulated over 50 yr after a single acute intake, by an adult, of 1 pCi. D = daughters.

that reaches the organ (0.04 for bone), τ = effective half-life (1.6×10^4 days), and T = duration of ingestion in days.

For uptake of ^{226}Ra by the skeleton in 50 yr, q (0.99) = (1) (0.04) (1.6×10^4)(1 - 0.454)/0.693 and the body burden q = 510 pCi for T = 18,250 days. It has been suggested that the effective half-life of ^{226}Ra is 17.1 yr (Miller and Finkel, 1968); the calculated body burden in the above example would then be somewhat smaller, 315 pCi.

In the case of the power function, the body burden, q, after an amount, a, of a long-lived radionuclide has been ingested per day for T days is given by:

$$q = \frac{Aaf_1}{1-n} T^{1-n}$$

where f_1 = fraction of ingested radioactivity that transfers from the gut to the blood (0.3), and A and n are the power-function constants for the fraction (R) retained at t days after a single injection ($R = At^{-n}$). Norris *et al.* (1952) give the values A = 0.54 and n = 0.52.

Hence, for uptake of ^{226}Ra in 50 yr,

$$q = \frac{(0.54)(1)(0.3)(18{,}250)^{0.48}}{0.48}$$

and the body burden q = 37 pCi. It should be noted that the power function, in the form given here, deals only with the total body burden; it is silent on the question of organ distribution.

Since 1959, additional data have tended to support a power-function model for bone seekers. In 1972, a task group of Committee II of the ICRP presented a detailed model of alkaline earth metabolism that evolved from the power function (ICRP, 1973). For a constant rate of intake into the blood for 50 yr, the newer model predicts a whole-body content that is only 5% less than the simple power function given above.

Measurements of radium-226 body burdens and dietary intake at environmental levels also indicate that the ICRP exponential model predicts long-term retentions that are too high. The average body burden of radium-226 in areas of normal radioactivity is about 50 pCi (40 pCi in the skeleton and 10 pCi in soft tissue; UNSCEAR, 1972, p. 32). Intake of radium in food appears to be the main source at normal levels, because the average daily intake in the United States is about 1 to 2 pCi in food and less than 0.1 pCi in water (NCRP, 1975, p. 92).

A quantitative relationship between the body burden of radium-226 and the concentration of radium in drinking water was found by Lucas

(1961). He measured the radium content of samples of bone and soft tissue from individuals with lifetime (or at least 30 yr) residence in their communities. He also measured the radium content of the water supply of each community. The average body burden of radium-226 was 36 pCi (42 persons) in cities with less than 0.1 pCi/liter, and higher body burdens (33 persons) were found in cities with 0.13-10.5 pCi/liter. With the assumption that intake of radium in food contributed 36 pCi to the total body burden of each person measured, the following relationship was found: $B = 36 + 50C_w$, where B is the total body burden (pCi) and C_w is the concentration of radium-226 in drinking water (pCi/liter). This relationship was confirmed in later work on 19 other persons of known and stable residence (Lucas *et al.*, 1964).

It should be emphasized that the Lucas equation is an empirical relationship between body burden and the concentration of radium-226 in the local water supply. Daily rates of intake, transfer from gut to blood, etc., were not known nor taken into account. If one assumes daily ingestion of 1-2 liters of local water for the persons analyzed, then the long-term accumulation of body radium from radium in water was 25 to 50 times the daily intake of radium in water. These values are compatible with ratios of body burden to daily intake that were estimated in other work (Stehney and Lucas, 1956; ICRP, 1973).

Combining the Lucas equation with the standard rate of water consumption, 2 liters/day (NCRP, 1963; ICRP, 1974), gives good agreement with the new model of alkaline earth metabolism (ICRP, 1973). According to the model, f_1 has a value of 0.21 and the body burden accumulated from daily ingestion of 2 pCi of ^{226}Ra for 50 yr is 50 pCi, of which 41.5 pCi is in bone.

Since the relevant metabolic parameters for radium-228 are the same as for radium-226, the ICRP power-function model may also be used to calculate long-term retention of radium-228. For ingestion of 2 pCi/day for 50 yr, the calculated body burden of radium-228 is 21 pCi (14.2 pCi in bone). The dose factors given in Table VII-2 are based on effective absorbed energies per disintegration of 106 MeV for radium-226, and 301 MeV for radium-228 (NCRP, 1975).

The metabolic model of ICRP Publication 20 (1973) was also used to calculate the retention of radiostrontium from continuous ingestion in water. For strontium-90, the calculated body burden from ingestion of 2 pCi/day for 50 yr is 229 pCi, of which 222 pCi are in bone; for strontium-89, the corresponding values are 7.6 pCi and 5.0 pCi. The effective absorbed energies of the strontium isotopes in bone and total body given in ICRP 1959 were used to calculate the dose factors shown in Table VII-2.

TABLE VII-3 Activity in a Hypothetical Water Supply

Nuclide	Concentration, pCi/liter	Potential Doses (mrem/yr)	
		Total Body	Bone Dose
Beta activity			
^{3}H	250	0.02	—
^{40}K	2.3	0.046	—
^{90}Sr	0.5	0.001	2.3
^{137}Cs	0.1	0.005	—
^{228}Ra	0.2	—	—
Total beta (without ^{3}H)	3.1	0.072	2.3
Alpha activity			
^{226}Ra & daughters	0.2	0.054	3.2
^{228}Ra daughters	0.2	0.118	3.2
Total alpha	0.4	0.172	6.4
Grant total		0.244	8.7

DOSES FROM WATER OF SPECIFIED COMPOSITION

To illustrate the doses to be expected from drinking water that may be typical of the United States generally, a hypothetical water supply was postulated to have the amounts of radioactivity shown in Table VII-3. Also tabulated are the corresponding annual doses to be expected in the fiftieth year of constant consumption of 2 liters/day of this water, as calculated with the dose factors of Table VII-2.

The concentrations in Table VII-3 were chosen to represent the average tritium concentration, beta activity, and alpha activity of the water analyses reported in the Environmental Protection Agency's 1975 Report to Congress (EPA, 1975). The average tritium concentration was found to be 250 pCi/liter (p. IV-4). The average beta activity (excluding tritium) from all interstate carrier water supplies—for which figures were reported for gross beta, gross alpha, strontium-90, and radium-226 activity—was 3.1 pCi/liter. The gross alpha activities for the same samples were less than 2 pCi/liter in all but one case. The reported detection limit for gross alpha was 2 pCi/liter, and for strontium-90 beta activity, 0.5 pCi/liter. In these samples, many of the entries were below this detection limit. Almost all samples were below 1 pCi/liter. A reasonable concentration of strontium was therefore taken to be 0.5 pCi/liter. Radium-226 concentration in these samples averaged about 0.2 pCi/liter (two of the entries in the EPA report were incorrectly given as 9.12 and 9.10, instead of 0.12 and 0.10).

In addition to the tritium and strontium-90 concentrations noted above, it was assumed that the other major beta-contributors would be potassium-40, cesium-137, and radium-228. Cesium-137 in drinking water in the United States is currently derived primarily from fallout from atmospheric weapons testing. As "surface" depositions, the concentrations vary. They are likely to be higher in surface water than in groundwater. Values for this nuclide are not available for all the states; and even within a single state (e.g., California), concentrations are variable. A plausible concentration of this nuclide was estimated to be 0.1 pCi/liter. Equally variable, but for reasons related more to geology than to anything else, is the concentration of radium-228. It was assumed that the radium-228 concentration is approximately equal to that of radium-226, and for this hypothetical example a value of 0.2 pCi/liter was adopted (Stehney and Krause, 1960). Finally, potassium-40, which is ubiquitous in water supplies, is also variable; in the absence of any nationwide surveys of its concentration, it was concluded, from the range of concentrations in California (Goldberg, 1976), that 2.3 pCi/liter would be a reasonable estimate for the hypothetical water composition.

Calculating a gonadal dose for bone-seeking radionuclides is difficult. Strontium-90, for example, when fed continuously to dogs, was found to be one thousand times less concentrated in gonadal tissue than in bone. It could then be estimated that a bone dose of 0.1 mrem/yr might be accompanied by a gonadal dose of about 0.1 μrem/yr (Della Rosa *et al.*, 1972).

Unfortunately, extensive analyses of specific radionuclides other than radium-226, strontium-90, and tritium in water are not available. Dose factors for the majority of known radionuclides, derived from NCRP Report 22 (1963), are given in Soldat *et al.* (1975) and may readily be used to calculate annual doses when new analytical results are obtained.

A spectrometric analysis of a 1974 drinking water composite from Los Angeles became available (Goldberg, 1976), and was used to construct another illustrative example as shown below. The potential doses, assuming 50-yr constant intake at 2 liters/day, were calculated as in the previous example.

Nuclide	Concentration, pCi/liter	Potential Doses (mrem/yr)	
		Total Body	Organ
^{40}K	5.20	0.09	
^{54}Mn	0.48	0.004	0.005 GI(LLI)
^{90}Sr	0.09	0.0002	0.4 (Bone)
^{95}Zr–^{95}Nb	0.61	0.000003	0.1 GI(LLI)
^{137}Cs	0.05	0.003	
^{144}Ce	0.21	0.000004	0.03 GI(LLI)
^{226}Ra	0.05	0.014	0.8 (Bone)

In this case, a total bone dose of 2 mrem/yr would be calculated (although not separately determined in this analysis, an amount of α-activity from radium-228 daughters nearly equal to that of the radium-226 would also be expected). For all other tissues, including the gonads, the annual dose would be about 0.12 mrem.

ESTIMATION OF RISK

Developmental and Teratogenic Effects

On the basis of numerous studies on the effects of external radiation, it has become generally accepted that developing mammals (intrauterine and juvenile) are more radiosensitive than adults (BEIR Committee, 1972; Sikov and Mahlum, 1969). Since the basic interactions of radiation do not differ with age, it appears that the increased sensitivity follows from the high rates of cell proliferation and the complex interactions associated with development. Also, the variety of integrated developmental stages, through which the immature organism must progress to attain maturity, increases the chance that derangements will occur.

In general, these deleterious effects may be divided into three categories: increased tumor incidence, death, and developmental abnormalities. The first category is discussed later and will not be considered here. In the broad sense, the last category includes physiological and biochemical deficits and deviations, as well as malformations. Most of the quantitative dose-effect relationships have been derived from studies using relatively high radiation doses from external photon beams.

The doses required for embryolethality change during development, and vary by more than a factor of 10. There are also short "critical periods" for most, if not all, malformative events. Most of the available data suggest an *apparent* threshold at about 10 rad of acute exposure and a sigmoid dose–response relation for production of lethality and developmental abnormalities (BEIR Committee, 1972; Brent and Gorson, 1972). It is possible, however, that this value may be overestimated since there are relatively few observations at low doses and there is a lack of satisfactory methods for detecting minimal defects. Many of the observed morphological malformations have been hypothesized to involve a reduction in cell number to a value below some critical level as an early step in the pathogenic process. These considerations would offer a theoretical explanation for the apparent threshold for radiation teratogenesis.

The difficulties inherent in extrapolating the results of experiments at high doses and high dose rates to low doses and low dose rates include those applicable to the adult as well as some that are specific to the immature organism. In general, protracting the dose from low-LET radiation results in a decreased biological effect. For developmental effects, the influence of protraction of exposure is even greater because only a small fraction of the life span is spent in the susceptible prenatal and neonatal stages. Only radiation that is absorbed during the critical period of hours or days would be effective in altering the particular processes occurring at that time.

Because of the apparent existence of thresholds, nonlinearity, and critical periods, risk estimates calculated in terms of events per rem are not meaningful at low doses and dose rates. Because of this and because of the available data, it may be expected that low doses of radiation delivered at low dose rates would have a small likelihood of being embryotoxic (embryocidal or teratogenic). Despite these limitations, the most pessimistic case for embryotoxicity can be calculated from the estimated threshold dose of 10 rad of acute radiation. If the 10 rad were protracted over the 9 months of gestation and the first year of life a daily dose of about 15 mrad would result. The conservatism of this estimate is suggested by the fact that the lowest dose of protracted external radiation for which confirmed deleterious effects have been reported (defective development of some organs and decreased life span, but no acute mortality) is slightly over 1 rad per day throughout late gestation and early postnatal life (BEIR Committee, 1972). It has been recently reported (Cahill *et al.*, 1976), however, that a radiation dose of 3 mrad per day to the conceptus from continuous ingestion of tritium by pregnant rats produced a slight, but statistically significant, delay in eye-opening and development of the righting reflex.

It should be noted that the water intake of the neonate is initially minimal, increasing with time. Even in the juvenile period, milk (from commercial or maternal sources) is often the major source of fluid, and it reflects, to some extent, the radionuclide content of the water supplies and food.

The exposure of the fetus to radionuclides depends on the maternal body burden, and particularly on the concentrations of radionuclides in the maternal circulation; the fraction available to cross the placenta depends on the rate of removal from the circulation. The amount of activity to which the conceptus may be exposed is also a function of the facility with which the nuclide crosses the placenta. Radioisotopes of normal dietary constituents generally behave as do the stable isotopic species, and there are extensive data on many contaminant radionuclides (Sikov and Mahlum, 1969; Brent and Gorson, 1972). Availability is influenced also by the chemical and physicochemical form of the nuclide and changes with the stage of gestation. Most elements, in their usual forms, fall into three broad categories relative to cross-placental transfer. The first category includes materials—such as phosphorus and iodine—that freely cross the placenta, either by rapid diffusion or by active transport, and reach fetal blood concentrations approximating those of the mother. Tissue concentrations depend on metabolic considerations and may influence the rate of removal from the blood. These processes are age-dependent, in that it is not until thyroid function or skeletal calcification begins that significant quantities of iodine or strontium are removed from the circulation. At these times, the fetal concentrations in the target organs may slightly exceed those in the mother, although they are often smaller. The second category encompasses the many elements that diffuse relatively slowly and may include those for which there appear to be placental barriers to their transfer. The third category consists of the elements that themselves or in their usual chemical form are poorly transferred to the conceptus. The average concentration of such a material in the fetus is only a small fraction of that in the mother, although specific tissue concentrations occasionally approach maternal values (Wrenn, 1975). For some of these elements (e.g., ^{239}Pu) it appears from rodent studies that most of the embryotoxicity early in gestation is attributable to material localized in the villus yolk sac (Sikov and Mahlum, 1972). Because this structure is vestigial in man, it is uncertain whether this finding has significance for exposure of humans.

On the basis of the foregoing, and the calculations of potential radiation doses, we anticipate that no measurable developmental and teratogenic effects of radionuclides in drinking water will be found at the levels studied.

Genetic Effects

Many national and international groups (BEIR, NCRP, ICRP) revise from time to time our understanding of the genetic risks to human populations from ionizing radiation. The estimates of genetic effects of low levels of radiation due to ingestion of radioactive isotopes in drinking water that follow this section are based on their work.

Mutations—changes in the genetic information—can occur at any time in any cell of the body. Geneticists, however, are concerned primarily with mutations that occur in the genes and chromosomes of *germ* cells, sperm and eggs, or the cells from which they are derived. Sperm and egg cells, after fertilization, give rise to the individuals of the next and later generations. Thus, a mutation originating in germ cells could, in time, spread through the population.

From the earliest studies on mutation, it was recognized that the vast majority of newly arising mutations were, in varying degrees, detrimental. If this seems paradoxical in an evolutionary sense, it should be noted that evolution proceeds by selection of individuals with the highest reproductive fitness, fixing beneficial mutations, and generally eliminating less favorable ones. This selection process is not perfect, and harmful mutants do spread into the population until they are eventually eliminated through death, sterility, or reduced fertility. In some cases, on the other hand, unusual selective phenomena have led to the maintenance of genetically determined diseases, such as sickle cell anemia, in which the genetic carriers are resistant to malaria. In general, however, the more severe the mutation, the more rapid is its elimination; indeed, a substantial proportion is most likely eliminated without notice in early pregnancy. Conversely, mutations that impair the vigor of individuals only slightly may penetrate a population over a long period of time before selection occurs.

Mutations arising in nongerminal or somatic cells are limited to expression in the individual and cannot be transmitted to future generations. They are nevertheless of considerable importance, in that the induction of many cancers may be related to mutation induction. For instance, studies indicate that approximately 90% of organic compounds that are carcinogens are also mutagens (McCann *et al.*, 1975; McCann and Ames, 1976).

Mutations fall into three major categories of genetic alteration: gene mutations, chromosome aberrations, and changes in chromosome number. Gene mutations, in which the genetic change is restricted to a submicroscopic region of a chromosome, affect only a rather restricted amount of the cell's information content. For example, mutations in the gene controlling the production of hemoglobin in red blood cells may be manifested as an altered or missing hemoglobin. Such a mutation may have no bearing on the manner in which the hemoglobin functions or it may be the cause of severe anemia, as in sickle cell anemia.

In the fertilized egg, chromosomes and genes (with the exception of sex chromosomes and their genes) are inherited in pairs, one member of the pair coming from each parent. Mutant genes are usually described by the manner in which their activity is manifested. A dominant mutation or gene is one that gives an altered effect (or phenotype) in the presence of a normal partner gene. A recessive mutant gene is one whose effect is apparent in the individual only if both members of the pair of genes are mutant; when the recessive and normal are both present, the mutant trait does not appear. Sex-linked recessive genes—those on the X-chromosome—govern traits more commonly observed in males than in females. Males have only one X-chromosome, whereas females have two; thus, the phenotype resulting from a recessive gene on the male's X can be expressed, whereas, in females, unless both X-chromosomes contain the recessive, it cannot. Some gene mutations are caused by the deletion of a single base pair within the gene. In practice, it is usually difficult or impossible to discriminate between gene mutations and deletions that extend beyond the borders of a single gene to neighboring genes. If the deletions are microscopically invisible, they will usually be classified as simple gene mutations.

Deletions may vary in scale from the loss of a single base pair to larger losses that extend into the second major category of genetic change: chromosome aberrations. This category encompasses alterations in chromosomal structure that are visible under the microscope. Recognizable aberrations include deletions of chromosomal segments, additions of segments, and changes in the position of segments, either within a single chromosome or between two or more chromosomes. These changes can have considerable biological consequences in that the health, survival, and reproduction of individuals with such altered chromosomes may be impaired. Although these individuals may appear to be normal, their offspring could be severely afflicted as a result of the reshuffling of the genetic information that routinely occurs in the formation of new germ cells.

The third category of mutation consists of changes in the number of whole chromosomes in the genetic set carried in the germinal cells. In man, each germ cell contains 23 chromosomes; the fertilized egg and the individual produced therefrom have 23 distinctly recognizable pairs of chromosomes in each somatic cell. With the exception of the X- and Y-chromosomes of the male, the members of each pair are morphologically alike.

During meiosis, the process of germ-cell formation, the chromosomes are redistributed, so that each germ cell will contain only one member of each pair. During this redistribution, mistakes sometimes occur, and some cells receive two members of a pair. Correspondingly other cells receive neither member. When these aneuploid cells (cells with abnormal numbers of chromosomes) are involved in fertilization, the most commonly observed consequence is prenatal death. In a small number of cases, survival associated with severe congenital abnormality occurs. Examples of this are Down's syndrome, Edwards' and Patau's syndromes, and various sex-chromosome anomalies. About 0.5% of all live-born children contain an improper chromosome number and since more than 3 million babies are born in the United States each year, this is a substantial number of severely handicapped children.

It should be mentioned that many cases of genetic disease in man result, not from single genes, but from the concerted actions of many genes (multifactorial traits). Strictly speaking, a mutation in one of the many genes does not necessarily influence the manifestation of disease. Because of the complexity of the genetics associated with these diseases, our understanding both of their nature and of their response to mutation is very limited.

All the forms of genetic change described above (see Table VII-4 for examples) are known to occur spontaneously, i.e., in the absence of known causative agents. They also can be produced by various physical agents, such as ultraviolet light and ionizing radiation, and by chemical agents. Whether or not naturally occurring mutagens in our environment are responsible for the "spontaneous" mutation rate is moot. Certainly no single agent can readily be implicated as the sole cause. Present evidence indicates that natural background radiation levels (from cosmic rays and natural terrestrial radioactivity) are able to account for only part of the spontaneous incidence.

Although there is no definitive proof that any single mutant human individual resulted from exposure of the parents to a known mutagen (radiation or chemical), and thus no direct proof that these agents are indeed mutagenic in man, radiation has been demonstrated to be mutagenic in so many organisms that it seems very unlikely that it is not mutagenic in man. In fact, all the various types of mutations described above have been induced in cultured human somatic cells. The question, therefore, is not whether mutations will be induced, but rather how many will be introduced into the population.

Basis for Estimating Genetic Risk in Man

Three major principles of particular relevance to human risk estimates have emerged from studies of induced mutation.

1. Radiation or other mutagens appear to produce genetic changes that are qualitatively the same as those that occur naturally. Different mutagens, however, may not increase all types of mutations in quantitatively the same manner.

TABLE VII-4 Some Selected Types of Human Diseases Caused by "Mutation"

Dominant	*Chromosomal*
Neurofibromatosis	Down's syndrome
Chondrodystrophy	Edwards' syndrome
Hereditary chorea	Patau's syndrome
Congenital cataract	Sex chromosome anomalies
Osteogenesis imperfecta	Cri du chat syndrome
Sex-linked	*Multifactorial*
Hemophilia A & B	Diabetes mellitus
Progressive muscular dystrophy	Idiopathic mental retardation
Hypogammaglobulinemia	Myopia
	Asthma
Recessive	Schizophrenia, several types
Cystic fibrosis	Epilepsy, several types
Phenylketonuria	Strabismus, convergent
Amaurotic idiocy	
Cystic kidney disease	
Albinism	
Deafness	

2. At low doses and low dose rates of low-LET radiation, mutations are induced in direct proportion to the dose. No threshold dose is evident in the experiments testing this (with a few exceptions that are presently the subject of reevaluation).

3. In the low dose range of irradiation to which human populations are normally exposed from natural background or man-made sources, the manner in which the dose is received will not affect the yield of induced mutations. The same number of mutations will result if 100 millirem are received all at once or spread out over weeks, months, or even years.

As mentioned earlier, national and international groups (ICRP, NCRP, UNSCEAR) have periodically evaluated the data and provided recommendations based on their assessments of radiation hazards. In the United States, the National Academy of Sciences in 1972 published a major document, *The Effects on Populations of Exposure to Low Levels of Ionizing Radiation.* This report (BEIR Committee, 1972) serves as a principal source of guidance for such governmental agencies as the Environmental Protection Agency, and the Nuclear Regulatory Commission, which are charged with protecting the public from unnecessary exposure.

The BEIR Committee report is the major basis for the risk estimates reached here. In addition, because of evidence that has become available since the publication of that report, some modifications will be considered.

The Subcommittee on Genetics of the BEIR Committee used four ways to estimate the risk:

1. *Risk Relative to That from Natural Background Radiation*

The average natural background radiation level in the United States is about 100 mrem/yr. The Committee noted that by keeping the additional radiation dose to the population from man-made sources below this level "we are assured that the additional consequences will neither differ in kind from those which we have experienced throughout human history nor exceed them in quantity." Thus, the BEIR Committee recommended that the natural background radiation be used as a standard of comparison.

2. *Risk Estimates for Specific Genetic Conditions*

To determine the risk, the BEIR Committee made estimates of the doubling dose for human mutation rates, i.e., the dose required to double the spontaneous mutation rate. These values were obtained by dividing the best estimates of human spontaneous gene mutation rates by the average induced mutation rate per gene (or locus) per Roentgen, which was obtained from mouse germ-cell studies. The average human rate was taken to be between 0.5×10^{-6} and 0.5×10^{-5} per gene per generation. The induced average gene mutation rate for spermatogonia was taken as 0.5×10^{-7} per rem, while that for oocytes was taken as zero and the two were averaged as 0.25×10^{-7}. The doubling dose for gene mutation was therefore taken to be between 20 and 200 rem ($0.5 \times 10^{-6}/0.25 \times 10^{-7}$ and $0.5 \times 10^{-5}/0.25 \times 10^{-7}$). The genetic conditions and their spontaneous incidences were taken from studies carried out in Northern Ireland up to 1958. Thus, the estimates of risk are themselves based on three separate estimates, each of which has some degree of uncertainty. The results of the BEIR analysis are presented in Table VII-5. The estimates are presented in terms of effects in the first generation and effects at equilibrium when the maximum permissible dose (5 rem over a 30-yr generation time) is given for many generations.

The BEIR Committee based its estimates of the number of radiation-induced chromosome anomalies resulting from unbalanced chromosome rearrangements on the frequency of balanced translocations recorded as semisterility in the offspring of male mice whose spermatogonia had been irradiated. For chronic irradiation at low LET and low dose rates, this frequency was taken to be 1.5×10^{-5} per rem. To convert to human terms, this value was multiplied by 2 to correct for the greater sensitivity of human chromosomes, multiplied by 4 to estimate the number of

TABLE VII-5 Estimated Effects of 5 rem per Generation on a Population of 1 Million Live Births (Figures from BEIR Committee, 1972)

Disease Classification	Current Incidence	Effect of 5 rem per Generation: First Generation	Effect of 5 rem per Generation: Equilibrium	Generations to Equilibrium
Dominant diseases	10,000	50–500[a]	250–2,500	5
X-linked recessive diseases	400	0–15[a]	10–100	6
Recessive diseases	1,500	very few	very slow increase	
Chromosomal anomalies				
Unbalanced rearrangements	1,000	60	75	2–3
Aneuploidy	4,000	5	5	0
Congenital anomalies	15,000	} 5–500	} 50–5,000	} 10
Anomalies expressed later	10,000			
Constitutional and degenerative diseases	15,000			
Total	56,900	120–1,100	390–7,700	

[a]Based on a doubling dose of 20–200 rem.

unbalanced translocations, and multiplied again by 2 to include an equivalent rate induced in females (since that value was unknown). This product, multiplied by 5, the maximum permissible dose in rem per 30-yr reproductive generation, gave 1200 zygotes per million with unbalanced translocations ($1.5 \times 10^{-5} \times 2 \times 4 \times 2 \times 5 = 1.2 \times 10^{-3} = 1{,}200 \times 10^{-6}$). A further adjustment for the 5% of these zygotes that were thought to survive, gave $1{,}200 \times 0.05 \times 10^{-6} = 60 \times 10^{-6}$ unbalanced translocations appearing in the first generation.

By a similar calculation, survival of 5% of the offspring of the 300 zygotes per million carrying balanced translocations ($1.5 \times 10^{-5} \times 2 \times 2 \times 5 = 3 \times 10^{-3} = 300 \times 10^{-6}$), was expected to contribute an additional 15 unbalanced translocations per million to equlibrium. These values are shown in Table VII-5.

For induced aneuploidy the BEIR Committee relied exclusively on the rate of X-chromosome loss obtained from female mice (6×10^{-6} losses per gamete per rad of chronic low-LET radiation). This rate was used to estimate the frequency of viable aneuploids induced in man, leading to the number 5 entered in Table VII-5.

3. *Risk Relative to Current Incidence of Serious Disabilities*

The BEIR Committee also made estimates from the evidence of diseases of complex etiology, described in the Northern Ireland study (Stevenson, 1959). These diseases make up the bulk of the 56,900 cases per million live births in Table VII-5. About 70% of the total are congenital anomalies, anomalies expressed after birth, and constitutional and degenerative diseases. A considerable uncertainty is associated with the radiosensitive mutational component of these diseases. The mutational component, which is the proportion of the incidence that is directly proportional to the mutation rate, was estimated to lie between 5% and 50%. It was also assumed that under equilibrium conditions only 10% of the disorders would be manifest in the first generation. The values are listed in Table VII-5.

4. *Risk in Terms of Ill-Health*

The BEIR Committee assumed that an independent measure of risk could be obtained from the component of ill health that results from mutationally dependent genetic disorders. It considered that perhaps 20% of all ill health had a mutationally dependent origin and therefore, by using the estimates of the doubling dose (20 rem to 200 rem), arrived at the suggestion that 5 rem per generation would increase the incidence of ill health by 0.5 to 5% (5 rem × 20%/20 rem = 5%, or 5 rem × 20%/200 rem = 0.5%).

RECONSIDERATION OF THE BEIR COMMITTEE'S ESTIMATES

Since the publication of the BEIR report, Trimble and Doughty (1974) have published a large-scale study of genetically determined diseases in children in British Columbia. In the interval between the 1958 study by Stevenson and that of Trimble and Doughty, understanding of the mode of transmission of many human genetic diseases has improved considerably, and this has led to a revision of the diagnostic categories originally used in the Stevenson study. The new study showed that a larger proportion of disease—approximately 9% (instead of approximately 6%)—had a genetic basis, but that the dominant gene class was reduced. In Trimble and Doughty's study, this class was lower by an order of magnitude. Their study did not present any information on the frequency of dominant gene diseases that show late onset (i.e., become manifest after childhood) and those with variable levels of penetrance. The frequency of the last two types of dominant disease is about twice the frequency of dominant diseases measured by Doughty and Trimble. Therefore, the suggested incidence of dominant disorders is believed to be approximately 3,000 cases per million (Table VII-6) rather than the 10,000 cases per million used by the BEIR Committee (Table VII-5).

The suggestion by human geneticists that there is no mutational component associated with the diseases classified as congenital anomalies, anomalies expressed later in life, and constitutional and degenerative diseases (Newcombe, 1975) has great significance for estimating the contribution of radiation to these diseases. The argument suggests that these categories are maintained exclusively by selection mechanisms, as was described in the simple case of sickle cell anemia, and that changes in the mutation rate will not greatly affect their numbers. Under these circumstances, the radiation-induced increase will be approximately zero. The numbers in brackets in Table VII-6 would represent the contribution from a 50% mutational component. Many geneticists believe this percentage to be unrealistically high (see Newcombe, 1975). Because of this and because these numbers are not based on experimental data, less confidence should be attached to them.

Another area of reappraisal results from studies of induced chromosome aberrations. A recent analysis of translocations induced in spermatogonial cells of both humans and marmosets (primates) suggests that after 100 R of acutely delivered radiation, the frequency of translocations observed in spermatocytes is 0.077 per cell (Brewen, Preston, and Gengozian, 1975). The same authors have also demonstrated that induced translocations (Y) in mouse germ cells, as well as dicentrics in human and marmoset lymphocytes, are best related to dose (D) by a quadratic equation $Y = C + \alpha D + \beta D^2$. They calculated that for acute X-ray doses the expected frequency of transmissible translocations is between 1×10^{-4} and 2×10^{-4} translocations per gamete per rem. This calculation, however, includes both the dose and dose-squared components expected for acute high-dose irradiation and thus is likely to be too high by a factor of 2 when chronic low-dose irradiation is considered. We shall thus assume the value per rem to be 0.5×10^{-4} to 1.0×10^{-4} transmissible translocations. The BEIR Committee's previous analysis used a rate of 3×10^{-5} (*viz.* $1.5 \times 10^{-5} \times 2$, the correction factor for humans). Correcting for this difference, we adopt the same approach. Thus, with exposure of 5 rem per generation, the expected number of liveborn chromosomally unbalanced offspring in a million live births would be 100–200 in the first generation and 125–250 at equilibrium (see Table VII-6).

Jacobs *et al.* (1972) stated that a realistic estimate of the spontaneous rate of reciprocal translocations is between 0.5 and 1.0×10^{-3} per gamete. Dividing by the radiation-induced rate obtained by Brewen, Preston, and Gengozian gives a doubling dose of 5–20 rem for this category of genetic event. Jacobs *et al.* (1974, p. 376) also reported data indicating that the

TABLE VII-6 Estimated Effect of 5 rem per Generation on a Population of 1 Million Live Births (BEIR Committee Estimates Modified to Account for New Data and Approaches)

		Effect of 5 rem per Generation	
Disease Classification	Incidence	First Generation	Equilibrium
Dominant diseases	3,000	60–600[a]	300–3,000[a]
X-linked recessive diseases	400	7–70[a]	40–400[a]
Recessive diseases	1,500	very few	very slow to increase
Chromosomal anomalies			
Unbalanced rearrangements	500	100–200	125–250
Aneuploidy	4,000	5–130	5–130
Congenital anomalies; Anomalies expressed later; Constitutional and degenerative diseases	85,000	(0–43)–[4,250][a,b]	(0–425)–[42,500][a,b]
Total	94,400	(172–215)–[5,250][b]	(474–900)–[46,300][b]

[a]Based on a doubling dose of 5–50 rem.
[b]The numbers in brackets are likely to be unreasonably high (see text).

current incidence of live-born suffering from unbalanced chromosome rearrangements is about 500 cases per million rather than 1,000 cases per million as estimated by the BEIR Committee (see Table VII-5).

Since publication of the BEIR report, data have appeared on radiation-induced nondisjunction in meiosis in the female mouse. After an average dose of 20 rad, Uchida and Lee (1974) found six oocytes out of 1,149 contained an extra chromosome. After 5 rad, only one-quarter (5/20) as many will be expected. Since irradiation of males does not seem to give nondisjunction (UNSCEAR, 1972, pp. 256–257), there will be a further reduction of one-half, and since the mouse has 20 pairs of chromosomes, the estimated rate per chromosome for 5 rads would then be $6/1149 \times 5/20 \times 1/20 \times 1/2 = 32$ per million. Only four types of chromosomal aneusomy have been found to be viable in humans, which leads to an estimate of 130 cases per million instead of the 5 originally given by the BEIR Committee.

A final area of reassessment involves the induced mutation rate estimates obtained from mouse studies. The BEIR Committee assumed a zero mutation rate for females based on the fact that, in the mouse female, no mutations appear to be induced by irradiation of the immature oocyte (the most persistent stage). When the United Nations Committee (UNSCEAR, 1972, p. 252) reviewed these results they concluded that use of mutation rate estimates based on immature oocytes in the female mouse could lead to a serious error because of major differences between human and mouse oocytes both in morphology and in their response to cell killing. They felt, however, that use of risk estimates from the genetically most sensitive stage in the mouse should not result in an underestimate of the hazard to man. Nonetheless, scientific controversy exists as to what figures should be applied here. Taken at face value, chronic irradiation of "mature" oocytes leads to a mutation rate estimate 1/20 of that obtained from acute exposure, or a rate of about 0.25×10^{-7} mutations per gene per rem ($5.4 \times 10^{-7} \times 1/20$). One recent analysis (Abrahamson and Wolff, 1976) suggests that this value might be too low, since the radiation procedures lead to recovery of mouse cells that were irradiated to a substantial extent during their insensitive immature stage—a stage that may not be applicable to human risk estimates. If the latter viewpoint is shown to be correct, the risk estimate for the female is likely to be in the range of 1.2×10^{-7} mutations per rem. Since a male rate of 0.7×10^{-7} was obtained from a regression analysis of all the data from chronically irradiated spermatogonia (Searle, 1974), the average for both sexes would be 1×10^{-7} rather than the value of 0.25×10^{-7} used by the BEIR Committee. This would mean that the doubling dose would be in the range of 5–50 rem for those genetic effects that are proportionally increased by irradiation. This value is used as the basis for the calculations presented in Table VII-6, even though some would argue that it is too low.

Thus, there is new evidence on the genetic basis of disease that would tend to lower the mutationally dependent contribution to future generations as well as studies and calculations that would raise the induced risk per rem of radiation for those mutationally dependent diseases. The results of combining these effects are shown in Table VII-6. Although the use of these figures can lead to a somewhat higher estimate of the genetic risk from radiation than will the use of the BEIR Committee's figures, in view of the uncertainties involved, the use of the figures in Table VII-6 seems to be a responsible and prudent way to establish risks.

Somatic Effects

The somatic effects of concern at the low dose rates associated with natural background radiation are those that might conceivably result from alterations in individual cells, singly or in small numbers, in the absence of extensive cell killing or tissue disorganization. The most important such effect is considered to be the induction of cancer (BEIR Committee, 1972).

Another effect of potential concern, possibly because it may prove to have preneoplastic significance, is the induction of chromosomal abnormalities in somatic cells, the pathological importance of which is unknown at present (UNSCEAR, 1969; NAS–NRC, 1974). Other effects that are also of potential concern include infant mortality, disturbances in the growth and development of the embryo, shortening of the life span from causes other than cancer, and effects on the nervous system. To date, however, neither the available dose–response data on these effects nor our knowledge of their mechanisms suggests that they deserve to be included with cancer as risks warranting evaluation in relation to natural background radiation levels (BEIR Committee, 1972).

For the above reasons, we will confine our attention here to the possible risk of carcinogenic effects.

RADIOBIOLOGICAL BASIS FOR EVALUATION OF CANCER RISK

As has been discussed extensively elsewhere (ICRP, 1969; BEIR Committee, 1972; UNSCEAR, 1972), there is no conclusive evidence that ionizing radiation exerts carcinogenic effects at the low dose rates commensurate with natural background. Evaluation of the potential risks at such levels must depend, therefore, on extrapolation from observations at higher doses and dose rates. Because the dose-rate characteristic of background radiation (approximately 100 mrem/yr) is several orders of magnitude lower than the lowest rates at which carcinogenic effects have been documented unequivocally, the extrapolation involves assumptions that are highly tentative in our present state of knowledge.

Among the major factors complicating the extrapolation is uncertainty about the shapes of the dose-incidence curves for cancers of different types, about the relevant mechanisms of carcinogenesis, and about the influence of biological and physical variables (e.g., spatial and temporal distribution of the radiation dose, age at irradiation, sex, and physiological state) that have been observed to affect the induction of malignancy at higher dose rates in human and animal populations. The problem is further complicated by the multiplicity and diversity of effects through which radiation is thought to influence the probability of cancer development. These effects include mutagenic changes in DNA, induction of chromosomal aberrations, activation or enhancement of occult tumor viruses, alteration in the dynamics of cell populations, disturbances in hormonal regulation, impairment of immunological defenses, and other effects interfering with homeostasis. Any or all of these effects may conceivably be implicated in a given situation, depending on the dose, dose rate, and other circumstances. Some of the effects, such as disturbances in hormonal regulation and impairment of immunological defenses, are likely to be minimal or absent at low doses and low rates, since their induction requires extensive killing of cells. The other types of effects also should be reduced in frequency per rad at low doses and low dose rates, because of the action of various repair processes, at least in the case of low-LET radiation. Furthermore, if the time required to accumulate a given dose is a sufficient fraction of the life span, then, in the absence of age-dependent changes in susceptibility, the carcinogenicity per rad of the total cumulative dose can be expected to diminish, because the latent period for carcinogenesis will ultimately exceed the life expectancy of some members of the population at risk (NCRP, 1976).

Also complicating the evaluation of carcinogenic effects are the confounding effects of other forms of radiation damage. At high doses and high dose rates, the cytotoxic effects of radiation may interfere drastically with tumor induction, presumably because too few cells remain capable of proliferation to express the carcinogenic changes that might otherwise be manifest (BEIR Committee, 1972; Mole, 1975; NCRP, 1976).

For the reasons indicated, the combined effects of the various types of radiation-induced carcinogenic changes must depend heavily on the dose, dose rate, quality of radiation, and other variables; hence, it is not astonishing that the dose-incidence relationship has been observed to vary with these factors, at least in those instances where cogent data are available (BEIR Committee, 1972; UNSCEAR, 1972; NCRP, 1976). The relationship differs quantitatively, however, from one type of cancer to another, and in no instance are the parameters known well enough to enable confident prediction of the carcinogenic effects to be expected at the low dose rates associated with background radiation levels. These limitations notwithstanding, the pattern of relationships in general implies that any simple linear interpolation on dose from observations at higher doses and dose rates, without allowance for the influence of the aforementioned variables, is likely to overestimate the risks of low-level, low-LET radiation (BEIR Committee, 1972; UNSCEAR, 1972; NCRP, 1976).

It may be concluded, therefore, from all available data, that for carcinogenic effects, just as for the induction of mutations, chromosome aberrations, cell killing, teratogenic effects, and most other effects on mammalian cells and tissues, the dose–response curves for low-LET radiation will tend to be concave upward (see Fig. II-1 in Chapter II).

Characteristically, the curves tend to increase in slope with increasing dose and dose rate, until they reach the point where, with high doses accumulated at high dose rates, they pass through a maximum and eventually turn downward, owing, presumably, to excessive cell killing or to other forms of injury. In comparison, the dose–response curves for high-LET radiation tend to be steeper, more nearly linear, and less dependent on dose rate (BEIR Committee, 1972; UNSCEAR, 1972; NCRP, 1976).

Because of these variations in the biological effectiveness of radiation with changes in the spatial and temporal distribution of dose, various weighting factors have been introduced for use in risk estimation. These include the quality factor (*Q*), which has long been used to adjust for differences in linear energy transfer, or LET (ICRP, 1963; NCRP, 1967). More recently, other dose-effectiveness factors have been introduced to adjust for the reduced effectiveness of low-LET radiation at low doses and low dose rates, both with respect to genetic effects (BEIR Committee, 1972; UNSCEAR, 1972) and carcinogenic effects (NRC, 1975; NCRP, 1976).

Although the dose-effectiveness factors for carcinogenic effects are based largely on empirical observations of radiation carcinogenesis in experimental animals, they are concordant with the data on man and with the bulk of radiobiological experience on the induction of mutations, chromosome aberrations, cell killing, cell transformation in culture, and other effects that may be involved in carcinogenesis (NCRP, 1976). The dose–response relation envisaged can be represented by a function of the form:

$$Y = (c + aD + bD^2)e^{-(\alpha D + \beta D^2)}$$

where Y is the frequency of cancers in the population at risk, C the control incidence, D the dose, and a, b, α, and β are constants. The model of carcinogenesis represented by the formula is that cancers are induced by changes that increase both linearly with dose and as the square of the dose in those cells that are not killed by radiation. The values of the constants are not known precisely for any neoplasm, and they may be presumed to vary somewhat from one type of neoplasm to another and under the influence of other variables. The data imply that for low-LET radiation the linear contribution (aD) is equal to the quadratic contribution (bD^2) at about 50 to 100 rad, i.e., a/b = 50 to 100. According to this interpretation, the linear dose term (aD) would be expected to predominate over the quadratic dose term (bD^2) at low doses and low dose rates, whereas the reverse would be true at high doses and high dose rates. As a result, the carcinogenic risks per rad would be expected to increase with dose and dose rate, until overridden by excessive cell and tissue damage, the total risks per rad being as much as 4 to 6 times higher after an acutely delivered dose of 300 rad than after a dose of 10 rad (NCRP, 1976). To allow for such differences in dose-effectiveness, weighting factors have been proposed that range in magnitude from 0.2, for doses of less than 10 rad, or for larger doses received at dose rates of less than 1 mrad per minute, to 1 for doses of 200 rad or more received at dose rates in excess of 1 mrad/min (Tables VII-7 and VII-8).

The values tabulated have been introduced for use in estimating the overall carcinogenic risk of low-level low-LET radiation for all malignancies combined, and are not intended for use in estimating the risk per rad for every type of cancer individually, there being indications that the dose–response relation may differ among malignancies. At best, therefore, the values can be taken to represent no more than crude approximations, based on an approach that is necessarily simplified for practical purposes. For estimating the risk of carcinogenesis in any one organ, it may be more appropriate to use other dose–response functions and weighting factors, depending on whether they may be indicated by the available data (NRC, 1975; NCRP, 1976). For example, evidence has been presented elsewhere that the dose-incidence relations for cancers of the breast and thyroid may be influenced less by dose rate (BEIR Committee, 1972; NRC, 1975; NCRP, 1976) and thus deserve to be treated differently. The values tabulated are also not intended for application to high-LET radiations, the effectiveness of which is generally assumed to be relatively invariant with dose and dose rate throughout the low-to-intermediate dose region (NCRP, 1976).

TABLE VII-7 Dose-Effectiveness Factors for Carcinogenic Effects of Low-LET Radiation, in Relation to Dose Rate and Dose Magnitude, as Proposed by NCRP, Scientific Committee 40 (NCRP, 1976)

Yearly Dose, rad	Effect-to-Dose Ratio At < 1 mrad/min	At > 1 mrad/min
0–5	0.2	0.2
5–50	0.2	0.3
50–100	0.2	0.5
100–200	0.2	0.7
200+	0.2	1.0

The values tabulated represent the assumed comparative effectiveness per rad of low-LET radiation in the ranges of dose and dose rate indicated, for purpose of risk estimation.

TABLE VII-8 Dose-effectiveness Factors for Carcinogenic Effects of Low-LET Radiation, as Used in the Reactor Safety Study (NRC,1975)

Total Dose, rem	Effect-to-Dose Ratio		
	At < 1 rem/day	At 1–10 rem/day	At >10 rem/day
10	0.2	0.2	0.2
10–25	0.2	0.4	0.4
25–300	0.2	0.4	1.0

Risk Estimates for Specific Cancers

Review of the available data on human and animal populations indicated that radiation may conceivably cause cancer of virtually any type or site, given appropriate conditions of irradiation and host susceptibility (BEIR Committee, 1972; UNSCEAR, 1972). At the same time, however, the data indicate that tissues vary widely in susceptibility to radiation-induced malignancy, cancers of a relatively small number of types and sites predominating during the first 25–30 yr after doses of a few hundred rem or less (ICRP, 1969; BEIR Committee, 1972; UNSCEAR, 1972).

The types of cancer that may conceivably result from low-level irradiation, the time required for their development following exposure ("latent period"), the time during which they are expected to occur in the excess among irradiated individuals ("plateau period"), and the average magnitude of the excess during the plateau period have been estimated by the BEIR Committee (1972). They assumed a linear nonthreshold dose-incidence relationship fitted to the observed human data and interpolated to pass through the control incidence at the intercept (Table VII-9). In presenting the estimates tabulated, the BEIR Committee qualified the values on the basis of the following sources of uncertainty:

1. None of the irradiated human populations studied to date has been followed throughout its entire life span, with the result that the duration and ultimate magnitude of the cancer excess attributable to a given exposure remain to be fully ascertained; by the same token, it is conceivable that additional types of radiation-induced cancers with unusually long latent periods are still to become manifest.

2. The relation between the radiation-induced risk and the natural risk is not clear from the existing data; that is, it is uncertain whether the excess resulting from a given dose more nearly approximates a constant percentage of the natural incidence (and thus varies with age at time of

TABLE VII-9 Values Assumed by BEIR Committee (1972) in Estimating Risks of Low-Level Irradiation

Type of Cancer	Age at Time of Irradiation (yr)	Latent Period (yr)	Plateau Period (yr)	Risk Estimate: Absolute (deaths/10^6/yr/rem)	Risk Estimate: Relative (% incr. in deaths/rem)
Leukemia	*In utero*	0	10	25	50
Leukemia	0–9.9	2	25	2	5.0
Leukemia	10+	2	25	1	2.0
Lung	10+	15	30[a]	1.3	0.3
GI tract, including stomach	10+	15	30[a]	1.0	0.2
Breast	10+	15	30[a]	1.5[b]	0.8
Bone	10+	15	30[a]	0.2	1.0
All other[c]	*In utero*	0	10	25[d]	50
All other[c]	0–9.9	15	30[a]	1[d]	2.0
All other[c]	10	15	30[a]	1[e]	0.1

[a]Alternatively, the remaining life expectancy could be considered as the plateau period.
[b]Includes males and an assumed 50% cure rate.
[c]Includes thyroid and skin. It is noteworthy that the mortality from thyroid cancer was inferred to be low, as compared with the morbidity from the disease, which was estimated to approximate 1.6–9.3 cases/10^6/yr/rem in persons irradiated during childhood.
[d]"All other" denotes all cancers except leukemia.
[e]"All other" denotes all cancers except those specified in table.

irradiation and other susceptibility factors) or a constant number of additional cases (irrespective of the natural incidence).

3. The existence of various kinds of homeostatic and repair processes argues strongly that the risk per rad of background radiation is likely to be smaller than that at the higher doses and dose rates where effects have been observed; in fact, the possibility that the risk may approach zero at background levels is not excluded by the data.

4. The killing of susceptible cells at high doses and high dose rates can be expected to counteract the carcinogenic effects of radiation to some extent, with the result that linear extrapolation based on effects observed under these circumstances may, conceivably, underestimate the risk of irradiation at lower doses and dose rates (BEIR Committee, 1972).

Although the values tabulated (Table VII-9) may ultimately prove to be underestimates, for the reasons given above, most observers have considered them more likely to be overestimates, owing to their failure to make any allowance for the effects of repair at low doses and dose rates, effects that have been amply documented in experimental animals. Thus, more recent evaluations of the risks of low-level low-LET irradiation have recommended the use of the aforementioned dose-effectiveness factors (Tables VII-7 and VII-8) in arriving at estimates for low doses and low dose rates by extrapolation from observations at higher doses and higher dose rates (NRC, 1975; NCRP, 1976).

In the Reactor Safety Study (NRC, 1975), while the upper bound estimates were derived from absolute risk values obtained by the BEIR Committee, the central estimates (Table VII-10) were small fractions of these values, derived by the use of dose-effectiveness factors (Table VII-8) intended to correct the estimates for the influence of repair at low doses and low dose rates of low-LET radiation. The lower bound estimates were based on the assumption that below a threshold of 10-25 rem the risk per rad is zero.

The dose-effectiveness factors proposed by NCRP Scientific Committee 40 (Table VII-7) are similar in direction and range to those used in the Reactor Safety Study, but they differ in magnitude at low doses, especially over the region between 10 and 100 rad. Because of this difference, and the fact that most of the human data on radiation carcinogenesis come from populations in which the average dose received

TABLE VII-10 Values Assumed in Reactor Safety Study for Use in Estimating Risks of Low-Level Low-LET Irradiation (NRC, 1975)

				Risk Estimate	
Type of Cancer	Age at Time of Irradiation (yr)	Latent Period (yr)	Plateau Period (yr)	Upper Bound (deaths/10^6/yr/rem)	Central Estimate (deaths/10^6/yr/rem)
Leukemia	*In utero*	0	10	15	3
Leukemia	0–9.9	2	25	2	0.4
Leukemia	10+	2	25	1	0.2
Lung	10+	15	30	1.3	0.5
Stomach	10+	15	30	0.6	0.12
Rest of GI tract	10+	10	30	0.2	0.04
Pancreas	10+	15	30	0.2	0.04
Breast	10+	15	30	1.5[a]	1.5
Bone	0–19.9	10	30	0.4	0.08
Bone	20+	10	30	0.2	0.04
All other	*In utero*	0	10	15[b]	3
All other	0–9.9	15	30	0.6[c]	0.12
All other	10+	15	30	1[d]	0.2

[a]Includes males and an assumed 50% cure rate.
[b]"All other" includes all cancers except leukemia.
[c]"All other" includes all cancers except leukemia and bone.
[d]"All other" includes all cancers except those specified in table.

in any one exposure has not greatly exceeded 100 rad, estimates derived with the NCRP factors should be intermediate between those calculated in the Reactor Safety Study and those reported by the BEIR Committee (Table VII-11). From the values tabulated, it will be noted that the number of cancers attributed hypothetically to continuous low-level irradiation of the U.S. population at a rate approximating natural background radiation levels (100 mrem per year) ranges from 0 to roughly 9,000 depending on the method used to arrive at the risk estimate. The larger of the values (9,000) corresponds to about 2.9% of the total number of cancer deaths from all causes recorded annually in the United States (BEIR Committee, 1972).

The enormous variation among estimates yielded by different extrapolation models (Table VII-11) reflects the large uncertainty about dose–response relationships that complicates current attempts to estimate the carcinogenic risks of low-level irradiation. The criteria for selecting one method of risk estimation in preference to another must thus depend in large measure on other than purely scientific considerations. To the extent that the estimates are intended for purposes of limiting risks to populations, it is desirable that they should include a margin of safety large enough to compensate for any uncertainty as to their reliability. On the other hand, if the estimates are to be used for purposes of cost–benefit analysis, it is desirable that they not be exaggerated, since overestimation of the risks may prompt decisions in favor of alternatives that could involve greater hazards or burdens to society.

RISKS FROM RADIOACTIVE DRINKING WATER

The average amount of background radiation to which the U.S. population is exposed is about 0.1 of a rem (100 mrem) per year. Part of this background comes from drinking water that contains radioactive materials.

The dose commitment from radioisotopes in U.S. drinking water supplies is very low. In a hypothetical water supply that was constituted in such a way as to contain either average or likely amounts of radioactivity, a total-body dose of less than one-thousandth of a rem (0.244 mrem) per year would be accumulated. This is less than 1% of background. Although the dose to bone would be considerably higher, because strontium and radium are bone seekers, even this dose would constitute less than 10% of the total average natural background.

Estimates were made of three possible types of risk that could be

TABLE VII-11 Comparative Estimates of the Number of Cancer Deaths per Year in the U.S. Population Attributable to Continuous Exposure at Rate of 0.1 rem per Year

		Estimated Excess Cancer Deaths Resulting from 0.1 rem per Year[a]						
Age at Time of Irradiation	Duration of Plateau Period (yr)	BEIR Estimates[b]		NRC Estimates[c]			NCRP Estimates[d]	
		Absolute Risk Model	Relative Risk Model	Upper Bound	Central Estimates	Lower Bound	Absolute Risk Model	Relative Risk Model
In utero	10	150	110	90	20	0	150	110
0–9 yr	25–30	240	800	240	50	0	100	320
	life	290	6,000	—	—	—	120	2,400
10+ yr	25–30	1,300	2,200	1,300	500	0	520	880
	life	1,600	3,000	—	—	—	640	1,200
Total	25–30	1,700	3,200	1,650	600	0	770	1,310
	life	2,000	9,000	—	—	—	910	3,710

[a]Values in table have been rounded to facilitate comparison.

[b]From BEIR Committee, 1972, p. 169, based on vital statistics for U.S. population, 1967.

[c]Values are rough calculations, based on application of NRC (1975) risk models to U.S. population, 1967.

[d]Values are rough calculations, based on application of NCRP (1976) risk model to U.S. population, 1967. The values for irradiation *in utero* are the same as the BEIR Committee's estimates, without adjustment for dose or dose rate, since they are based on data from populations exposed to doses averaging 5 rad or less. The values for postnatal irradiation, on the other hand, have been derived by adjusting the BEIR estimates for dose and dose rate by application of the appropriate dose-effectiveness factors set forth in Table VII-7. Since the BEIR Committee's estimates are based largely on data from populations in which the average dose received in any one exposure did not greatly exceed 100 rad, and a dose rate corresponding to a dose-effectiveness factor of 0.5 (Table VII-7), the BEIR values have been multiplied by a factor of 0.2/0.5 to adjust them for the conditions of low-dose low-dose-rate irradiation in question.

induced by the radiation: developmental and teratogenic risks, genetic risks, and somatic risks.

Developmental and Teratogenic Risks

Although the developing fetus is sensitive to radiation, the total low-dose-rate doses that would be delivered during the sensitive periods of gestation are so small that no measurable effects of the radiation from drinking water will be found. The lowest dose level at which any effect has been reported is 3 mrem/day or 1,100 mrem/yr in contrast to the 0.244 mrem per year described above.

Genetic Risks

For the general population, the maximum permissible dose of man-made radiation is 170 mrem/yr, excluding medical uses of radiation. This amounts to a 5 rem genetic dose in each 30-yr generation. This dose would increase the current incidence of genetic diseases, which is about 94,400 per million live births, by about 200 per million in the first generation. The estimate of 200, however, is so uncertain that there are very large limits about the value. The gonadal dose of 0.244 mrem/yr calculated for the hypothetical drinking water is expected to increase the genetic diseases from the $94,000/10^6$ live births by 200×0.244 mrem/30×170 mrem = 0.0098 additional genetic diseases per million live births per year. Since there are approximately 3.6 million live births in the United States each year, this is an increase of 0.035 total genetic diseases in the United States per year. If one takes the unlikely extreme limits of the estimated genetic hazards of radiation (about 4,000) instead of the value 200, the increase is 0.7 cases per year.

Somatic Risks

The natural background of radiation can be estimated to cause 4.5 to 45 fatal cases of cancer per year per million people, depending on the risk model used to make the calculation (Table VII-11). Less than 1% of this will be contributed by the radionuclides in drinking water.

Variations in the radium content of drinking water, however, may cause appreciable differences in the radiation dose to the skeleton and, in turn, in the risks of associated carcinogenic effects. Under average conditions, the annual dose to bone from radium amounts to approximately 6.4 mrem/yr, which represents about 6% of the total dose to the skeleton from all sources of natural background radiation (roughly 100 mrem annually). The highest radium levels in drinking water (25 pCi/liter of ^{226}Ra and an additional 12.5 pCi/liter of ^{228}Ra), however, may be expected to deliver a dose to the skeleton of about 600 mrem/yr, which would represent a sixfold increase in the total dose to bone from all natural sources combined. If the carcinogenic risks associated with skeletal irradiation are assumed to be 0.2 fatal cases of bone cancer per million persons per year per rem (Table VII-9), then for a period up to 30 yr, in a population with a typical distribution of ages, the risks attributable to natural background radiation can be estimated to range up to about 0.6 per million persons per year under average conditions,* and to 4.2 per million per year under conditions of maximal intake of radium in the drinking water (about 600 mrem/yr from the radium).

In addition to these risks, the possibility of carcinogenic effects from radium on cells adjacent to bone, such as those in epithelia lining cranial sinuses and those in the bone marrow, should also be mentioned. However, the risks of such effects are likely to be appreciably smaller and cannot be estimated precisely from existing data. In comparison with the overall risks of cancers of all sites combined, of which 4.5 to 45 (i.e. 9000/200) fatal cases per million per year can be attributed to natural background radiation at average levels (Table VII-11), the additional 3.6 fatal bone malignancies per million per year ascribable to maximal intakes of radium in drinking water constitute a significant increment. It should be noted that only about 120,000 people drink water estimated to contain between 9 and 25 pCi/liter. Thus the excess bone cancers in this group would be between 0.16 and 0.43 per year; that is to say, one excess bone cancer every 2 to 6 yr. Since about 113,000 of the 120,000 people drink water containing less than 20 pCi/liter, the true number of excess bone cancers will lie somewhere towards the lower end of the range.

When interpreting the above estimates, it must be remembered that they depend on dose–response models that remain highly uncertain. For example, the value given for the combined frequency of deaths from all types of cancer attributable to natural background radiation— namely, 45 deaths per million per year— is higher by a factor of three or more than estimates derived with any of the other risk models cited (Table VII-11). Likewise, the corresponding risk estimates for skeletal cancer could vary widely, depending on the postulated dose–response relationship. Although the value yielded by the BEIR Committee's absolute risk model (0.2 fatal cancers per million per year per rem) is not greatly different from the value yielded by the BEIR Committee's relative risk model (since 9 out of the 1,704 fatal cancers per million per year are bone

*(0.2 fatal cases × 0.1 rem/yr × 30 yr)/(10^6 persons per yr per rem)

cancers, this would be approximately 0.09 fatal bone cancers per million per year per rem), both models, in postulating a linear nonthreshold dose–response relationship, give substantially higher estimates than do models postulating dose-dependent and dose-rate-dependent variations in the risk per rem. Given the uncertainties in present knowledge, the BEIR Committee's absolute risk model as used in the foregoing would seem to provide an acceptably conservative approach for the purposes at hand.

SUMMARY—RADIOACTIVITY IN DRINKING WATER

Everyone is exposed to some natural radiation that comes from both cosmic rays and terrestrial sources. Although there are large geographic variations in the amount of natural background radiation, the average background dose in the United States is about 100 mrem/yr. A small proportion of this unavoidable background radiation comes from drinking water that contains radionuclides.

By far the largest contribution to the radioactivity in drinking water comes from potassium-40, which is present as a constant percentage of total potassium. Only a small percentage of the total potassium-40 body burden, however, comes from drinking water. The total body dose from other possible radioactive contaminants of water constitutes a small percentage of the background radiation to which the population is exposed. Although the amounts of individual radioactive contaminants fluctuate from place to place, calculations made for a hypothetical water supply that might be typical for the United States have shown that a total soft-tissue dose of only 0.24 mrem/yr would be contributed by all the radionuclides found in the water. Even with rather wide fluctuations in the concentrations, the total contribution of the radionuclides will remain very small.

However, bone-seeking radionuclides—such as strontium-90, radium-226, and radium-228—account for a somewhat larger proportion of the total bone dose. This is particularly true for the two isotopes of radium because they, or their daughters, emit high-linear-energy-transfer (LET) radiation, and because certain restricted localities have been found to have rather high concentrations of radium in drinking water. Nevertheless, in the hypothetical typical water supply, less than 10% of the annual background dose comes from such radiation. It has also been estimated that the total population exposed to levels of radium greater than 3 pCi/liter is about a million people. About 120,000 people are exposed to radium at levels greater than 9 pCi/liter.

Risk estimates were made of three kinds of adverse health effects that radiation could produce: developmental and teratogenic effects, genetic effects, and somatic (chiefly carcinogenic) effects.

Developmental and Teratogenic Effects

The developing fetus is exposed to radiation from radionuclides in drinking water for nine months. Thus, the total dose accumulated by the fetus will be very small. Furthermore, although the fetus is sensitive to the effects of radiation in some stages of development, these periods are sharply limited and extremely short. For this reason, too, the total dose administered that could possibly have developmental and teratogenic effects would be extremely small. Current concentrations of radionuclides in drinking water lead to doses of about one five-thousandth of the lowest dose at which a developmental effect has been found in animals. Therefore, the developmental and teratogenic effects of radionuclides would not be measurable.

Genetic Effects

It has been estimated that there are about 94,400 genetic diseases per million live births in the United States. The maximum permissible dose of man-made radiation for the general population (170 mrem/yr) has been estimated to increase this number in the first generation by 170–215, with an unlikely upper limit of 4,250. On the basis of a 30-yr generation and 3.6 million live births per year in the United States, we would expect the 0.24 mrem soft-tissue dose, or gonad dose, to lead to 0.0098 additional cases of genetic disease per million live births per year or 0.035 additional cases of genetic disease in the United States per year. Even at the unlikely extreme upper limit of possible genetic effects of radiation of around 4,000 extra cases in the first generation, there would still be less than one additional case per year in the $94{,}400 \times 3.6 = 340{,}000$ live births with genetic defects. The wide fluctuation in bone dose caused by fluctuations in the radium concentration of drinking water would not have any sensible effect on the genetically significant dose, because radium is predominantly a bone seeker and will deliver very little radiation to the gonads.

Somatic and Carcinogenic Effects

The natural background of radiation can be estimated to cause 4.5 to 45 cases of cancer per million people, depending on the risk model used. The per year amount of whole-body radiation from radionuclides in typical drinking water contributes less than 1% of this amount, and thus, for cancers other than those in bone, may cause a negligible increase in the total. Radium, however, can contribute somewhat less than 7% of the total bone dose received from background radiation in areas of "normal" radium concentration. The average carcinogenic risk associated with skeletal irradiation by radium in a population with a typical distribution of ages is estimated to approximate 0.2 fatal cases of bone cancer per million persons per year per rem. Therefore, over a period from 10 to 40 yr after the beginning of skeletal irradiation, the average risk attributable to natural background radiation is estimated to range from 0.6 per million persons per year, under typical conditions, to as much as 4.2 per million per year, in regions where 25 pCi/liter of radium-226 are found in the drinking water. It has been noted that in the United States 120,000 people are estimated to drink water containing between 9 and 25 pCi/liter of radium-226, and only a small number lie near the upper end of this range. The number of excess cancers in this group would therefore lie between 0.16 and 0.43 per year. Since not all the 120,000 people drink water containing 25 pCi/liter of radium-226, the latter number is inordinately high.

CONCLUSIONS

The radiation associated with most water supplies is such a small proportion of the normal background to which all human beings are exposed, that it is difficult, if not impossible, to measure any adverse health effects with certainty. In a few water supplies, however, radium can reach concentrations that pose a higher risk of bone cancer for the people exposed.

FUTURE NEEDS

The precision of estimation of the health risks associated with radioactivity in drinking water could be enhanced if several water systems were analyzed to determine the complete distributions of beta and alpha radiation that constitute the gross counting measurements.

Because the precise ratio of radium-228 to radium-226 in water has not been measured extensively, an attempt should be made to determine the ratio in several ground and surface waters whose content of radium-226 is known. Activity concentrations of the waters to be analyzed should range from about 0.1–50 pCi/liter. The percentage of the daughter radionuclides present should be determined.

Because radon is a noble gas that is quickly released from water, it is possible that, in some areas of high radon content, water vapor containing radon might constitute an inhalation hazard when such water is used, for example, in humidifiers or for showers. A determination should be made whether or not radon emanations from water do indeed constitute an inhalation hazard.

The models used in this report do not take into account the possibility that the finely divided solid particles that occur in water may alter the uptake of radionuclides. The effects of the solids in drinking water on the metabolism and uptake of radionuclides merit investigation.

GLOSSARY

Absolute risk. Excess or incremental risk due to exposure to a toxic or injurious agent (e.g., to radiation). Difference between the risk (or incidence) of disease or death in the exposed population, and the risk in the unexposed population. Usually expressed as number of excess cases in a population of a given size, per unit time, per unit dose (e.g., cases/10^6 exposed population/year/rem).

Curie (Ci). Unit of radioactivity. 1 Curie = 3.7×10^{10} nuclear transformations per second. Some fractions are: millicurie (1 mCi = 10^{-3} Ci), microcurie (1 μCi = 10^{-6} Ci), nanocurie (1 nCi = 10^{-9} Ci), picocurie (1 pCi = 10^{-12} Ci), femtocurie (1 fCi = 10^{-15} Ci).

Latent period. Period between time of exposure to a toxic or injurious agent and appearance of a biological response.

LET. Linear energy transfer. Average amount of energy lost by an ionizing particle or photon per unit length of track in matter.

Plateau period. Period of above-normal, relatively uniform, incidence of disease or death in response to a toxic or injurious agent.

Rad. Unit of dose or radiation (energy) absorbed in any medium, except air. 1 Rad = 100 erg/g.

Relative risk. Ratio of the risk in the exposed population to that in the unexposed population. Usually given as a multiple of the natural risk.

Rem. Unit of radiation dose equivalence. Numerically equal to absorbed dose in rad multiplied by a quality factor that expresses the biological effectiveness of the radiation of interest, and other factors. Equal doses expressed in rem produce the same biological effects, independently of the type of radiation involved.

Roentgen (R). Unit of radiation (energy) absorbed in air. 1 R = 2.58×10^{-4} coulomb/kg of air.

REFERENCES

Abrahamson, S., and S. Wolff. 1976. Reanalysis of radiation-induced specific locus mutations in the mouse. Nature 264:715-719.

AEC. 1974. Plutonium and other transuranium elements: Sources, environmental distribution and biomedical effects. WASH-1359, U.S. Atomic Energy Commission.

BEIR Committee. 1972. The effects on populations of exposure to low levels of ionizing radiation. Advisory Committee on the Biological Effects of Ionizing Radiations, National Academy of Sciences, National Research Council, Washington, D.C.

Batchelor, A.L., R.J.S. Phillips, and A.G. Searle. 1969. The ineffectiveness of chronic irradiation with neutrons and gamma rays in inducing mutations in female mice. Br. J. Radiol. 42:448-451.

Brent, R.L., and R.O. Gorson. 1972. Radiation exposure in pregnancy. Curr. Probl. Radiol., vol. 2, no. 5.

Brewen, J.G., R.J. Preston, and N. Gengozian. 1975. Analysis of X-ray-induced chromosomal translocations in human and marmoset stem cells. Nature 253:468-470.

Cahill, D.F., L.W. Reiter, J.A. Santolucito, G.T. Rehnberg, M.E. Ash, M.J. Fauor, S.J. Bursian, J.F. Wright, and J.W. Laskey. 1976. Biological assessment of continuous exposure to tritium and lead in the rat. *In* Symposium on Biological Effects of Low-Level Radiation Pertinent to Protection of Man and His Environment, Chicago, 1975. International Atomic Energy Agency, Vienna.

Cavalli-Sforza, L.L., and W.F. Bodmer. 1971. The Genetics of Human Populations. W.H. Freeman and Company, San Francisco.

Della Rosa, R.J., M. Goldman, H.G. Wolf, and L.S. Rosenblatt. 1972. Application of canine metabolic data to man. *In* Biomedical Implications of Radiostrontium Exposure. AEC Symposium Series No. 25. CONF-710201:52-67. U.S. Atomic Energy Commission.

EPA. 1975. Preliminary Assessment of Suspected Carcinogens in Drinking Water. Report to Congress, U.S. Environmental Protection Agency, Washington, D.C.

Gesell, T.F., H.M. Pritchard, E.M. Othel, L. Prittle, and W. Di Pietro. 1975. Nuclear Medicine Environmental Discharge Measuremets. Final report to EPA, University of Texas, Houston, Office of Radiation Programs, U.S. Environmental Protection Agency.

Goldberg, J. 1976. California Department of Health, Radiologic Health Section. Personal communication.

Hickey, J.L.S., and S.D. Campbell. 1968. High radium-226 concentrations in public water supplies. Public Health Rep. 83:551-557.

ICRP. 1959. Permissible Dose for Internal Radiation. International Commission on Radiological Protection. Publication No. 2. Pergamon Press, New York.

ICRP. 1963. Report of the RBE Committee to the International Commissions on Radiological Protection and on Radiological Units and Measurements. International Commission on Radiological Protection. Health Phy. 9:357-386.

ICRP. 1969. Radiosensitivity and Spatial Distribution of Dose. International Commission on Radiological Protection. ICRP Publication No. 14. Pergamon Press, New York.

ICRP. 1973. Alkaline Earth Metabolism in Adult Man. International Commission on Radiological Protection. Publication No. 20. Pergamon Press, New York.

ICRP. 1974. Reference Man: Anatomical, Physiological and Metabolic Characteristics. International Commission on Radiological Protection. ICRP Publication No. 23. Pergamon Press, New York.

Jacobs, D.G. 1968. Sources of Tritium and Its Behavior upon Release to the Environment. U.S. Atomic Energy Commission. Available from National Technical Information Service as Report 24635.

Jacobs, P.A., M. Melville, S. Ratcliffe, A.J. Keay, and J. Syme. 1974. A cytogenetic survey 11,680 newborn infants. Ann. Hum. Genet. (Lond.) 37:359-376.

Kaul, A., and W. Loose. 1975. Experiences with the release of radioactive sewage from a medical area. Kerntechnik 17(2):81-88.

Klement, A.W., Jr., C.R. Miller, R.P. Miux, and B. Schleien. 1972. Estimates of ionizing radiation doses in the United States 1960-2000. Report no. ORD/CSD/72-1. U.S. Environmental Protection Agency.

Lucas, H.F., Jr. 1971. Correlation of the natural radioactivity of the human body to that of the environment: uptake and retention of Ra^{226} from food and water. *In* Radiological Physics Division. Semiannual Report, July-Dec. ANL-6297:55-56. Argonne National Laboratories.

Lucas, H.F., Jr., R.B. Holtzman, and D.C. Dahlin. 1964. Radium-226, radium-228, lead-210, and fluorine in persons with osteogenic sarcoma. Science 144:1573-1575.

Lucas, H.F., Jr., and D.P. Krause. 1960. Preliminary survey of radium-226 and radium-228 (MsThI) contents of drinking water. Radiology 74:114.

Lyon, M.F., and R.J.S. Phillips. 1975. Specific locus mutation rates after repeated small radiation doses to mouse oocytes. Mutat. Res. 30:375-382.

Marshall, J.F., and P.G. Groer. 1975. Theory of the induction of bone cancer by radiation: a preliminary report. I. A three-stage alpha particle model and the data for radium in man. *In* Radiological and Environmental Research Division Annual Report, Center for Human Radiobiology. ANL-75-60, Part II:1-38, Argonne National Laboratory, Argonne, Illinois.

McCann, J., E. Choi, E. Yamasaki, and B.N. Ames. 1975. Detection of carcinogens as mutagens in the *Salmonella*/microsome test: Assay of 300 chemicals. Proc. Nat. Acad. Sci. USA 72:5135-5139.

McCann, J., and B.N. Ames. 1976. Detection of carcinogens as mutagens in the *Salmonella*/microsome test: Assay of 300 chemicals: Discussion. Proc. Nat. Acad. Sci. USA 73:950-954.

Miller, C.E., and A.J. Finkel. 1968. Radium retention in man after multiple injections: The power function re-evaluated. Am. J. Roentgenol. 103:871-880.

Mole, R.H. 1975. Ionizing radiation as a carcinogen: practical questions and academic pursuits. Br. J. Radiol. 48:157-169.

NAS-NRC. 1973. Radionuclides in Foods. Food Protection Committee, National Academy of Sciences, National Research Council, Washington, D. C.

NAS-NRC. 1974. Research Needs for Estimating the Biological Hazards of Low Doses of Ionizing Radiations. Committee on Nuclear Science, National Research Council, National Academy of Sciences, Washington, D.C.

NCRP. 1963. Maximum Permissible Body Burdens and Maximum Permissible Concentrations of Radionuclides in Air and Water for Occupational Exposure. National Commission on Radiation Protection, Report No. 22. National Bureau of Standards Handbook 69. U.S. Department of Commerce, Washington, D.C.

NCRP. 1967. Dose–effect modifying factors in radiation protection. Report of Subcommittee M-4 (Relative Biological Effectiveness). BNL-50073 (T-471). National Commission on Radiation Protection. Brookhaven National Laboratory.

NCRP. 1975. Natural Background Radiation in the United States. NCRP Report No. 45. National Council on Radiation Protection and Measurements, Washington, D.C.

NCRP. 1976. Influence of dose rate and LET on dose–effect relationships: Implications for estimation of risks of low-level irradiation. Report prepared by NCRP Scientific Committee 40. National Council on Radiation Protection and Measurements, Washington, D.C. To be published.

Newcombe, H.B. 1975. Mutation and the amount of human ill health. *In* O.F. Nygaard, H.I. Adler, and W.K. Sinclair, eds. Radiation Research, Proceedings of the Fifth International Congress of Radiation Research. Academic Press, New York.

Norris, W.P., T.W. Speckman, and P.F. Gustafson. 1955. Studies of the metabolism of radium in man. Am. J. Roentgenol. 73:785-802.

Norris, W.P., S.A. Tyler, and A.M. Brues. 1958. Retention of radioactive bone-seekers. Science 128:456-462.

NRC. 1975. Reactor safety study; an assessment of accident risks in U.S. commercial nuclear power plants. WASH-1400, NUREG-75/014. U.S. Nuclear Regulatory Commission, Washington, D.C.

NRC. 1976. Standards for Protection Against Radiation. Nuclear Regulatory Commission, Title 10 Code of Federal Regulations, Part 20. U.S. Government Printing Office, Washington, D.C.

Peterson N.J., L.D. Samuels, H.F. Lucas, and S.P. Abrahams. 1966. An epidemiologic approach to low-level radium-226 exposure. Public Health Rep. 81:805-814.

Rowland, R.E., H.F. Lucas, Jr., and A.F. Stehney. 1977. High radium levels in the water supplies of Illinois and Iowa. *In* T.L. Cullen and L.P. Franca, eds. Proc. Int. Symp. Areas of High Natural Radioactivity. Academia Brasileira de Ciencias, Rio de Janeiro.

Rowland, R.E., H.F. Lucas, Jr., and A.F. Stehney. 1976. Personal communication.

Russell, L.B. 1971. Definition of functional units in a small chromosomal segment of the mouse and its use in interpreting the nature of radiation-induced mutations. Mutat. Res. 11:107-123.

Searle, A.G. 1974. Mutation induction in mice. Adv. Radiat. Biol. 4:131-207.

Sikov, M.R., and D.D. Mahlum, eds. 1969. Radiation Biology of the Fetal and Juvenile Mammal. AEC Symposium Series no. 17. CONF-690501. U.S. Atomic Energy Commission

Sikov, M.R., and D.D. Mahlum. 1972. Plutonium in the developing animal. Health Phys. 22:707-712.

Sodd, V.J., R.J. Velten, and E.L. Saenger. 1975. Concentrations of the medically useful radionuclides technetium-99m and iodine-131 at a large metropolitan waste water treatment plant. Health Phys. 28:355-359.

Soldat, J.K., N.M. Robinson, and D.A. Baker. 1975. Models and computer codes for evaluating environmental radiation doses. U.S. Atomic Energy Commission Report BNWL-1754 (Feb. 1975, as revised 10/31/75).

Soldat, J.K. 1976. Radiation doses from iodine-129 in the environment. Health Physics 30:61-70.

Stehney, A.F. 1960. Radioisotopes in the skeleton: Naturally occurring radioisotopes in man. *In* R.S. Caldecott and L.A. Snyder, eds. Symposium on Radioisotopes in the Biosphere. Center for Continuation Study, University of Minnesota. 366-381.

Stehney, A.F., and H.F. Lucas, Jr. 1956. Studies on the radium content of humans arising from the natural radium of their environment. *In* Proc. First Int. Conf. on Peaceful Uses of Atomic Energy, United Nations, 11:49-54.

Trimble, B.K., and J.H. Doughty. 1974. The amount of hereditary disease in human populations. Ann. Hum. Genet. (Lond.) 38:199-223.

Uchida, I.A., and C.P.V. Lee. 1974. Radiation-induced nondisjunction in mouse oocytes. Nature 250:601-602.

UNSCEAR. 1958. Report of the United Nations Scientific Committee on the Effects of Atomic Radiation. General Assembly, Official Records, 13th. Session, Suppl. 17 (A/3838). United Nations, New York.

UNSCEAR. 1962. Report of the United Nations Scientific Committee on the Effects of Atomic Radiation. General Assembly, Official Records, 17th. Session, Suppl. 17 (A/5216). United Nations, New York.

UNSCEAR. 1966. Report of the United Nations Scientific Committee on the Effects of Atomic Radiation. General Assembly, Official Records, 21st. Session, Suppl. 14 (A/6314). United Nations, New York.

UNSCEAR. 1969. Report of the United Nations Scientific Committee on the Effects of Atomic Radiation. General Assembly, Official Records, 24th. Session, Suppl. 13 (A/7613). United Nations, New York.

UNSCEAR. 1972. Ionizing Radiation: Levels and Effects. Report of the United Nations Scientific Committee on the Effects of Atomic Radiation. General Assembly, Official Records, 27th. Session, Suppl. 25 (A/8725). United Nations, New York.

Wrenn, M.E. 1976. Internal dose estimates. *In* T.L. Cullen and E.P. Franca eds. First Int. Symp. on Areas of High Natural Radioactivity. Academia Brasileira de Ciencias, Rio de Janeiro.

APPENDIX

A

Legislation and Terms of Reference of the Study

THE SAFE DRINKING WATER ACT OF 1974 AND THE NAS STUDY
(Public Law 93-523)

PURPOSE OF LEGISLATION

The purpose of the legislation is to assure that the public is provided with an adequate quantity of safe drinking water. It is to assure that water supply systems serving the public meet minimum national standards for protection of public health.

Until passage of the Act, the Federal Government was authorized to prescribe drinking water standards only for water supplies used by interstate carriers, and they were enforceable only with respect to contaminants capable of causing communicable diseases. Public Law 93-523 authorized the Environmental Protection Agency to establish Federal standards for protection from all harmful contaminants and established a joint Federal-State system for assuring compliance with these standards and for protecting underground sources of drinking water.

ABRIDGED SUMMARY OF THE LEGISLATION

a. Required the Administrator of EPA to prescribe national drinking water regulations for contaminants that may adversely affect health.

b. Provided that such regulations apply to public water systems and protect health to the maximum extent feasible.

c. Provided that interim primary regulations be prescribed initially and that, after a study by the National Academy of Sciences, health goals were to be established and revised primary regulations promulgated. That portion of the Act pertaining to the NAS study and the scope of work is detailed below.

d. Provided for a number of other requirements and administrative authorizations not directly related to the NAS study.

NEED FOR LEGISLATION

Congressional hearings, EPA studies, and evidence from a number of sources found that Federal legislative authority prior to passage of the Act was inadequate to assure that water supplied to the public was safe to drink.

This conclusion was based on evidence that waterborne disease outbreaks still occur in this country. Examples include an epidemic at Riverside, California, in 1965 that affected 18,000 people, an outbreak of gastroenteritis in Angola, New York, in 1968 affecting 30% of the population, and an epidemic of giardiasis in Rome, New York, in 1974 affecting almost 5,000 people. According to a 1970 EPA survey of 969 drinking water supply systems, approximately 8 million people in this country are served water that is potentially dangerous in that it failed to meet the mandatory standards set by the Federal Government with respect to interstate carrier systems. The deficiencies in the majority of cases were in smaller systems.

Until passage of the Act there was no provision in Federal law to protect the public from toxic chemicals, and none to protect those not traveling on interstate conveyances from being supplied with drinking water that might cause communicable or noncommunicable illness.

Several extensive surveys have shown serious deficiencies in the number of water samples examined and in the bacteriological and chemical quality of drinking water. Many systems had physical deficiencies, including poorly protected groundwater sources, inadequate disinfection and clarification capacity. In addition, plant operators were inadequately trained. Plants were not being inspected by State or local authorities. In one survey, 50% of plant officials did not remember when, if ever, they had been surveyed by a State or local health department.

House of Representatives Report No. 93-1185 and Senate Report No. 93-231 and Public Law 93-523 are the sources of information for the foregoing.

THE NATIONAL ACADEMY OF SCIENCES STUDY

Public Law 93-523 [Section 1412(e)] mandated the NAS study as follows:

1. The Administrator shall enter into appropriate arrangements with the National Academy of Sciences (or with another independent scientific organization if appropriate arrangements cannot be made with such Academy) to conduct a study to determine:

A. The maximum contaminant levels which should be recommended in order to protect the health of persons from any known or anticipated adverse effects, and

B. The existence of any contaminants the levels of which in drinking water cannot be determined but which may have an adverse effect on the health of persons.

2. The result of the study shall be reported to Congress no later than 2 years after the date of enactment of this title. The report shall contain:

A. A summary and evaluation of relevant publications and unpublished studies;

B. A statement of methodologies and assumptions for estimating the levels at which adverse health effects may occur;

C. A statement of methodologies and assumptions for estimating the margin of safety that should be incorporated in the national primary drinking water regulations;

D. Proposals for recommended maximum contaminant levels for national primary drinking water regulations;

E. A list of contaminants the level of which in drinking water cannot be determined but which may have an adverse effect on the health of persons; and

F. Recommended studies and test protocols for future research on the health effects of drinking water contaminants, including a list of the major research priorities and estimated costs necessary to conduct such priority research.

3. In developing its proposals for recommended maximum contaminants levels, the National Academy of Sciences shall evaluate and explain the impact of the following considerations:

A. The existence of groups or individuals in the population that are more susceptible to adverse effects than the normal healthy adult.

B. The exposure to contaminants in other media than drinking water (including exposures in food, in the ambient air, and in occupational settings) and the resulting body burden of contaminants.

C. Synergistic effects resulting from exposure to or interaction by two or more contaminants.

D. The contaminant exposure and body burden levels that alter physiological function or structure in a manner reasonably suspected of increasing the risk of illness.

4. In making the study under this subsection, the National Academy of Sciences (or other organization) shall collect and correlate:

A. Morbidity and mortality data and

B. Monitored data on the quality of drinking water. Any conclusions based on such correlation shall be included in the report of the study.

5. Neither the report of the study under this subsection nor any draft of such report shall be submitted to the Office of Management and Budget or to any other Federal agency (other than the Environmental Protection Agency) prior to its submission to Congress.

6. Of the funds authorized to be appropriated to the Administrator by this title, such amounts as may be required shall be available to carry out the study and make the report.

SCOPE OF WORK

The following definition of the scope of the study was elaborated jointly by the National Academy of Sciences and the Environmental Protection Agency.

The Academy will undertake to complete the study and report described in Section 1412(e) of the Public Health Service Act, as amended by the Safe Drinking Water Act, with the following understanding: The Academy considers that the intent of Congress in using the phrase "maximum contaminant levels which should be recommended . . . in order to protect the health of persons from any known or anticipated adverse effects" is to provide for recommendations that are consistent with the best scientific knowledge. It is the Academy's judgment that from a scientific point of view, the absolute guarantee of safety implied by this language cannot be made for most or all of the contaminants to be studied. The Academy report will explain and discuss this point. Accordingly, with respect to recommended levels, taking only health effects into account, the Academy's report will provide the following:

(1) Where there are sufficient data from which a human dose-response relationship can be projected with some degree of precision, a projection will be made. The projection will be explained and its qualifications will be made explicit.

(2) For contaminants for which the data are of sufficient quantity and quality, the Academy will exercise its scientific judgment and identify and propose contaminant levels for which it anticipates the risk of adverse health effects to be specifiable and very small. The risks at the proposed levels will be described, with an explanation as to why no "safe" level has been identified.

(3) For contaminants for which the evidence provides no scientific basis or methodology for recommending levels, the Academy will describe the available data, and its significance in terms of known or anticipated adverse health effects.

APPENDIX

B

List of Participants

SAFE DRINKING WATER COMMITTEE

GERARD A. ROHLICH, University of Texas, Austin, *Chairman*
J. CARRELL MORRIS, Harvard University, *Vice Chairman*
JOSEPH F. BORZELLECA, Medical College of Virginia
THOMAS D. BROCK, University of Wisconsin
JOHN DOULL, University of Kansas
PAUL KOTIN, Johns-Manville Corporation
CORNELIUS W. KRUSÉ, Johns Hopkins University
RUTH H. NEFF, Tennessee Environmental Council
PAUL M. NEWBERNE, Massachusetts Institute of Technology
VAUN A. NEWILL, Exxon Corporation
DAVID P. RALL, National Institute of Environmental Health Sciences
CLAYTON O. RUUD, University of Denver
MARVIN A. SCHNEIDERMAN, National Cancer Institute
SHELDON WOLFF, University of California, San Francisco

NAS-NRC Staff

RILEY D. HOUSEWRIGHT, *Project Director*
J. P. T. PEARMAN, *Assistant Project Director*
ROBERT J. GOLDEN
YI-NING K. CHEN
RALPH C. WANDS, *Director, Advisory Center on Toxicology*

Subcommittee on Particulate Contaminants

CLAYTON O. RUUD, University of Denver, *Chairman*
ARNOLD L. BROWN, Mayo Clinic
BROOKS D. CHURCH, University of Denver
JOHN M. DEMENT, National Institute of Occupational Safety and Health
EDWARD CUYLER HAMMOND, American Cancer Society
BRUCE B. HANSHAW, U. S. Geological Survey
JAMES R. KRAMER, McMaster University
MAX M. MORTLAND, Michigan State University
CHARLES R. O'MELIA, University of North Carolina
RAYMOND E. SHAPIRO, National Institute of Environmental Health Sciences
ROBERT L. WERSHAW, U. S. Geological Survey

Subcommittee on Radioactivity

SHELDON WOLFF, University of California, San Francisco, *Chairman*
MARVIN GOLDMAN, University of California, Davis, *Vice Chairman*
SEYMOUR ABRAHAMSON, University of Wisconsin
A. BERTRAND BRILL, Vanderbilt University School of Medicine
JAMES F. CLEAVER, University of California, San Francisco
MELVIN R. SIKOV, Battelle Pacific Northwest Laboratory
ANDREW F. STEHNEY, Argonne National Laboratory
ARTHUR C. UPTON, State University of New York, Stony Brook

Subcommittee on Special Ions

J. CARRELL MORRIS, Harvard University, *Chairman*
EDWARD J. CAFRUNY, Sterling-Winthrop Research Institute
THURSTON E. LARSON, Illinois State Water Survey
LOT BATES PAGE, Tufts University School of Medicine
THURSTON E. LARSON, Illinois State Water Survey
KENNETH E. SHULL, Philadelphia Suburban Water Company
DONALD R. TAVES, University of Rochester
STEVEN R. TANNENBAUM, Massachusetts Institute of Technology
RICHARD L. WOODWARD, Camp, Dresser and McKee

Subcommittee on Trace Metals

CORNELIUS W. KRUSÉ, Johns Hopkins University, *Chairman*
J. JULIAN CHISOLM, Baltimore City Hospitals

TSAIHWA J. CHOW, University of California, San Diego
RICHARD S. ENGELBRECHT, University of Illinois
FRANCIS E. GARTRELL, Chattanooga, Tennessee
JACK E. MCKEE, California Institute of Technology
JAMES O. PIERCE, University of Missouri

Subcommittee on Metalloids

PAUL M. NEWBERNE, Massachusetts Institute of Technology, *Chairman*
WILLIAM B. BUCK, Iowa State University
WILLIAM W. CARLTON, Purdue University
RONALD C. SHANK, University of California, Irvine

Subcommittee on Organic Contaminants

JOSEPH F. BORZELLECA, Medical College of Virginia, *Chairman*
DAVID AXELROD, New York State Department of Health
HERBERT H. CORNISH, University of Michigan
HANS P. DROBECK, Sterling-Winthrop Research Institute
PERRY J. GEHRING, Dow Chemical Company
HERMAN F. KRAYBILL, National Institutes of Health
STANLEY M. KURTZ, Parke, Davis and Company
FRANK L. LYMAN, North Beach, New Jersey
JOHN R. MCCOY, Rutgers Medical School
FREDERICK W. OEHME, Kansas State University
JACK L. RADOMSKI, University of Miami
FARRELL R. ROBINSON, Purdue University
ROBERT L. ROUDABUSH, Rochester, New York
THOMAS E. SHELLENBERGER, National Center for Toxicological Research
CLARENCE J. TERHAAR, Eastman Kodak Company

Subcommittee on Pesticides

JOHN DOULL, University of Kansas Medical Center, *Chairman*
DONALD R. BUHLER, Oregon State University
WENDELL W. KILGORE, University of California, Davis
ROBERT E. MENZER, University of Maryland
ROBERT L. METCALF, University of Illinois
JOSEPH C. STREET, Utah State University

Subcommittee on Microbiology

THOMAS D. BROCK, University of Wisconsin, *Chairman*
DEAN O. CLIVER, University of Wisconsin
WALTER GINSBURG, Chicago Bureau of Water
ARNOLD E. GREENBERG, California Department of Health
LEON JACOBS, National Institutes of Health
WALTER N. MACK, Michigan State University
THEODORE G. METCALF, University of New Hampshire
SUMNER M. MORRISON, Colorado State University
RUTH H. NEFF, Tennessee Environmental Council

Subcommittee on Margin of Safety and Extrapolation

DAVID P. RALL, National Institute of Environmental Health Sciences, *Chairman*
J. MARTIN BROWN, Stanford University School of Medicine
DAVID G. HOEL, National Institute of Environmental Health Sciences
EDWIN H. LENNETTE, California Department of Health
SHELDON D. MURPHY, Harvard University
MARVIN A. SCHNEIDERMAN, National Cancer Institute

Subcommittee on Morbidity and Mortality

PAUL KOTIN, Johns-Manville Corporation, *Co-chairman*
VAUN A. NEWILL, Exxon Corporation, *Co-chairman*
BENJAMIN G. FERRIS, Harvard University
BERNARD G. PASTERNACK, New York University
ARTHUR H. WOLFF, University of Illinois Medical Center

Advisers, Consultants, and Contributors

CHARLES C. BROWN, National Cancer Institute
FLORENCE M. CARLETON, Washington, D.C.
PENELOPE FENNER-CRISP, Georgetown University
EUGENE GANGAROSA, Center for Disease Control
JOSEPH HASEMAN, National Institute of Environmental Health Services
FRED LI, University of California, Davis
L. R. MUENZ, National Cancer Institute
KENNETH OLSON, Dow Chemical Company
LANA R. SKIRBOLL, Georgetown University
FRANK G. STANDAERT, Georgetown University

EPA Project Officers

JOSEPH COTRUVO and
EDGAR A. JEFFREY, Office of Water Supply, Washington, D.C.

EPA Liaison Representatives

ERVIN BELLACK
NORMAN A. CLARK
GUNTER F. CRAUN
EDWARD E. GELDREICH
CHARLES HENDRICKS
LELAND J. MCCABE
JUDITH L. MULLANEY
LIBBEY SMITH
JAMES M. SYMONS
ROBERT G. TARDIFF

APPENDIX

C

Executive Summary

The Safe Drinking Water Act of 1974 (PL93-523) required the Administrator of the Environmental Protection Agency to arrange for a study that would serve as a scientific basis for revising the primary drinking-water regulations that were promulgated under the Act. The Study was conducted by the Safe Drinking Water Committee of the National Research Council.

A thorough study of the scientific literature was undertaken in order to assess the implications for human health of the constituents of drinking water in the United States. Assessment of the health benefits and the economic or technological feasibility of achieving a given level of contaminant control was outside the scope of the study, although the beneficial effects of some constituents of drinking water were considered.

The risk to man of contaminants ingested in drinking water was evaluated on the basis of both epidemiological studies and studies of toxicity in laboratory animals. The theoretical and experimental bases for extrapolating estimations of risk to low levels of dose were reviewed, and some principles to guide the conduct of this and future studies were defined.

Five classes of contaminants were examined: Microorganisms, Particulate Matter, Inorganic Solutes, Organic Solutes, and Radionuclides.

A great reduction in the incidence of gastroenteric diseases has resulted from the control of pathogenic microorganisms by the standard drinking-water treatments (coagulation, sedimentation, filtration, and disinfection) adopted early in this century. However, in 1975, more than 10,000 cases of waterborne enteric disease were reported, but in only about 10% of these cases were causal agents identified. There are reasons to believe that many cases go unreported. Improved detection and reporting systems are needed to determine more accurately the nationwide incidence and causes of these diseases. Chlorine is the standard disinfectant against which others are compared. While it is not ideal in every respect, much more research is required before any of the proposed substitutes can be recommended to replace it in water treatment. Questions concerning effectiveness of disinfection, toxicity of by-products, and residual in the distribution system must be answered for proposed substitutes, as well as for chlorine.

Finely divided solid particles are found suspended in many drinking-water supplies, particularly in those not treated by coagulation and filtration. While certain particles may indirectly reduce the efficiency of disinfection treatments, and act as carriers of some other contaminants, only in the case of particles derived from asbestos minerals are there grounds for suspecting that direct effects on human health may result. Inhalation of asbestos dust for long periods of time has been shown to produce toxic effects, but evidence of the toxicity of ingested particles of abestos minerals is not conclusive. Further research is necessary to resolve this problem.

Health effects associated with 22 inorganic solutes were reviewed. Most were judged to present little or no threat to human health, either because of low concentration in drinking water, minimal potential toxicity, or both. Thirteen are essential nutrients. Their potential toxicity at high levels and nutritional role at lower levels complicate the issue, but none of them poses a threat to health at the concentrations normally found in drinking water. The inorganic contaminant with the greatest potential for toxicity is lead. The present standard may not provide an adequate margin of safety, especially for infants and young children. The data presented justify reexamination of the current standards for arsenic and selenium. The preponderance of evidence supports an inverse correlation between the incidence of cardiovascular disease and water hardness, but the underlying causal relationships are not clear.

On the basis of their relevance to the purpose of the study, 129 organic compounds (including 55 pesticides) were selected for detailed examination.

A list of the compounds in drinking water that are known or suspected carcinogens was prepared after a detailed analysis of the available data. Estimates of cancer risk to man from a lifetime exposure were made when sufficient data were available to permit a statistical extrapolation. These projections were made for 22 compounds judged to be either known or suspected human or animal carcinogens. Of these only vinyl chloride is confirmed to be a human carcinogen. The available data on mutagenicity and teratogenicity also were summarized.

Although the carcinogenic effects of the compounds were of primary concern, evidence of other effects was considered. An "Acceptable Daily Intake" (ADI) was calculated for 45 compounds that were judged to be potentially toxic but not carcinogenic. The ADI is an empirically derived value that reflects a particular combination of both knowledge and uncertainty about the relative safety of a chemical. It is the level at which exposure to a single chemical is not anticipated to produce an observable toxic response in man. The ADI does not represent a safe level in drinking water because it does not specify what fraction of the potential contaminant intake may come from water. Data were insufficient to calculate an ADI for 61 of the compounds that were considered.

The radiation associated with most water supplies is a small proportion of the normal background to which all human beings are exposed. Consequently, it is difficult, if not impossible, to measure with certainty any adverse health effects that may be due to radionuclides in water. In a few water supplies, however, radium can reach concentrations that pose a higher risk of bone cancer for the people exposed.

Subgroups within the population have been identified that are more susceptible to the adverse effects of certain constituents of drinking water than would normally be expected of the population-at-large.

Index